VOLUME ONE

Diagnostic Ultrasound

VOLUME ONE

Diagnostic Ultrasound

Carol M. Rumack, M.D.

Professor of Radiology and Pediatrics
University of Colorado Health Sciences Center
Denver, Colorado

Stephanie R. Wilson, M.D.

Associate Professor of Radiology
University of Toronto
Head, Division of Ultrasound
The Toronto Hospital
Toronto, Ontario

J. William Charboneau, M.D.

Professor of Radiology
Mayo Clinic
Rochester, Minnesota

with 2020 illustrations and 110 color illustrations

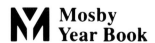 **Mosby Year Book**

St. Louis   Baltimore   Boston   Chicago   London   Philadelphia   Sydney   Toronto

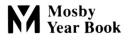
Mosby Year Book
Dedicated to Publishing Excellence

Editor: Anne S. Patterson
Developmental Editor: Elaine Steinborn
Assistant Editors: Jo Salway, Maura Leib
Project Manager: John A. Rogers
Production Editor: Celeste Clingan
Book Design: Jeanne Wolfgeher
Production: Jeanne Genz

Printed in the United States of America

Mosby–Year Book, Inc. Company
11830 Westline Industrial Drive
St. Louis, Missouri 63146

Library of Congress Cataloging-in-Publication Data

Diagnostic ultrasound / [edited by] Carol M. Rumack, Stephanie R. Wilson, J. William Charboneau.
    p.   cm.
   Includes index.
   ISBN (invalid) 0-8016-2209-7 (set)
   1. Diagnosis, Ultrasonic. I. Rumack, Carol M. II. Wilson, Stephanie. III. Charboneau, J. William.
   [DNLM: 1. Ultrasonography.   WB 289 D536]
RC78.7.U4D514 1991
616.07'543—dc20
DNLM/DLC   91-27608
for Library of Congress   CIP

C/WA/WA 9 8 7 6 5 4 3 2

CONTRIBUTORS

Mostafa Atri, M.D. F.R.C.P. (C)
Assistant Professor of Radiology,
McGill University;
Director of the Division of Ultrasound,
Department of Radiology;
Montreal General Hospital,
Montreal, Quebec, Canada

Diane S. Babcock, M.D.
Professor of Radiology and Pediatrics,
Children's Hospital Medical Center,
University of Cincinnati College of Medicine,
Cincinnati, Ohio

Beryl R. Benacerraf, M.D.
Clinical Associate Professor of Radiology and
    Obstetrics and Gynecology;
Harvard Medical School,
Consultant, Ultrasound;
Brigham and Women's Hospital,
Boston, Massachusetts

Carol B. Benson, M.D.
Assistant Professor of Radiology,
Harvard Medical School;
Co-director, Division of Ultrasound;
Department of Radiology,
Brigham and Women's Hospital,
Boston, Massachusetts

William E. Brant, M.D.
Assistant Professor of Radiology,
University of California, Davis,
School of Medicine,
Sacramento, California

Robert L. Bree, M.D.
Associate Professor of Radiology,
University of Michigan Medical School;
Chief, Radiology Service;
Ann Arbor Veterans Administration Medical Center,
Ann Arbor, Michigan

Linda K. Brown, M.D.
Staff Radiologist,
Cobb Hospital and Medical Center,
Austell, Georgia

Barbara A. Carroll, M.D.
Associate Professor of Radiology,
Duke University Medical Center,
Durham, North Carolina

William F. Chandler, M.D.
Professor of Surgery,
Section of Neurosurgery,
University of Michigan,
Ann Arbor, Michigan

J. William Charboneau, M.D.
Professor of Radiology,
Mayo Clinic,
Rochester, Minnesota

Christine H. Comstock, M.D.
Assistant Professor of Obstetrics and Gynecology,
Wayne State University School of Medicine,
Detroit, Michigan;
Director, Division of Fetal Imaging;
William Beaumont Hospital,
Royal Oak, Michigan

Peter L. Cooperberg, M.D.
Professor of Radiology,
University of British Columbia;
Head, Department of Radiology;
St. Paul's Hospital,
Vancouver, British Columbia, Canada

Dale R. Cyr, R.D.M.S.
Chief Sonographer,
Department of Radiology;
Division of Ultrasound;
University of Washington School of Medicine,
Seattle, Washington

Sidney M. Dashefsky, M.D., F.R.C.P. (C)
Lecturer,
Department of Diagnostic Radiology;
University of Manitoba Health Sciences Centre,
Winnipeg, Manitoba, Canada

Michael A. DiPietro, M.D.
Associate Professor of Radiology,
University of Michigan,
Ann Arbor, Michigan

Peter M. Doubilet, M.D., Ph.D.
Associate Professor of Radiology,
Harvard Medical School;
Co-director, Division of Ultraosound;
Department of Radiology,
Brigham and Women's Hospital,
Boston, Massachusetts

Julia A. Drose, BA, RT, R.D.M.S.
Instructor,
Department of Radiology;
University of Colorado Health Sciences Center,
Denver, Colorado

Paul W. Finnegan, M.D., C.M., F.R.C.P. (C)
Fellow,
Gastrointestinal and Interventional Radiology;
University of Toronto,
Toronto, Ontario, Canada

Katherine W. Fong, M.B., B.S., F.R.C.P. (C)
Assistant Professor of Radiology,
University of Toronto;
Head, Division of Ultrasound;
Women's College Hospital,
Toronto, Ontario, Canada

Bruno Fornage, M.D.
Professor of Radiology,
Chief, Section of Ultrasound;
The University of Texas M.D. Anderson
    Cancer Center,
Houston, Texas

Charles M. Glasier, M.D.
Associate Professor of Radiology,
University of Arkansas for Medical Sciences,
Arkansas Children's Hospital,
Little Rock, Arkansas

Albert Goldstein, Ph.D.
Associate Professor of Radiology and Obstetrics and
    Gynecology,
Wayne State University School of Medicine,
Detroit, Michigan

Gretchen A. W. Gooding, M.D.
Professor and Vice-Chairman of Radiology,
University of California, San Francisco:
Chief, Radiology Service;
Department of Veteran Affairs Medical Center,
San Francisco, California

Lawrence P. Gordon, M.D.
Associate Professor of Pathology,
State University of New York,
Health Science Center at Syracuse:
Attending Pathologist,
Crouse Irving Memorial Hospital,
Syracuse, New York

Leslie E. Grissom, M.D.
Assistant Professor of Radiology,
Jefferson Medical College,
Philadelphia, Pennsylvania;
Attending Radiologist,
Alfred I. duPont Institute,
Wilmington, Delaware

H. Theodore Harcke, M.D.
Professor of Radiology,
Jefferson Medical College,
Philadelphia, Pennsylvania;
Director of Medical Imaging,
Alfred I. duPont Institute,
Wilmington, Delaware

Curtis L. Harlow, M.D.
Assistant Professor of Radiology,
University of Colorado Health Sciences Center,
Denver, Colorado

Chris R. Harman, M.D., F.R.C.S (C)
Associate Professor of Obstetrics and Gynecology,
University of Manitoba;
Director, Fetal Assessment Unit,
Women's Hospital,
Winnipeg, Manitoba, Canada

Ian D. Hay, M.B., Ph.D.
Professor of Medicine,
Department of Metabolism and Internal Medicine,
Mayo Clinic,
Rochester, Minnesota

Thomas C. Hay, D.O.
Assistant Professor of Radiology,
University of Colorado Health Sciences Center,
Children's Hospital,
National Jewish Center of Immunology and Respiratory
    Disease,
Denver, Colorado

C. Keith Hayden, Jr., M.D.
Clinical Professor of Radiology,
University of Texas Medical Branch at Galveston,
Galveston, Texas;
Deputy Director,
Pediatric Radiology,
Cook-Ft. Worth Children's Medical Center,
Fort Worth, Texas

Pamela L. Hilpert, M.D., Ph.D.
Assistant Professor of Radiology,
Pennsylvania Hospital,
Philadelphia, Pennsylvania

J. Gerard Horgan, M.B., M.R.C.P., F.R.C.R.
Associate Professor of Pediatric Radiology and Imaging,
University of Colorado Health Sciences Center,
Children's Hospital,
Denver, Colorado

E. Meredith James, M.D.
Associate Professor of Radiology,
Vice Chairman, Department of Radiology;
Mayo Clinic,
Rochester, Minnesota

Jo-Ann Johnson, M.D., F.R.C.S. (C)
Assistant Professor of Obstetrics and Gynecology,
Division of Maternal Fetal Medicine,
University of Toronto,
The Toronto Hospital,
Toronto, Ontario, Canada

Bernard F. King, M.D.
Assistant Professor of Radiology,
Mayo Clinic,
Rochester, Minnesota

Janet S. Kirk, M.D.
Assistant Director,
Division of Fetal Imaging;
William Beaumont Hospital,
Royal Oak, Michigan

Frederick W. Kremkau, Ph.D.
Professor and Director,
Center for Medical Ultrasound;
Bowman Gray School of Medicine,
Wake Forest University,
Winston-Salem, North Carolina

J. Scott Kriegshauser, M.D.
Assistant Professor of Radiology,
Mayo Clinic-Scottsdale,
Scottsdale, Arizona

Faye C. Laing, M.D.
Clinical Professor of Radiology,
University of Washington Medical Center;
Staff Radiologist, Swedish Hospital Medical Center,
Seattle, Washington

Robert A. Lee, M.D.
Staff Radiologist,
Mayo Clinic,
Rochester, Minnesota

Richard E. Leithiser, Jr., M.D.
Associate Professor of Radiology,
University of Arkansas for Medical Sciences,
Arkansas Children's Hospital,
Little Rock, Arkansas

Clifford S. Levi, M.D., F.R.C.P. (C)
Associate Professor of Radiology,
University of Manitoba Health Sciences Centre,
Winnipeg, Manitoba, Canada

Bernard J. Lewandowski, M.D.
Associate Professor of Radiology,
University of Ottawa,
Ottawa Civic Hospital,
Ottawa, Ontario, Canada

Gregory J.S. Lewis, M.D.
Staff Radiologist,
Riverside Radiology,
North Little Rock, Arkansas

Edward A. Lyons, M.D., F.R.C.P. (C), F.A.C.R.
Professor and Chairman,
Department of Diagnostic Radiology;
University of Manitoba Health Sciences Centre,
Winnipeg, Manitoba, Canada

Laurence A. Mack, M.D.
Professor of Radiology, Obstetrics and Gynecology and
   Orthopedics,
Director of Ultrasound,
University of Washington School of Medicine,
Seattle, Washington

Frank A. Manning, M.D.
Professor of Obstetrics and Gynecology,
University of Manitoba;
Head of Obstetrics and Gynecology,
Women's Hospital,
Winnipeg, Manitoba, Canada

John R. Mathieson, M.D.
Assistant Professor of Radiology,
University of British Columbia,
Vancouver, British Columbia, Canada

Frederick A. Matsen III, M.D.
Professor and Chairman,
Department of Orthopedics;
University of Washington Medical Center,
Seattle, Washington

John P. McGahan, M.D.
Professor of Radiology,
Chief of Abdominal Imaging and Ultrasound,
University of California Davis Medical Center,
Sacramento, California

Ellen B. Mendelson, M.D.
Clinical Associate Professor of Radiology,
University of Pittsburgh School of Medicine;
Chief, Mammography and Women's Imaging,
The Western Pennsylvania Hospital,
Pittsburgh, Pennsylvania

Savas M. Menticoglou, M.D.
Assistant Professor of Obstetrics and Gynecology,
University of Manitoba,
Winnipeg, Manitoba, Canada

Christopher R.B. Merritt, M.D.
Chairman,
Department of Radiology;
The Oschner Clinic and Alton Oschner Medical
    Foundation,
New Orleans, Louisiana

Berta Maria Montalvo, M.D.
Associate Professor of Radiology,
University of Miami School of Medicine,
Miami, Florida

Khanh T. Nguyen, M.D., M.Sc., F.R.C.P. (C)
Associate Professor of Radiology,
Queen's University,
Kingston, Ontario, Canada

Stuart Nicholson, M.D., F.R.C.P. (C)
Clinical Assistant Professor of Radiology,
University of Calgary,
Department of Radiological Sciences and Diagnostic
    Imaging,
Foothills Hospital,
Calgary, Alberta, Canada

Carl A. Nimrod, M.D., F.R.C.P. (C)
Professor of Obstetrics and Gynecology,
University of Ottawa;
Director, Division of Perinatology;
Ottawa General Hospital,
Ottawa, Ontario, Canada

Robert L. Nolan, M.D., F.R.C.P. (C)
Associate Professor of Radiology,
Queen's University,
Kingston, Ontario, Canada

David A. Nyberg, M.D.
Associate Clinical Professor of Radiology and Obstetrics
    and Gynecology,
University of Washington Medical Center;
Co-Director of Obstetric Ultrasound,
Swedish Hospital Medical Center,
Seattle, Washington

Heidi B. Patriquin, M.D.
Professor of Radiology,
University of Montreal,
Hopital Sainte-Justine,
Montreal, Quebec, Canada

Randall M. Patten, M.D.
Clinical Assistant Professor of Radiology,
University of Washington School of Medicine;
Medical Director,
Ranier Medical Imaging,
Seattle, Washington

Joseph F. Polak, M.D.
Associate Professor of Radiology,
Harvard Medical School;
Director, Noninvasive Vascular Imaging;
Brigham and Women's Hospital,
Boston, Massachusetts

Carl C. Reading, M.D.
Associate Professor of Radiology,
Mayo Clinic,
Rochester, Minnesota

Martin H. Reed, M.D., F.R.C.P (C)
Professor of Radiology,
University of Manitoba Health Sciences Centre,
Winnipeg, Manitoba

Henrietta Kotlus Rosenberg, M.D.
Professor of Radiology;
University of Pennsylvania School of Medicine,
Senior Radioologist and Director of Ultrasound,
Children's Hospital of Philadelphia,
Philadelphia, Pennsylvania

Jonathan M. Rubin, M.D., Ph.D.
Professor of Radiology,
University of Michigan,
Ann Arbor, Michigan

Carol M. Rumack, M.D.
Professor of Radiology and Pediatrics,
University of Colorado Health Science Center,
Denver, Colorado

Shia Salem, M.D., F.R.C.P. (C)
Associate Professor of Radiology,
University of Toronto,
Head, Division of Ultrasound,
Department of Radiology;
Mount Sinaii Hospital,
Toronto, Ontario, Canada

Eric E. Sauerbrei, M.D., F.R.C.P. (C)
Professor of Radiology,
Queen's University,
Kingston General Hospital,
Ontario, Canada

Joanna J. Seibert, M.D.
Professor of Radiology,
Medical Director, Pediatric Radiology;
University of Arkansas for Medical Sciences,
Arkansas Children's Hospital,
Little Rock, Arkansas

Robert W. Seibert, M.D.
Associate Professor of Otolaryngology—HNS;
University of Arkansas for Medical Sciences,
Chief, Department of Otolaryngology;
Arkansas Children's Hospital,
Little Rock, Arkansas

Nancy H. Sherman, M.D.
Clinical Assistant Professor of Radiology,
University of Pennsylvania School of Medicine;
Attending Radiologist,
Alfred I. duPont Institute,
Willmington, Delaware

Beverly A. Spirt, M.D.
Professor of Radiology,
Chief of Ultrasound;
State University of New York,
Health Science Center at Syracuse,
Syracuse, New York

Elizabeth R. Stamm, M.D.
Assistant Professor of Radiology,
University of Colorado Health Sciences Center,
Denver, Colorado

Rhonda Stewart, M.D.
Staff Radiologist,
Alexandria Hospital,
Alexandria, Virginia

Leonard E. Swischuk, M.D.
Professor of Radiology;
Director, Pediatric Radiology;
University of Texas Medical Branch at Galveston,
Galveston, Texas

David I. Thickman, M.D.
Associate Professor of Radiology,
University of Colorado Health Sciences Center,
Denver, Colorado

Ants Toi, M.D., DMR, F.R.C.P. (C)
Associate Professor of Radiology, Obstetrics and
    Gynecology;
University of Toronto,
The Toronto Hospital,
Toronto, Ontario, Canada

Keith Y. Wang, M.D.
Assistant Professor of Radiology, Obstetrics and
    Gynecology;
University of Washington School of Medicine,
Seattle, Washington

Stephanie R. Wilson, M.D., F.R.C.P. (C)
Associate Professor of Radiology,
University of Toronto,
Head, Division of Ultrasound;
The Toronto Hospital,
Toronto, Ontario, Canada

David A. Wiseman, M.D.
Associate Professor of Radiology,
Foothills Hospital,
Calgary, Alberta, Canada

Cynthia E. Withers, M.D.
Assistant Professor of Radiology,
Sunnybrook Medical Centre,
University of Toronto,
Toronto, Ontario, Canada

To my husband, Barry, and my children, Becky and Marc, for their understanding and support through a stimulating and productive year. Also, to my parents for giving me the strength to enjoy the challenge.

CMR

To Ken, Jessica, and Jordon. Your independence and continuous encouragement were my inspiration.

SRW

To Cathy, Nicholas, Ben, and Laurie for all the love and joy they bring to my life.

JWC

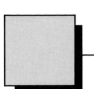

PREFACE

Sonography has expanded rapidly over the last two decades on a world-wide basis. Despite the explosive growth of this field and the extensive applications of sonographic techniques, few comprehensive reference texts are available. To this end, we undertook the task of producing a state-of-the-art text on ultrasonography.

The authors who have contributed chapters to this book are recognized experts in their fields. We believe that they have provided the most up-to-date information available, making the book current and comprehensive. We hope that it will become a trusted primary reference for all who are interested in this exciting field of medical imaging.

This book is intended for practicing physicians, residents, medical students, and sonographers. It is organized into six parts, covering all aspects of sonography except cardiac and ophthalmologic applications. The information in Volume One, Part I, covers the physics of sonography; Part II, abdominal, pelvic, and thoracic imaging; Part III, intraoperative imaging; and Part IV,

small parts imaging, including carotid and peripheral vessels. The contents of Volume Two include Part V, obstetric and fetal topics and Part VI, pediatric applications. Every effort was made to cover the broad scope of ultrasound practice without redunduancy.

We greatly appreciate the efforts of the contributing authors. Without their experience, expertise, and commitment, we could not have achieved the goal of a comprehensive and authoritative textbook. We are indebted to them.

The high-quality images are the product of many talented sonographers, and to them we offer our sincere thanks. Their dedication to sonography has contributed substantially to its rapid growth and acceptance.

We also thank Janine Jacobson, our talented manuscript coordinator, whose patience and care with multiple manuscript revisions has led to a first-class product. Further, we acknowledge the support of Elaine Steinborn, Jo Salway, Jim Ryan, and Anne Patterson of Mosby-Year Book for encouraging us in this endeavor.

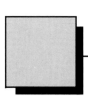

CONTENTS

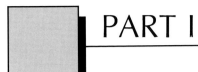

PART I

Physics

CHAPTER 1

Physics of Ultrasound

- Albert Goldstein, Ph.D.

Ultrasound waves are mechanical pressure waves similar to audible sound waves and must have a medium in which to propagate. The **frequency (f)** is the number of high- or low-pressure regions crossing each area of tissue each second. The frequencies of the sound waves used in medical ultrasound are much higher than the human audible range (20 to 16,000 hertz); hence, the waves are called **ultrasound.**

The **acoustic velocity (c)** of an ultrasound wave is the wave velocity of the pressure waves traveling through the propagation medium. Acoustic velocity is essentially frequency independent with an average value of 1540 meters per second. Most soft tissues in the body have acoustic velocities within 3% of this average.[1,2]

Longitudinal acoustic waves are waves in which the direction of particle motion is parallel or antiparallel to the wave velocity. **Transverse acoustic waves** are waves in which the direction of particle motion is perpendicular to the wave velocity. **Longitudinal acoustic waves** are the only waves that will propagate in a fluid (liquid or gas), so only longitudinal acoustic waves can propagate in the soft-tissue structures of the body.

The **acoustic wavelength** is the basic repetition distance in space for a single frequency wave, joining points of equal phase. In ultrasound the term **phase** refers to the time an event occurs, such as the exact point in the acoustic cycle when a certain pressure is attained. Due to their definitions, the wavelength and frequency of acoustic waves are related to each other by the following standard equation (true for all propagating waves).

$$c = \lambda f \tag{1}$$

$$\text{Acoustic velocity} = \text{Acoustic wavelength} \times \text{Frequency}$$

The **acoustic pressure amplitude** at a point in space **P** is the particle pressure, which is the difference between the pressure when the wave is present and the ambient pressure. The acoustic intensity **I** is defined as the energy (power) propagating through a unit area in the medium per unit time.

The **acoustic impedance (Z)** of the propagation medium is important in predicting the magnitudes of the reflected echoes at interfaces between two different tissues. It is given by the relation

$$Z = \rho c \tag{2}$$

$$\text{Acoustic impedance} = \frac{\text{Tissue density}}{\text{g/cm}^3} \times \frac{\text{Acoustic velocity}}{\text{cm/sec}}$$

Because both tissue density and acoustic velocity are independent of frequency, acoustic impedance is also frequency independent and relies only on the tissue's mechanical properties.

PULSE-ECHO DISTANCE MEASUREMENTS

The slowness of acoustic velocity in tissue permits distance measurements to be made in a novel manner. The time it takes for a pulsed sound wave to travel from a transducer to a reflector and back can be measured and then, along with the known acoustic velocity, can be used to calculate their separation with the equation

$$R = \frac{1}{2} ct \qquad (3)$$

$$\text{Distance} = \frac{1}{2} \frac{\text{Acoustic}}{\text{velocity}} \times \frac{\text{Time of flight}}{\text{of sound wave}}$$

The factor of one half in this equation comes from the fact that the sound waves have actually traversed the range twice, once as transmitted sound and once as reflected sound.

ECHO GENERATION
Reflection

Ultrasound echoes are produced by two types of reflectors: specular and diffuse. **Specular reflectors** are large mirrorlike interfaces in the body between two different soft tissues, such as the liver capsule or the kidney capsule. If a sound ray (direction of travel of the short sound pulse) is incident on an interface, two rays are produced: a transmitted ray that propagates into the second soft tissue and a reflected ray that propagates back into the first soft tissue.

The direction of the reflected ray (echo) is governed by the law of reflection that states that the angle of incidence equals the angle of reflection. For single transducer pulse-echo equipment to register the reflected echo, it must be backscattered at an angle of 180 degrees and back to the front face of the transducer. So only when the incident beam is perpendicular to the interface will the reflected beam be received by the transducer (the angles of incidence and reflection are both 0).

The **reflection coefficient** is defined as the fraction of sound intensity reflected from the reflector (target).

At normal incidence on a specularly reflecting interface, the reflection coefficient is given by the expression

$$R = \frac{(Z_2 - Z_1)^2}{(Z_2 + Z_1)^2} \qquad (4)$$

where the wave is propagating in medium 1 and meets a specular interface with medium 2. The strength of the reflection coefficient is governed uniquely by the acoustic impedances of the two different tissues at the interface. The strength of the reflection coefficient really depends on the ratio of the acoustic impedances at the boundary, and not on their absolute magnitude. The reflection coefficient is of the same magnitude for both the ratio of the acoustic impedance and its reciprocal (if the ratio of the acoustic impedances at a boundary is either 1:4 or 4:1, the magnitude of the reflection coefficient is the same). The reflection coefficient is zero (no reflection) if the ratio of acoustic impedances at the boundary is unity. This is known as **impedance matching** and maximum energy transmission results with no reflection. The larger the difference in acoustic impedances at the boundary, the larger the magnitude of the reflection coefficient. This is known as **impedance mismatching** and the more the acoustic impedance mismatch, the larger the reflection coefficient.

Table 1-1 lists acoustic velocities and impedances for several nonbiologic and biologic materials. The biologic tissues fall into three distinct groups. **Fat** has an acoustic velocity that is about 6% lower than soft tissue; most **soft tissues** have an acoustic velocity close to the average value of 1540 m/s; **bone** has a much higher acoustic velocity than soft tissue. The acoustic impedances of these tissues fall into the same three groups because fat has a lower mass density than soft tissue, and

■ **TABLE 1-1**
Acoustic Velocities, Impedances, and Ultrasonic Attenuation Coefficients for Body Components

	Velocity (m/s)	Acoustic Impedance (10^5 Rayls)	Attenuation (dB/cm at 1 MHz)	HVL† (at 1 MHz) (cm)
Air	330	0.0004	12 (f^2)*	0.25
Water	1480	1.48	0.002 (f^2)*	1500
Fat	1450	1.38	0.63	4.76
Blood	1570	1.61	0.18	16.67
Kidney	1560	1.62	1.0	3.00
Soft tissue, average	1540	1.63	0.70	4.29
Liver	1550	1.65	0.94	3.19
Muscle	1580	1.70		
along fibers			1.3	2.31
across fibers			3.3	0.91
Bone	4080	7.80	5	0.21

*The f^2 notation indicates a quadratic frequency dependence of these attenuation coefficients.
†The *HVL* (half value layer) is the tissue thickness required to reduce the acoustic intensity by one half in transmission.
STP, Standard temperature and pressure.

bone has a much higher mass density than soft tissue. Thus, we would expect high amplitude specular echoes from fat-soft tissue and soft tissue-bone interfaces, and lower amplitude specular reflections from the various soft-tissue interfaces in the body, due to their almost matched acoustic impedances at these interfaces.

Diffuse reflectors have physical dimensions that are much smaller than the acoustic wavelength. Point reflectors and interface roughness are common examples of diffuse reflectors. Diffuse reflectors scatter ultrasound in all directions, producing low-amplitude echoes. Slight local variations in acoustic impedance inside body organs act as diffuse reflectors. Modern ultrasonic scanners use a gray scale presentation in which image shades of gray represent the received range of echo amplitudes. High-amplitude echoes are usually due to specular reflectors; low-amplitude echoes are due to diffuse reflectors.

Attenuation

Attenuation refers to the loss of strength of the acoustic waves as they travel through a medium.

Attenuation = Beamwidth + Scatter + Absorption

After being emitted from the transducer, the sound energy travels into tissue confined along a pathway known as the **beam pattern.** In a nonscattering and nonabsorbing medium the energy in the acoustic pulse remains constant. However, as the beam pattern beomes wider, the acoustic intensity decreases because this energy must be distributed over a larger area. This change of intensity as the beam widens causes depth variations in the amplitudes of the received echoes from identical reflectors.

While propagating through soft tissue, ultrasound waves are scattered by either specular or diffuse reflectors and a small portion of the ultrasound energy is removed from the transmitted beam. As the ultrasound wave moves through the tissue, the tissue particles are set into motion. In a nonabsorbing medium, as the wave passes by, the particles give back their vibrational energy and the wave-particle combination conserves energy. In tissue, however, the particles lose some of their vibrational energy to frictional effects or to other internal modes of tissue motion and energy is absorbed as tissue heat energy.

The average value of tissue attenuation is usually taken to be -1 dB/cm MHz. As the ultrasound frequency increases the tissue attenuation gets stronger. A 3.5 MHz beam will be attenuated at the rate of 3.5 dB for every centimeter of propagation. For a target inside the body, ultrasound waves actually travel twice the depth, once as the transmitted pulse and once as the scattered echo. Thus, in terms of centimeters of depth, the 3.5 MHz beam is attenuated at the rate of 7 dB for every centimeter of range. So a 3.5 MHz beam is being reduced by more than a factor of one quarter in intensity for every centimeter of tissue depth.

Ultrasonic attenuation coefficients (Table 1-1) show that fat has the lowest value. Liver, kidney, and muscle are intermediate in value. Bone has the highest value of attenuation. Due to its high impedance and attenuation, very little ultrasound energy transmits through bone and is represented in the ultrasonic image.

Whenever there is a difference in acoustic velocity across an interface, the direction of the transmitted ray shifts as it crosses the interface. This phenomenon is known as **refraction.** The focusing property of eyeglasses is due to the refraction that occurs at the curved lens surface. As in optics, the magnitude of the directional change may be calculated from Snell's law

$$\frac{\sin \theta_1}{\sin \theta_2} = \frac{C_1}{C_2} \qquad (5)$$

The angles θ_1 and θ_2 are defined as the angle between the normal and the interface and the directions of the incident and transmitted rays, respectively. There will be no refraction (bending) of the ultrasound ray when it is incident normal to the interface ($\theta_1 = \theta_2 = 0°$).

TRANSDUCER BEAM PATTERN

The beam pattern of the transducer is identical in transmission and reception for point reflector targets. The most fundamental transducer element is the plane circular piston radiator, a flat disk shaped piezoelectric element that resonates in a thickness changing mode. For continuous-wave (CW) ultrasound, the beam pattern from this unfocused transducer is made up of a near field and a far field (Fig. 1-1). In the near field, diffraction effects, caused by the finite size of the transducer aperture, cause spatial varying intensity. In the far field, the transducer aperture is sufficiently distant to be approximated by a point source. The intensity is spatially uniform and at far distances decreases from the source with the inverse square law.

The beam pattern of a plane circular piston radiator is known to be complex.[3] Usually, a simple geometric approximation suffices to describe the near and far fields. The near field is taken to be a circular cylinder with the diameter of the piezoelectric disk whose height (depth into the transmission medium) is given by

$$\text{Height} = \frac{\text{Radius}^2}{\text{Acoustic wavelength}} \qquad (6)$$

The far field is taken to be a circular cone whose vertex is located at the center of the transducer front face. The half angle of divergence of the cone is given by

$$\sin \theta = \frac{0.61 \text{ Acoustic wavelength}}{\text{Radius}} \qquad (7)$$

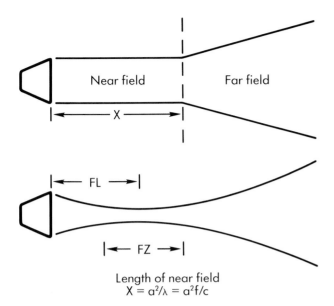

Length of near field
$$X = a^2/\lambda = a^2 f/c$$

FIG 1-1. Unfocused and focused transducers. Unfocused and focused (bottom) circular single element transducers beam patterns with same frequency. Focal length *(FL)* in focused case cannot extend beyond near field length of unfocused case. *FZ,* Focal zone.

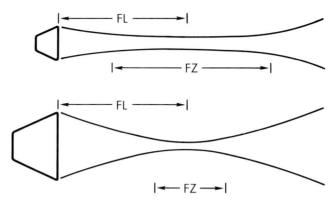

FIG 1-2. Aperture size effect on focal properties. Two single-element transducers have same frequency and focal length *(FL).* As element diameter increases, degree of focus increases but focal zone *(FZ)* decreases.

Keeping the transducer radius constant, as frequency is increased, wavelength decreases and the near zone increases in length. The half-angle of divergence of the far zone decreases with increasing frequency; thus the unfocused beam pattern becomes more uniform in depth. If frequency is decreased, the length of the near zone decreases, producing a much wider beam pattern. If the frequency is lowered sufficiently, the beam pattern will become almost uniformly distributed at all angles and the transducer is known as a **hydrophone,** an ideal receiver of acoustic signals.

All transducers follow very specific rules in focusing (Fig. 1-1). The **focal length (FL)** is the distance from the transducer face to the narrowest portion of the beam pattern. The **focal zone (FZ)** is the range of axial distances over which the beam pattern is sufficiently narrow to produce good image spatial resolution. The focal length cannot be longer than the near zone length in the unfocused case.[4] Because the near zone length increases as the square of the transducer radius, focusing at depth requires a larger transducer aperture diameter than shallow focusing.

The transducer focus gets stronger (its beam pattern gets narrower) as the aperture increases (Fig. 1-2). However, the advantage of stronger focus can only be realized over a reduced focal zone length, since increasing transducer diameter reduces the focal zone extent.[5]

Image Spatial Resolution

Axial resolution (parallel to the beam central ray) is determined by the pulse length of the ultrasonic signal (Fig. 1-3). An underdamped transducer produces long transmission pulses and echoes. When the transducer receives echoes from two-point reflectors at slightly different depths, their combined signal resembles an echo from a single strong reflector at their depth. If the transducer output pulse were short, due to heavy transducer damping the echoes received from these two point reflectors would also have (reflect) short pulse lengths, which permit the identification of the individual point reflectors in the combined received signal.

Lateral resolution (perpendicular to the beam central ray) is governed by the beamwidth of the transducer at the depth of the point reflectors and is a consequence of the transducer scanning motion (Fig. 1-4). Lateral resolution difficulties really occur because of uncertainties in the lateral position of point reflectors in the beam. When generating an image the ultrasonic equipment must, by necessity, make certain simplifying assumptions. These are:

- all tissue has the same acoustic velocity (1540 m/s)
- the ultrasonic pulse travels in a straight line in tissue
- all detected targets are on the central ray of the transducer beam pattern

Lateral blurring or misregistration of the reflector position in the image occurs when the third assumption is not valid (Fig. 1-4). When a point reflector is inside the beam pattern, an echo is received by the transducer but its horizontal position is always assumed to be at the center of the beam pattern. A single-point reflector in the medium will be represented as a horizontal rectangle in the image. The vertical dimension of the rectan-

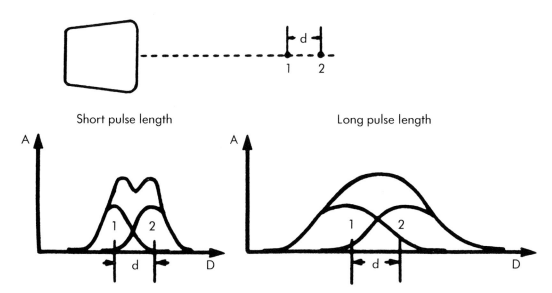

FIG 1-3. Axial resolution. The ability to resolve two point reflectors (*1* and *2*) a distance *d* apart in depth depends upon the transmitted pulse length. *A,* Amplitude; *D,* depth.

gle is governed by axial position uncertainties and is an indicator of the pulse length at this depth. The horizontal dimension of the rectangle is governed by lateral position uncertainties and is an indicator of the beamwidth at this depth. If two adjacent point reflectors are closer together than the beamwidth at their depth, their respective images will overlap and they will not be identified in the image. However, if they are separated by a dis-

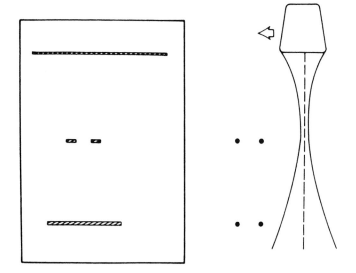

FIG 1-4. Lateral resolution. The ability of a focused transducer to resolve two point reflectors separated laterally (perpendicular to) the beam axis depends upon the beamwidth at their depth. The real space scan is shown on the right and the resultant image on the left. The top horizontal line in the image is caused by the (electrical transmission pulse) main bang echo, which is also "picked up" by the receiver.

tance larger than the beamwidth, they will be easily separated (resolved) in the image.

Lateral resolution blurring is usually 3 to 4 times greater than axial resolution blurring and is the prime cause of spatial resolution difficulties in ultrasonic images. The lateral blur decreases with higher-frequency transducers because they have narrower beam patterns. Thus, if optimum spatial resolution is desired, the high frequencies should always be chosen for imaging. However, penetration into the patient decreases at higher frequencies because of frequency-dependent attenuation; the selection of the transducer frequency for each clinical imaging situation is a compromise between patient penetration and spatial resolution. The general rule is to choose the highest frequency that will penetrate adequately to the depths required.

Even in the image regions where the transducer is well focused, the beam profile will affect the image spatial resolution (Fig. 1-5). The transmit/receive beam profile of a weakly focused transducer is so wide that both reflectors are shown in its main lobe and will be spatially unresolved in the resultant image (Fig. 1-5, *A*). A wider aperture improves the focus of this transducer (Fig. 1-5, *B*). With only one reflector in the main lobe, the two reflectors will be spatially resolved in the image (Fig. 1-5, *C*).

For a focused circular single-crystal transducer used in pulse-echo imaging, the first side lobe of the transmit/receive beam pattern is typically 40 to 45 dB lower than the main lobe signal, regardless of the degree of focusing. When equal amplitude point reflectors are located both at the maxima of the main lobe and the first side lobe (Fig. 1-5, *B*), the addition of the side lobe sig-

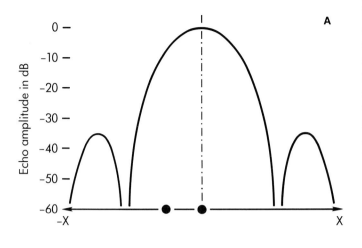

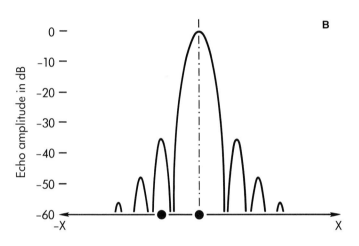

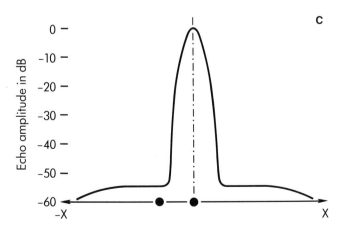

FIG 1-5. Spatial resolution. Effect of focus on spatial resolution. **A,** Weak focus does not resolve closely spaced point reflectors. **B,** Stronger focus (larger aperture) permits spatial resolution of point reflectors. **C,** Apodization reduces side lobe amplitude so that tissue fill-in effects caused by off-axis reflectors are reduced.

nal to the main lobe signal will not seriously distort the echo amplitude. However, if the reflector at the center of the main lobe is removed, then the mapping of this image point will be distorted. This is because the adjacent reflector would cause a low-amplitude fill-in signal. These fill-in image side lobe artifacts are commonly seen when cysts or other anechoic structures are imaged. These artifacts are also possible, although not as readily identifiable, at all image points. The presence of side lobes thus limits the dynamic range of received echo amplitudes that can be uniquely identified as being caused by reflectors in the main lobe of the focused transducer beam pattern.

ULTRASOUND INSTRUMENTATION

At present, gray scale imaging equipment uses only time delay and echo amplitude information in creating the image. Most equipment contains the same basic building-block circuits: transmitter, receiver, display, and scan converter.

Transmitter

The first circuit building block, the **transmitter circuit,** produces either a high-amplitude, short-duration voltage shock pulse or a driving voltage waveform. Then an **output control** attenuates the amplitude of the shock pulse or the driving voltage waveform before it is applied to the transducer (Fig. 1-6).

After each transmission pulse the transducer then receives its returning echoes. The repetition rate of the transmitted pulses is called the **pulse repetition frequency (PRF).**

Receiver

After the received echoes are converted into weak voltage waveforms by the transducer, they are processed by the next circuit building block, which is called the **receiver.** The receiver actually is made up of many smaller sub-blocks or circuits, each one performing a specific signal processing function (Fig. 1-6).

The first sub-block is the **limiter.** Its function is to protect the rest of the receiver from the high-transmitter voltages. Because both the transmitter and the receiver must be connected to the transducer, the transmitter is connected directly into the receiver. If the high-transmission voltages were to enter the receiver unattenuated, it would be saturated for a long period of time, obscuring shallow echoes (because the receiver is specifically designed to handle very weak signals). The limiter is a circuit that passes low-amplitude signals (echoes) unaffected but in order to protect the receiver, it limits or clips any high-amplitude signal that is above a certain threshold.

The next sub-block is the **log amplifier** that amplifies the weak echo signals by 50 to over 100 dB. In this

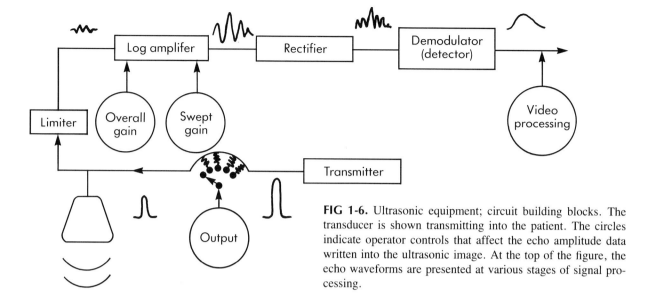

FIG 1-6. Ultrasonic equipment; circuit building blocks. The transducer is shown transmitting into the patient. The circles indicate operator controls that affect the echo amplitude data written into the ultrasonic image. At the top of the figure, the echo waveforms are presented at various stages of signal processing.

type of amplifier the output voltage is proportional to the logarithm of the input voltage. By using a log amplifier, small relative differences in both low-amplitude and high-amplitude echoes may be seen in the same image.

Next, the echo signals enter the **rectifier sub-block,** where the negative half-cycles in the echo voltage waveforms are converted into positive half-cycles. Then, with **demodulation,** the fundamental frequency signal on which the echo amplitude information has been riding (transported) is eliminated. All that is left is the so-called **envelope** (magnitude) of the echo signal. The demodulator circuit is really just a circuit with a very slow time response (smoothing circuit) that can only respond to the envelope of the pulse and not to the oscillations at the transducer center frequency. (If the rectification had not been performed, the output of the demodulator circuit would have been the average value of the oscillating RF signal, which is zero.)

The output of the demodulator is the amplitude of the echo signal and its time delay from the transmission pulse. Operator control of the echo amplitude signal is necessary because of the large variability of patient anatomy and acoustic parameters of normal tissues. Homogeneous soft tissues in the body should appear uniform in the ultrasonic image. However, echo amplitudes received from deeper soft tissue structures have lower amplitudes because of the attenuation of the overlying tissue. This leads to a graded appearance of the tissue gray-scale image. The **overall gain** control changes the gain of the log amplifier. This change of gain affects all echoes by the same amount (in dB) and does not compensate for the lower echo amplitudes received from larger depths.

This problem is solved by a very ingenious method called **swept gain** or **time gain compensation** (TGC).

The swept gain is a method of time-increasing the gain of the log amplifier in synchrony with the arrival of lower and lower amplitude echoes from deeper and deeper in the body. The voltage that controls the gain of the log amplifier is usually varied linearly with an operator selectable slope. Thus, by proper selection of the operator selectable slope of the swept gain, the effects of tissue attenuation in the image may be compensated.

Display

Cathode Ray Tubes. **Cathode ray tubes** (CRT) or broadcast TV tubes are used as the display in most ultrasonic images. The face of the CRT is a two-dimensional surface that can display the echo data (as brightness) in a two-dimensional format.

The simplest ultrasonic display mode is called the **A-mode (amplitude mode)** display (Fig. 1-7), in which the horizontal axis of the CRT tube represents distance into the patient (depth) and the vertical axis represents the amplitude of the amplified and demodulated echoes. The horizontal axis is calibrated in distance, which means that the equipment, even though it is always making time measurements of the returning echoes, is converting the measured times into depths in the patient. A-mode displays give a great deal of echo amplitude information but along only one transducer line of sight. They are useful with fairly simple patient anatomy, as seen in ophthalmologic scans.

Another method of presenting echo data on the two-dimensional CRT face is called **B-Mode display (brightness mode),** in which the brightness of the CRT spot represents the amplitude of the received echoes (Fig. 1-8). A set of B-mode image lines scanned through a linear plane in the patient (**scan plane**) is called a B-scan and presents a cross-sectional image of the scan plane called a **gray scale image,** in which the

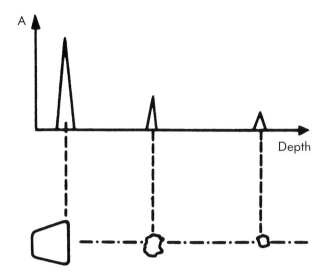

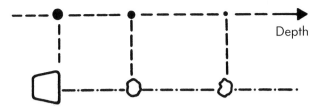

FIG 1-8. B-mode display. The echoes are registered along the B-mode display line at the depth corresponding to their respective reflectors. The brightness of the B-mode spot on the CRT face is proportional to the amplified echo amplitude.

FIG 1-7. A-mode display. The amplitudes *(A)* of the received echoes are demonstrated at the depths of their respective reflectors. This display mode presents the echo amplitude information received from only one transducer line of sight. The first "echo" on the horizontal axis is called the "main bang" and is produced by the reception of a clipped transmission pulse. It indicates the spatial position of the transducer front face.

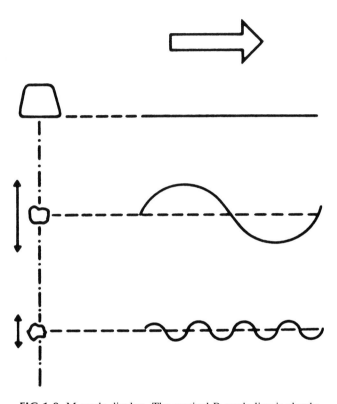

echo amplitudes are encoded in image shades of gray. Gray scale displays present both specular and diffuse echoes for diagnosis. The tissue parenchyma information contained in the low amplitude diffuse echo signals has proved to be of great value in diagnosing many different disease states from ultrasonic images.

The last display mode to be discussed is called the **M-mode** (**motion mode;** Fig. 1-9). On a B-mode display the distance into the patient is represented by the vertical B-mode display line on the CRT and the echo amplitudes are represented by the beam brightness. The vertical B-mode display line is swept slowly in a horizontal direction across the display with a known constant velocity. The main bang echo (which is due to the transmission pulse) (Fig. 1-7) presents as a straight horizontal line. As internal reflectors move toward and away from the transducer, their echoes are displayed higher or lower on the vertical B-mode line. The amplitude of their motion and velocities can be quite easily obtained from their M-mode traces. The vertical base line is swept across the display with a known slow velocity, so the calculated slope of the M-mode trace yields the reflector velocity.

FIG 1-9. M-mode display. The vertical B-mode line is slowly swept in a horizontal direction across the CRT face with a known velocity. The slope of the reflector M-mode (motion) trace gives a quantitative measure of its velocity toward or away from the transducer and the extent of displacement. **A,** R_1. **B,** R_2.

Scan Converter

The received echoes are stored in a scan converter (which stores both echo position and amplitude information) and then passed on to the display for viewing and hardcopy generation. A scan converter is a memory

that accepts data in one scan format and outputs it at a later time in a different scan format. The receiver outputs the echo position information in the same format in which the patient was scanned, a preprogrammed scan motion in a real-time image. Thus, memory input format is different from the display format, which is a broadcast TV format (525 horizontal display lines/frame at 30 frames/sec).

Historically, two types of scan converters, analog and digital, were developed. The **analog scan converters** presented a gray scale analog image that appeared spatially continuous, much like a photograph. The analog scan converter was basically a CRT with the output phosphor replaced by a semiconductor storage grid containing a 1000×1000 matrix of tiny capacitor-like structures. The use of analog scan converters in ultrasonic imaging was of short duration because of the expense, fragility, and electronic drifting inherent in the analog scan converters. **Digital scan converters** proved to be relatively inexpensive, reliable, and flexible in data handling capabilities.[6] Before the ultrasonic image can be handled digitally, the echo, spatial, and amplitude information must be quantified into discrete units or pixels (picture elements) that can be represented by numbers. In dividing the patient cross-section into pixels, the tacit assumption has been made that inside each pixel in the patient the tissue is homogeneous and can, therefore, be represented by a single number in the scan converter memory or a single shade of gray in the image. The received echo amplitudes from each pixel are quantified (analog to digital conversion), and then numbers representing these ranges of echo amplitudes are stored in the computer memory locations that correspond to each pixel.

One common clinical task in ultrasonic imaging is the identification of small focal lesions with slightly different acoustic properties from the background normal tissue. The focal lesion might be large enough to be perceived if it had high contrast with the background tissue, but its identification in the low-contrast case depends on the echo amplitude resolution of the image. Echo amplitude resolution depends on the quantization scheme used in digitizing the echo amplitudes.[7] When the analog echo amplitude dynamic range is digitized it is divided into a number of smaller intervals displayed as multiple shades of gray. All echo amplitudes that fall into a given interval will be assigned the same number in digital memory. The key for good echo amplitude resolution is to have very small intervals so that a slight difference in analog echo amplitude will cause two echoes to fall into adjacent intervals and to be assigned different numbers in computer memory. To increase the echo amplitude resolution without increasing the memory size and thus the cost, one can use unequal intervals arranged so that they are the closest together in the echo amplitude range of interest. The most diagnostically useful echo amplitude digitization schemes have closely spaced intervals in the low amplitude (diffuse echoes) range and widely spaced intervals in the high amplitude (specular echoes) range.[7]

REAL-TIME ULTRASOUND
Mechanical Sector Scanners

Mechanical sector scanners generally use single element transducers. The transducers are angled back and forth in an oscillatory motion such that the transducer beam defines a pie-shaped sector in the patient cross-section with a limited field of view for anterior structures and a widening field of view for more posterior structures. Some mechanical sector scanners use multiple transducers (usually three) rotating continuously around a common axis. As the beam of each transducer enters the sector field of view, its return echoes are processed to form the image. The mechanical sector scanner transducer has a small contact area with the skin, and its diverging field of view fits between the ribs, thus preventing their reverberation artifacts and the distortion of the image caused by bending of the beam. At the depth of the heart valves, the sector field of view is sufficiently wide to show the anatomy of interest.

Phased Array Scanners

Phased arrays are sector scanners with no moving parts. A set of thin piezoelectric elements are arranged in a line, with their length along the slice thickness direction (perpendicular to the scan plane) and their thinnest dimension along the multi-element array axis. The length of the array is small so that it can fit between the ribs for cardiac scanning. In sector array scanners, the focusing and beam angulation are accomplished by electronic circuits.

If a single-element piezoelectric crystal is spherically curved, then all of the ultrasound energy in the transmitted waves is directed toward the center or curvature of the spherical element (focal point). Because the acoustic path lengths to this point are identical, all the waves arrive in phase (at the same time). Due to the simultaneous arrival times, constructive interference occurs and the amplitude of the transmitted ultrasound wave is maximal at this focal point. The same result can occur with an unfocused piezoelectric element and an acoustic lens.

It is easy to approximate a curved single element with an array of individual elements by placing them along a curved arc section with their individual beams pointed at the center of curvature of the arc section (Fig. 1-10, A). However, this is not a practical solution. To go one step further toward our goal, the individual elements are kept on the arc section but rotated so that they are all parallel and pointing horizontally (Fig. 1-10, B). The focus, which is formed when the individual elements are then fired simultaneously, is almost as good as with the first arrangement. The reason is that the beam patterns of the individual elements (with small apertures) are almost omnidirectional, so that the magnitude of the acoustic energy each individual element directs toward the center of curvature of the arc section is almost the same as before. Because the individual elements are still on the arc section, the condition of "in phase" arrival at the focal point is still obeyed. But this new arrangement still is not a practical solution.

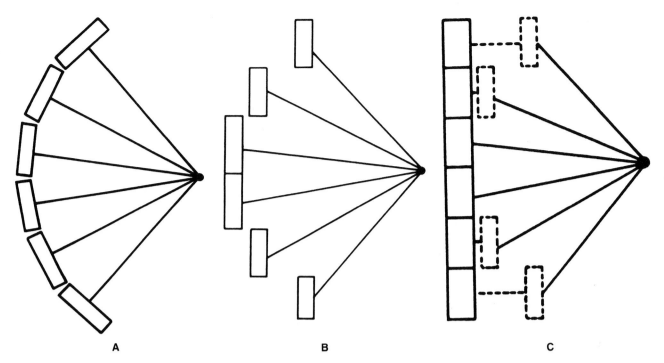

FIG 1-10. Principles of multi element array focusing. **A,** The elements lie along an arc section and are all aimed at its center of curvature. **B,** The elements are still on the arc section but now point to the right. **C,** Firing the elements from a linear multi element array at different times simulates the arrangement shown in **B** by Huygens' principle.

If the individual elements were arranged in a line then the array would be much easier to fabricate and much more flexible in use. However, if the individual elements are in a line and fired simultaneously, then the array beam pattern would be focused at infinity, which essentially means an unfocused beam pattern. In firing the individual elements at different times, we make use of Huygens' principle, which in very simple terms states that a sound wavefront (a surface of constant phase) propagating in a medium may at any time be considered as a source (new transducer) of ultrasound waves. The individual elements are fired with suitable time delays so that when the last elements fire, the positions of the wavefronts in the tissue from the previous firings all lie on a curved arc (Fig. 1-10, C). From Huygens' principle we see that this is equivalent to having the individual elements on the curved section of arc fired simultaneously. This is a very powerful tool in practice because:

- it permits one multi element array structure to select beam patterns of different focal properties by simply changing the firing time delays
- it permits the replacement of failure prone mechanical components by much more reliable and less expensive electronic circuits
- the multi element arrays have the capability for parallel processing (and other sophisticated signal

processing) of the return echo data to improve image quality and increase information throughput[8]

The procedure for changing the beam direction from a multi-element array is called **beam steering** and is also accomplished by phasing the firings of the individual elements. A basic rule for longitudinal plane acoustic waves propagating in a fluid is that the direction of propagation is always perpendicular to the wavefront. If all of the elements are fired simultaneously, then the individual wavefronts (due to individual elements) will combine in the tissue to form a wavefront parallel to the front face of the multi-element array. If the elements are fired in sequence from one side to the other with the same time delay between each sequential firing, their individual wavefronts combine in the tissue to form a single wavefront that is straight (a plane wave) and tilted at an angle to the linear array front face in the scan plane (Fig. 1-11). The angle of tilt depends on the time delay (phase difference) between the element firings and may be changed simply by varying the time delay. By firing the elements in the reverse order the beam may be steered in the opposite direction. So by controlling the phasing (timing) of the firings of the individual elements the ultrasound beam can be steered as well as focused for each transmission and reception of the multi-element array.

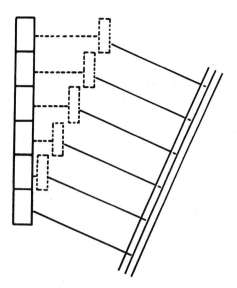

FIG 1-11. Beam steering. By firing the elements of a linear multi element array in sequence with the same time delay between firings, their individual wave fronts combine in tissue to form a straight wavefront at an angle to the array front face. Because the direction of ultrasonic energy propagation is perpendicular to the straight wavefront, this sequential firing method effectively "steers" the beam at selectable angles to the array normal by varying the time delays used.

Linear Arrays

A linear array is also a linear arrangement of individual elements, but it is much longer and fires in a different manner from the sector array. Linear arrays form real-time images with a **rectangular field of view.** They are especially useful in obstetrics where their large field of view is useful in studying the fetus and where the large distended abdominal surface may be readily coupled acoustically to the entire length of the transducer surface. Because a rectangular field of view is desired from this long array of individual elements, the elements must be fired sequentially in subgroups along the length of the array without beam steering. This generates a set of parallel lines of sight (perpendicular to the array front face) forming a rectangular field of view. To attain good spatial resolution of the image, two criteria must be met. The first is narrow beamwidths to minimize the lateral resolution blurring in the image; the second is closely spaced lines of sight in order to interrogate as much of the tissue as possible in the patient scan plane. If a small number of elements is chosen in the subgroup, then the requirement for closely spaced lines in the image will be met but the narrow subgroup aperture produces a divergent beam pattern that causes a great deal of lateral resolution blurring (even if some form of focusing is used).

To obtain a large subgroup aperture that may be focused to narrow beamwidths at large depths in the pa-

tient, a larger number of elements should be chosen in each subgroup. However, now the lines from adjacent large subgroup apertures are much farther apart in the image and a loss of image resolution (or information imaged) occurs due to these widely spaced lines. Actually, the solution to this dilemma of conflicting requirements is quite simple and elegant. A large number of elements is chosen for the subgroup so that they combine to have a sufficiently large aperture to attain a reasonably narrow focused beamwidth. But when the next subgroup is chosen for the sequential image line, it is made up of almost the same elements except that they are shifted over one element's width. For example, if four elements are used for the subgroup then the firing order would be elements 1, 2, 3, 4, then 2, 3, 4, 5, then 3, 4, 5, 6, and so on. Thus, the subgroup is large enough for a proper focus at depth and the image lines are close (one element's width apart). It is even possible to have lines closer together in the image by alternatively firing even and odd numbers of elements. When the elements in the subgroup are fired, they are time-delayed to obtain a focused transducer beam pattern. There is just one circuit used to generate the time-delayed high-voltage signals used to fire each subgroup. By means of electronic switches this circuit is sequentially connected to all the elements in the proper order. This use of one circuit with many switches is called **multiplexing.** Because the ultrasonic measurement is a pulse-echo ranging measurement, each subgroup must also be connected (multiplexed) to a receiving circuit that contains the same time delays used in transmission in order to have the transducer focused in reception.

To decrease **side lobe artifact,** the array elements that make up the transmit/receive aperture can be controlled individually with digital circuits, and the signal strength can be varied across the aperture to be maximum in the center and reduced at the edges. This process, known as **apodization,** results in reduction of the beam pattern side lobe amplitude. The improved beam profile (Fig. 1-5, C) is shown with the same two equal-amplitude reflectors. The side lobes have been replaced by a low-amplitude off-axis signal known as **clutter.** Clutter is caused by the combined effects of side, grating, spurious lateral, and phase quantization lobes. The off-axis clutter can be reduced to approximately 55 dB lower than the main lobe signal in an optimum pulse-echo multi-element array configuration. Then the displayed echo amplitude dynamic range can be increased to 55 dB without causing excessive noise pickup in the image. Also, since tissue fill-in caused by adjacent strong reflectors has been reduced, low-contrast small focal lesion detection is potentially enhanced in some instances.

If the array width is too small, then the slice thickness diverges into the patient and any advantage gained by focusing the beam in the scan plane is lost. So it is also important to focus the multi-element beam pattern in the slice thickness direction as well by using a cylindric acoustic lens on the multi-element array front surface.

Convex Arrays

Convex arrays are a variant of the linear array design. They attain large sector type fields of view at depth without side lobe difficulties and a loss of focus at the image edges. They also couple more effectively into the patient because of their curved surface. The divergence of the image lines causes some loss of image spatial information at depth. Tightly curved convex arrays have a small effective aperture and a large line divergence due to their limited number of elements; they are, therefore, not useful for imaging at depth.

Annular Arrays

Annular arrays are an improvement on focused single crystal transducers. The transducer face is divided into a set of concentric ring elements. The rings can be electronically focused in much the same manner as the individual elements in a linear multi-element array. Because of the circular symmetry of both the concentric rings and the resultant beam pattern, beam steering is not possible. Mechanical means must be provided for scanning the patient cross-section. Because of the cylindrically symmetric beam pattern, focusing in the slice thickness direction is identical to the in-plane focusing. When properly designed the side lobes are almost equal in amplitude to a single-crystal circular transducer focused at the same depth.

The phased array has the disadvantage of a limited field of view for anterior structures, but its advantage is that its sector-shaped field of view can avoid superficial reflecting structures such as ribs or pockets of bowel gas. The advantage of the linear array is its large field of view for anterior structures but it has the disadvantage of being affected by superficial reflecting structures and of needing a long contact area with the transducer, which is sometimes impaired by scars or body curvature. Convex arrays have a larger field of view that is useful in many instances.

Velocity Constraints

In the generation of real-time images, the slowness of the acoustic velocity becomes a disadvantage. After each transmission pulse, the transducer must wait for echoes from the farthest depths to be received before it can send out another transmission pulse. The PRF of the transmission pulses thus depends on the depth of the image field of view. This constraint limits the information that can be displayed in the real-time images. The relation between the real-time image variables is

$$PRF = F\,N = \frac{77,000}{P} \qquad (8)$$

$$\frac{\text{Image frames}}{\text{per second}} \times \frac{\text{Lines per}}{\text{frame}} = \frac{77,000}{\text{Penetration distance}}$$

If there is a low number of lines/frame (**N**), spatial resolution will suffer. If the frame rate (**F**) is too low, then fast-moving structures in the body will not be properly visualized or resolved in the real-time images. When the image depth (**P**) is selected by the operator, the **F** times **N** product is determined by Equation 8. Because frame rate and lines per frame are inversely proportional, there is a tradeoff between spatial and temporal resolution. Depending on the imaging task one or the other will be maximized. For example,

P = 20 cm
F N = 3850 lines per second
30 frames per second—128 lines per frame
15 frames per second—256 lines per frame

Cardiac real-time scanners have a frame rate of 30 frames/s in order to resolve the motion of the cardiac valves. At this high frame rate the number of image lines per frame is low and spatial resolution is not optimum. However, the heart is a high-contrast tissue structure with relatively simple anatomy so the loss of spatial resolution is not too serious. In abdominal scanning spatial resolution is a crucial factor, so the frame rate is lowered to about 15 frames/s in order to have an increased line density in each frame.

Zone Focusing

A serious disadvantage of focused single-crystal transducers is that the lateral blurring is only minimized over the length of the fixed focal zone, which can never cover the entire image field of view. With modern multi-element arrays and their complex supporting digital electronics, this disadvantage can be overcome.[9] Three different ways to form the beam pattern of one image line of a linear array transducer are demonstrated (Fig. 1-12, *A*). On the left, an aperture of four elements was chosen and the time delays (in transmit and receive) were selected to focus the beam in the upper third of the image field of view. In the middle, a larger six-element aperture was chosen and the time delays were selected to focus the beam in the middle third. On the right, an eight-element aperture was chosen with appropriate time delays for focusing in the bottom third. In this "selectable transmit-receive zone focus" mode, the user can choose the image depths that will be in sharp focus. The PRF is governed by the full depth of the image field of view and is the same for all three choices.

Modern imaging equipment incorporates a variation of this scheme called **multizone transmit-receive focusing,** which enables all depths to be in focus in the same image. For example, using the focusing demon-

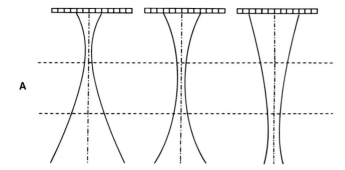 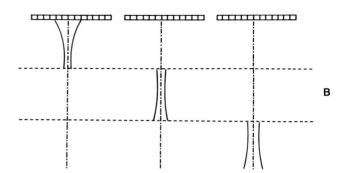

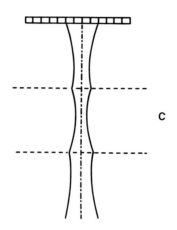

FIG 1-12. Zone focusing. **A,** Selectable zone focusing in which different sets of time delays may be selected to obtain best focus (focal zones) in the near, middle, or far regions of the image field of view. **B** and **C,** Multiple zone focusing is illustrated where several lines of sight are used to generate one image line. Only the echo information from the focal zone of each transducer line of sight is used in the image line. The effective compound transducer beam pattern is illustrated in **C.** Note that, besides different time delays, different numbers of array elements are used to obtain focuses at near, middle, and far depths in the image.

strated (Fig. 1-12, *A*), for each image line the transducer can be fired three separate times, focusing successively in transmit and receive for each of the three image zones. For each transmission only the echoes coming from the focal zone would be acquired in receive; the rest would be ignored (Fig. 1-12, *B*). When the results of these three separate transmissions are combined, a single "effective" beam pattern with good focus at all depths is achieved (Fig. 1-12, *C*). Improved spatial resolution is accomplished with multizone transmit-receive focusing at the expense of temporal resolution because multiple transmissions are required for each image line.

High quality real-time scanners use an even more complicated focusing scheme called **dynamic focus,** which takes advantage of the fact that receive focus time delays can be continuously varied so that as echoes are being received they are in focus.[10] The transmit beam pattern cannot be changed once the ultrasonic energy is launched so optimum focusing can only be realized if a multizone mode in transmission focusing is used along with dynamic receive focus.

Another advantage of real-time multi-element arrays over single-crystal transducers is that acquisition of the image lines need not be performed in sequence. This permits better time sharing between the gray scale image and the M-mode line being acquired in cardiac

equipment, or the Doppler signal being analyzed in duplex scanners. Also, it aids in reducing image ambiguity artifacts[11] and permits higher frame rates in multizone focusing modes.[9]

Special Probes

High-frequency transducers are useful in superficial small-parts imaging. Image spatial resolution is governed by the density of image lines in each frame, beamwidth, and pulse length.[12] With shallow fields of view the transducer can be fired more often, resulting in more closely spaced image lines. With this shorter penetration, higher-frequency transducers may be used, resulting in tighter beam focusing (narrower beams) and better axial resolution. Carotid imaging, along with breast, testes, and thyroid scans, yields better images when these new transducers are used.

By mounting a small transducer on a transvaginal probe, all of the advantages of small-parts scanning can be applied to scans of the female reproductive organs without requiring a full bladder so there is less patient discomfort and better quality pelvic images.[13] Prostate imaging is now possible because of the advent of transrectal ultrasound probes. Detection of early prostatic cancer can be done and the potential for mass screening for this disease is being investigated.[14] Small intraoperative probes are frequently used in surgery. Recently, both very small single-crystal transducers and multi-element arrays have been used to obtain very high frequency (20 MHz) scans of the arterial wall.[15] These intraluminal scans may prove to be effective in the detection and treatment of vascular disease.

DOPPLER ULTRASOUND

The Doppler effect is a change in frequency of received echoes (from that of the transmission pulse) due to target motion relative to the front face of the transducer (toward or away). If both the source and the receiver are stationary (at rest), then the received frequency (which we will call the effective frequency f_{eff}) is equal to the transmitted frequency f_o. If the source is moving toward or away from the stationary receiver, then the received frequency is given by

$$f_{eff} = \frac{C\, f_o}{C \pm V_s} \qquad (9)$$

where the sign is negative if the source is moving toward the receiver and the sign is positive if the source is moving away from the receiver. In the usual clinical case where the source is stationary but the receiver is moving, the received frequency is given by

$$f_{eff} = \frac{(C \pm V_r)}{C}\, f_o \qquad (10)$$

where the sign is negative when the receiver is moving away from the source and the sign is positive when the receiver is moving toward the source. In general, when the relative motion between source and receiver is toward each other, the received frequency is higher than the transmitted frequency. When the relative motion between source and receiver is away from each other, the received frequency is lower than the transmitted frequency.

In a pulse-echo ultrasonic measurement with the source and receiver being the same, the reflector motion causes a frequency difference between the received and transmitted frequencies

$$\Delta f = \frac{2\, V\, f_o}{C} \cos \theta \qquad (11)$$

where:

Δf = Doppler shift frequency
f_o = Transmitted frequency
V = Reflector velocity
θ = Angle between beam axis and V
C = Acoustic velocity

The Doppler shift is greatest when the reflector is moving either directly toward or away from the transducer. When the reflector is moving toward the transducer the Doppler shift is positive (the received frequency is greater than the transmitted frequency). When the reflector is moving away from the transducer, the Doppler shift is negative (the received frequency is lower than the transmitted frequency). When the reflector is moving in a direction perpendicular to the beam axis, there is no Doppler shift of the received echoes.

Continuous-Wave (CW) Doppler Ultrasound

In CW Doppler ultrasonic equipment the transmitted bandwidth of frequencies is very narrow, so very small reflector velocities with correspondingly small Doppler shifted frequencies can be detected. Because the output is continuous and not pulsatile, two separate transducer crystals must be used for transmission and reception. These two semicircular transducer crystals are housed together, pointing in the same direction with their beam patterns overlapping.

Because of the CW waveform, echo ranging cannot be used and, theoretically, the Doppler signals from reflectors at all depths in the overlapping beam patterns will be detected. The size of the sampling volume (overlap region) depends on the angle between the two crystals. A relatively large angle results in an overlap region that is closest from the transducer and shorter in depth extent. A relatively small angle will result in an overlap region that is farther from the transducer and longer in depth extent. The prime use for CW Doppler equipment is peripheral vascular studies where echoes from the red blood cells give a measure of blood velocities in blood vessels.

An advantage of the CW Doppler equipment is the relatively simple signal processing required to present the Doppler information to the operator. An oscillator generates the CW frequency, which is amplified and used to drive the transmission crystal. The received echoes are amplified and then combined with the transmission frequency in a circuit called a **mixer.** The mixer effectively multiplies the two signals together producing a resultant signal, which contains their sum and difference frequencies. If the output of the mixer is low pass filtered, only the difference frequency remains, which is the Doppler shifted frequency caused by the velocity of the moving reflectors. For a transmitted frequency of 5 MHz, an angle of 45 degrees, an acoustic velocity of 1540 meters per second and a reflector velocity of 100 centimeters per second, we may calculate a Doppler shift of 4.59 KHz (Equation 11). This frequency is within the audible range of frequencies. For the range of reflector velocities found in the body (up to several hundred centimeters per second), the Doppler shift frequencies are all within the audible range. The low pass filtered output of the mixer is used to drive an audio loudspeaker. Then the Doppler shifts may be analyzed by one of the best computers in the world, the human brain. The operator simply moves the transducer beam until he hears the Doppler shift frequencies that correspond to the moving red blood cells.

The amplitude of the audible Doppler signal is related to the number of reflectors in the sample volume. The pitch (frequency) of the audible Doppler signal is related to the velocities of the reflectors in the sample volume.

One great practical difficulty with CW Doppler is that if there are several blood vessels close to one another, the operator cannot be certain which vessel he is "listening to." Sometimes one vessel is below the other and the CW Doppler sampling volume picks up signals from both of them at the same time. One way out of this difficulty is to use pulsed Doppler equipment where the Doppler shift frequencies are detected from a much smaller sampling volume.

Pulsed Doppler Ultrasound

In pulsed Doppler equipment a single transducer is time shared in transmission and reception. A finite duration transmission pulse (tone burst) is emitted by the transducer, which will generate a continuous stream of echoes backscattered to the transducer. The received echo signals are then time-gated so that only a selected short distance along the transducer beam axis (range gate) is "listened to" by the equipment. This time gate may be placed at any depth along the transducer beam axis. Along with beamwidth at its depth, it determines the sampling volume of any moving reflectors.

Clinically, in coherent pulsed Doppler equipment, the phase of the echo signal is compared to the phase of the transmitted signal in order to detect any Doppler shifts. To make this phase comparison meaningful, the onsets of the transmitted tone burst and the range gate are both synchronized precisely with the phase of the transmitted signal. For every transmitted pulse the phase comparison circuit takes one sample of the Doppler shifted signal from the range-gated sampling volume. Repeat samples from the sampling volume are needed to determine the time dependence of the echo phase changes and, thus, the Doppler shift frequencies. These samples are taken at the equipment PRF and this causes some difficulties.

In any pulsed type of ultrasonic measurement, in order to avoid range ambiguities, it is important to wait for the echoes from the deepest part of the patient to be received before sending out the next transmission pulse. In pulsed Doppler the depth of interest is the position of the range gate. Thus the maximum PRF that can be used is related to the range R of the range gate as follows:

$$PRF_{max} = \frac{C}{2R} \qquad (12)$$

In most pulsed Doppler equipment the PRF is automatically set at its maximum value for the depth of the range gate selected in order to increase the amount of Doppler data received per second; this improves the Doppler signal-to-noise ratio. The highest frequency that can be measured unambiguously by a sampling process is governed by the **sampling (Nyquist) theorem.** This theorem states that to unambiguously measure a frequency F_r the sampling rate must be at least $2F_r$. If the sampling is $2F_r$ and there are frequencies larger than F_r contained in the signal being sampled, then the energy at these frequencies will be erroneously assigned to other frequencies. This error in measuring frequencies is called **aliasing.** The sampling rate is determined from Equation 12, so the maximum Doppler shift frequency that can be unambiguously determined by the equipment is given by the equation:

$$PRF_{max} = \frac{C}{4R} \qquad (13)$$

and, combining Equations 12 and 13, the maximum reflector velocity that can be measured is given by the equation:

$$V_{max} = \frac{C^2}{8} f_o R \cos\theta \qquad (14)$$

In using this equation to predict the performance of pulsed Doppler equipment it is important to verify that the equipment is programmed to change its PRF according to Equation 12.

In digital pulsed Doppler equipment the sampled signal is digitized upon acquisition (after each transmission pulse). A finite number of samples are then combined and analyzed to determine the "instantaneous" reflector velocity distribution in the sampling volume. A typical collection of samples might have a 10 millisecond time span. One method of analyzing the collection of samples (time variation of the phase signal) is by using a fast Fourier transform (FFT) on the digitized data. The output of the FFT is the frequency spectrum of the Doppler shifts (the relative number of reflectors at each Doppler frequency) during this time interval. By using Equation 11, the Doppler shift frequency may be converted to a velocity if the value of θ is known.

The standard display format of the Doppler frequency spectrum has a horizontal time axis (which is continuously updated until the operator "freezes" it) and a vertical axis on which the Doppler shift frequencies are presented with the positive frequencies up (toward) and the negative frequencies down (away) from the transducer. The number of reflectors at each Doppler shift frequency is represented by the shades of gray or colors in each "instantaneous" spectrum displayed (vertical column at each time interval of 10 milliseconds).

One clinical application of Doppler ultrasound is in the peripheral vascular system. By measuring the Doppler shift frequencies from the red blood cells, the spatial distribution of blood velocities inside the vessel may be determined if the sampling volume is much smaller than the lumen of the vessel. In the case of laminar blood flow, the velocity is greatest at the center of the lumen and decreases to zero at the lumen wall because of viscosity effects. In the case of an artery, the time variation of the blood flow (velocities) with the cardiac cycle may be determined. If plaque or other constrictions of the vessel lumen exist, then the Doppler measurement detects an increased velocity at the constriction. The presence of plaque sometimes causes nonlaminar turbulent flow, which can be easily detected from the "instantaneous" Doppler shift frequency spectrum. Severe turbulence sometimes causes reverse inflow, which is also easily detected.

Duplex Scanner

Some Doppler equipment combines a real-time imaging mode with a pulsed Doppler range-gated mode. The operator first surveys the patient anatomy until a scan plane is found that contains the vessels or structures of interest. Then the line of sight of the Doppler measurement is adjusted until it intersects the point of interest. The range gate indicator is then moved along the Doppler line of sight until it is over the point of interest. When the standard Doppler shift frequency spectrum display is enabled, it appears on the display screen along with a frozen gray scale image. The equipment then converts the Doppler shift frequency axis into a velocity axis.

Color Flow Doppler Imaging

Although duplex scanners provide a great deal of velocity information concerning one small region (sample volume) in the gray scale image, there is no velocity information provided concerning the other image points. Thus the operator cannot be certain that the most diagnostically relevant Doppler information has been acquired. With color-coded Doppler, all (or most of) the imaged vascularity is surveyed and estimates are obtained of the blood velocity. Then a range gate may be placed at the most relevant image positions and detailed blood flow Doppler data obtained.

Both gray scale and velocity information must be acquired and processed over all of the image, so there is not sufficient time to make accurate velocity measurements. As a result, two general methods of obtaining estimates of mean velocity were developed. One is called **frequency estimation,** in which the Doppler line of sight is divided into a multitude of range gates and the signal from each range gate is analyzed separately. Because the measurement time for each range is limited, the resultant Doppler shift frequency is only an estimate of its mean Doppler shift. Using the Doppler equation (with a zero Doppler angle), estimates of the mean velocity can be obtained. The other method is called **velocity estimation** and uses gray scale echo position information. Each of the gray scale image lines is acquired multiple times and the resultant echo wavetrains are analyzed to detect targets that have changed depth between acquisitions. Moving target indicator or cross correlation techniques are commonly used in these measurements. From the depth change and the timing between acquisitions, the target velocity toward or away from the transducer can be estimated.

Both of these methods lead to a two-dimensional pixel map of estimated mean velocity. (The velocity map pixel size is larger, in general, than the gray scale pixel size). To present both the gray scale and the velocity data on the same display, use is made of colors. The tissue gray scale information is coded in the usual manner with shades of gray. Velocity information is coded into colors so that the operator can view the two unambiguously on the same display. The color schemes are typically two-color (red and blue) using brightness, hue, or saturation to differentiate between the different velocity magnitudes toward or away from the transducer.

Another piece of information presented in the color flow image is the variance of the velocity (or frequency) measured. The variance (or distribution of velocities around the mean value) is an indicator of turbulent flow. It is calculated from the acquired data and also presented in the color flow image using a different color, usually green.

At present, the clinical gain using color flow Doppler imaging over duplex scanners is similar to the gain obtained when real-time scanners replaced static gray scale imagers.

REFERENCES

1. Chivers RC, Parry RJ: Ultrasonic velocity and attenuation in mammalian tissues. *J Acoust Soc Am* 1978; 63:940-953.
2. Goss SA, Johnston RL, Dunn F: Comprehensive compilation of empirical ultrasonic properties of mammalian tissues. *J Acoust Soc Am* 1978; 64:423-457.

Transducer beam pattern

3. Zemanek J: Beam behavior within the nearfield of a vibrating piston. *J Acoust Soc Am* 1971; 49:181-191.
4. Kossoff G: Analysis of focusing action of spherically curved transducers. *Ultrasound Med Biol* 1979; 5:359-365.
5. Christensen DA: *Ultrasonic bio-instrumentation.* New York: John Wiley & Sons, Inc; 1988.

Ultrasound instrumentation

6. Goldstein A, Ophir J, Templeton AW: A computerized ultrasound processing, acquisition and display (CUPAD) system: Research in ultrasound image generation. *Ultrasound Med* 1974; 1:475-480.
7. Goldstein A: *Quality assurance in diagnostic ultrasound: A manual for the clinical user.* HHS Pub, FDA 81-08139, DC: Food and Drug Administration, 1980.

Real-time ultrasound

8. Maslak SH: Computed sonography. In: Sanders RC, Hill MC, editors. *Ultrasound annual,* New York: Raven Press; 1985.

9. Goldstein A, Ranney D, McLeary RD: Linear array test tool. *J Ultrasound Med* 1989; 8:385-397.

10. Goldstein A: Ultrasonic imaging. In: Webster JG, editor. *Encyclopedia of medical devices and instrumentation,* vol 4, New York: John Wiley & Sons Inc; 1988.

11. Goldstein A: Range ambiguities in real-time ultrasound. *J Clin Ultrasound* 1981; 9:83-90.

12. Goldstein A: Pertinent physics of an optimal examination. In: Lee F, McLeary RD, editors. *The use of transrectal ultrasound in the diagnosis and management of prostate cancer.* New York: Alan R Liss, Inc; 1987.

13. Fleischer AC: TVS claims diagnostic role in ovarian CA. *Diagn Imaging* 1988; 10:124-128.

14. Lee F, Littrup PJ, et al: The use of transrectal ultrasound in the diagnosis, guided B biopsy, staging and screening of prostate cancer. *Radiology* 1987; 7:627-644.

15. Yucel EK, Waltman AC: Ultrasound-tipped catheter views arteries from inside. *Diagn Imaging* 1990; 4:108-111.

CHAPTER 2

Biologic Effects and Safety

▪ Frederick W. Kremkau, Ph.D.

RISK VERSUS BENEFIT

As with any diagnostic test, there may be some risk (some probability of damage or injury) with the use of diagnostic ultrasound. This risk, if known, must be weighed against benefit to determine the appropriateness of the diagnostic procedure. Knowledge of how to minimize the risk (even if it is unidentified) is useful to everyone involved in diagnostic ultrasound. Multiple sources of information have been used to develop policies regarding the use of diagnostic ultrasound. They include bioeffects data from experimental systems, output data from diagnostic instruments, and knowledge and experience regarding how the diagnostic information obtained is of benefit in patient management.[1-4] It seems reasonable to assume that there is some risk (however small) in the use of diagnostic ultrasound because ultrasound is a form of energy and has at least the potential to produce a biologic effect that could constitute risk.

It is difficult to make firm statements about the clinical safety of diagnostic ultrasound. However, much work has been done with no evidence of clinical harm.[1-8] Patients should be informed that there currently is no basis for judging that diagnostic ultrasound produces any harmful effects in humans. However, ultrasound should not be used indiscriminately. Even if this risk is so minimal that it is difficult to identify, prudent practice dictates that routine measures be implemented to minimize the risk while obtaining the necessary information to achieve the benefit. Prudence in practice is exercised by minimizing exposure time and output. Display of instrument outputs in the form of amplitudes or intensities and the display of thermal and mechanical indexes will greatly facilitate this approach to prudent use.

ULTRASOUND PARAMETERS

In discussions of bioeffects experiments and instrument outputs, various parameters descriptive of continuous and pulsed ultrasound are used.[9] **Sound** is a traveling wave of acoustic variables such as pressure. **Frequency,** given in megahertz (MHz), describes how many cycles of pressure variation occur in a second; **megahertz** means millions of cycles per second. **Duty factor** is the fraction of time that pulsed ultrasound is on and is the pulse duration divided by the pulse repetition period (the time from the beginning of one pulse to the beginning of the next).

Amplitude is the maximum variation that occurs in an acoustic variable during a cycle. The most common amplitude given is that for pressure. Because the amplitudes of the positive and negative half-cycles in an ultrasound pulse are not normally equal, they are expressed separately as peak compressional (positive) and peak rarefactional (negative) pressures, p_c and p_r, respectively (Fig. 2-1). Pressure amplitudes are commonly given in megapascals (mPa). **Power** (given in watts [W] or milliwatts [mW]) is the energy emitted by the transducer per second. **Intensity** is the power in a wave or pulse divided by the area over which the power is spread; intensity is proportional to the amplitude squared. Because intensity is not uniform across a sound beam (Fig. 2-2) and, in the case of pulsed ultrasound, is not uniform in time (Fig. 2-3), several intensities result. With regard to spatial nonuniformity, either the spatial peak (SP) or the spatial average (SA) value may be used. For temporal nonuniformity considerations in pulsed beams, the temporal-average (TA) value or pulse-average (PA) value may be used. The **temporal average intensity** is equal to the **pulse-average intensity** times the duty factor. If the sound is continuous instead of pulsed, the duty factor is equal to one, and the pulse-average and temporal-average intensities are equal to each other. The four intensities resulting from spatial and temporal considerations are **spatial-**

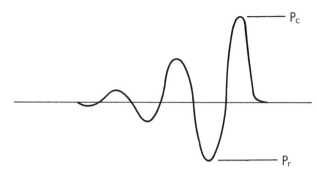

FIG 2-1. A three cycle pulse of ultrasound. p_c indicates the peak compressional pressure and p_r indicates peak rarefactional pressure.
(Modified from Kremkau with permission.)

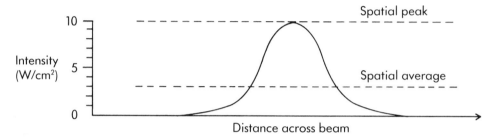

FIG 2-2. Intensity as a function of distance across the beam. In this figure, the spatial peak intensity (at the beam center) is 10 W/cm^2, and the spatial average is 3 W/cm^2.
(Reprinted from Kremkau with permission.)

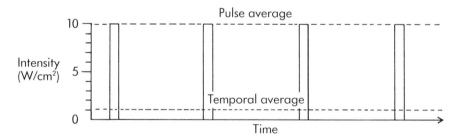

FIG 2-3. Intensity as a function of time for pulsed ultrasound. Pulse average intensity (10 W/cm^2) is the intensity over the time the sound is actually on. Temporal average intensity (1 W/cm^2) is the intensity that results when averaged over the time from one pulse to the next. In this figure, the duty factor is 0.1 or 10 percent.
(Reprinted from Kremkau with permission.)

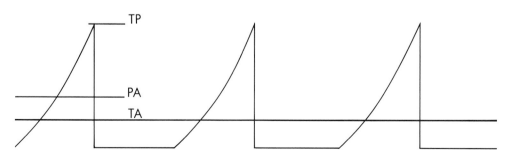

FIG 2-4. Intensity for three pulses similar to that in Fig. 2-1. Indicated intensities are *TP*, temporal peak; *PA*, pulse average; and *TA*, temporal average.
(Reprinted from Kremkau with permission.)

average temporal-average (SATA) intensity, **spatial-peak temporal-average (SPTA)** intensity, **spatial-average pulse-average (SAPA)** intensity and **spatial-peak pulse-average (SPPA)** intensity. Other intensities are the **temporal-peak (TP)** intensity, which is the peak intensity occurring within a pulse (Fig. 2-4), and the **maximum intensity (I_m),** which is the average intensity over the largest half cycle in the pulse.

Attenuation is an important consideration in the subject of bioeffects. It is a reduction in amplitude and intensity as sound travels. It includes absorption (conversion of sound to heat), reflection, and scattering of sound. Absorption is normally the dominant contribution to attenuation in soft tissue. Absorption is commonly given in decibels (dB). The attenuation of the sound as it travels from the transducer to the site of interest is determined by the attenuation coefficient for the intervening tissue (given in dB/cm), which is frequency dependent. Clearly, the longer the path is, the greater the attenuation will be. It is also true that the greater the frequency is, the greater the attenuation will be. Tissue attenuation coefficients are approximately proportional to frequency. For "average" tissue, attenuation coefficient can be expressed in frequency-normalized form as 0.5 dB/cm/MHz.

BIOEFFECTS

Our knowledge of bioeffects resulting from ultrasound exposure comes from several sources. These include experimental observations in cell suspensions and cultures, plants, and experimental animals, epidemiologic studies with humans, and information about interaction mechanisms such as heating and cavitation.

Cells

Several endpoints have been used in studies of the effects of ultrasound on cells in suspension or in culture. Liebeskind et al[10] reported ultrastructural changes and altered motility patterns in fibroblasts. Miller et al[11] failed to confirm these results in their study of ultrasound and fibroblast motility and morphology. Miller et al[12] studied single strand breaks in the DNA of human leukocytes after exposure to ultrasound. Various continuous- and pulsed-exposure frequencies and intensities were used, some involving cavitation and some not. Only one (94 W/cm^2 SPTA at 8 MHz CW) yielded significantly increased frequency of breaks, which may have resulted from the chemical activity associated with transient cavitation. It appears that for virtually all bioeffects found in cell suspensions, cavitation is involved.

The most extensively studied endpoint with ultrasound exposure of cells is **sister-chromatid exchange** (Fig. 2-5). Over a ten-year period, about two dozen reports have been published on this subject.[13-23] Most studies have yielded negative results, while a few have

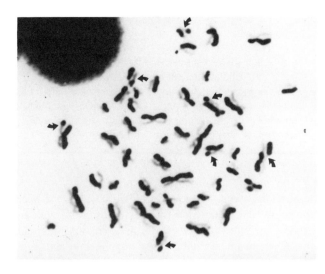

FIG 2-5. Sister-chromatid exchange indicated by arrows. These chromosomal effects usually have no genetic effect and therefore do not constitute a risk. Bromodeoxyuridine (BUdR)-substituted, Giemsa stained human lymphocyte metaphase.
(Courtesy Morton W. Miller.)

reported positive results. Of importance is the fact that there is no independent confirmation of a published positive effect. Attempts to do so have led to the conclusion that the cause for small but statistically significant effects is unknown, but it seems clear that the ultrasound exposure either does not produce increased exchanges or the effect is not reproducible and is too small to be consistently produced.[13-20] Even if ultrasound had consistently been shown to produce increased exchanges with all this activity, sister-chromatid exchanges usually have no genetic effect and, therefore, do not constitute a risk.[21-23]

Because cells in suspension or in culture are so different from those in the intact patient in a clinical environment, restraint must be exercised in extrapolating in vitro results to clinical significance. Cellular studies are useful in determining mechanisms of interaction and guiding the design of experimental animal and epidemiologic studies. The American Institute of Ultrasound in Medicine (AIUM) Official *Statement on In Vitro Biological Effects* follows.[1]

It is difficult to evaluate reports of ultrasonically induced in vitro biological effects with respect to their clinical significance. The predominant physical and biological interactions and mechanisms involved in an in vitro effect may not pertain to the in vivo situation. Nevertheless, an in vitro effect must be regarded as a real biological effect.

Results from in vitro experiments suggest new endpoints and serve as a basis for design of in vivo experiments. In vitro studies provide the capability to control experimental variables and thus offer a means to explore and evaluate specific mechanisms. Although they may have limited applicability to in vivo biological effects, such studies can disclose fundamental intercellular or intracellular interactions.

While it is valid for authors to place their results in context and to suggest further relevant investigations, reports of in vitro studies which claim direct clinical significance should be viewed with caution.

Plants

The primary components of plant tissues—stems, leaves, and roots—contain gas-filled channels between the cell walls. Plants have thus served as useful biologic models for studying the effects of cavitation. Through this mechanism, normal cellular organization and function can be disturbed. Irreversible effects appear to be limited to cell death.[24] Reversible effects include chromosome abnormalities, mitotic index reductions, and growth-rate reduction. Membrane damage induced by microstreaming shear stress appears to be the cause of cell death in leaves.[25] Intensity thresholds for the lysis of leaf cells are much higher with pulsed ultrasound than they are with continuous ultrasound; apparently the response of bubbles within the tissues to continuous ultrasound and pulsed fields is different.[26]

Animals

With experimental animals, mostly mice and rats, reported in vivo effects include fetal weight reduction, postpartum fetal mortality, fetal abnormalities, tissue lesions, hind limb paralysis, blood flow stasis, wound repair enhancement, and tumor regression. Recent negative studies include B-cell development, ovulatory response, and teratogenicity, all in mice.[27-31]

Many studies have been performed on fetal weight reduction in mice and rats.[32] All rat and several mouse studies yielded negative results. O'Brien[33] reported a linear dose-effect dependence of exposure condition versus average fetal weight in which the dose parameter was defined as I_2t, where I is spatial-average exposure intensity and t is the exposure time. Child et al[34] failed to confirm this exposure dependence. In their study, no effect on fetal weight was found at values of the dose parameter large enough to produce measurable heating in the fetal and maternal tissues.

Focal lesion production is a well-documented bioeffect from at least three laboratories.[35] It has been observed over a wide range of intensity and exposure duration conditions (Fig. 2-6). The lesion threshold follows an intensity exposure time relation $It^{0.5} = x$, where x is approximately 200 W/cm^2·s$^{0.5}$ for brain and 460 for liver.

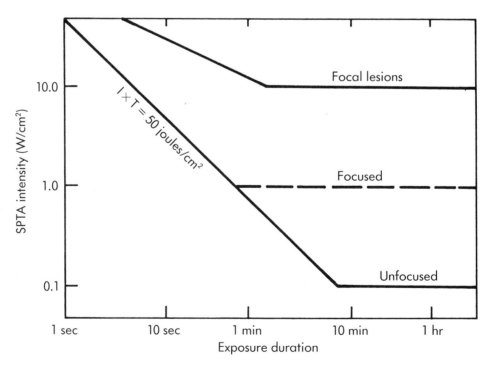

FIG 2-6. Comparison of the minimum SPTA intensities required for ultrasonic bioeffects specified in the AIUM Statement on Mammalian Bioeffects. The minimum levels required for focal lesions are also shown on the figure for comparison. Note that logarithmic scaling has been used for the axes of this figure so that the horizontal lines are separated by factors of ten in intensity.
(Reprinted from AIUM with permission.)

The AIUM has summarized the conditions under which mammalian bioeffects have been reported in its statement on *In Vivo Mammalian Bioeffects*.[1]

> In the low megahertz frequency range there have been (as of this date) no independently confirmed significant biological effects in mammalian tissues exposed *in vivo* to unfocused ultrasound with intensities* below 100 mW/cm², or to focused† ultrasound intensities below 1 W/cm². Furthermore, for exposure times‡ greater than 1 second and less than 500 seconds for unfocused ultrasound or 50 seconds for focused ultrasound, such effects have not been demonstrated even at higher intensities, when the product of intensity and exposure time is less than 50 joules/cm².

A graphic presentation of the statement is given in Fig. 2-6. In the latest revision of this statement, the sentence on focused beams was added to indicate their importance and the current knowledge relevant to them. The difference between the unfocused and focused levels for bioeffects is consistent with a thermal mechanism where, for a given intensity, a more focused beam produces a smaller temperature rise. In summary, no independently confirmed significant biological effects have been observed below 100 mW/cm². Focal lesions occur at intensities greater than 10 W/cm².

Mechanisms

Mechanisms of action by which ultrasound could produce biological effects can be characterized into two groups: heating and mechanical. Attenuation in tissue is primarily caused by absorption, that is, conversion of ultrasound to heat. Thus, ultrasound produces a temperature rise as it propagates through tissues. The heating produced depends on the applied intensity and frequency of sound (since the absorption coefficient is approximately proportional to frequency) and on the beam focusing and tissue perfusion. Heating increases as intensity or frequency is increased. For a given transducer output intensity, at greater tissue depths, heating is decreased at higher frequencies because of the increased attenuation, which reduces the intensity arriving at depth. Temperature rises are considered significant if greater than 1° C.[1] Intensities greater than a few hundred mW/cm² can produce such temperature rises. Absorption coefficients are higher in bone than they are in soft tissues. Bone heating, particularly in the fetus, therefore, should receive special consideration.

Heating has been shown to be an important consid-

eration in some bioeffects reports.[36] Mathematical models have been developed for calculating temperature rises in tissues.[1,37-42] These have been used, for example, to calculate estimated intensities required for a given temperature rise (e.g., 1° C). The AIUM has summarized these calculations in its *Conclusions Regarding Thermal Bioeffects Mechanism:*[1]

- A thermal criterion is one reasonable approach to specifying potentially hazardous exposures for diagnostic ultrasound.
- Based solely on a thermal criterion, a diagnostic exposure that produces a maximum temperature rise of 1° C above normal physiological levels may be used without reservation in clinical examinations.
- An in situ temperature rise to or above 41° C is considered hazardous in fetal exposures; the longer this temperature elevation is maintained, the greater is the likelihood for damage to occur.
- Analytical models of ultrasonically induced heating have been applied successfully to in vivo mammalian situations. In those clinical situations where local tissue temperatures are not measured, estimates of temperature elevations can be made by employing such analytical models.
- Calculations of ultrasonically induced temperature elevation, based on a simplified tissue model and a simplified model of stationary beams, suggest the following. For examinations of fetal soft tissues with typical perfusion rates, employing center frequencies between 2 and 10 MHz and beam widths* less than 11 wavelengths, the computed temperature rise will not be significantly above 1° C if the in situ SATA intensity† does not exceed 200 mW/cm². If the beam width does not exceed eight wavelengths the corresponding intensity is 300 mW/cm². However, if the same beam impinges on fetal bone, the local temperature rise may be much higher.

Experimental measurements have been performed,[36,43-45] which have shown reasonable confirmation of the mathematical calculations. Bone heating has not been found to be significantly greater than that calculated for soft tissues. Biologic consequences of hyperthermia include[36,46] fetal absorption or abortion, growth retardation, microphthalmia, cataract production, abdominal wall defects, renal agenesis, palate defects, reduction in brain wave, microencephaly, anencephaly, spinal cord defects, amyoplasia, forefoot hypoplasia, tibial and fibular deformations, and abnormal tooth genesis. Miller and Ziskin[46] have compiled a table that includes about 80 biologic effects of hyperthermia. None has occurred at temperatures less than 39° C. Above that, the occurrence of a biologic effect

---

*Free-field spatial peak, temporal average (SPTA) for continuous-wave exposure, and for pulsed-mode exposures with pulses repeated at a frequency greater than 100 Hz.

†Quarter-power (−6 dB) beamwidth smaller than four wavelengths or 4 mm, whichever is less at the exposure frequency.

‡Total time including off-time as well as on-time for repeated pulse exposures.

---

*−6 beam width, according to AIUM/NEMA definition.

†SATA intensity refers to spatial average value over the focal area.

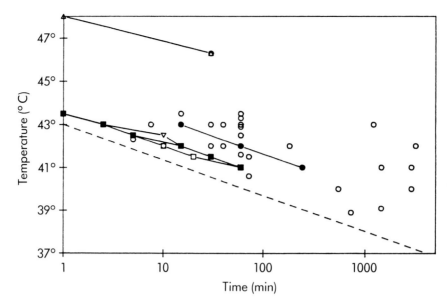

FIG 2-7. Thermal bioeffects. A plot of thermally produced biologic effects that have been reported in the literature in which the temperature elevation and exposure durations are provided. Each data point represents either the lowest temperature reported for any duration or the shortest duration for any temperature reported for a given effect. The solid lines represent multiple data points relating to a single effect. The dashed line represents a lower boundary ($t_{43} = 1$) for observed thermally induced biologic effects.
(Reprinted from Miller with permission.)

depends on temperature and exposure time as shown in Fig. 2-7.

Cavitation is the production and dynamics of bubbles in a liquid medium.[1,47,48] A propagating sound wave is one means by which cavitation can occur. Two types of cavitation are recognized to occur. **Stable cavitation** is the term used to describe bubbles that oscillate in diameter with the passing pressure variations of the sound wave. Streaming of surrounding liquid can occur in this situation and result in shear stresses on suspended cells or intracellular organelles. Detection of cavitation in tissues under continuous-wave high-intensity conditions has been reported.[49] **Transient (collapse) cavitation** occurs when bubble oscillations are so large that the bubble collapses (Fig. 2-8,*A*), producing pressure discontinuities (shock waves), localized extremely high temperatures and light emission in clear liquids (Fig. 2-8, *B*). Transient cavitation has the potential for significant destructive effects. It is the means by which laboratory cell disruptors operate. Theoretically, ultrasound could produce transient cavitation under diagnostically relevant conditions in water.[50-53] Another theory[54] incorporates a range of bubble sizes and yields a predicted dependence of the cavitation threshold on pressure and frequency. Experimental verification of this dependence was carried out with stabilized microbubbles in water. Thresholds for cavitation in soft tissue and body liquids have not been determined. The

AIUM has summarized information on the cavitation mechanism in its *Conclusions Regarding Cavitation*:[1]

- Acoustic cavitation may occur with short pulses and has the potential for producing deleterious biological effects.
- Currently available information indicates that pulses with peak pressures greater than 10 MPa (3300 W/cm^2) can induce cavitation in mammals.*
- With the limited data available, it is not possible to specify *threshold* pressure amplitudes at which acoustic cavitation will occur in mammals, with diagnostically relevant pulse lengths and repetition rates.

SAFETY

Information from in vitro and in vivo experimental studies has yielded no known risk in the use of diagnostic ultrasound. Thermal and mechanical mechanisms have been considered but do not appear to be operating significantly at diagnostic intensities. Currently there is no known risk associated with the use of diagnostic ultrasound. Experimental animal data have helped to define the intensity-exposure time region in which bioeffects can occur. However, differences, both physical and biologic, between the two situations make it difficult to apply results from one to risk assessment in the

---

*Evidence from observations with lithotripters.

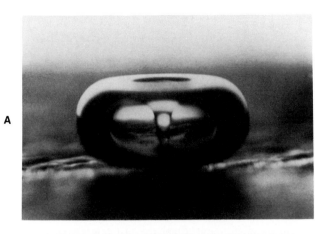

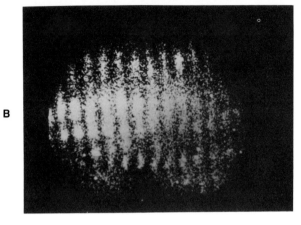

FIG 2-8. A, Photograph of liquid jet produced by collapsing cavitation bubble. Width of bubble is approximately 1 mm. **B,** Photograph taken from TV monitor of image intensifier system showing light emission from an acoustic standing wave produced in amniotic fluid at 37° C. The vertical bands are separated by approximately 0.75 mm or ½ the wavelength for the applied acoustic frequency of 1.0 MHz. The light emission is caused by transient cavitation in the standing wave.
(Courtesy of Lawrence A. Crum.)

other. In the absence of known risk, but recognizing the possibility that bioeffects could be occurring subtly, be of low incidence, or delayed, we recommend a conservative approach to the medical use of ultrasound.

Instrument Outputs

Intensities cited in previous sections included 100 mW/cm² SPTA and 1 W/cm² SPTA from the AIUM *In Vivo Mammalian Bioeffects Statement;* 200 and 300 mW/cm² SATA from AIUM *Conclusions Regarding Thermal Bioeffects Mechanism;* and 3300 W/cm² SPTP from the AIUM *Conclusions Regarding Cavitation.* Measurements of output intensities from commercial diagnostic instruments may be presented in several ways.[9] SPTA intensity is used in the AIUM *Statement*

■ TABLE 2-1
SPTA Output Intensities* (mW/cm²)

All instruments	0.01-2500
Imaging instruments	0.01-680
Scanning	0.01-440
linear array	0.01-48
phased array	0.1-85
mechanical	0.1-440
Stopped	0.5-680
linear array	3.8-332
phased array	10.1-240
mechanical	1.6-680
static	0.5-200
Doppler instruments	0.6-2500
CW obstetrics	0.6-80
CW cardiac/PV	20-2500
pulsed	40-1945

*Measured in water bath.

on Mammalian Bioeffects and relates well to a thermal mechanism of interaction. It is the output intensity most commonly presented. Table 2-1 gives a compilation of ranges of SPTA intensities from several sources. It can be seen that output intensities have a large range, with the highest being 250,000 times the lowest. Imaging instruments dominate the lower portion of the range while Doppler instruments dominate the higher portion. Within specific classes of instruments, intensity ranges vary by factors as small as 24 (phased array-stopped) and as large as 4800 (linear array-scanning).

These output intensity measurements are usually made with the use of hydrophones and radiation-force balances located in the beam in a water bath. Attenuation in water is low compared to that in tissues so that an intensity at a comparable location within tissue would be less than that in water. Models for accounting for the tissue attenuation have been proposed.[55,56] These approaches have yielded the following somewhat conflicting conclusions:

- Total attenuation to the human fetus averages approximately 11 dB at 3.5 MHz.
- A realistic estimate of the minimum expected attenuation in early pregnancy is, in dB, one or two times the frequency in megahertz.

The United States Food and Drug Administration (FDA) in its *Guide for Measuring and Reporting Acoustic Output of Diagnostic Ultrasound Medical Devices*[57] and *Diagnostic Ultrasound Guidance Update of 1987* for the "fetal imaging and other" category, lists the following as the highest known spatial-peak temporal-average intensities emitted from pre-1976 diagnostic ultrasound devices:

- 94 mW/cm² (calculated in situ value)
- 180 mW/cm² (water value)

■ **TABLE 2-2**
Upper Limits of Attenuated* SPTA Output
Intensities† from Table 2-1

All instruments	500
Imaging instruments	136
Scanning	88
Stopped	136
Doppler instruments	500
CW	500
Pulsed	389

*7 dB subtracted from water bath measurements to account for human tissue path.
†mW/cm^2

■ **TABLE 2-3**
SPTA 510(k) Guide SPTA In Situ Intensity Upper
Limits (mW/cm^2)

Cardiac	430
Peripheral vessel	720
Ophthalmic	17
Fetal imaging and other*	94

*Abdominal; intraoperative; pediatric; small organ (breast, thyroid, testes); neonatal cephalic, adult cephalic.

There is a 2.8 dB difference between these two values.

To compare instrument output intensities with bioeffects knowledge (AIUM *Statement on In Vivo Mammalian Bioeffects*), let us assume a frequency of 3.5 MHz and a 7 dB attenuation. This corresponds to an intensity reduction of 80%. Reducing the values in Table 2-1 by 80% yields upper limits as given in Table 2-2. Because most of the bioeffects studies were done in small animals such as mice and rats, the attenuation would be negligible and the values in Table 2-2 can be compared to the AIUM Statement value of 1 W/cm^2 for focused beams because virtually all diagnostic ultrasound uses focused beams. It can be seen from this comparison that on the basis of experimental animal studies, clinical bioeffects would not be expected to occur from outputs of current and past diagnostic instrumentation.

Regulatory Activities

Manufacturers are required to submit premarket notifications to the FDA before marketing a device for a specific application. The FDA then reviews this notification to determine if the device is substantially equivalent, with regard to safety and effectiveness, to instruments on the market before the enactment of the act (1976). If the device is determined to be substantially equivalent, the manufacturer may then market it for that application. Part of the FDA evaluation involves output data for the instrument; the data are then compared to maximum values found for pre-1976 devices. These values are given in the 510(k) *Guide for Measuring and Reporting Acoustic Output of Diagnostic Ultrasound Medical Devices*[57] and are presented here in Table 2-3. Some of the values have been updated since the 1985 publication of this guide. The current values are shown in the table. Until recently fetal Doppler imaging was not approved by the FDA primarily because of efficacy considerations. However, some devices are now approved for this application. One of the requirements for this approval is the real-time display of output information on the instrument. Over the last few years, a voluntary output display standard has been developed by a joint committee involving the AIUM, FDA, National Electrical Manufacturers Association (NEMA), and several other ultrasound-related professional societies. The goal of this activity is to develop a voluntary standard that will provide a parallel pathway to the current regulatory 510(k) process. It would allow exemption from the upper limits given in the 510(k) guide in exchange for presenting output information on the instrument (probably on the display). The current draft of this standard includes two indexes, thermal and mechanical, that would be displayed. The **thermal index** is defined as the transducer acoustic output power divided by the estimated power required to raise tissue temperature by one degree Celsius. The **mechanical index** is equal to the peak rarefactional pressure divided by the square root of the center frequency of the pulse bandwidth. In the case of both indexes, display would not be required if the instrument were incapable of exceeding index values of 1. At this time the development of this voluntary standard is still in progress. However, it is hoped that a standard will be approved by the organizations involved and be implemented quickly by the FDA.

Epidemiology

Several studies of an epidemiologic nature have been conducted and published. These have been reviewed by Ziskin and Petitti[58] who concluded that "epidemiologic studies and surveys in widespread clinical usage over 25 years have yielded no evidence of any adverse effect from diagnostic ultrasound." The most recent of these studies are those of Stark et al[59] and Lyons et al.[60] Stark et al studied 806 children, half of whom had been exposed to diagnostic ultrasound in utero, and measured Apgar scores, gestational age, head circumference, birth weight, length, congenital abnormalities, neonatal infection, congenital infection at birth, conductive and nerve measurements of hearing, visual acuity and color vision, cognitive function, behavior, and complete and detailed neurologic examinations from ages 7 to 12 years. No biologically significant differences between exposed and unexposed children were found. Lyons studied head circumference, height, and weight of 149 sibling pairs of the same sex, one of whom had been exposed to diagnostic ultrasound in utero. No statistically significant differences of head circumference at birth or of height and weight between birth and 6 years of age were found between ultrasound-exposed and unexposed siblings.

Although these studies have limitations and some flaws, they have not revealed risk in clinical use of diagnostic ultrasound. The AIUM developed and approved in 1987 the following *Statements Regarding Epidemiology:*[1]

- Widespread clinical use over 25 years has not established any adverse effect arising from exposure to diagnostic ultrasound.
- Randomized clinical studies are the most rigorous method for assessing potential adverse effects of diagnostic ultrasound. Studies using this methodology show no evidence of an effect on birthweight in humans.*
- Other epidemiologic studies have shown no causal association of diagnostic ultrasound with any of the adverse fetal outcomes studied.*

Prudent Use

Epidemiologic studies have yielded no known risk in the use of diagnostic ultrasound. Experimental animal studies show bioeffects to be occurring at intensities higher than those expected at relevant tissue locations during ultrasound imaging and flow measurements. Thus, comparison of instrument output data adjusted for tissue attenuation with experimental bioeffects data does not indicate any risk. However, we must be open to the possibility that unrecognized risk may exist. Such risk, if it does exist, may have eluded detection up to this point because it is subtle, delayed, or of incidence rates close to normal values. As more sensitive endpoints are studied over longer periods of time or on larger populations, such risk may be identified. On the other hand, future studies may not yield any positive effects, thus strengthening the possibility that medical ultrasound imaging is without detectable risk. In the meantime, with no known risk and with known benefit to the procedure, a conservative approach to imaging should be followed.[1,61,62] That is, ultrasound imaging should be used when medically indicated with minimum exposure of the patient and fetus. Exposure is maximally reduced by minimizing both instrument output intensity and by minimizing exposure time during a study. Doppler instrument outputs can be significantly higher than those required for imaging (Table 2-1). It thus seems most likely that the greatest potential for

*The acoustic exposure levels in these studies may not be representative of the full range of current exposures.

risk in ultrasound diagnosis (although no specific risk has been identified even in this case) is for fetal Doppler studies. These combine potentially high output intensities with stationary geometry and the presumably more sensitive fetus.

Ultrasound should be used for imaging only when medically indicated. A controversial area relating to this is whether pregnancy constitutes a medical indication. The NIH Consensus Development Panel[63] concluded that "the data on clinical efficacy and safety do not allow a recommendation for routine screening at this time." The Royal College of Obstetricians and Gynaecologists,[64] concentrating on the safety aspect, has stated "the present evidence for the safety of ultrasound based on over 20 years of experience and research is sufficiently convincing for us not to recommend a change in the common practice of routine ultrasound examination between 16-18 weeks of pregnancy." The European Federation of Societies for Ultrasound in Medicine and Biology[65] has stated that "routine clinical scanning of every woman during pregnancy is not contra-indicated by the evidence currently available from biological investigations and its performance should be left to clinical judgement."

The diagnostic methods committee of the British Institute of Radiology in 1984 created a working group to review the scientific evidence relevant to the safety of diagnostic ultrasound.[62] The working group concluded that there is no reason to suspect that any hazard exists.

The AIUM[1] issued the following *Statement On Clinical Safety* (October 1982, revised October 1983 and March 1988):

Diagnostic ultrasound has been in use since the late 1950's. Given its known benefits and recognized efficacy for medical diagnosis, including use during human pregnancy, the AIUM herein addresses the clinical safety for such use:

"No confirmed biological effects on patients or instrument operators caused by exposure at intensities typical of present diagnostic ultrasound instruments have ever been reported. Although the possibility exists that such biological effects may be identified in the future, current data indicate that the benefits to patients of the prudent use of diagnostic ultrasound outweigh the risks, if any, that may be present."

Clinicians in academic settings have the additional responsibility of ensuring that the use of ultrasound in training and research is conducted in a prudent manner with regard to risk consideration. The AIUM[1] approved a statement on this subject in March 1983 (revised March 1988):

Diagnostic ultrasound has been in use since the late 1950's. No confirmed biological effects on patients resulting from its usage have ever been reported. Although no hazard has been identified that would pre-

clude the prudent and conservative use of diagnostic ultrasound in education and research, experience from
normal diagnostic practice may or may not be relevant
to extended exposure times and altered exposure conditions. It is therefore considered appropriate to make the
following recommendations:

*"In those special situations in which examinations
are to be carried out for purposes other than direct
medical benefit to the individual being examined, the
subject should be informed of the anticipated exposure
conditions, and how these compare with conditions for
normal diagnostic practice."*

REFERENCES
Risk versus benefit

1. AIUM: Bioeffects considerations for the safety of diagnostic ultrasound. *J Ultrasound Med* 1988; 7(suppl 9): s1-s38.
2. National Council on Radiation Protection and Measurements:
   *NCPR report no. 74: biological effects of ultrasound: mecha-
   nisms and clinical implications,* Bethesda, Md, 1983; 74.
3. World Health Organization: Environmental health criteria 22. *Ultrasound* 1982; 65.
4. Nyborg WL, Ziskin MC: *Biological effects of ultrasound,* New
   York: Churchill Livingstone Inc; 1985.
5. Williams AR: *Ultrasound: biological effects and potential hazards.* New York: Academic Press; 1983.
6. Repacholi MH, Grandolfo M, Rindi A: *Ultrasound: medical applications, biological effects, and hazard potential.* New York:
   Plenum Press; 1987.
7. Suslick KS: *Ultrasound: Its chemical, physical, and biological
   effects.* New York: VCH Publishers Inc; 1988.
8. World Health Organization: *Nonionizing radiation protection* ed
   2, Geneva, 1989.

Ultrasound parameters

9. Kremkau FW: *Diagnostic ultrasound: principles, instruments
   and exercises,* ed 3, Philadelphia: WB Saunders Inc; 1989.

Bioeffects

10. Liebeskind D, Padawer J, Wolley R, et al: Diagnostic ultra-
    sound: time-lapse and transmission electron microscopic studies
    of cells insonated in vitro. *Bri J Cancer* 1982; 45 (suppl V):176-
    186.
11. Miller MW, Church CC, Ciaravino V: Time-lapse and micro-
    scopic examinations of insonated in vitro cells, *Ultrasound Med
    Biol* 1990; 16(1):73-79.
12. Miller DL, Reese JA, Frazier ME: Single strand DNA breaks in
    human leukocytes induced by ultrasound in vitro. *Ultrasound
    Med Biol* 1989; 15(8):765-771.
13. Ciaravino V, Brulfert A, Miller MW, et al: Diagnostic ultra-
    sound and sister-chromatid exchanges: failure to reproduce posi-
    tive findings. *Science* 1985; 227:1349-1351.
14. Ciaravino V et al: Lack of effect of high-intensity pulsed ultra-
    sound on sister-chromatid exchanges and in vitro Chinese ham-
    ster ovary cell viability. *Ultrasound Med Biol* 1985; 11(3):491-
    495.
15. Ciaravino V, Miller MW, Carstensen EL: Sister-chromatid ex-
    changes in human lymphocytes exposed in vitro to therapeutic ul-
    trasound. *Mutat Res* 1986; 172:185-188.
16. Henderson LM, Aghamohammadi SZ, Arlett CF, et al: Lack of
    discernible effect of diagnostic ultrasound on the chromosomes
    of cord blood lymphocytes exposed in utero. *Br J Radiol* 1986;
    59:499-503.
17. Barnett SB: Sister-chromatid exchanges in laboratory cultured

cells after repeated exposures to pulsed ultrasound. *J Ultrasound
    Med* 1987; 6:377-383.
18. Barnett SB, Miller MW, Cox C, et al: Increased sister-chromatid
    exchanges in Chinese hamster ovary cells exposed to high-intensity
    pulsed ultrasound, *Ultrasound Med Biol* 1988; 14(5):397-
    403.
19. Miller MW, Azadniv M, Pettit SE, et al: Sister-chromatid ex-
    changes in Chinese hamster ovary cells exposed to high-intensity
    pulsed ultrasound: inability to confirm previous positive results.
    Ultrasound Med Biol 1989; 15(3):255-262.
20. Miller MW: Does ultrasound induce sister-chromatid exchanges?
    Ultrasound Med Biol 1985; 11(4):561-570.
21. Stahl FW: Genetic recombination. *Sci Am* 1987; 256(2):91-101.
22. Jacobson-Kram D: The effects of diagnostic ultrasound on sister-
    chromatid exchanges frequencies: a review of the recent litera-
    ture. *J Clin Ultrasound* 1984; 12:5-10.
23. Martin AO: Can ultrasound cause genetic damage? *J Clin Ultra-
    sound* 1984; 12:11-20.
24. Miller DL: The botanical effects of ultrasound: a review. *Environ
    Exp Bot* 1983; 23(1):1-27.
25. Miller DL: Microstreaming shear as a mechanism of cell death in
    elodea leaves exposed to ultrasound, *Ultrasound Med Biol* 1985;
    11(2):285-292.
26. Carstensen EL, Child SZ, Crane C, et al: Lysis of cells in elodea
    leaves by pulsed and continuous wave ultrasound. *Ultrasound
    Med Biol* 1990; 16(2):167-173.
27. Desai BB, Sosolik RC, Ciaravino V, et al: Effect of fetal expo-
    sure to ultrasound on B cell development in balb/c mice. *Ultra-
    sound Med Biol* 1989; 15(6):567-573.
28. Desai BB, Sosolik RC, Ciaravino V, et al: Effect of fetal exposure
    to ultrasound on the development of functional, antigen-specific B
    lymphocytes in fetal and neonatal balb/c mice. *Ultrasound Med
    Biol* 1989; 15(6):575-580.
29. Sosolik RC, Desai BB, Ciaravinov, et al: Effect of fetal exposure
    to ultrasound on B lymphocyte function and antibody class pro-
    duction. *Ultrasound Med Biol* 1989; 15(6):581-587.
30. Gates AH, Carstensen EL, Child SZ, et al: Murine ovulatory re-
    sponse to ultrasound exposure and its gynecological relevance.
    Ultrasound Med Biol 1988 14(6):485-491.
31. Child SZ, Cartensen EL, Gates AH, et al: Testing for the terato-
    genicity of pulsed ultrasound in mice. *Ultrasound Med Biol*
    1988; 14(6):493-498.
32. O'Brien WD Jr: Safety of ultrasound with selective emphasis of
    obstetrics. *Semin Ultrasound, CT, MR* 1984; 5(2):105-120.
33. O'Brien WD Jr: Dose-dependent effect of ultrasound on fetal
    weight in mice. *J Ultrasound Med* 1983; 2:1-8.
34. Child SZ, Hoffman D, Strassner D, et al: A test of I^2t as a dose
    parameter for fetal weight reduction from exposure to ultrasound.
    Ultrasound Med Biol 1989; 15(1):39-44.
35. Frizzell LA: Threshold dosages for damage to mammalian liver
    by high-intensity focused ultrasound. *IEEE Trans Ultrasonics,
    Ferroelectrics, Frequency Control* 1988; 35(5):578-581.
36. Lele PP: Ultrasonic teratology in mouse and man. *Excerpta Med-
    ica Intern'l Congress Series No. 363* 1975; pp 22-27.
37. Nyborg WL: Temperature elevation in a beam of ultrasound. *Ul-
    trasound Med Biol* 1983; 9(6):611-620.
38. Nyborg WL: Sonically produced heat in a fluid with bulk viscos-
    ity and shear viscosity. *J Acoust Soc Am* 1986; 80(4):1133-1139.
39. Lizzi FL, Ostromogilsky M: Analytical modelling of ultrasoni-
    cally induced tissue heating. *Ultrasound Med Biol* 1987;
    13(10):607-618.
40. Nyborg WL: Solutions of the bio-heat transfer equation. *Phys
    Med Biol* 1988; 33(7):785-792.
41. Nyborg WL: NCRP-AIUM models for temperature calculations.
    Ultrasound Med Biol 1989; Suppl 1:37-40.
42. Wu J, Du G: Temperature elevation generated by a focused

Gaussian ultrasonic beam at a tissue-bone interface. *J Acoust Soc Am* 1990; 87(6):2748-2755

43. Abraham V, Ziskin MC, Heyner S: Temperature elevation in the rat fetus due to ultrasound exposure. *Ultrasound Med Biol* 1986; 15(5):443-449.

44. Drewniak JL, Carnes KI, Dunn F: In vitro ultrasonic heating of fetal bone. *J Acoust Soc Am* 1989; 86(4)1254-1258.

45. Carstensen EL, Child SZ, Norton S, et al: Ultrasonic heating of the skull. *J Acoustic Soc Am* 1990; 87(3):1310-1317.

46. Miller MW, Ziskin MC: Biological consequences of hyperthermia. *Ultrasound Med Biol* 1989; 15(8):707-722.

47. Carstensen EL: Acoustic cavitation and the safety of diagnostic ultrasound. *Ultrasound Med Biol* 1987; 13(10):597-606.

48. Miller DL: A review of the ultrasonic bioeffects of microsonation, gas-body activation, and related cavitation-like phenomena. *Ultrasound Med Biol* 1987; 13(8):443-470.

49. ter Haar G, Daniels S: Evidence for ultrasonically induced cavitation in vivo. *Phys Med Biol* 1981; 26:1145-1149.

50. Flynn HG: Generation of transient cavities in liquids by microsecond pulses of ultrasound, *J Acoust Soc Am* 1982; 72:1926-1932.

51. Apfel RE: Possibility of microcavitation from diagnostic ultrasound. *IEEE Trans Ultrasonics, Ferroelectrics, Frequency Control* 1986; 33(2):139-142.

52. Flynn HG, Church CC: Transient pulsations of small gas bubbles in water. *J Acoust Soc Am* 1988; 84(3):1863-1876.

53. Holland CK, Apfel RE: An improved theory for the prediction of microcavitation thresholds, *IEEE Trans* 1989; 30(2):204-208.

54. Apfel RE, Holland CK: Gauging the likelihood and degree of cavitational activity from diagnostic ultrasound, *Ultrasound Med Biol,* 1991; 17(2):179-185.

Safety

55. Smith SW, Stewart HF, Jenkins DP: A plane layered model to estimate in situ ultrasound exposures. *Ultrasonics* 1985; 23: 31-40.

56. National Council on Radiation Protection and Measurements: *NCRP Report no. 74, Biological effects of ultrasound: mechanisms and clinical implications.* Bethesda, Md: 1983; 37-39.

57. Center for Devices and Radiology Health—Food and Drug Administration: *510(k) guide for measuring and reporting acoustic output of diagnostic ultrasound medical devices,* Rockville, Md, 1985.

58. Ziskin MC, Petitti DB: Epidemiology of human exposure to ultrasound: a critical review. *Ultrasound Med Biol* 1988; 14:91.

59. Stark CR, Orleans M, Haverkamp AD, et al: Short- and long-term risks after exposure to diagnostic ultrasound in utero. *Obstet Gynecol* 1984; 63:194.

60. Lyons EA, Dykes C, Toms M: In utero exposure to diagnostic ultrasound: a 6-year follow-up. *Radiology* 1988; 166:687.

61. Kremkau FW: Safety and long-term effects of ultrasound: what to tell your patients. *Clin Obstet Gynecol* 1984; 27:269.

62. Wells PNT: The safety of diagnostic ultrasound. *Br J Radiol* 1987; Suppl. 20.

63. National Institutes of Health—Department of Health and Human Services: *Diagnostic ultrasound imaging in pregnancy,* 1984.

64. Royal College of Obstetricians and Gynaecologists: *Report of the RCOG working party on routine ultrasound examination in pregnancy.* London, 1984.

65. Watchdog group's evaluation of the safety of ultrasound. *Eur Med Ultrasonics* 1984; 6:5.

CHAPTER 3

Contrast Agents in Diagnostic Ultrasound

• Pamela L. Hilpert, M.D., Ph.D.

FREE GAS BUBBLES
ENCAPSULATED GAS BUBBLES
COLLOIDAL SUSPENSIONS
  Collagen or Gelatin Spheres
  IDE Particles
  Perflurochemicals
LIPID EMULSIONS
AQUEOUS SOLUTIONS
FUTURE DIRECTIONS

Great strides have been made both in the development and in the method of administration of contrast agents to opacify the lumen of bowel, veins, arteries, bile ducts, and ureters. Contrast agents are routinely administered orally and intravenously to enhance the small differences in roentgenographic attenuation between normal and abnormal tissues, and to assess organ function for intravenous urography, computed tomography, nuclear medicine and magnetic resonance imaging.

Administered contrast is not new to the field of ultrasound. Nonvascular applications are common in day to day practice. Water can be introduced into the bowel lumen orally to distinguish a fluid-filled stomach from a left upper quadrant collection[1] and rectally to distinguish a large-bowel collection from a pelvic collection.[2] Microbubbles produced by the injection of small quantities of agitated saline can be used to confirm the location of biopsy needles and catheters during interventional procedures.[3,4] Intravenous contrast agents were first introduced to ultrasound more than two decades ago,[5,6] but progress has been slow and sporadic, limited to right-sided cardiovascular imaging by the lack of a clinically suitable agent for other vascular or abdominal uses.

Intravenous ultrasound contrast agents are substances introduced into the vascular system to enhance contrast differences between normal and abnormal tissue or to enhance arterial or venous Doppler signal. Contrast agents may be specifically devised to best address certain clinical situations. For imaging of the liver and spleen, preferential biodistribution or tissue uptake by the reticuloendothelial system or by hepatocytes is advantageous. Contrast agents may aid in tissue characterization with the development of tissue-specific or tumor-specific agents. An agent may also be designed for use in a functional study to measure uptake and clearance of the organ-specific agent. For Doppler interrogation, identification of tumor vasculature may be an arduous task and a long-lived agent that is capable of recirculating in the bloodstream is required. For determination of vascular patency or for venous imaging, an agent with a relatively short half-life can be used. Contrast agents may also be introduced into the lumen of an organ (e.g., uterus and fallopian tubes) to outline a cavity, determine patency, or identify a fistula.

To be effective, the contrast agent must be stable for a sufficient period to be imaged. The substance must be metabolized or removed from the circulation in a prompt fashion. It must have low toxicity, so that a quantity sufficient to produce the desired effect can be administered. Finally, the physical properties of the contrast agent must produce an identifiable alteration in acoustic parameters of the tissue under examination.

Contrast agents can be classified into several groups, including free gas bubbles, encapsulated gas bubbles, colloidal suspensions, lipid emulsions, and aqueous solutions.[7,8] These agents may improve contrast resolution among various tissues by alteration of one or more of the acoustic parameters of tissue:
- the backscatter or echogenicity
- the attenuation or degree of beam penetration
- the speed of sound propagation through tissue

FREE GAS BUBBLES

Free gas bubbles are excellent scatterers of the ultrasound beam because of the large impedance mismatch between gas and surrounding body tissues. Gas bubbles may pre-exist in solutions,[9,10] result from vigorous shaking during preparation,[10] or occur with a change in temperature of the solution (e.g., the vaporization of ether at body temperature),[11] through cavitation at the catheter tip following a rapid, high-volume injection,[9] or through ultrasonic microcavitation.[12-14] The uses of free gas bubbles are limited because free bubbles are relatively large (10 to 100 μm), short-lived, and effectively removed by the pulmonary capillary circulation.[15,16] Smaller bubbles, capable of traversing the pulmonary bed (<8 μm), have high surface tension and high internal pressures, leading to dissolution before the pulmonary bed is reached.[17] For these reasons, free gas bubbles are only suitable for the delineation of right sided cardiac structures and intracardiac shunts.

Gramiak et al[5,6] first described the use of solutions containing free gas bubbles as ultrasound contrast agents. Rapid injections directly into the aortic root or cardiac chambers allowed specific anatomic validation of the origin of M-mode ultrasound images by the production of an intense cloud of echoes at the site of injection. These microbubbles were produced in various solutions (indocyanine green, 5% dextrose, saline or autologous blood), probably during the injection phase as a result of cavitation occurring at the catheter tip. Cavitation bubbles refer to solubilized gases that transiently come out of solution because of the large pressure changes produced during rapid high-volume injections.[9] Meltzer et al[10] later found that with clinically used catheter sizes (19- to 23-gauge) and forceful hand injections, cavitation bubbles played no significant role in echo enhancement. The amount of microbubbles contained in the solution before injection was responsible for the ultrasound contrast effect. Later studies supported this notion in that hand agitation of solutions before injection produced a more striking contrast effect, probably because of the larger number of microbubbles in the fluid.[13,14,16,18]

Ziskin et al[11] demonstrated enhanced Doppler signal from arteries following intra-arterial injections of a variety of substances, including Renografin, carbonated water, and ether. Ether, which boils at body temperature, releasing gas bubbles, produced the most intense Doppler enhancement.

Since that time, sonication of solutions has been used to produce smaller, more uniform microbubbles.[12-14,18] **Sonication,** or the deposition of ultrasound energy to produce transient cavitation bubbles in solutions, is able to produce microbubbles of less than 10 μm in high-osmolarity, high-viscosity solutions such as 70% sorbitol or dextrose. More dilute, less viscous solutions produce larger microbubbles, ranging in size from 10 to 23 μm. The high surface tension of these small microbubbles can be reduced through the use of surfactants or other stabilizers. These microbubbles are more resistant to intravascular collapse[12,19] and have less tendency to coalesce.[10,20]

Opacification of the left atrium and left ventricle has been reported following injection of sonicated Renografin or sorbitol from the pulmonary capillary wedge position, probably resulting from transit time being short enough for the microbubbles to survive.[21,22] Otherwise, free gas bubbles produced by hand agitation or sonication play little role in left-sided cardiac imaging or opacification of the systemic arterial tree because of the short life span and instability of smaller bubbles. Intraarterial injections are possible, but may cause the embolization of larger particles and are contrary to the noninvasive nature of the abdominal ultrasound examination.

SH U 454* is a gas-containing contrast agent that shows great promise for both intravenous and intracavitary uses. This agent is a powdered polysaccharide that, when mixed with a diluent, forms a crystalloid-microbubble suspension.[23-25] The crystals have varied shapes and range in size from 1 to 10 μm (medium 3.5 μm).

The mechanism of increased echogenicity is currently unknown, but trapping of gas bubbles between crystals, vaporization of water as the materials dissolve in the blood, and enhanced reflectance of the crystals have been postulated. The carrier substance, galactose, which is quickly metabolized by the liver, is tolerated well without severe side effects or toxicity. Initial work with SH U 454 has been limited to the imaging of right heart structures[23-25] and intracavitary injections[25-30] because of particle instability. Following injection, the particles dissolve within several seconds because of the concentration and temperature gradient within the bloodstream. A more stable agent, SH U 508, is currently under investigation and shows great promise for left-sided cardiovascular imaging[31,32] and systemic arterial Doppler after intravenous injection.[33]

SH U 454[34] has shown improved detection of liver tumors in rats following hepatic arterial or portal venous injections. Only 21% of induced hepatomas were visible on noncontrast sonography while 71% were detected as a hypoechoic mass with contrast administration. Contrast-enhanced sonography may improve hepatic tumor detection during intraoperative procedures.

Intracavitary uses of SH U 454 have also been described. Fallopian tube patency could be well assessed by contrast-enhanced transvaginal ultrasound-guided hysterosalpingography.[26-30] In human trials, a hysterosalpingogram was performed with SH U 454 as the agent and vaginal sonography for imaging. Fallopian tube patency was accurately determined following transcervical instillation of SH U 454 by visualizing the echogenic material fill the uterine cavity and flow through the tubes[8] (Fig. 3-1). Color or duplex Doppler ultrasound allowed direct assessment of flow of the contrast agent within the uterine cavity and tubes with improved accuracy over traditional radiographic hysterosalpingography imaging alone[27,30] (Fig. 3-2). Results

---

*Echovist, Schering AG, Berlin, Federal Republic of Germany

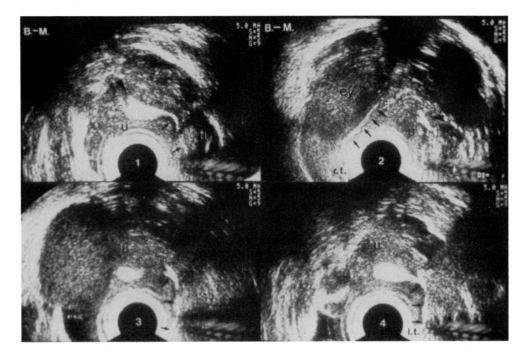

FIG 3-1. Transvaginal hysterosalpingo-contrast-sonography using SH U 454 through the cervical canal. *(1)* Longitudinal section of the uterus *(U)* filled with SH U 454; *(2)* Lumen of right tube *(RT)* perfused *(arrow),* cross-section of fundus uteri *(arrowhead); (3)* Lumen of left tube perfused *(arrows),* cross section of fundus uteri; *(4)* Transfer of contrast medium from cavum uteri *(cross-section)* to the pars intramularis of left tube *(LT).*
(From Deichert U, Schlief R, van de Sandt M, et al, with permission.)

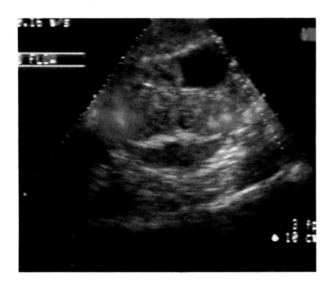

FIG 3-2. Color Doppler-assisted transvaginal-hysterosalpingo-contrast-sonography using SH U 454. Transverse image of the uterus shows enhanced color Doppler signal in the area of both tubes.
(Courtesy of Reinhard Schlief, Berlin, Federal Republic of Germany.)

were highly correlated with conventional radiographic hysterosalpingography and laparoscopy, without the risks of radiation exposure, anesthesia or a laparoscopy. Transvaginal ultrasound-guided hysterosalpingography may be a simple method of screening for tubal patency.

Real-time ultrasound and Doppler have revolutionized the diagnosis of peripheral venous disease. However, the varied appearance of venous thrombosis poses difficulty in the identification of intraluminal filling defects. Slow flow, low signal-to-noise ratios, and inability to compress central veins such as the inferior and superior vena cava, limit the evaluation of venous hemodynamics. SH U 454 has been used to increase the echogenicity of blood, producing improved diagnosis of venous thrombosis (residual lumen, recanalization), venous valvular insufficiency, and varicosities[35] (Fig. 3-3).

ENCAPSULATED GAS BUBBLES

To overcome the size and stability limitations of free gas bubbles, encapsulation of bubbles was proposed. Although initial attempts at encapsulation produced large bubbles that clogged the capillary tree, the utility of this notion was clearly demonstrated. Carroll et al[36,37] produced nitrogen microbubbles encapsulated within a thin gelatin coating (**gelatin encapsulated nitrogen**

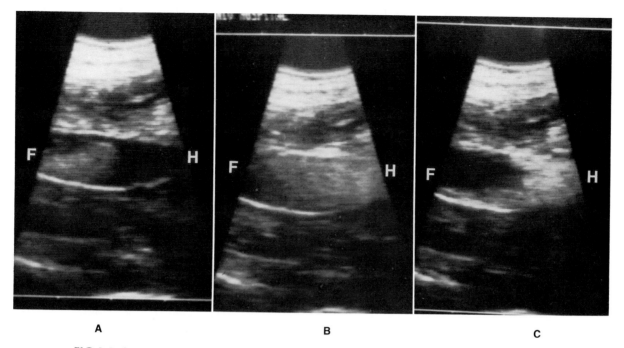

FIG 3-3. SH U 454 outlining the caudal vena cava. **A,** Following a femoral venous injection of SH U 454, the bolus of echogenic contrast agent is noted to arrive in the caudal vena cava of a dog. **B,** Several seconds later, the echogenic contrast agent fills entirely the lumen of the vena cava. **C,** Still later, nonopacified blood enters the caudal vena cava as the bolus of contrast agent travels towards the heart. *H,* Head; *F,* Feet.

microspheres [GENM]). The echogenicity of this gas containing contrast agent is based on the presence of multiple solid-gas interfaces with a large acoustic impedance mismatch. Several sizes of GENM (80, 76, and 12 μm) were injected intra-arterially while imaging over normal organs (liver and kidney) and VX2 tumors implanted within the rabbit thigh or kidney. Intravenous injections were prohibited because of the large size of the particles. GENM are seen as highly echogenic particles flowing through large vessels. Because of their size, the particles are trapped within normal parenchyma and at the vascular margins of tumors, producing enhancement that persists for several minutes.

Sonication of 5% human serum albumin* produces a gas-filled microbubble that is small (3 to 5 μm) and stable enough to allow free passage through the pulmonary capillary circulation. Particle concentration is high (4 × 10^8 spheres/ml). The agent is available prepackaged in ready-to-use 4 ml vials. It has a clinically useful shelf life of 6 months. Albunex has caused no clinically significant hemodynamic effect or toxicity in animal or patient studies.[38-40] Following intravenous administration, the agent's microbubbles rapidly dissolve (half-life less than 1 minute), and the residual free albumin is taken up by the Kupffer cells of the liver.

Cardiac applications of Albunex are the most promising. Albunex crosses the pulmonary bed and opacifies the left atrial and ventricular cavities[38,39,41] (Fig. 3-4). Following intracoronary injections, perfused myocardium increases markedly in echogenicity, allowing quantification of myocardial perfusion.[40,42] Many potential cardiac applications can be proposed, including delineation of endocardial borders, calculation of left-ventricular ejection fraction, quantification of regurgitant and shunt lesions, and enhancement of low-intensity Doppler signals.[43] Although Albunex arrives intact in the systemic arterial tree, the concentration of the agent is far less in the left ventricle than in the right ventricle. A significant amount of agent is trapped and/or destroyed during its passage through the lungs, cardiac chambers, and valves. Quantitative studies of the loss of the agent as it traverses the heart and lungs are not, as yet, available.

Albunex has been studied with abdominal imaging in small animals. It is not yet approved for human use. With conventional gray-scale imaging, visualization of the contrast agent within large and small arteries or a change in the tissue echogenicity of the liver and kidney has not been identified following intravenous injection.[44,45]

---

*Albunex, Molecular Biosystems, Inc., San Diego, California

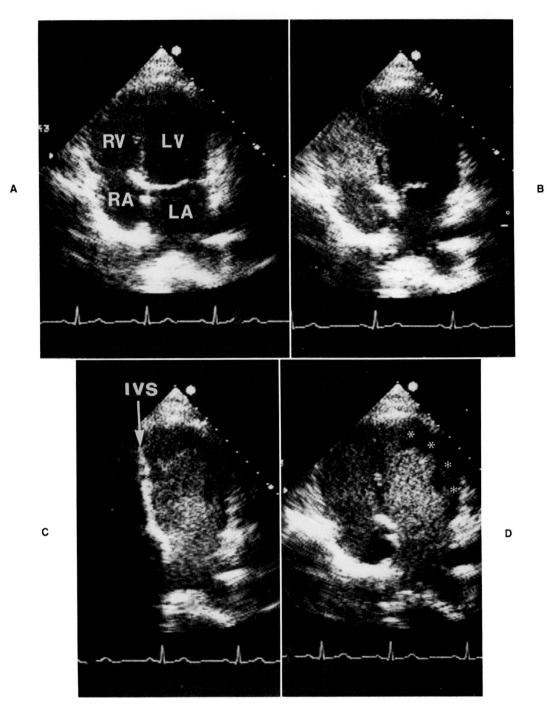

FIG 3-4. Opacification of the cardiac chambers using Albunex. **A,** Four chamber view of the heart before administration of intravenous Albunex. *RV,* Right ventricle; *RA,* Right atrium; *LV,* Left ventricle; *LA,* Left atrium. **B,** The echogenic microspheres first opacify the right atrium and right ventricle. **C,** Several seconds later, Albunex opacifies the left atrial and left ventricle chambers. Note that the high concentration of microbubbles within the right-sided cardiac chambers produce significant attenuation of the sound beam. *IVS,* Interventricular septum. **D,** The concentration of Albunex decreases in the right ventricle and increases in the left ventricle, improving delineation of the hypoechoic myocardial borders (*).

(Courtesy of Joel R. Raichlen, Philadelphia, PA.)

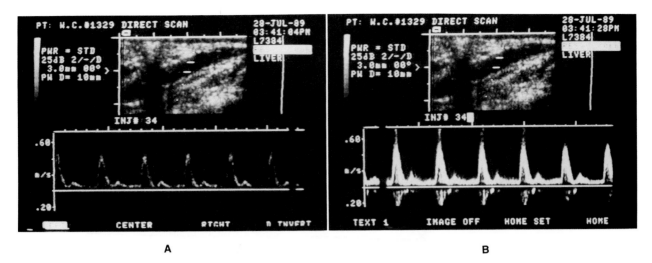

FIG 3-5. Spectral Doppler enhancement with Albunex. Sagittal image of the woodchuck aorta, **A,** before, and **B,** after the intravenous administration of 0.2 ml/kg Albunex shows marked of the septral Doppler signal intensity.

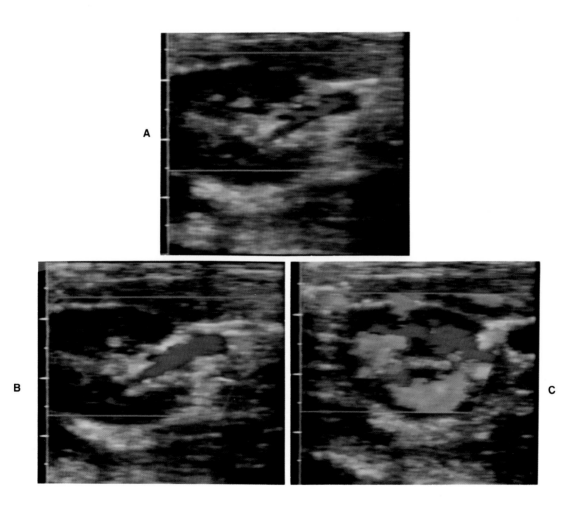

FIG 3-6. Renal cortical color Doppler enhancement following Albunex administration. Transverse images through the renal hilum of a woodchuck kidney, **A,** before, and after, **B,** the intravenous administration of 0.2 ml/kg Albunex shows enhancement of the central renal arteries (coded in red). Two seconds later, at a lower transverse image of the kidney, **C,** dense cortical color Doppler enhancement is present lasting 5 to 6 seconds.

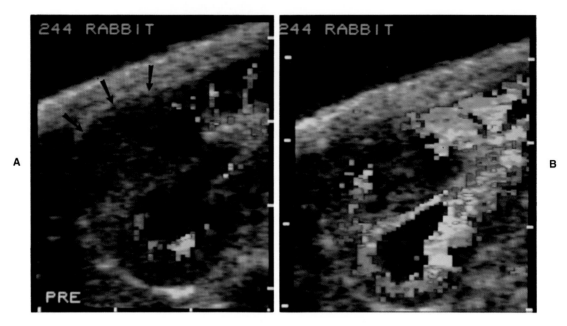

FIG 3-7. Cortical color Doppler enhancement improves the delineation of a renal mass. **A,** Color Doppler preinjection image through the upper pole of the right kidney in a rabbit with an implanted VX2 tumor shows a slight cortical bulge and loss of the normal cortical medullary distinction *(arrows)*. **B,** Following 0.3 ml/kg of Albunex, dense color Doppler enhancement of the normal renal cortex occurs. The hypovascular mass does not enhance, improving detectability of the mass.

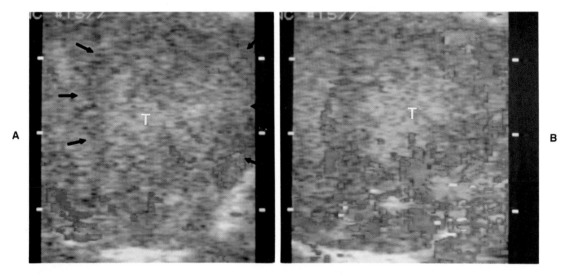

FIG 3-8. Peripheral vascular enhancement of a woodchuck hepatoma using Albunex. **A,** Transverse image through the hepatoma shows the ill-defined tumor to be of mildly increased echogenicity *(arrows)* relative to the adjacent normal parenchyma. Minimal color Doppler signal from the peripheral vessels is noted. **B,** After the intravenous injection of 0.2 ml/kg of Albunex, dramatic color Doppler enhancement of the peripheral vessels of the tumor occurs.
(From Goldberg BD, Hilpert PL, Burns PN et al, with permission.)

However, pronounced Doppler signal enhancement is produced in arteries of all sizes by both qualitative[44] and quantitative[45] methods (Fig. 3-5). Significant dose-related Doppler signal enhancement can be documented by both pulsed and color Doppler. The degree of signal augmentation is such that, with larger doses, parenchymal color Doppler enhancement, reflecting capillary blood flow, can be identified (Fig. 3-6). Typically, such signals are below the power threshold for conventional Doppler equipment. Use of a Doppler-enhancing agent with color Doppler technology, providing a global picture of organ vascularity, may allow the identification of perfusion abnormalities caused by vascular occlusions, vascular displacement, tissue replacement by masses of altered vascularity (Fig. 3-7), and tumor neovascularity (Fig. 3-8).

COLLOIDAL SUSPENSIONS

Colloidal suspensions consist of solid particles suspended in a liquid carrier. These agents are selectively taken up by the reticuloendothelial system and lead to an increase in backscatter or attenuation of tissues. Many factors affect particle backscatter; among these are, primarily, the radius of the particle and, less so, the frequency of the imaging transducer, the density difference between the particle and the surrounding tissue, and the particle concentration.[7,8]

Collagen or Gelatin Spheres

Ophir et al examined the backscatter properties of 2 to 3 μm collagen[46] or gelatin[47] spheres in both in vitro and in vivo models. Backscatter measurements from suspensions of collagen microspheres and human blood standards showed that those containing collagen microspheres have a significantly greater (29.6 dB) echogenicity. Subsequent in vivo measurements, following intravenous injections into dogs, confirmed an increase liver echogenicity. The degree of backscatter enhancement in the in vivo preparation was much greater than predicted by the in vitro data, suggesting that other mechanisms may also play a role. One such mechanism may be particle reaction with circulating proteins to produce larger aggregates of particles within the Kupffer cells of the liver.[48]

IDE Particles

In vitro and ex vivo corroboration of initial work by Ophir et al[46,47] was performed by Violante et al,[49] using iodipamide ethyl ester (IDE) particles, which increase backscatter in the livers of rate. This is thought to be caused by colloid particles that are phagocytized by Kupffer cells present in normal liver but absent in tumors. Thus, detection of lesions that are hypoechoic or isoechoic to normal surrounding tissue should improve with IDE particles.

Perfluorochemicals (PFC)

Perfluorochemicals are a class of compounds composed entirely of carbon and fluorine atoms. These compounds were first introduced to the medical research community by Clark and Gollan,[50] who demonstrated their oxygen-carrying capacity by submerging mice in the liquid for an extended period of time without ill effect.

Perfluorooctylbromide (PFOB)* is a type of PFC in which a bromine atom is substituted for a fluorine atom, resulting in a compound that is radiopaque[51-55] and nearly twice as dense as water, with a specific gravity of 1.9 gm/ml. It is emulsified in lecithin to produce a 100% weight-per-volume emulsion. The particles, 0.1 to 0.2 μm in size, are unable to leak out of normal capillaries, thus initially limiting the contrast to the intravascular space (Fig. 3-9). PFOB is removed from the bloodstream by the phagocytic function of the reticuloendothelial system of the liver and spleen, and later excreted by evaporation through the lungs without significant breakdown of the compound. The kidneys play no role in concentration or excretion of the compound.[56] The half-life of intravenous PFOB given to rats at a dose of 1.5 g/kg is 3 days, long enough to allow thorough radiologic investigation. Toxicity is low,[56] but not insignificant.[55] There are no cardiovascular or systemic hemodynamic effects following intravenous administration.[57,58] In a human clinical trial, side effects included pain in the lower back, fever and chills, reduced platelet count, mild cholestasis, and modification of blood lipid levels.[55]

PFOB-containing tissues are more echogenic, which is related to an increase in the number and brightness of reflectors. The increased echogenicity of PFOB is related to its high density (1.9 g/ml) and low acoustic velocity (600 m/s). This yields an acoustic impedance difference of 30% with non-PFOB-containing tissues, much greater than the typical impedance differences of 1% to 5% among various normal tissues and between normal and abnormal tissues. Although the particle size of PFOB falls well below the calculated optimum size for obtaining enhanced backscatter (0.8 to 2 μm at 5 MHz), agglomeration to other particles or to proteins within the vascular system or within the reticuloendothelial system may produce a larger effective particle size, resulting in altered echogenicity.[7,8]

Perfluorochemicals, particularly PFOB, have shown great promise as ultrasound and Doppler contrast agents.[59,60] Proposed applications of PFOB have been spearheaded by R.F. Mattrey et al, and include hepatic[61-63] and renal[64,65] ultrasound and computed tomography for detection of focal lesions, Doppler imaging for tumor blood flow,[65] blood pool ultrasound im-

---

*Alliance Pharmaceuticals, San Diego, California.

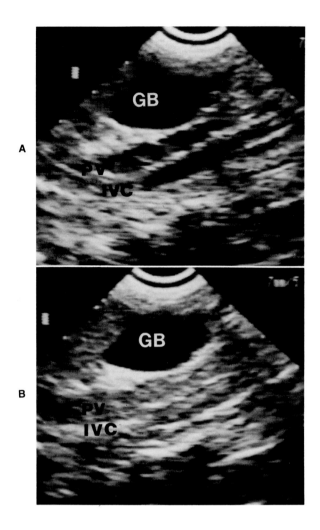

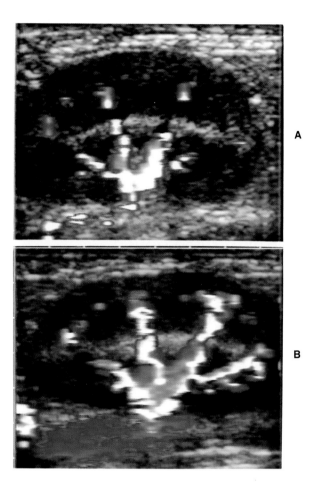

FIG 3-9. A PFC opacifies venous blood flow. **A,** In a prein-jection sagittal image of the right upper quadrant of a wood-chuck, the portal vein *(PV)* and inferior vena cava *(IVC)* are anechoic due to the presence of flowing blood. **B,** Shortly af-ter the administration of 5 ml/kg of a PFC solution, dense and persistent echoes are identified within the *PV* and *IVC. GB,* Gallbladder.

FIG 3-10. PFOB produces vascular enhancement. **A,** Base-line color Doppler image of a rabbit kidney. **B,** Shortly after intravenous administration of 2 ml/kg of PFOB, there is pro-found enhancement of the vascular signal, including visual-ization of the accurate ring and small cortical vessels.
(From Coley BD, Mattrey RF, Roberts A, et al: The potential role of PFOB enhanced sonography of the kidney. Part II—Detection of partial infarction. *Kidney International,* in press, with permission.)

aging for organ perfusion,[66] and assessment of renal concentrating ability.[67]

Following the intravenous injection of PFOB, the stages of parenchymal and tumor enhancement on ultra-sound vary with time. Initially, as PFOB is contained within the intravascular space, the degree of enhance-ment of an organ is related to the degree of organ per-fusion (Fig. 3-10). For example, relatively hypovascu-lar renal tumors that are isoechogenic with the kidney become more apparent (relatively less echogenic) after the administration of PFOB because the normal kidney increases in echogenicity in proportion to its blood sup-ply.[64] As the contrast agent is fixed by the reticuloen-dothelial system, the normal liver and spleen increase in

echogenicity.[61-63] Hepatic tumors and abscesses, which were typically less echogenic or isoechogenic with nor-mal surrounding parenchyma, appear relatively more hypoechoic after the administration of PFOB. These fo-cal lesions, which lack reticuloendothelial system func-tion, do not take up the contrast agent as normal sur-rounding parenchyma, resulting in increased contrast differences between normal and abnormal tissues and improved lesion detection.[61-63] With both ultrasound and computed tomography, enhancement of the margin of VX2 tumors in rabbits has been identified as a late finding (1 to 2 days following administration) and at-tributed to the deposition of PFOB-containing macro-phages at the tumor periphery.[61,68] Additionally, PFOB

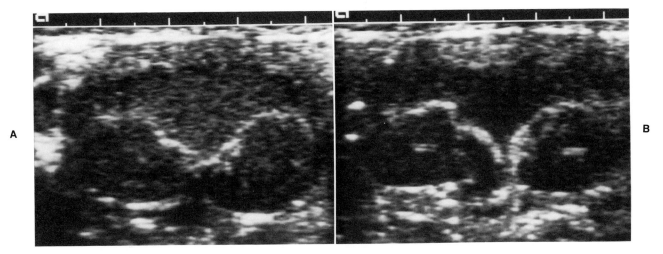

FIG 3-11. PFOB enhances diagnosis of acute tubular necrosis (ATN). **A,** After the intravenous administration of 5 ml/kg of PFOB, there is enhancement of the medullary portion of the normal kidney. The intact osmotic gradient across the medulla results in an increased concentration of PFOB in the vasa rectal. **B,** In the kidney with ischemia-induced ATN, the osmotic gradient is disrupted, resulting in lack of medullary enhancement.
(From Munzing D, Mattrey RF, Reznick VM, et al: The potential role of PFOB enhanced sonography of the kidney. Part I - Detection of renal function and acute tubular necrosis. *Kidney International,* in press, with permission.)

has been shown to accumulate in other immunologically active lesions, such as abscesses[69,70] and infarcted tissue.[71]

The normal osmotic gradient in the renal medulla causes hemoconcentration in the vasa recta, which causes increased concentration of PFOB and, therefore, increased echogenicity in the medullary portion of the kidney compared to the cortex. To study this process, Mattrey et al[67] subjected a group of rabbits to unilateral transient renal ischemia. The resulting acute tubular necrosis disrupted the normal concentration gradient of the renal medulla. The disruption of the concentration gradient was not apparent on precontrast images, but was identified by a lack of medullary enhancement after the administration of PFOB.

Because PFOB can be used as a blood-pool sonographic imaging agent, perfusion defects within an organ may also be mapped. Rabbits were subjected to partial renal embolization. Before the administration of PFOB, gray-scale imaging did not detect the infarcted kidneys and color Doppler imaging correctly detected only 10% of renal infarcts. After the administration of PFOB, gray-scale imaging and color Doppler imaging allowed correct detection of all infarcted kidneys, since the perfused areas were significantly enhanced by the contrast (Fig. 3-11).[66]

Advantages of PFOB include its long half-life, allowing thorough imaging, gray-scale changes in echogenicity proportional to blood flow, both color and spectral Doppler enhancing properties, reticuloendothelial system update, and potential to be used in conjunction with computed tomography. The major limitations of PFOB include possible side effects and the complex relation of preinjection sonographic appearance of parenchymal lesions to the dynamic role of PFOB, including perfusion imaging, reticuloendothelial system deposition, and macrophage imaging.

LIPID EMULSIONS

Because excess fat deposition in hepatocytes produces enhanced backscatter,[72,73] lipid emulsions have been evaluated as ultrasound contrast agents.[74] It was hypothesized that transient hepatic lipid accumulation would lead to increased echogenicity of normal liver parenchyma compared to abnormal parenchyma. However, preliminary studies using intravenous lipid emulsions suggest that a perceptible difference in echogenicity between control and lipid-containing livers has not been readily achieved, apparently because of their small particle size and relatively low concentration within the liver.

AQUEOUS SOLUTIONS

The introduction of solutions into the bloodstream to enhance ultrasound backscatter and reflectivity from tissues was first proposed by Ophir et al.[75] Some aqueous solutions show a linear increase in the speed of sound propagation and density as a function of the molar concentration.[76] Therefore the acoustic impedance, the product of density and velocity (the speed of sound through tissue), is a function of concentration. Ophir et al[75] have shown that a transient acoustic impedance

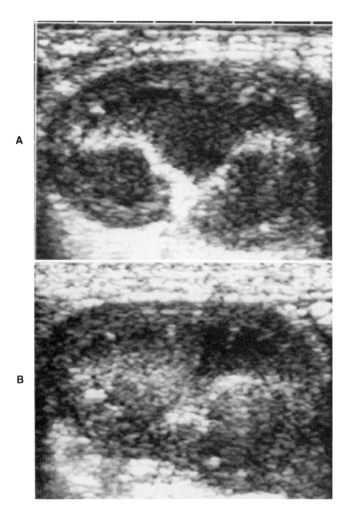

FIG 3-12. . Partial renal infarction detected with PFOB. **A,** Precontrast coronal image of a rabbit kidney, following segmental infarction is normal. **B,** Following the intravenous administration of 3 ml/kg PFOB, a hypoechoic, wedge-shaped infarct is identified because of enhancement of the remainder of the kidney.

(From Coley BD, Mattrey RF, Roberts A, et al: The potential role of PFOB enhanced sonography. Part II — Detection of partial infarction. *Kideny International,* in press, with permission.)

mismatch is created between the vascular and nonvascular beds in the time immediately following an intravenous injection of an agent with a significantly different acoustic impedance from normal body tissues. Materials that bear a strong dependence of the speed of sound on concentration and have a low toxicity include buffered sodium citrate, calcium gluconate, and calcium disodium EDTA.[77] In vitro and in vivo investigations[75,77] have supported these assumptions, showing transient renal cortical echo enhancement following intravenous injections of these solutions.

FUTURE DIRECTIONS

Several contrast agents offer great promise for improved diagnostic accuracy. Each agent offers slightly different applications, tailored to its physical characteristics. SH U 454 is an agent that because of its short half-life is suited for venous imaging and for intracavitary uses. With the development of SH U 508, which is more stable agent capable of transpulmonary passage, alterations in parenchymal echogenicity or systemic arterial Doppler enhancement may be identified. Encapsulated human albumin microspheres (Albunex), which also have a short half-life are most useful for flow imaging with color Doppler, allowing improved detection of small or deep vessels, distinction between high-grade stenosis and complete occlusion, and identification of neovascularity. Basic research shows PFOB to be a useful contrast agent for sonographic tumor and abscess detection in the liver and tumor detection in the kidney. Presently, PFOB is undergoing clinical trials in Europe. Because PFOB enhances the Doppler signal of normal vascular structures, vascular displacement, occlusion, and tumor vascularity are more easily appreciated by both duplex and color Doppler imaging. Additionally, PFOB may be used as a blood-pool agent to assess, in a dynamic fashion, the concentration gradient of the tubules in the renal medulla.

To date, ultrasound contrast agents are essentially experimental. Given the lower cost and greater worldwide availability of sonography over other imaging modalities (computed tomography and magnetic resonance imaging), the need for a contrast agent is great.

REFERENCES

1. Yeh HC, Wolf BS: Ultrasonic contrast study to identify stomach using tap water microbubbles. *J Clin Ultrasound* 1977; 5(3):170-174.
2. Rubin C, Kurtz A, Goldberg BB: Water enema: A new technique for defining pelvic anatomy. *J Clin Ultrasound* 1978; 6:28-33.
3. Goldberg BB: Ultrasonic cholangiography. *Radiology* 1976; 118:401-404.
4. Widder DJ, Simeone JF: Microbubbles as a contrast agent for neurosonography and ultrasound-guided catheter manipulation: in vitro studies. *Am J Roentgenol* 1986; 147:347-352.
5. Gramiak R, Shah PM: Echocardiography of the aortic root. *Invest Radiol* 1968; 3:356-366.
6. Gramiak R, Shah PM, Kramer DH: Ultrasound cardiography: Contrast studies in anatomy and function. *Radiology* 1969; 92:939-948.
7. Gobuty AH: Perspectives in ultrasound contrast agents. In: Parvez Z, editor: *Contrast media: biologic effects and clinical application.* Boca Raton, Fla: CRC Press; 1987.
8. Ophir J, Parker KJ: Contrast agents in diagnostic ultrasound. *Ultrasound Med Biol* 1989; 15(4):319-333.

Free gas bubbles

9. Kremkau FW, Gramiak R, Carstensen EL, et al: Ultrasonic detection of cavitation at catheter tips. *Am J Roentgenol* 1970; 110(1):177-183.
10. Meltzer RS, Tickner EG, Sahines TP, et al: The source of ultrasound contrast effect. *J Clin Ultrasound* 1980; 8:121-127.
11. Ziskin MC, Bonakdarpour A, Weinstein DP, et al: Contrast agents for diagnostic ultrasound. *Invest Radiol* 1972; 7(6):500-505.

12. Feinstein SB, Ten Cate FJ, Zwehl W, et al: Two-dimensional contrast echocardiography. Part I. In vitro development and quantitative analysis of echo contrast agents. *JACC* 1984; 3(1):14-20.

13. Keller MW, Feinstein SB, Briller RA, et al: Automated production and analysis of echo contrast agents. *J Ultrasound Med* 1986; 5:493-498.

14. Reisner SA, Shapiro JR, Schwarz KQ, et al: Sonication of echo-contrast agents: a standardized and reproducible method. *J Cardiovasc Ultrasonography* 1988; 7(3):273-276.

15. Meltzer RS, Vered Z, Roelandt J, et al: Systemic analysis of contrast echocardiograms. *Am J Cardiol* 1983; 52:375-380.

16. Feinstein SB, Shah PM. Bing RJ, et al: Microbubble dynamics visualized in the intact capillary circulation. *J Am Coll Cardiol* 1984; 4(3):595-600.

17. Meltzer RS, Tickner EG, Popp RL: Why do the lungs clear ultrasonic contrast? *Ultrasound Med Biol* 1980; 6:263-269.

18. Feinstein SB, Maurer G, Tei C, et al: In vitro comparisons of echo contrast agents (abstract). *Circulation* 1982; 66(Suppl II):II-188.

19. Bommer WJ, Miller L, Takeda P, et al: Contrast echo-cardiography: Pulmonary transmission and myocardial perfusion imaging using surfactant stabilized microbubbles (abstract). *Circulation* 1981; 64(Suppl IV): IV-203.

20. Butler BD: Production of microbubbles for use as echo contrast agents. *J Clin Ultrasound* 1986; 14:408-412.

21. Serruys PW, Meltzer RS, McGhie J, et al: Factors affecting the success for attaining left heart echo contrast after pulmonary wedge injection. In: Meltzer RS, Roelandt J, editors: *Contrast echocardiography* Boston, London, The Hague: Martinus Nijhoff; 1982.

22. Ten Cate FJ, Feinstein S, Zwehl W, et al: Two-dimensional contrast echocardiography. Part II. Transpulmonary studies. *J Am Coll Cardiol* 1984; 3(1):21-27.

23. Smith MD, Kwan OL, Reiser J, et al: Superior intensity and reproducibility of SH U 454, a new right heart contrast agent. *J Am Coll Cardiol* 1984; 3(4):992-998.

24. Lange L, Fritzsch T, Hilmann J, et al: Right-heart echocontrast in the anesthetized dog after i.v. administration of a new standardized sonographic contrast agent. Comparison of various contrast agents employed in contrast echocardiography. *Drug Res* 1986; 36(II):1037-1040.

25. Fritzsch T, Schartl M, Siegert J: Preclinical and clinical results with an ultrasonic contrast agent. *Invest Radiol* 1988; 23(Suppl 1):S302-S305.

26. Henkel B, Schlief R, Hamm MK: Transvaginal contrast-sonographic assessment of fallopian tube patency. *Proceedings of the Sixth Congress of the European Federation of Societies for Ultrasound in Medicine and Biology* 1987; p 223.

27. Huneke B, Lindner C, Braendle W: Untersuchung der tubenpassage mit der vaginalen gepulsen kontrastmittel-Doppler sonographie. *Ultraschall Klin Prax* 1989; 4:192-198.

28. Deichert U, Schlief R, van de Sandt M, et al: Transvaginal hysterosalpingo-contrast-sonography (Hy-Co-Sy) compared with conventional tubal diagnostics. *Human Reproduction* 1989; 4(4):418-424.

29. Schlief R, Deichert U: Hysterosalpingo-contrast-sonography: Results of a clinical trial with a novel ultrasound contrast medium in 120 patients. Paper presented at the meeting of the Radiologic Society of North America, Chicago, 1989.

30. Fobbe F, Becker R, Siegart J, et al: Fallopian tube patency demonstrated with color-coded duplex sonography and ultrasound contrast medium. Paper presented at the meeting of the Radiologic Society of North America, Chicago, 1989.

31. Schlief R, Staks T, Mahler M, et al: Successful opacification of the left heart chambers on echocardiographic examination after intravenous injection of a new saccharide based contrast agent. *Echocardiography* 1990; 7(1):61-64.

32. Fritzsch T, Scharti M, Siegert J, et al: Detection of mitral regurgitation with contrast-enhanced color Doppler echocardiography. Paper presented at the meeting of the Radiologic Society of North America, Chicago, 1989.

33. Fobbe F, Siegert J, Wolf KJ, et al: Arterial perfusion imaging after intravenous injection of a transpulmonary ultrasound contrast agent in color-coded duplex sonography: preclinical results. Paper presented at the meeting of the Radiologic Society of North America, Chicago, 1989.

34. El-Moussouy A, Becker HD, Schlief R, et al: Rat liver model for testing intraoperative echo contrast sonography. Paper presented at the meeting of the Radiologic Society of North America, Chicago, 1989.

35. Schlief R: Sonographic imaging of venous hemodynamics by use of a new ultrasound contrast medium (SH U 454). Paper presented at the *Fourth European-American Symposium on Venous Diseases,* Washington, DC, 1987.

Encapsulated gas bubbles

36. Carroll BA, Turner RJ, Tickner EG, et al: Gelatin encapsulated nitrogen microbubbles as ultrasonic contrast agents. *Invest Radiol* 1980; 15(3):260-266.

37. Carroll BA, Young SW, Rasor JS, et al: Ultrasonic contrast enhancement of tissue by encapsulated microbubbles. *Radiology* 1982; 143:747-750.

38. Keller MW, Feinstein FB, Watson DD: Successful left ventricular opacification following peripheral venous injection of sonicated contrast agent: an experimental evaluation. *Am Heart J* 1987; 114:570-575.

39. Feinstein SB, Heidenriech PA, Dick CD, et al: Albunex: A new intravascular contrast agent: preliminary safety and efficacy results (abstract). *Circulation* 1988; 78(suppl II):565.

40. Keller MW, Glasheen WP, Teja K, et al: Myocardial contrast echocardiography without significant hemodynamic effects or hyperemia: a major advantage in the imaging of regional myocardial perfusion. *J Am Coll Cardiol* 1988; 12:1039-1047.

41. Armstrong WF, Sawada S, Felisky J, et al: Left ventricular echocardiographic contrast via transpulmonary passage of Albunex (abstract). *Circulation* 1988; 78(suppl II):565.

42. Keller MW, Glasheen W, Kaul Sanjiv: Albunex: A safe and effective commercially produced agent for myocardial contrast echocardiography. *J Am Soc Echo* 1989; 2:48-52.

43. Shapiro JR, Reisner SA, Meltzer RS: Prospects for trans-pulmonary contrast echocardiography. *J Am Coll Cardiology* 1989; 13:1629-1630.

44. Hilpert PL, Mattrey RF, Mitten R, et al: IV injection of air-filled human-albumin microspheres to enhance arterial Doppler signal: a preliminary study in rabbits. *Am J Roentgenology* 1989; 153:613-616.

45. Goldberg BB, Hilbert PL, Burns PN, et al: intravenous injection of Hepatic tumors: signal enhancement at Doppler US after contrast agent. *Radiology* 1990; 177:713-717.

Colloidal suspensions

46. Ophir J, Gobuty A, McWhirt RE, et al: Ultrasonic backscatter from contrast producing collagen microspheres. *Ultrasonic Imaging* 1980; 2:67-77.

47. Ophir J, Gobuty A, Maklad N, et al: Quantitative assessment of in vivo backscatter enhancement from gelatin microspheres. *Ultrasonic Imaging* 1985; 7:293-299.

48. Bloch EH, McCuskey RS: Biodynamics of phagocytosis: an analysis of the dynamics of phagocytosis in the liver by in vivo microscopy in Kupffer cells and other sinusoidal cells. In: Wisse E, Knock OL, editors: *Kupffer cells and other liver sinusoidal cells.* Amsterdam: Elsevier Biomedical Press; 1977.

49. Violante MR, Parker KJ, Fischer HW: Particulate suspensions as ultrasonic contrast agents for liver and spleen. *Invest Radiol* 1988; 23(suppl 1):S294-S297.

50. Clark LC, Gollan F: Survival of mammals breathing organic liquids equilibrated with oxygen at atmospheric pressure. *Science* 1966; 152:1755-1756.

51. Liu MS, Long DM: Perfluorooctylbromide as a diagnostic contrast medium in gastroenterography. *Radiology* 1977; 122:71-76.

52. Long DM Jr, Lasser EC, Sharts CM, et al: Experiments with radiopaque perfluorocarbon emulsions for selective opacification of organs and total body angiography. *Invest Radiol* 1980; 15(3):242-247.

53. Mattrey RF, Long DM, Peck WW, et al: Perfluorooctylbromide as a blood pool contrast agent for liver, spleen, and vascular imaging in computed tomography. *J Comput Assist Tomogr* 1984; 8(4):739-744.

54. Mattrey RF, Peck WW, Slutsky RA, et al: Perfluorooctylbromide as a blood pool imaging agent for computed tomography. *Invest Radiol* 1983; 18(4):515.

55. Bruneton JN, Falewee MN, Francois E, et al: Liver, spleen and vessels: preliminary clinical results of computed tomography with perfluorooctylbromide. *Radiology* 1989; 170:179-183.

56. Burgan AR, Long DM, Mattrey RF, et al: Results of pharmacokinetic and toxicologic studies with PFOB emulsions. Presented at the *International Symposium on Artificial Blood Substitutes,* Montreal, Canada, May 1987.

57. Peck WW, Mattrey RF, Slutsky RA, et al: Perfluorooctylbromide: acute hemodynamic effects in pigs, of intravenous administration compared with the standard ionic contrast media. *Invest Radiol* 1984; 19(2):129-132.

58. Mattrey RF, Hilpert PL, Long CD, et al: Hemodynamic effects of intravenously administered lecithin-based perfluorocarbon emulsions in dogs. *Critical Care Med* 1989; 17:652-656.

59. Mattrey RF: Perfluorooctylbromide: a new contrast agent for computed tomography, sonography and magnetic resonance imaging. *Am J Roentgenology* 1989; 152:247-252.

60. Mattrey RF: Potential role of perfluorooctylbromide in the detection and characterization of liver lesions with computed tomography. *Radiology* 1989; 170:18-20.

61. Mattrey RF, Scheible FW, Gosink BB, et al: Perfluorooctylbromide: a liver/spleen-specific and tumor-imaging ultrasound contrast material. *Radiology* 1982; 145(3):759-762.

62. Mattrey RF, Strich G, Shelton RE, et al: Perfluorochemicals as ultrasound contrast agents for tumor imaging and hepatosplenography: Preliminary clinical results. *Radiology* 1987; 163:339-343.

63. Behan M, O'Connell DJ, Carney DN, et al: Perfluorooctylbromide as an ultrasound contrast agent for liver metastases: preliminary findings and clinical tolerance. Paper presented at the meeting of the Radiologic Society of North America, Chicago, 1989.

64. Mattrey RF, Mitten R, Peterson T, et al: Vascular ultrasonic enhancement of tissues with perfluorooctylbromide for renal tumor detection (abstract). *Radiology* 1987; 156(suppl):76.

65. Hilpert PL, Mattrey RF, Mitten R, et al: Intravenous ultrasonic contrast agent to enhance systemic arterial Doppler signal (abstract). *Invest Radiol* 1988; 23-S9.

66. Coley BD, Roberts A, Keane S, et al: PFOB aided sonography can detect partial renal infarction. Paper presented at the meeting of the *American Roentgen Ray Society,* Washington, DC, 1990.

67. Mattrey RF, Munzing D, Reznik VM: Sonographic imaging of renal concentrating ability with PFOB. Paper presented at the meeting of the *American Roentgenology Ray Society,* Washington, DC, 1990.

68. Mattrey RF, Long DM, Multer F, et al: Perfluorooctylbromide: a reticuloendothelial specific and a tumor imaging agent for computed tomography. *Radiology* 1982; 145:759.

69. Mattrey RF, Andre M, Campbell J, et al: Specific enhancement of intra-abdominal abscesses with perfluorooctylbromide for computed tomography. *Invest Radiol* 1984; 19:438-446. scesses with perfluorooctylbromide for computed tomography. *Invest Radiol* 1984; 19:438-446.

70. Miller ML, Stinnett D, Clark LC Jr: Ultrastructure of tumoricidal peritoneal exudate cells stimulated in vivo by perfluorochemical emulsions. *Reticuloendothel Soc* 1980; 27:105-118.

71. Mattrey RF, Andre MP: Ultrasonic enhancement of myocardial infarction with perfluorocarbon compounds. *Am J Cardiol* 1984; 54:206-210.

Lipid emulsions

72. Shawker TH, Moran B, Linzer M, et al: B-scan amplitude measurements in patients with diffuse infiltrative liver disease. *J Clin Ultrasound* 1981; 9:293-301.

73. Scatarige JC, Scott WW, Donavan PJ, et al: Fatty infiltration of the liver: Ultrasonographic and computed tomographic correlation. *J Ultrasound Med* 1984; 3:9-14.

74. Fink IJ, Miller DL, Shawker TH, et al: Lipid emulsions as contrast agents for hepatic sonography: An experimental study in rabbits. *Ultrason Imaging* 1985; 7:191-197.

Aqueous solutions

75. Ophir J, McWhirt RE, Maklad NF: Aqueous solutions as potential ultrasonic contrast agents. *Ultrason Imaging* 1979; 1:265-279.

76. McWhirt RE: Speed of sound measurements in potential contrast agents for use in diagnostic ultrasound, Master's thesis, Lawrence, University of Kansas, 1979.

77. Tyler TD, Ophir J, Maklad NF: In vivo enhancement of ultrasonic image luminance by aqueous solutions with a high speed of sound. *Ultrason Imaging* 1981; 3:323-329.

PART II

Abdominal, Pelvic, and Thoracic Sonography

CHAPTER 4

The Liver

- Cynthia E. Withers, M.D.
- Stephanie R. Wilson, M.D.

The liver is the largest organ in the human body, weighing approximately 1500 g in the adult.[1] Because the liver is frequently involved in systemic and local disease, sonographic examination is often requested to assess hepatic abnormality.

TECHNIQUE

The liver is best examined with real-time sonography. Ideally, the patient should fast a minimum of 6 hours before the examination so that bowel gas is limited and the gallbladder is not contracted. Both supine and right anterior oblique views should be obtained if the patient can move or be moved. Because many patients have livers that are tucked beneath the lower right ribs, a transducer with a small scanning face, allowing an intercostal approach, is invaluable. Suspended inspiration enables examination of the dome of the liver, frequently an ultrasound "blind spot."

NORMAL ANATOMY

The liver lies in the right upper quadrant of the abdomen, suspended from the right hemidiaphragm. Functionally it can be divided into **three lobes,** the right, left, and caudate lobes. The **right lobe** of the liver is separated from the left by the main lobar fissure, which passes through the gallbladder fossa and the inferior vena cava (Fig. 4-1, *A*). The right lobe of the liver can be further divided into anterior and posterior segments by the right intersegmental fissure. The left intersegmental fissure divides the **left lobe** into medial and lateral segments. The **caudate lobe** is situated on the posterior aspect of the liver, having as its posterior border the inferior vena cava and as its anterior border the fissure for the ligamentum venosum (Fig. 4-1, *B*). The papillary process is the anteromedial extension of the caudate lobe, which may appear separate from the liver and mimic lymphadenopathy (Fig. 4-1, *C*).[2]

Understanding the vascular anatomy of the liver is essential to an appreciation of the relative positions of the hepatic segments. The major **hepatic veins** course between the lobes and segments (interlobar and intersegmental). They are ideal segmental boundaries but are visualized only when scanning the superior liver

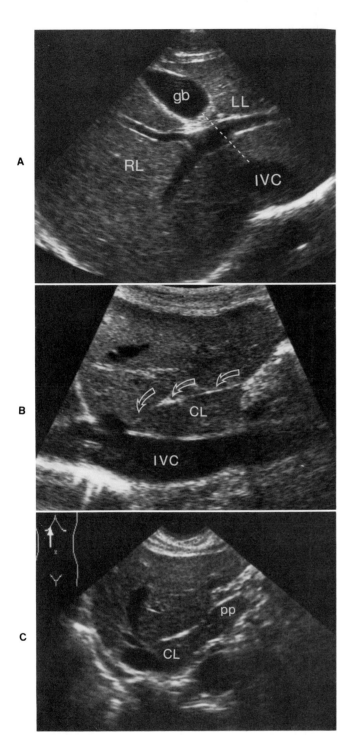

FIG 4-1. Normal lobar anatomy. **A,** Subcostal oblique sonogram shows right lobe *(RL)* of liver is separated from left lobe *(LL)* by plane *(dashed line),* which passes through gallbladder fossa *(gb)* and inferior vena cava *(IVC).* **B,** Boundaries of caudate lobe *(CL)* are fissure for the ligamentum venosum *(arrows)* anteriorly and inferior vena cava *(IVC)* posteriorly. **C,** Papillary process *(pp)* is tonguelike projection of caudate lobe *(CL).*

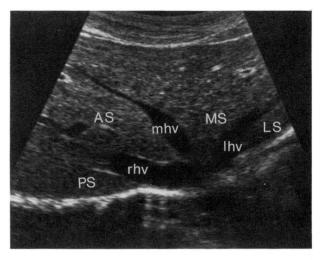

FIG 4-2. Normal segmental anatomy. Subcostal oblique sonogram shows confluence of three hepatic veins. Middle hepatic vein *(mhv)* divides liver into right and left lobes. Right hepatic vein *(rhv)* divides right lobe into anterior segment *(AS)* and posterior segment *(PS).* Left lobe is divided into medial *(MS)* and lateral segment *(LS)* by left hepatic vein *(lhv).*

(Fig. 4-2). The middle hepatic vein courses within the main lobar fissure and separates the anterior segment of the right lobe from the medial segment of the left. The right hepatic vein runs within the right intersegmental fissure and divides the right lobe into anterior and posterior segments. In more caudal sections of the liver, the right hepatic vein is no longer identified, therefore the segmental boundary becomes a more ill-defined division between the anterior and posterior branches of the right portal vein.[3] The major branches of the right and left **portal veins** run centrally within the segments (intrasegmental), with the exception of the ascending portion of the left portal vein, which runs in the left intersegmental fissure. The left intersegmental fissure, which separates the medial segment of the left lobe from the lateral segment, can be divided into cranial, middle, and caudal sections. The left hepatic vein forms the boundary of the cranial third, the ascending branch of the left portal vein represents the middle third, and the fissure for the ligamentum teres acts as the most caudal division of the left lobe (Table 4-1).[4]

Because of recent surgical advances in segmental liver resection, the sonologist needs to be familiar with **modern hepatic anatomy** as defined by Couinaud in 1957.[5] This description is based on portal segments and is of both functional and pathologic importance. Each segment has its own blood supply (arterial, portal, hepatic venous), lymphatics, and biliary drainage. Thus the surgeon may resect a segment of a hepatic lobe, providing the vascular supply to the remaining lobe is left intact. Couinaud's functional description also en-

■ **TABLE 4-1**
Normal Hepatic Anatomy: Anatomic Structures Useful for Identifying the Hepatic Segments

Structure	Location	Usefulness
RHV	Right intersegmental fissure	Divides cephalic aspect of anterior and posterior segments of right lobe
MHV	Main lobar fissure	Separates right and left lobes
LHV	Left intersegmental fissure	Divides cephalic aspect of medial and lateral segments of left lobe
RPV (anterior branch)	Intrasegmental in anterior segment of right lobe	Courses centrally in anterior segment of right lobe
RPV (posterior branch)	Intrasegmental in posterior segment of right lobe	Courses centrally in posterior segment of right lobe
LPV (horizontal segment)	Anterior to caudate lobe	Separates caudate lobe posteriorly from medial segment of left lobe anteriorly
LPV (ascending segment)	Left intersegmental fissure	Divides medial from lateral segment of left lobe
GB fossa	Main lobar fissure	Separates right and left lobes
Fissure for the ligamentum teres	Left intersegmental fissure	Divides caudal aspect of left lobe into medial and lateral segments
Fissure for the ligamentum venosum	Left anterior margin of the caudate lobe	Separates caudate lobe posteriorly from left lobe anteriorly

RHV indicates right hepatic vein; *MHV*, middle hepatic vein; *LHV*, left hepatic vein; *RPV*, right portal vein; *LPV*, left portal vein; *GB*, gallbladder.
(Modified from Marks WM, Filly RA, Callen PW. Ultrasonic anatomy of the liver: a review with new applications, *J Clin Ultrasound* 1979; 7:137-146.)

corporates the distribution of the three hepatic veins. The right, middle, and left hepatic veins divide the liver longitudinally into four sections. Each of these sections is further divided transversely by an imaginary plane through the right main and left main portal pedicles. Thus segment I is the caudate lobe, II and III are the left superior and inferior lateral segments, respectively, and segment IV, which is further divided into IVa and IVb, is the medial segment of the left lobe. The right lobe consists of segments V and VI, located caudal to the transverse plane, and segments VII and VIII, which are cephalad (Fig. 4-3).[6]

Ligaments

The liver is covered by a thin connective tissue layer called **Glisson's capsule.** The capsule surrounds the entire liver and is thickest around the inferior vena cava and the porta hepatis. At the porta hepatis the main portal vein, the proper hepatic artery, and the common bile duct are contained within investing peritoneal folds known as the **hepatoduodenal ligament** (Fig. 4-4). The **falciform ligament** conducts the umbilical vein to the liver during fetal development (Fig. 4-5). After birth, the umbilical vein atrophies, forming the **ligamentum teres.** As it reaches the liver, the leaves of the falciform ligament separate. The right layer forms the upper layer of the **coronary ligament;** the left layer forms the upper layer of the **left triangular ligament.**

The most lateral portion of the coronary ligament is known as the **right triangular ligament** (Fig. 4-6). The peritoneal layers that form the coronary ligament are widely separated, leaving an area of the liver not covered by peritoneum. This posterosuperior region is known as the "bare area" of the liver. The ligamentum venosum carries the obliterated ductus venosus, which—until birth—shunts blood from the umbilical vein to the inferior vena cava (Fig. 4-7).

HEPATIC CIRCULATION
Portal Veins

The liver receives a dual blood supply from both the portal vein and the hepatic artery. Although the portal vein carries incompletely oxygenated (80%) venous blood from the intestines and spleen, it supplies up to half the oxygen requirements of the hepatocytes because of its greater flow. This dual blood supply explains the low incidence of hepatic infarction.

The **portal triad** contains a branch of the portal vein, hepatic artery, and bile duct. These are contained within a connective tissue sheath that gives the portal vein an echogenic wall on sonography and allows for its distinction from the hepatic veins, which have an almost imperceptible wall. The main portal vein divides into right and left branches. The right portal vein has an anterior branch that lies centrally within the anterior segment of the right lobe and a posterior branch that

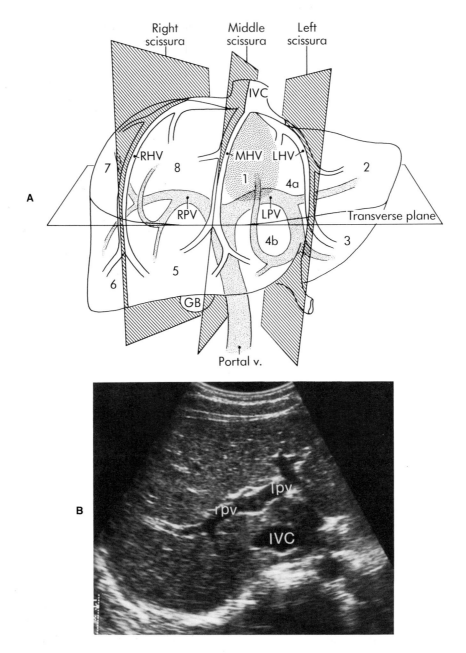

FIG 4-3. Couinaud's functional segmental anatomy. **A,** Liver is divided into nine segments. Longitudinal boundaries (right, middle, and left scissurae) are three hepatic veins. Transverse plane is defined by right main and left main portal pedicles. Segment 1, caudate lobe (stippled region), is situated posteriorly. *RHV* indicates right hepatic vein; *MHV,* middle hepatic vein; *LHV,* left hepatic vein. *RPV* indicates right portal vein; *LPV,* left portal vein; *IVC,* inferior vena cava; *GB,* gallbladder. **B,** Subcostal oblique sonogram at level of major branches of right *(rpv)* and left *(lpv)* portal veins. Cephalad to this level lie segments II, IVa, VII, and VIII. Caudally located are segments III, IVb, V, and VI. *IVC* indicates inferior vena cava.
(**A** Modified from Sugarbaker PH. *Neth J Surg* 1988; PO:100.)

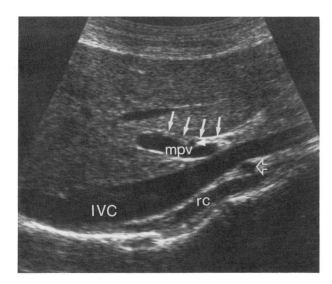

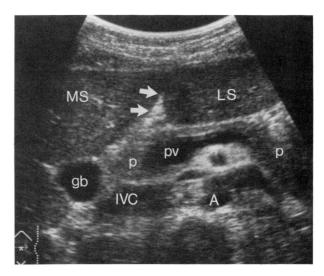

FIG 4-4. Porta hepatis. Sagittal sonogram shows that common duct *(arrows)*, hepatic artery *(arrowhead)*, and main portal vein *(mpv)* run within hepatoduodenal ligament. *IVC* indicates inferior vena cava; *rc*, right diaphragmatic crus; *open arrow*, right renal artery.

FIG 4-5. Falciform ligament. Transverse scan through midabdomen shows echogenic falciform ligament *(arrows)*, which separates lateral segment *(LS)* of left lobe from medial segment *(MS)*. *IVC* indicates inferior vena cava; *A*, aorta; *gb*, gallbladder, *p*, pancreas; *pv*, portal vein.

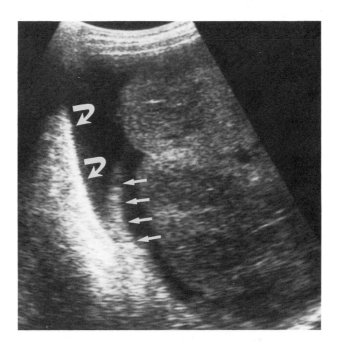

FIG 4-6. Right triangular ligament. Subcostal oblique scan near dome of right hemidiaphragm *(curved arrows)*. Note lobulated contour and inhomogeneity of liver in this patient with cirrhosis. Right triangular ligament *(straight arrows)* is visualized because of ascites.

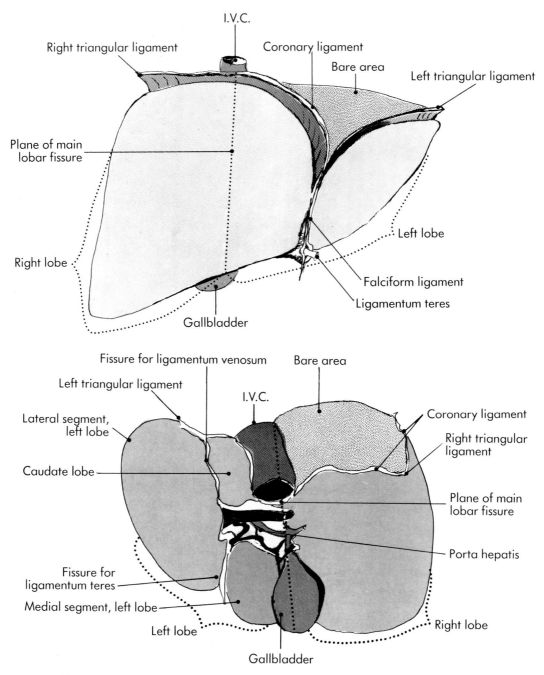

FIG 4-7. Hepatic ligaments. Diagram of anterior (**A**) and posterior (**B**) surfaces of liver. (Courtesy of Jocelyne Salem.)

lies centrally within the posterior segment of the right lobe. The left portal vein initially courses anterior to the caudate lobe. The ascending branch of the left portal vein then travels anteriorly in the left intersegmental fissure to divide the medial and lateral segments of the left lobe (Fig. 4-8).

Arterial Circulation

The branches of the hepatic artery accompany the portal veins. The terminal branches of the portal vein

and their accompanying hepatic arterioles and bile ducts are known as the acinus.

Hepatic Venous System

Blood perfuses the liver parenchyma through the sinusoids and then enters the terminal hepatic venules. These terminal branches unite to form sequentially larger veins. The hepatic veins vary in number and position. However, in the general population, there are three major veins: the right, middle, and left hepatic

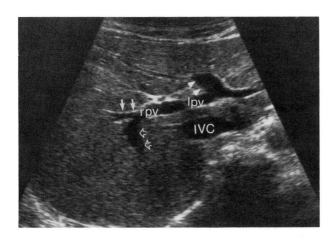

FIG 4-8. Normal portal venous anatomy. Subcostal oblique sonogram shows junction of right *(rpv)* and left *(lpv)* portal veins. Right portal vein has anterior branch *(closed arrows)* and posterior branch *(open arrows)*. Ascending branch of left portal vein *(arrowheads)* runs in left intersegmental fissure. *IVC* indicates inferior vena cava.

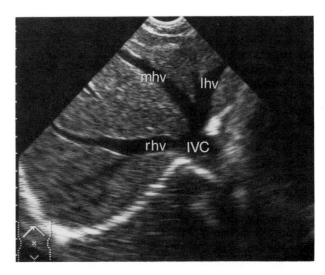

FIG 4-9. Normal hepatic venous anatomy. In majority of patients, middle hepatic vein *(mhv)* and left hepatic vein *(lhv)* form a common trunk before emptying into inferior vena cava *(IVC)*. Right hepatic vein *(rhv)* empties directly into inferior vena cava.

veins. All drain into the inferior vena cava and, like the portal veins, are without valves. The right hepatic vein is usually single and runs in the right intersegmental fissure, separating the anterior and posterior segments of the right lobe. The middle hepatic vein, which courses in the main lobar fissure, forms a common trunk with the left hepatic vein in the majority of individuals (Fig. 4-9).[7] The left hepatic vein forms the most cephalad boundary between the medial and lateral segments of the left lobe.

NORMAL LIVER SIZE AND ECHOGENICITY

The upper border of the liver lies approximately at the level of the fifth intercostal space at the midclavicular line. The lower border extends to or slightly below the costal margin. An accurate assessment of liver size is difficult with real-time ultrasound equipment because of the limited field of view. Gosink proposed measuring the liver length in the midhepatic line. In 75% of patients with a liver length of greater than 15.5 cm, hepatomegaly is present.[8] Niederau et al. measured the liver in a longitudinal and anteroposterior diameter in both the midclavicular line and midline and correlated these findings with gender, age, height, weight, and body surface area.[9] They found that organ size increases with height and body surface area and decreases with age. The mean longitudinal diameter of the liver in the midclavicular line in this study was 10.5 ± 1.5 (standard deviation) cm and the mean midclavicular anteroposterior diameter was 8.1 ± 1.9 (standard deviation) cm. In most patients, measurement of the liver length suffices to measure liver size. In heavy or asthenic individuals,

the anteroposterior diameter should be added to avoid underestimations or overestimations, respectively. Reidel's lobe is a tonguelike extension of the inferior tip of the right lobe of the liver, which is frequently found in asthenic women.

The normal liver is homogeneous, contains fine-level echoes, and is either minimally hyperechoic or isoechoic compared to the normal renal cortex (Fig. 4-10, *A*). The liver is hypoechoic compared to the spleen. This relationship is evident when the lateral segment of the left lobe is elongated and wraps around the spleen (Fig. 4-10, *B*).

DEVELOPMENTAL ANOMALIES
Agenesis

Agenesis of the liver is incompatible with life. Agenesis of both the right and left lobes has been reported.[10-12] In three of five recently reported cases of agenesis of the right lobe, the caudate lobe was also absent.[11] Compensatory hypertrophy of the remaining lobes normally occurs, and liver function tests are normal.

Anomalies of Position

In situs inversus totalis, the liver is found in the left hypochondrium. In congenital diaphragmatic hernia or omphalocele, varying amounts of liver may herniate into the thorax or outside the abdominal cavity.

Accessory Fissures

Although invaginations of the dome of the diaphragm have been called accessory fissures,[13] strictly

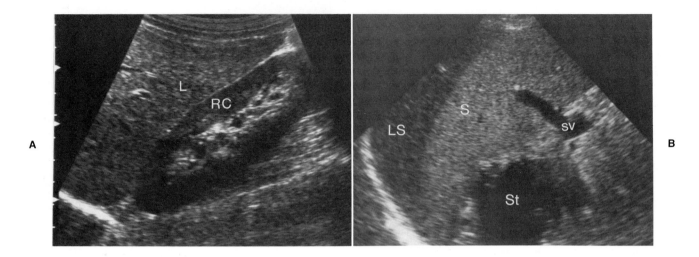

FIG 4-10. Normal liver echogenicity. **A,** Normal liver *(L)* is either minimally hyperechoic or iso-echoic to normal renal cortex *(RC).* **B,** Sagittal sonogram of left upper quadrant shows elongated lateral segment of liver *(LS)* wrapping around spleen *(S).* Liver is normally hypoechoic compared to spleen. *St* indicates stomach; *sv,* splenic vein.

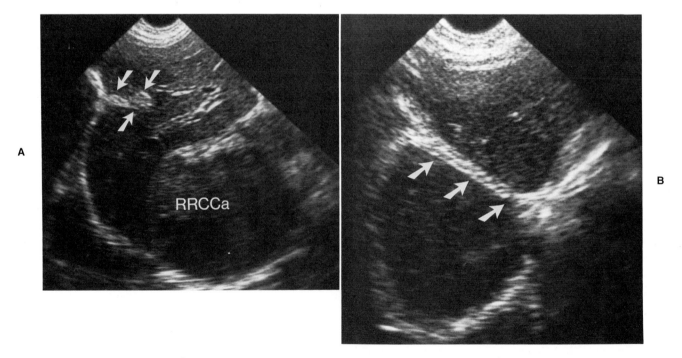

FIG 4-11. Diaphragmatic slip. **A,** Sagittal sonogram shows echogenic "mass" *(arrows)* adjacent to right hemidiaphragm in this patient with right renal cell carcinoma *(RRCCa).* **B,** Subcostal oblique image reveals "mass" is diaphragmatic slip *(arrows).*

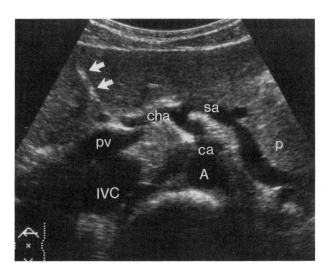

FIG 4-12. Normal celiac axis. Transverse sonogram at origin of celiac artery *(ca)* shows common hepatic artery *(cha)* and splenic artery *(sa)*. *A* indicates aorta; *IVC*, inferior vena cava; *pv*, portal vein; *p*, pancreas; *arrows*, falciform ligament.

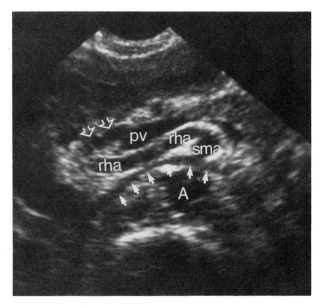

FIG 4-13. Replaced right hepatic artery. Transverse sonogram at level of left renal vein *(closed arrows)* shows right hepatic artery *(rha)* arising from superior mesenteric artery *(sma)*. *Pv* indicates portal vein; *A*, aorta; *open arrows*, left hepatic artery.

speaking, these are not fissures but rather diaphragmatic slips. They are a cause of pseudomasses on sonography if the liver is not carefully examined in both sagittal and transverse planes (Fig. 4-11). True accessory fissures are uncommon and are caused by an infolding of peritoneum. The inferior accessory hepatic fissure is a true accessory fissure that stretches inferiorly from the right portal vein to the inferior surface of the right lobe of the liver.[14]

Vascular Anomalies

The **common hepatic artery** arises from the celiac axis (Fig. 4-12) and divides into right and left branches at the porta hepatis. This classic textbook description of the hepatic arterial anatomy occurs in only 55% of the population.[15] The remaining 45% have some variation of this anatomy, of which the main patterns are (1) replaced left hepatic artery originating from the left gastric artery (10%); (2) replaced right hepatic artery originating from the superior mesenteric artery (11%); and (3) replaced common hepatic artery (2.5%) originating from the superior mesenteric artery (Fig. 4-13).[15]

Congenital anomalies of the **portal vein** include atresias, strictures and obstructing valves—all of which are uncommon. Sonographic variations include absence of the right portal vein with anomalies of branching from the main and left portal veins and absence of the horizontal segment of the left portal vein.[16]

In contrast, variations in the branching of the hepatic

veins and accessory hepatic veins are relatively common. The most common accessory vein drains the superoanterior segment of the right lobe (segment VIII) and is seen in approximately one third of the population. It usually empties into the middle hepatic vein, although occasionally it joins the right hepatic vein.[17] An inferior right hepatic vein, which drains the inferoposterior portion of the liver (segment VI), is observed in 10% of individuals. This inferior right hepatic vein drains directly into the inferior vena cava and may be as large as or larger than the right hepatic vein (Fig. 4-14, *A*).[18] Left and right marginal veins, which drain into the left and right hepatic veins, occur in approximately 12% and 3% of individuals, respectively (Fig. 4-14, *B*). Absence of the main hepatic veins is relatively less common, occurring in approximately 8% of people.[18] Awareness of the normal variations of the hepatic venous system is helpful in accurately defining the location of focal liver lesions and aids the surgeon in segmental liver resection.

CONGENITAL ABNORMALITIES
Liver Cyst

A liver cyst is defined as a fluid-filled space having an epithelial lining. Abscesses, parasitic cysts, and posttraumatic cysts are therefore not true cysts. The frequent presence of columnar epithelium within simple hepatic cysts suggests they have a ductal origin, although their precise cause is unclear.[19] Nor is it clear

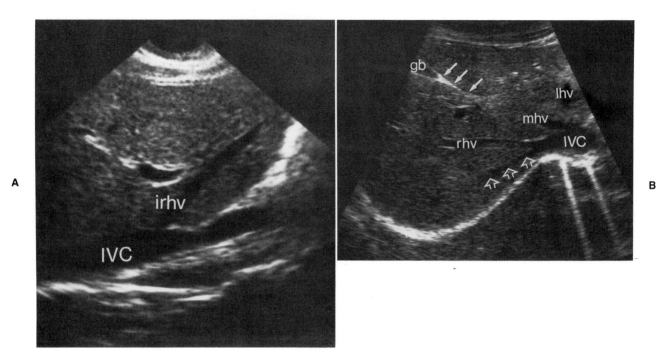

FIG 4-14. Accessory hepatic veins. **A,** Sagittal sonogram of right lobe of liver. Inferior right hepatic vein *(irhv)* drains directly into inferior vena cava *(IVC)*. **B,** Right marginal vein *(open arrows)*, which drains Couinaud's segment VII, empties into right hepatic vein *(rhv)*. *Mhv* indicates middle hepatic vein; *lhv*, left hepatic vein; *gb*, gallbladder; *closed arrows*, major fissure. *IVC*, inferior vena cava.

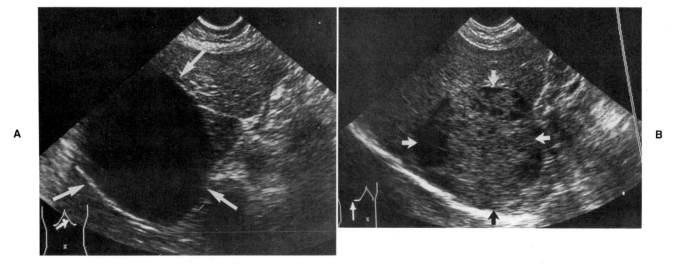

FIG 4-15. Hemorrhagic hepatic cyst. **A,** Subcostal oblique sonogram shows large hepatic cyst *(arrows)*. **B,** Six months later, patient returned with right upper quadrant pain and fever. Note internal echoes and septations within cyst *(arrows)*. Aspiration yielded sanguinous fluid.

why these lesions do not appear until middle age. Although thought at one time to be relatively uncommon, ultrasound examination has shown that liver cysts occur in 2.5% of the general population, increasing to 7% in the population older than 80 years of age.[20]

On sonographic examination, benign hepatic cysts are anechoic with a well-demarcated, thin wall and posterior acoustic enhancement. Occasionally the patient may develop pain and fever secondary to cyst hemorrhage or infection. In this situation, the cyst may contain internal echoes and septations, a thickened wall, or all three (Fig. 4-15). Active intervention is recommended only in the symptomatic patient. Although aspiration will yield fluid for evaluation, the cyst with an epithelial lining will recur. Cyst ablation with alcohol can be performed using ultrasound guidance.[21] Alternatively, surgical excision is indicated.

Adult Polycystic Disease

The adult form of polycystic kidney disease is inherited in an autosomal dominant pattern. The frequency of liver cysts in association with this condition varies between 57% to 74%.[22,23] No correlation exists between the severity of the renal disease and the extent of liver involvement (Fig. 4-16).[22] Liver function tests are usually normal and, unlike the infantile autosomal recessive form of polycystic kidney disease, there is no association with hepatic fibrosis and portal hypertension. Indeed, if liver function tests are abnormal, complications of polycystic liver disease such as tumor, cyst infection, or biliary obstruction should be excluded.[22]

INFECTIOUS DISEASES
Viral

Jaundice was recognized to be infectious by Hippocrates more than 2000 years ago. To this day, viral hepatitis remains a common disease. Type A hepatitis is transmitted largely by the fecal-oral route, whereas hepatitis B is transmitted parenterally. Hepatitis that is not caused by hepatitis A, B, or other recognized viruses, such as cytomegalovirus and Epstein-Barr virus, is currently referred to as non-A, non-B hepatitis.

Acute hepatitis has a spectrum of severity ranging from a mild subclinical form to fulminant liver failure. Histologically, there is diffuse swelling of the hepatocytes, proliferation of Kupffer cells lining the sinusoids, and infiltration of the portal areas by lymphocytes and monocytes. In regeneration, the normal lobular architecture is replaced by a cobblestone pattern. The sonographic features parallel the histologic findings. The liver parenchyma may have a diffusely decreased echogenicity, with accentuated brightness of the portal triads (Fig. 4-17).[24] Thickening of the gallbladder wall is an associated finding.[25]

Chronic hepatitis exists when there is clinical or biochemical evidence of hepatic inflammation for at least 3 to 6 months. Chronic active hepatitis (CAH) is the severe form and often progresses to cirrhosis and liver failure. Chronic persistent hepatitis (CPH) is benign, and many patients with CPH are asymptomatic. The sonographic features of chronic hepatitis are a coarse liver echopattern and decreased brightness of the portal triads, reflecting progressive periportal fibrosis (Fig. 4-18).[24]

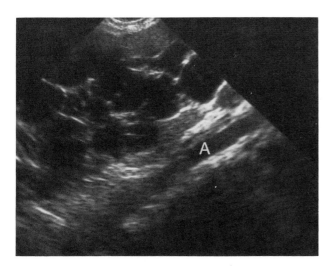

FIG 4-16. Liver cysts associated with adult polycystic kidney disease. Liver parenchyma is almost completely replaced by multiple cysts. Liver function test results were normal. *A* indicates aorta.

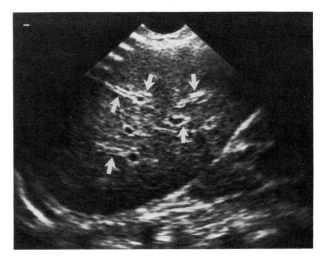

FIG 4-17. Acute viral hepatitis. Sagittal sonogram shows increased echogenicity of portal triads *(arrows)*.

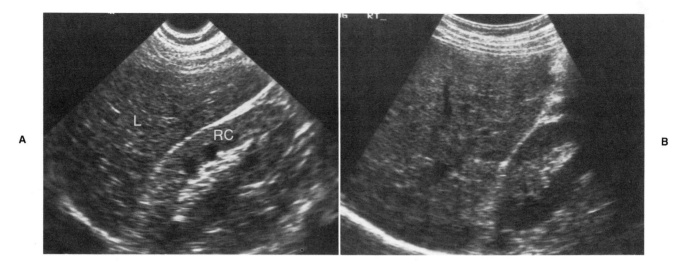

FIG 4-18. Chronic active hepatitis. **A,** At presentation, liver *(L)* is minimally hypoechoic compared with normal renal cortex *(RC)*. **B,** Eight months later, clinical deterioration. Liver texture is inhomogeneous and coarse. Repeat liver biopsy confirmed worsening disease.

Bacterial

Pyogenic bacteria reach the liver by several routes, the most common being direct extension from the biliary tract in patients with suppurative cholangitis and cholecystitis. Other routes are through the portal venous system in patients with diverticulitis or appendicitis and through the hepatic artery in patients with osteomyelitis and subacute bacterial endocarditis. Pyogenic bacteria may also be present in the liver as a result of blunt or penetrating trauma. No cause can be found in approximately half the cases of hepatic abscesses. Most of this latter group are due to anaerobic infection.[26] Diagnosis of bacterial liver infection is often delayed. The most common presenting features of pyogenic liver abscess are fever, malaise, anorexia, and right upper quadrant pain. Jaundice may be present in one quarter to one half of these patients. The most common physical finding is hepatomegaly. Prompt diagnosis of pyogenic liver abscesses significantly decreases mortality, which is reported to be 100% in untreated cases.[27]

Sonography has proved to be extremely helpful in the detection of abdominal abscesses. The ultrasound features of pyogenic liver abscesses are varied. Frankly purulent abscesses appear cystic, with the fluid ranging from echo free to highly echogenic. Regions of early suppuration may appear solid and echogenic, related to the presence of necrotic hepatocytes.[28] Occasionally gas-producing organisms give rise to echogenic foci with a posterior reverberation artifact (Fig. 4-19, *A*).[29,30] Fluid-fluid interfaces, internal septations, and debris have all been observed. The abscess wall can vary from well defined to irregular and thick (Fig. 4-19, *B*).[30]

The **differential diagnosis** of pyogenic liver abscess includes amebic or echinococcal infection, simple cyst with hemorrhage, hematoma, and necrotic or cystic neoplasm. Ultrasound-guided liver aspiration is an expeditious means to confirm the diagnosis. Specimens should be sent for both aerobic and anaerobic culture. Fifty percent of abscesses in the past were considered sterile. This was almost certainly due to failure to transport the specimen in an oxygen-free container, and thus anaerobic organisms were not identified.[31] Once the diagnosis of liver abscess is made by the presence of pus or a positive Gram stain and culture, the collection can be drained percutaneously using ultrasound or computed tomography (CT) guidance.

Fungal

Candidiasis. The liver is frequently involved secondary to hematogenous spread of mycotic infections in other organs, most commonly the lungs. Patients are generally immunocompromised, although systemic candidiasis may occur in pregnancy or following hyperalimentation.[32]

The ultrasound features of hepatic candidiasis include:[33]

- **"Wheel within a wheel"**—Peripheral hypoechoic zone with an inner echogenic wheel and central hypoechoic nidus. Central nidus represents focal necrosis in which fungal elements are found. This is seen early in the disease.
- **"Bull's eye"**—1 to 4 cm lesion having a hyperechoic center and a hypoechoic rim. It is present when neutrophil counts return to normal.

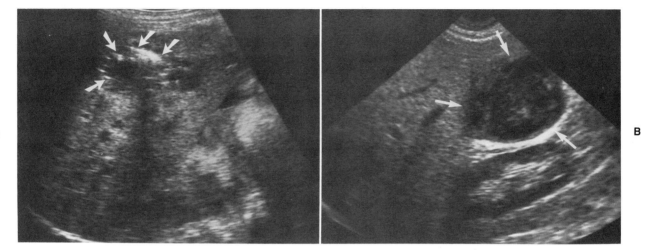

FIG 4-19. Pyogenic liver abscesses. **A,** Echogenic regions *(arrows)* within abscess cavity correspond to gas. **B,** Purulent material was aspirated from this abscess *(arrows)* with poorly defined wall and internal debris.

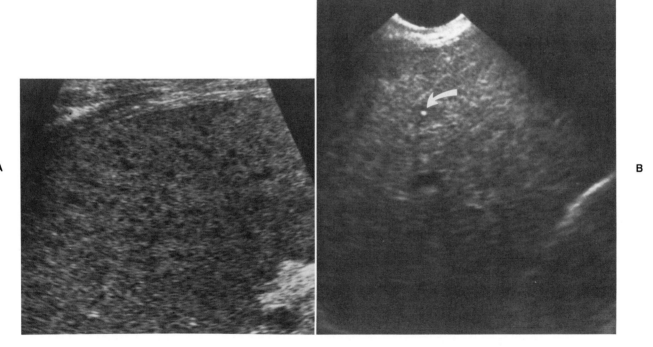

FIG 4-20. Candidiasis. **A,** Uniformly hypoechoic pattern. Multiple hypoechoic hepatic lesions are present in this young patient with acute myelogenous leukemia. **B,** Echogenic pattern, following medical therapy. Small calcified lesion *(arrow)* is visualized in a second immunocompromised patient.

- **"Uniformly hypoechoic"**—Most common. This corresponds to progressive fibrosis (Fig. 4-20, *A*).
- **"Echogenic"**—Variable calcification representing scar formation (Fig. 4-20, *B*).

It is interesting to note that, although percutaneous liver aspiration is of great benefit in obtaining the organism in pyogenic liver abscesses, it frequently yields falsely negative results for the presence of *Candida* organisms.[33]

Parasitic

Amebiasis. Hepatic infection by the parasite *Entamoeba histolytica* is the most common extraintestinal manifestation of amebiasis. Transmission is by the fecal-oral route. The protozoan reaches the liver by penetrating through the colon, invading the mesenteric venules, and entering the portal vein. However, in more than one half of patients with amebic abscesses of the liver, the colon appears normal and stool culture results are negative, thus delaying diagnosis.[32] The most common presenting symptom in patients with amebic abscess is pain, which occurs in 99% of patients. Approximately 15% of patients have diarrhea at the time of diagnosis.

Sonographic features include a round or oval-shaped lesion, absence of a prominent abscess wall, hypoechogenicity compared to normal liver, fine low-level internal echoes, distal sonic enhancement, and contiguity with the diaphragm (Fig. 4-21).[34,35] These features, however, can all be found in pyogenic abscesses.

In a recent review of 112 amebic lesions by Ralls et

al., two sonographic patterns were significantly more prevalent in amebic abscesses: (1) round or oval shapes in 82% versus 60% of pyogenic abscess (*P* < .01) and (2) hypoechoic appearance with fine internal echoes at high gain in 58% versus 36% of pyogenic abscesses (*P* < .04).[36] Most amebic abscesses occur in the right lobe of the liver. Practically speaking, the **diagnosis** of amebic liver abscess is made using a combination of the clinical features, the ultrasound findings and results of serologic testing. The indirect hemagglutination test is positive in 94% to 100% of patients.[37]

Amebicidal drugs are effective therapy. The indications for percutaneous drainage are somewhat controversial.[38,39] It seems reasonable that catheter drainage is warranted in abscesses of the left lobe that abut the heart and those that are adjacent to the hemidiaphragm because of the risk of intrapericardial and intrathoracic rupture. Patients on medical therapy who exhibit clinical deterioration may also benefit from catheter drainage. If pyogenic superinfection is suspected, percutaneous aspiration is indicated, followed by drainage if bacteria are present. The majority of hepatic amebic abscesses disappear with adequate medical therapy. The time from termination of therapy to resolution varies from 1½ to 23 months (median 7 months).[40] A minority of patients have residual hepatic cysts and focal regions of increased or decreased echogenicity.

Hydatid Disease. The most common cause of hydatid disease in humans is infestation by the parasite *Echinococcus granulosus*. *E. granulosus* has a worldwide distribution. It is most prevalent in sheep- and cat-

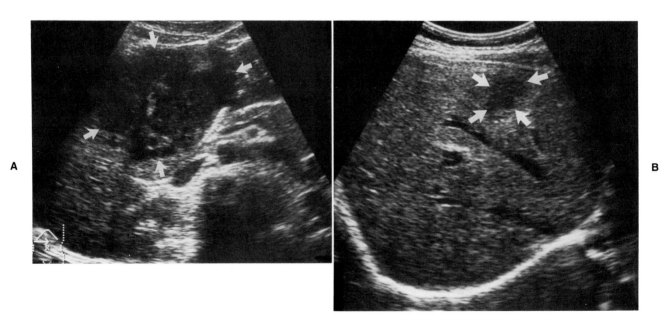

FIG 4-21. Amebiasis. **A,** Large hypoechoic abscess *(arrows)* is present in liver. **B,** Six weeks following amebicidal therapy, abscess *(arrows)* has dramatically decreased in size.

tle-raising countries, notably in the Middle East, Australia, and the Mediterranean. Endemic regions are also present in the United States (the central valley in California, the lower Mississippi valley, Utah, and Arizona) and northern Canada. *E. granulosus* is a tapeworm, 3 to 6 mm in length, which lives in the intestine of the definitive host, usually the dog. Its eggs are excreted in the dog's feces and swallowed by the intermediate hosts—sheep, cattle, goats, or humans. The embryos are freed in the duodenum and pass through the mucosa to reach the liver through the portal venous system. Most of the embryos remain trapped in the liver, although the lungs, kidneys, spleen, central nervous system, and bone may become secondarily involved. In the liver, the right lobe is most frequently involved. The surviving embryos form slow-growing cysts. The cyst wall consists of an external membrane that is approximately 1 mm thick, which may calcify (the **ectocyst**). The host forms a dense connective tissue capsule around the cyst (the **pericyst**). The inner germinal layer (the **endocyst**) gives rise to brood capsules that enlarge to form protoscolices. The brood capsules may separate from the wall and form a fine sediment called hydatid sand. When hydatid cysts within the organs of a herbivore are eaten, the scolices attach to the intestine and grow to adult tapeworms, thus completing the life cycle.

Several reports describe the **sonographic features** of hepatic hydatid disease (Figs. 4-22 and 4-23).[41-43] Lewall proposed four groups[42]:

- Simple cysts containing no internal architecture except sand
- Cysts with detached endocyst secondary to rupture
- Cysts with daughter cysts, matrix (echogenic material between the daughter cysts), or both
- Densely calcified masses

Surgery is accepted as the **treatment** of choice in echinococcal disease, although recent reports describe success with percutaneous drainage.[44,45] If neither surgery nor percutaneous catheter drainage are deemed possible because of the high risk of anaphylaxis from spillage of viable scolices, medical therapy is an alternative. Ultrasound has been used to monitor the course of medical therapy in patients with abdominal hydatid disease.[46] Changes noted in the resolution of the disease were a gradual reduction in cyst size (43%), membrane detachment (30%), progressive increase in echogenicity of the cyst cavity (12%), and wall calcification (6%). No change was identified in 26% of patients.

Hepatic alveolar echinococcus is a rare parasitic infestation by the larvae of *E. multilocularis*. The fox is the main host. The sonographic features include echogenic lesions, which may be single or multiple; necrotic irregular lesions without a well-defined wall; clusters of calcification within lesions; and dilated bile ducts.[47] The differential diagnosis is that of primary or metastatic tumors. Diagnosis is made using immunologic tests, percutaneous biopsy, or angiography.[47]

Schistosomiasis. Schistosomiasis is one of the most common parasitic infections in humans, estimated to affect 200 million people worldwide.[48] Hepatic schistosomiasis is caused by *Schistosoma mansoni*, *S. japonicum*, *S. mekongi*, and *S. intercalatum*. Hepatic involvement by *S. mansoni* is particularly severe. *S. mansoni* is prevalent in Africa, Egypt, and South America, particularly in Venezuela and Brazil. The ova reach the liver through the portal vein and incite a chronic granulomatous reaction first described by Symmers as claypipestem fibrosis.[49] The terminal portal vein branches become occluded, leading to presinusoidal portal hypertension, splenomegaly, varices, and ascites.

The **sonographic features** of schistosomiasis are widened echogenic portal tracts, sometimes reaching a thickness of 2 cm.[50,51] The porta hepatis is the region most often affected. Initially the liver size is enlarged; however, as the periportal fibrosis progresses, the liver becomes contracted and the features of portal hypertension prevail.

Pneumocystis carinii. *Pneumocystis carinii* is the most common organism causing opportunistic infection in patients with acquired immunodeficiency syndrome (AIDS). Pneumocystis pneumonia affects nearly 80% of AIDS patients.[52] Extrapulmonic *P. carinii* infection is being reported with increasing frequency.[53-56] It is postulated that the use of maintenance aerosolized pentamidine achieves lower systemic levels than the intravenous form, allowing subclinical pulmonary infections and systemic dissemination of the protozoa. Extrapulmonary *P. carinii* infection has been documented in the liver, spleen, renal cortex, thyroid gland, pancreas, and lymph nodes. The **sonographic findings** of *P. carinii* involvement of the liver range from diffuse, tiny, nonshadowing echogenic foci to extensive replacement of the normal hepatic parenchyma by echogenic clumps representing dense calcification (Fig. 4-24). Recently, a similar sonographic pattern was identified with hepatic infection by *Mycobacterium avium intracellulare* and cytomegalovirus.[57]

DISORDERS OF METABOLISM
Fatty Liver

Fatty liver is an acquired, reversible disorder of metabolism, resulting in an accumulation of triglycerides within the hepatocytes. Probably the most common **cause** of a fatty liver is obesity. Excessive alcohol intake produces a fatty liver by stimulating lipolysis, as does starvation. Other causes of fatty infiltration include poorly controlled hyperlipidemia, diabetes, excess exogenous or endogenous corticosteroids, pregnancy, total parenteral hyperalimentation, severe hepatitis, gly-

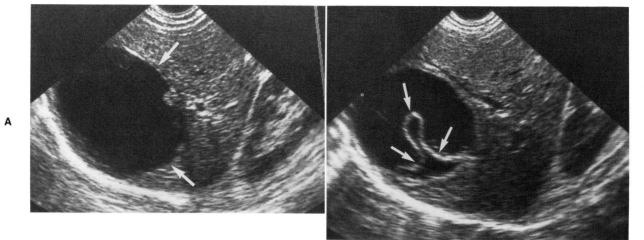

FIG 4-22. Hydatid disease. **A,** Longitudinal sonogram shows large cystic mass within right lobe of liver *(arrows)*. **B,** Three weeks later, patient presented with right upper quadrant pain and elevated serum eosinophil count. Endocyst *(arrows)* has ruptured.

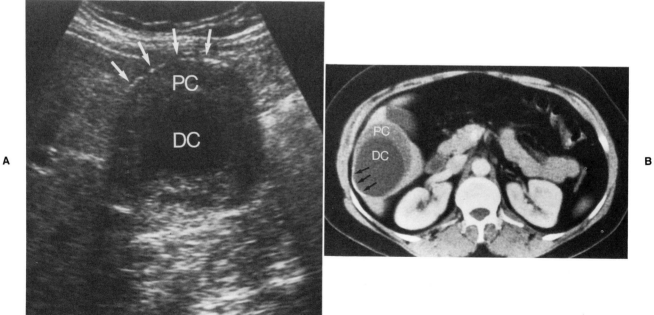

FIG 4-23. Hydatid disease. **A,** Sonogram shows complex liver mass with subtle calcified wall. **B,** Confirmatory CT scan. *Straight arrows* indicate calcification; *DC,* daughter cyst; *PC,* parent cyst.

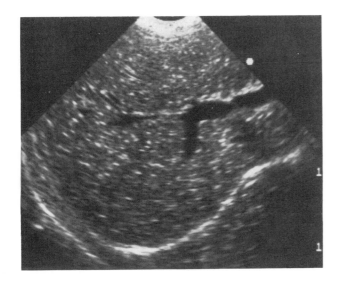

FIG 4-24. *Pneumocystis carinii.* Subcostal oblique sonogram shows multiple hyperechoic foci throughout liver in this young patient with AIDS.

cogen storage disease, jejunoileal bypass procedures for obesity, cystic fibrosis, congenital generalized lipodystrophy, several chemotherapeutic agents including methotrexate, and toxins such as carbon tetrachloride and yellow phosphorus.[58] The presence of excess fat in the liver has no harmful effect on liver function. Correction of the primary abnormality will reverse the process.

Sonographically, fatty infiltration leads to increased liver echogenicity and attenuation of the ultrasound beam.[59-61] It is important that the inexperienced sonographer not adjust the time gain compensation (TGC)

settings and power to make the fatty liver appear normal. Three grades have been described for fatty infiltration (Fig. 4-25):[59]

Mild   Minimal diffuse increase in hepatic echogenicity; normal visualization of diaphragm and intrahepatic vessel borders

Moderate   Moderate diffuse increase in hepatic echogenicity; slightly impaired visualization of intrahepatic vessels and diaphragm

Severe   Marked increase in echogenicity; poor penetration of the posterior segment of the right lobe of the liver and poor or nonvisualization of the hepatic vessels and diaphragm

Focal fatty infiltration and **focal fatty sparing** may mimic neoplastic involvement. In focal fatty infiltration, regions of increased echogenicity are present within a background of normal liver parenchyma. Features of focal fatty change include (Fig. 4-26):

- Lack of mass effect: Hepatic vessels are not displaced.
- Geometric margins are present, although focal fat may appear round, nodular, or interdigitated with normal tissue.
- Rapid change with time: Fatty infiltration may resolve as early as within 6 days.[62-66]

CT scans of the liver will demonstrate corresponding regions of low attenuation (Fig. 4-27). Radionuclide liver and spleen scintigraphic examination will yield normal results, indicating adequate numbers of Kupffer cells within the fatty regions.[62] Conversely, islands of normal liver parenchyma may appear as hypoechoic masses within a dense, fatty infiltrated liver. It has been postulated that these focal spared areas are caused by a regional decrease in portal blood flow as demonstrated by CT scans during arterial portographic examinations.[67]

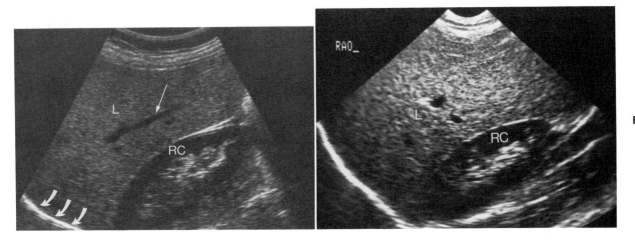

FIG 4-25. Fatty infiltration. **A,** Mild. Liver parenchyma *(L)* is minimally hyperechoic compared with normal renal cortex *(RC).* Hepatic vein *(straight arrow)* and diaphragm *(curved arrows)* are well seen. **B,** Moderate. Hepatic echogenicity *(L)* is more marked. *RC* indicates renal cortex.

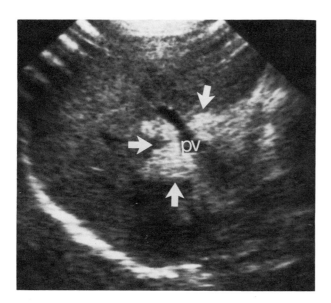

FIG 4-26. Focal fatty infiltration, nodular pattern. Irregular echogenic "mass" *(arrows)* is seen centrally. Portal vein *(pv)* runs unaltered through abnormality.

Focal fatty sparing most commonly involves the periportal region of the medial segment of the left lobe.[68,69] Knowledge of this pattern and use of CT scans and nuclear medicine scintigraphy will avoid the necessity for biopsy in the majority of cases.

Glycogen Storage Disease (Glycogenosis)

Recognition of glycogen storage disease (GSD) affecting the kidneys and liver was first made by von Gierke in 1929. Type 1 GSD (von Gierke's disease, glucose 6-phosphatase deficiency) is manifested in the neonatal period by hepatomegaly, nephromegaly, and hypoglycemic convulsions. Because of the enzyme deficiency, large quantities of glycogen are deposited in the hepatocytes and proximal convoluted tubules of the kidney.[70] With dietary management and supportive therapy, more patients currently are surviving to childhood and young adulthood. As a result, several patients have developed benign adenomas or, less commonly, hepatocellular carcinoma.[71] Sonographically, type 1 GSD appears indistinguishable from other causes of diffuse fatty infiltration. Secondary hepatic adenomas are well-demarcated, solid masses of variable echogenicity (Fig. 4-28). Malignant transformation can be recognized by rapid growth of the lesions, which may become more poorly defined.[71]

Cirrhosis

Cirrhosis is defined by the World Health Organization (WHO) as a diffuse process characterized by fibrosis and the conversion of normal liver architecture into

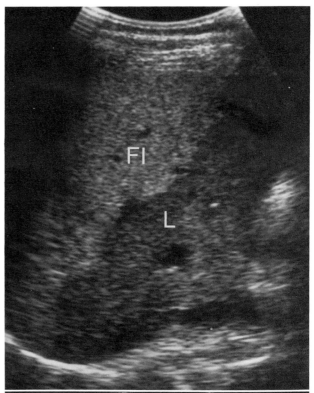

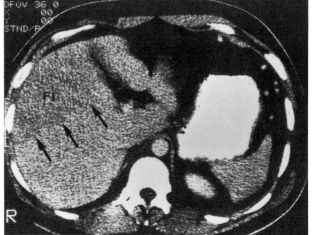

FIG 4-27. Focal fatty infiltration *(FI)*, geometric pattern. **A,** Sagittal sonogram of right lobe of liver. Normal liver parenchyma *(L)* appears hypoechoic. **B,** Corresponding CT image. Note relatively straight line of demarcation *(arrows)* between regions of fatty infiltration and normal liver.

structurally abnormal nodules.[72] There are three major **pathologic** mechanisms which, in combination, create cirrhosis: cell death, fibrosis, and regeneration.[73] Cirrhosis has been classified as **micronodular,** in which nodules are 0.1 to 1 cm in diameter, and **macronodular,** characterized by nodules of varying size, up to 5

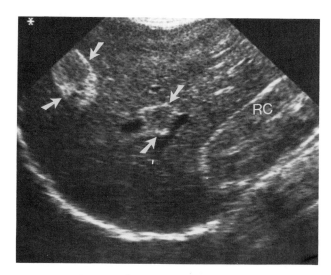

FIG 4-28. Adenomas in type 1 glycogen storage disease. Sagittal sonogram shows nonspecific echogenic hepatic masses *(arrows)*. Renal cortex *(RC)* is hyperechoic secondary to chronic renal disease.

cm in diameter. Alcohol consumption is the most common cause of micronodular cirrhosis, and chronic viral hepatitis is the most frequent cause of the macronodular form.[74] Other causes are biliary cirrhosis (primary and secondary), Wilson's disease, and hemochromatosis. The classic **clinical presentation** of cirrhosis is hepatomegaly, jaundice, and ascites. However, serious liver injury may be present without any clinical clues. In fact, only 60% of patients with cirrhosis have signs and symptoms of liver disease.

Because liver biopsy is invasive, there has been great clinical interest in the ability to detect cirrhosis by noninvasive means, such as sonography. The sonographic patterns associated with cirrhosis include:

- **Volume redistribution**—In the early stages of cirrhosis the liver may be enlarged, whereas in the advanced states the liver is often small, with relative enlargement of the caudate, left lobe, or both in comparison with the right lobe (Fig. 4-29, *A*). Several studies have evaluated the ratio of the caudate lobe width to the right lobe width (C/RL) as an indicator of cirrhosis.[75-77] A C/RL value of 0.65 is considered indicative of cirrhosis. The specificity is high (100%) but the sensitivity is low (ranging from 43% to 84%), indicating that the C/RL ratio is a useful measurement if it is abnormal.[75,76] It should be noted, however, that there were no patients in these studies with Budd-Chiari syndrome, which may also cause caudate lobe enlargement.
- **Coarse echotexture**—Increased echogenicity and coarse echotexture are frequent observations in dif-

fuse liver disease (Fig. 4-29, *B* and *C*). These are subjective findings, however, and may be confounded by inappropriate TGC settings and overall gain. Two techniques are available to assess in vivo ultrasound attenuation, based on (1) amplitude change and (2) frequency change.[61,78,79] Liver attenuation is correlated with the presence of fat and not fibrosis.[78] Cirrhotic livers without fatty infiltration had attenuation values similar to those of controls. This accounts for the relatively low accuracy in distinguishing diffuse liver disease[60,80] and for the conflicting reports regarding attenuation values in cirrhosis.[61,81,82]

- **Nodular surface**—Irregularity of the liver surface during routine scanning has been appreciated as a sign of cirrhosis when the appearance is gross or when ascites is present (Fig. 4-29, *D*).[83]
- **Regenerating nodules**—Regenerating nodules have been identified using a high-frequency (5 or 7.5 MHz) probe to examine the liver surface.[83,84] The ability of ultrasound to define regenerating nodules is controversial, and their sonographic appearance is nonspecific (Fig. 4-29, *E*). They tend to be hypoechoic and have a thin echogenic border that corresponds to fibrofatty connective tissue.[83] It is suspected that, with the increased use of high-resolution ultrasound to screen patients with chronic liver disease who are at risk of developing hepatocellular carcinoma, regenerating nodules will be identified more frequently. Diagnosis is established by biopsy.

VASCULAR ABNORMALITIES
Portal Hypertension

Normal portal vein pressure is 5 to 10 mm Hg (14 cm H_2O). Portal hypertension is defined by a wedged hepatic vein pressure or direct portal vein pressure of more than 5 mm Hg greater than inferior vena cava pressure, splenic vein pressure of greater than 15 mm Hg, or portal vein pressure (measured surgically) of greater than 30 cm H_2O. **Pathophysiologically,** portal hypertension can be divided into presinusoidal and intrahepatic groups, depending on whether the hepatic vein wedged pressure is normal (presinusoidal) or elevated (intrahepatic).

Presinusoidal portal hypertension can be subdivided into extrahepatic and intrahepatic forms. The causes of **extrahepatic presinusoidal portal hypertension** include thrombosis of the portal or splenic veins. This should be suspected in any patient who presents with clinical signs of portal hypertension—ascites, splenomegaly, and varices—and a normal liver biopsy. Thrombosis of the portal venous system occurs in children secondary to umbilical vein catheterization, omphalitis, and neonatal sepsis. In adults the causes of

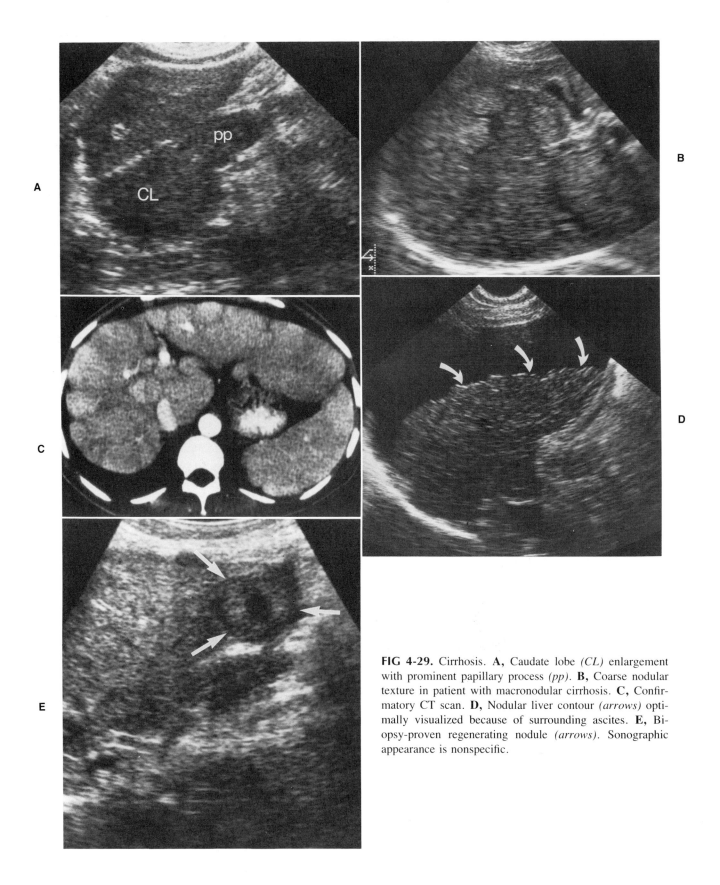

FIG 4-29. Cirrhosis. **A,** Caudate lobe *(CL)* enlargement with prominent papillary process *(pp).* **B,** Coarse nodular texture in patient with macronodular cirrhosis. **C,** Confirmatory CT scan. **D,** Nodular liver contour *(arrows)* optimally visualized because of surrounding ascites. **E,** Biopsy-proven regenerating nodule *(arrows).* Sonographic appearance is nonspecific.

portal vein thrombosis include trauma, sepsis, hepatocellular carcinoma, pancreatitis, portacaval shunts, splenectomy, and hypercoagulable states.[85] The intrahepatic presinusoidal causes of portal hypertension are due to lesions within the portal zones of the liver, notably schistosomiasis, primary biliary cirrhosis, congenital hepatic fibrosis, and toxic substances such as polyvinyl chloride and methotrexate.[85]

Cirrhosis is the most common cause of **intrahepatic portal hypertension** and accounts for greater than 90% of all cases of portal hypertension in the West.[74] In cirrhosis, most of the normal liver architecture is replaced by distorted vascular channels that provide increased resistance to portal venous blood flow and obstruction to hepatic venous outflow. Diffuse metastatic liver disease also produces portal hypertension by the same mechanism. Thrombotic diseases of the inferior vena cava and hepatic veins, as well as constrictive pericarditis and other causes of severe right-sided heart failure, over time will lead to centrilobular fibrosis, hepatic regeneration, cirrhosis, and finally portal hypertension.

Sonographic findings of portal hypertension include the secondary signs of splenomegaly, ascites, and portosystemic venous collaterals. When the resistance to blood flow in the portal vessels exceeds the resistance to flow in the small communicating channels between the portal and systemic circulations, portosystemic collaterals form. Thus, although the caliber of the portal vein initially may be increased (≥ 1.3 cm) in portal hypertension,[86] with the development of portosystemic shunts, the portal vein caliber will decrease.[87] Five major sites of **portosystemic venous collaterals** are visualized by ultrasound (Fig. 4-30)[88-90]:

- **Gastroesophageal junction**—Between the coronary and short gastric veins and the systemic esophageal veins. These varices are of particular importance as they may lead to life-threatening or fatal hemorrhage. Dilation of the coronary vein (> 0.7 cm) is associated with severe portal hypertension (portohepatic gradient > 10 mm Hg).[87]
- **Paraumbilical vein**—Runs in the falciform ligament and connects the left portal vein to the systemic epigastric veins near the umbilicus (Cruveilhier-Baumgarten syndrome).[91] Several authors have suggested that, if the hepatofugal flow in the patent paraumbilical vein exceeds the hepatopetal flow in

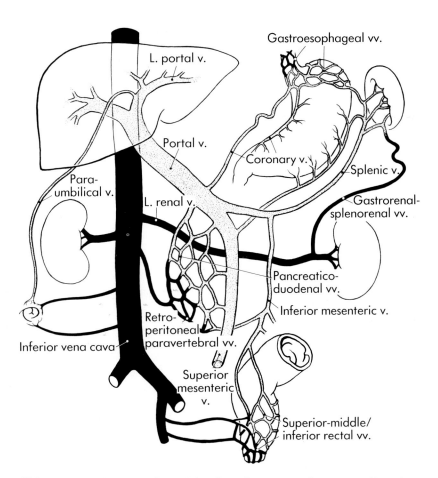

FIG 4-30. Portal hypertension. Major sites of portosystemic venous collaterals.
(Modified from Subramanyam BR, Balthazar EJ, Madamba MR, et al. *Radiology* 1983; 146:161–166.)

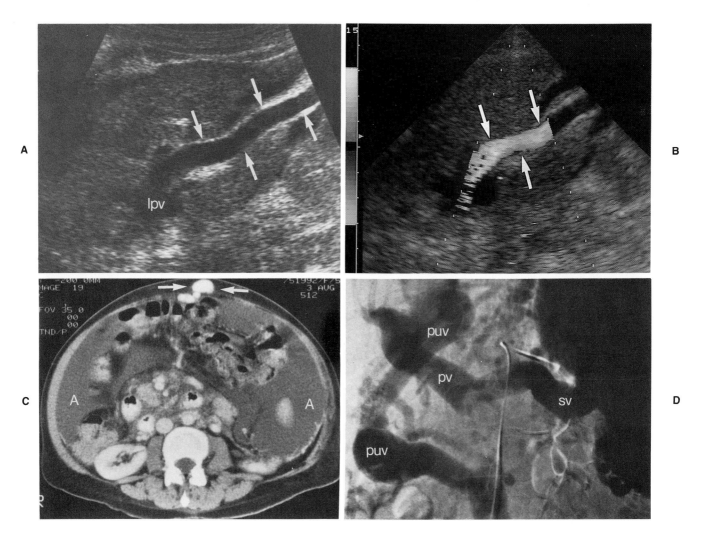

FIG 4-31. Portosystemic venous collaterals. Patent paraumbilical vein. Sagittal gray-scale **(A)** and color-flow Doppler **(B)** sonograms show recanalized paraumbilical vein *(arrows)*. Flow is hepatofugal. *lpv* indicates left portal vein. **C,** Postcontrast CT scan. Communication of paraumbilical vein with systemic epigastric vein *(arrows)* is evident. *A* indicates ascites). **D,** Venous phase of selective splenic arterial injection shows the large paraumbilical vein *(puv)*, equal in size to main portal vein *(pv)*. *Sv* indicates splenic vein.

the portal vein, patients may be protected from developing esophageal varices (Fig. 4-31).[92,93]

- **Splenorenal and gastrorenal**—Tortuous veins may be seen in the region of the splenic and left renal hilus, which represent collaterals between the splenic, coronary, and short gastric veins and the left adrenal or renal veins (Fig. 4-32).
- **Intestinal**—Regions in which the gastrointestinal tract becomes retroperitoneal so that the veins of the ascending and descending colon, duodenum, pancreas, and liver may anastomose with the renal, phrenic, and lumbar veins (systemic tributaries).

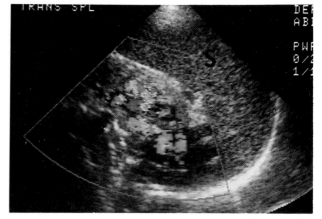

FIG 4-32. Portosystemic venous collaterals. Transverse color-flow Doppler sonogram of splenorenal varices at splenic hilus.

(Courtesy of J. William Charboneau, MD, Mayo Clinic, Rochester, Minn.)

- **Hemorrhoidal**—The perianal region where the superior rectal veins, which extend from the inferior mesenteric vein, anastomose with the systemic middle and inferior rectal veins.

Duplex **Doppler sonography** provides additional information regarding direction of portal flow. False results may occur, however, when sampling is obtained from periportal collaterals in patients with portal vein thrombosis or hepatofugal portal flow.[94] The current limitations of duplex sonography in the evaluation of portal hypertension are the inability to accurately determine vascular pressures and flow rates. Normal portal venous flow rates will vary in the same individual: increasing postprandially and during inspiration[86,95] and decreasing following exercise or when the patient is in the upright position.[96] Because many patients with portal hypertension are ill and have contracted cirrhotic livers, technical measurement errors also limit flow-rate determinations. Angiographic examination remains the gold standard for evaluating the portal venous system.[94] Duplex sonographic examination provides a valuable, noninvasive means of assessing the presence and direction of portal venous flow and of detecting clinically significant portosystemic collaterals such as gastroesophageal varices.

Portal Vein Thrombosis

Portal vein thrombosis has been associated with malignancy, including hepatocellular carcinoma, metastatic liver disease, carcinoma of the pancreas, and primary leiomyosarcoma of the portal vein; as well as chronic pancreatitis; hepatitis; septicemia; trauma; splenectomy; portocaval shunts; hypercoagulable states such as pregnancy; and in neonates, omphalitis; umbilical vein catheterization; and acute dehydration.[97,98]

Sonographic findings in portal vein thrombosis include an echogenic thrombus within the lumen of the vein (67%), portal vein collateral channels (48%), enlargement of the thrombosed segment of vein (38%), and cavernous transformation of the portal vein (19%) (Figs. 4-33 and 4-34).[97] **Cavernous transformation** of the portal vein refers to numerous wormlike vessels at the porta hepatis, which represent periportal collateral circulation.[99] This pattern is observed in long-standing portal vein thrombosis, requiring up to 12 months to occur, and thus is more likely to develop with benign disease.[100] The sonographic appearance of the endoluminal thrombus is nonspecific and cannot be used to distinguish between a benign and a malignant process. Portal vein thrombosis associated with a liver mass, however, is more likely the result of invasion by hepatocellular carcinoma than of tumor extension from metastatic liver disease.[97]

Portal Vein Aneurysm

Aneurysms of the portal vein are rare. Their origin is thought to be either congenital or acquired secondary to portal hypertension.[101] Portal vein aneurysms have been described proximally at the junction of the superior mesenteric and splenic veins and distally involving the portal venous radicles. The **sonographic appearance** is that of an anechoic cystic mass, which connects with the portal venous system. Pulsed Doppler sonographic examination demonstrates turbulent venous flow.[101]

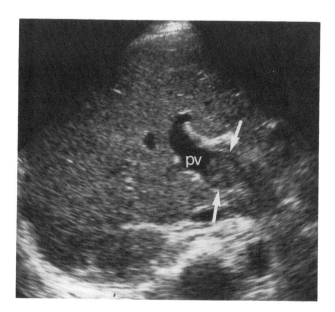

FIG 4-33. Portal vein thrombosis. Echogenic thrombus (arrows) expands lumen of portal vein (pv).

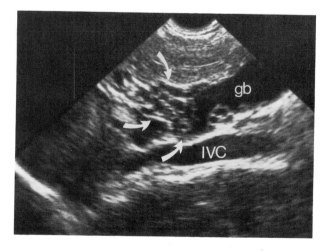

FIG 4-34. Cavernous transformation of portal vein. Numerous periportal collateral vessels (arrows) are present. gb indicates gall bladder; IVC, inferior vena cava.

Intrahepatic Portosystemic Venous Shunts

Intrahepatic **arterial-portal fistulas** are well-recognized complications of large-gauge percutaneous liver biopsy and trauma. Conversely, intrahepatic **portohepatic venous shunts** are rare. Their cause is controversial and thought to be either congenital or related to portal hypertension.[102,103] Patients typically are middle aged and present with hepatic encephalopathy. Anatomically, portohepatic venous shunts are more common in the right lobe.[102] **Sonography** demonstrates a tortuous tubular vessel or complex vascular channels, which connect a branch of the portal vein to an hepatic vein or the inferior vena cava.[102-104] The diagnosis is confirmed angiographically.

Hepatic Artery Aneurysm and Pseudoaneurysm

The hepatic artery is the fourth most common site of an intraabdominal aneurysm, following the infrarenal aorta, iliac, and splenic arteries. Eighty percent of patients with an hepatic artery aneurysm experience catastrophic rupture into the peritoneum, biliary tree, gastrointestinal tract, or portal vein.[105] Hepatic artery pseudoaneurysm secondary to chronic pancreatitis has been described. The duplex Doppler sonographic examination revealed turbulent arterial flow within a sonolucent mass.[105]

Hereditary Hemorrhagic Telangiectasia

Hereditary hemorrhagic telangiectasia, or Osler-Weber-Rendu disease, is an autosomal dominant disorder that causes arteriovenous malformations in the liver, hepatic fibrosis, and cirrhosis. Patients present with multiple telangiectasias and recurrent episodes of bleeding. **Sonographic findings** in hereditary hemorrhagic telangiectasia include: a large feeding common hepatic artery measuring up to 10 mm, multiple dilated tubular structures representing arteriovenous malformations, and large draining hepatic veins secondary to arteriovenous shunting.[106]

Budd-Chiari Syndrome

The Budd-Chiari syndrome is caused by thrombosis of the main hepatic veins. Patients present with ascites (90%), hepatomegaly, right upper quadrant pain, and to a lesser degree, splenomegaly (30%). Causes of Budd-Chiari syndrome include coagulation abnormalities such as polycythemia rubra vera and paroxysmal nocturnal hemoglobinuria; trauma; oral contraceptives; tumor extension from primary hepatocellular carcinoma, renal carcinoma, and adrenal cortical carcinoma; pregnancy; and obstructing membranes.[85] In 50% to 75% of cases, no etiologic factor is found.

There have been numerous recent reviews in the radiology literature outlining the **sonographic evaluation** of Budd-Chiari syndrome.[107-116] In the acute or suba-cute stage, hemorrhagic infarction may be seen as hypoechoic regions. As the infarcted areas become more fibrotic, the echogenicity increases.[116] The caudate lobe is often spared in Budd-Chiari syndrome because the emissary veins drain directly into the inferior vena cava at a level lower than the main hepatic veins. The increased blood flow through the caudate lobe leads to caudate enlargement. Real-time scanning allows the radiologist to evaluate the inferior vena cava and hepatic veins noninvasively. Sonographic features of hepatic venous involvement include stenosis with proximal dilation, thickened walls, thrombosis, and intrahepatic collaterals (Fig. 4-35).[109,110] Membranous webs may be identified as echogenic or focal obliteration of the lumen.[110] Real-time ultrasonography, however, underestimates the presence of thrombosis and webs[109] and may be inconclusive in a cirrhotic patient in whom the hepatic veins cannot be imaged.

Duplex and **color-flow Doppler imaging** have considerable potential in the evaluation of patients with suspected Budd-Chiari syndrome. Both determine the presence and direction of flow. The middle and left hepatic veins are best scanned in the transverse plane at the level of the xiphoid process. From this angle, the veins are almost parallel to the Doppler beam, allowing optimal reception of their Doppler signals. The right hepatic vein is best evaluated from a right lateral intercostal approach.[112]

The normal blood flow in the inferior vena cava and hepatic veins is phasic in response to both the cardiac and respiratory cycles.[117] In Budd-Chiari syndrome, flow in the inferior vena cava, hepatic veins, or both

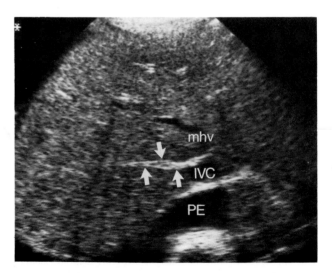

FIG 4-35. Budd-Chiari syndrome. Transverse subcostal oblique sonogram shows echogenic, obliterated right hepatic vein *(arrows)* and attenuated, irregular middle hepatic vein *(mhv).* Left hepatic vein could not be seen. *IVC* indicates inferior vena cava; *PE,* right pleural effusion.

changes from phasic to absent, reversed, turbulent, or continuous.[114] Continuous flow has been called the pseudoportal Doppler signal and appears to reflect either partial inferior vena cava obstruction or extrinsic inferior vena cava compression.[113] The portal blood flow also may be affected and is characteristically either slowed or reversed.[114]

Hepatic venoocclusive disease causes progressive occlusion of the small hepatic venules. The disease is endemic in Jamaica, secondary to alkaloid toxicity from bush tea. In North America, most cases are iatrogenic secondary to hepatic irradiation and chemotherapy used in bone marrow transplantation.[115] Patients with hepatic venoocclusive disease are clinically indistinguishable from those with Budd-Chiari syndrome. Duplex Doppler sonography demonstrates normal caliber, patency, and phasic forward (toward the heart) flow of the main hepatic veins and inferior vena cava.[115] Flow in the portal vein, however, may be abnormal showing either reversed or "to and fro" flow.[115,118] In addition, the diagnosis of hepatic venoocclusive disease can be suggested in a patient with decreased portal blood flow (as compared with a baseline measurement performed before ablative therapy).[115]

BENIGN HEPATIC NEOPLASMS
Cavernous Hemangioma

Cavernous hemangiomas are the most common benign tumors of the liver, occurring in approximately 4% of the population. They occur in all age groups but are more common in adults, particularly women. The female to male ratio is about 5:1.[119] The vast majority of hemangiomas are small, asymptomatic, and discovered incidentally. Large lesions may produce symptoms of acute abdominal pain caused by hemorrhage or thrombosis within the tumor. Thrombocytopenia, caused by sequestration and destruction of platelets within a large cavernous hemangioma (Kasabach-Merritt syndrome), occasionally occurs in infants and is rare in adults. Once hemangiomas are identified in the adult, they usually have reached a stable size and change in appearance or size is uncommon.[120] Hemangiomas may enlarge, however, during pregnancy or with the administration of estrogens, suggesting the tumor is hormone-dependent. Histologically, hemangiomas consist of multiple vascular channels that are lined by a single layer of endothelium and separated and supported by fibrous septa. The vascular spaces may contain thrombi.[119]

The **sonographic appearance** of cavernous hemangioma varies (Figs. 4-36 to 4-38). Typically the lesion is small, less than 3 cm in diameter, well defined, homogeneous and hyperechoic.[121] The increased echogenicity has been related to the numerous interfaces between the walls of the cavernous sinuses and the blood

within them.[122] Posterior acoustic enhancement has been correlated with hypervascularity on angiography.[123] It is estimated that approximately 67% to 79% of hemangiomas are hyperechoic,[124,125] and of these 58% to 73% are homogeneous.[121,123] Larger lesions tend to be heterogeneous with central hypoechoic foci corresponding to fibrous collagen scars, large vascular spaces, or both. A hemangioma may appear hypoechoic within the background of a fatty infiltrated liver.[126]

When a hyperechoic lesion typical of a cavernous hemangioma is incidentally discovered, no further examination is usually necessary, or at most, a repeat ultrasound is performed in 3 to 6 months to document lack of change. In a patient with a known malignancy, abnormal results of liver function tests, clinical symptoms referable to the liver, or an atypical sonographic pattern, one of the following additional imaging techniques is recommended:

- **Computed tomography**—Using the strict CT criteria of (1) hypodense lesion on precontrast scan, (2) peripheral contrast enhancement during the dynamic bolus phase, and (3) complete isodense fill-in of the lesion on delayed scans up to 60 minutes after contrast material administration, between 55% to 79% of hepatic hemangiomas are specifically diagnosed.[127,128]
- **Red blood cell scintigraphy**—Technetium-99m labeled red blood cell (RBC) scintigraphy using single-photon emission CT (SPECT) has achieved a positive predictive value and specificity of almost 100% in evaluating hemangiomas.[127,129,130] The classic appearance is decreased activity on early dynamic images with increased activity on delayed blood pool scanning.
- **Magnetic resonance imaging (MRI)**—Hemangiomas demonstrate marked hyperintensity on T2-weighted images, regardless of field strength.[131] MR imaging is more accurate than SPECT in diagnosing hemangiomas <2 cm and those ≤2.5 cm that are adjacent to the heart and major intrahepatic vessels.[132]

In a minority of patients, imaging will not allow a definitive diagnosis of hemangioma to be made. **Percutaneous biopsy** of hepatic hemangiomas has been safely performed.[121,133,134] Cronan et al. performed biopsies on 15 patients (12 of whom were outpatients) using a 20-gauge Franseen needle.[134] In all cases the histologic sample was diagnostic and was characterized by large spaces with an endothelial lining. It is recommended that normal liver be interposed between the abdominal wall and the hemangioma to allow hepatic tamponade of any potential bleeding.

The best approach to the **diagnosis** of hemangiomas will depend on the clinical situation, the size and location of the lesion, the availability of imaging modalities

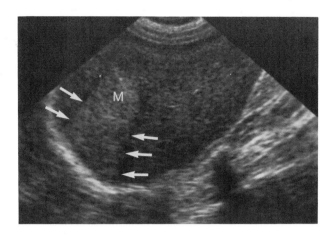

FIG 4-36. Cavernous hemangioma. Sagittal sonogram of right lobe of liver shows echogenic mass *(M)* with posterior acoustic enhancement *(arrows)*.

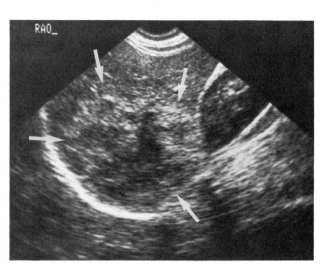

FIG 4-37. Cavernous hemangioma. Large inhomogeneous mass in right lobe of the liver *(arrows)*.

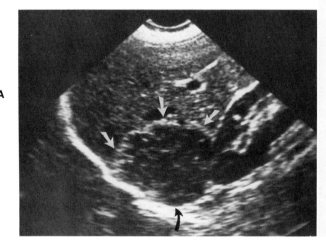

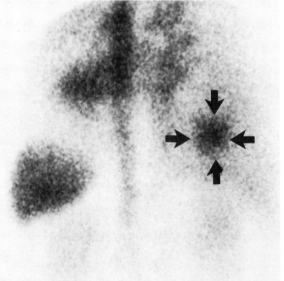

FIG 4-38. Cavernous hemangioma. **A,** Atypical sonographic appearance. Hypoechoic mass in right lobe of liver *(arrows)*. **B,** Delayed RBC scintigraphy (posterior view) confirms diagnosis of hemangioma. Note increased uptake of pharmaceutical within lesion *(arrows)*.

such as MRI and SPECT, and the experience of the imager. In general, the combination of two confirmatory studies is diagnostic of hemangioma.[135] If the lesion is greater than 2.5 cm in diameter, a Tc-99m RBC study with SPECT is recommended. If the lesion is less than 2.5 cm in diameter, MRI with T2-weighting (TE > 120 msec) is recommended.[132,135] Dynamic contrast-enhanced CT scans, although less specific than both Tc-99m RBC scintigraphy and MRI, is useful if these two modalities are unavailable. If the imaging investigation provides indeterminate results, either percutaneous biopsy or follow-up at 6 months is recommended.

Focal Nodular Hyperplasia

Focal nodular hyperplasia (FNH) is a rare hepatic neoplasm that occurs in individuals of all ages, but most frequently in young women. Most patients are asymptomatic and the lesion is discovered incidentally. Whether or not FNH is linked etiologically to oral contraceptives has been debated throughout the years. The current consensus is that it is not. There is, however, evidence to support that FNH may be hormone dependent because several reports describe regression following discontinuation of the birth control pill.[136,137]

Pathologically, the lesion is a nodular mass that frequently contains a central stellate scar and radiating fibrous septa, which divide the lesion into lobules. Histologically, FNH resembles an inactive cirrhosis. Normal appearing hepatocytes, Kupffer cells, bile ducts, and blood vessels are present. However, they lack the normal arrangement.[136]

The **sonographic appearance** of FNH is nonspecific (Fig. 4-39 and 4-40).[138-141] The tumor may be isoechoic, hypoechoic, or hyperechoic. The size ranges from 1 cm to over 20 cm in diameter. Approximately 13% are multiple.[138] A central fibrous scar is infrequently demon-

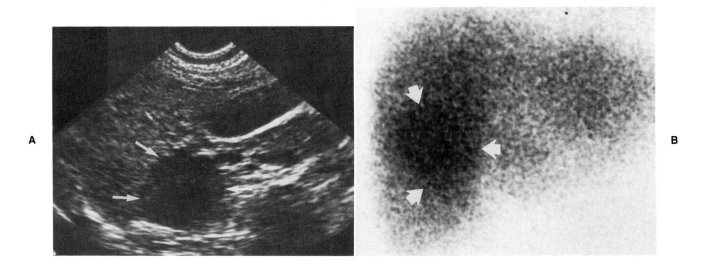

FIG 4-39. Focal nodular hyperplasia—hypoechoic pattern. **A,** Hypoechoic mass present in right lobe of liver *(arrows)*. **B,** ^{99m}Tc-sulfur colloid liver scan shows corresponding region of increased uptake *(arrows),* which is virtually diagnostic of benign focal nodular hyperplasia.

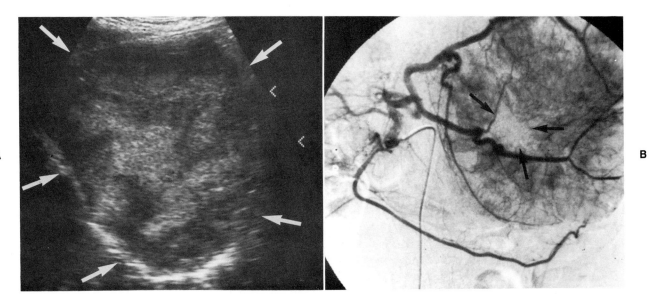

FIG 4-40. Focal nodular hyperplasia—central scar. **A,** Transverse sonogram of left lobe of liver shows large heterogeneous mass *(arrows)* with irregular hyperechoic center. **B,** Angiogram, performed because ^{99m}Tc-sulfur colloid liver scan was indeterminate, shows hypervascular left lobe mass with central nonenhancing scar *(arrows),* which is typical of FNH.

(Courtesy V Ozolins, M.D.; The Mississauga Hospital, Mississauga, Canada.)

strated.[140] Because FNH contains Kupffer cells, **[99m]Tc-sulfur colloid** imaging is most helpful in confirming the diagnosis. In the study by Welch et al.,[140] 70% of their patients had either increased or normal radionuclide uptake compared with the uptake of normal livers. Thirty percent were cold. Angiography or percutaneous biopsy is reserved for the cold lesions. Angiography characteristically shows a hypervascular lesion with a central blood supply and intense capillary staining.[138,141] Because FNH rarely leads to clinical problems and does not undergo malignant transformation, conservative management is recommended.[142]

Hepatic Adenoma

Hepatic adenomas are less common than FNH. Since the 1970s, however, there has been a dramatic rise in their incidence and a link clearly established to the usage of oral contraceptive agents. The tumor may be asymptomatic, but often the patient or the physician feels a mass in the right upper quadrant. Pain may occur as a result of bleeding or infarction within the lesion. The most alarming manifestation is shock caused by tumor rupture and hemoperitoneum. Hepatic adenomas have also been reported in association with glycogen storage disease. In particular, the frequency of adenoma for type 1 GSD (von Gierke's disease) is 40%.[143]

Pathologically, the hepatic adenoma is usually solitary and well encapsulated, and ranges in size from 8 to 15 cm. Microscopically, the tumor consists of normal or slightly atypical hepatocytes. Bile ducts and Kupffer cells are either few in number or absent.[144]

The **sonographic appearance** of hepatic adenoma is nonspecific (Fig. 4-41). The echogenicity may be hyperechoic, hypoechoic, isoechoic, or mixed.[140,141] The majority of adenomas are cold on ^{99m}Tc-sulfur colloid imaging as a result of absent or markedly decreased numbers of Kupffer cells. Isolated cases of radiocolloid uptake by the adenoma have been reported.[145] Hepatic adenomas may undergo malignant transformation to hepatocellular carcinoma.[142] Surgical resection is thus recommended.

Hepatic Lipomas

Hepatic lipomas are extremely rare, and only isolated cases have been reported in the radiologic literature.[146,147] There is an association between hepatic lipomas and renal angiomyolipomas and tuberous sclerosis. The lesions are asymptomatic. Ultrasound demonstrates a well-defined echogenic mass, indistinguishable from a hemangioma, echogenic metastasis, or focal fat. The diagnosis is confirmed using CT scanning, which reveals the fatty nature of the mass by the negative Hounsfield units (< -30 HU).[146]

MALIGNANT HEPATIC NEOPLASMS
Hepatocellular Carcinoma

Hepatocellular carcinoma is one of the most common malignant tumors, particularly in Southeast Asia, sub-Saharan Africa, Japan, Greece, and Italy. It occurs predominantly in men, with a sex ratio of about 5:1.[144] Etiologic factors contributing to the development of hepatocellular carcinoma depend on the geographic distri-

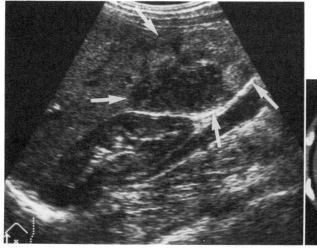
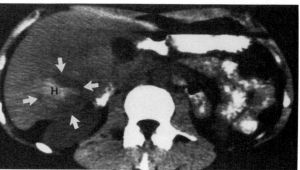

FIG 4-41. Hepatic adenoma. Young female with several years' history of oral contraceptive use, presented with severe right upper quadrant pain and dizziness. **A,** Sagittal sonogram shows inhomogeneous mass (arrows) in right lobe of liver. **B,** CT scan without intravenous contrast. Liver lesion (arrows) has central hyperdense region (H) indicative of recent hemorrhage. Surgery confirmed benign hepatic adenoma.

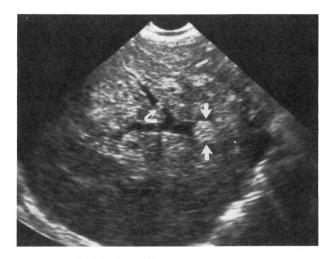

FIG 4-42. Hepatocellular carcinoma–diffuse infiltration. Thrombi are present in main right portal vein *(straight arrows)* and anterior branch of right portal vein *(curved arrow).*

*Alcoholic Cirhosis
Chronic Hbp. B
Alfatoxins*

bution. In the West, **alcoholic cirrhosis** is the most common condition predisposing to hepatoma. Chronic hepatitis B infection accounts for the high incidence of hepatocellular carcinoma in sub-Saharan Africa, Southeast Asia, China, Japan, and the Mediterranean. Aflatoxins, which are toxic metabolites produced by fungi in certain foods, have also been implicated in the pathogenesis of hepatomas in developing countries.[144] The clinical presentation is often delayed until the tumor reaches an advanced stage. Symptoms include right upper quadrant pain, weight loss, and abdominal swelling when ascites is present.

Pathologically, hepatocellular carcinoma occurs in three forms:[74]

- Solitary tumor
- Multiple nodules
- Diffuse infiltration

There is a propensity towards venous invasion. The portal vein is involved more commonly than the hepatic venous system, occurring in 30% to 60% of cases.[148-150]

Ultrasound is the screening method of choice for detection of hepatomas. The **sonographic appearance** is variable (Figs. 4-42 to 4-45). The masses may be hypoechoic, complex, or echogenic. Most small (< 5 cm) hepatocellular carcinomas are hypoechoic, corresponding histologically to a solid tumor without necrosis.[151,152] With time and increasing size, the masses tend to become more complex and inhomogeneous as a result of necrosis and fibrosis. Calcification is uncommon but has been reported.[153] Small tumors may appear diffusely hyperechoic secondary to fatty metamorphosis or sinusoidal dilation, making them indistinguishable from focal fatty infiltration, cavernous hemangiomas, and lipo-

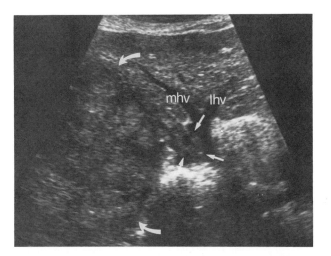

FIG 4-43. Hepatocellular carcinoma—invasion of hepatic venous system. Large minimally hypoechoic mass in right lobe of liver *(curved arrows)* obliterates right hepatic vein and extends into inferior vena cava *(straight arrows). mhv* indicates middle hepatic vein; *lhv,* left hepatic vein.

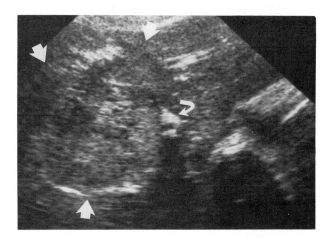

FIG 4-44. Fibrolamellar hepatocellular carcinoma seen as ill-defined echogenic mass *(straight arrows)* with focal calcification *(curved arrow).* Calcification is more common in fibrolamellar subtype of hepatoma.

mas.[151,152,154] Intratumoral fat also occurs in larger masses. However, because it tends to be focal, it is unlikely to cause confusion in diagnosis.

Fibrolamellar carcinoma is a histologic subtype of hepatocellular carcinoma that is found in younger patients (adolescents and young adults) without coexisting liver disease. It is often resectable, resulting in a better prognosis than the more common hepatocellular carcinoma. Fibrolamellar hepatocellular carcinoma tends to be solitary, ranging in size from 6 to 20 cm. The echogenicity is variable and has been described as isoechoic, mixed, and hyperechoic. Punctate calcification

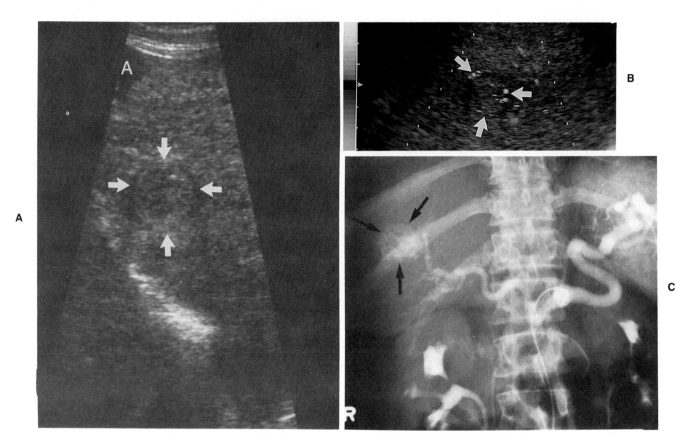

FIG 4-45. Hepatocellular carcinoma—solitary tumor. **A,** Subtle isoechoic mass with hypoechoic rim *(arrows)* is present in dome of liver. *A* indicates ascites. **B,** Color-flow sonography shows increased blood flow at periphery of mass *(arrows)*. **C,** Angiography, performed before surgery, confirmed hypervascularity *(arrows)*.

and a central echogenic scar—features which are distinctly unusual in hepatomas—are more common in the fibrolamellar subtype (Fig. 4-44).[155,156]

Preliminary studies in evaluating focal liver lesions with **duplex** and **color flow Doppler ultrasound** suggests that hepatocellular carcinoma has characteristic high-velocity signals.[157,158] In the study by Taylor et al., which used a frequency of 3 MHz for both imaging and Doppler examinations, 10 to 12 hepatocellular carcinomas (all > 4 cm) exhibited Doppler shifts of 5 KHz or above.[157] The high-velocity Doppler signals were associated with large pressure gradients caused by arteriovenous shunting. None of the other benign and malignant focal hepatic masses had Doppler shifts greater than 4 KHz.[157] Color-flow Doppler imaging has demonstrated increased vascularity surrounding and branching within the hepatoma, which corresponded on angiography to the feeding tumor vessels (see Fig. 4-45).[158]

Hemangiosarcoma (Angiosarcoma)

Hepatic hemangiosarcoma is an extremely rare malignant tumor. It occurs almost exclusively in adults, reaching its peak incidence in the sixth and seventh decades of life. Hemangiosarcoma is of particular interest because of its association with specific carcinogens—thorotrast, arsenic, and polyvinyl chloride.[144] Very few cases of hepatic hemangiosarcoma have been reported in the radiologic literature. The **sonographic appearance** is that of a large mass of mixed echogenicity (Fig. 4-46).[159,160]

Hepatic Epithelioid Hemangioendothelioma

Hepatic epithelioid hemangioendothelioma (EHE) is a rare malignant tumor of vascular origin that occurs in adults. Soft tissues, lung, and liver are affected. The prognosis is variable. Many patients survive longer than 5 years with or without treatment.[161] Hepatic EHE begins as multiple hypoechoic nodules. Over time the

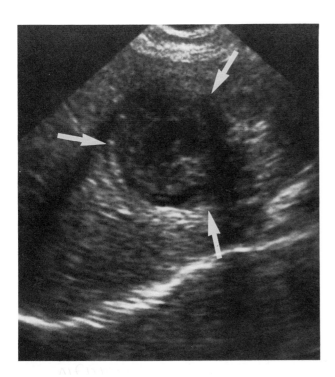

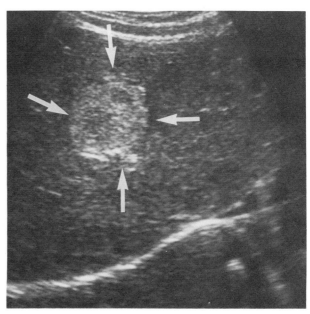

GI
RENAL
CARCINOID
ENDOCRINE
PANCREAS

FIG 4-47. Echogenic metastasis—carcinoid *(arrows)*. Sonographic appearance is identical to that of benign hemangioma.

FIG 4-46. Hemangiosarcoma. Solid hepatic mass of mixed echogenicity *(arrows)* is seen in this patient with history of polyvinyl chloride exposure.

nodules grow and coalesce, forming larger confluent hypoechoic masses, which tend to involve the periphery of the liver. Foci of calcification may be present.[161,162] The diagnosis is made by percutaneous liver biopsy, providing immunohistochemical staining is performed.

Metastatic Disease

In the United States, metastatic disease to the liver is 18 to 20 times more common than hepatocellular carcinoma. Ultrasound is an excellent screening modality because of its relative accuracy (compared with scintigraphy and liver function tests), speed, lack of ionizing radiation, and availability. It is evident that the detection of metastatic liver disease greatly alters the patient's prognosis and very often the management. The incidence of hepatic metastases depends on the type of tumor and its stage at initial detection. Patients with short survival rates (< 1 year) after initial detection of liver metastases are those with hepatocellular carcinoma and carcinomas of the pancreas, stomach, and esophagus. Patients with a more prolonged survival are those with head and neck carcinomas and carcinoma of the colon. Most patients with melanoma have an extremely low incidence of hepatic metastases at diagnosis. Liver involvement at autopsy, however, may be as high as 70%.

The following **sonographic patterns** of metastatic liver disease have been described: echogenic, hypoechoic, target, calcified, cystic, and diffuse. Although the ultrasound appearance is not specific for determining the origin of the metastasis, certain generalities apply.

Echogenic metastases tend to arise from a gastrointestinal origin or from hepatocellular carcinoma. Also the more vascular the tumor, the more likely the lesion is to be echogenic.[152,163] Therefore metastases from renal cell carcinoma, carcinoid, choriocarcinoma and islet cell carcinoma tend to be hyperechoic (Fig. 4-47).

Hypoechoic metastases are generally hypovascular. Lymphomatous involvement of the liver may manifest as hypoechoic masses. Although at autopsy the liver is often a secondary site of involvement by Hodgkin and non-Hodgkin lymphoma, the disease tends to be diffusely infiltrative and undetected by sonographic examination and CT scanning.[164] The pattern of multiple hypoechoic hepatic masses is more typical of primary non-Hodgkin lymphoma of the liver or lymphoma associated with AIDS.[164,165] The lymphomatous masses may appear anechoic and septated, mimicking hepatic abscesses (Fig. 4-48).

The **bull's eye** or **target pattern** is characterized by a peripheral hypoechoic zone (Fig. 4-49). The appearance is nonspecific, although it is frequently identified in metastases from bronchogenic carcinoma.[166] Radiologic–histologic correlation has revealed that, in the majority of cases, the hypoechoic rim corresponds to normal liver parenchyma, which is compressed by the rapidly expanding tumor. Less commonly, the hypoechoic rim represents tumor fibrosis or vascularization.[167]

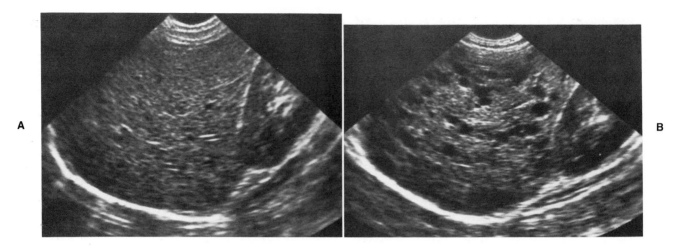

FIG 4-48. Non-Hodgkin lymphoma associated with AIDS. **A,** Liver parenchyma appears normal. **B,** Three weeks later, multiple hypoechoic lesions are present. Differential diagnosis includes hepatic abscesses. Percutaneous biopsy confirmed non-Hodgkin lymphoma.

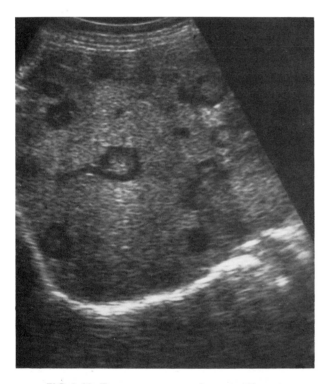

FIG 4-49. Target metastases—breast carcinoma.

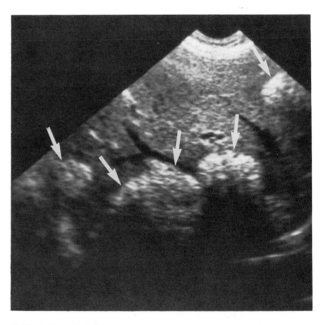

FIG 4-50. Calcified metastases—rectal carcinoma. Echogenic metastases *(arrows)* with posterior acoustic shadowing are present in this patient with primary mucinous adenocarcinoma of rectum.

Calcified metastases are distinctive by virtue of their marked echogenicity and distal acoustic shadowing (Fig. 4-50). Mucinous adenocarcinoma of the colon is most frequently associated with calcified metastases. Other primary malignancies that give rise to calcified metastases are endocrine pancreatic tumors, leiomyosarcoma, adenocarcinoma of the stomach, neuroblastoma, osteogenic sarcoma, chondrosarcoma, and ovarian cystadenocarcinoma and teratocarcinoma.[168]

Cystic metastases are fortunately uncommon and generally exhibit features that enable them to be distinguished from the ubiquitous benign hepatic cyst—for example, mural nodules, thick walls, fluid-fluid levels, and internal septations (Fig. 4-51).[169,170] Primary neoplasms having a cystic component, such as cystadenocarcinoma of the ovary and pancreas and mucinous carcinoma of the colon, may produce cystic lesions. Extensive necrosis, seen most commonly in metastatic sar-

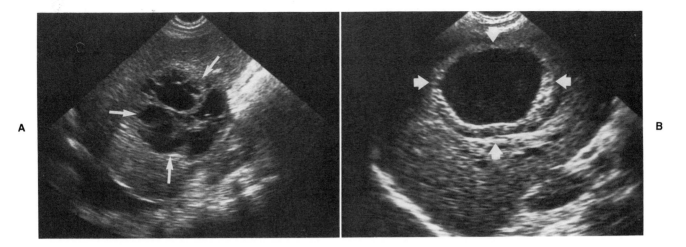

FIG 4-51. Cystic metastases. **A,** Myxomatous liposarcoma. Irregular cystic mass *(arrows)* with thick internal septations is present in right lobe of liver. Differential diagnosis includes infected or hemorrhagic cyst and abscess. **B,** Necrotic metastasis *(arrows)* from gastric leiomyosarcoma.

comas, gives rise to sonolucent metastases, which typically have low-level echoes and a shaggy, thickened wall.

Diffuse disorganization of the hepatic parenchyma reflects an infiltrative form of metastatic disease and is the most difficult to appreciate. In our experience, breast and lung carcinoma and malignant melanoma are the most common primary tumors to give this pattern. The diagnosis can be even more difficult if the patient has a fatty liver from chemotherapy. In these patients, CT scanning may be helpful.

Hepatic involvement by Kaposi sarcoma, although frequent in patients with AIDS at autopsy, is rarely diagnosed by imaging studies.[171] Sonography has demonstrated periportal infiltration and multiple, small, peripheral hyperechoic nodules (Fig. 4-52).[172]

Because of the nonspecific appearance of metastatic liver disease, ultrasound-guided biopsy is widely used to establish a primary tissue diagnosis. In addition, ultrasound is an excellent means to monitor the response to chemotherapy in oncology patients.

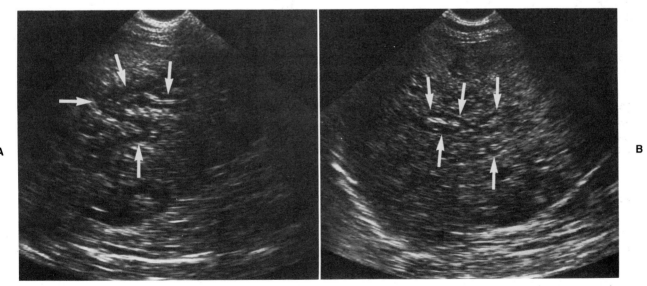

FIG 4-52. Diffuse metastases—Kaposi sarcoma. Sagittal **(A)** and transverse **(B)** sonograms show hypoechoic periportal tumor infiltration *(arrows)*.
(From Towers MJ, Withers CE, Rachlis AR, et al. Ultrasound diagnosis of hepatic kaposi sarcoma. *J Ultrasound Med.* In press.)

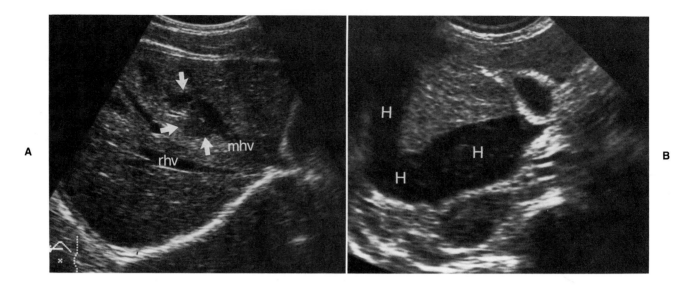

FIG 4-53. Blunt hepatic trauma. **A,** Perivascular laceration. Subcostal oblique sonogram shows hypoechoic hematoma *(arrows)* lateral to middle hepatic vein *(mhv)*. *rhv* indicates right hepatic vein. **B,** Perihepatic hematoma. Hypoechoic blood *(H)* surrounds right lobe of liver.

HEPATIC TRAUMA

The approach to the management of blunt hepatic injury is becoming increasingly more conservative. Operative exploration is indicated for patients in shock or for those who are hemodynamically unstable.[173] In the hemodynamically stable patient, many institutions initially perform abdominal CT scans to assess the extent of liver trauma. Ultrasound may be used to serially monitor the pattern of healing.

The predominant site of hepatic injury in blunt trauma is the right lobe—in particular, the posterior segment.[174] In the study series by Foley et al., the most common type of injury was a perivascular laceration paralleling branches of the right and middle hepatic veins and the anterior and posterior branches of the right portal vein. Other findings were subcapsular, pericapsular, or isolated hematomas, liver fracture (which was defined as a laceration extending between two visceral surfaces), lacerations involving the left lobe, and hemoperitoneum (Fig. 4-53).[175] Hepatic infarcts are rarely identified following blunt abdominal trauma because of the liver's dual blood supply.

vanSonnenberg et al. evaluated the **sonographic findings** of acute trauma to the liver (< 24 hours following injury or transhepatic cholangiogram) and determined that fresh hemorrhage was echogenic.[176] Within the first week, the hepatic laceration becomes more hypoechoic and distinct as a result of resorption of devitalized tissue and ingress of interstitial fluid. At 2 to 3 weeks later, the laceration becomes increasingly indistinct as a result of resorption of the fluid and filling of the spaces with granulation tissue.[175]

HEPATIC SURGERY
Liver Transplantation

Orthotopic liver transplantation is performed to eliminate irreversible disease when more conservative medical and surgical treatments have failed.[177] The procedure has the potential to restore the patient's normal life-style. The common indications for transplantation in adults are cirrhosis, especially secondary to chronic active hepatitis; fulminant acute hepatitis; inborn errors of metabolism; sclerosing cholangitis; Budd-Chiari syndrome; and unresectable but local hepatoma.[177,178] As a treatment for metastatic disease, transplantation is controversial and usually not performed.

The **surgical procedure** in the recipient includes hepatectomy, revascularization of the new liver, hemostasis, and biliary reconstruction.[178] Although details of the surgery are beyond the scope of this textbook, it is relevant to sonography to note that both venous and arterial grafts, harvested from the donor, may be used to obtain vascular anastomoses in complicated situations. Following transplantation, immunosuppression is necessary to prevent rejection of the liver. Optimal immunosuppression minimizes rejection without potentiating infection.

Complications of liver transplantation include rejection, vascular thrombosis or leak, biliary stricture or leak, infection, and neoplasia. The clinical manifestations of each are not always distinct. Biliary stricture and rejection, in particular, may cause similar manifestations including abnormal liver function.

Rejection is the most common cause of hepatic dysfunction following transplantation and affects over one half of transplant recipients. Rejection is a clinical diagnosis confirmed by liver biopsy. Sonographic examinations and Doppler evaluations have not proved to be sensitive or specific in suggesting this diagnosis, and their role in patients with hepatic dysfunction is to eliminate causes other than rejection.[179,180]

Vascular thrombosis may affect the hepatic artery, the portal vein, or less commonly, the inferior vena cava and aorta. **Hepatic arterial thrombosis** affects approximately 3% to 10% of transplant recipients and may cause parenchymal ischemia and infarction or biliary stricture and necrosis.[181] Early occlusion of the hepatic artery before the development of collateral circulation is a life-threatening occurrence with a high mortality, necessitating immediate retransplantation. **Inferior vena caval thrombosis** occurs most commonly in patients with an initial diagnosis of Budd-Chiari syndrome.

Biliary complications, including stricture and leak, affect approximately 15% of transplant recipients.[182] Because the hepatic artery is the sole supply of blood to the bile ducts in transplant patients, identification of a stricture of the bile duct is an indication for assessment of hepatic arterial patency.

Infection is potentiated in liver transplant patients by immunosuppression and a long operative procedure. An altered immune response minimizes the overt clinical manifestations of sepsis. Therefore all sonographically identified fluid collections should be viewed with suspicion and percutaneous aspiration performed as indicated.

Neoplasia may affect liver transplant patients either as a recurrent tumor, especially hepatocellular carcinoma, or a new neoplasia potentiated by immunosuppression (Fig. 4-54).[183] Neoplastic development should be considered in all transplant patients if new masses are identified in the abdomen or in the liver. Frequently, these tumors have a fulminant, rapidly progressive course.

Sonographic examination and **Doppler evaluation** are critical to both preoperative and postoperative noninvasive evaluation of liver transplant recipients. The **preoperative sonographic** assessment is aimed at appropriate patient selection and transplant timing and includes a general assessment of the abdomen to detect any findings that might alter patient selection, such as a large abdominal aortic aneurysm or extrahepatic malignant disease. Liver size and morphologic features are evaluated to determine the nature and extent of the liver disease. Vascular evaluation is critical, including assessment of portal vein patency; portal vein caliber; the direction of portal vein flow; the presence of venous collaterals, cavernous transformation of the portal vein, or both; hepatic arterial anatomy; and inferior vena caval size and patency. Of the preceding, identification

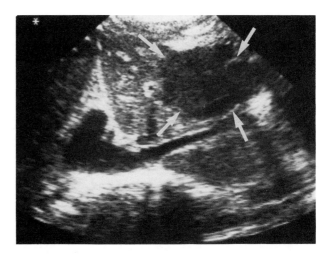

FIG 4-54. Cyclosporine-induced lymphoma, 5 months after liver transplantation. Sagittal sonogram shows large hypoechoic mass *(arrows)* in porta hepatis region.

of portal vein thrombosis or a very tiny portal vein calibre, for example, would not prevent transplantation. However, the surgeon would harvest donor veins to allow for adequate anastomosis. If the portal vein is not assessed adequately by sonography, an arteriographic examination is recommended.

Postoperative assessment includes a baseline sonogram, which is usually performed shortly after surgery. Further sonograms are performed for specific indications—most commonly, abdominal pain, fever, and abnormal liver function test results. Knowledge of the surgical procedure is essential, including the specifics of vascular anastomoses and the use of grafts, any reduction of donor liver caused by size incompatibility, details of the biliary-enteric anastomosis, and intraoperative complications such as bleeding.

Sonography should include[184]:

■ **Evaluation of the liver parenchyma** with assessment of any diffuse or focal abnormalities, the appearance of the periportal areas, and liver volume. Vascular occlusion, complicated by liver ischemia or gangrene, may produce a variable picture, although typically hypoechoic regions, which progress to large areas of liquefactive necrosis, are seen (Fig. 4-55). Liver infection, abscesses, and tumors have an identical appearance in the transplanted and normal liver. Liver shrinkage may occur with chronic rejection, vascular occlusion, or chronic inflammation.

■ **Evaluation of vascular patency** with both direct inspection of the vessels (portal vein, hepatic artery, and inferior vena cava) for thrombus and Doppler interrogation (Fig. 4-56). The hepatic artery and main portal vein, as well as their major

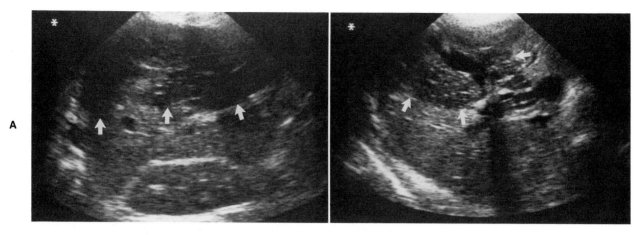

FIG 4-55. Massive liver necrosis from hepatic arterial occlusion 4 weeks after transplantation. Sagittal **(A)** and transverse **(B)** sonograms show fairly well-demarcated zone of inhomogeneous hypoechogenicity *(arrows),* which corresponded at pathologic examination to a large zone of liver necrosis. No hepatic arterial Doppler signal could be obtained in porta hepatis or liver parenchyma.

right and left branches, should be studied to avoid missing segmental occlusions.

- **Bile duct evaluation,** evaluating for the presence of dilated intrahepatic or extrahepatic bile ducts, evidence of a bile duct stricture, or both (Fig. 4-57).

- **Assessment of intraabdominal fluid collections** for size, morphologic features, and location. These may be hematomas, abscesses, bilomas, or seromas. In questionable cases, ultrasound-guided aspiration is most helpful to determine the nature of an identified fluid collection.

Portosystemic Shunts

Surgical portosystemic shunts are performed to decompress the portal system in patients with portal hypertension. The most commonly created surgical shunts

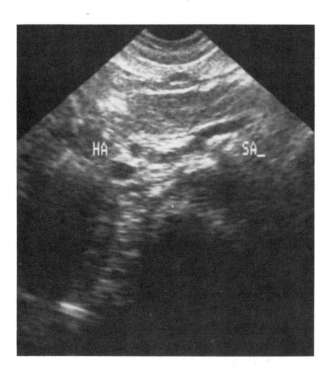

FIG 4-56. Hepatic artery occlusion. Transverse sonogram of celiac axis shows unremarkable celiac trunk and splenic arterial branch *(SA).* Hepatic artery *(HA)* is filled with echogenic thrombus. No Doppler arterial signal could be obtained.

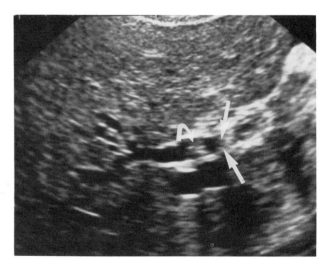

FIG 4-57. Bile duct stricture. Right anterior oblique sonogram shows dilated bile ducts with abrupt narrowing *(straight arrows)* in region of biliary anastomosis. Small nonshadowing echogenic mass *(curved arrow)* is seen within duct, presumably representing debris.

include mesocaval, distal splenorenal (Warren), mesoatrial, and portacaval. **Duplex Doppler sonography** and, more recently, **color Doppler imaging** appear to be reliable noninvasive methods of assessing shunt patency or thrombosis.[185-188] Both modalities are effective in assessing portacaval, mesoatrial, and mesocaval shunts.[187] Shunt patency is confirmed by demonstrating flow at the anastomotic site. If the anastomosis cannot be visualized, hepatofugal portal flow is an indirect sign of patency (Fig. 4-58).[185,186]

Distal splenorenal communications are particularly difficult to examine with duplex Doppler sonography because overlying bowel gas and fat hinder adequate placement of the Doppler cursor.[187,189] Color Doppler imaging more readily locates the splenic and renal limbs of Warren shunts. The splenic limb is best imaged from a left subcostal approach, whereas the left renal vein is optimally scanned through the left flank. In the study by Grant et al., color Doppler sonography correctly inferred patency or thrombosis in all 14 splenorenal communications by evaluating the flow in both limbs of the shunt.[187]

PERCUTANEOUS LIVER BIOPSY

Percutaneous biopsy of malignant disease involving the liver has a sensitivity greater than 90% in most study series.[190,191] Relative contraindications to percu-

taneous biopsy are an uncorrectable bleeding diathesis, an unsafe access route, and a patient who cannot adequately cooperate.[191] Ultrasound guidance allows real-time observation of the needle tip as it is advanced into the lesion. Several biopsy attachments have been developed that allow continuous observation of the needle as it follows a predetermined path. Alternatively, many experienced radiologists prefer a "free-hand" technique. Even small masses ($\leq$ 3 cm) can undergo successful biopsy using sonographic guidance.[191] CT guidance is superior for lesions located deep to the bowel or bone or for masses in obese patients in whom ultrasound visualization is limited by sound attenuation. Ultrasound guidance may also be used in percutaneous aspiration and drainage of complicated fluid collections in the liver. Recent studies have proposed ultrasound-guided percutaneous ethanol injection for the treatment of hepatocellular carcinoma and hepatic metastases.[192,193]

INTRAOPERATIVE ULTRASOUND

Intraoperative ultrasound is a relatively new application of ultrasound technology. The exposed liver is scanned with a 7.5 MHz transducer, covered by a sterile sheath. Intraoperative ultrasound has been found to change the operative strategy in 31% to 49% of patients undergoing hepatic resection, either by allowing more precise resection or by indicating inoperability because of unsuspected masses or venous invasion.[194,195]

REFERENCES

1. Jones AL. Anatomy of the normal liver. In: Zakim D, Boyer TD eds. *Hepatology: A Textbook of Liver Disease*. Philadelphia: W.B. Saunders Co; 1982:3-31.

Normal anatomy

2. Donoso L, Martinez-Noguera A, Zidan A, Lora F. Papillary process of the caudate lobe of the liver: sonographic appearance. *Radiology* 1989;173:631-633.
3. Sexton CC, Zeman RK. Correlation of computed tomography, sonography, and gross anatomy of the liver. *AJR* 1983;141:711-718.
4. Marks WM, Filly RA, Callen PW. Ultrasonic anatomy of the liver: a review with new applications. *J Clin Ultrasound* 1979;7:137-146.
5. Couinaud C. Le foie. In: *Etudes anatomiques et chirugicales*. Paris: Masson et Cie; 1957.
6. Sugarbaker PH. Toward a standard nomenclature for the surgical anatomy of the liver. *Neth J Surg* 1988;PO:100.

The hepatic circulation

7. Nakamura S, Tsuzuki T. Surgical anatomy of the hepatic veins and the inferior vena cava. *Surg Gynecol Obstet* 1981;152:43-50.

Normal liver size and echogenicity

8. Gosink BB, Leymaster CE: Ultrasonic determination of hepatomegaly. *J Clin Ultrasound* 1981;9:37-41.
9. Niederau C, Sonnenberg A, Muller JE, et al. Sonographic measurements of the normal liver, spleen, pancreas, and portal vein. *Radiology* 1983;149:537-540.

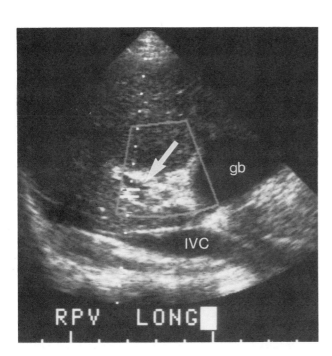

FIG 4-58. Surgical mesocaval shunt. Sagittal duplex Doppler sonogram shows hepatofugal flow in portal vein *(arrow)*, which is indirect sign of shunt patency. Note phasic Doppler waveform, which reflects transmitted right atrial pressure. *IVC* indicates inferior vena cava; *gb*, gall bladder. (Courtesy of J. William Charboneau, MD, Mayo Clinic, Rochester, Minn.)

Developmental anomalies

10. Belton R, Van Zandt TF. Congenital absence of the left lobe of the liver: a radiologic diagnosis. *Radiology* 1983;147:184.
11. Radin DR, Colletti PM, Ralls PW, et al. Agenesis of the right lobe of the liver. *Radiology* 1987;164:639-642.
12. Yamamoto S, Kojoh K, Saito I, et al. Computer tomography of congenital absence of the left lobe of the liver. *J Comput Assist Tomogr* 1988;12:206-208.
13. Auh YH, Rubenstein WA, Zirinsky K, et al. Accessory fissures of the liver: CT and sonographic appearance. *AJR* 1984; 143:565-572.
14. Lim JH, Ko YT, Han MC, et al. The inferior accessory hepatic fissure: sonographic appearance. *AJR* 1987;149:495-497.
15. Michels NA. Newer anatomy of the liver: variant blood supply and collateral circulation. *JAMA* 1960;172:125-132.
16. Fraser-Hill MA, Atri M, Bret PM, et al. Intrahepatic portal venous system: variations demonstrated with duplex and color Doppler US. *Radiology* 1990;177:523-526.
17. Cosgrove DO, Arger PH, Coleman BG. Ultrasonic anatomy of hepatic veins. *J Clin Ultrasound* 1987;15:231-235.
18. Makuuchi M, Hasegawa H, Yamazaki S, et al. The inferior right hepatic vein: ultrasonic demonstration. *Radiology* 1983;148:213-217.

Congenital abnormalities

19. Witzleben CL. Cystic diseases of the liver. In: Zakim D, Boyer TD, eds. *Hepatology: A Textbook of Liver Disease.* Philadelphia: WB Saunders Co; 1982:1193-1212.
20. Gaines PA, Sampson MA. The prevalence and characterization of simple hepatic cysts by ultrasound examination. *Br J Radiol* 1989;62:335-337.
21. Bean WJ, Rodan BA. Hepatic cysts: treatment with alcohol. *AJR* 1985;144:237-241.
22. Levine E, Cook LT, Granthem JJ. Liver cysts in autosomal-dominant polycystic kidney disease: clinical and computed tomographic study. *AJR* 1985;145:229-233.
23. Segal AJ, Spataro RF. Computed tomography of adult polycystic disease. *J Comput Assist Tomogr* 1982;6:777-780.

Infectious diseases

24. Kurz AB, Rubin CS, Cooper HS, et al. Ultrasound findings in hepatitis. *Radiology* 1980;136:717-723.
25. Juttner H-U, Ralls PW, Quinn MF, Jenney JM. Thickening of the gallbladder wall in acute hepatitis: ultrasound demonstration. *Radiology* 1982;142:465.
26. Lee JF, Block GE. The changing clinical pattern of hepatic abscesses. *Arch Surg* 1972;104:465-470.
27. Altemeier WA III, Schowengerdt CG, Whitely DH. Abscesses of the liver: surgical considerations. *Arch Surg* 1970;101:258-265.
28. Wilson SR, Arenson AM. Sonographic evaluation of hepatic abscesses. *J Can Assoc Radiol* 1984;35:174-177.
29. Kressel HY, Filly RA. Ultrasonographic appearance of gas-containing abscesses in the abdomen. *AJR* 1978;130:71-73.
30. Kuligowska E, Connors SK, Shapiro JH. Liver abscess: sonography in diagnosis and treatment. *AJR* 1982;138:253-257.
31. Sabbaj J, Sutter VL, Finegold SM. Anaerobic pyogenic liver abscess. *Ann Intern Med* 1972;77:629-638.
32. Simson IW, Gear JHS. Other viral and infectious diseases. In: MacSween RNM, Anthony PP, Scheuer PJ, eds. *Pathology of the Liver.* 2nd ed. New York: Churchill Livingstone; 1987:224-264.
33. Pastakia B, Shawker TH, Thaler M, et al. Hepatosplenic candidiasis: wheels within wheels. *Radiology* 1988;166:417-421.
34. Ralls PW, Colletti PM, Quinn MF, et al. Sonographic findings in hepatic amebic abscess. *Radiology* 1982;145:123-126.

35. Berry M, Bazaz R, Bhargava S. Amebic liver abscess: sonographic diagnosis and management. *J Clin Ultrasound* 1986;14:239-242.
36. Ralls PW, Barnes PF, Radin DR. Sonographic features of amebic and pyogenic liver abscesses: a blinded comparison. *AJR* 1987;149:499-501.
37. Patterson M, Healy GR, Shabot JM. Serologic testing for amebiasis. *Gastroenterology* 1980;78:136-141.
38. vanSonnenberg E, Mueller PR, Schiffman HR, et al. Intrahepatic amebic abscesses: indications for and results of percutaneous catheter drainage. *Radiology* 1985;156:631-635.
39. Ralls PW, Barnes PF, Johnson MB, et al. Medical treatment of hepatic amebic abscess: rare need for percutaneous drainage. *Radiology* 1987;165:805-807.
40. Ralls PW, Quinn MF, Boswell WD, et al. Patterns of resolution in successfully treated hepatic amebic abscess: sonographic evaluation. *Radiology* 1983;149:541-543.
41. Gharbi HA, Hassine W, Brauner MW, et al. Ultrasound examination of the hydatic liver. *Radiology* 1981;139:459-463.
42. Lewall DB, McCorkell SJ. Hepatic echinococcal cysts: sonographic appearance and classification. *Radiology* 1985;155:773-775.
43. Beggs I. Radiology of hydatid disease. *AJR* 1985;145:639-648.
44. Mueller PR, Dawson SL, Ferrucci JT Jr, et al. Hepatic echinococcal cyst: successful percutaneous drainage. *Radiology* 1985;155:627-628.
45. Bret PM, Fond A, Bretagnolle M, et al. Percutaneous aspiration and drainage of hydatid disease of the liver. *Radiology* 1988;168:617-620.
46. Bezzi M, Teggi A, De Rosa F, et al. Abdominal hydatid disease: ultrasound findings during medical treatment. *Radiology* 1987;162:91-95.
47. Didier D, Weiler S, Rohmer P, et al. Hepatic alveolar echinococcus: correlative ultrasound and computed tomography study. *Radiology* 1985;154:179-186.
48. McCully RM, Barron CM, Cheever AW. Schistosomiasis, in Binford CH, Connor DH, eds. *Pathology of Tropical and Extraordinary Disease.* Washington, DC: Armed Forces Institute of Pathology; 1976:482-508.
49. Symmers W St C. Note on a new form of liver cirrhosis due to the presence of the ova of *Bilharzia hematobilia. J Pathol* 1904;9:237-239.
50. Cerri GG, Alves VAF, Magalhaes A. Hepatosplenic schistosomiasis mansoni: ultrasound manifestations. *Radiology* 1984;153:777-780.
51. Fataar S, Bassiony H, Satyanath S, et al. Characteristic sonographic features of schistosomal periportal fibrosis. *AJR* 1984;143:69-71.
52. Pentamidine aerosol to prevent *Pneumocystis carinii* pneumonia. *Med Lett Drugs Ther* 1989;31:91-92.
53. Radin DR, Baker EL, Klatt EC, et al. Visceral and nodal calcification in patients with AIDS-related *Pneumocystis carinii* infection. *AJR* 1990;154:27-31.
54. Spouge AR, Wilson SR, Gopinath N, et al. Extrapulmonary *Pneumocystis carinii* in a patient with AIDS: sonographic findings. *AJR* 1990;155:76-78.
55. Telzak EE, Cote RJ, Gold JWM, et al. Extrapulmonary *Pneumocystis carinii* infections. *Rev Infect Dis* 1990;12:380-386.
56. Lubat E, Megibow AJ, Balthazar EJ, et al. Extrapulmonary *Pneumocystis carinii* infection in AIDS: computed tomography findings. *Radiology* 1990;174:157-160.
57. Towers MJ, Withers CE, Hamilton PA, et al. Visceral calcification in AIDS may not be always due to *Pneumocystis carinii. AJR.* 1991; 156:745-747.

Disorders of metabolism

58. Zakim D. Metabolism of glucose and fatty acids by the liver. In: Zakim D, Boyer TD, eds: *Hepatology: A Textbook of Liver Disease*. Philadelphia: WB Saunders Co; 1982:76-109.

59. Scatarige JC, Scott WE, Donovan PJ, et al. Fatty infiltration of the liver: ultrasonographic and computed tomographic correlation. *J Ultrasound Med* 1984;3:9-14.

60. Gosink BB, Lemon SK, Scheible W, Leopold GR. Accuracy of ultrasonography in diagnosis of hepatocellular disease. *AJR* 1979;133:19-23.

61. Garra BS, Insana MF, Shawker TH, et al. Quantitative estimation of liver attenuation and echogenicity: normal state versus diffuse liver disease. *Radiology* 1987;162:61-67.

62. Wilson SR, Rosen IE, Chin-Sang HB, et al. Fatty infiltration of the liver: an imaging challenge. *J Can Assoc Radiol* 1982;227-232.

63. Scott WW, Sanders RC, Siegelman SS. Irregular fatty infiltration of the liver, diagnostic dilemmas. *AJR* 1980;135:67-71.

64. Quinn SF, Gosink BB. Characteristic sonographic signs of hepatic fatty infiltration. *AJR* 1985;145:753-755.

65. Yates CK, Streight RA. Focal fatty infiltration of the liver simulating metastatic disease. *Radiology* 1986;159:83-84.

66. Yoshikawa J, Matsui O, Takashima T, et al. Focal fatty change of the liver adjacent to the falciform ligament: computed tomography and sonographic findings in five surgically confirmed cases. *AJR* 1987;149:491-494.

67. Arai K, Matsui O, Takashima T, et al. Focal spared areas in fatty liver caused by regional decreased blood flow. *AJR* 1988;151:300-302.

68. Sauerbrei EE, Lopez M. Pseudotumor of the quadrate lobe in hepatic sonography: a sign of generalized fatty infiltration. *AJR* 1986;147:923-927.

69. White EM, Simeone JF, Mueller PR, et al. Focal periportal sparing in hepatic fatty infiltration: a cause of hepatic pseudomass on ultrasound. *Radiology* 1987;162:57-59.

70. Ishak KG, Sharp HL. Metabolic errors and liver disease. In: MacSween RNM, Anthony PP, Scheuer PJ, eds. *Pathology of the Liver*. 2nd ed. New York: Churchill Livingstone; 1987:99-180.

71. Grossman H, Ram PC, Coleman RA, et al. Hepatic ultrasonography in type 1 glycogen storage disease (von Gierke disease). *Radiology* 1981;141:753-756.

72. Anthony PP: The morphology of cirrhosis: definition, nomenclature, and classification. *Bull WHO* 1977;55:521.

73. Millward-Sadler GH: Cirrhosis. In: MacSween RNM, Anthony PP, Scheuer PJ, eds. *Pathology of the Liver*. 2nd ed. New York: Churchill Livingstone; 1987:342-363.

74. Cotran RS, Kumar V, Robbins SL. The liver and biliary tract. In: Cotran RS, Kumar V, Robbins SL, eds. *Robbins' Pathologic Basis of Disease*. 4th ed. Philadelphia: WB Saunders Co; 1989:911-980.

75. Harbin WP, Robert NJ, Ferrucci JT. Diagnosis of cirrhosis based on regional changes in hepatic morphology. *Radiology* 1980;135:273-283.

76. Giorgio A, Amoroso P, Lettiri G, et al. Cirrhosis: value of caudate to right lobe ratio in diagnosis with ultrasound. *Radiology* 1986;161:443-445.

77. Hess CF, Schmiedl U, Koelbel G, et al. Diagnosis of liver cirrhosis with ultrasound: receiver-operating characteristic analysis of multidimensional caudate lobe indexes. *Radiology* 1989;171:349-351.

78. Taylor KJW, Riely CA, Hammers L, et al. Quantitative ultrasound attenuation in normal liver and in patients with diffuse liver disease: importance of fat. *Radiology* 1986;160:65-71.

79. Ralls PW, Johnson MB, Kanel G. FM sonography in diffuse liver disease: prospective assessment and blinded analysis. *Radiology* 1986;161:451-454.

80. Sandford N, Walsh P, Matis C, et al. Is ultrasonography useful in the assessment of diffuse parenchymal liver disease? *Gastroenterology* 1985;89:186-191.

81. Kuc R, Taylor KJW. Variation of acoustic attenuation coefficient slope estimates for in vivo liver. *Ultrasound Med Biol* 1982;8:403-412.

82. Wilson LS, Robinson DE, Doust BD. Frequency domain processing for ultrasonic measurement in liver. *Ultrason Imaging* 1984;6:117-125.

83. Freeman MP, Vick CW, Taylor KJW, et al. Regenerating nodules in cirrhosis: sonographic appearance with anatomic correlation. *AJR* 1986;146:533-536.

84. Di Lelio A, Cestari C, Lomazzi A, et al. Cirrhosis: diagnosis with sonographic study of the liver surface. *Radiology* 1989;172:389-392.

Vascular abnormalities

85. Boyer TD. Portal hypertension and its complications. In: Zakim D, Boyer TD, eds. *Hepatology: A Textbook of Liver Disease*. Philadelphia: WB Saunders Co; 1982:464-499.

86. Bolondi L, Gandolfi L, Arienti V, et al. Ultrasonography in the diagnosis of portal hypertension: diminished response of portal vessels to respiration. *Radiology* 1982;142:167-172.

87. Lafortune M, Marleau D, Breton G, et al. Portal venous system measurements in portal hypertension. *Radiology* 1984; 151:27-30.

88. Juttner H-U, Jenney JM, Ralls PW, et al. Ultrasound demonstration of portosystemic collaterals in cirrhosis and portal hypertension. *Radiology* 1982;142:459-463.

89. Subramanyam BR, Balthazar EJ, Madamba MR, et al. Sonography of portosystemic venous collaterals in portal hypertension, *Radiology* 1983;146:161-166.

90. Patriquin H, Lafortune M, Burns PN, et al. Duplex Doppler examination in portal hypertension. *AJR* 1987;149:71-76.

91. Lafortune M, Constantin A, Breton G, et al. The recanalized umbilical vein in portal hypertension: a myth. *AJR* 1985;144:549-553.

92. DiCandio G, Campatelli A, Mosca F, et al. Ultrasound detection of unusual spontaneous portosystemic shunts associated with uncomplicated portal hypertension. *J Ultrasound Med* 1985;4:297-305.

93. Mostbeck GH, Wittich GR, Herold C, et al. Hemodynamic significance of the paraumbilical vein in portal hypertension: assessment with duplex ultrasound. *Radiology* 1989;170:339-342.

94. Nelson RC, Lovett KE, Chezmar JL, et al. Comparison of pulsed Doppler sonography and angiography in patients with portal hypertension. *AJR* 1987;149:77-81.

95. Bellamy EA, Bossi MC, Cosgrove DO. Ultrasound demonstration of changes in the normal portal venous system following a meal. *Br J Radiol* 1984;57:147-149.

96. Ohnishi K, Saito M, Nakayama T, et al. Portal venous hemodynamics in chronic liver disease: effects of posture change and exercise. *Radiology* 1985;155:757-761.

97. Van Gansbeke D, Avni EF, Delcour C, et al. Sonographic features of portal vein thrombosis. *AJR* 1985;144:749-752.

98. Wilson SR, Hine AL. Leiomyosarcoma of the portal vein. *AJR* 1987;149:183-184.

99. Kauzlaric D, Petrovic M, Barmeir E. Sonography of cavernous transformation of the portal vein. *AJR* 1984;142:383-384.

100. Aldrete JS, Slaughter RL, Han SY. Portal vein thrombosis resulting in portal hypertension in adults. *Am J Gastroenterol* 1976;65:3-11.

101. Vine HS, Sequira JC, Widrich WC, Sacks BA. Portal vein aneurysm. *AJR* 1979;132:557-560.

102. Chagnon SF, Vallee CA, Barge J, et al. Aneurysmal portahepatic venous fistula: report of two cases. *Radiology* 1986; 159:693-695.

103. Mori H, Hayashi K, Fukuda T, et al. Intrahepatic portosystemic venous shunt: occurrence in patients with and without liver cirrhosis. *AJR* 1987;149:711-714.

104. Park JH, Cha SH, Han JK, Han MC. Intrahepatic portosystemic venous shunt. *AJR* 1990;155:527-528.

105. Falkoff GE, Taylor KJW, Morse S. Hepatic artery pseudoaneurysm: diagnosis with real-time and pulsed Doppler ultrasound. *Radiology* 1986;158:55-56.

106. Cloogman HM, DiCapo RD. Hereditary hemorrhagic telangiectasia: sonographic findings in the liver. *Radiology* 1984;150:521-522.

107. Stanley P. Budd-Chiari syndrome. *Radiology* 1989;170:625-627.

108. Makuuchi M, Hasegawa H, Yamazaki S, et al. Primary Budd-Chiari syndrome: ultrasonic demonstration. *Radiology* 1984;152:775-779.

109. Menu Y, Alison D, Lorphelin J-M, et al. Budd-Chiari syndrome: ultrasound evaluation. *Radiology* 1985;157:761-764.

110. Park JH, Lee JB, Han MC, et al. Sonographic evaluation of inferior vena caval obstruction: correlative study with vena cavography. *AJR* 1985;145:757-762.

111. Murphy FB, Steinberg HV, Shires GT, et al. The Budd-Chiari syndrome: a review. *AJR* 1986;147:9-15.

112. Grant EG, Perrella R, Tessler FN, et al. Budd-Chiari syndrome: the results of duplex and color Doppler imaging. *AJR* 1989;152:377-381.

113. Keller MS, Taylor KJW, Riely CA. Pseudoportal Doppler signal in the partially obstructed inferior vena cava. *Radiology* 1989;170:475-477.

114. Hosoki T, Kuroda C, Tokunaga K, et al. Hepatic venous outflow obstruction: evaluation with pulsed Duplex sonography. *Radiology* 1989;170:733-737.

115. Brown BP, Abu-Youssef M, Farner R, et al. Doppler sonography: a non-invasive method for evaluation of hepatic venocclusive disease. *AJR* 1990;154:721-724.

116. Becker CD, Scheidegger J, Marincek B. Hepatic vein occlusion: morphologic features on computed tomography and ultrasonography. *Gastrointest Radiol* 1986;11:305-311.

117. Taylor KJW, Burns PN, Woodcock JP, et al. Blood flow in deep abdominal and pelvic vessels: ultrasonic pulsed Doppler analysis. *Radiology* 1985;154:487-493.

118. Kriegshauser SJ, Charboneau JW, Letendre L. Hepatic venocclusive disease after bone marrow transplantation: diagnosis with duplex sonography. *AJR* 1988;150:289-290.

Benign hepatic neoplasms

119. Edmondson HA: Tumors of the liver and intrahepatic bile ducts. In: *Atlas of Tumor Pathology.* Washington, DC: Armed Forces Institute of Pathology; 1958; sect VII (Fasc 25): 113.

120. Gibney RG, Hendin AP, Cooperberg PL. Sonographically detected hemangiomas: absence of change over time. *AJR* 1987;149:953-957.

121. Bree RL, Schwab RE, Neiman HL. Solitary echogenic spot in the liver: is it diagnostic of a hemangioma? *AJR* 1983;140:41-45.

122. McCardle CR. Ultrasonic appearances of a hepatic hemangioma. *J Clin Ultrasound* 1978;6:122-123.

123. Taboury J, Porcel A, Tubiana J-M, Monnier J-P. Cavernous hemangiomas of the liver studied by ultrasound. *Radiology* 1983;149:781-785.

124. Itai Y, Ohnishi S, Ohtomo K, et al. Hepatic cavernous hemangioma in patients at high risk for liver cancer. *Acta Radiol* 1987;28:697-701.

125. Itai Y, Ohtomo K, Araki T, et al. Computed tomography and sonography of cavernous hemangioma of the liver. *AJR* 1983;141:315-320.

126. Marsh JI, Gibney RG, Li DKB. Hepatic hemangioma in the presence of fatty infiltration: an atypical sonographic appearance. *Gastrointest Radiol* 1989;14:262-264.

127. Freeny PC, Marks WM. Hepatic hemangioma: dynamic bolus computed tomography. *AJR* 1986;147:711-719.

128. Scatarige JC, Kenny JM, Fishman EK, et al. Computed tomography of hepatic cavernous hemangioma. *J Comput Assist Tomogr* 1987;11:455-460.

129. Brunetti JC, Van Heertum RL, Yudd AP. SPECT in the diagnosis of hepatic hemangioma. *J Nucl Med* 1985;26:8. Abstract.

130. Birnbaum BA, Weinreb JC, Megibow AJ, et al. Blinded retrospective comparison of MR imaging and Tc-99m-labeled red blood cell SPECT for definitive diagnosis of hepatic hemangiomas. *Radiology* 1989;173:270. Abstract.

131. Ohmoto K, Itai Y, Yoshikawa K, et al. Hepatocellular carcinoma and cavernous hemangioma: differentiation with MR imaging— efficacy of T2 values at 0.35 and 1.5 T. *Radiology* 1988;168:621-623.

132. Birnbaum BA, Weinreb JC, Megibow AJ, et al. Definitive diagnosis of hepatic hemangiomas: magnetic resonance imaging versus Tc-99m-labeled red blood cell SPECT. *Radiology* 1990;176:95-101.

133. Solbiati L, Livraghi T, DePra L, et al. Fine-needle biopsy of hepatic hemangioma with sonographic guidance. *AJR* 1985;144:471-474.

134. Cronan JJ, Esparza AR, Dorfman GS, et al: Cavernous hemangioma of the liver: role of percutaneous biopsy. *Radiology* 1988;166:135-138.

135. Nelson RC, Chezmar JL. Diagnostic approach to hepatic hemangiomas. *Radiology* 1990;176:11-13.

136. Knowles DM, Casarella WJ, Johnson PM, et al. The clinical, radiologic and pathologic characterization of benign hepatic neoplasms: alleged association with oral contraceptives. *Medicine* 1978;57:223-237.

137. Ross D, Pina J, Mirza M, et al. Regression of focal nodular hyperplasia after discontinuation of oral contraceptives. *Ann Intern Med* 1976;85:203-204.

138. Rogers JY, Mack LA, Freenyu PC, et al. Hepatic focal nodular hyperplasia: angiography, computed tomography, sonography, and scintigraphy. *AJR* 1981;137:983-990.

139. Scatarige JC, Fishman EK, Sanders RC. The sonographic "scar sign" in focal nodular hyperplasia of the liver. *J Ultrasound Med* 1982;1:275-278.

140. Welch TJ, Sheedy PF, Johnson CM, et al. Focal nodular hyperplasia and hepatic adenoma: comparison of angiography, computed tomography, ultrasound and scintigraphy. *Radiology* 1985;156:593-595.

141. Mathieu D, Bruneton JN, Drouillard J, et al. Hepatic adenomas and focal nodular hyperplasia: dynamic computed tomography study. *Radiology* 1986;160:53-58.

142. Kerlin P, Davis GL, McGill DB, et al. Hepatic adenoma and focal nodular hyperplasia: clinical, pathologic and radiologic features. *Gastroenterology* 1983;84:994-1002.

143. Brunelle R, Tammam S, Odievre M, Chaumont P. Liver adenomas in glycogen storage disease in children: ultrasound and angiographic study. *Pediatr Radiol* 1984;14:94-101.

144. Kew MC: Tumors of the liver. In: Zakim D, Boyer TD, eds. *Hepatology: A Textbook of Liver Disease.* Philadelphia: WB Saunders Co; 1982:1048-1084.

145. Lubbers PR, Ros PR, Goodman ZD, et al. Accumulation of Technetium-99m sulfur colloid by hepatocellular adenoma: scintigraphic-pathologic correlation. *AJR* 1987;148:1105-1108.

146. Roberts JL, Fishman E, Hartman DS, et al. Lipomatous tumors of the liver: evaluation with computed tomography and ultrasound. *Radiology* 1986;158:613-617.

147. Marti-Bonmati L, Menor F, Vizcaino I, et al. Lipoma of the liver: ultrasound, computed tomography and magnetic resonance imaging appearance. *Gastrointest Radiol* 1989;14:155-157.

Malignant hepatic neoplasms

148. Jackson VP, Martin-Simmerman P, Becker GJ, et al. Real-time ultrasonographic demonstration of vascular invasion by hepatocellular carcinoma. *J Ultrasound Med* 1983;2:277-280.
149. Subramanyam BR, Balthazar EJ, Hilton S, et al. Hepatocellular carcinoma with venous invasion: sonographic-angiographic correlation. *Radiology* 1984;150:793-796.
150. LaBerge JM, Laing FC, Federle MP, et al. Hepatocellular carcinoma: assessment of resectability by computed tomography and ultrasound. *Radiology* 1984;152:485-490.
151. Sheu J-C, Chen D-S, Sung J-L, et al. Hepatocellular carcinoma: ultrasound evaluation in the early stage. *Radiology* 1985;155:463-467.
152. Tanaka S, Kitamura T, Imaoka S, et al. Hepatocellular carcinoma: sonographic and histologic correlation. *AJR* 1983;140:701-707.
153. Teefey SA, Stephens DH, Weiland LH. Calcification in hepatocellular carcinoma: not always an indicator of fibrolamellar histology. *AJR* 1987;149:1173-1174.
154. Yoshikawa J, Matsui O, Takashima T, et al. Fatty metamorphosis in hepatocellular carcinoma: radiologic features in 10 cases. *AJR* 1988;151:717-720.
155. Friedman AC, Lichtenstein JE, Goodman Z, et al. Fibrolamellar hepatocellular carcinoma. *Radiology* 1985;157:583-587.
156. Brandt DJ, Johnson CD, Stephens DH, et al. Imaging of fibrolamellar hepatocellular carcinoma. *AJR* 1988;151:295-299.
157. Taylor KJW, Ramos I, Morse SS, et al: Focal liver masses: differential diagnosis with pulsed Doppler ultrasound. *Radiology* 1987;164:643-647.
158. Tanaka S, Kitamura T, Fujita M, et al. Color Doppler flow imaging of liver tumors. *AJR* 1990;154:509-514.
159. Mahony B, Jeffrey RB, Federle MP. Spontaneous rupture of hepatic and splenic angiosarcoma demonstrated by computed tomography. *AJR* 1982;138:965-966.
160. Fitzgerald EJ, Griffiths TM. Computed tomography of vinyl-chloride-induced angiosarcoma of liver. *Br J Radiol* 1987;60:593-595.
161. Furui S, Itai Y, Ohtomo D, et al. Hepatic epithelioid hemangioendothelioma: report of five cases. *Radiology* 1989;171:63-68.
162. Radin R, Craig JR, Colletti PM, et al. Hepatic epithelioid hemangioendothelioma. *Radiology* 1988;169:145-148.
163. Rubaltelli L, Del Mashio A, Candiani F, et al. The role of vascularization in the formation of echographic patterns of hepatic metastases: microangiographic and echographic study. *Br J Radiol* 1980;53:1166-1168.
164. Sanders LM, Botet JF, Straus DJ, et al. Computed tomography of primary lymphoma of the liver. *AJR* 1989;152:973-976.
165. Townsend RR, Laing FC, Jeffrey RB, et al. Abdominal lymphoma in AIDS: evaluation with ultrasound. *Radiology* 1989;171:719-724.
166. Yoshida T, Matsue H, Okazaki N, et al. Ultrasonographic differentiation of hepatocellular carcinoma from metastatic liver cancer. *J Clin Ultrasound* 1987;15:431-437.
167. Marchal GJ, Pylyser K, Tshibwabwa-Tumba EA. Anechoic halo in solid liver tumors: sonographic, microangiographic, and histologic correlation. *Radiology* 1985;156:479-483.
168. Bruneton JN, Ladree D, Caramella E, et al. Ultrasonographic study of calcified hepatic metastases: a report of 13 cases. *Gastrointest Radiol* 1982;7:61-63.

169. Wooten WB, Green B, Goldstein HM. Ultrasonography of necrotic hepatic metastases. *Radiology* 1978;128:447-450.
170. Federle MP, Filly RA, Moss AA. Cystic hepatic neoplasms: complementary roles of computed tomography and sonography. *AJR* 1981;345-348.
171. Nyberg DA, Federle MP. AIDS-related Kaposi sarcoma and lymphomas. *Sem Roentgenol* 1987;22(1):54-65.
172. Luburich P, Bru C, Ayuso MC, et al. Hepatic Kaposi sarcoma in AIDS: ultrasound and computed tomography findings. *Radiology* 1990;175:172-174.

Hepatic trauma

173. Anderson CB, Ballinger WF. Abdominal injuries. In: Zuidema GD, Rutherford RB, Ballinger WF, eds. *The Management of Trauma.* 4th ed. Philadelphia: WB Saunders Co; 1985:449-504.
174. Moon KL, Federle MP. Computed tomography in hepatic trauma. *AJR* 1983;141:309-314.
175. Foley WD, Cates JD, Kellman GM, et al. Treatment of blunt hepatic injuries: role of computed tomography. *Radiology* 1987;164:635-638.
176. vanSonnenberg E, Simeone JF, Mueller PR, et al. Sonographic appearance of hematoma in the liver, spleen, and kidney: a clinical, pathologic, and animal study. *Radiology* 1983;147:507-510.

Hepatic surgery

177. Tzakis AG, Gordon RD, Makowka L, et al. Clinical considerations in orthotopic liver transplantation. *Radiol Clin North Am* 1987;25(2):289-297.
178. Starzl TE, Iwatsuki S, Shaw BW Jr. Transplantation of the human liver. In: Swarts SI, ed. *Maingot's Abdominal Operations.* 8th ed. Connecticut: Appleton-Century-Crofts; 1985: 1687-1722.
179. Longley DG, Skolnick ML, Sheahan DG. Acute allograft rejection in liver transplant recipients: lack of correlation with loss of hepatic artery diastolic flow. *Radiology* 1988;169:417-420.
180. Marder DM, DeMarino GB, Sumkin JH, Sheahan DG. Liver transplant rejection: value of the resistive index in Doppler US of hepatic arteries. *Radiology* 1989;173:127-129.
181. Tzakis AG, Gordon RD, Shaw BW Jr, et al. Clinical presentation of hepatic artery thrombosis after liver transplantation in the cyclosporine era. *Transplantation* 1986;40:667-671.
182. Lerut J, Gordon RD, Iwatsuki S, et al. Biliary tract complications in human orthotopic liver transplantation. *Transplantation* 1987;43:47-51.
183. Honda H, Franken Jr EA, Barloon TJ, et al. Hepatic lymphoma in cyclosporine-treated transplant recipients: sonographic and computed tomography findings. *AJR* 1989;152:501-503.
184. Letourneau JG, Day DL, Ascher NL, et al. Abdominal sonography after hepatic transplantation. *AJR* 1987;149:229-303.
185. Lafortune M, Patriquin H, Pomier G, et al. Hemodynamic changes in portal circulation after portosystemic shunts: use of duplex sonography in 43 patients. *AJR* 1987;149:701-706.
186. Chezmar JL, Bernardino ME. Mesoatrial shunt for the treatment of Budd-Chiari syndrome: radiologic evaluation in eight patients. *AJR* 1987;149:707-710.
187. Grant EG, Tessler FN, Gomes AS et al. Color Doppler imaging of portosystemic shunts. *AJR* 1990;154:393-397.
188. Ralls PW, Lee KP, Mayekawa DS, et al. Color Doppler sonography of portocaval shunts. *J Clin Ultrasound* 1990;18:379-381.
189. Foley WD, Gleysteen JJ, Lawson TL, et al. Dynamic computed tomography and pulsed Doppler sonography in the evaluation of splenorenal shunt patency. *J Comput Assist Tomogr* 1983;7:106-112.

Percutaneous liver biopsy

190. Charboneau JW, Reading CC, Welch TJ. CT and sonographically guided needle biopsy: current techniques and new innovations. *AJR* 1990;154:1-10.
191. Reading CC, Charboneau JW, James EM, et al. Sonographically guided percutaneous biopsy of small (3 cm or less) masses. *AJR* 1988;151:189-192.
192. Livragi T, Festi D, Monti F, et al. US-guided percutaneous alcohol injection of small hepatic and abdominal tumors. *Radiology* 1986;161:309-312.
193. Shiina S, Yasuda H, Muto H, et al. Percutaneous ethanol injection in the treatment of liver neoplasms. *AJR* 1987;149:949-952.

Intraoperative ultrasound

194. Rifkin MD, Rosato FE, Mitchell Branch H, et al. Intraoperative ultrasound of the liver: an important adjunctive tool for decision making in the operating room. *Ann Surg* 1987;205:466-471.
195. Parker GA, Lawrence Jr J, Horsley JS, et al. Intraoperative ultrasound of the liver affects operative decision making. *Ann Surg* 1989;209:569-577.

CHAPTER 5

The Spleen

- John R. Mathieson, M.D.
- Peter L. Cooperberg, M.D.

In patients with palpable splenomegaly or left upper quadrant trauma, sectional imaging techniques are indispensable to diagnose or rule out splenic abnormalities. Although in many centers computed tomography is the technique of choice for evaluation of the spleen and surrounding structures, ultrasound can be particularly useful in the first stage of the investigation and also in the follow-up of suspected or confirmed abnormalities. Particularly by the use of the real-time sector format, the spleen and other structures in the left upper quadrant can easily be examined without having to move the patient. If necessary, examination can even be done portably.

In that the normal spleen is uniform in echogenicity, abnormalities stand out clearly. Similarly, perisplenic fluid collections and other abnormalities usually are identified easily. Inadequate sonographic assessment of the spleen and surrounding structures is rare. Occasionally, because the spleen is located high in the left upper quadrant, difficulties can be encountered. Shadowing from ribs, overlying bowel gas, and overlying lung in the costophrenic angle can obscure visualization of the deeper structures. Expertise and persistence may be required to overcome these obstacles.

EMBRYOLOGY AND ANATOMY

Embryologically, the spleen arises from a mass of mesenchymal cells located between the layers of the dorsal mesentery, which connects the stomach to the posterior peritoneal surface over the aorta (Fig. 5-1, *A*). These mesenchymal cells differentiate to form the splenic pulp, the supporting connective tissue structures and capsule of the spleen. The splenic artery penetrates the primitive spleen and arterioles branch through the connective tissue into the splenic sinusoids.

As the embryonic stomach rotates 90 degrees along its longitudinal axis, the spleen and dorsal mesentery are carried to the left along with the greater curvature of the stomach (Fig. 5-1, *B*). The base of the dorsal mesentery fuses with the posterior peritoneum over the left kidney, giving rise to the splenorenal ligament. This explains why, although the spleen is intraperitoneal, the splenic artery enters from the retroperitoneum via the splenorenal ligament (Fig. 5-1, *C*). In most adults, a portion of the splenic capsule is firmly adherent to the fused dorsal mesentery anterior to the upper left kidney, giving rise to the so-called "bare area" of the spleen. The size of the splenic bare area is variable, but usually involves less than half of the posterior splenic surface (Fig. 5-2). This anatomic feature is analogous to the bare area of the liver, and similarly can be helpful in distinguishing intraperitoneal from pleural fluid collections.[1]

The normal adult spleen is convex superolaterally, concave inferomedially, and has a very homogeneous echo pattern. The spleen lies between the fundus of the stomach and the diaphragm, with its long axis in the line of the left tenth rib. The diaphragmatic surface is convex and is usually situated between the ninth to eleventh ribs. The visceral or inferomedial surface has gentle indentations where it comes in contact with the stomach, left kidney, pancreas, and splenic flexure. The spleen is suspended by the splenorenal ligament, which is in contact with the posterior peritoneal wall and left phrenicocolic ligament, and by the gastrosplenic ligament. The gastrosplenic ligament is composed of the two layers of the dorsal mesentery, which separate the lesser sac posteriorly from the greater sac anteriorly.

The average adult spleen measures 12 cm in length, 7 cm in breadth, and 3 to 4 cm in thickness and has an average weight of 150 g, varying between 80 and 300

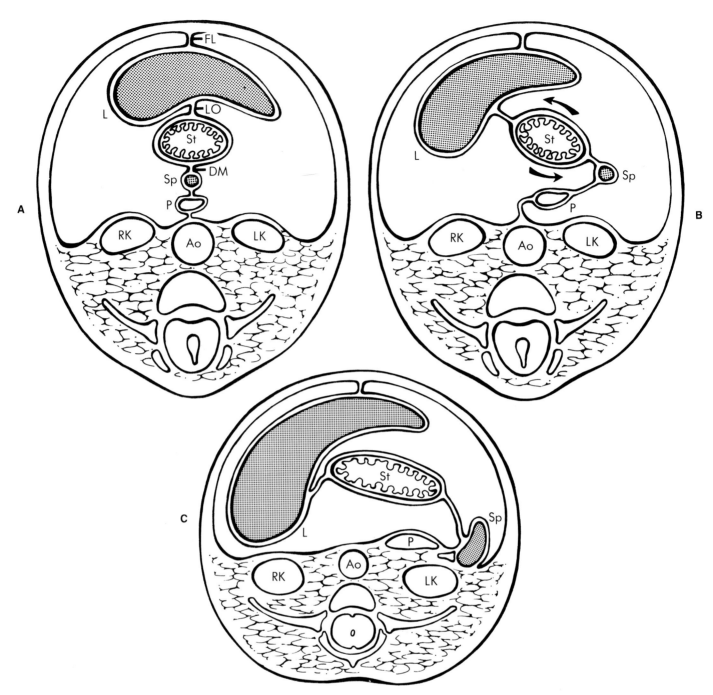

FIG 5-1. The embryologic development of the spleen. Schematic axial drawings of the upper abdomen. **A,** A 4- to 5-week embryo. The mesentery anterior to the stomach *(ST)* is the ventral mesentery divided into the falciform ligament *(FL)* anteriorly and the gastrohepatic ligament or lesser omentum *(LO)* posteriorly by the liver *(L)*. Posterior to the stomach is the dorsal mesentery *(DM)*, which contains the developing spleen *(Sp)* and pancreas *(P)*. The dorsal mesentery is divided into two portions by the spleen: the splenogastric ligament anteriorly, and the splenorenal ligament posteriorly. The pancreas has not yet become retroperitoneal and remains within the dorsal mesentery. **B,** An 8-week embryo. The stomach rotates counterclockwise, displacing the liver to the right and the spleen to the left. The portion of the dorsal mesentery containing the pancreas, the splenic vessels, and the spleen begins to fuse to the anterior retroperitoneal surface, giving rise to the splenogastric ligament and the bare area of the spleen. If fusion is incomplete, the spleen will be attached to the retroperitoneum only by a long mesentery, giving rise to a mobile or "wandering" spleen. **C,** Newborn baby. Fusion of the dorsal mesentery is now complete. The pancreas is now completely retroperitoneal, and a portion of the spleen has fused with the retroperitoneum. Note the close relation of the tail of the pancreas to the splenic hilum. *L,* Liver; *ST,* stomach; *SP,* spleen; *P,* pancreas; *FL,* falciform ligament; *LO,* lesser omentum or gastrohepatic ligament; *LK,* left kidney; *RK,* right kidney; *Ao,* aorta.

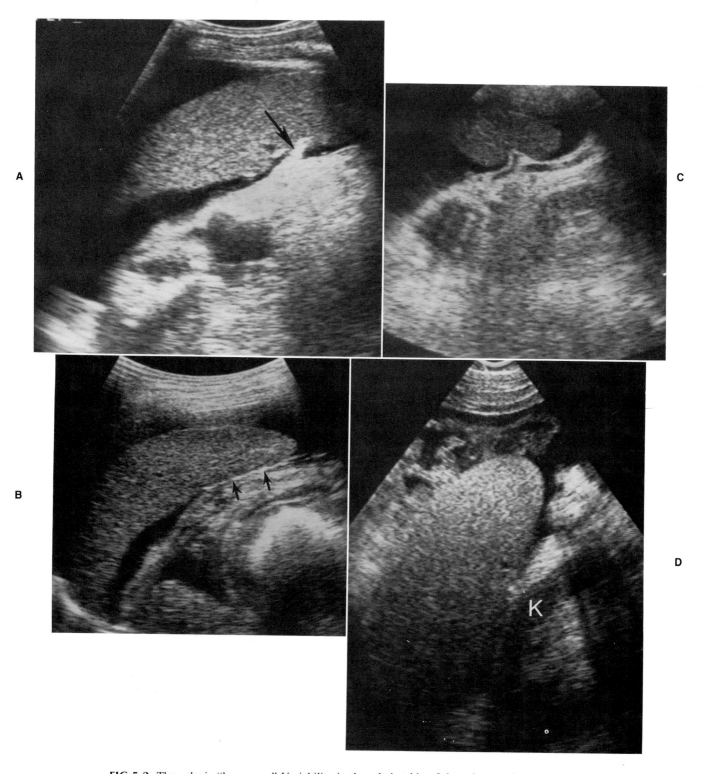

FIG 5-2. The splenic "bare area." Variability in the relationship of the spleen to the anterior retroperitoneal surface shows patients with **A,** This patient has no "bare area." The splenorenal ligament *(arrow)* is outlined on both sides by ascitic fluid. **B,** Part of the lower pole of the spleen is fused posteriorly. **C,** The lower pole of the spleen is fused to the retroperitoneum *(arrows)*. **D,** A large proportion of this patient's spleen is fused posteriorly. Note the close relationship of the spleen to the left kidney *(K)*.

g. A normal spleen decreases in size and weight with advancing age. It also increases slightly during digestion and can vary in size in accordance with the nutritional status of the body.

Splenic functions include phagocytosis, fetal hematopoiesis, adult lymphopoiesis, immune response, and erythrocyte storage. Under a variety of conditions, including surgical misadventure, the spleen may be removed. Most commonly, people can live successfully without a spleen. However, particularly in childhood, the immune response may be impaired, particularly to encapsulated bacteria. Recently, the surgical trend is towards splenic preservation wherever possible.

EXAMINATION TECHNIQUE

All routine abdominal sonographic examinations, regardless of the indication, should include at least one coronal view of the spleen and upper pole of the left kidney. This view is easy to obtain with real-time scanning, particularly by the sector format. The most common approach to visualizing the spleen is to maintain the patient in the supine position and place the transducer in the coronal plane of section posteriorly in one of the lower left intercostal spaces. The patient then can be examined in various degrees of inspiration to maximize the window to the spleen. Excessive inspiration introduces air into the lung in the lateral costophrenic angle and may obscure visualization. A modest inspiration depresses the central portion of the left hemidiaphragm and spleen inferiorly so that they can be visualized (Fig. 5-3). The plane of section should then be

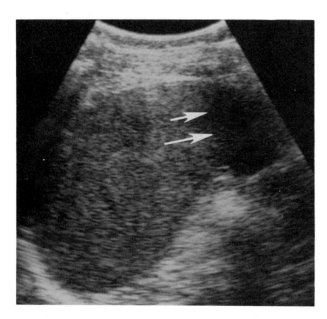

FIG 5-3. Normal spleen, coronal scan. The lower pole is partially obscured by a rib shadow (arrows). The echo texture is homogenous.

swept posteriorly and anteriorly to view the entire volume of the spleen. We generally find that a thorough examination in the coronal plane of section is highly accurate for ruling out any lesion within or around the spleen and for documenting approximate splenic size. If an abnormality is discovered within or around the spleen, other planes of section can be used. An oblique plane of section along the intercostal space can avoid rib shadowing (Fig. 5-4). Because the long axis of the spleen lies obliquely, this oblique plane of section is also convenient with the upper pole located posterior to the lower pole. A transverse plane from a lateral, usually intercostal, approach may help to localize a lesion within the spleen anteriorly and posteriorly. In this regard, especially for beginners, it must be emphasized that the apex of the sector image is always placed at the top of the screen. However, on a left lateral intercostal transverse image, the top of the screen (apex of the sector) is actually to the patient's left, the right side of the sector image is posterior, and the left side of the image is anterior. To look at the image appropriately, one would have to rotate it 90 degrees in a clockwise direction or turn one's head in a 90 degrees counterclockwise direction.

If the spleen is not enlarged and is not surrounded by a large mass, scanning from an anterior position (as one would for imaging the liver) is not helpful because of the interposition of gas within the stomach and splenic flexure of the colon.[2] However, if the patient has a relatively large liver, one may be able to see the spleen through the left lobe of the liver and the collapsed stomach, analogous to the image seen on the transverse CT scan of the upper abdomen. Also, if the spleen is enlarged or if there is a mass in the left upper quadrant, the spleen may be visualized from an anterior approach. If there is free intraperitoneal fluid around the spleen or a left pleural effusion, the spleen may even be better visualized from an anterolateral approach.

Often, it is beneficial to have the patient roll onto his or her right side as much as 45 or even 90 degrees, so that a more posterior approach can be used to visualize the spleen. We no longer use the prone position.

Generally, the same technical settings for gain, time-gain compensation, and power are used for examination of the spleen as for examination of the other organs in the upper abdomen. Because the spleen is a superficial structure and there is generally little absorption of sound within the spleen, a 5-MHz internally focused transducer of medium length is recommended. Although mechanical sector scanners, with or without annular array focusing, or phased array sector scanners can be used, we most commonly use curvilinear transducers now. There is a slight disadvantage in intercostal scanning with the larger transducer face, but the image quality is significantly improved with these transducers.

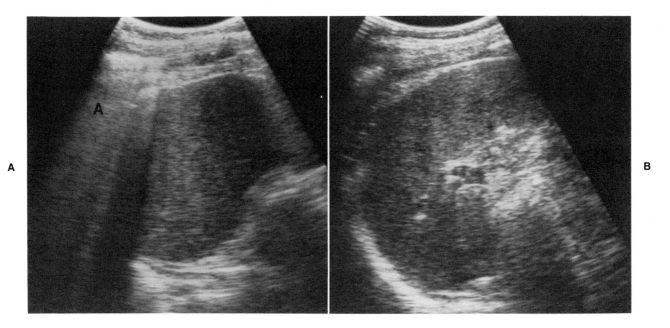

FIG 5-4. Importance of scan plane. **A,** Coronal scan showing partial obscuring of the spleen by air *(A)* in the lung and by a rib shadow. **B,** Oblique coronal scan, aligned with the tenth interspace, shows improved visualization of the spleen.

It is important to appreciate that often the ribs may be broader and flatter than expected and may encroach on the intercostal spaces, making them particularly narrow. This can severely impair the quality of the image seen from an intercostal space.

SONOGRAPHY OF THE SPLEEN

The shape of the normal spleen is variable. The spleen consists of two components joined at the hilum: a superomedial component and an inferolateral component. More superiorly, on transverse scanning, the spleen has a typical fat "inverted comma" shape with a thin component extending anteriorly and another component extending medially, either superior to or adjacent to the upper pole of the kidney. This is the component that can be seen to indent the gastric fundus on plain films of the abdomen or barium studies. As one moves the scan plane inferiorly, only the inferior component of the spleen is seen. This is the component that can be outlined by a thin rim of fat above the splenic flexure on a plain film of the abdomen. It may extend inferiorly to the costal margin and present as a palpable spleen clinically. However, either component can enlarge independently without enlargement of the other component.

It is important to recognize the normal structures that are anatomically related to the spleen. The diaphragm cradles the spleen posteriorly, superiorly, and laterally. The normal liver usually does not touch the spleen. If the left lobe is enlarged, it may extend into the left up-

per quadrant anterior to the spleen. The fundus of the stomach and lesser sac are medial and anterior to the splenic hilum. It is important to appreciate that the fundus may contain gas or fluid. The tail of the pancreas lies posterior to the stomach and lesser sac and also approaches the hilum of the spleen, in close relation to the splenic artery and vein. The left kidney generally lies inferior and medial to the spleen. A useful landmark in identifying the spleen and splenic hilum is the splenic vein, which can generally be demonstrated, especially in splenic enlargement.

The splenic parenchyma is extremely homogeneous and therefore the spleen has a uniform mid- to low-level echogenicity. It is generally considered that the liver is more echogenic than the spleen but, in fact, the echogenicity of the parenchyma is higher in the spleen than in the liver. It is difficult to directly compare the echogenicity of these two organs. The impression that the liver has increased echogenicity is because of its large number of reflective vessels. When the spleen enlarges, it can become more echogenic. Unfortunately, one cannot differentiate between the different types of enlargement on the basis of the degree of echogenicity.

PATHOLOGIC CONDITIONS OF THE SPLEEN
Splenomegaly

Frequently, sonography is performed to determine the presence or absence of splenomegaly. If there is gross enlargement of the spleen, confirmation of splenomegaly is easy. However, if there is only mild en-

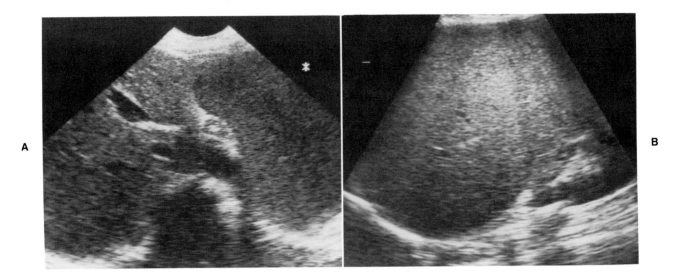

FIG 5-5. Splenomegaly. **A,** Transverse scan in the upper abdomen shows the liver touching the large spleen in the epigastrium. **B,** Coronal scan shows only the mid-portion of the large spleen with the superior and inferior aspects beyond the sector format.

largement it can be difficult to make the decision based on a sonographic study. Techniques have been developed to measure serial sections of the spleen by planimetry, and then compute the volume of the spleen by adding the values for each section.[3] However, these techniques are cumbersome and not popular. The most commonly used method is the "eyeball" technique: if it looks big, it is (Fig. 5-5). Unfortunately, this method of assessment requires considerably more experience than is necessary with other imaging techniques. Furthermore, it is relatively inaccurate. As with all other structures in the body, it is helpful to have measurements that establish the upper limits of normal. The wide range of what a normal sized adult spleen is combined

with its complex three-dimensional shape makes it particularly difficult to establish a normal range of sonographic measurements. Nonetheless, a study of almost 800 normal adults found that in 95% of patients, the length of the spleen was less than 12 cm, the breadth less than 7 cm and the thickness less than 5 cm.[4] These measurements may be useful for borderline cases.

The spleen is capable of growing to an enormous size. It may extend inferiorly into the left iliac fossa. It can cross the midline and present as a mass inferior to the left lobe of the liver on longitudinal section (Fig. 5-6).

The differential diagnosis of splenomegaly is exceedingly long and includes infection, neoplasia, infil-

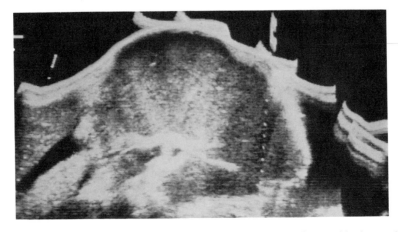

FIG 5-6. Splenomegaly. Sagittal scan through the left lobe of the liver, with the markedly enlarged spleen extending below the liver.

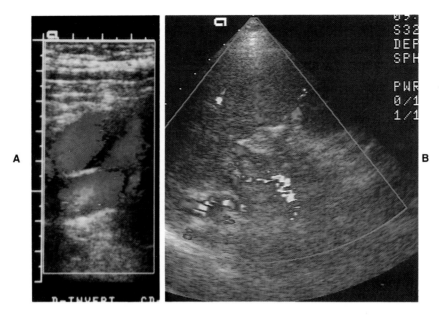

FIG 5-7. Portal systemic collaterals. **A,** Color Doppler scan of the left upper quadrant showing distended veins with high flow in a lienorenal shunt. Hepatofugal flow was noted in the portal vein. **B,** Color Doppler scan of the left upper quadrant showing flow in splenic vein varices, due to portal hypertension.

tration, trauma, blood dyscrasias, storage disorders, and portal hypertension. Sonography usually is not helpful in the specific diagnosis of splenomegaly. However, the degree of splenomegaly can help to narrow the differential diagnosis. Mild to moderate splenomegaly is most often caused by infection, portal hypertension, and AIDS. More marked splenomegaly is usually the result of hematologic disorders including leukemia and lymphoma as well as infectious mononucleosis. Massive splenomegaly can be seen in myelofibrosis. In addition, focal lesions within the spleen may suggest lymphomatous involvement, metastatic disease, cysts, or hematomas. Nonsplenic abnormalities such as lymph node enlargement or liver involvement may suggest lymphoma whereas recanalization of the umbilical vein or other evidence of portal systemic collaterals, such as lienorenal shunts, splenic vein varices, or ascites, establish portal hypertension as the cause of splenomegaly (Fig. 5-7). However, in most cases, splenomegaly may be the only one or one of several nonspecific sonographic findings.

Several investigators have attempted to quantify the degree of diffuse splenic fibrosis or tumor infiltration by analyzing various parameters of the reflected ultrasound signal. Speed and attenuation measurements have been studied, but to date, these parameters are not regarded as clinically useful.[5-7]

Focal Abnormalities

Cysts. Like cysts located elsewhere in the body, splenic cysts characteristically appear as echo-free areas with smooth, sharp borders and enhancement of the echoes deep to the lesions. When small, they may be located within the splenic parenchyma. Occasionally, these cysts can grow very large, and become mainly exophytic. It may then be difficult to appreciate their intrasplenic origin (Fig. 5-8).

Cystic lesions of the spleen can be divided into four categories:

- Infectious cysts
- Posttraumatic cysts
- Primary congenital cysts
- Intrasplenic pancreatic pseudocysts

Infectious cysts are usually caused by echinococcus. However, the spleen is one of the least common sites for the development of hydatid cysts. Calcification may be identified in the wall of the cyst (Fig. 5-9). The diagnosis is made with a combination of appropriate history, geographic background, serologic testing and ultrasound appearance.[8,9] Percutaneous fine needle aspiration can be diagnostic provided the pathologist has been alerted to search for the scolices.

Posttraumatic cysts have no cellular lining and are also called **pseudocysts.**[10] The walls of these cysts, like echinococcal cysts, may become calcified. These cysts may contain low-level echoes that can be cholesterol crystals or debris.[11] Hemorrhage into any cyst also can give rise to echogenic fluid (Fig. 5-10).[12]

Primary congenital cysts, also called **epidermoid cysts,** can be differentiated from posttraumatic cysts by the presence of an epithelial or endothelial lining in the former. Congenital cysts are thought to arise from

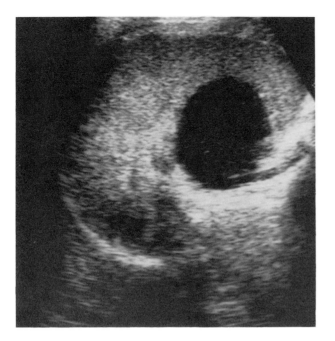

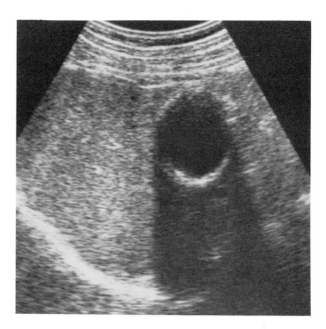

FIG 5-8. Splenic cyst. Coronal scan of the spleen showing a cyst with a 5-cm diameter in the hilar region of the spleen adjacent to the splenic vein. This patient suffered trauma to the left upper quadrant several years ago.

FIG 5-9. Calcified splenic cyst. Note the shadowing from the near side of the splenic cyst. The calcification is incomplete in the near wall, so that echoes from the deep wall can be seen through the shadow. Both "burned out" hydatid cysts and posttraumatic cysts can look like this.

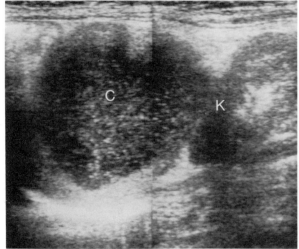

A

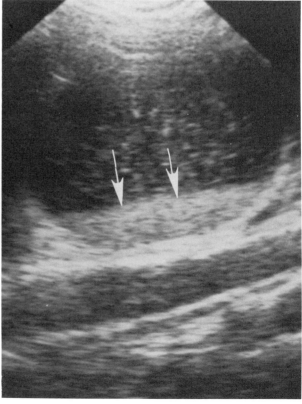

B

FIG 5-10. Splenic cyst. **A,** Composite linear array images. Note the splenic cyst *(C)* with a 8-cm diameter. A small rim of spleen is noted superiorly and medially. The left kidney *(K)* is displaced inferiorly. The echoes from the cholesterol crystals and debris within the cyst mimic a solid lesion. **B,** The sector image shows a more echogenic dependent layer *(arrows)*.

embryonal rests of primitive mesothelial cells within the spleen. Endothelial-lined cysts are rare and include lymphangiomas and, very rarely, cystic hemangiomas.[13]

Pancreatic **pseudocysts** extending into the spleen can be diagnosed by the associated features of pancreatitis. Splenic abscesses may have an appearance similar to simple cysts, but the diagnosis can easily be made in conjunction with the clinical findings. Frequently, there may be gas within an abscess cavity in the spleen, which should point to an infectious cause. Gas can cause a confusing picture if only an area of increased echogenicity is seen in the spleen (Fig. 5-11). However, there may be acoustic shadowing and/or a ring

down artifact. In questionable cases, aspiration can be useful for diagnosis.[14] Furthermore, catheter drainage guided by sonography can be safely and successfully performed.[15]

Solid Masses. Solid focal lesions in the spleen are uncommon, but may be caused by a large number of diseases. The most common focal lesions result from previous granulomatous infections, typically seen as focal bright echogenic lesions, with or without shadowing. Histoplasmosis and tuberculosis are the most common causes, although granulomas may rarely occur in the spleen in patients with sarcoidosis (Fig. 5-12).[16,17] Calcification in the splenic artery is common, and should not be confused with calcification in a lesion (Fig. 5-13).

Primary malignancies of the spleen are extremely rare, but primary lymphoma and angiosarcoma have been reported.[19] Metastatic involvement of the spleen generally occurs as a late phenomenon rather than as a presenting feature. Splenic metastases occur most commonly in malignant melanoma, lymphoma, and leukemia, but can also occur with carcinoma of the ovary, breast, lung, and stomach (Fig. 5-14).[16,19] Metastases are most commonly hypoechoic, but may be echogenic or of mixed echogenicity.

Hemangiomas of the spleen have been reported in up to 14% of patients undergoing autopsy,[20,21] but the typ-

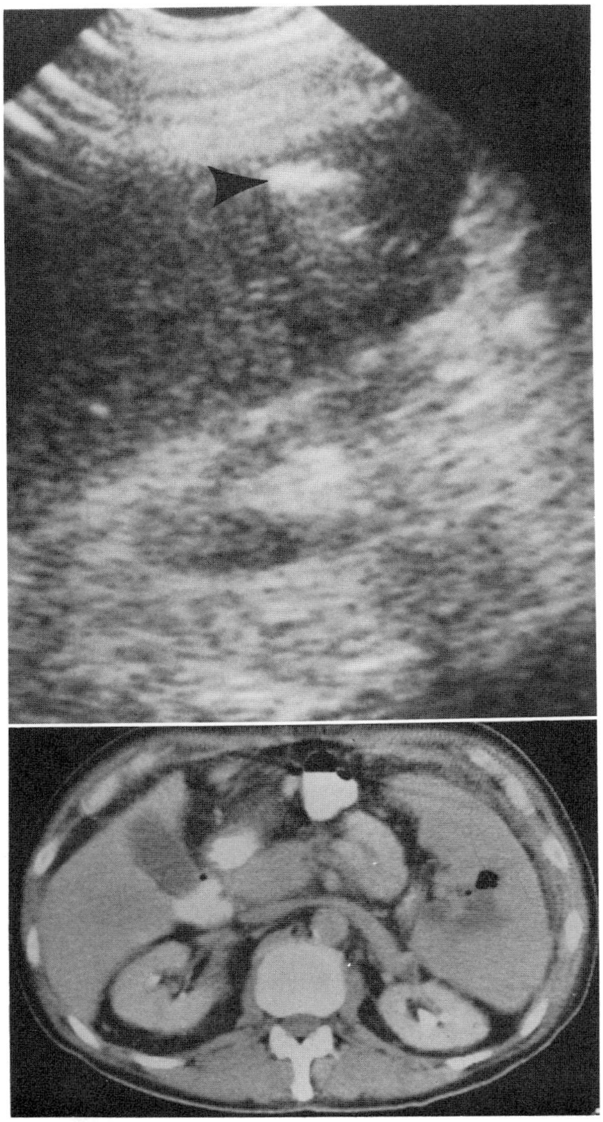

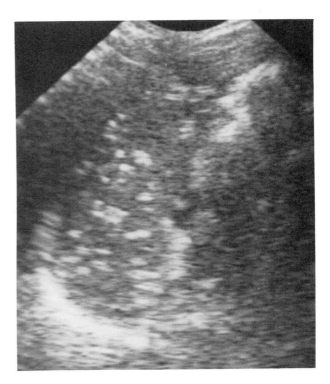

FIG 5-11. Splenic abscess. **A,** Coronal scan shows a gas collection with "dirty shadowing" *(arrowhead).* **B,** CT scan confirms the presence of gas and fluid within the spleen.

FIG 5-12. Granulomatous disease (typical histoplasmosis). Coronal scan showing tiny bright echoes measuring 2 to 3 mm throughout the spleen.

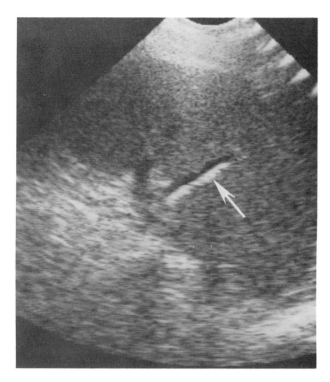

FIG 5-13. Calcified splenic artery. Transverse scan of the spleen showing calcification *(arrow)*, coursing parallel to the splenic vein.

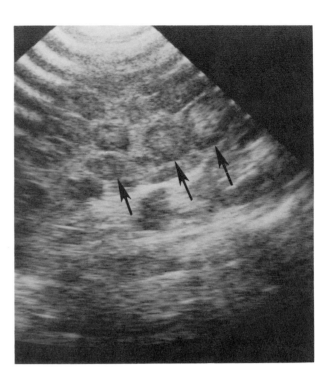

FIG 5-14. Splenic metastases from malignant melanoma. Longitudinal sonogram shows multiple target lesions *(arrows)* in the spleen.

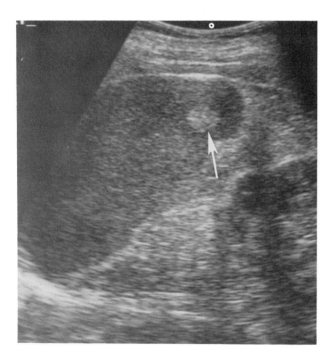

FIG 5-15. Splenic hemangioma. Note the small well-defined, rounded echogenic lesion *(arrow)* measuring 1.4 cm in diameter (similar to typical liver hemangiomas).

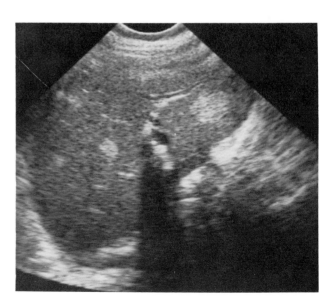

FIG 5-16. Multiple splenic hemangiomas. Coronal scan shows multiple echogenic lesions of different sizes in the spleen. Note the calcified splenic artery adjacent to the vein in the splenic hilum.

ical appearance of hemangioma is seen far less frequently in the spleen than in the liver. Hemangiomas are usually an isolated phenomenon but may occur in association with other stigmata of the Klippel-Trenaunay-Weber syndrome.[22] The sonographic appearance of hemangiomas is variable. The lesions may have a well-defined echogenic appearance, similar to the typical appearance of hemangiomas in the liver (Figs. 5-15 and 5-16). However, lesions of mixed echogenicity with cystic spaces of variable sizes have been reported. Occasionally, foci of calcification have been found.[23-25] Lymphangiomas may also occur in the spleen and have an appearance similar to hemangiomas.[26] It remains to be shown whether MRI will be as helpful for confirming the diagnosis of hemangioma in the spleen as it is in the liver.

Splenic infarction is one of the more common causes of focal splenic lesions. If a typical, peripheral, wedge-shaped hypoechoic lesion is noted, splenic infarction should be the first diagnostic consideration (Figs. 5-17 and 5-18). However, splenic infarctions do not always have this typical appearance and may have a nodular appearance or, as fibrosis progresses, a hyperechoic appearance. Ultrasound, CT, and MRI have a similar sensitivity in the diagnosis of splenic infarction, but the wedge-shaped morphology of the lesion may be more

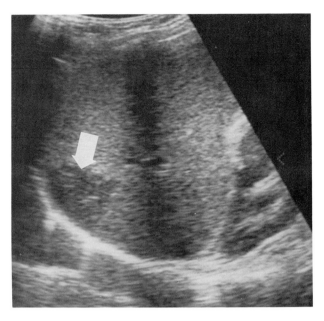

FIG 5-17. Splenic infarct, seen as a triangular echo-poor area (*arrow*) in the superior aspect of the spleen. The wedge-shaped area extends to the splenic capsule, analogous to the pleural wedge-shaped density seen in pulmonary infarction.

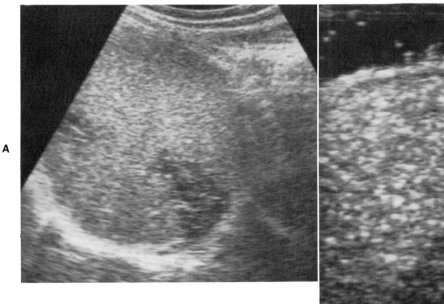

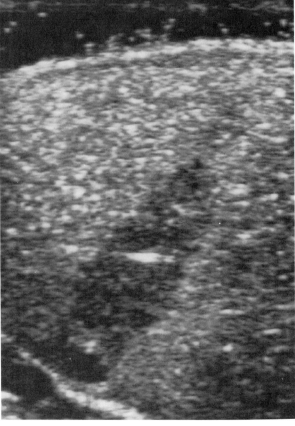

FIG 5-18. Splenic infarct in acute myelogenous leukemia. **A,** In vivo, and **B,** in vitro (postsplenectomy) scans show echo-poor wedge-shaped area with its base on the splenic capsule.

easily appreciated with the multiplanar imaging capability of ultrasound than with CT or MRI.[17] The temporal evolution of the ultrasonic appearance of splenic infarctions has been studied, showing that the echogenicity of the lesion is related to the age of the infarction. Infarctions are hypoechoic or echo-free in early stages and progress to hyperechoic lesions over time.[27,28]

Several relatively rare diseases have a high frequency of associated splenic abnormalities. For example in Gaucher's disease, splenomegaly occurs almost universally, and approximately one third of patients have multiple splenic nodules. These nodules are most frequently well-defined hypoechoic lesions, but may be irregular, hyperechoic, or of mixed echogenicity.[29,30] Pathologically, these nodules represent focal areas of Gaucher's cells associated with fibrosis and infarction. Rarely the entire spleen may be involved, with ultrasound showing diffuse inhomogeneity.[29]

In patients with schistosomiasis, splenomegaly is found universally, and focal hyperechoic nodules are seen in 5% to 10% of patients.[31]

Multiple nodules may also be found in patients with splenic infections, particularly in immunocompromised patients. The so-called "wheels within wheels" appearance has been described in patients with hepatosplenic candidiasis. The outer "wheel" is thought to represent a ring of fibrosis, surrounding the inner echogenic "wheel" of inflammatory cells and a central hypoechoic necrotic area. However, this appearance is not universally seen in splenic candidiasis, as some patients may have a "bull's eye" appearance or may present with hypoechoic or hyperechoic nodules[32] (Fig. 5-19).

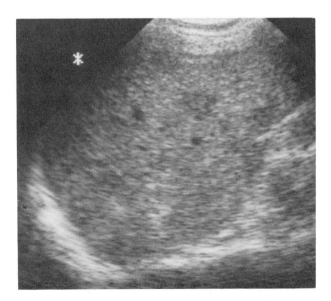

FIG 5-19. Candida abscesses of the spleen in an AIDS patient. There are several characteristic lesions with an echogenic center and a hypoechoic rim.

Miliary spread can occur with both typical and atypical mycobacterial infection, and is more commonly seen in immunocompromised patients. Innumerable tiny echogenic foci can be seen diffusely throughout the spleen (Fig. 5-20). In active tuberculosis, echo-poor or cystic lesions representing tuberculous abscesses may be seen (Fig. 5-21).

In summary, although ultrasound is very helpful in finding focal splenic lesions, there is so much overlap in the appearance of the different pathologies that it is rarely possible to make a specific diagnosis. If a typical appearance of splenic infarction is found, serial observations may be used to confirm the diagnosis and avoid a biopsy. If a very well-defined echogenic lesion is found in an asymptomatic patient, the lack of change on serial ultrasound examinations may be used to confirm the diagnosis of hemangioma. Calcified lesions in the spleen may be safely followed with serial ultrasound scanning, as they are unlikely to represent any condition requiring treatment. Otherwise, most other focal splenic lesions will require a biopsy for diagnosis.

Splenic Trauma

Ultrasound can be very useful and highly accurate in the diagnosis of subcapsular and pericapsular hematomas of the spleen. Nonetheless, this is one area in which CT has proven particularly useful because more upper-abdominal pathology can be identified in one examination.[33,34] However, splenic trauma from blunt nonpenetrating injuries of the left upper quadrant is not always an emergency and ultrasound can be useful. In addition, if the patient is in extreme distress, the CT scanner often cannot be made available quickly enough, so ultrasound can again play an important role. Furthermore, now that nonoperative management is preferred, ultrasound is preferable for numerous follow-up examinations.

If the spleen is involved in blunt abdominal trauma, two outcomes are possible. If the capsule remains intact, the outcome may be an intraparenchymal or subcapsular hematoma (Figs. 5-22 and 5-23). If the capsule ruptures, a focal or free intraperitoneal hematoma may result. With capsular rupture, it might be possible to demonstrate fluid surrounding the spleen in the left upper quadrant. Although blood may spread within the peritoneal cavity and be found in the flanks or in Morrison's pouch, most commonly it becomes walled off in the left upper quadrant (Figs. 5-24 and 5-25). It is important to consider the timing of the sonographic examination relative to the trauma. Immediately after the traumatic incident, the hematoma is liquid and can easily be differentiated from splenic parenchyma. However, after the blood clots, and for the subsequent 24 to 48 hours, the echogenicity of the perisplenic clot may closely resemble the echogenicity of normal splenic pa-

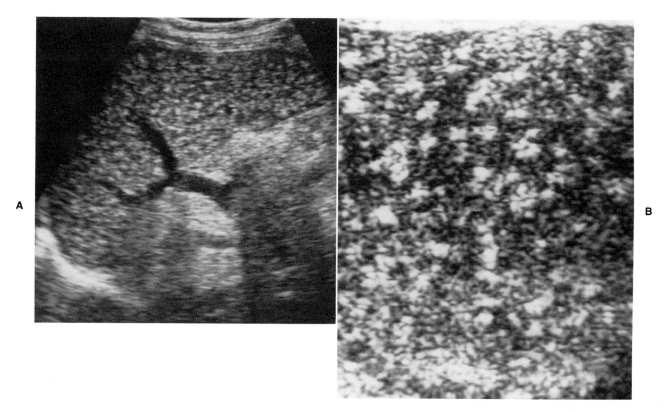

FIG 5-20. Active miliary tuberculosis (TB) of the spleen. **A,** Coronal. **B,** High-resolution linear array images show multiple tiny echogenic foci of tuberculous granulomata. This was active TB throughout the entire spleen.

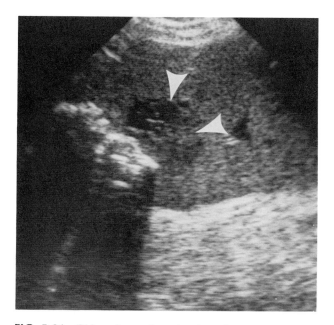

FIG 5-21. Old and reactivated tuberculosis (TB) in the spleen. The coronal image shows old calcified granulomas with shadowing in the superior aspect of the spleen, and active echo-poor lesions *(arrowheads)* in the midportion.

renchyma. The appearance may mimic that of an enlarged spleen. Subsequently, the blood reliquefies and the diagnosis becomes easy again. Usually, by the time the patient has been admitted and has settled down, one only sees an irregularly marginated echogenic mass that is larger than one would expect for a normal spleen. Furthermore, there are often focal areas of inhomogeneity within the spleen to indicate that there is an abnormality. Because current therapy for stable patients with suspected splenic trauma consists of nonintervention and temporization, a follow-up sonogram is suggested in 2 or 3 days to demonstrate reliquefaction of the hematoma. With time, one may clearly see the subcapsular hematoma differentiated from the pericapsular walled-off hematoma by the capsule itself.[35] However, the splenic capsule is very thin and is frequently not visualized separately from adjacent fluid. In these cases, the shape of the fluid collection can provide an important clue to the location of the hematoma. If the collection is crescentic and conforms to the contour of the spleen, the hematoma should be assumed to be subcapsular. More irregularly shaped collections are seen with perisplenic hematomas.

Perisplenic fluid may persist for weeks or even

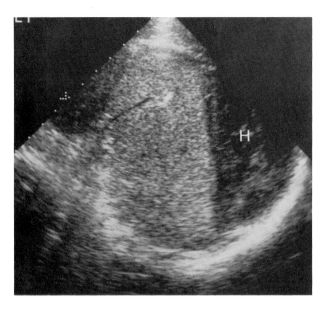

FIG 5-22. Spontaneous subcapsular hematoma *(H)* of the spleen. Transverse scan shows a crescentic area filled with fluid and debris in the lateral aspect of the spleen.

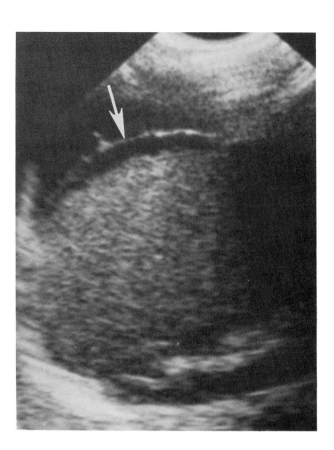

FIG 5-23. Subcapsular and perisplenic hematomas. The thin brightly echogenic crescentic line *(arrow)* represents the splenic capsule.

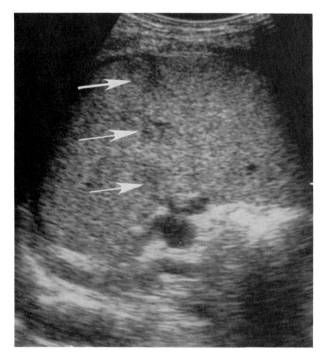

FIG 5-24. Splenic laceration. Coronal scan shows irregular discontinuous echo-poor area *(arrows)* through the midportion of the spleen. There is a small amount of perisplenic blood. This improved and was not visible on a subsequent scan 2 weeks later.

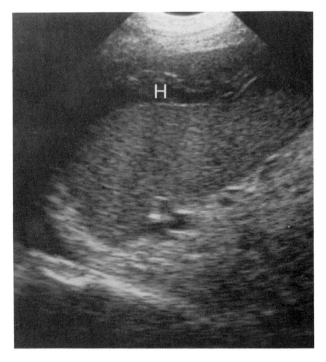

FIG 5-25. Posttraumatic perisplenic hematoma *(H)*. Coronal scan shows fluid around the convexity of the spleen and a left pleural effusion.

months following the trauma. Although there may actually be a condition of delayed rupture of the spleen, it is possible that all ruptures of the spleen occur at the time of injury and are walled off initially. Delayed rupture may only be the extension of a perisplenic hematoma into the peritoneal cavity.

Aside from splenic capsule rupture, there may be internal damage to the spleen with an intact splenic capsule. This can result in intraparenchymal or subcapsular hematoma of the spleen, which initially appears only as an inhomogeneous area in the otherwise uniform splenic parenchyma. Subsequently, the hematoma may resolve and repeat scans can show the cyst at the site of the original injury.

Sonographically, a perisplenic hematoma can closely mimic a perisplenic abscess. The hematoma can become infected easily and transform into a left subphrenic abscess.[37] Generally, the distinction can be made clinically. If it is not clinically obvious, fine-needle aspiration can differentiate easily between hematoma and abscess. Catheter drainage can then be performed under ultrasound or CT guidance for definitive therapy.

Acquired Immune Deficiency Syndrome (AIDS)

The most common splenic ultrasound finding in patients with AIDS is moderate splenomegaly, reported in 50% to 70% of patients referred for abdominal ultra-sound.[37,38] Splenomegaly has been noted more frequently in patients with sexually transmitted HIV infection than in patients acquiring the disease through intravenous drug use. Focal lesions can occur in patients with AIDS. These may be caused by opportunistic infections such as *Candida* (Fig. 5-19), pneumocystis, or mycobacterium. There have been reports of disseminated pneumocystis appearing as tiny focal echoes throughout the liver, spleen, and kidneys.[39] We have seen an additional identical case caused by atypical mycobacteria (Fig. 5-26). The spleen may also be involved in Kaposi's sarcoma or lymphoma.

Congenital Anomalies

Supernumerary spleens are common normal variants found in up to 30% of autopsies. These are also referred to as **splenunculi.** These may be confused with enlarged lymph nodes around the spleen, or with a mass in the tail of the pancreas (Fig. 5-27). Furthermore, when the spleen enlarges, the accessory spleens may also enlarge. Ectopic accessory spleens may be confused with an abnormal mass, or may undergo torsion and may present with acute abdominal pain.[40-43] The vast majority of accessory spleens, however, are easy to recognize sonographically as small rounded masses, less than 5 cm in diameter (Fig. 5-28). They are located near the splenic hilum and have identical echogenicity

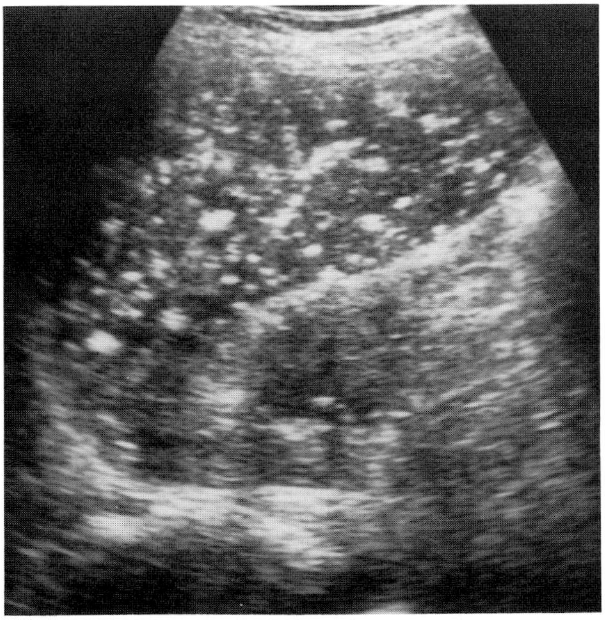

FIG 5-26. Atypical tuberculosis of the spleen in an AIDS patient. Tiny calcifications throughout the spleen were also seen throughout the liver and isolated foci in the kidney. Several core liver biopsies confirmed *Mycobacterium avium intracellulare* granulomas.

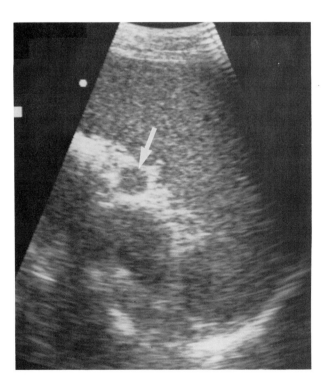

FIG 5-27. Accessory spleen splenunculus. Coronal scan shows a small "mass" *(arrow)* in the splenic hilum with homogeneous echogenicity identical to the spleen.

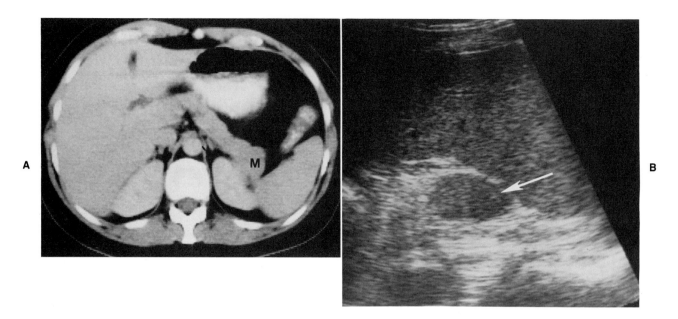

FIG 5-28. Accessory spleen presenting as possible mass in the tail of the pancreas. **A,** CT scan was done first. An ultrasound-guided biopsy of the mass *(M)* of the pancreatic tail was requested. **B,** Coronal sonogram clearly shows that the apparently enlarged pancreatic tail is actually an accessory spleen *(arrow)* lying adjacent to the tail of the pancreas.

to the adjacent spleen. A nuclear scan with heat-damaged red cells can confirm the diagnosis, if necessary.

The spleen may have a long, mobile mesentery if the dorsal mesentery fails to fuse with the posterior peritoneum. The "wandering" spleen can be found in unusual locations and may be mistaken for a mass. It may undergo torsion and result in acute or chronic abdominal pain.[44-46] If the diagnosis of a wandering spleen is made in a patient with acute abdominal pain, the diagnosis of torsion may be supported by a color-flow Doppler examination showing absence of blood flow.

The other two major congenital splenic anomalies are asplenia and polysplenia syndromes. These conditions are best understood if viewed as part of the spectrum of anomalies known as **visceral heterotaxy.** A normal arrangement of asymmetric body parts is known as **situs solitus.** The mirror image condition is called **situs inversus.** In between these two extremes is a wide spectrum of abnormalities called **situs ambiguous.** Splenic abnormalities in patients with visceral heterotaxy consist of polysplenia and asplenia. Interestingly, patients with polysplenia have bilateral left-sidedness, or a dominance of left-sided over right-sided body structures. They may have two morphologically left lungs, left-sided azygous continuation of an interrupted inferior vena cava, biliary atresia, absence of the gall bladder, gastrointestinal malrotation, and frequent cardiovascular abnormalities. Conversely, patients with asplenia may have bilateral right-sidedness. They may

have two morphologically right lungs, midline location of the liver, reversed position of the abdominal aorta and inferior vena cava, anomalous pulmonary venous return, and horseshoe kidneys. The wide variety of possible anomalies obviously accounts for a wide variety of presenting symptoms, but absence of the spleen per se causes impairment of immune response, and such patients can present with serious infections such as bacterial meningitis.

Polysplenia must be differentiated from posttraumatic splenosis. Following splenic rupture, splenic cells may implant throughout the peritoneal cavity and increase in size resulting in multiple ectopic splenic rests.[48-50] Nuclear studies with technetium-labelled heat-damaged red blood cells are the most sensitive studies for both posttraumatic splenosis and congenital polysplenia. Accessory spleens as small as 1 cm can be demonstrated by this method.[50]

INTERVENTIONAL ULTRASOUND AND THE SPLEEN

Despite the fact that ultrasound-guided fine-needle aspiration biopsy and catheter drainage have been established as safe and successful techniques for most areas of the abdomen, many interventional radiologists have been reluctant to apply these techniques to the spleen. The main concern has been fear of bleeding due to the highly vascular nature of the organ. Reluctance also exists because of the frequent necessity to transgress the pleural space or colon to reach the spleen. However, in recent years a number of reports have appeared of ultrasound-guided interventional procedures in the spleen, with safety and success records similar to those obtained elsewhere in the abdomen.[14,51-55] Fine- and core-cutting needle biopsies have been performed for the diagnosis of focal lesions, including abscesses, sarcoidosis, primary splenic malignancies, metastases, and lymphoma. Successful catheter drainage of abscesses, cysts, hematomas, and infected necrotic tumors have been reported. However, only very small numbers of cases have been reported and further experience will be needed to verify the safety and efficacy of these procedures.

Pitfalls

There are several sonographic pitfalls that one must be wary of when scanning the left upper quadrant and spleen. The first of these is the crescentic echo-poor area superior to the spleen that can be caused by the left lobe of the liver in thin individuals (Fig. 5-29).[56-59] This can mimic the appearance of a subcapsular hematoma or subphrenic abscess. The correct interpretation can be made by noting the hypoechoic liver slide over the more echogenic spleen during quiet respiration. It would be desirable to follow the liver from the anterior axillary line in the midline over to the posterior axillary line in the coronal plane, but this is usually not possible because of the presence of gas in the stomach.

Hepatic and/or portal veins may help to identify this structure as the liver.

The tail of the pancreas may look large and simulate a mass adjacent to the hilum of the spleen. This is particularly true if the plane of section is aimed along the long axis of the tail of the pancreas. Identifying the splenic artery and vein may be helpful to confirm this as the normal tail of the pancreas.

Similarly, the fundus of the stomach may nestle in the hilum of the spleen. A particular oblique plane of section may pass through the spleen and include the hilum with an echogenic portion of the stomach simulating an intrasplenic lesion. Sometimes this is just the fat around the stomach. Occasionally, fluid in the fundus of the stomach can simulate an intrasplenic fluid collection or an abscess in the hilum of the spleen. This can usually be resolved by scanning transversely, and, if necessary, giving the patient water to drink.

An occasional anatomic variant can occur if the inferior portion of the spleen lies posterolateral to the upper pole of the left kidney. This variant has been called the retrorenal spleen. Knowledge of this variant can prevent the misdiagnosis of an abnormal mass. Furthermore, if visualized sonographically, it should be avoided in any interventional procedure on the left kidney.[60]

Finally, it can be very difficult to determine the site of origin of large, left upper quadrant masses, arising from the spleen, left adrenal gland, left kidney, tail of the pancreas, stomach, or retroperitoneum. Differential

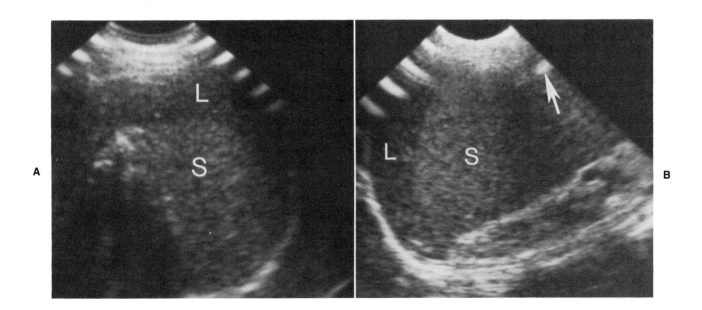

FIG 5-29. Potential pitfall. **A,** Transverse scan. **B,** Sagittal scan. Both scans show the crescentic echo-poor enlarged left lobe of the liver *(L)* anterior and superior to the more echogenic spleen *(S)*. This should not be mistaken for a fluid collection. Gas *(arrow)* within the stomach.

motion observed during shallow respiration can sometimes be helpful. Additionally, the identification of the splenic vein entering the splenic hilum can be definitive. CT or MRI can usually solve difficult cases.

REFERENCES
Embryology and anatomy

1. Vibhakar SD, Bellon EM: The bare area of the spleen: a constant computed tomography feature of the ascitic abdomen. *AJR* 1984;141(5):953-955.

Examination technique

2. Hicken P, Sauerbrei EE, Cooperberg PL: Ultrasonic coronal scanning of left upper quadrant. *J Can Assoc Radiol* 1981;32:107-110.

Pathologic conditions of the spleen

3. Briarman RS, Beck JW, Corobkin M, et al: *AJR* 1982;138:329-333.
4. Frank K, Linhart P, Kortsik C, et al: Sonographic determination of spleen size: normal dimensions in adults with a healthy spleen. *Ultraschall Med* 1986;7(3):134-137.
5. Manoharan A, Chen CF, Wilson LS, et al: Ultrasonic characterization of splenic tissue in myelofibrosis: further evidence for reversal of fibrosis with chemotherapy. *Eur J Haematol* 1988;40(2):149-154.
6. Wilson LS, Robinson DE, Griffiths KA, et al: Evaluation of ultrasonic attenuation in diffuse diseases of spleen and liver. *Ultrasound Imaging* 1987;9(4):236-247.
7. Robinson DE, Gill RW, Kossoff G: Quantitative sonography. *Ultrasound Med Biol* 1986;12(7):555-565.
8. Franquet T, Montes M, Lecumberri FJ, et al: Hydatid disease of the spleen: imaging findings in nine patients. *AJR* 1990;154(3):525-528.
9. Al-Moyaya S, Al-Awami M, Vaidya MP, et al: Hydatid cyst of the spleen. *Am J Trop Med Hyg* 1986;35(5):995-999.
10. Bhimji SD, Cooperberg PL, Naiman S: Ultrasound diagnosis of splenic cysts. *Radiology* 1977;122:787-789.
11. Thurber LA, Cooperberg PL, Clemente JG, et al: Echogenic fluid: a pitfall in the ultrasonographic diagnosis of cystic lesions. *JCU* 1979;7:273-278.
12. Propper RA, Weinstein BJ, Skolnick ML, et al: Ultrasonography of hemorrhagic splenic cysts. *JCU* 1979;7:18-20.
13. Duddy MJ, Calder CJ: Cystic hemangioma of the spleen: findings on ultrasound and computed tomography. *Br J Radiol* 1989;62(734):180-182.
14. Quinn SF, van Sonnenberg E, Casola G, et al: Interventional radiology in the spleen. *Radiology* 1986;161:289-291.
15. Learner RM, Spataro RF: Splenic abscess:percutaneous drainage. *Radiology* 1984;153:643-645.
16. Hess CF, Griebel J, Schmiedl U, et al: Focal lesions of the spleen: preliminary results with fast magnetic resonance imaging at 1.5 T. *J Comput Assist Tomogr* 1988;12(4):569-574.
17. Schaeffer A, Vasile N: Computed tomography of sarcoidosis (case report). *J Comput Assist Tomogr* 1986;10(4):679-680.
18. Iwasaki M, Hiyama Y, Myojo S, et al: Primary malignant lymphoma of the spleen: report of a case. *Rinsho Hoshasen* 1988;33(3):405-408.
19. Costello P, Kane RA, Oster J, et al: Focal splenic disease demonstrated by ultrasound and computed tomography. *J Can Assoc Radiol* 1985;36:22-28.
20. Sammis AF Jr, Weitzman S, Arcomano JP: Hemangiolymphangioma of spleen and bone. *NY State J Med* 1971;71:1762-1764.
21. Manor A, Starinsky R, Gorfinkel D, et al: Ultrasound features of a symptomatic splenic hemangioma. *J Clin Ultrasound* 1984;12:95-97.
22. Pakter RL, Fishman EK, Nussbaum A, et al: Computed tomography findings in splenic hemangiomas in the Klippel-Trenaunay-Weber syndrome. *J Comput Assist Tomogr* 1987;11(1):88-91.
23. Ross PR, Moser RP, Dackman AH, et al: Hemangioma of the spleen: radiologic-pathologic correlation in ten cases. *AJR* 1987;162:73-77.
24. Moss CN, Van Dyke JA, Koehler RE, et al: Multiple cavernous hemangiomas of the spleen: computed tomography findings. *J Comput Assist Tomogr* 1986;10(2):338-340.
25. Kagalwala TY, Vaidya VU, Bharucha BA, et al: Cavernous hemangiomas of the liver and spleen. *Indian Pediatr* 1987;24(5):427-430.
26. Pistoia F, Markowitz SK: Splenic lymphangiomatosis: computed tomography diagnosis. *AJR* 1988;150:121-122.
27. Maresca G, Mirk P, DeGaetano AM, et al: Sonographic patterns in splenic infarction. *J Clin Ultrasound* 1986;14:23-28.
28. Balcar I, Seltzer SE, Davis S, Geller S: Computed tomography patterns of splenic infarction: a clinical and experimental study. *Radiology* 1984;151:723-729.
29. Hill SC, Reinig JW, Barranger JA, et al: Gaucher's disease: sonographic appearance of spleen. *Radiology* 1986; 160:631-634.
30. Stevens PG, Kumari-Subaiya SS, Kahn LB: Splenic involvement in Gaucher's disease: sonographic findings. *J Clin Ultrasound* 1987;15:397-400.
31. Cerri GG, Alvis VAF, Magalhaes A: Hepatosplenic schistosomiasis Mansoni: ultrasound manifestations. *Radiology* 1984; 153:777-780.
32. Pastakia B, Shawker TH, Thalar M, et al: Hepatosplenic Candidiasis: wheels within wheels. *Radiology* 1988;166:417-421.
33. Jeffrey RB, Laing FC, Federle MP et al: Computed tomography of splenic trauma. *Radiology* 1981;141:729-732.
34. Koropkin M, Moss AA, Callan PW, et al: Computed tomography of subcapsular splenic hematoma. *Radiology* 1978;129:441-445.
35. Lupien C, Sauerbrie EE: Healing in the traumatized spleen: Sonographic investigation. *Radiology* 1984;150:181-185.
36. Epstein NB, Omar GM: Infective complications of splenic trauma. *Clin Radiol* 1983;34:91-94.
37. Langer R, Langer M, Schutze B, et al: Ultrasound findings in patients with AIDS. *Digitale Bilddiagn* 1988;8(2):93-96.
38. Yee JM, Raghavendra BN, Horii SC, et al: Abdominal sonography in AIDS: a review. *J Ultrasound Med* 1989;8(12):705-714.
39. Spouge AR, Wilson SR, Gopinath N, et al: Extrapulmonary pneumocystis carinii in a patient with AIDS: sonographic findings. *AJR* 1990;155(1):76-78.
40. Hansen S, Jarhult J: Accessory spleen imaging: radionuclide, ultrasound and computed tomography investigations in a patient with thrombocytopenia 25 years after splenectomy for ITP. *Scand J Haematol* 1986;37(1):74-77.
41. Mostbeck G, Sommer G, Haller J, et al: Accessory spleen: presentation as a large abdominal mass in an asymptomatic young woman. *Gastrointest Radiol* 1987;12(4):337-339.
42. Muller H, Schneider H, Ruckauer K, et al: Accessory spleen torsion: clinical picture, sonographic diagnosis and differential diagnosis. *Klin Pediatr* 1988;200(5):419-421.
43. Nino-Murcia M, Friedland GW, Gross D: Imaging the effects of an ectopic spleen on the urinary tract. *Urol Radiol* 1988;10(4):195-197.
44. Plaja Ramon P, Aso Puertolas C, Sanchis Solera L: Wandering spleen: discussion apropos of a case. *An Esp Pediatr* 1987;26(1):69-70.
45. Scicolone G, Contin I, Bano A, et al: Wandering spleen: preoperative diagnosis by echotomography of the abdomen. *Chir Ital* 1986;38(1):72-79.

46. Azoulay D, Gossot D, Sarfati E, et al: Volvulus of a mobile spleen: apropos of a case diagnosed in the preoperative period by ultrasonography. *J Chir* 1987;124(10):520-522.

47. Maillard JC, Menu Y, Scherrer A, et al. Intraperitoneal splenosis: diagnosis by ultrasound and computed tomography. *Gastrointest Radiol* 1989;14(2):179-180.

48. Delamarre J, Capron JP, Drouard F, et al: Splenosis: ultrasound and computed tomography findings in a case complicated by an intraperitoneal implant traumatic hematoma. *Gastrointest Radiol.* 1988;13(3):275-278.

49. Turk CO, Lipson SB, Brandt TD: Splenosis mimicking a renal mass. *Urology.* 1988;31(3):248-250.

50. Nishitani H, Hayashi T, Onitsuka H, et al. Computed tomography of accessory spleens. *Radiat Med.* 1984;2(4):222.

51. Vyborny CJ, Merrill TN, Reda J, et al. Subacute subcapsular hematoma of the spleen complicating pancreatitis: successful percutaneous drainage. *Radiology.* 1989;169:161-162.

Interventional ultrasound and the spleen

52. Suzuki T, Shibuya H, Yoshimatsu S, et al. Ultrasonically guided staging splenic tissue core biopsy in patients with non-Hodgkin's lymphoma. *Cancer.* 1987;60:879-882.

53. Taavitsainen M, Koivuniemi A, Helminen J, et al. Aspiration biopsy of the spleen in patients with sarcoidosis. *Acta Radiol.* 1987;28:723-725.

54. Suzuki T, Shibuya H, Yoshimatsu S, et al. Ultrasonically guided staging splenic tissue core biopsy in patients with non-Hodgkin's lymphoma. *Cancer.* 1987; 60(4):879-882.

55. Suzuki T. Ultrasonically guided splenic biopsy in patients with malignant lymphoma. *Nippon Igaku Hoshasen Gakkai Zasshi.* 1988;48(8):982-987.

56. Rao MG. Enlarged left lobe of the liver mistaken for a mass in the splenic region. *Clin Nucl Med.* 1989;14(2):134.

57. Li DK, Cooperberg PL, Graham MF, et al. Psuedo peri-splenic "fluid collections": a clue to normal liver and spleen echogenic texture. *J Ultrasound Med* 1986;5(7):397-400.

58. Crivello MS, Peterson IM, Austin RM: Left lobe of the liver mimicking perisplenic collections. *JCU* 14(9):697-701.

59. Arenson AM, McKee JD: Left upper quadrant pseudolesion secondary to normal variants in liver and spleen. *JCU* 1986; 14(7):558-561.

60. Dodds WJ, Darweesh RMA, Lawson TL, et al: The retroperitoneal spaces revisited. *AJR* 1986; 174:1155-1161.

The Gallbladder and Bile Ducts

■ Faye C. Laing, M.D.

Despite the availability of sophisticated imaging modalities, especially CT and, more recently, MRI, sonography remains the initial screening modality of choice for evaluating the appearance of the gallbladder and bile ducts. The advantages of sonography include:

- High sensitivity and accuracy for detecting gallstones as well as intrahepatic and extrahepatic bile duct dilatation
- Lack of ionizing radiation; no need for contrast material
- Speed, safety, flexibility, and portability
- Independence of gastrointestinal, hepatic, and biliary function
- Multiple organ examination

Indications for performing sonography of the gallbladder and biliary tree include signs and symptoms of acute or chronic cholecystitis and jaundice, abnormal liver function tests, and pancreatitis.

GALLBLADDER
Normal Anatomy

A normal gallbladder should be visible in virtually all patients if it is physiologically distended following an 8- to 12-hour fast. Rarely, massive obesity or overlying distended bowel loops preclude a satisfactory examination. The anatomic position of the gallbladder fundus can vary dramatically from one patient to another. It may even vary quite markedly in a single patient depending upon the patient's position. The neck of the gallbladder, however, bears a fixed anatomic relationship to the main lobar fissure and the undivided right portal vein.[1] In approximately 70% of patients a linear echo, thought to represent a portion of the main lobar fissure, can be identified connecting the gallbladder to the right or main portal vein (Fig. 6-1).[2] This anatomic consideration becomes important for conclusively identifying the gallbladder in patients with pathologic conditions such as small contracted gallbladders or gallbladders filled with calculi.

Because the **size** and **shape** of the normal gallbladder vary widely in individual patients, it is difficult to formulate precise size criteria. In general, if its transverse diameter exceeds 5 cm and if it is no longer ovoid but rounded in shape, the gallbladder is likely to be hydropic.[3] Conversely, if its diameter is less than 2 cm despite adequate fasting, the gallbladder is likely to be abnormally contracted. Gallbladder volume measurements may be useful for physiologic evaluation of gallbladder contractility. Calculation of gallbladder volume can be obtained most easily by assuming the gallbladder has an ellipsoid shape and using the formula

$$V = .52 (L \times W \times H)$$

or by using a sonic digitizer and a digital computer.[4, 5]

Although the shape of a typical gallbladder is oval or gourdlike, it frequently varies from this configuration because of apparent folding or kinking. True septations

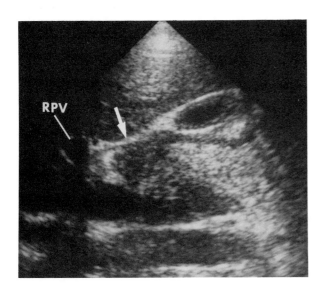

FIG 6-1. The interlobar hepatic fissure, a useful anatomic landmark for identifying the gallbladder fossa is seen on longitudinal scan through the right hepatic lobe as a linear echo *(arrow)* extending between the right portal vein *(RPV)* and the gallbladder neck. Thickening of the gallbladder wall has resulted from physiologic contraction.

(From Laing FC, Filly RA, Gooding GAW: Ultrasonography of the liver and biliary tract. In: Margulis AR, Burhenne HJ, eds: *Alimentary Tract Radiology.* 4th ed. St. Louis: CV Mosby Co; 1989.)

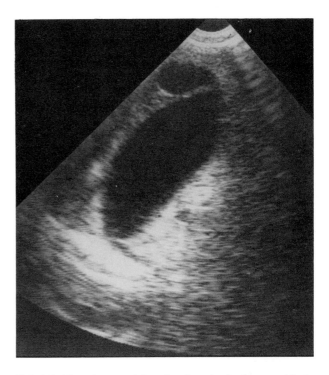

FIG 6-2. Phrygian cap deformity. Longitudinal scan with the gallbladder fundus appearing to be folded on the body.

(From Laing FC: Ultrasonography of the gallbladder and biliary tree. In: Sarti DA, ed: *Diagnostic Ultrasound: Text and Cases.* 2nd ed. Chicago: Yearbook Medical Publishers; 1987.)

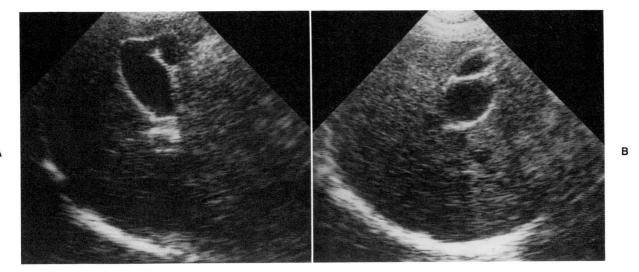

FIG 6-3. Phrygian cap. **A,** Longitudinal scan shows a typical appearance. **B,** On transverse image, a confusing picture is present, suggesting that the sonolucency anterior to the gallbladder could be caused by an abscess, hematoma, or liver cyst.

(From Laing FC: Ultrasonography of the gallbladder and biliary tree. In: Sarti DA, ed: *Diagnostic Ultrasound: Text and Cases.* 2nd ed. Chicago: Yearbook Medical Publishers; 1987.)

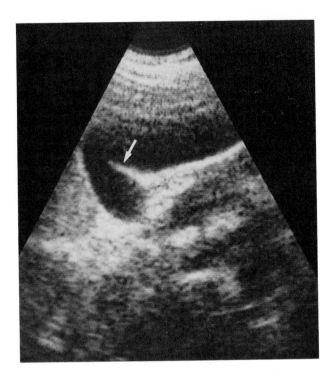

FIG 6-4. Junctional fold *(arrow)*, a common anatomic variant between the body and infundibulum of the gallbladder seen on longitudinal scan.
(From Laing FC: Ultrasonography of the gallbladder and biliary tree. In: Sarti DA, ed: *Diagnostic Ultrasound: Text and Cases.* 2nd ed. Chicago: Yearbook Medical Publishers; 1987.)

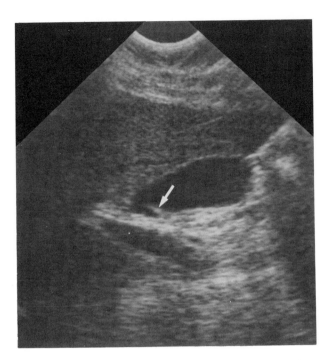

FIG 6-5. Junctional fold *(arrow)* seen on longitudinal scan as a small linear echo in the proximal portion of the gallbladder. This appearance could be confused with a small calculus, especially if shadowing is present. A repeat scan following a deep inspiratory effort often eliminates the junctional fold.
(From Laing FC: Ultrasonography of the gallbladder and biliary tree. In: Sarti DA, ed: *Diagnostic Ultrasound: Text and Cases.* 2nd ed. Chicago: Yearbook Medical Publishers; 1987.)

are rare but in approximately 4% of patients a **phrygian cap deformity** is present in which the gallbladder fundus appears to be folded upon the body (Figs. 6-2 and 6-3).[6,7] A more frequent variation is the presence of a fold between the body and infundibulum of the gallbladder, known as a junctional fold (Fig. 6-4).[7] Any fold in the gallbladder can produce high-amplitude echoes that occasionally may be associated with posterior acoustic shadowing caused by refractive effects (Fig. 6-5). This appearance can cause folds to be mistaken for polyps and/or calculi. An awareness of these variations as well as meticulous scanning technique should minimize diagnostic errors.

The normal **gallbladder wall** is visible as a pencil-thin echogenic line that is less than 3 mm thick. Although the gallbladder may be normally indented by adjacent bowel loops, focal impressions upon it from the liver suggest the presence of an hepatic mass. Because bile does not contain particulate material, the gallbladder lumen is normally echo free.

Scanning Techniques

To ensure adequate gallbladder distension, the examination should be performed after an overnight fast of 8 to 12 hours. Fasting is necessary to avoid diagnostic er-

rors. Physiologic gallbladder contraction causes the gallbladder to appear small and thick-walled; this could be misinterpreted as a pathologic condition. Real-time equipment minimizes operator dependency and allows rapid and complete display of the entire gallbladder. For most patients, a sector transducer is better than a linear array, because the smaller sector transducer can be more optimally positioned subcostally or within rib interspaces. The highest-frequency transducer that can satisfactorily image the gallbladder should be used. For most patients, a 3.5-MHz transducer is necessary. In thin patients or in those with an anteriorly positioned gallbladder, a 5-MHz transducer should be used to provide superior resolution. Optimal images usually require the patient to suspend respiration following a deep inspiratory effort.

A thorough examination of the gallbladder can usually be accomplished in 5 to 10 minutes. The scans are performed from a lower intercostal, or preferably a subcostal approach with the patient supine or in a left posterior oblique position. Occasionally, however, scans should be performed with the patient in an erect or prone position in order to convincingly demonstrate calculi mobility.[8] Cholecystosonography requires meticulous scanning technique to avoid overlooking small calculi. Special attention should be directed to the most dependent region of the gallbladder, where most calculi are found. In most patients this is the region of the gallbladder neck and the cystic duct.

Pathology

Cholelithiasis.   Detection of cholelithiasis is the primary role of gallbladder sonography. Since Hublitz et al[9] first reported the ultrasonographic detection of gallstones in 4 of 8 patients, cholecystosonographic visualization of calculi has improved dramatically. As a result of reported sensitivities and accuracies of greater than 95%,[10-12] ultrasonography has essentially replaced oral cholecystography as the examination of choice for detecting cholelithiasis. Furthermore, not infrequently, ultrasound detects gallstones that are not visualized on technically adequate oral cholecystograms.[10,13] Although a recently reported comparative study between oral cholecystography and cholecystosonography suggested that the sensitivity of these two examinations for detecting gallbladder disease was similar,[14] close scrutiny of the statistics reveals that oral cholecystography detected stones in 65% of patients with cholelithiasis whereas ultrasound detected stones in 93% of patients with cholelithiasis.[15] Nonetheless, renewed interest in oral cholecystography has recently occurred as a result of the development of nonsurgical therapy for gallstone removal. Although ultrasound may be superior for gallstone detection, oral cholecystography may be superior for evaluating the number and size of stones, as well as demonstrating cystic duct patency.[16]

Because gallstones both absorb and reflect the ultrasound beam, the net sonographic effect is a **highly reflective echo** originating from the anterior surface of the calculus with a prominent **posterior acoustic shadow.** The demonstration of a posterior acoustic shadow is important. Shadowing echo densities that originate within the gallbladder correlate with cholelithiasis virtually 100% of the time, whereas nonshadowing echo densities correlate with calculi in only 50% of cases.[11] To visualize a posterior acoustic shadow optimally, it is important to use a transducer with the highest possible frequency that is focused maximally at the depth of the stone (Fig. 6-6). The combination of a narrow sound beam with the stone centrally positioned in the beam is optimal for creating an acoustic shadow. In vitro studies have shown that all gallstones whose diameters exceed 1 mm should cast an acoustic shadow, regardless of composition, surface characteristics, or shape of the calculus.[17,18] Because very small calculi may fail to demonstrate acoustic shadowing, it is sometimes advantageous to reposition the patient in an attempt to pile small stones upon one another (Fig. 6-7). The effect of

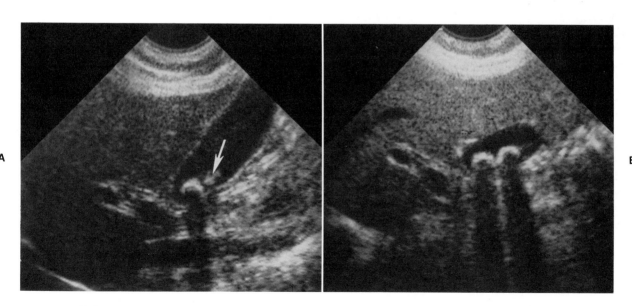

A   B

FIG 6-6. Cholelithiasis. **A,** Two stones are located near the gallbladder neck. One has acoustic shadowing. Lack of shadowing from the second stone *(arrow)* is due to its position, which is slightly off center with respect to the transducer beam. **B,** A repeat scan performed with both stones in the central portion of the beam shows two acoustic shadows.

(From Laing FC: Ultrasonography of the gallbladder and biliary tree. In: Sarti DA, ed: *Diagnostic Ultrasound: Text and Cases.* 2nd ed. Chicago: Yearbook Medical Publishers; 1987.)

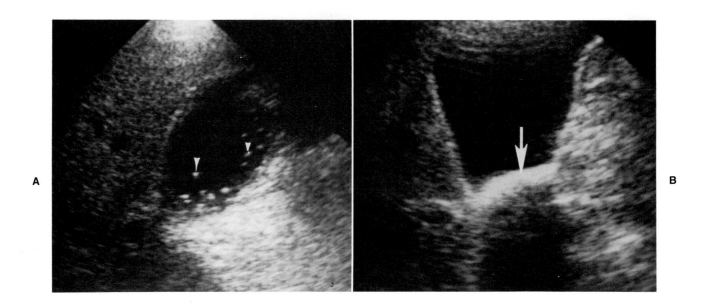

FIG 6-7. Cholelithiasis. **A,** Multiple small nonshadowing echogenic foci *(arrowheads)* are seen in the gallbladder lumen immediately after turning the patient in an attempt to demonstrate mobility of calculi. **B,** Subsequent settling of the stones to the dependent region of the gallbladder *(arrow)* shows a prominent acoustic shadow below the stones that is caused by the additive effect of multiple small stones lying upon one another.

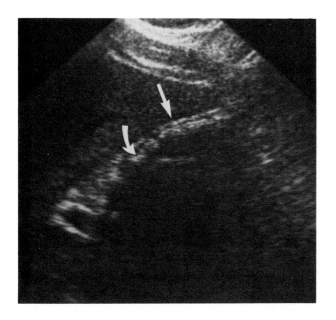

FIG 6-8. Wall-echo shadow (WES) triad. The gallbladder is filled with multiple stones and may not be visible. Instead, one may see the anterior gallbladder wall *(straight arrow)* with an adjacent superficial layer of calculi *(curved arrow).*
(From Laing FC, Filly RA, Gooding GAW: Ultrasonography of the liver and biliary tract. In: Margulis AR, Burhenne HJ, eds: *Alimentary Tract Radiology.* 4th ed. St. Louis: CV Mosby Co; 1989.)

this maneuver is to form an aggregate of small stones that acoustically behaves like a larger stone in that it casts a posterior acoustic shadow. In addition, the time–gain compensation curve should be adjusted so that acoustic enhancement behind the gallbladder does not obliterate a faint acoustic shadow.

The diagnosis of calculus disease can also be made confidently when gravity-dependent **movement** of a stone is demonstrated. Except when a stone is impacted in the gallbladder neck or is adherent to the gallbladder wall, calculi should be mobile. On rare occasions, **sludge balls**[19] or **tumefactive biliary sludge**[20] can appear as mobile masses within the gallbladder lumen. The nature of this material varies from case to case and includes parasites, blood clots, aggregated pus, sludge, and contrast material. In contradistinction to calculi, this material is evanescent and is not associated with posterior acoustic shadowing.

As the gallbladder becomes **filled with stones,** its ultrasound appearance changes dramatically. Instead of visualizing the outline of the gallbladder, a high-amplitude reflection with a prominent acoustic shadow emanates from the gallbladder fossa (Fig. 6-8). The echoshadow complex originates from the most superficial layer of stones. The deeper calculi as well as the intraluminal bile and outline of the gallbladder are rendered invisible.[21] Close scrutiny of these images usually reveals characteristic findings that have been described as the **wall-echo-shadow (WES triad),**[22] or the **double arc shadow sign.**[23] These signs consist of two parallel curved echogenic lines separated by a thin anechoic space with distal acoustic shadowing. The proximal echogenic line is the result of the near wall of the gallbladder whereas the deeper echogenic line is the result of the anterior surface of the gallstone that causes the acoustic shadow. A similar appearance can also occur with calcification in the gallbladder wall **(porcelain gallbladder)**[24] or air in the gallbladder wall.[25,26] In patients with emphysematous cholecystitis, reverberation echoes from the air suggest the correct diagnosis.

Wall Changes. The most frequent gallbladder-wall abnormality detected by sonography is **diffuse thickening,** which is diagnosed when the wall is greater than 3 mm thick (Fig. 6-9). Wall thickening typically appears as a hypoechoic region between two echogenic lines. Although initially described as highly specific for cholecystitis, diffuse wall thickening is now recognized as neither sensitive nor specific for an inflammatory process. Approximately 50% to 75% of patients with acute cholecystitis have diffusely thickened gallbladder walls whereas fewer than 25% of patients with chronic cholecystitis have this finding.[3,27,28]

Other conditions associated with diffuse gallbladder wall thickening include hepatic dysfunction (associated with alcoholism, hypoalbuminemia, ascites, and hepati-

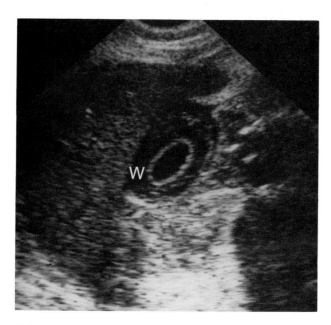

FIG 6-9. Diffuse gallbladder wall thickening *(W)* presents as hypoechoic ring associated with severe hypoalbuminemia.
(From Laing FC: Ultrasonography of the gallbladder and biliary tree. In: Sarti DA, ed: *Diagnostic Ultrasound: Text and Cases.* 2nd ed. Chicago: Yearbook Medical Publishers; 1987.)

tis), congestive heart failure, renal disease, AIDS, and sepsis.[29-33] Although a unifying pathophysiologic mechanism may not explain these diverse disease processes, many of these patients have decreased intravascular osmotic pressure and elevated portal venous pressure. In addition, because of the underlying disease processes, many patients with diffuse gallbladder wall thickening also have ascites. Several recent investigations have suggested that ultrasound may be useful for distinguishing benign from malignant ascites by measuring the thickness of the gallbladder wall.[34-36] Malignant ascites is usually associated with normal gallbladder wall thickness whereas many benign causes are associated with an abnormally thickened gallbladder wall (Fig. 6-10). In the study by Huang et al[34], a normal gallbladder wall thickness could predict malignant ascites with a sensitivity of 81% and a specificity of 94%.

Another cause of generalized gallbladder wall thickening is partial contraction caused by eating (Fig. 6-1). If the maximum diameter of the gallbladder is less than 2 cm and if diffuse wall thickening is present, the sonographer should inquire as to whether or not the patient fasted appropriately before the ultrasound examination.

In contrast to diffuse gallbladder wall thickening, **focal gallbladder wall thickening** strongly suggests primary gallbladder disease (Fig. 6-11). **Gallbladder carcinoma** is most often visualized as a mass that fills or replaces the gallbladder lumen. In approximately 40% of cases, it is seen as either a focal mass that protrudes into the gallbladder lumen or as an asymmetrically thickened wall.[37] Additional findings include variable degrees of gallbladder wall calcification, liver metastases, evidence for direct hepatic invasion, adenopathy, bile duct dilatation, and cholelithiasis (80% to 90% of cases) (Figs. 6-12 and 6-13). Other causes of focal gallbladder wall thickening are polyps (adenomatous, cholesterol), papillary adenomas, metastatic nodules (melanoma, pancreatic),[38,39] adenomyomatosis, and occasionally, tumefactive sludge (Fig. 6-14). In patients with **adenomyomatosis,** anechoic or echogenic foci may sometimes be visible within the thickened gallbladder wall. **Intraluminal diverticula (Rokitansky-Aschoff sinuses or RAS)** that contain bile are most likely to be responsible for the anechoic areas whereas biliary sludge or gallstones within the diverticula are most likely to responsible for echogenic foci.[40] Not infrequently, a V-shaped reverberation artifact is seen to emanate from small cholesterol stones that are lodged within the RAS (Fig. 6-15).[41] This artifact occurs as a result of sound reverberating within or between cholesterol crystals and may be similar in appearance to comet-tail artifacts that occur when there is air in the gallbladder wall. In the latter condition, however, the reverberation artifact is usually longer (more comet-tail

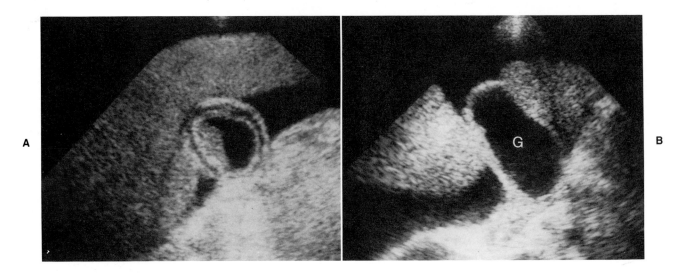

FIG 6-10. Ascites and gallbladder wall thickening. **A,** Gallbladder wall is abnormally thickened; the patient had chronic liver disease and benign ascites. **B,** The gallbladder *(G)* wall is of normal thickness in this patient with malignant ascites.

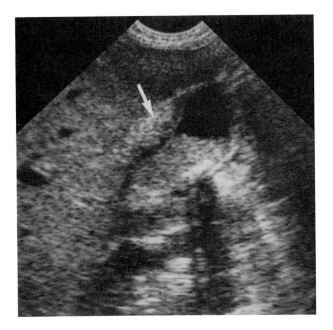

FIG 6-11. Primary gallbladder carcinoma *(arrow)* seen as localized thickening of the anterior gallbladder wall. The dependent portion of the gallbladder is filled with sludge and numerous small stones.

(From Laing FC: Ultrasonography of the gallbladder and biliary tree. In: Sarti DA, ed: *Diagnostic Ultrasound: Text and Cases.* 2nd ed. Chicago: Yearbook Medical Publishers; 1987.)

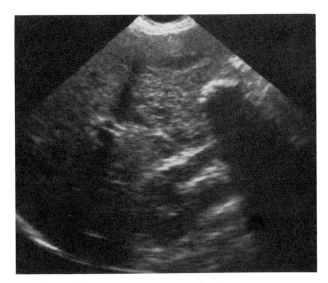

FIG 6-12. Carcinoma of the gallbladder. Sagittal sonogram shows a large gallstone that is trapped by a solid mass that completely fill the gallbladder.

(Courtesy Wilson SR, MD, Toronto Hospital, Canada.)

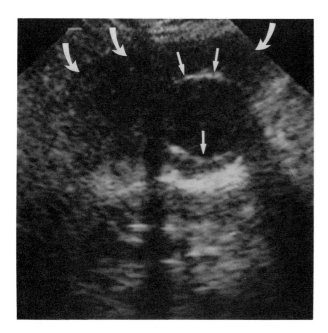

FIG 6-13. Gallbladder carcinoma. A thin echogenic line appears to outline the gallbladder wall *(arrows)* and is caused by calcification within the wall. In addition, a poorly defined hypoechoic mass surrounds the gallbladder anteriorly and is caused by direct invitation of tumor into the liver *(curved arrows)*.

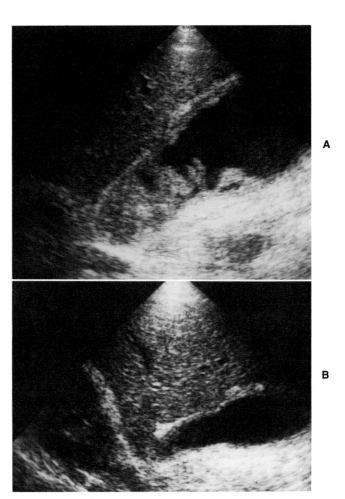

FIG 6-14. Tumefactive sludge simulating neoplasm. **A,** Nonshadowing echogenic material is visible in the gallbladder and the gallbladder wall appears to be mildly thickened. **B,** Scan obtained 10 days later shows disappearance of this echogenic material.

in appearance as opposed to V-shaped) and the patient is acutely ill. Focal gallbladder wall irregularities may also be seen in patients with gangrenous cholecystitis. These irregularities correspond to areas of mucosal ulceration, hemorrhage, necrosis, and/or microabscess formation.[42]

Sludge. Echogenic bile or sludge is a term used to describe the presence of particulate material (specifically calcium bilirubinate and/or cholesterol crystals) in bile.[43] Unlike gallstones, which generate strong echoes, sludge characteristically displays low- to mid-level echoes (Fig. 6-16). It is never accompanied by posterior acoustic shadowing unless stones are also present (Fig. 6-17). Because of its viscous nature, sludge moves sluggishly after the patient has been repositioned.

The most frequent predisposing factor associated with sludge is bile stasis. This can occur in patients who undergo prolonged fasting or hyperalimentation, as well as in patients with biliary obstruction at the level of the gallbladder, cystic duct, or common bile duct. In a series of fasting patients, ultrasound detected gallbladder sludge in 4% of patients within 5 days after surgery and in 31% of patients within 10 days after surgery.[44] In patients receiving total parenteral nutrition, sludge was uniformly present after 6 weeks of treatment.[45]

Although gallbladder sludge suggests an underlying abnormality, its presence does not necessarily imply primary gallbladder pathology. The clinical significance of sludge remains uncertain. In rare instances sludge or sludge balls have been observed to develop into gallstones.[46] Follow-up ultrasound studies performed on 12 postoperative patients with gallbladder sludge revealed the presence of gallstones in 3 patients who were examined 6 months after their initial surgery.[44] These studies involve a limited numbers of patients; further investigation is required to determine whether or not sludge can irritate the gallbladder mucosa and act as a precursor to stone formation.

Pericholecystic Fluid. Localized pericholecystic fluid is most often attributable to acute cholecystitis, complicated by gallbladder perforation and abscess formation. Ultrasound can diagnose this condition by visu-

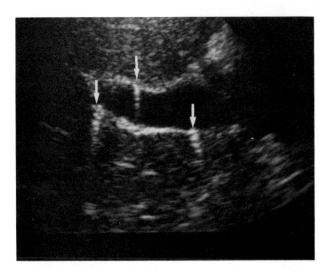

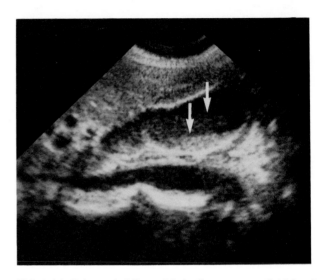

FIG 6-15. Adenomyomatosis with small cholesterol crystals lodged within Rokitansky-Aschoff sinuses. V-shaped reverberation artifacts emanate from the anterior and posterior walls of the gallbladder *(arrows).*

FIG 6-16. Echogenic bile or "sludge" creates two fluid levels *(arrows)* in this gallbladder. The most dependent layer of sludge has the highest concentration of crystalline material; the second layer (centrally located) is less echogenic.
(From Laing FC: Ultrasonography of the gallbladder and biliary tree. In: Sarti DA, ed: *Diagnostic Ultrasound: Text and Cases.* 2nd ed. Chicago: Yearbook Medical Publishers; 1987.)

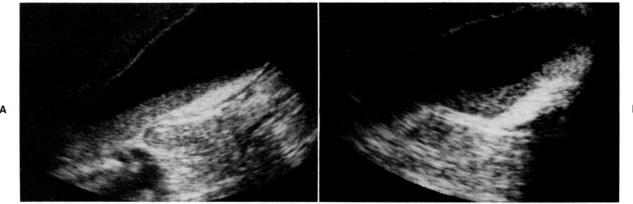

FIG 6-17. Biliary sludge and stones. **A,** The gallbladder contains what appears to be two different layers of echogenic bile. **B,** After placing the patient into a decubitus position, acoustic shadowing becomes visible from the dependent echogenic material because of aggregation of small stones.

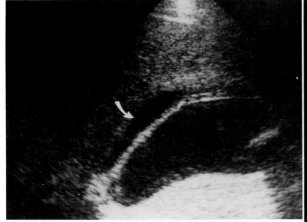

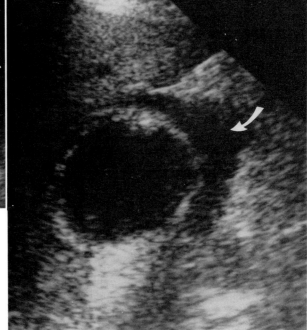

FIG 6-18. Localized pericholecystic fluid *(curved arrow)*, caused by gangrenous cholecystitis and fundic gallbladder perforation seen on longitudinal (**A,**) and transverse (**B,**) scans. A gallstone is seen in the fundus of the gallbladder.
(From Laing FC, Jeffrey RB, Federle MP: Gallbladder and bile ducts. In: Jeffrey RD, ed: *Computed Tomography and Sonography of the Acute Abdomen.* New York: Raven Press; 1989: 59-62.)

alizing an anechoic or complex fluid collection adjacent to or surrounding the gallbladder (Fig. 6-18).[47]

Rarely, an isolated pericholecystic fluid collection can be seen in patients with pancreatitis, peptic ulcer disease, or both (Fig. 6-19).[48] This fluid presumably results from extension of the primary inflammatory process along the hepatoduodenal ligament into the main lobar fissure, where it comes to rest adjacent to the gallbladder neck.

Acute Cholecystitis. Acute cholecystitis occurs in approximately one third of patients who have gallstones and is caused by persistent calculous obstruction of the gallbladder neck or cystic duct. This results in inflammation of the gallbladder wall with variable degrees of necrosis and infection. The physical findings in these patients range from mild to dramatic. Typically, there is some degree of right upper-quadrant tenderness and guarding, although with advanced gallbladder inflammation or in elderly patients the findings may suggest diffuse peritonitis, or there may be deceptively few signs and symptoms, respectively.

In western countries, cholesterol stones predominate (as opposed to pigment stones, which are composed of calcium bilirubinate). The incidence of cholesterol gallstones is almost three times higher in women than in men and increases with age and possibly, multiparity. The differential diagnosis for acute cholecystitis is extensive and includes pancreatitis, appendicitis, peptic disease, hepatitis, perihepatitis (Curtis Fitz-Hugh syndrome), liver abscess, or liver neoplasm, as well as re-

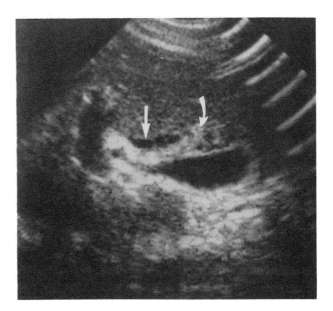

FIG 6-19. Localized pericholecystic fluid anterior to the gallbladder neck *(arrow)* is caused by inflammation in association with pancreatitis seen on longitudinal sonogram. The gallbladder wall *(curved arrow)* is thickened and irregularly sonolucent.
(From Nyberg DA, Laing FC: Ultrasonographic findings in peptic ulcer disease and pancreatitis that simulate primary gallbladder disease. *J Ultrasound Med.* 1983;2:303-307.)

nal and even intrathoracic conditions (pneumonia and cardiac disease).

Acute cholecystitis is associated with cholelithiasis in approximately 90% to 95% of patients. In the remaining 5% to 10% of patients in whom acalculous cholecystitis occurs, morbidity and mortality is much greater because this disease frequently complicates a prolonged critical illness. Although many patients with acute right upper quadrant pain are suspected of having acute cholecystitis, only one third are subsequently proved to have this disease.[27] Sonography can be used to confirm the diagnosis of acute cholecystitis[3,27,49]; it can distinguish acute from chronic cholecystitis with an accuracy of 95% to 99%[10-12], and it can frequently suggest nonbiliary causes for the patient's symptoms. Tests using technetium-tagged IDA and IDA-like compounds are also sensitive and accurate for determining whether or not acute cholecystitis is present,[50] by demonstrating patency of the cystic duct. Because the majority of symptomatic patients do not have acute cholecystitis and because nuclear imaging is not as sensitive as ultrasound for making a nonbiliary diagnosis, many authors suggest that nuclear imaging be reserved for patients with equivocal ultrasonograms for the diagnosis of acute cholecystitis.[3,27,49] The most sensitive sonographic criterion for diagnosing acute cholecystitis is the presence of gallstones in association with focal gallbladder tenderness. A **sonographic Murphy's sign** is present when maximal tenderness is elicited over the sonographically localized gallbladder.[51] A positive sonographic Murphy's sign is superior to a positive clinical Murphy's sign because real-time sonography can precisely localize the gallbladder, which is not generally feasible by the clinical examination alone. In the evaluation by Ralls et al[52] of 497 patients with acute cholecystitis, a positive sonographic Murphy's sign in conjunction with cholelithiasis had a positive predictive value of 92% for diagnosing acute cholecystitis. In addition, as part of the sonographic examination for acute cholecystitis, an effort should be made to determine if a stone is impacted in the gallbladder neck or cystic duct (Fig. 6-20). This frequently necessitates positioning the patient in the prone, decubitus, or other positions to determine whether or not a calculus moves with gravitational maneuvers. Cystic duct stones are particularly difficult to detect because they are not surrounded by bile, can mimic the appearance of duodenal gas, and may be located several centimeters away from the bile-filled gallbladder.

Other **secondary sonographic criteria** that are sensitive but less specific for diagnosing acute cholecystitis include gallbladder dilatation, sludge, and diffuse wall thickening. Cohan et al[53] reported that **striated** diffuse wall thickening was highly specific (100% in their series) for acute cholecystitis. This appearance consists of

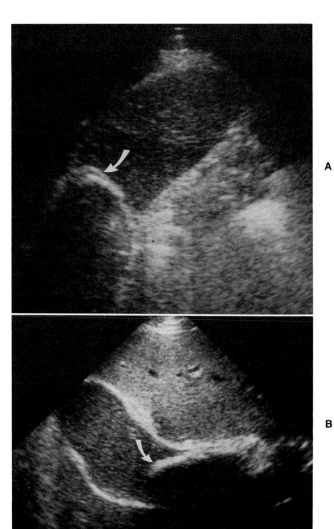

FIG 6-20. Acute cholecystitis. **A,** Supine sagittal scan of the gallbladder shows a large gallstone in the neck of the gallbladder *(curved arrow)* and low-level intraluminal echoes because of sludge. **B,** After the patient was placed in a right lateral decubitus position, the stone failed to move, indicating stone impaction. H, Head; R, right.
(From Laing FC, Jeffrey RB, Federle MP: Gallbladder and bile ducts. In: Jeffrey RD, ed: *Computed Tomography and Sonography of the Acute Abdomen.* New York: Raven Press; 1989;59-62.)

several alternating, irregular, discontinuous, lucent, and echogenic bands in the gallbladder wall. A more recent investigation[54] refutes the conclusion reached by Cohan et al and emphasizes that striated gallbladder thickening is nonspecific and may be seen in many nonbiliary conditions.

As previously mentioned, acute cholecystitis occurs in only one third of patients with gallstones. The remaining patients are either asymptomatic or develop chronic cholecystitis. On pathologic examination, however, every gallbladder that contains stones will show changes of chronic inflammation (unless it is acutely inflamed). The term **chronic cholecystitis** when used clinically refers to symptomatic but nonacute cholecystolithiasis. These patients complain of recurrent biliary colic that usually lasts for several hours and is caused by transient obstruction of the gallbladder neck or cystic duct by a stone. The diagnosis is based on the clinical findings; however, if the ultrasound examination shows gallbladder wall thickening that cannot be attributed to nonbiliary causes, the diagnosis can be confirmed on the basis of the sonogram.

Complications of acute cholecystitis include emphysematous and gangrenous cholecystitis as well as perforation. Each of these sequelae is associated with significantly increased morbidity and mortality. Large research series are not available to determine the overall sensitivity and specificity of ultrasound to detect these complications; however, ultrasound can frequently suggest the correct diagnosis.

Emphysematous cholecystitis is a relatively rare form of acute cholecystitis associated with the presence of gas-forming bacteria in the gallbladder. It differs from the usual type of acute cholecystitis in that cholelithiasis is often absent, 38% of patients are diabetic, the male to female ratio is 7:3, and gangrene with associated perforation is five times more common.[55] Gasforming organisms invade and devitalize the gallbladder wall and release gas into the gallbladder lumen and wall. Emphysematous cholecystitis is a surgical emergency and the diagnosis can be suggested by its characteristic ultrasound appearance. If the gas is intraluminal, the sonographic image consists of a prominent nondependent hyperechoic focus with an associated ring down or comet-tail artifact (Fig. 6-21). Intramural gas usually has a semicircular or arc-like configuration.[56,57] The differential diagnosis is limited although calcification in the gallbladder wall or a gallbladder filled with stones may bear a superficial resemblance to emphysematous cholecystitis. Strong reverberative echoes should not be visible in these conditions, however. Nonetheless, suspected gas collections detected by sonography should be confirmed by either plain film radiography or CT. A rare and dramatic appearance for emphysematous cholecystitis consists of tiny echogenic foci rising from the dependent portion of the gallbladder, reminiscent of rising champagne bubbles.[58] Presumably the rising echoes are due to tiny bubbles of gas as they are released from organisms within the infected gallbladder wall.

The incidence of **gangrenous cholecystitis** ranges from 2% to 38% in patients with acute cholecystitis and is associated with gallbladder perforation in up to 10% of cases.[42] Because of the increased morbidity and mortality with perforation, specific sonographic findings

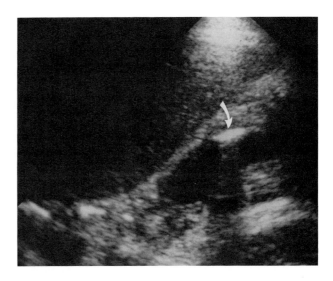

FIG 6-21. Emphysematous cholecystitis. Intraluminal gas creates a prominent hyperechoic focus with a ring-down artifact *(curved arrow)* in a nondependent position.
(From Laing FC, Jeffrey RB, Federle MP: Gallbladder and bile ducts. In: Jeffrey RD, ed: *Computed Tomography and Sonography of the Acute Abdomen.* New York: Raven Press; 1989:59-62.)

that suggest gangrenous cholecystitis should be sought. In a symptomatic patient, marked irregularity or asymmetric thickening of the gallbladder wall should be viewed with suspicion (Fig. 6-22). According to Jeffrey et al,[42] this finding was present in approximately 50% of patients and was due to ulceration, hemorrhage, necrosis, and/or micro-abscesses in the gallbladder wall. Intraluminal membranes may also be present and are due to either fibrinous strands or exudate, or necrosis and sloughing of the gallbladder mucosa (Fig. 6-23). As the gallbladder becomes devitalized by the ravages of gangrenous cholecystitis, the patient's clinical findings paradoxically may shift away from the gallbladder. In a review by Simeone et al[59] of 18 patients with pathologically proven gangrenous cholecystitis, the sonographic Murphy's sign was positive in only 6 patients (33%) possibly because of denervation of the gallbladder by gangrenous changes. Diffuse abdominal pain was more common (50% of patients), possibly because of generalized peritonitis with inflammation of the parietal peritoneum.

Although additional clinical studies are necessary, at least one investigative group has attempted to assign an ultrasonographic risk score in order to time optimally operative intervention in patients with acute cholecystitis.[60] This approach was undertaken in an effort to surgically intercede prior to gallbladder necrosis and perforation. Pericholecystic fluid, intraluminal membranes, and a rounded appearance to the gallbladder were findings associated with an increased incidence of gangrenous cholecystitis.

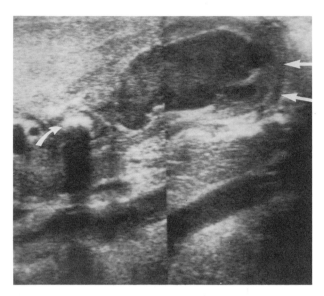

FIG 6-22. Gangrenous cholecystitis. The gallbladder wall is markedly thickened and irregular in contour in the fundus *(arrows)*. A large amount of sludge is also present. The gallbladder neck contains a high-amplitude echo with acoustic shadowing caused by an impacted cystic duct stone *(curved arrow)*.
(From Laing FC: Ultrasonography of the gallbladder and biliary tree. In: Sarti DA, ed: *Diagnostic Ultrasound: Text and Cases.* 2nd ed. Chicago: Yearbook Medical Publishers; 1987.)

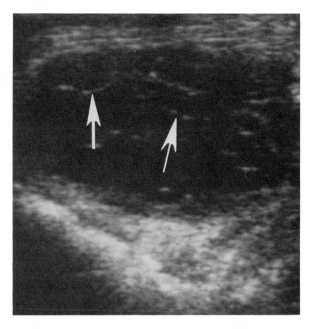

FIG 6-23. Gangrenous cholecystitis. Prominent intraluminal membranes *(arrows)* are present in the gallbladder.

Gallbladder perforation complicates acute cholecystitis in 5% to 10% of cases and is associated with a mortality of 19% to 24%.[61] Niemeier[62] has classified gallbladder perforation into three categories:

- Acute, resulting in generalized peritonitis
- Subacute, resulting in a pericholecystic abscess
- Chronic, resulting in an internal biliary fistula

Most perforations are subacute and result in a pericholecystic abscess adjacent to the fundus (the region with the sparest blood supply) (Fig. 6-24). Similar to abscesses elsewhere, these collections have a variety of sizes and appearances.[63] They may be primarily anechoic or highly echogenic, especially if they are caused by gas-forming organisms.

As interventional and imaging techniques become more sophisticated, ultrasound is assuming an increasingly important role in the classification and treatment of pericholecystic abscesses. Recent work by Takada et al[64] suggests that ultrasound can successfully predict which collections require immediate surgical intervention, as opposed to collections that can be treated conservatively with antibiotics and/or catheter drainage. Their experience, which involved 15 patients with pericholecystic abscesses, suggests that abscesses located in either the gallbladder bed or intramurally respond satisfactorily to conservative management, while intraperitoneal abscesses require emergent surgical drainage.

Initial reports by McGahan et al indicate that percutaneous bile aspiration could be useful in patients suspected of acute cholecystitis.[65] Despite initial optimism for detecting leukocytes and bacteria in infected bile, a more recent study by this group reveals that this technique is limited by the fact that a negative result does not exclude acute cholecystitis and that culture results are not available for a minimum of 24 to 48 hours following aspiration.[66]

Because critically ill patients with suspected acute cholecystitis may not be suitable candidates for surgery, and because of the limitations of percutaneous bile aspiration, McGahan now advocates that emergency percutaneous cholecystostomy be performed on these patients.[67] In his experience ultrasound was able to successfully guide transhepatic placement of a drainage catheter into the gallbladder 97.5% of the time (39 of 40 attempted procedures). This approach may be life saving and should be considered as an alternative in patients who are unable to tolerate emergency cholecystectomy.

Acalculous cholecystitis is a difficult diagnosis to establish both clinically and by imaging modalities. The accuracy of ultrasound and radionuclide imaging for making the correct diagnosis is significantly less for acalculous than calculous disease. Two major limitations of ultrasound are that gallstones are absent and many patients have severe intercurrent illnesses that limit the evaluation of the sonographic Murphy's sign. The sonographic diagnosis, therefore, depends on gall-

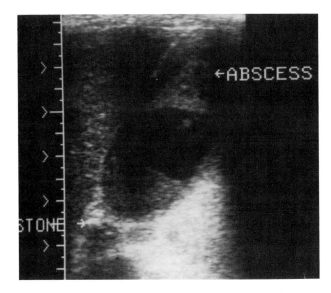

FIG 6-24. Pericholecystic abscess. A longitudinal scan shows very subtle cystic duct stone and gallbladder sludge. An echogenic collection adjacent to the fundus of the gallbladder is surgically proven abscess.

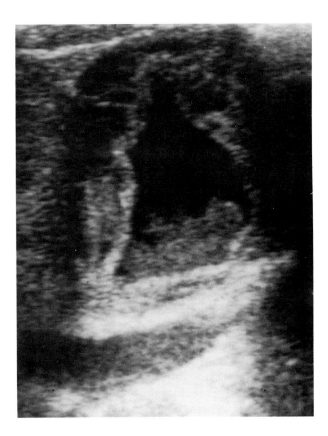

FIG 6-25. Acalculous cholecystitis. Irregular gallbladder wall thickening and tumefactive sludge are seen.

bladder wall thickening (in the absence of hypoalbuminemia, ascites, congestive heart failure, etc.), pericholecystic fluid or subserosal edema, intraluminal or intramural gas, or sloughed mucosal membranes (Fig. 6-25). Although one investigator has suggested that a complete lack of response to cholecystokinin (CCK) should suggest the diagnosis,[68] this finding is of limited usefulness in postoperative patients because their gallbladders (proven to be normal at surgery) not infrequently also fail to contract following CCK administration.[69] Personal experience also suggests that patients who are critically ill and whose gallbladders contain sludge frequently fail to show a positive response to CCK administration.

Although cholescintigraphy has a reported sensitivity of 90% to 95% for diagnosing acalculous cholecystitis on the basis of functional cystic duct obstruction,[68,70] the reported specificity of only 38% has limited the usefulness of this study.[68] False-positive examinations (nonvisualization of a noninflamed gallbladder) are common and occur with prolonged hyperalimentation, severe intercurrent illness, and hepatocellular dysfunction, conditions that are frequently concurrent in patients who are at risk for developing acalculous cholecystitis. Although a negative cholescintigraphic examination (gallbladder visualization) strongly suggests that acalculous cholecystitis is absent, a positive study should be interpreted with caution. Because of the difficulty in diagnosing acalculous cholecystitis, in selected patients biliary aspiration should be performed, which, if positive for leukocytes and bacteria, confirms

the diagnosis. If the aspirate is negative but clinical suspicion is very high, consideration should be given to percutaneous placement of a cholecystostomy tube using ultrasonographic guidance.

Biliary Lithotripsy

In 1985, **extracorporeal shock wave lithotripsy (ESWL)** was first used in Germany to fragment gallstones. In 1988, the FDA began clinical trials in the United States and currently this procedure is being performed in centers throughout Western Europe and Japan. To date, ESWL has been used to treat symptomatic gallstones in over 20,000 patients worldwide. Different manufacturers use a variety of techniques to generate a succession of shock waves that are aimed at the gallstones.

Ultrasound is used as an integral part of this procedure in several ways. Most often, it is used initially for diagnosing of cholelithiasis. In order for patients to qualify for lithotripsy in the United States, stringent selection criteria have been formulated. These include:

- Up to three gallstones
- Each gallstone must be less than 30 mm in diameter

- Stones should appear noncalcified on a plain abdominal x-ray
- Evidence that the gallbladder functions on **oral cholecystography (OCG)**

It has been estimated that on the basis of these criteria, approximately 85% of patients with gallstones are excluded as candidates for ESWL.[71]

ESWL treatment is usually performed under ultrasound **monitoring** using a side arm transducer and in some cases an in-line transducer as well. During the procedure, the stone(s) change in appearance such that as they fragment, their echogenic focus becomes increasingly large and broad, and their acoustic shadow may diminish. At the end of the treatment, the ultrasound images may look like a cloud of dust that is caused by the swirling of the fragmented gallstones.[72] This appearance can sometimes cause problems in that it may limit visualization of residual stone fragments that are not apparent until settling occurs.

In order to differentiate large residual fragments versus clumps of small fragments that can mimic an intact stone on sonography, Laufer et al have developed a "roll over maneuver" whereby rolling the patient 360 degrees allows dispersion of small fragments.[72] If large fragments remain, retreatment is often performed. Ultrasound, and often OCG are used to evaluate patients who have undergone ESWL to look for retained or recurrent stones, as well as to evaluate gallbladder function. Torres et al have recently noted that 14% of patients studied 6 weeks to 6 months after ESWL had abnormal-appearing gallbladders (not present before lithotripsy). This was manifested by a collapsed or contracted gallbladder on ultrasound examination, or faint visualization or nonvisualization by OCG.[73] Usually this is a temporary condition with 64% of these patients having normal-appearing sonogram 12 months after treatment.[73] Patients with persistent contraction or nonvisualization are likely to be symptomatic. Other sonographic abnormalities seen following this therapy include fluid surrounding the gallbladder or an echogenic focus in the liver that is thought to be caused by hemorrhage.

In a comparison with OCG, ultrasound has been shown to be more sensitive for detecting small residual fragments.[74] In these cases, it is recommended that adjuvant therapy with bile salts be administered until 3 months after ultrasound has shown that the fragments no longer exist.

Another role for ultrasound is the long-term **follow-up** of patients undergoing ESWL to detect recurrent stones. These patients also would be treated medically by dissolution therapy in an effort to dissolve the newly forming stones. Because of limited number of patients and the fact that this is a relatively new therapeutic modality, experience in this area is limited.

Pitfalls

Real-time equipment has facilitated ultrasound's ability to examine the gallbladder, but occasional problems still arise.[75] One source of confusion involves the definitive diagnosis of cholelithiasis. **Shadows** that appear to arise from the gallbladder neck are a common source of diagnostic confusion. Because refraction from the edge of the gallbladder is associated with shadowing, it is mandatory to visualize the stone (not merely the shadow) before diagnosing cholelithiasis. Similarly, shadowing posterior to the gallbladder that originates from within the bowel should not be misinterpreted as being suggestive of primary gallbladder pathology (Figs. 6-26 and 6-27). Scanning after repositioning the patient in the prone or right lateral decubitus position often makes it technically easier to prove the presence of a stone. This is because repositioning causes the stone to move away from the adjacent bowel gas.

Anatomic variations in the appearance and shape of the gallbladder can also create diagnostic difficulties. Folds that are present normally in the gallbladder can cause confusing echoes that may be associated with posterior acoustic shadowing. The junctional fold, located between the body and infundibulum of the gallbladder, and folds from the valves of Heister located in the region of the gallbladder neck are two common anatomic sites that can cause echoes that mimic stones (Figs. 6-5 and 6-28). Scanning following deep inspiration will often make these folds less apparent, especially those in the region of the junctional zone. In addition, if the patient is not acutely symptomatic and if the gallbladder is not distended, echoes that arise from the neck and the region of the valve of Heister should be viewed with suspicion because they are not likely to represent impacted gallstones.

A false-positive diagnosis of cholelithiasis can also be made if the gallbladder is physiologically contracted and the gastric antrum/duodenum contains material that mimics the appearance of a gallbladder filled with stones (Fig. 6-29). This can cause a **false-positive appearance for the WES triad or double arc shadow sign.** Careful observation using real-time equipment and the administration of water is often required to evaluate these questionable cases. Other disorders that can mimic this appearance include a porcelain gallbladder, emphysematous cholecystitis, milk of calcium bile, and gallbladder wall micro-abscesses.[75] Clinical correlation, plain film radiology, and even CT may be necessary to determine the etiology for these sonographic findings. Very rarely, particulate material may enter the gallbladder through a spontaneous or surgically created gastrointestinal fistula and may be responsible for a false-positive diagnosis of cholelithiasis.[76,77]

Although the great majority of gallstones have a classic sonographic appearance, sometimes **atypical**

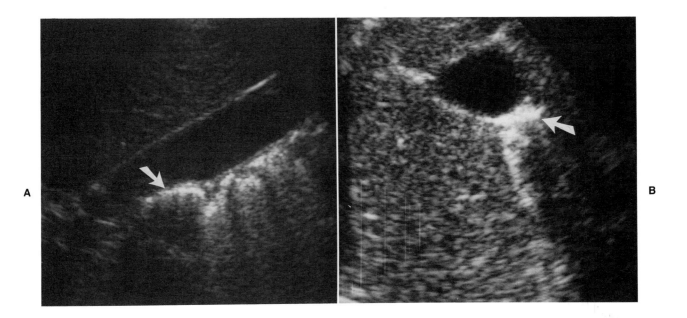

FIG 6-26. Pitfall—bowel gas. **A,** Longitudinal scan shows echogenic shadowing region near the gallbladder neck *(arrow)*. This appearance, caused by bowel gas, may resemble subtle stones. **B,** Transverse scan with the patient in a right lateral decubitus position shows that the echogenic material is not in the dependent portion of the gallbladder and is now seen posterior to the medial aspect of the gallbladder *(arrow)*.

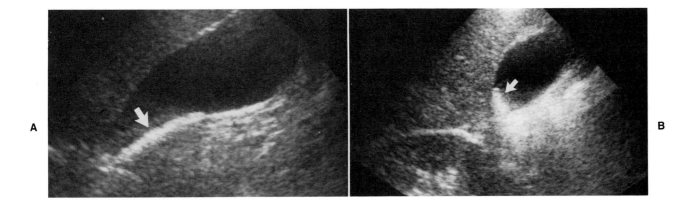

FIG 6-27. Subtle cholelithiasis mimicking bowel gas artifact. **A,** An echogenic region *(arrow)* is seen on this longitudinal scan near the neck of the gallbladder. **B,** Transverse scan, obtained with the patient into a right lateral decubitus position, confirms dependent gallstones with mild acoustic shadowing.

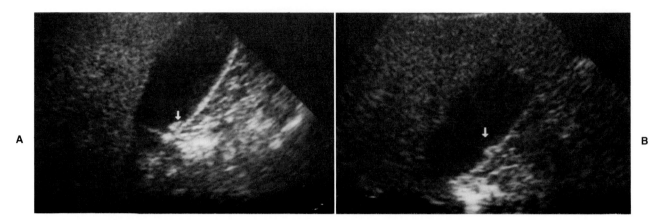

FIG 6-28. Nonshadowing stone mimicking a junctional fold. **A,** Supine longitudinal scan reveals an echogenic focus near the gallbladder neck *(arrow)* without acoustic shadowing. **B,** After repositioning the patient into an erect position, the echogenic focus demonstrated mobility *(arrow)* confirming the presence of a small nonshadowing gallstone.

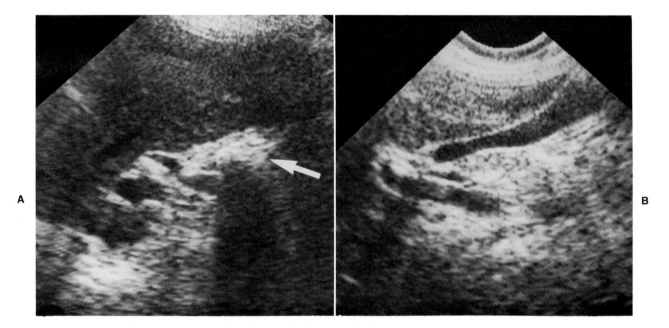

FIG 6-29. Pitfall—food-filled duodenum mimicking stone-filled gallbladder. **A,** Emergency longitudinal scan in a nonfasting patient with acute right upper quadrant pain reveals a region of acoustic shadowing *(arrow)* suggestive of a gallbladder filled with stones. **B,** A repeat study following an overnight fast confirmed a normal-appearing gallbladder.
(From Laing FC: Ultrasonography of the gallbladder and biliary tree. In: Sarti DA, ed: *Diagnostic Ultrasound: Text and Cases.* 2nd ed. Chicago; Yearbook Medical Publishers; 1987.)

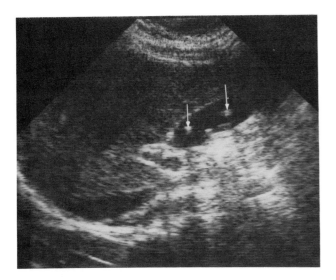

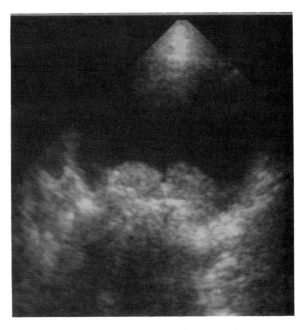

FIG 6-30. Floating gallstones *(arrows)* seen on a supine longitudinal scan.

(From Laing FC, Filly RA, Gooding GAW: Ultrasonography of the liver and biliary tract. In: Margulis AR, Burhenne HJ, eds: *Alimentary Tract Radiology.* 4th ed. St. Louis; CV Mosby Co: 1989.)

FIG 6-31. Cholelithiasis—stones with unusual morphology. These gallstones cast acoustic shadows but are less echogenic than usual. Although this appearance may occur with soft, calcium bilirubinate pigment stones, in this patient computed tomography suggested the stones were composed primarily of cholesterol.

(From Laing FC, Filly RA, Gooding GAW: Ultrasonography of the liver and biliary tract. In: Margulis AR, Burhenne HJ, eds: *Alimentary Tract Radiology.* 4th ed. St. Louis; CV Mosby Co: 1989.)

calculi are encountered. Stones either adherent to or within the gallbladder wall can mimic focal air or calcification within the gallbladder wall or cholesterol polyps (cholesterolosis). These entities can sometimes be distinguished from one another by plain film radiographs, although in special circumstances CT may be required.

Normally, calculi are located in a dependent position within the gallbladder because their specific gravity exceeds that of bile. Rarely, however, the specific gravity of bile exceeds that of calculi causing gallstones to float in bile (Fig. 6-30). The nondependent position for calculi was initially attributed to the presence of oral cholecystographic contrast material within bile.[78] Recently, cholesterol stones and those containing gas fissures have also been observed to float.[79-81]

Echoes produced by gallstones are usually high in amplitude. Occasionally, however, they are less echogenic than expected (Fig. 6-31). This appearance occurs most often in patients with soft pigment stones that have a mud-like consistency. These calculi are unusual in the gallbladder, but are common in the intrahepatic and extrahepatic biliary tree. In addition, they are seen in patients with Oriental cholangiohepatitis.[82] These stones may have an appearance that is identical to tumefactive sludge[20] or even to the focal masses that protrude into the gallbladder lumen. The degree to which pigment stones cast acoustic shadows also ranges widely from none to dramatic.

In a small percentage of patients, despite the use of optimal equipment and scanning techniques, neither the gallbladder nor shadowing from its fossa is seen. In most of these cases the gallbladders are abnormal with an obliterated lumen (Fig. 6-32). Rarely, the gallbladder may be difficult to detect because it is filled with sludge that is iso-echoic with liver parenchyma (Fig. 6-33).[83] Other causes for **gallbladder nonvisualization** include physiologic contraction, contractions associated with acute hepatitis, congenital absence of the gallbladder, an unusually positioned gallbladder, or technical error.[84,85] In these situations, oral cholecystography or technetium-IDA imaging should be done as a confirmatory examination because the gallbladder will sometimes prove normal despite nonvisualization by sonography.

Sludge-like intraluminal echoes can also be a source of confusion. Both pus and blood within the gallbladder lumen can appear identical to biliary sludge. Patient history may be critical in evaluating the source of these echoes. Tumefactive sludge also may cause diagnostic difficulty because it can resemble either soft pigment stones or an intraluminal mass. Unlike true stones, it does not shadow and moves slowly when the patient is repositioned. Gravity dependence should be a distinguishing feature between sludge and neoplasm,

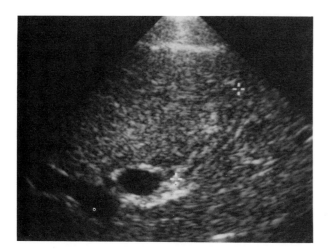

FIG 6-32. Abnormally contracted gallbladder with an obliterated lumen (between cursors). The anatomic position, shape, and the fact that it did not appear to communicate with the bowel following the administration of water suggest that the cause of this unusual echogenic region is an abnormally contracted gallbladder.

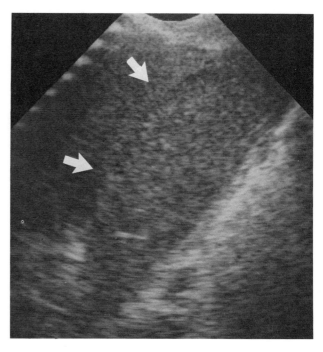

FIG 6-33. Gallbladder—sludge isoechoic with hepatic parenchymal tissue makes the gallbladder difficult to detect *(arrows)*. This appearance has been termed *hepatization* of the gallbladder.
(From Laing FC: Ultrasonography of the gallbladder and biliary tree. In: Sarti DA, ed: *Diagnostic Ultrasound: Text and Cases.* 2nd ed. Chicago: Yearbook Medical Publishers; 1987.)

but it is not always possible to demonstrate motion reliably in cases of tumefactive sludge (Fig. 6-14).[20] A repeat examination performed several days later can usually differentiate between these two entities because tumefactive sludge will either disappear or change in appearance, whereas a neoplasm will remain unchanged.

Milk of calcium or **limy bile** results in a variety of sonographic appearances.[86,87] Both an echogenic flat fluid-fluid level and a convex shadowing meniscus pattern have been reported. Occasionally, the echogenicity of milk of calcium resembles sludge, although it can be distinguished from sludge by the presence of gradual acoustic shadowing (Fig. 6-34).

Occasionally, **artifacts** may be responsible for intraluminal, dependent, low-level echoes. Most often, these are due to either slice-thickness or side-lobe artifacts (Fig. 6-35).[88,89] Slice-thickness artifacts result from a partial volume effect and occur when a portion of the ultrasound beam interacts with the fluid-filled gallbladder lumen, while an adjacent portion of the beam interacts with a true-echo reflector. These artifactual echoes can be minimized by using a narrow sound beam focused at the level of the gallbladder and by scanning through the gallbladder's central portion.[88]

Side-lobe artifacts are caused by transducer side lobes interacting with highly reflective acoustic surfaces, such as duodenal gas located adjacent to the gallbladder. These echoes, which appear to originate within the main ultrasound beam, can be minimized by repositioning the patient so the gallbladder falls away from the adjacent gas-filled structures, by changing the angu-

lation of the transducer, or by decreasing machine intensity.[89] Because slice-thickness and side-lobe artifacts are independent of gravity, "pseudo-sludge" will not layer with changes in patient position, unlike true sludge.

Gallbladder wall thickening is usually categorized as diffuse or focal. As previously discussed, diffuse thickening may or may not be associated with primary gallbladder disease, whereas focal wall changes are usually caused by underlying gallbladder pathology. Occasionally, however, focal gallbladder wall changes occur in patients who do not have gallbladder disease. Dilatation of the cystic veins in association with portal hypertension or extrahepatic portal vein obstruction can make the gallbladder wall look unusual because of varices located in its outer layers.[90] Real-time images reveal dilated tortuous vessels in the adventitial layers surrounding the gallbladder. These vessels are visible on both the peritoneal surface of the gallbladder as well as in the gallbladder bed adjacent to the liver and may protrude into the gallbladder lumen. The vascular nature of the abnormality is usually evident and color Doppler can readily confirm the presence of varices.[91]

Edema localized to the gallbladder fossa (Fig. 6-36)

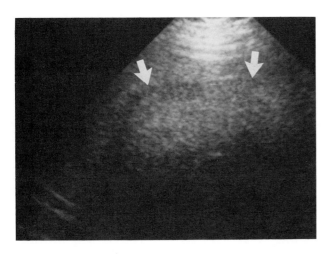

FIG 6-34. Milk of calcium bile. The gallbladder is filled with isoechoic material *(arrows)*, and posterior acoustic shadowing is present.

may be erroneously diagnosed as gallbladder wall thickening. Careful scanning reveals that the only portion of the gallbladder wall that appears thickened is in contact with the undersurface of the liver. This appearance is nonspecific, and in our experience is usually caused by pancreatitis with inflammation that ascends the hepatoduodenal ligament. As a result, edematous changes occur in the region of the portahepatis[48] or in the gallbladder fossa.

INTRAHEPATIC BILE DUCTS
Normal Anatomy

Because sonography can be used to identify and trace tubular fluid-filled structures, it is an ideal modality for evaluating dilated intrahepatic bile ducts. Until recently it was believed that only portal veins are visible within the portal triads of the hepatic parenchyma. With the advent of newer electronically focused equipment, it is now possible to see intrahepatic structures

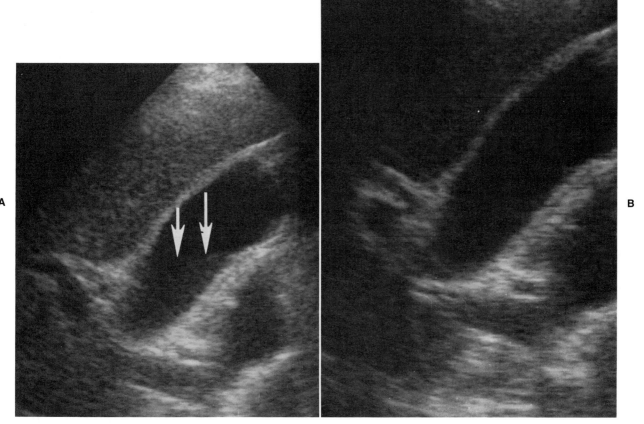

FIG 6-35. Side-lobe artifacts. **A,** Longitudinal scan of the gallbladder shows diffuse echoes *(arrows)* in the dependent portion, closely mimicking biliary sludge. **B,** The artifactual echoes disappear when the output setting is decreased. Alternative methods to eliminate this side-lobe artifact include changing the angle of the transducer and repositioning the patient such that the gallbladder falls away from adjacent gas-filled structures.

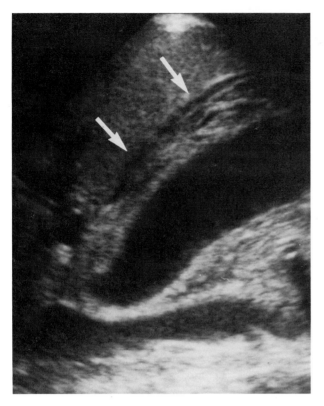

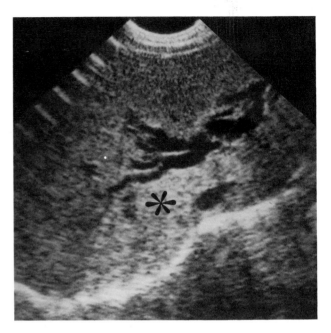

FIG 6-37. Dilated intrahepatic bile ducts. Transverse scan of the right lobe of the liver and porta hepatis shows irregular, tortuous appearing tubular structures with acoustic enhancement (*).
(From Laing FC: Ultrasonography of the gallbladder and biliary tree. In: Sarti DA, ed: *Diagnostic Ultrasound: Text and Cases.* 2nd ed. Chicago: Yearbook Medical Publishers; 1987.)

FIG 6-36. Pseudo-gallbladder wall thickening caused by edema in the gallbladder fossa in a patient with acute pancreatitis. The apparent gallbladder thickening is localized to that portion of the gallbladder wall that is in contact with the undersurface of the liver *(arrows)*.

that represent either normal bile ducts or hepatic arteries.[92] As the sensitivity of color Doppler improves, it probably will be possible to determine if these structures represent vessels or biliary structures. These tubular structures are considered normal if they are 2 mm or less in diameter, or not more than 40% of the diameter of the accompanying portal vein.[92] It is also routinely possible to visualize the normal right and left hepatic ducts, which are extrahepatic and do not lie within hepatic parenchyma. They course in the porta hepatis with the undivided portion of the right portal vein or initial segment of the left portal vein respectively.

Dilated Intrahepatic Bile Ducts

Four criteria enable intrahepatic bile ducts to be easily differentiated from portal veins.[93] The first and most reliable differentiating feature is detection of an **alteration in the normal appearance of the portal triads.** When intrahepatic bile ducts dilate, two or more tubular structures become readily visible in the expected position of the portal vein (Figs. 6-37 and 6-38). Dilated bile ducts are greater than 2 mm in diameter and are more than 40% of the diameter of the accompanying

portal vein; normal hepatic arteries and/or bile ducts are very small and are barely perceptible with 3.5 MHz transducers. This alteration of anatomy, which occurs in virtually all patients with generalized intrahepatic bile duct dilatation, is best seen on transverse scans of the right hepatic lobe, where the dilated intrahepatic bile ducts accompany the anterior and posterior divisions of the right portal vein. It is traditionally believed that intrahepatic bile ducts lie anterior to the corresponding portal vein branches; however, recent anatomic correlation obtained by careful ultrasound scanning of patients with intrahepatic bile duct dilatation as well as correlation with cadaver livers (studied by sectioning or CT imaging) clearly document that bile ducts may be anterior, posterior, or tortuous relative to the corresponding portal vein branches.[94,95]

The second sonographic feature of intrahepatic bile duct dilatation is **irregularity of the walls** of dilated bile ducts. Similar to changes seen on cholangiograms, progressive biliary dilatation is accompanied by an alteration in the course and caliber of bile ducts such that they become increasingly tortuous and irregular. In contrast, the walls of portal veins, even when dilated, remain smooth and gradually tapering.

In patients with moderate to marked intrahepatic biliary dilatation, a **stellate confluence** of tubular struc-

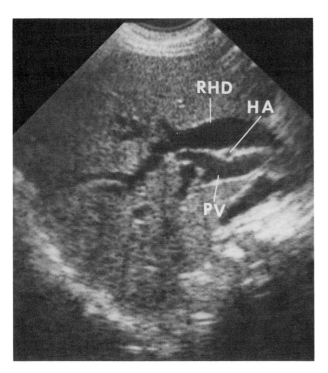

FIG 6-38. Dilated intrahepatic bile ducts. Oblique scan parallel to the long axis of the right portal vein shows the convergence of dilated intrahepatic bile ducts entering the dilated right hepatic duct *(RHD)*. The portal vein *(PV)* is posterior and seen as a separate structure. Between the right hepatic duct and portal vein is a small circular lucency, the right hepatic artery (HA).
(From Laing FC: Ultrasonography of the gallbladder and biliary tree. In: Sarti DA, ed: *Diagnostic Ultrasound: Text and Cases.* 2nd ed. Chicago: Yearbook Medical Publishers; 1987.)

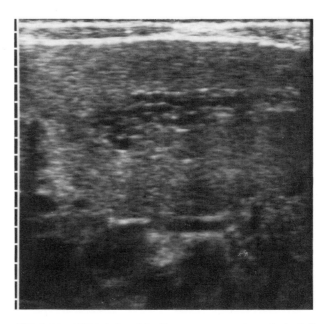

FIG 6-39. AIDS cholangitis. Transverse scan through the left lobe of the liver shows irregular thickening of the walls of the intrahepatic bile ducts.
(From Dolmatch BL, Laing FC, Federle MP, et al: AIDS-related cholangitis: radiographic findings in nine patients. *Radiology* 1987;163:313-316.)

tures may be seen that has been likened to the spokes of a wheel. This finding, which is evident in approximately two thirds of patients, occurs at points of convergence of several large ducts.

The final distinguishing feature of dilated intrahepatic bile ducts is **acoustic enhancement behind dilated ducts.** This occurs in approximately 55% to 60% of cases and is usually not seen behind portal veins. Acoustic enhancement is visible in association with biliary structures because bile does not attenuate the sound beam. Blood, however, because of its high protein content dramatically attenuates the acoustic beam.[96]

Pathology

In the great majority of cases, changes in the intrahepatic bile ducts occur secondary to extrahepatic bile duct obstruction. Occasionally, however, intrahepatic pathology is responsible for the biliary changes.

Intrahepatic Biliary Neoplasms. These are relatively rare and almost without exception are limited to cystadenoma and its malignant counterpart, cystadenocarci-

noma (primary bile duct carcinoma is rarely confined to the intrahepatic ducts). These tumors usually occur in middle-aged women who present with abdominal pain, mass, and/or jaundice. Their typical appearance is similar to ovarian cystadenoma (cystadenocarcinoma) in that the tumors are cystic masses with multiple septae and frequently, papillary excrescences.[97] Variations can occur with occasional tumors described as unilocular, calcified, or multiple. The **differential diagnosis** includes cysts complicated by hemorrhage or infection, echinococcal cyst, abscess, hematoma, or cystic metastasis. Cyst aspiration should be considered to differentiate a primary biliary neoplasm from other causes, but surgical resection is necessary to distinguish a benign cystadenoma from a cystadenocarcinoma.

Sclerosing and AIDS Cholangitis. These two entities can have intrahepatic bile duct changes that are virtually identical on sonography. Clinically more than 50% of patients with sclerosing cholangitis have ulcerative colitis. In both of these conditions, the walls of the intrahepatic bile ducts may be thickened in a smooth or irregular fashion (Fig. 6-39).[98-100] The wall thickening may be marked, such that it compromises the lumen of the bile duct. This is often reflected clinically by markedly obstructive liver chemistries (increased alkaline phosphatase and bilirubin) with only mild luminal bile duct dilatation. Although in theory primary or metastatic tumors may have a similar appearance, cholangitis per se usually involves the bile ducts in a more generalized fashion.

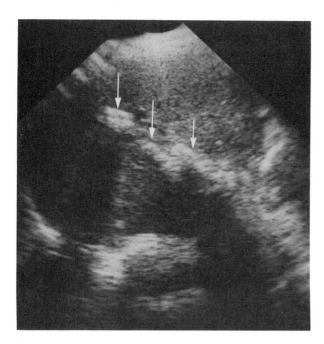

FIG 6-40. Recurrent pyogenic cholangiohepatitis (RPC). Longitudinal scan shows multiple high-amplitude echoes *(arrows)* with acoustic shadowing caused by intrahepatic biliary calculi.

(From Laing FC: Ultrasound diagnosis of choledocholithiasis. *Sem Ultrasound, CT and MR* 1987;8:103-113.)

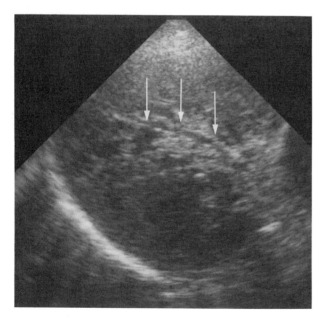

FIG 6-41. Recurrent pyogenic cholangiohepatitis. Nonshadowing intraductal echogenic material *(arrows)* is due to soft pigment stones. Biliary sludge could have an identical appearance.

(From Laing FC: Ultrasound diagnosis of choledocholithiasis. *Sem Ultrasound, CT and MR* 1987;8:103-113.)

Intrahepatic Biliary Calculi. Intrahepatic biliary calculi are uncommon in patients with gallstones, but characteristically occur in patients with **recurrent pyogenic cholangitis (RPC).**[101] This condition has a variety of names including **Oriental cholangiohepatitis, intrahepatic pigment stone disease,** and **biliary obstruction syndrome of the Chinese.** Although extremely common in Asia, RPC can occur in any patient with prolonged bile stasis. This contributes to infection (especially with coliform organisms), which causes bile to deconjugate and results in precipitates of calcium bilirubinate pigment crystals that form soft, mud-like stones. In contrast to extrahepatic cholesterol stones seen in the western hemisphere, in Asia intrahepatic pigment stones tend to form in younger patients, with no sexual preference. The stones are usually multiple and develop in the intrahepatic and extrahepatic ductal system (Figs. 6-40 and 6-41).[102] Not infrequently, they form a cast of the biliary tree. Sonographic examination usually reveals these stones to be of medium echo intensity with variable degrees of acoustic shadowing. Although the anterior surfaces of the stones are usually rounded, their appearance can mimic sludge, pus, blood, or even a neoplasm in the biliary tree. In patients with very large stones, the acoustic shadow can predominate and can cause a dramatic appearance that obliterates visualization of the bile ducts in a manner similar to a gallbladder filled with small stones (Fig. 6-42).[102] Because ultrasound is often used as the initial examination in these patients, it is important for sonographers to recognize the varied appearances of this disease process. In contrast to patients with choledocholithiasis caused by gallstone disease, surgical treatment differs considerably in these patients. If this preoperative diagnosis is suggested by sonography, computed

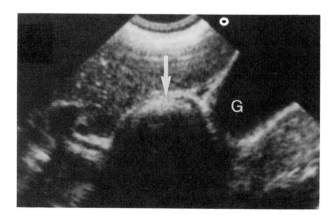

FIG 6-42. Choledocholithiasis. Large calculus is present in the CBD *(arrow).* The profound acoustic shadow causes nonvisualization of the posterior bile duct. *G,* Gallbladder.

(From Laing FC: Ultrasound diagnosis of choledocholithiasis. *Sem Ultrasound, CT and MR* 1987;8:103-113.)

tomography should usually be obtained because its results may complement those of sonography and allow more precise delineation of the ductal system. Recent evidence also suggests that biliary ascariasis may be associated with intrahepatic calculi.[103,104]

Sonography is limited in patients with RPC who have undergone biliary-enteric anastomoses. This is because reflux of gas into the biliary tree can obscure and/or mimic intrahepatic calculi. In addition, gas-containing abscesses, a rather common sequelae in patients with this condition, may also be obscured.

Caroli's Disease. Caroli's disease is characterized by segmental nonobstructive saccular dilatation of intrahepatic bile ducts. This rare disease is frequently associated with infantile polycystic kidney disease and congenital hepatic fibrosis. Biliary complications include the development of pyogenic cholangitis, liver abscesses, and intrahepatic stones within the dilated ducts. Sonography of the liver and bile ducts reveals localized irregular dilatation of intrahepatic bile ducts.[105,106] In addition, an unusual feature seen in patients with Caroli's disease consists of complete or partial bridging of the ductal walls, and unusual intraluminal soft-tissue protrusions into the bile ducts and portal radicals.[105,106]

The differential diagnosis for this appearance is limited (especially in the presence of infantile polycystic kidney disease), but to the unwary the dilated bile ducts might suggest polycystic disease. Close examination of patients with multiple liver cysts, however, reveals that the cysts do not communicate with one another, whereas in Caroli's disease the dilated bile ducts do intercommunicate.

Pitfalls

Although dilated intrahepatic bile ducts are specific for active biliary obstruction, this finding is not highly sensitive because up to 23% of patients with biliary obstruction have intrahepatic bile ducts that are normal size.[107] In the study by Sample et al,[107] neither the level of hyperbilirubinemia nor the duration of jaundice bore any relation to the presence or absence of intrahepatic biliary dilatation. **False-negative results,** therefore, are common and are usually due to lack of intrahepatic dilatation despite obstruction that is usually distal in location.

Segmental biliary obstruction can also cause a false-negative ultrasound examination. This may be due to intrahepatic calculi (especially in patients with RPC), strictures, or neoplasm. Although detecting dilated intrahepatic ducts usually and reliably can be made by scanning the region of the right portal vein, it is important to observe the entire portal venous system when the liver is being scanned.

Because blood clot can be iso-echoic with hepatic parenchymal tissue, it may be very difficult to detect di-

lated bile ducts in the presence of **hemobilia.**[108,109] Hemobilia occurs in at least 13% to 14% of patients who undergo percutaneous biliary drainage procedures. In most instances the bleeding is transient and mild.[109] The sonographic appearance for acute intraductal clot consists of diffuse, homogeneous echoes that may make it difficult to distinguish the ductal system from surrounding liver parenchyma. Within 24 to 48 hours after the onset of hemobilia, the clot forms a soft-tissue mass within a portion of the duct. After 48 hours, the clot retracts and appears as a discrete tubular soft-tissue mass. The varying appearances of intraductal clot may be identical to intraductal sludge, pus, or pigment stones.

Occasionally, the sonolucent portion of the duct immediately adjacent to the retracted clot can be misconstrued as the entire duct; this can cause a false-negative result with regard to ductal dilatation.[108]

Shadowing from either the biliary tree or adjacent structures can also limit sonographic ability to evaluate the ductal system. **Pneumobilia** can be due to a surgically created biliary-enteric anastomosis, incompetence of the sphincter of Oddi, or wall erosion by a gallstone or ulcer into the common bile duct (Fig. 6-43). On ultrasound, pneumobilia is characterized by variable

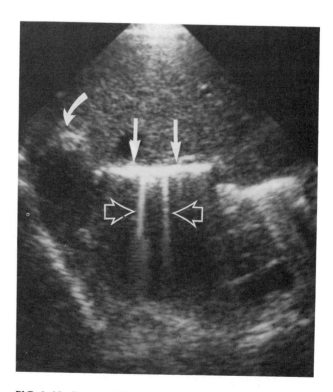

FIG 6-43. Pneumobilia *(arrows)* caused by a surgically created biliary enteric anastomosis is seen as intensely echogenic linear foci in the distribution of the biliary tree. Comet-tailed artifacts *(open arrows)* are also present. This patient (with recurrent pyogenic cholangitis) also has intrahepatic biliary calculi *(curved arrow).* Pneumobilia may mask the presence of intrahepatic stones.

length echogenic foci in the distribution of the biliary tree. Intermittent acoustic shadowing, especially of the comet-tail variety, typically is seen.[110] Because of the geometry of the bile ducts, when a patient is supine, the gas usually rises to the most anterior structure, which is the left ductal system. Occasionally, intrahepatic arterial calcification has been reported to mimic pneumobilia.[111] In difficult cases, plain film radiography should be performed so that a definitive diagnosis can be made.

Intrahepatic parenchymal calcifications may be difficult to differentiate from intrahepatic biliary stones.[112] This is especially true in patients with peripherally impacted intrahepatic ductal stones that do not appear to be continuous with the biliary tree. Criteria that may be useful for suggesting intrahepatic calculi as opposed to parenchymal calcification include the presence of bile duct dilatation, multiple lesions, left lobe involvement, and elevated alkaline phosphatase.[112]

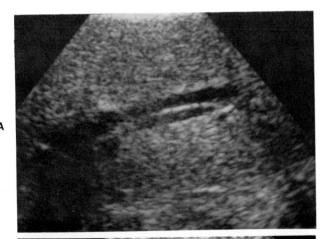

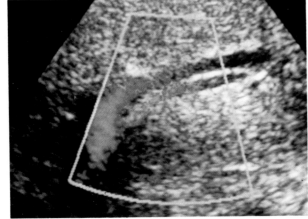

FIG 6-44. Pitfall—large hepatic artery mimicking dilated intrahepatic bile ducts. **A,** Transverse scan over the left lobe of the liver demonstrates two parallel tubular structures. **B,** Color Doppler shows blood flowing within both tubular structures.

Although false-negative diagnoses for intrahepatic bile duct dilatation are common, **false-positive diagnoses** are very unusual. They can be made, however, in patients with abnormally large hepatic arteries, in which case the dilated intrahepatic arteries mimic dilated intrahepatic bile ducts (Fig. 6-44).[113] This situation occurs most often in patients with severe cirrhosis and portal hypertension. Pseudodilated intrahepatic bile ducts can usually be distinguished from truly dilated bile ducts; in the former, the extrahepatic hepatic artery is large whereas the common bile duct is normal in size. The changes are manifest primarily in the left hepatic lobe, and there is evidence of portal hypertension (recanalized umbilical vein, varices, splenomegaly, ascites). The recent introduction of color Doppler sonography has also greatly simplified differentiating between dilated intrahepatic bile ducts and vascular structures.[114]

EXTRAHEPATIC BILE DUCTS
Normal Anatomy

The most easily visualized portion of the extrahepatic ductal system is the **common hepatic duct,** which results from the union of the right and left intrahepatic bile ducts. This structure, which is present in the porta hepatis, is visible in virtually all patients regardless of body size or habitus. The anatomic position of the common hepatic duct is constant, and it can be readily detected as it crosses anterior to the undivided right portal vein. At this level, the right hepatic artery is usually visible in cross section between the posteriorly positioned portal vein and the anteriorly positioned bile ducts. As the common hepatic duct leaves the porta hepatis, it joins the cystic duct and forms the **common bile duct** (CBD) (Fig. 6-45).[2] In a recent report by Parulekar, the normal distal cystic duct whose average diameter was 1.8 mm, was visible 51% of the time.[115] In 95% of patients, the distal cystic duct was posterior to the CBD, and in 5% of patients it was anterior to the CBD.

After its union with the cystic duct, the CBD descends within the hepatoduodenal ligament in a fixed but somewhat confusing anatomic relationship with two other tubular structures, the main portal vein and the proper hepatic artery. Recognition of these three tubular structures requires an understanding of their fixed and reproducible anatomic relationship. Proximally within the hepatoduodenal ligament the portal vein is posterior; the bile duct is anterior and somewhat laterally positioned (on the same side as the gallbladder). The proper hepatic artery is anteriorly and medially positioned (on the same side as the aorta) relative to the portal vein. As these three structures descend within the hepatoduodenal ligament, their anatomic relationship changes in accordance with their sites of termination. Because the

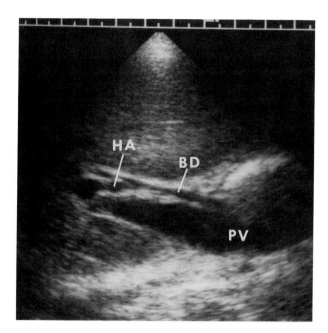

FIG 6-45. Normal portal hepatis. Parasagittal oblique scan shows the portal vein *(PV)* is posterior, the bile duct *(BD)* is anterior, and the right hepatic artery *(HA)* is interposed.
(From Laing FC, Filly RA, Gooding GAW: Ultrasonography of the liver and biliary tract. In: Margulis AR, Burhenne HJ, eds: *Alimentary Tract Radiology.* 4th ed. St. Louis: CV Mosby Co; 1989.)

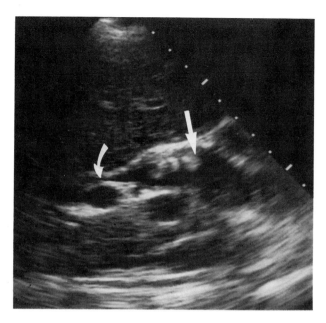

FIG 6-46. Disparate CBD dilatation. The extrahepatic duct *(arrow)* is much larger than the common hepatic duct *(curved arrow)*. This funnelled appearance was caused by an acute obstruction from choledocholithiasis. Many nonobstructing stones are also visible.

CBD terminates in the retroperitoneally located second part of the duodenum, it courses posteriorly as it descends. The portal vein descends in a relatively anterior direction to form the splenic and superior mesenteric veins. The third component of this tubular triad, the proper hepatic artery, remains anterior as it gives off the gastroduodenal artery, which enters the anterior aspect of the pancreatic head. Proper identification of these similar-appearing but very differently functioning anatomic structures is crucial to analyze the extrahepatic biliary tree correctly. The recent addition of duplex and color Doppler has greatly simplified their anatomic identification.

The **size** of the extrahepatic bile duct is the most sensitive means of distinguishing medical from surgical jaundice. There are discrepant reports in the literature about the maximal diameter of the CBD that is normal in size. Measurements as small as 4 mm or as large as 8 mm have been reported.[116,117] The literature is similarly unclear as to whether or not the CBD dilates postcholecystectomy. Articles can be found which both support[116,118] and refute[119,120] the claim that CBD dilatation occurs after cholecystectomy.

Studies have also suggested that the diameter of the CBD may increase slightly with aging and that 10 mm should be considered the upper normal value in elderly patients.[121] A simple rule of thumb is to consider as normal a 4-mm mean duct diameter at age 40, a 5-mm mean duct diameter at age 50, a 6-mm mean duct diameter at age 60, and so on.

It is generally accepted that the diameter of the CBD is normally slightly greater in its distal than its proximal portion. In most patients this discrepancy in size is barely perceptible but occasionally the duct becomes funneled and the distal diameter is several millimeters wider than the proximal diameter (Fig. 6-46). In this situation, if the duct is measured solely in the porta hepatis, it may be of normal caliber. When measured more distally, it may be borderline or even frankly enlarged. The significance of the funneled appearance is that it may indicate early extrahepatic bile duct obstruction. This finding is nonspecific, however, because a similar appearance may be seen in patients whose obstruction has been relieved.

Sonographic measurements are somewhat smaller than corresponding ductal measurements made during radiographic procedures such as transhepatic cholangiography, intravenous cholangiography, or endoscopic retrograde cholangiopancreatography, because the ultrasonograms do not include the effects of radiographic magnification or the choleretic effect of contrast agents.

The size of the common hepatic or common bile duct may be somewhat larger in patients who have undergone previous biliary surgery. Postoperatively, the common hepatic duct may measure up to 10 mm in diameter.[119] Unless baseline postoperative scans are obtained, however, a single measurement of 10 mm should be followed with sequential scans and liver function tests (especially alkaline phosphatase) in order to evaluate the possibility of early obstruction. If a symptomatic postoperative patient has a large or equivocal duct measurement (by nonoperated size criteria), further evaluation should be undertaken.

Scanning Techniques

The CBD is most commonly examined by means of parasagittal scans obtained with the patient in a supine **left posterior oblique (LPO)** position. This approach is based on the widely quoted article reported in 1978 by Behan and Kazam.[117] Scans obtained by this method are acceptable for evaluating the common hepatic duct or proximal CBD but they are frequently suboptimal for visualizing the distal CBD, which is the most common site of biliary obstruction. Because the duodenum often contains gas when the patient is supine or in an LPO position, the distal bile duct is usually obscured as it passes behind this gas-filled bowel loop. A superior scanning method is to examine the proximal and distal portions of the CBD separately (Fig. 6-47).[6]

Initially, the **distal CBD** should be examined. This is most satisfactorily accomplished by performing scans with the patient in an erect RPO position and by relying on transverse as opposed to parasagittal scans.[122] The erect RPO position minimizes gas in the antrum and duodenum whereas the transverse scan plane maximizes the ability to trace the course of the intrapancreatic distal duct. If overlying bowel gas obscures this region, the patient should be given 16 ounces of water to drink, placed in a right lateral decubitus position for 2 to 3 minutes, and rescanned in the erect RPO position.

Although the **proximal CBD** can also be evaluated in this position, it is usually seen to better advantage in the parasagittal plane after the patient has been repositioned in the conventional supine LPO position.[122] In most patients examination of the proximal and distal bile ducts can be completed in 5 to 10 minutes. In difficult cases, the study may take as long as 15 to 30 minutes.

Pathology

As a screening modality, the primary function of ultrasound is to determine whether or not biliary obstruction is present. A secondary function is to determine the level and cause of the obstruction.

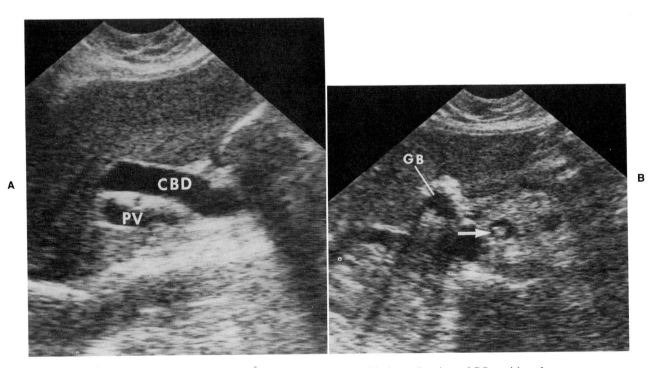

FIG 6-47. Dilated CBD. **A,** Longitudinal oblique scan with the patient in an LPO position shows a markedly dilated proximal common bile duct *(CBD)* anterior to the portal vein *(PV)*. **B,** Transverse scan with the patient in an erect position reveals a stone *(arrow)* in the distal common bile duct. This calculus was not visible with the patient in supine LPO position. *GB,* Gallbladder.
(From Laing FC: Ultrasonography of the gallbladder and biliary tree. In: Sarti DA, ed: *Diagnostic Ultrasound: Text and Cases.* 2nd ed. Chicago: Yearbook Medical Publishers; 1987.)

Diagnosing Obstruction. Because bile ducts expand centrifugally from the point of obstruction, extrahepatic dilatation occurs before intrahepatic dilatation.[123] It is not unusual, therefore, to see isolated or disparate dilatation of the extrahepatic duct in patients with obstructive jaundice (Fig. 6-46). There are two possible explanations for this phenomenon. The first involves La-Place's law, according to which expansion of a fluid-containing structure is proportional to its diameter. Because the gallbladder and CBD have the largest diameters in the biliary system, they dilate preferentially after an obstruction.[123] The second explanation for disparate dilatation is that in patients with fibrosed or infiltrated livers, intrahepatic dilatation cannot readily occur due to lack of compliance of the hepatic parenchyma. Because intrahepatic bile ducts may not always dilate in patients with surgical jaundice, most authorities consider the diameter of the common hepatic duct as the most sensitive indicator for diagnosing biliary obstruction.

In our laboratory, biliary obstruction is suggested if the common hepatic duct diameter is 8 mm or greater.[107] A diameter of 6 to 7 mm is equivocal, and smaller diameters are not suggestive of this diagnosis. Dilated intrahepatic ducts also suggest obstruction.

Level and Cause of Obstruction. Localizing the anatomic site and cause for biliary obstruction is important for determining what other examinations, if any, should be performed for further diagnostic evaluation. This information may also be useful for determining whether further procedures such as surgery, endoscopy, or percutaneous drainage are necessary. In cases of biliary obstruction, the ultrasonographer should attempt to place the level of obstruction at one of three sites: the intrapancreatic common duct, the suprapancreatic common duct, or the porta hepatis.

Initial reports on the ability of ultrasound to display the level of dilatation and suggest the cause of obstruction were rather dismal, with the level of dilatation correctly predicted 27% of the time, and the cause of obstruction correctly predicted 23% of the time.[124] With refinements in real-time equipment, and improved scanning techniques, ultrasound has been reported to define the level of dilatation in up to 92% of cases and suggest the correct cause in up to 71% of cases.[125]

Intrapancreatic Obstruction. The most common site of biliary obstruction is distal, at the level of the pancreatic head. In affected patients the extrahepatic bile duct should be dilated throughout its course (Fig. 6-48). Depending on the severity and duration of the obstruction, the intrahepatic bile ducts may or may not be dilated. Tumor, calculi, and inflammatory strictures commonly cause distal obstruction.

In a technically adequate examination, solid **pancreatic masses** larger than 2.5 cm in diameter should be

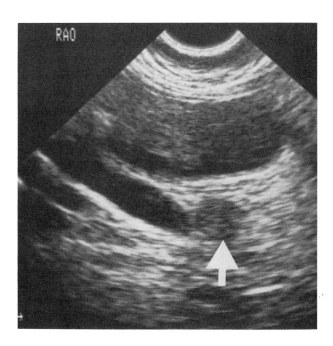

FIG 6-48. Pancreatic head carcinoma. Longitudinal scan shows CBD dilatation and a mass in the head of the pancreas *(arrow)*. At surgery, a 2-cm pancreatic carcinoma was confirmed.

readily visible. Because of their anatomic location within the head and/or uncinate process, the pancreatic duct is frequently obstructed and dilated. Masses smaller than 2.5 cm in diameter are often not visible, but their presence may be inferred if a double duct sign is present. Neoplasm and focal pancreatitis may be indistinguishable causes of distal biliary obstruction unless secondary findings such as adenopathy or distant metastases are visible.

When using the scanning techniques outlined above, distal **CBD calculi** can now be visualized in approximately 70% of patients.[122] Other new techniques introduced in an effort to improve stone detection in the extrahepatic ductal system include scanning after administering a fatty meal and scanning after positioning the patient in a knee-chest or Trendelenberg position.[126] Using these approaches, Dong et al reported a sensitivity of 86% for detecting distal choledocholithiasis.[126] As with gallstones, acoustic shadowing is almost always present. Choledocholithiasis may be detected in a normal-sized bile duct but calculi are more readily identified in a dilated system. Not surprisingly, ultrasound's sensitivity for diagnosing choledocholithiasis diminishes dramatically if the region over the head of the pancreas is obscured due to overlying bowel gas or obesity.

Strictures, the third most common cause for distal obstruction, are a problem for sonography. Apart from abrupt termination of the dilated distal CBD, the stricture per se is not usually visible and the precise cause of obstruction is not usually apparent. If a patient is known to have AIDS, careful scanning will sometimes reveal echogenic thickening of the distal duct wall, indicative of a stricture due to AIDS cholangitis (Fig. 6-49).[100] In most patients, however, after ultrasound indicates a distal site of obstruction, endoscopic retrograde cholangiopancreatography should be performed for precise diagnosis.

Suprapancreatic Obstruction. Suprapancreatic obstruction is defined as obstruction that originates between the pancreas and the porta hepatis. Sonographically, the head of the pancreas is normal, as are the diameters of the intrapancreatic bile duct and pancreatic duct. **Malignancy** (both primary and secondary) is the most common cause of these obstructions (Fig. 6-50).[2] Ultrasound may reveal a mass or adenopathy at this level. Rarely, a mass may be visible within the intraluminal portion of the duct. **Calculi** and **inflammatory strictures** are uncommon causes of suprapancreatic obstruction.

Porta Hepatis Obstruction. Obstruction at the level of the porta hepatis is also usually due to **neoplasm,** either primary or secondary. In a prospective study that included 40 patients with hilar lesions, 31 (78%) had lesions caused by neoplasms. Of the 65 patients included in the entire study, ultrasound was able to define the level of obstruction in 95% of cases, and predict tumor

unresectability 71% of the time.[127] Criteria used to evaluate resectability included the presence of hepatic metastases, remote or marked lymphadenopathy, the level of bile duct involvement, venous invasion, and lobar liver atrophy.

In patients with obstruction at the level of the porta, sonography discloses intrahepatic ductal dilatation and a normal-sized CBD. The gallbladder may or may not be obstructed, depending on the level of the lesion relative to the position of the cystic duct. In patients with secondary neoplasms, adenopathy is often present in the region of the porta hepatis. Occasionally, pathology may involve the right or left ductal system separately. In these instances, only one side of the biliary system will be dilated while the other side and CBD will be normal.

Unusual Causes for Bile Duct Dilatation. **Bile duct carcinoma (cholangiocarcinoma)** is a relatively rare malignancy, accounting for fewer than 1% of all cancers.[128] Predisposing conditions include ulcerative colitis, Caroli's disease, *Clonorchis sinensis* infestation, and exposure to a variety of chemicals. This tumor originates within the larger bile ducts and in more than two thirds of cases is located in either the CBD or CHD. Involvement of the right or left intrahepatic ducts is reported to occur in 13% of cases.[129] A Klatskin tumor is a specific type of cholangiocarcinoma that occurs in 10% to 25% of cases and is named after the physi-

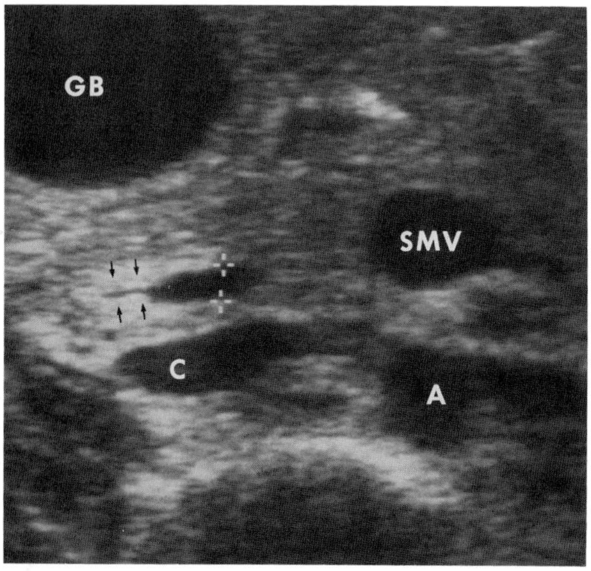

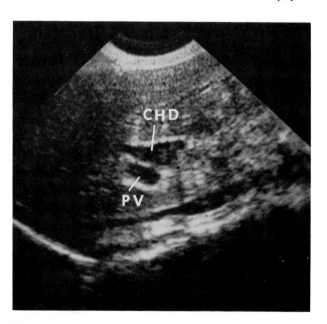

FIG 6-49. AIDS cholangitis—stricture of CBD. Transverse scan through the head of the pancreas shows abrupt distal tapering of the duct as well as echogenic thickening of the distal duct wall *(arrows)*. A, Aorta; C, inferior vena cava; *SMV,* superior mesenteric vein; *GB,* gallbladder.
(From Dolmatch BL, Laing FC, Federle MP, et al: AIDS-related cholangitis: radiographic findings in nine patients. *Radiology* 1987;163:313-316.)

FIG 6-50. Gastric carcinoma invading the porta hepatis. Longitudinal scan shows a dilated common hepatic duct *(CHD)* with an echogenic mass in the duct. Note the irregular margin at the interface of the duct and mass. CHD, Common hepatic duct; *PV,* portal vein.
(From Laing FC: Ultrasonography of the gallbladder and biliary tree. In: Sarti DA, ed: *Diagnostic Ultrasound: Text and Cases.* 2nd ed. Chicago: Yearbook Medical Publishers; 1987.)

cian who described its anatomic location at the hepatic hilum.[130] This neoplasm clinically presents with signs and symptoms of biliary obstruction while the tumor is relatively small. Because sonography is often the initial examination in evaluating patients with suspected biliary obstruction, the sonographic features of this tumor should be recognized.[131,132] The primary features seen in all 17 reported cases include dilated intrahepatic ducts with a normal-sized extrahepatic biliary tree (Fig. 6-51). Meyer et al emphasize that the dilated intrahepatic ducts do not appear to join one another at the hilum.[131] Because of the tumor's small size, an intraductal mass at the confluence of the right and left ducts has only been reported in 5 of 17 cases.[131,132] Additional features that may be used to suggest this diagnosis include absent intraductal calculi, normal pancreas, local invasion of the liver and porta hepatis, and absence of a primary tumor.[131] The differential diagnosis includes sclerosing or suppurative cholangitis, benign stricture, benign bile duct tumor, metastasis, and proximal spread of distal bile duct carcinoma.[132]

Mirizzi's Syndrome. Mirizzi's syndrome is an uncommon cause for extrahepatic biliary obstruction due to an impacted stone in the cystic duct causing extrinsic mechanical compression of the common hepatic duct.[133] Not uncommonly, the stone penetrates into the common hepatic duct or the gut, resulting in a cholecystobiliary or cholecystenteric fistula. In most cases the cystic duct inserts unusually low into the common hepatic duct.

This results in the two ducts having parallel alignment, which geometrically allows for the development of the syndrome. The sonographic findings include intrahepatic bile duct dilatation, a normal-sized CBD, and a large stone in the neck of the gallbladder or cystic duct (Fig. 6-52).[133] Failure to recognize these changes can lead to surgical complications that include ligation and transection of the CBD. Unfortunately, ultrasound findings are not always classic, and in suspicious cases CT and especially cholangiography should be performed for confirmation and for detection of the extrinsic compression of the CBD or a cholecystobiliary fistula.[134]

Choledochal Cyst. Choledochal cyst is a third uncommon lesion that may cause bile duct dilatation. This congenital anomaly has been subdivided into various types, including:

- Type I—Cystic fusiform dilatation of the CBD (the most common form)
- Type II—A diverticulum protruding from the wall of the CBD (rare)
- Type III—A choledochocele or herniation of the CBD into the duodenum (rare)[135]

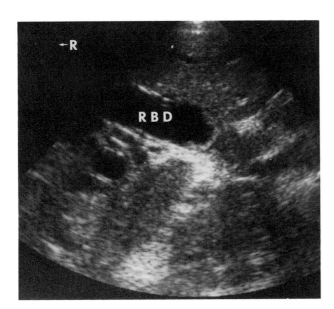

FIG 6-51. Cholangiocarcinoma (Klatskin tumor). Transverse scan through the porta hepatis shows marked dilatation of the right intrahepatic bile duct *(RBD)*. Although a mass was not visible, the irregular narrowing of the medial portion of the duct suggests the existence of a neoplasm. *R*, Right.

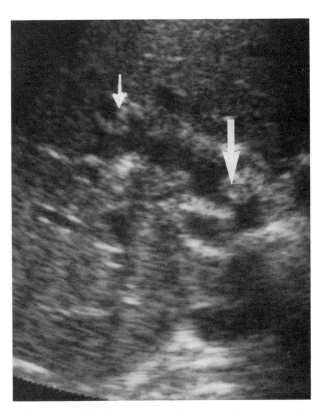

FIG 6-52. Mirizzi's syndrome. Large cystic duct calculus *(large arrow)* caused intrahepatic bile duct obstruction *(small arrow)*. Although the appearance of this scan suggests the stone may be in the common hepatic duct, careful scanning and surgery confirmed that the calculus was in the cystic duct.

This entity usually occurs in Oriental women whose symptoms vary from none to the classic triad of pain, jaundice, and an abdominal mass.[136] The sonographic findings will reflect the specific type of choledochal cyst that is present, although typically a cystic extrahepatic mass will be present. Not infrequently, a portion of the dilated proximal bile duct can be seen extending into the choledochal cyst. Despite reports to the contrary, intrahepatic bile duct dilatation is also commonly present.[136] The differential diagnosis includes other fluid-filled masses such an hepatic cyst, pancreatic pseudocyst, or enteric duplication cyst. Ultrasound can often suggest the correct diagnosis by accurately localizing the cyst to the biliary tree and showing its relationship to less distended portions of the biliary system and intrahepatic ducts.

Biliary Parasites. Occasionally, symptoms that result from biliary parasites may lead to an ultrasound examination. It has been estimated that one quarter of the world's population is infested with **ascariasis.** High-risk populations are in the Far East, the USSR, Latin America, and Africa.[137] Because the adult worm is greater than 10 cm in length, 3 to 6 mm thick, and has a propensity to enter the biliary tree, it may be visible by sonography (Fig. 6-53) where it may cause biliary obstruction. Characteristic sonographic findings include visualizing the worm(s) in the bile duct or gallbladder as one or more nonshadowing tube-like structures that may either be straight or coiled.[138,139] Aggregates of multiple worms have been described as having an appearance like spaghetti.[139] In addition to diagnosing ascariasis, ultrasound can also be used to document disappearance of the worm(s) following treatment.

Clonorchis sinensis, a liver fluke that is endemic to populations living in the Far East, frequently infests medium or small intrahepatic bile ducts. In some patients, the extrahepatic bile ducts and/or gallbladder may be affected.[140] Although the diagnosis of clonorchiasis depends on detecting eggs or adult worms in the feces or bile, ultrasound can suggest the diagnosis. Characteristic sonographic findings include diffuse dilatation of small intrahepatic ducts with minimal or absent dilatation of the extrahepatic ductal system. Increased echogenicity and thickening of the involved bile duct walls are also present. Because these parasites are 8 to 15 mm long and 1.5 to 5 mm thick, they are not usually visible as they obstruct the intrahepatic bile ducts. Aggregates of adult worms or individual worms may occasionally be seen in the extrahepatic bile duct and gallbladder, respectively.[140] Their appearance can be distinguished from gallstones on the basis of their fusiform outline and the fact that they may show spontaneous floating movement. In addition, they are less echogenic than typical gallstones and do not cause acoustic shadowing.

A consequence of chronic biliary infestation by this liver fluke is an increased incidence of cholangiocarcinoma and possibly recurrent pyogenic cholangitis.[141]

Pitfalls

To maximize the use of ultrasound in evaluating the extrahepatic duct, sonographers must have a clear understanding of the problems and pitfalls pertaining to examining the CBD.

Anatomic Problems. Variations in the course of the extrahepatic bile duct can occasionally occur. In approximately 20% of patients with CBD dilatation, the course of the duct is more transverse than vertical.[142] In these cases the sonogram can be confusing with respect to distinguishing the bile duct from the oblique to horizontal courses of the portal and splenic veins. Variations in the course of the CBD can also occur in the presence of a pancreatic mass, particularly within the uncinate process. This may result in anterior elevation of the distal duct, such that it mimics the course of the gastroduodenal artery. In addition, patients who have undergone biliary surgery may have anatomic deviations in the position of the extrahepatic bile ducts.

In approximately 8% of patients, redundancy, elongation, or folding of the gallbladder neck on itself can each cause a pattern that mimics dilatation of either the common hepatic or proximal CBD (Fig. 6-54).[2,143] To avoid misinterpreting a redundant or elongated gallbladder neck for a dilated CBD, real-time equipment is essential. Emphasis should be placed on scanning the region of the gallbladder neck in an effort to note redundancy. The CBD can usually be located by angling the transducer along its expected course, just medial to the gallbladder neck.

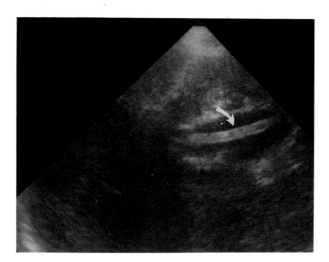

FIG 6-53. Ascaris worm in CBD. Echogenic tubular structure *(curved arrow)* is visible in a markedly dilated CBD.
(From Laing FC: Ultrasonography of the gallbladder and biliary tree. In: Sarti DA, ed: *Diagnostic Ultrasound: Text and Cases.* 2nd ed. Chicago: Yearbook Medical Publishers; 1987.)

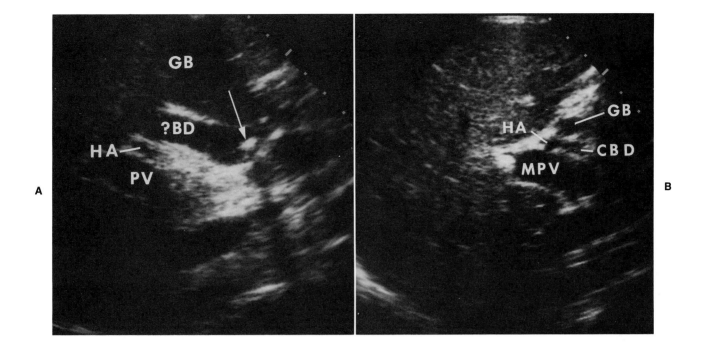

FIG 6-54. Pitfall—stone in a redundant gallbladder neck mimicking choledocholithiasis. **A,** Calculus with acoustic shadowing (arrow) is visible in what might be mistaken for a dilated bile duct. The gallbladder *(GB)* is anterior, the portal vein *(PV)* and hepatic artery *(HA)* are posterior to this structure. **B,** Longitudinal scan obtained in a slightly more medial direction confirms a normal-size bile duct *(CBD)* posterior to the gallbladder neck *(GB)*. *MPV,* Main portal vein; *HA,* hepatic artery.

(From Laing FC, Filly RA, Gooding GAW: Ultrasonography of the liver and biliary tract. In: Margulis AR, Burhenne HJ, eds: *Alimentary Tract Radiology.* 4th ed. St. Louis: CV Mosby Co; 1989.)

Variations in the anatomic position of the hepatic artery, which occur in approximately 30% of patients, can also cause diagnostic problems.[144] Because the diameters of both the aberrant artery and duct are usually small, in most circumstances it is not necessary to determine which structure is the duct and which the artery. A problem may develop, however, if the hepatic artery (aberrant or normally positioned) dilates and becomes larger in diameter than the CBD. This has been reported to occur in 59% of cases and may result in the hepatic artery being mistaken for an enlarged CBD.[144]

Although duplex Doppler sonography has been used to help discriminate bile ducts from vessels in the porta hepatis,[144] it is technically difficult to position the sample volume within these relatively small structures that rapidly change position with respiration. Since the introduction of color Doppler, it is no longer necessary to depend on morphology to distinguish biliary from vascular strictures.

Atypical Cases. Although ultrasound can distinguish medical from surgical jaundice in more than 90% of cases, atypical cases will be encountered. Infrequently, **dilatation** of the biliary tree can occur **without jaundice.**[145,146] In these patients, partial or incomplete biliary obstruction may be present, or only one hepatic duct may be dilated. Rarely, complete obstruction can occur with a significant time delay from the onset of obstruction to the development of clinical signs. In patients with anicteric dilatation, the ultrasound findings and the serum alkaline phosphatase level appear to be more sensitive than the serum bilirubin for suggesting obstruction. Occasionally, anicteric dilatation of the extrahepatic bile duct may be seen in postcholecystectomy patients or in patients with prior obstruction who exhibit dilatation without obstruction. Intestinal hypomotility is also felt to be responsible for some cases of nonobstructed bile duct dilatation as it relates to factors that inhibit the relaxation of the sphincter of Oddi or prolongs its contraction.[147]

The converse situation can also occur. A patient with obstructive jaundice may fail to exhibit dilatation of either the intrahepatic or extrahepatic bile ducts.[107,148] Cholangitis, partial obstruction, or intermittent obstruction from choledocholithiasis are usually responsible for these cases (Fig. 6-55). Finally, an occasional patient may have an extrahepatic duct that changes

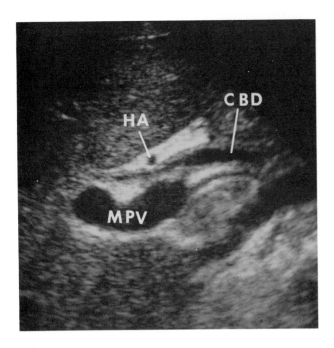

FIG 6-55. AIDS cholangitis. Longitudinal scan of the CBD reveals diffuse wall thickening without dilatation. Note the aberrant location of the hepatic artery *(HA)*. *CBD*, Common bile duct; *MPV*, main portal vein.

rapidly in size (over a period of several minutes to several days).[149,150] These prominent fluctuations most probably relate to the elasticity and associated distensibility of the duct.

The literature suggests that biliary dynamics can be assessed in questionable cases by repeating the scan after administering a **fatty meal** (Fig. 6-56). Indications for administering a fatty meal include:

- Equivocal extrahepatic duct diameter
- Mildly abnormal caliber duct with normal laboratory values
- Normal caliber duct with abnormal laboratory values
- A persistent question of choledocholithiasis
- Asymptomatic bile duct dilatation[151]
- An attempt to detect choledocholithiasis[126]

In true-negative cases, a normal-sized duct remains unchanged or decreases in size following a fatty meal whereas an initially enlarged duct decreases in caliber. In true-positive cases, an initially normal or slightly dilated duct increases in size.[151-153] The literature is discrepant with regard to interpreting an initially dilated duct that fails to change in size following a fatty meal. According to Simeone et al, this is an abnormal finding suggestive of obstruction.[151] Willson et al[152] claim that

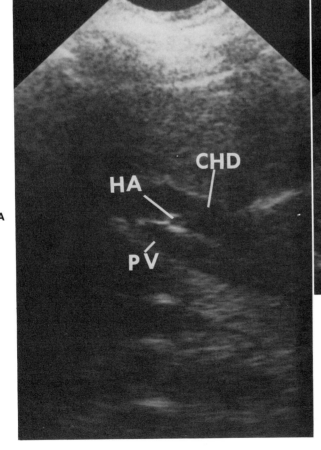

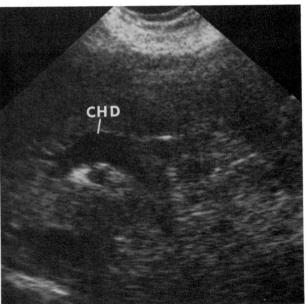

FIG 6-56. Fatty meal. **A,** Longitudinal scan over the porta hepatis shows mild dilatation of the common hepatic duct (diameter of 9 mm). **B,** A repeat scan performed 45 minutes after a fatty meal shows progressive dilatation of the common hepatic duct *(CHD)* (diameter of 11 mm), indicating active obstruction. The cause was a distal bile duct stricture in a patient with AIDS cholangitis. *CHD*, Common hepatic duct; *PV*, portal vein; *HA*, hepatic artery.

a dilated CBD that does not decrease in size following a fatty meal is not a specific indicator of obstruction, because in their experience 84% of such cases fail to show obstruction. In general, this test has been most useful for detecting patients with partial CBD obstruction; in the experience of Darweesh et al[153] it had a sensitivity of 74% and a specificity of 100% for detecting partial common duct obstruction. When performing this test it is important to measure the duct before and after the fatty meal at precisely the same location. Simeone et al[151] consider a 1-mm size change significant; other investigators conclude that differences in duct diameters of ±1 mm are within the range of measurement error; therefore, they consider changes of 2 mm or greater as significant.[153] Furthermore, in our laboratory, many critically ill patients often fail to show any biliary response following the administration of either oral fat (Lipomul) or intravenous cholecystokinin (Sincalide). Because gallbladder contraction fails to occur, the test loses its validity in these patients.

Detecting Choledocholithiasis. Modern ultrasound equipment and careful scanning techniques currently allow approximately 75% of CBD stones to be visualized.[122,126] Although experienced sonographers can usually diagnose choledocholithiasis with confidence, there are several possible sources of confusion. Dis-

tally, gas or particulate material in the adjacent duodenum may mimic a CBD stone. Transverse scanning with fluid in the duodenum can minimize this problem. Pancreatic calcification can also be confused for a distal calculus. Careful transverse scanning over the distal duct can usually differentiate between these two entities but CT or a radiographic contrast examination of the bile duct may be required for definitive diagnosis.

Occasionally, soft pigment stones will be difficult if not impossible to distinguish from intrabiliary sludge, pus, blood, or even neoplasm (Figs. 6-57 and 6-58). Gas anywhere in the biliary tree will also limit ultrasound's ability to detect and diagnose biliary calculi confidently (Fig. 6-59). Patients known to have biliary gas as a result of prior surgery or biliary-enteric fistula should probably undergo CT or cholangiography for bile duct evaluation.

Ultrasound will also be limited in its ability to detect choledocholithiasis in the absence of bile duct dilatation. Because patients with impacted distal calculi frequently seek medical help soon after the onset of their symptoms, it is not surprising that one third of CBD calculi are found in nondilated bile ducts (Fig. 6-60).[154,155] In our limited experience for detecting choledocholithiasis in normal-sized ducts, our sensitivity was 60% (3 of 5 patients).[122] In Cronan's series of 78 patients with choledocholithiasis, 26 patients (33%) had normal-sized ducts and the detection rate for calculi in this group was only 12% (3 of 26 patients).[156]

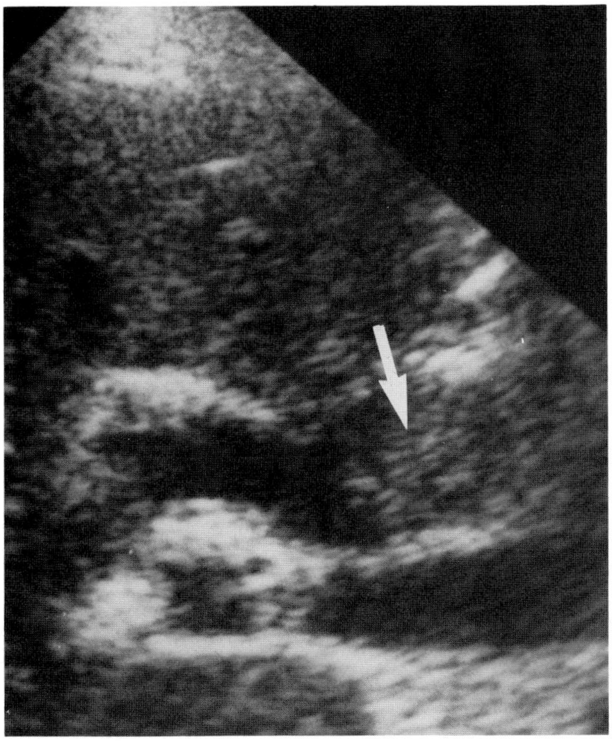

FIG 6-57. Biliary obstruction due to soft pigment stone in the distal CBD *(arrow)*.

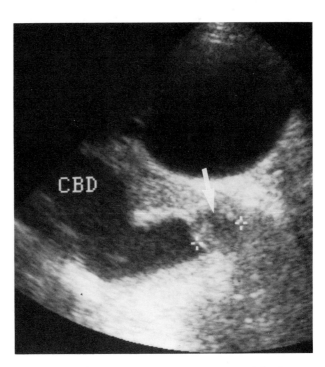

FIG 6-58. Biliary obstruction due to a primary bile duct tumor *(arrow)*. *CBD,* Common bile duct.

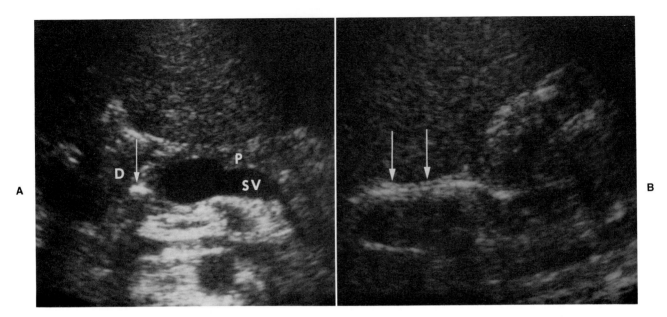

FIG 6-59. Gas in common bile duct mimicking choledolithiasis. **A,** Transverse scan over the body and head of the pancreas obtained with the patient in an erect position reveals an echogenic shadowing focus that suggests distal choledocholithiasis *(arrow).* **B,** Longitudinal scan of the same patient reveals a linear area of echogenicity *(arrows)* in the expected position of the common bile duct (CBD), suggesting air. Choledocholithiasis was not present. *SV,* Splenic vein; *P,* pancreas; *D,* duodenum.

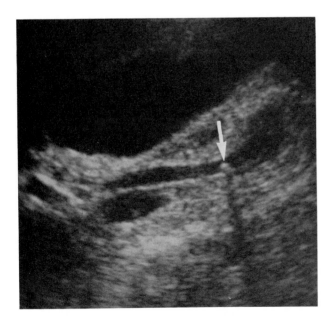

FIG 6-60. Choledocholithias *(arrow).* Parasagittal scan shows an echogenic focus with acoustic shadowing in a normal size bile duct.

The sensitivity of ultrasound for detecting calculi in the proximal CBD approximates 90%.[122] Despite this high sensitivity, there are several pitfalls that can cause problems for the unwary. Sources of this confusion include: the right hepatic artery, postcholecystectomy surgical clips, the cystic duct, tortuosity of the duct, and reverberation echoes within the bile duct. It must be emphasized that appropriate equipment and scanning technique, as well as familiarity with these causes of echogenic foci within the common duct, should minimize false-positive diagnoses of choledocholithiasis.

REFERENCES
The gallbladder

1. Callen PW, Filly RA: Ultrasonographic localization of the gallbladder. *Radiology* 1979;133:687-691.
2. Laing FC, Filly RA, Gooding GAW: Ultrasonography of the liver and biliary tract. In: Margulis Ar, Burhenne HJ, eds: *Alimentary Tract Radiology,* 4th ed. St. Louis, CV Mosby Co; 1989.
3. Worthen NJ, Uszler JM, Funamura JL: Cholecystitis: prospective evaluation of sonography and 99 mTc-HIDA cholescintigraphy. *AJR* 1981;137:973-978.
4. Dodds WJ, Groh WJ, Darweesh RMA, et al: Sonographic measurement of gallbladder volume. *AJR* 1985;145:1009-1011.
5. Hopman WPM, Brouwer WFM, Rosenbusch G, et al: A computerized method for rapid quantification of gallbladder volume from real-time sonograms. *Radiology* 1985;154:236-237.

6. Laing FC: Ultrasonography of the gallbladder and biliary tree. In: Sarti DA, ed: *Diagnostic Ultrasound: Text and Cases,* 2nd ed. Chicago, Yearbook Medical Publishers, 1987.

7. Sukov RJ, Sample WF, Sarti DA, et al: Cholecystosonography: the junctional fold. *Radiology* 1979;133:435-436.

8. Parulekar SG: Evaluation of the prone view for cholecystosonography. *J Ultrasound Med* 1986;5:617-624.

9. Hublitz UF, Kahn PC, Sell LA: Cholecystosonography: an approach to the nonvisualized gallbladder. *Radiology* 1972;103:645-649.

10. Cooperberg PL, Burhenne HJ: Real-time ultrasonography. Diagnostic technique of choice in calculus gallbladder disease. *New Engl J Med* 1980;302:1277-1279.

11. Crade M, Taylor KJW, Rosenfield AT, et al: Surgical and pathologic correlation of cholecystosonography and cholecystography. *AJR* 1978;131:227-229.

12. McIntosh DMF, Penney HF: Gray scale ultrasonography as a screening procedure in the detection of gallbladder disease. *Radiology* 1980;136:725-727.

13. de Graff CS, Dembner AG, Taylor KJW: Ultrasound and false normal oral cholecystogram. *Arch Surg* 1978;113:877-879.

14. Gelfand DW, Wolfman NT, Ott DJ, et al: Oral cholecystography vs gallbladder sonography: a prospective, blinded reappraisal. *AJR* 1988;151:69-72.

15. Amberg JR, Leopold GR: Is oral cholecystography still useful? *AJR* 1988;151:73-74.

16. Simeone JF, Mueller PR, Ferrucci JT: Nonsurgical therapy of gallstones: implications for imaging. *AJR* 1989;152:11-17.

17. Carroll BA: Gallstones: in vitro comparison of physical, radiographic, and ultrasonic characteristics. *AJR* 1978;131:223-226.

18. Filly RA, Moss AA, Way LW: In vitro investigation of gallstone shadowing with ultrasound tomography. *J Clin Ultrasound* 1979;7:255-262.

19. Jeanty P, Ammann W, Cooperberg P, et al: Mobile intraluminal masses of the gallbladder. *J Ultrasound Med* 1983;2:65-71.

20. Fakhry J: Sonography of tumefactive biliary sludge. *AJR* 1982;139:717-719.

21. Laing FC, Gooding GAW, Herzog KA: Gallstones preventing ultrasonographic visualization of the gallbladder. *Gastrointest Radiol* 1977;1:301-303.

22. MacDonald FR, Cooperberg PL, Cohen MM: The WES triad: a specific sonographic sign of gallstones in the contracted gallbladder. *Gastrointest Radiol* 1981;6:39-41.

23. Raptopoulos V, D'Orsi C, Smith E, et al: Dynamic cholecystosonography of the contracted gallbladder: the double-arc-shadow sign. *AJR* 1982; 138:275-278.

24. Kane RA, Jacobs R, Katz J, et al: Porcelain gallbladder: ultrasound and computed tomography appearance. *Radiology* 1984;152:137-141.

25. Hunter ND, Macintosh PK: Acute emphysematous cholecystitis: an ultrasonic diagnosis. *AJR* 1980;134:592-593.

26. Parulekar SG: Sonographic findings in acute emphysematous cholecystitis. *Radiology* 1982;145:117-119.

27. Laing FC, Federle MP, Jeffrey RB, et al: Ultrasonic evaluation of patients with acute right upper quadrant pain. *Radiology* 1981;140:449-455.

28. Sanders RC: The significance of sonographic gallbladder wall thickening. *J Clin Ultrasound* 1980;8:143-146.

29. Shlaer WJ, Leopold GR, Scheible FW: Sonography of the thickened gallbladder wall: a nonspecific finding. *AJR* 1981;136:337-339.

30. Ralls PW, Quinn MF, Juttner HU: Gallbladder wall thickening: patients without intrinsic gallbladder disease. *AJR* 1981;137:65-68.

31. Wegener M, Borsch G, Schneider J, et al: Gallbladder wall thickening: a frequent finding in various nonbiliary disorders—a prospective ultrasonographic study. *J Clin Ultrasound* 1987;15:307-312.

32. Romano AJ, VanSonnenberg E, Casola G, et al: Gallbladder and bile duct abnormalities in AIDS: sonographic findings in eight patients. *AJR* 1988;150:123-127.

33. Maresca G, De Gaetano AM, Mirk P, et al: Sonographic patterns of the gallbladder in acute viral hepatitis. *J Clin Ultrasound* 1984;12:141-146.

34. Huang Y-S, Lee S-D, Wu J-C, et al: Utility of sonographic gallbladder wall patterns in differentiating malignant from cirrhotic ascites. *J Clin Ultrasound* 1989;17:187-192.

35. Tsujimoto F, Miyamoto Y, Tada S: Differentiation of benign from malignant ascites by sonographic evaluation of gallbladder wall. *Radiology* 1985;157:503-504.

36. Marti-Bonmati L, Andres JC, Aguado C: Sonographic relationship between gallbladder wall thickness and the etiology of ascites. *J Clin Ultrasound* 1989;17:497-501.

37. Weiner SN, Koenigsberg M, Morehouse H, et al: Sonography and computed tomography in the diagnosis of carcinoma of the gallbladder. *AJR* 1984;142:735-739.

38. Bundy AL, Ritchie WGM: Ultrasonic diagnosis of metastatic melanoma of the gallbladder presenting as acute cholecystitis. *J Clin Ultrasound* 1982; 10:285-287.

39. Phillips G, Pochaczevsky R, Goodman J, et al: Ultrasound patterns of metastatic tumors in the gallbladder. *J Clin Ultrasound* 1982;10:379-383.

40. Raghavendra BN, Subramanyam BR, Balthazer EJ, et al: Sonography of adenomyomatosis of the gallbladder: radiologic-pathologic correlation. *Radiology* 1983;146:747-752.

41. Lafortune M, Gariepy G, Dumont A, et al: The V-shaped artifact of the gallbladder. *AJR* 1986;147:505-508.

42. Jeffrey RB, Laing FC, Wong W, et al: Gangrenous cholecystitis: diagnosis by ultrasound. *Radiology* 1983;148:219-221.

43. Filly RA, Allen B, Minton MJ, et al: In vitro investigation of the origin of echoes within biliary sludge. *J Clin Ultrasound* 1980;8:193-200.

44. Bolondi L, Gaiani S, Testa S, et al: Gallbladder sludge formation during prolonged fasting after gastrointestinal tract surgery. *Gut* 1985;26:734-738.

45. Messing B, Bories C, Kustlinger F, et al: Does total parenteral nutrition induce gallbladder sludge formation and lithiasis? *Gastroenterology* 1983;84:1012-1019.

46. Britten JS, Golding RH, Cooperberg PL: Sludge balls to gallstones. *J Ultrasound Med* 1984; 3:81-84.

47. Laing FC, Jeffrey RB, Federle MP: Gallbladder and bile ducts. In: Jeffrey RB, ed: *Computed Tomography and Sonography of the Acute Abdomen.* New York: Raven Press; 1989:59-62.

48. Nyberg DA, Laing FC: Ultrasonographic findings in peptic ulcer disease and pancreatitis that simulate primary gallbladder disease. *J Ultrasound Med* 1983;2:303-307.

49. Shuman WP, Mack LA, Rudd TG, et al: Evaluation of acute right upper quadrant pain: sonography and 99mTc-PIPIDA cholescintigraphy. *AJR* 1982;139:61-64.

50. Weissman HS, Frank MS, Bernstein LH, et al: Rapid and accurate diagnosis of acute cholecystitis with 99mTc-HIDA cholescintigraphy. *AJR* 1979;132:523-528.

51. Sherman M, Ralls PW, Quinn M, et al: Intravenous cholangiography and sonography in acute cholecystitis: prospective evaluation. *AJR* 1980;135:311-313.

52. Ralls PW, Colletti PM, Lapin SA, et al: Real-time sonography in suspected acute cholecystitis. *Radiology* 1985;155:767-771.

53. Cohan RH, Mahony BS, Bowie JD, et al: Striated intramural gallbladder lucencies on ultrasound studies: predictors of acute cholecystitis. *Radiology* 1987;164:31-35.

54. Teefey SH, Baron RL, Bigler SA: Sonography of the gallbladder: the significance of striated (layered) thickening of the gallbladder wall. *AJR* 1991; 156:945-947

55. Mentzer RM, Golden CT, Chandler JC, et al: A comparative appraisal of emphysematous cholecystitis. *Am J Surg* 1975;129:10-15.

56. Bloom RA, Libson E, Lebensart PD, et al: The ultrasound spectrum of emphysematous cholecystitis. *J Clin Ultrasound* 1989;17:251-256.

57. Parulekar SG: Sonographic findings in acute emphysematous cholecystitis. *Radiology* 1982;145:117-119.

58. Nemcek AA Jr, Gore RM, Vogelzang RL, et al: The effervescent gallbladder: a sonographic sign of emphysematous cholecystitis. *AJR* 1988;150:575-577.

59. Simeone JF, Brink JA, Mueller PR, et al: The sonographic diagnosis of acute gangrenous cholecystitis: importance of the Murphy sign. *AJR* 1989;152:289-290.

60. Miyazaki K, Uchiyama A, Nakayama F: Use of ultrasonographic risk score in the time of operative intervention for acute cholecystitis. *Arch Surg* 1988;123:487-489.

61. Strohl EL, Diffenbaugh WG, Baker JH, et al: Collective reviews: gangrene and perforation of the gallbladder. *Int Obstet Surg* 1962; 114:1-7.

62. Niemeier OW: Acute free perforation of the gallbladder. *Ann Surg* 1934;99:922-924.

63. Madrazo BL, Francis I, Hricak H, et al: Sonographic findings in perforation of the gallbladder. *AJR* 1982;139:491-496.

64. Takada T, Yasuda H, Uchiyama K, et al: Pericholecystic abscess: classification of ultrasound findings to determine the proper therapy. *Radiology* 1989;172:693-697.

65. McGahan JP, Walter JP: Diagnostic percutaneous aspiration of the gallbladder. *Radiology* 1985;155:619-622.

66. McGahan JP, Lindfors KK: Acute cholecystitis: diagnostic accuracy of percutaneous aspiration of the gallbladder. *Radiology* 1988;167:669-671.

67. McGahan JP, Lindfors KK: Percutaneous cholecystostomy: an alternative to surgical cholecystostomy for acute cholecystitis? *Radiology* 1989;173:481-485.

68. Mirvis SE, Vainright JR, Nelson AW, et al: The diagnosis of acute acalculous cholecystitis: a comparison of sonography, scintigraphy, and computed tomography. *AJR* 1986;147:1171-1175.

69. Raduns K, McGahan JP, Beal S: Cholecystokinin sonography: lack of utility in diagnosis of acute calculous cholecystitis. *Radiology* 1990;175:463-466.

70. Swayne LC: Acute acalculous cholecystitis: sensitivity in detection using technetium-99m iminodiacetic acid cholescintigraphy. *Radiology* 1986;160:33-38.

71. Ferrucci JT: Biliary lithotripsy. *AJR* 1989;153:15-22.

72. Lauffer I: Imaging stones in era of nonsurgical therapy. *Diagn Imaging Clin Med* 1989; 11:101-111.

73. Torres WE, Baumgartner BR, Casarella WJ: The abnormal appearing gallbladder following ESWL. *Radiology* 1990;submitted for publication.

74. Gleeson D, Ruppin DC: Discrepancies between cholecystography and ultrasonography in the detection of recurrent gallstones. *J Hepatol* 1985;1:597-607.

75. Fitzgerald EJ, Toi A: Pitfalls in the ultrasonographic diagnosis of gallbladder diseases. *Postgrad Med J* 1987;63:525-532.

76. White M, Simeone JF, Mueller PR: Imaging of cholecystocolic fistulas. *J Ultrasound Med* 1983;2:181-185.

77. Gooding GAW: Food particles in the gallbladder mimic cholelithiasis in a patient with a cholecystojejunostomy. *J Clin Ultrasound* 1981;9:346-347.

78. Scheske GA, Cooperberg PL, Cohen MM: Floating gallstones: the role of contrast material. *J Clin Ultrasound* 1980;8:227-231.

79. Rubaltelli L, Talenti E, Rizzatto G, et al: Gas-containing gallstones: their influence on ultrasound images. *J Clin Ultrasound* 1984;12:279-282.

80. Mitchell DG, Needleman L, Frauenhoffer S, et al: Gas containing gallstones: the sonographic "double echo sign". *J Ultrasound Med* 1988;7:39-43.

81. Yeh HC, Goodman J, Rabinowitz JG: Floating gallstones in bile without added contrast material. *AJR* 1986;146:49-5O.

82. Federle MP, Cello JP, Laing FC, et al: Recurrent pyogenic cholangitis in Asian immigrants. *Radiology* 1982;143:151-156.

83. Reinig JW, Stanley JH: Sonographic hepatization of the gallbladder: a cause of nonvisualization of the gallbladder by cholecystosonography. *J Clin Ultrasound* 1984;12:234-236.

84. Hammond DI: Unusual causes of sonographic nonvisualization or nonrecognition of the gallbladder: a review. *J Clin Ultrasound* 1988;16:77-85.

85. Ferin P, Lemer RM: Contracted gallbladder: a finding in hepatic dysfunction. *Radiology* 1985;154:769-770.

86. Childress MH: Sonographic features of milk calcium cholecystitis. *J Clin Ultrasound* 1986;14:312-314.

87. Chun GH, Deutsch AL, Scheible W: Sonographic findings in milk of calcium bile. *Gastrointest Radiol* 1982;7:371-373.

88. Fiske CE, Filly RA: Pseudo-sludge: a spurious ultrasound appearance within the gallbladder. *Radiology* 1982;144:631-632.

89. Laing FC, Kurtz AB: The importance of ultrasonic side-lobe artifacts. *Radiology* 1982;145:763-768.

90. Marchal GJ, Holsbeeck MV, Tshibwabwa-Ntumba E: Dilatation of the cystic veins in portal hypertension: sonographic demonstration. *Radiology* 1985;154:187-189.

91. Ralls PW, Mayekawa DS, Lee KP, et al: Gallbladder wall varices: diagnosis with color flow doppler sonography. *J Clin Ultrasound* 1988;16:595-598.

Intrahepatic bile ducts

92. Bressler EL, Rubin JM, McCracken S, et al: Sonographic parallel channel sign: a reappraisal. *Radiology* 1987;164:343-346.

93. Laing FC, London LA, Filly RA: Ultrasonographic identification of dilated intrahepatic bile ducts and their differentiation from portal venous structures. *J Clin Ultrasound* 1978;6:90-94.

94. Bret PM, de Stempel JV, Atri M, et al: Intrahepatic bile duct and portal vein anatomy revisited. *Radiology* 1988;169:405-407.

95. Lim JH, Ryu KN, Ko YT, et al: Anatomic relationship of intrahepatic bile ducts to portal veins. *J Ultrasound Med* 1990;9:137-143.

96. Filly RA, Sommer FG, Minton MJ: Characterization of biological fluids by ultrasound and computed tomography. *Radiology* 1980;134:167-171.

97. Byung IC, Lim JH, Han MC, et al: Biliary cystadenoma and cystadenocarcinoma: computed tomography and sonographic findings. *Radiology* 1989;171:57-61.

98. Carroll BA, Oppenheimer DA: Sclerosing cholangitis: sonographic demonstration of bile duct wall thickening. *AJR* 1982;139:1016-1018.

99. Singcharoen T, Baddeley H, Benson M, et al: Primary sclerosing cholangitis: sonographic findings. *Aust Radiol* 1986;30:99-102.

100. Dolmatch BL, Laing FC, Federle MP, et al: AIDS-related cholangitis: radiographic findings in nine patients. *Radiology* 1987;163:313-316.

101. Federle MP, Cello JP, Laing FC, et al: Recurrent pyogenic cholangitis in Asian immigrants. *Radiology* 1982;143:151-156.

102. Laing FC: Ultrasound diagnosis of choledocholithiasis. *Sem Ultrasound, CT and MR* 1987;8:103-113.

103. Schulman A: Non-Western patterns of biliary stones and the role of ascariasis. *Radiology* 1987;162:425430.

104. Chen HH, Zhang WH, Wang SS: Twenty-two year experience with the diagnosis and treatment of intrahepatic calculi. *Surg Gynecol Obstet* 1984;159:519-524.

105. Marchal GJ, Desmer VJ, Proesmans WC, et al: Caroli's disease: high-frequency ultrasound and pathologic findings. *Radiology* 1986;158:507-511.

106. Mittelstaedt CA, Volberg FM, Fisher GJ et al: Caroli's disease: sonographic findings. *AJR* 1980;136:585-587.

107. Sample WF, Sarli DA, Goldstein Ll, et al: Gray-scale ultrasonography of the jaundiced patient. *Radiology* 1978;128:719-725.

108. Laffey PA, Teplick SK, Haskin PH: Hemobilia: a cause of false-negative ductal dilatation. *J Clin Ultrasound* 1986;14:636-638.

109. Laffey PA, Brandon JC, Teplick SK, et al: Ultrasound of hemobilia: a clinical and experimental study. *J Clin Ultrasound* 1988;16:167-170.

110. Lewandowski BJ, Withers C, Winsberg F: The air-filled left hepatic duct: the saber sign as an aid to the radiographic diagnosis of pneumobilia. *Radiology* 1984;153:329-332.

111. Desai RK, Paushter DM, Armistead J: Intrahepatic arterial calcification mimicking pneumobilia. *J Ultrasound Med* 1989;8:333-335.

112. Lin HH, Changchien CS, Lin DY: Hepatic parenchymal calcifications: differentiation from intrahepatic stones. *J Clin Ultrasound* 1989;17:411-415.

113. Wing VW, Laing FC, Jeffrey RB: Sonographic differentiation of enlarged hepatic arteries from dilated intrahepatic bile ducts. *AJR* 1985;145:57-61.

114. Ralls PW, Mayekawa, Lee KP, et al: The use of color doppler sonography to distinguish dilated intrahepatic ducts from vascular structures. *AJR* 1988;152:291-292.

Extrahepatic bile ducts

115. Parulekar SG: Sonography of the distal cystic duct. *J Ultrasound Med* 1989;8:367-373.

116. Niederau C, Muller J, Sonnenberg A, et al: Extrahepatic bile ducts in healthy subjects, in patients with cholelithiasis, and in postcholecystectomy patients: a prospective ultrasonic study. *J Clin Ultrasound* 1983;11:23-27.

117. Behan M, Kazam E: Sonography of the common bile duct: value of the right anterior oblique view. *AJR* 1978;130:701-709.

118. Paruleker SG: Ultrasound evaluation of common bile duct size. *Radiology* 1979;133:703-707.

119. Graham MF, Cooperberg PL, Cohen MM, et al: The size of the normal common hepatic duct following cholecystectomy: an ultrasonographic study. *Radiology* 1980;135:137-139.

120. Mueller PR, Ferrucci JT, Simeone JF, et al: Postcholecystectomy bile duct dilatation: myth or reality? *AJR* 1981;136:355-358.

121. Wu CC, Ho YH, Chen CY: Effect of aging on common bile duct diameter: a real-time ultrasonographic study. *J Clin Ultrasound* 1984;12:473-478.11

122. Laing FC, Jeffrey RB, Wing VW: Improved visualization of choledocholithiasis by sonography. *AJR* 1984;143:949-952.

123. Shawker TH, Jones BL, Girton ME: Distal common bile duct obstruction: an experimental study in monkeys. *J Clin Ultrasound* 1981;9:77-82.

124. Honickman SP, Mueller PR, Wittenberg J, et al: Ultrasound in obstructive jaundice: prospective evaluation of site and cause. *Radiology* 1983;147:511-515.

125. Laing FC, Jeffrey RB Jr, Wing VW: Biliary dilatation: defining the level and cause by real-time ultrasound. *Radiology* 1986;160:39-42.

126. Dong B, Chen M: Improved sonographic visualization of choledocholithiasis. *J Clin Ultrasound* 1987;15:185-190.

127. Gibson RN, Yeung E, Thompson J, et al: Bile duct obstruction: radiologic evaluation of level, cause, and tumor resectability. *Radiology* 1986;160:43-47.

128. Nesbit GM, Johnson CD, James EM, et al: Cholangiocarcinoma: diagnosis and evaluation of resectability by computed tomography and sonography as procedures complementary to cholangiography. *AJR* 1988;151:933-938.

129. Clemett AR: Radiology of the liver and biliary tree. In: Margulis AR, Burhenne HJ, eds: *Alimentary Tract Radiology*. 4th ed. St. Louis, CV Mosby Co; 1989;1275-1281.

130. Klatskin G: Adenocarcinoma of the hepatic duct at its bifurcation within the porta hepatis: an unusual tumor with distinctive clinical and pathologic features. *Am J Med* 1965;38:241-256.

131. Meyer DG, Weinstein BJ: Klatskin tumors of the bile ducts: sonographic appearance. *Radiology* 1983;148:803-804.

132. Machan L, Muller NL, Cooperberg PL: Sonographic diagnosis of Klatskin tumors. *AJR* 1986;147:509-512.

133. Jackson VP, Lappas JC: Sonography of the Mirizzi syndrome. *J Ultrasound Med* 1984;3:281-283.

134. Becker CD, Hassler H, Terrier F: Preoperative diagnosis of the Mirizzi syndrome: limitations of sonography and computed tomography. *AJR* 1984;143:591-596.

135. Kimura K, Ohto T, Ono T, et al: Congenital cystic dilatation of the common bile duct: relationship to anomalous pancreaticobiliary ductal union. *AJR* 1977;128:571-577.

136. Han BK, Babcock DS, Gelfand MH: Choledochal cyst with bile duct dilatation: sonography and 99mTc-IDA cholescintigraphy. *AJR* 1981;136:1075-1079.

137. Gabaldon A, Mofidi C, Moskovskij S, et al: Control of ascariasis. *World Health Organization*. Technical Report Series 1967;379:6-7.

138. Cerri GG, Leite GJ, Simoes JB, et al: Ultrasonographic evaluation of ascaris in the biliary tract. *Radiology* 1983;146:753-754.

139. Schulman A, Loxton AJ, Heydenrych JJ, et al: Sonographic diagnosis of biliary ascariasis. *AJR* 1982;139:485-489.

140. Lim JH, Ko YT, Lee DH: Clonchiasis: sonographic findings in 59 proved cases. *AJR* 1989;152:761-764.

141. Lim JH: Radiologic findings of clonorchiasis. *AJR* 1990;155(100):1000-1008.

142. Jacobson JB, Brody PA: The transverse common duct. *AJR* 1981;136:91-95.

143. Laing FC, Jeffrey RB. The pseudo-dilated common bile duct: ultrasonographic appearance created by the gallbladder neck. *Radiology* 1980;135:405-407.

144. Berland LL, Lawson TL, Foley WD: Porta hepatis: sonographic discrimination of bile ducts from arteries with pulsed Doppler with new anatomic criteria. *AJR* 1982;138:833-840.

145. Weinstein BJ, Weinstein DP: Biliary tract dilatation in the nonjaundiced patient. *AJR* 1980;134:899-906.

146. Zemen R, Taylor KJW, Burrell MI, et al: Ultrasound demonstration of anicteric dilatation of the biliary tree. *Radiology* 1980;134:689-692.

147. Raptopoulos V, Smith EH, Cummings T, et al: Bile-duct dilatation after laparotomy: a potential effect of intestinal hypomotility. *AJR* 1986;147:729-731.

148. Muhletaler CA, Gerlock AJ Jr, Fleischer AC, et al: Diagnosis of obstructive jaundice with nondilated bile ducts. *AJR* 1980;134:1149-1152.

149. Glazer GM, Filly RA, Laing FC: Rapid change in caliber of the nonobstructed common duct. *Radiology* 1981;140:161-162.

150. Mueller PR, Ferrucci JT Jr, Simeone JF, et al: Observations on the distensibility of the common bile duct. *Radiology* 1982;142:467-472.

151. Simeone JF, Butch RJ, Mueller PR, et al: The bile ducts after a fatty meal: further sonographic observations. *Radiology* 1986;160:29-31.

152. Willson SA, Gosink BB, vanSonnenberg E: Unchanged size of a dilated common bile duct after fatty meal: results and significance. *Radiology* 1986;160:29-31.

153. Darweesh RM, Dodds WJ, Hogan WJ: Fatty meal sonography for evaluating patients with suspected partial common duct obstruction. *AJR* 1988;151:63-68.

154. Cronan JJ, Mueller PR, Simeone JF, et al: Prospective diagnosis of choledocholithiasis. *Radiology* 1983;146:467-469.

155. Laing FC, Jeffrey RB Jr: Choledocholithiasis and cystic duct obstruction: difficult ultrasonographic diagnosis. *Radiology* 1983;146:475-479.

156. Cronan J: Ultrasound diagnosis of choledocholithiasis: a reappraisal. *Radiology* 1986;161:133-134.

CHAPTER 7

The Pancreas

- Mostafa Atri, M.D.
- Paul W. Finnegan, M.D.

Before 1970, imaging of the pancreas was limited to the assessment of its surrounding structures or assessment of its angiographic vascular tree. With the advent of real-time ultrasound imaging, compute tomography (CT), and magnetic resonance (MR), visualization of the pancreas itself has become a reality. Although CT has played a major role, ultrasound remains the most widely available and cheapest means to visualize the pancreas.

Although a spectrum of pathologic processes affect the pancreas, the major tasks of the sonographer are to distinguish a normal from an abnormal pancreas and to differentiate between pancreatitis and malignant neoplasms. With the development of ultrasound-guided percutaneous fine-needle aspiration (PFNA) biopsy, the ability to differentiate between the latter two conditions has significantly improved. Ultrasound guidance has also helped to promote percutaneous interventional procedures as an alternative to surgical treatment for a number of pathologic conditions related to the pancreas.

EMBRYOLOGY

The primitive pancreas consists of a dorsal and a ventral bud.[1] The dorsal bud arises as a diverticulum of the dorsal aspect of the duodenum, whereas the ventral bud originates as a common diverticulum with the primitive common bile duct (Fig. 7-1, *A*). At 6 weeks of gestation, the ventral bud rotates 270 degrees to lie posteroinferior to the dorsal bud (Fig. 7-1, *B*). Fusion of these two buds forms the final pancreas. The dorsal bud develops into the cephalad aspect of the head, neck, body, and the tail, whereas the caudad aspect of the head and the uncinate process originate from the ventral bud (Fig. 7-1, *C*). Initially, each pancreatic bud has its own duct, which drains separately into the duodenum at two different openings, the major and minor papillas. Following fusion of the two buds, the ventral duct in the head anastomoses with the proximal part of the dorsal duct in the body and tail to form the final main pancreatic duct (duct of Wirsung), which drains most of the pancreas (Fig. 7-1, *C*). This main duct empties into the duodenum through the major papilla in combination with the common bile duct. The remaining portion of

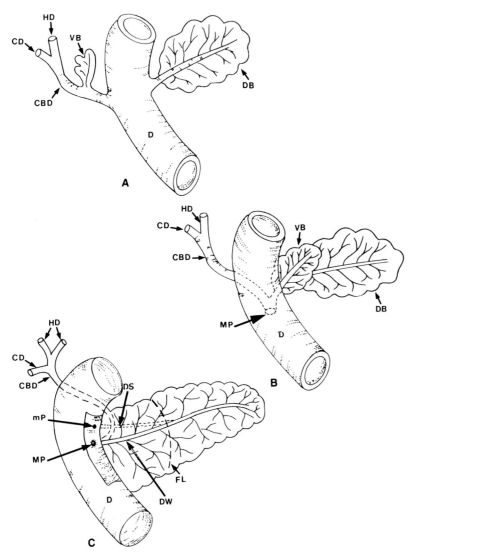

FIG 7-1. Stages in development of pancreas. **A,** Original pancreatic buds ventral and dorsal. **B,** 270 degree rotation of ventral bud. **C,** Fusion of two buds and formation of final pancreatic duct. *CBD,* Common bile duct; *CD,* cystic duct; *D,* duodenum; *DB,* dorsal bud; *DS,* duct of Santorini; *DW,* duct of Wirsung; *FL,* fusion line; *HD,* hepatic duct; *MP,* major papilla; *mP,* minor papilla; *VB,* ventral bud.

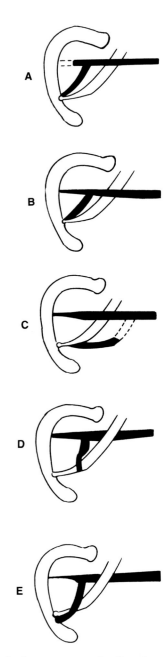

the dorsal pancreatic duct, called the accessory pancreatic duct (duct of Santorini), opens into the duodenum at the minor papilla. In most people, the terminal part of the dorsal duct in the head of the pancreas tends to completely or incompletely regress,[2] resulting in different variants of the pancreatic duct (Fig. 7-2).

ANATOMY

The pancreas can be localized with ultrasound by identifying its parenchymal architecture and the anatomic landmarks that surround the organ. The level of the pancreas is known to change slightly, depending on

FIG 7-2. Variations, pancreatic duct anatomy. **A,** Complete regression of duct of Santorini (40%-50%). **B,** Persistence of the duct of Santorini (35%). **C,** Persistence of both Santorini and Wirsung ducts without communication (5% to 10%). **D,** Communication of Santorini and Wirsung ducts, with duct of Wirsung entering common bile duct proximal to ampulla (5% to 10%). **E,** Separate entrance of duct of Wirsung and common bile duct with variable persistence of duct of Santorini (5%).

(From Berman LG, Prior JT, Abramow SM, et al: *Surg Gynecol Obstet* 1960; 11:391-403.)

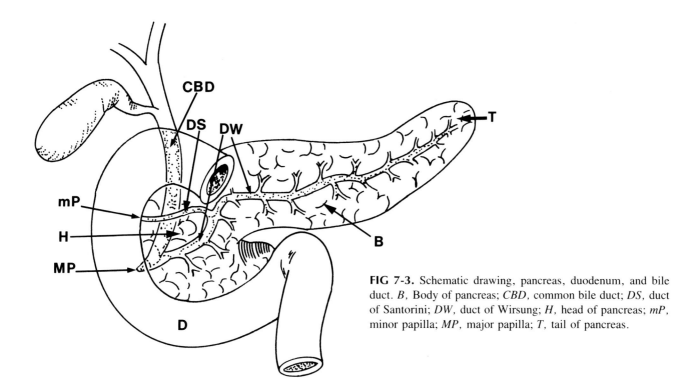

FIG 7-3. Schematic drawing, pancreas, duodenum, and bile duct. *B,* Body of pancreas; *CBD,* common bile duct; *DS,* duct of Santorini; *DW,* duct of Wirsung; *H,* head of pancreas; *mP,* minor papilla; *MP,* major papilla; *T,* tail of pancreas.

the phase of respiration. With maximal inspiration and expiration, the organ has been shown to shift 2 to 8 cm in the craniocaudad axis.[3] These respiratory migrations should be taken into consideration when imaging the pancreas and especially during ultrasound-guided biopsy.

The pancreas is a nonencapsulated, retroperitoneal structure that lies in the anterior pararenal space between the duodenal loop and the splenic hilum over a length of 12.5 to 15 cm.[1] The head, uncinate process, neck, body, and tail constitute the different parts of the pancreas (Fig. 7-3). The superior mesenteric vessels course posterior to the neck of the pancreas, separating the head from the body. The uncinate process represents the medial extension of the head and lies behind the superior mesenteric vessels. No anatomic landmark separates the body from the tail. The pancreas is divided into an exocrine and an endocrine component. The exocrine pancreas constitutes 80% of the pancreatic tissue and is made up of ductal and acinar cells. The endocrine islet cells of Langerhans form only 2% of the pancreatic substance. The remaining 18% consists of fibrous stroma that contains blood vessels, nerves, and lymphatics.[4]

Surrounding Structures

Gastrointestinal Tract, Ligaments, and Peritoneal Spaces. The antrum of the **stomach** lies transversely across the midline usually anterior to the pancreas with the gastric body located anterior to the pancreatic tail. However, depending on the patient's body habitus,

which alters the shape and orientation of the stomach, the pancreas may occupy a position cephalad or caudad to the stomach. The **duodenal loop,** except for the first segment, is retroperitoneal, encircling the pancreatic head.

The **transverse mesocolon** attaches to the anterior aspect of the head, body, and proximal tail of the pancreas posteriorly and to the greater omentum anteriorly. At the level of the head of the pancreas, the mesocolon joins midway between the superior and the inferior borders; at the level of the body, it suspends from the inferior border of the pancreas, dividing the organ into supra and inframesocolic portions. The stomach, omentum, and lesser sac lie anterior to the pancreas in the **supramesocolic portion.**[1]

The **lesser omentum,** a double layer of peritoneum, bridges the abdominal part of the esophagus, lesser curvature of the stomach, and first portion of the duodenum to the fissure for the ligamentum venosum of the liver. The **greater omentum,** also double-layered, hangs down from the greater curvature of the stomach and, after looping back on itself, attaches to the transverse colon. The lesser sac is a potential space situated between the lesser omentum, greater omentum, and the stomach anteriorly and the parietal peritoneum posteriorly. Depending on the position of the stomach, different parts of the lesser and greater omentum, stomach, and lesser sac are related to the pancreas anteriorly.[1] The **lesser sac** is frequently partially or completely obliterated by adhesions, and therefore the stomach and greater and lesser omentum come in close contact with the anterior surface of the pancreas. The jejunal loops, duodenojejunal junction, and splenic flexure of the colon lie anterior to the pancreas in the **inframesocolic space.**[1] The tip of the tail of the pancreas is intraperitoneal because it is ensheathed in the lienorenal ligament.[1]

Vessels

Arteries. The **abdominal aorta** runs posterior to the body of the pancreas. The **celiac axis** arises from the abdominal aorta at the superior border of the pancreas. It gives off the left gastric artery and then divides into the common hepatic artery (which proceeds anteriorly and to the right, cephalad to the head of the pancreas) and the splenic artery (which follows a tortuous course along the superior border of the body and the tail of the pancreas). At the inferior border of the epiploic foramen, the common hepatic artery divides into its two terminal branches, the hepatic proper and the gastroduodenal arteries. The hepatic artery proper travels superiorly toward the liver along the free edge of the lesser omentum anterior to the portal vein and to the left of the bile duct. A common normal variant, present in 25% of the population, consists of a completely or incompletely replaced hepatic artery, which arises from the right lateral aspect of the superior mesenteric artery. This accessory (or replaced hepatic artery) usually courses between the portal vein and the inferior vena cava as opposed to the normal hepatic artery that runs anterior to the portal vein. The gastroduodenal artery travels a short distance posterior to the junction of the pylorus and the first portion of the duodenum within a groove on the superior border of the pancreas lateral to the neck. Then, passing anterior to the head of the pancreas, it divides into its terminal branches, the right gastroepiploic and the superior pancreaticoduodenal arteries.[1] The **superior mesenteric artery** arises from the abdominal aorta just caudad to the inferior border of the pancreas, descending anterior to the uncinate process of the pancreas and the third portion of the duodenum to enter the mesentery.

Veins. The **inferior vena cava** lies posterior to the head of the pancreas. Depending on the level at which the renal veins drain into the inferior vena cava, the left renal vein may travel posterior to the head of the pancreas, although it is usually more caudal.

The **splenic vein** runs from its origin in the splenic hilum along the posteroinferior aspect of the pancreas to join the superior mesenteric vein. The **superior mesenteric vein** travels to the right of the superior mesenteric artery and ascends anterior to the third portion of the duodenum and the uncinate process of the pancreas. The superior mesenteric vein and the splenic vein join posterior to the neck of the pancreas to form the portal vein. The **portal vein** ascends towards the porta hepatis cephalad to the head of the pancreas.[1]

Common Bile Duct. The common bile duct passes inferiorly in the free edge of the lesser omentum to the level of the duodenum. It then travels posterior to the first portion of the duodenum and the head of the pancreas to lie to the right of the main pancreatic duct. The common bile duct then opens into the duodenum at the hepaticopancreatic ampulla on the summit of the major papilla after forming a common trunk with the pancreatic duct (80%). In 20% of people, the common bile duct has its own separate ampulla but still enters the duodenum at the major papilla.[5] In its course behind the head of the pancreas, it lies in a groove on the posterior aspect of the pancreas or is embedded in its substance.

PANCREATIC SONOGRAPHY

The classical planes for pancreatic sonographic examination include the transverse and sagittal planes. However, in practice, the orientation of the scan is seldom exact with respect to the true sagittal or transverse planes. Because the transducer is guided with reference to the sonographic display, the actual examination is conducted by recognizing the familiar landmark organs and vascular structures and therefore providing an unlimited number of planes, which is one of the advantages of sonography over CT.

Head

Transverse Plane. The pancreatic head may be quite long, extending over several centimeters. The sonographic appearance varies from the most cephalad to the most caudal image. **Cephalad to the pancreatic head,** the hepatic artery and bile duct are seen anterior to the portal vein. The air- or fluid-filled pylorus and the first portion of the duodenum may also be seen at this level. In the **superior aspect of the head,** two circular structures can be identified on the right lateral aspect of the head that represent a cross-sectional view of the gastroduodenal artery anteriorly and the common bile duct posteriorly. The latter structures demarcate the lateral aspect of the pancreatic head, allowing for separation of the head of the pancreas from the more laterally placed duodenum (Fig. 7-4, *A*). At this level the medial extent of the head merges with the neck of the pancreas. The inferior vena cava lies posterior to the head. However, the relation of the pancreas to the inferior vena cava and aorta is variable and can occasionally be off center to the left of the major vessels, especially in thin patients and in patients lying in the left decubitus position. The main pancreatic duct and its branches may be seen extending obliquely between the neck of the pancreas, more superiorly, and to the second portion of the duodenum, more inferiorly where it may or may not join the common bile duct before entering the duodenum. In its most **inferior aspect,** the medial portion of the pancreatic head tapers to form the uncinate process. At this level in cross-section, the superior mesenteric vein is seen to the right and the superior mesenteric artery to the left between the uncinate process and the neck of the pancreas (Fig. 7-4, *B*). A replaced hepatic artery is commonly shown by sonographic examination,[6] arising from the right lateral aspect of the superior mesenteric artery and running towards the liver between the portal

vein and inferior vena cava (Fig. 7-5). **Caudally to the head,** the third portion of the duodenum may be seen running transversely from right to left.

Sagittal Plane. On the right and lateral to the head, the second portion of the duodenum projects in a cephalocaudal direction. In the lateral aspect of the head in some patients, the gastroduodenal artery may be seen coursing in a cephalocaudal direction anterior to the pancreas with the common bile duct running parallel but more posteriorly (Fig. 7-6, *A*). The latter may lie posterior to the pancreas or embedded in its posterior aspect. The third portion of the duodenum is seen in cross-section views caudally to the pancreas. More medially, the longest cephalocaudal dimension of the head is displayed. A longitudinal view of the main portal vein projects superior to the head of the pancreas at this level (Fig. 7-6, *B*).

Neck, Body, and Tail

The pancreatic neck lies anterior to the portal venous confluence with the body to the left. There is no anatomic landmark separating the body and the tail of the pancreas, but the left lateral border of the vertebral column is considered the arbitrary plane demarcating these two segments. The level of the tail in relation to the body of the pancreas on the horizontal plane varies depending on the body habitus. It may be located cephalad, at the same level, or (rarely) lower than the body.

Transverse plane. The celiac axis is seen **cephalad** to the body of the pancreas at this level, dividing simi-

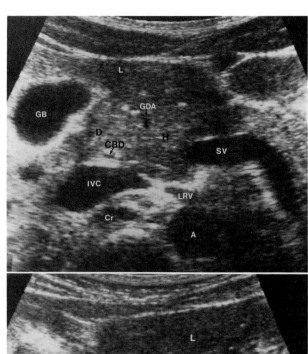

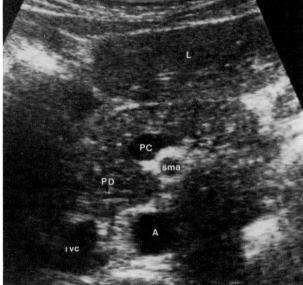

FIG 7-4. Head of pancreas, transverse scans. **A,** Superior aspect of head. Duodenum is as echogenic as pancreas and can only be distinguished from head because of visualization of gastroduodenal artery *(GDA)* and common bile duct *(CBD)*. **B,** Inferior aspect of head. Arrow points to branch of pancreatic duct (PD). *A,* Aorta; *CBD,* common bile duct; *Cr,* crus of diaphragm; *D,* duodenum; *GB,* gallbladder; *GDA,* gastroduodenal artery; *H,* head of pancreas; *IVC,* inferior vena cava; *L,* liver; *LRV,* left renal vein; *PC,* portal confluence; *PV,* portal vein; *sma,* superior mesenteric artery; *smv,* superior mesenteric vein; *sv,* splenic vein.

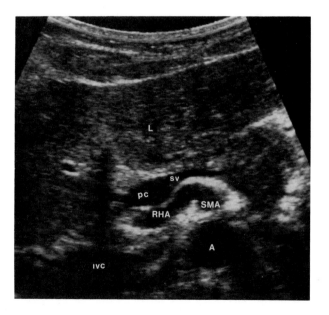

FIG 7-5. Replaced hepatic artery (RHA) running between portal confluence *(PC)* and inferior vena cava *(IVC)*. Transverse scan. *A,* Aorta; *L,* liver; *SMA,* superior mesenteric artery; *SV,* splenic vein

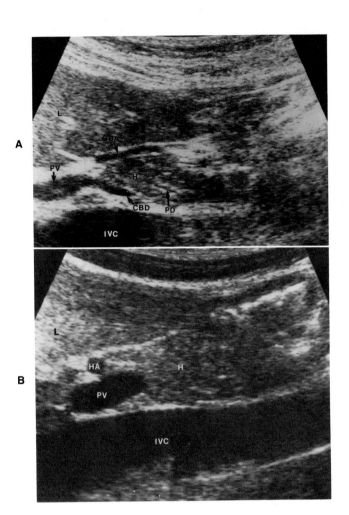

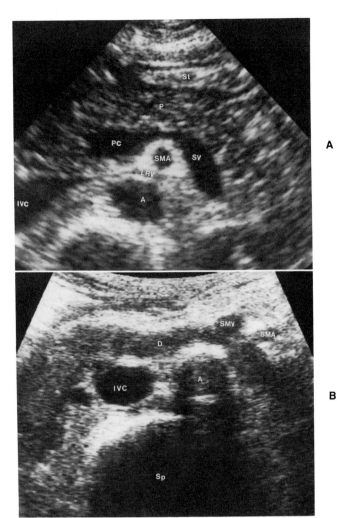

FIG 7-6. Head of pancreas, sagittal view. **A,** Lateral aspect of head. **B,** medial aspect of head. *CBD,* Common bile duct; *GDA,* gastroduodenal artery; *H,* head of pancreas; *HA,* hepatic artery; *IVC,* inferior vena cava; *L,* liver; *PD,* pancreatic duct; *PV,* portal vein.

FIG 7-7. Neck, body, and tail of pancreas, transverse view. **A,** Through pancreas. **B,** Caudad to pancreas. *A,* Aorta; *D,* duodenum; *IVC,* inferior vena cava; *L,* liver; *LRV,* left renal vein; *P,* pancreas; *PC,* portal confluence; *SMA,* superior mesenteric artery; *Sp,* spine; *St,* stomach; *SV,* splenic vein.

lar to a Y into the hepatic and splenic arteries. At the **level of the neck,** the confluence of the splenic and superior mesenteric veins is seen posterior to the pancreas. More laterally, the splenic vein runs posterior to the body and the tail. The abdominal aorta lies posterior to the proximal body of the pancreas. The left renal vein courses between the superior mesenteric artery and the aorta and posterior to the pancreas to drain into the inferior vena cava. The upper pole of the left kidney and the left renal vessels may also be seen posterior to the tail of the pancreas. Depending on the location of the stomach, its posterior wall may be visualized anterior to the pancreas (Fig. 7-7, *A*). **Caudad** to the pancreas lie the third and fourth portions of the duodenum (Fig. 7-7, *B*).

Sagittal Plane. At the level of the neck, the superior mesenteric vein is seen posterior to the pancreas (Fig. 7-8, *A*). The uncinate process of the head is seen posterior to the superior mesenteric vein. A longitudinal view of the aorta is identified with the **body** of the pancreas situated between the celiac axis and the superior mesenteric artery (Fig. 7-8, *B*). At the levels of the body and the tail, the stomach lies anteriorly (Fig. 7-8, *C*). A cross-section of the splenic vein is seen posteriorly, whereas a cross-section of the splenic artery appears cephalady. The third portion of the duodenum projects inferiorly. Using the spleen as an acoustic window, the **tail** of the pancreas is occasionally seen medial to that organ on both transverse and coronal planes (Fig. 7-8, *D*).

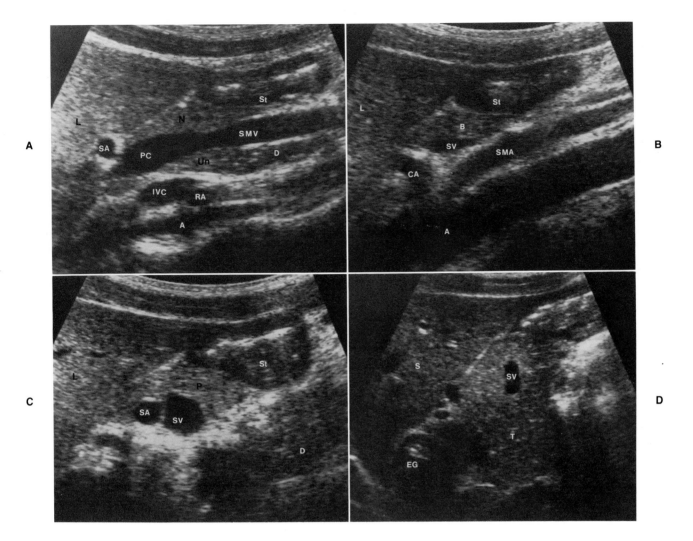

FIG 7-8. Neck, body, and tail of pancreas, sagittal view. **A,** Level of neck. **B,** Slightly to left of neck. **C,** Level of body. **D,** Level of tail on coronal plane through spleen. Projection of splenic vein *(SV)* in middle of tail of pancreas is due to averaging. *A,* Aorta; *B,* body of stomach; *CA,* celiac artery; *D,* third portion of duodenum; *EG,* esophagogastric junction; *IVC,* inferior vena cava; *L,* liver; *N,* neck of pancreas; *P,* body of pancreas; *PC,* portal confluence; *RA,* right renal artery; *S,* spleen; *SA,* splenic artery; *SMA,* superior mesenteric artery; *SMV,* superior mesenteric vein; *St,* stomach; *SV,* splenic vein; *T,* tail of pancreas; *Un,* uncinate process.

Pancreatic Duct

The normal pancreatic duct is seen at least partially in 86% of patients.[7] It is optimally visualized in the central portion of the body where the duct is perpendicular to the ultrasound beam. Based on the resolution of the ultrasound system, the patient's body habitus, and the angle of insonation, the pancreatic duct is seen as a single linear structure or as double-parallel lines (Fig. 7-9). The mean internal diameter on sonographic examination has been reported to measure 3 mm in the head, 2.1 mm in the body, and 1.6 mm in the tail.[8] The dimensions of the pancreatic duct obtained sonographically are smaller than the corresponding endoscopic retrograde cholangiopancreatogram (ERCP) measurements as a result primarily of x-ray magnification and overdistension of the duct.[9] With age, its diameter increases probably because of parenchymal atrophy. Although 2- to 2.5-mm[7,9] diameter has been reported as the upper limit of normal, for practical purposes, the pancreatic duct is probably normal as long as the walls maintain their parallel course and the duct can be followed along its whole length to the duodenum. When the pancreatic duct becomes dilated, its side branches may also be seen and may be mistaken for pancreatic cysts. Occa-

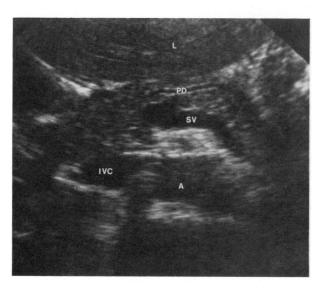

FIG 7-9. Pancreatic duct, transverse scan. Double-line pancreatic duct *(PD)*. *A*, Aorta; *IVC*, inferior vena cava; *L*, liver; *PD*, pancreatic duct; *SV*, splenic vein.

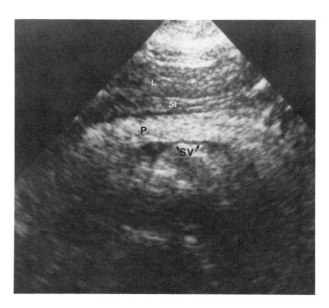

FIG 7-10. Echogenic pancreas, transverse scan. *L*, Liver; *P*, pancreas; *St*, stomach; *SV*, splenic vein.

sionally the accessory duct of Santorini and some normal branches of the main pancreatic duct can be identified in the pancreatic head.

Pancreatic Echotexture

The normal pancreas is usually homogeneous. The echogenicity, when compared with the normal liver, is either isoechoic or hyperechoic (Fig. 7-4, *B*). Sometimes a mottled appearance may be seen (Fig. 7-7, *A*). The contour of the pancreas is distinct when its echogenicity is less than the surrounding retroperitoneal fat. The gland usually appears smoothly contoured, although a lobulated contour occasionally is discerned. With aging and obesity, the pancreas becomes more echogenic as a result of the presence of **fatty infiltration** and in up to 35% of cases may be as echogenic as the adjacent retroperitoneal fat (Fig. 7-10).[10] The increased echogenicity resulting from excessive body fat is reversible.[11] Hyperechogenicity may account for difficulty in visualizing the pancreas as it blends with the adjacent retroperitoneal fat, making its contour and true size impossible to identify. In such patients, the gland can be assessed only by describing the pancreatic fossa using the vascular anatomy as landmarks. Because the size of the pancreas cannot be evaluated in these patients, pancreatic atrophy resulting in pancreatic insufficiency should not be excluded.[10] CT scans are indicated in these patients. **Causes of fatty infiltration** of the pancreas include: aging, obesity, chronic pancreatitis, dietary deficiency, viral infection, steroid therapy, cystic fibrosis, diabetes mellitus, hereditary pancreatitis, and obstruction caused by a stone or pancreatic carci-

noma.[11] In lipomatous pseudohypertrophy, the pancreas is massively enlarged as a result of fatty replacement.[12]

Dimensions

The normal head of the pancreas generally has the largest dimension with the neck having the smallest.[13] The body and most of the tail are both slightly smaller than the head. In one study[14] the anteroposterior dimension of the normal head measured 2.2 ± 0.3 cm with the body measuring 1.8 ± 0.3 cm. The cephalocaudal dimension of the head has been reported as 2.01 ± 0.39 cm and the body as 1.18 ± 0.36 cm.[13] The pancreas may appear larger in obese patients because it blends with the excessive retroperitoneal fat. The size of the pancreas diminishes with age.[15]

Pitfalls

Pancreas.   Structures that may be mistaken for the pancreas include:

- Posterior part (segment 2) of the lateral segment of the left lobe of the liver, when it is less echoic than the anterior part (segment 3) because of sound attenuation by perivascular fat.
- Papillary process of the caudate lobe, when it is completely separated from the liver (Fig. 7-11, *A*).
- Third part of the duodenum, when it is collapsed or filled with echogenic fluid (bowel wall layers and peristalsis differentiate).
- Retroperitoneal fibrosis, when seen as a midline band (It usually occurs inferior to the pancreas between the aorta and the mesenteric vessels.)
- Horseshoe kidney, which is usually inferior and

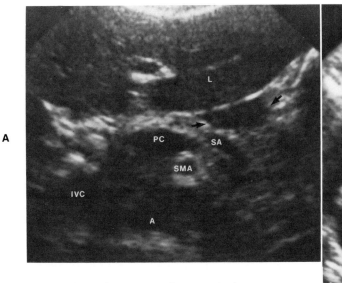

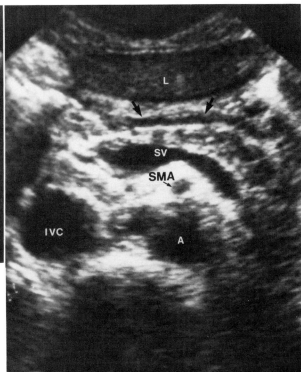

FIG 7-11. Pitfalls of pancreas and pancreatic duct, transverse scans. **A,** Papillary process of caudate lobe *(arrows)* simulating mass in pancreatic fossa. **B,** Muscular layer of posterior wall of stomach *(arrows)* simulating pancreatic duct. *A,* Aorta; *IVC,* inferior vena cava; *L,* liver; *PC,* portal confluence; *SMA,* superior mesenteric artery.

posterior to the mesenteric vessels, continuous with kidneys, and reniform in shape.
- Lymph nodes, which can simulate a bandlike pancreas (the associated aortocaval, retrocaval, or retroaortic lymphadenopathy help to differentiate them from the pancreas).

The relation of the structure to the splenic vein helps to differentiate most of the above from the pancreas.

Pancreatic Duct. Structures that are confused with the pancreatic duct and errors of interpretation include:
- The layers of the posterior wall of the stomach and the outline of the splenic vein (Fig. 7-11, *B*): No pancreatic parenchyma surrounds them and their course is not towards the second portion of the duodenum.
- A jejunal branch of the superior mesenteric vein may have a similar appearance and orientation as the pancreatic duct because it may be surrounded by retroperitoneal fat that can simulate pancreatic tissue on ultrasonograms. Following the vessel to its junction with the superior mesenteric vein and Doppler interrogation helps to differentiate a vascular structure from the pancreatic duct.
- Artifacts inherent to the ultrasound technology, such as beam width, can cause averaging of a tortuous splenic artery within the pancreas and may simulate a dilated pancreatic duct.
- With significant pancreatic atrophy caused by ob-

struction, no pancreatic tissue is seen around the dilated duct, potentiating an erroneous interpretation of a vascular structure. This is more likely to happen when the pancreas is very anterior as a result of significant emaciation caused by pancreatic carcinoma.
- Air in the pancreatic duct, usually secondary to pancreaticoenterostomy, should not be mistaken for ductal calculi.

Technical Aspects

Patient Preparation. Evaluation of the pancreas is usually performed as part of the ultrasound examination of the upper abdomen and especially in conjunction with assessment of the biliary system. Because optimal gallbladder distension requires fasting, ultrasound examination of the pancreas has been traditionally performed following a minimum fast of 6 hours. Theoretically, fasting also diminishes gaseous distension of the upper gastrointestinal tract, which can interfere with the visualization of the pancreas. However, in some patients in both pre- and postfasting states, evaluating the pancreas alone appears to be feasible.[16]

Considerations of Technique. There are two major factors preventing optimal visualization of the pancreas: fat and interfering gastrointestinal gas. As the pancreas is retroperitoneal, it is a deep structure in larger patients and a particular technical challenge because it is covered by the gas-filled gastrointestinal tract. **Scanning principles** used for the examination of the pancreas include the following:

- Place the area of interest within the **focal zone** of the transducer.
- **Alter the patients position** to include erect, supine, both obliques, both decubituses, and even prone positions, to displace the gas-containing structures or transfer the gas into another part of the gastrointestinal tract. The erect position displaces the gas-filled stomach or colon away from the pancreas and causes the liver to move down over the pancreas, becoming an acoustic window. The erect position appears to be most effective if used in the beginning of the examination because aerophagia caused by deep inspirations during the examination fills the stomach with gas.
- Furthermore, **breathing mechanisms,** including suspended inspiration or expiration, and a Valsalva maneuver may be helpful. Differentiation of a pancreatic mass from a lesion arising from surrounding structures may be helped by evaluating the mobility of the mass relative to these structures during respiration. The mobility of the pancreas is not as great as the intraperitoneal structures.[3]
- Last, **increasing stomach distention** with fluid when there is a large amount of interfering gas and when the upright position has failed to demonstrate

the pancreas may allow pancreatic visualization (Fig. 7-12). The fluid-filled stomach provides an acoustic window, causes movement of the intragastric gas and acts as a balloon, displacing the gas-filled colon and small bowel loops inferiorly. The patient should ingest a large volume of deonated water through a straw to minimize air swallowing. Some investigators have advocated the use of tubeless hypotonic duodenography with glucagon to facilitate visualization of the head of the pancreas.[17] Alternatively, some authors have shown that using agents such as metoclopramide which increases gastric and duodenal contractility can improve visualization of the pancreas.[18] However, in practice, ingestion of water alone is adequate for most patients and no additional medication is required. In patients who have had barium studies of the upper gastrointestinal tract, ultrasound evaluation of the pancreas with a water-filled stomach 1 hour after the upper gastrointestinal study has been shown to give better results than an ultrasound examination performed immediately after or 1 hour after the barium examination without a fluid-filled stomach.[19]

- **Sonographic examination of the pancreas** should begin with the patient in the erect position. Transverse scans in the midline below the xiphoid are made using the related vascular landmarks to iden-

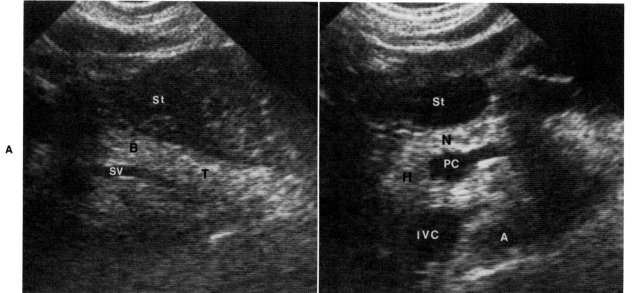

FIG 7-12. Stomach distension, transverse views. **A,** body and tail of pancreas are distinctly seen through fluid-filled stomach. Echogenicity of fluid is due to residual gas bubbles. **B,** Head and neck of pancreas are seen through fluid-filled antrum. *A,* Aorta; *B,* body of pancreas; *H,* head of pancreas; *IVC,* inferior vena cava; *N,* neck of pancreas; *PC,* portal confluence; *St,* stomach; *SV,* splenic vein; *T,* tail of pancreas.

tify the region of the pancreas. The probe may need to be oblique to visualize the gland in its entirety. Angling the transducer cephaladly and caudally from the level of the longitudinal view of the splenic vein appears to be adequate in most patients to scan through the entire gland.

- Sagittal scanning of the pancreas is initiated with the transducer in the midline below the xiphoid. The level of the pancreas is easily localized by identification of the portal splenic confluence. There should be minimal movement of the transducer to the left or right of the midline, and in practice, side-tilting of the probe has proved more effective than a lateral sliding displacement.
- Using the left kidney as an acoustic window, the tail of the pancreas may be visualized anterior to its upper pole with a left coronal view. In some thin patients, the tail of the pancreas can also be seen through the spleen from the left lateral intercostal approach using a coronal plane. The head can occasionally be seen through the right lateral approach on a coronal plane.

CONGENITAL ANOMALIES
Congenital Cysts

Epithelium-lined true cysts of the pancreas are believed to be congenital in origin, representing anomalous development of the pancreatic ducts.[20] Multiple congenital cysts, ranging in size from microscopic to 3 to 5 cm,[20] are associated with cystic disease of the pancreas, liver, spleen, and kidneys as part of the broad spectrum of adult type polycystic kidney disease. von Hippel-Lindau syndrome is another entity associated with multiple true pancreatic cysts.[20] Solitary congenital pancreatic cysts are rare and usually seen in infancy and childhood.[21]

Cystic Fibrosis

Cystic fibrosis is characterized by viscous secretions and dysfunction of multiple glands including the pancreas. It can lead to pancreatic insufficiency with the majority of patients showing evidence of exocrine pancreas dysfunction. When severely affected, the pancreas is shrunken with marked fibrosis, fatty replacement, and cysts secondary to the obstruction of small ducts.[22]

The most common **sonographic manifestation** is increased echogenicity caused by fibrosis or fatty replacement resulting from glandular atrophy.[23,24] In one study series, all patients demonstrated abnormal pancreatic echopatterns when compared with an age- and sex-matched normal population.[23] The pancreas may be small,[25] but this can only be appreciated in cases in which the pancreas is less echogenic than the adjacent retroperitoneal fat. If the pancreas is enlarged, it indicates the presence of complicating pancreatitis, and it is

usually associated with a hypoechoic parenchyma.[25] The pancreatic duct is less often visualized in patients with cystic fibrosis than in the normal population.[26] Small cysts of 1 to 3 mm that are seen on pathologic examination of the pancreas are uncommonly seen on sonography.[25] Individual larger cysts, less than 5 cm in diameter, have been reported on ultrasound examinations.[24] Rarely, pancreatic cytosis or multiple cysts can completely replace the pancreatic parenchyma. A high-amylase content has been shown on aspiration biopsy of these cysts.[27]

Pancreas Divisum

Pancreas divisum, which is caused by the lack of fusion of the dorsal and ventral pancreatic buds, occurs in 10% of the population on anatomic studies.[28,29] Drainage of the entire dorsal pancreas is through the minor papilla, with only the ventral part draining through the major papilla. There is controversy regarding the predisposition of patients with pancreas divisum to pancreatitis, which may be related to the drainage of most of the pancreatic secretions through the relatively small orifice of the minor papilla. In a group of patients with recurrent idiopathic pancreatitis, Cotton[28] reported an incidence of 25.6% with associated pancreas divisum.[29] Involvement of the pancreas with acute pancreatitis is usually limited to the dorsal part of the gland.[29] However, isolated ventral pancreatitis has also been documented.[30] Increased prominence of the ventral pancreas has been reported as an indication of pancreas divisum.[15]

von Hippel-Lindau Syndrome

Pancreatic cysts are common in von Hippel-Lindau syndrome and are described in 72% of autopsy results[31] and 25% of patients on sonographic examination.[31] Other associated lesions include apudomas, microcystic adenomas, ductal cell adenocarcinomas, ampullary cell carcinomas, and hemangioblastomas.[32]

INFLAMMATORY PROCESSES
Acute Pancreatitis

The diagnosis of acute pancreatitis is usually based on clinical and laboratory findings, with clinical severity best determined by Ranson's criteria.[33] Radiologic examinations are helpful for patients with a confusing history or clinical findings. The role of ultrasound lies in the detection, guidance for interventional procedures, and follow-up of complications arising from acute pancreatitis. Ultrasound is limited in its usefulness as part of the early investigation of acute pancreatitis or traumatic pancreatic injury,[34] whereas CT has been shown to be useful in helping to predict the outcome of acute pancreatic inflammation and to detect necrosis and fracture of the pancreas.[35]

Pathologic changes in acute pancreatitis depend on the severity of the disease, with mild forms showing only interstitial edema of the pancreas with or without a mild degree of peripancreatic inflammation or fat necrosis. Inflammation is associated with extravasation of enzymes into the surrounding tissues. More severe cases show fat necrosis, parenchymal necrosis, and necrosis of blood vessels with subsequent hemorrhage and more severe peripancreatic inflammatory changes appearing in 1 to 2 days.[36] If the patient survives, the necrotic tissue is replaced by diffuse or focal parenchymal or stromal fibrosis, calcifications, and irregular ductal dilations. Pseudocysts may form by the accumulation of enzyme-rich fluid and necrotic debris confined by a nonepithelialized capsule of retroperitoneal connective tissue.[20]

Acute pancreatitis has numerous causes; however, the precise pathophysiologic factors are yet to be elucidated. Congenital causes include hereditary pancreatitis and compression from a congenital choledochal cyst. The role of pancreas divisum as a predisposing factor to pancreatitis is controversial, with studies showing both an increased[29] and similar[37] incidence of acute pancreatitis in these patients. Acquired conditions such as alcohol abuse and biliary calculi account for the majority of the cases of acute pancreatitis. Trauma and many other less common entities can induce acute pancreatitis (see box below).[38]

Because the **natural history** of acute pancreatitis is variable, serial examination by ultrasound plays an important role in monitoring the inflammatory process of the pancreas after an initial attack. The process can take several directions: resolution, pseudocyst formation, or chronic pancreatitis. Cases of mild pancreatitis, or self-limiting disease, often revert to normal organ echotexture and size. More severe disease may result in increased echogenicity of the pancreas. This increase may be homogeneous and accompanied by scattered, random, bright reflections representing minute calcifications (often without acoustic shadowing) or inhomogeneous and a mottled appearance to the gland. These changes reflect the healing of the pancreas by fibrosis accompanied by calcifications deposited along the main pancreatic duct or in the branches within the parenchyma.

Pseudocyst formation is an attempt by the body to wall off the pancreatic secretions to prevent further autodigestion of the peripancreatic tissue. In many instances patients feel better at the time of pseudocyst formation because it acts as a cordon, enclosing the active inflammation.

Chronic pancreatitis usually results from repeated bouts of acute pancreatitis. This condition is progressive, with indolent destruction and fibrosis of the organ leading to functional exocrine and endocrine glandular failure.

Sonography. Ultrasound findings may be negative in the milder forms of acute pancreatitis. The examination may, however, find the cause of pancreatitis, such as choledocholithiasis, or an alternative diagnosis in questionable cases. In more severe cases CT is the primary early examination to identify necrotic parenchyma and extraparenchymal involvement because the associated ileus limits ultrasonographic visualization.[39] The technical success of the ultrasound examination improves 48 hours after the acute episode, as the paralytic ileus resolves.[40] **Complications** may be found, such as phlegmon, hemorrhage, intrapancreatic and extrapancreatic fluid collections, and pseudocyst formation. Sonograms may differentiate between phlegmonous inflammatory masses and fluid collections and can also be used to guide needle aspiration to differentiate between a phlegmon, an atypical pseudocyst, and noninfected and infected fluid.

Ultrasound findings of acute pancreatitis can be classified by distribution (focal or diffuse) and by severity (mild, moderate, and severe).[40]

Focal pancreatitis, presenting as focal isoechoic or hypoechoic enlargement of the pancreas without extrapancreatic manifestations, poses a dilemma to the

---

▢ CAUSES OF ACUTE PANCREATITIS

Biliary tract disease
Ethyl alcohol abuse
Peptic ulcer
Trauma, surgery (cardiopulmonary bypass surgery), hypotensive shock
Pregnancy
Hyperlipoproteinemias (types I, IV, and V)
Hypercalcemia (primary and secondary, hyperparathyroidism, multiple myeloma)
Drugs (azathioprime, estrogens, corticosteroids, and thiazides)
Hereditary pancreatitis, idiopathic fibrosing pancreatitis
Infectious agents (mumps, ascaris, *Campylobacter* and *Mycoplasma* spp infections, and hydatid)
Methyl alcohol, L-asparaginase
Scorpion bites
Carcinoma of pancreas (primary and metastatic); ductal obstruction by tumor
Endoscopic retrograde cholangiopancreatography, upper gastrointestinal endoscopy, percutaneous transhepatic biliary tract drainage
Posttransplantation
Legionnares' disease

Modified from Geokas MC, moderator: Acute pancreatitis. *Ann Intern Med* 1985;103:87.

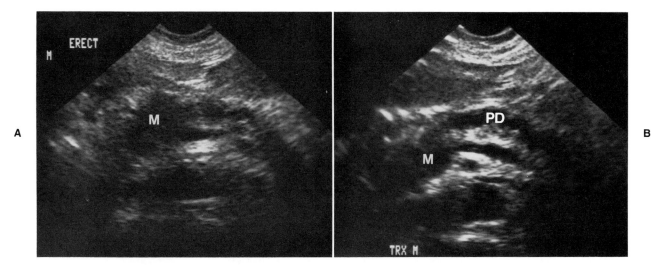

FIG 7-13. Focal pancreatitis. **A,** Transverse scan of lower head and, **B,** rest of pancreas in patient with large hypoechoic mass *(M)* in region of head of pancreas. Dilated pancreatic duct *(PD)* is seen extending to this mass. Multiple percutaneous and surgical biopsies yielded negative findings.

sonographer. This generally occurs in the pancreatic head (Fig 7-13).[41] Affected patients are usually alcoholic and have a previous history of pancreatitis or pain, suggesting that focal pancreatitis tends to occur with a background of chronic pancreatitis.[41] Differentiation from neoplasm may be difficult because both conditions create a focal hypoechoic mass on sonograms. If the serum amylase level is normal and the patient is asymptomatic, the mass is likely to represent a neoplasm. If the patient's symptoms and signs are severe, the focal hypoechogenicity is more likely to be caused by pancreatitis rather than a tumor. The presence of calcification within the mass and abnormal ductal changes outside the focal enlargement on ERCP also favor an inflammatory mass.[41] In addition, serial sonographic examination while the patient is undergoing treatment may differentiate focal pancreatitis from tumor. CT scans can be helpful by showing peripancreatic soft tissue inflammation. Percutaneous biopsy should be performed on patients whose diagnoses remain questionable, keeping in mind that a negative biopsy finding does not exclude malignancy. Focal pancreatitis may also be caused by an adjacent inflammatory process, such as a penetrating peptic ulcer (Fig. 7-14).

In **diffuse pancreatitis,** the pancreas becomes increasingly hypoechogenic relative to the normal liver and increases in size (Fig. 7-15). The assessment of relative pancreatic echogenicity may be difficult because of the alcohol-induced fatty liver present in a large number of these patients. Therefore comparison of the echogenicity of the pancreas with the liver may be of little practical value. In mild acute pancreatitis, sono-

grams show a normal pancreas with abnormal clinical and laboratory findings. As the condition worsens, decreased echogenicity and increased size are more evident as a result of the increased fluid content in the interstitium secondary to inflammation. The pancreas may also appear inhomogeneous (Fig. 7-16). The pancreatic duct may be compressed or dilated. Ductal dilation is usually caused by a focal pancreatic inflammation located upstream from the dilated pancreatic duct. Rarely, another cause of duct obstruction such as a calculus, tumor, or ascaris can be detected by high-resolution ultrasound.[42]

Complications of acute pancreatitis, seen in more severe cases, include phlegmon, hemorrhage, and pseudocyst formation. Focal areas of hypoechogenicity either represent fluid collection or phlegmon.[40] The former is better defined and shows more through transmission. Focal hemorrhage is detected as a focal echogenic mass. When acute inflammation of the pancreas becomes masslike and is accompanied by severe symptoms and clinical findings, the term *phlegmon* can be employed (Fig. 7-16). Conservative management with serial ultrasonographic imaging is advised because most phlegmons resolve without intervention.[43]

The **extrapancreatic manifestations** of acute pancreatitis are an important and difficult part of the ultrasonographic evaluation.[39] They consist of fluid collections and edema along the different soft tissue planes and are generally seen in severe cases. The common spaces for the extrapancreatic fluid to collect include the lesser sac, anterior pararenal spaces, mesocolon, perirenal spaces, and peripancreatic soft tissues.[39] Lesser sac

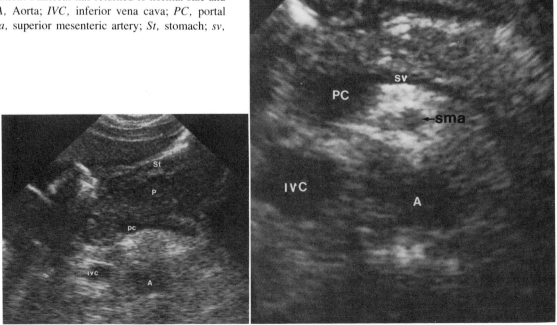

FIG 7-14. Focal pancreatitis caused by penetrating benign gastric ulcer. **A,** Transverse scan of pancreas shows hypoechoic mass-like enlargement *(M)* of body and tail. No fat plane is present between this mass and adjacent stomach *(St)*. *A*, Aorta; *GB*, gall bladder; *IVC*, inferior vena cava; *L*, liver; *P*, pancreas; *sma*, superior mesenteric artery; *smv*, superior mesenteric vein. **B,** Large ulcer of posterior wall of body of stomach *(arrow)*.

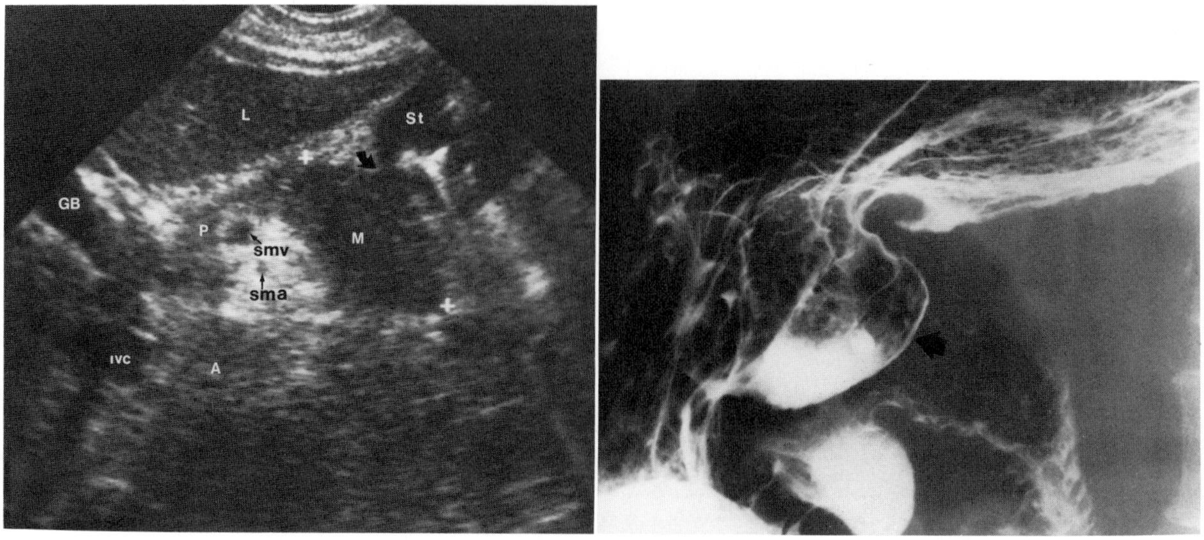

FIG 7-15. Acute pancreatitis with resolution. **A,** Transverse scan of enlarged hypoechoic pancreas *(P)*. **B,** Same patient following resolution. Pancreas has returned to normal size and echogenicity. *A*, Aorta; *IVC*, inferior vena cava; *PC*, portal confluence; *sma*, superior mesenteric artery; *St*, stomach; *sv*, splenic vein.

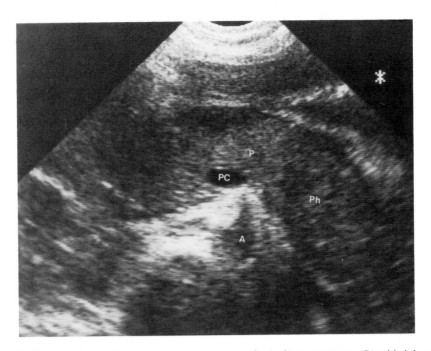

FIG 7-16. Severe acute pancreatitis. Transverse scan shows large pancreas *(P)* with inhomogeneous, hypoechoic area in tail, which represents phlegmon *(Ph)*. *A,* Aorta; *PC,* portal confluence.

fluid lying between the pancreas and the stomach is the easiest to visualize with ultrasonograph (Fig. 7-17, *A*). If the fluid is located in its superior recess, it tends to surround the caudate lobe (Fig. 7-17, *B*).[39] The free edge of the gastrohepatic ligament may be visualized with a combination of lesser sac and greater sac fluid (Fig. 7-17, *C*). Perirenal fluid is also easy to demonstrate but edema or fluid in the anterior pararenal space is more difficult to show and may require coronal scanning. When seen, it produces a hypoechoic band, separated from the kidney by the echogenic perirenal fat.[39] Fluid collections in the mesocolon are the most difficult to identify by ultrasonographic examination. They present in the midline just caudal to the pancreas. Peripancreatic soft tissue changes are seen as a hypoechoic bands adjacent to the pancreas or surrounding the portal venous system (Fig. 7-18).[39] Fluid or edema may be visualized around the ligamentum teres (Fig. 7-19).

Pancreatic fluid is either clear or septated as a result of associated hemorrhage or infection. Retroperitoneal collections, in particular, may be nonhomogeneous as a result of the nature of the edematous retroperitoneal tissues. Extrapancreatic fluid collections occur within 4 weeks from the onset of an acute attack and have a high incidence of spontaneous regression; therefore they can be treated conservatively in conjunction with serial ultrasonographic scanning. Therapeutic interventions are neither necessary nor recommended for pancreatic fluid collections found within a month of the onset of acute

pancreatitis.[44] The term *pseudocyst* can only be used when a pancreatic fluid collection has developed into a well-defined, thin-walled structure that persists on serial ultrasonographic imaging examinations for an interval of at least 4 weeks.[45]

Other extrapancreatic findings include ascites, thickening of the adjacent gastrointestinal tract (stomach, duodenum, and colon), and a thickened gallbladder wall associated with pericholecystic fluid, which may simulate acute cholecystitis.[44]

Complications

Pancreatic Pseudocysts. A pancreatic pseudocyst is a fluid collection that has developed a well-defined nonepithelialized wall in response to extravasated enzymes.[47] It is generally spherical in shape and distinct from other structures. Approximately 4 to 6 weeks are necessary for a fluid collection to enclose itself by forming a wall composed of collagen and vascular granulation tissue.[48] Pseudocysts occur in 10% to 20% of cases of acute pancreatitis,[49] most commonly, of alcoholic or biliary origin. However, they may also occur following blunt trauma or as a result of pancreatic malignancy. Persistent pain and elevation of amylase levels suggest the diagnosis; however, it is confirmed by imaging. Ultrasound is the initial imaging modality of choice to monitor a pseudocyst and provide guidance during intervention. Classically, a pseudocyst is seen on ultrasonographic examination as a well-defined, smooth-walled, anechoic structure with acoustic en-

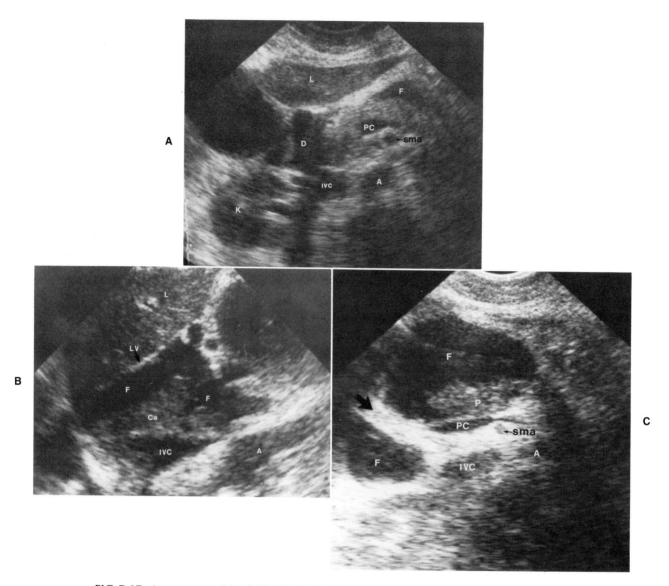

FIG 7-17. Acute pancreatitis, fluid collection in peripancreatic spaces. **A,** Fluid *(F)* anterior to pancreas in lower lesser sac. **B,** Fluid *(F)* surrounding caudate lobe *(Ca)* in sagittal plane. **C,** Fluid *(F)* on both sides of gastrohepatic ligament *(arrow)* in transverse plane. *A,* Aorta; *D,* duodenum; *IVC,* inferior vena cava; *K,* kidney; *L,* liver; *P,* pancreas; *PC,* portal confluence; *sma,* superior mesenteric artery.

hancement. Occasionally, they may also appear solid or complex, especially during formation.[47,50] As a pseudocyst matures, serial scanning will generally reveal gradual clearing of the internal echoes. Debris within a pseudocyst may occur with complications such as hemorrhage or infection (Fig. 7-20).[47] A pseudocyst may also remain multiloculated without complications and may develop calcifications within its walls (Fig. 7-20). A heavily calcified pseudocyst may be difficult to see on ultrasonograms because of the presence of shadowing (Fig. 7-21). Pseudocysts can migrate outside

the abdomen and have been reported to occur in the mediastinum and the thigh.[51,52]

Complications have been reported in 30% to 50% of the patients with a pancreatic pseudocyst.[53] These lesions may become large or may be strategically placed and cause **obstruction** of the stomach, small bowel (especially duodenum), colon, or the biliary duct.[54] The latter may progress from obstructive jaundice to obstructive cholangitis. Bowel obstruction may follow extrinsic compression or intramural extension of the pseudocyst between the serosa and muscularis or be-

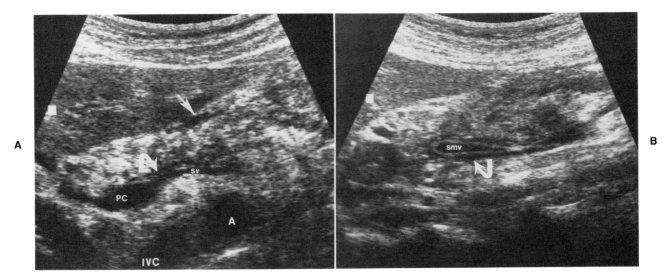

FIG 7-18. Acute pancreatitis, extrapancreatic soft tissue edema. **A,** Transverse scan. **B,** Longitudinal scan. Pancreas echotexture is inhomogeneous. Peripancreatic edema *(straight arrow)* and periportal system edema *(curved arrow)* are present. *A,* Aorta; *IVC,* inferior vena cava; *PC,* portal confluence; *smv,* superior mesenteric vein; *SV,* splenic vein.

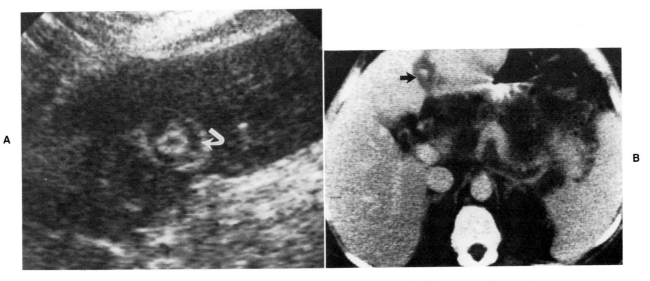

FIG 7-19. Acute pancreatitis, edema around ligamentum teres. **A,** Transverse ultrasound scan shows hypoechoic edema *(curved arrow)* around ligamentum teres. **B,** Hypodense edema *(arrow)* is seen in same area on CT scan.

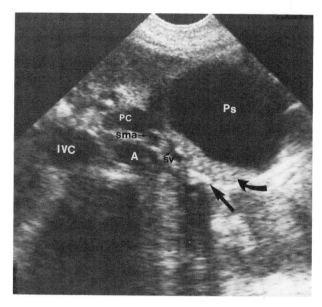

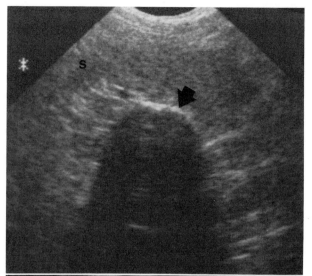

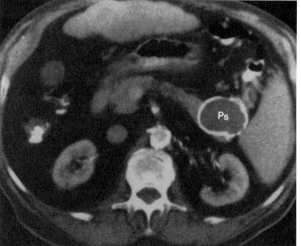

FIG 7-20. Complicated pseudocyst. Transverse scan of partially calcified *(straight arrow)* pseudocyst *(Ps)* containing debris *(curved arrow)* in tail of pancreas. *A,* Aorta; *IVC,* inferior vena cava; *PC,* portal confluence; *sma,* superior mesenteric artery; *SV,* splenic vein.

FIG 7-21. Calcified pseudocyst. **A,** Heavily calcified pseudocyst *(arrow)* in splenic hilum causing shadowing. **B,** Confirmatory CT scan. *Ps,* Pseudocyst; *S,* spleen.

tween the muscularis and mucosa (Fig. 7-22).[55] Pseudocysts can also **dissect** into the parenchyma of the adjacent organs such as the liver, spleen, and kidney (Fig. 7-23).[58]

Gastrointestinal hemorrhage may occur as a result of direct erosion of the pseudocyst into the stomach or from variceal bleeding from local hypertension caused by portosplenic venous compression or thrombosis.[53,57] A pseudocyst may erode into an adjacent visceral artery, most commonly the splenic, with resultant intracystic hemorrhage and formation of a pseudoaneurysm. Hemorrhage may also occur with pancreatic abscess and severe necrotizing pancreatitis without pseudocyst formation.[58,59] With vigilance, areas of increased echogenicity representing hemorrhage can be detected. With the addition of Doppler insonation, the presence of a **pseudoaneurysm** and **portosplenic thrombosis** can be revealed.[60] If thrombosis becomes chronic, cavernous transformation of the portal venous system may follow. This can be best assessed with the help of pulsed and color Doppler imaging.

Acute peritonitis can ensue with rupture of a pseudocyst into the peritoneal cavity. This serious complication should be differentiated clinically from pancreatic ascites, which is due to a slow leakage of fluid into the peritoneal cavity, not with peritonitis.

Pseudocysts that form during acute, necrotizing pancreatitis have a high propensity toward spontaneous regression. Pseudocysts that occur in patients with chronic pancreatitis do not generally resolve on their own, especially when calcifications are seen within the walls.[61] Spontaneous decompression of the pseudocyst may occur by rupturing into the pancreatic duct, the adjacent portion of the gastrointestinal tract (usually the stomach), or the common bile duct.[62] In general, pseudocysts that persist beyond 6 weeks require decompression because spontaneous resolution beyond this period occurs infrequently and the risk of complications rises significantly.[48] A pseudocyst will persist as long as disruption of the pancreatic ducts exist, whereas on healing of this disruption, spontaneous resorption will occur.[62] **Criteria for decompression** of a pancreatic pseudocyst include:

- Persistence greater than 6 weeks

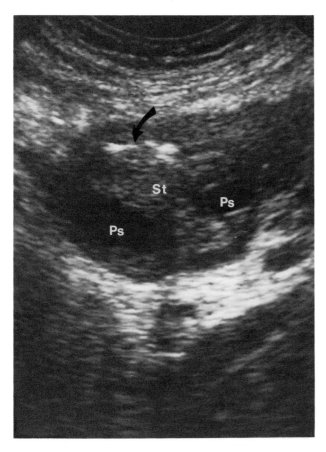

FIG 7-22. Intramural pseudocyst in wall of stomach *(St)*. Transverse view of antrum showing multiple pseudocysts *(Ps)* in thickened wall. *Curved arrow,* Gas in lumen.

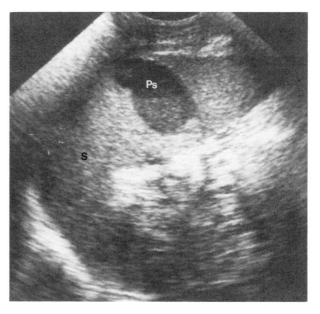

FIG 7-23. Pseudocyst of spleen. Sagittal view of spleen *(S)* shows cyst *(Ps)* containing a fluid level.

- Size larger than 5 cm in diameter without evidence of ongoing regression on follow-up ultrasonographic examination or CT
- Smaller pseudocysts causing symptoms
- Presence of complications such as infection, internal hemorrhage, or intraabdominal perforation

Nonsurgical decompression is becoming more popular with the more favorable results obtained in the past few years.[63] Controversy exists on the choice of approach, with some large study series advocating the transgastric approach as the primary route[64] and others advocating the direct approach if possible, with the transgastric or duodenal and transhepatic approaches reserved for more inaccessible pseudocysts.[63] Single aspiration has been abandoned because of the high-recurrence rate.[63] Percutaneous transgastric pseudocyst drainage is a combined technique of percutaneous gastrostomy with cystogastrostomy using a Mitty-Pollack needle* performed under fluoroscopy and ultrasonography.

*Cook, Bloomingdale, IND.

There is minimal chance of pseudocyst recurrence because of internal drainage to the stomach. In one study series using this technique, a success rate of 67% was observed with a recurrence rate of 12.5%.[64] This approach is considered the route of choice in pseudocysts associated with obstruction of the pancreatic duct. The direct approach is performed using the usual percutaneous technique. The reported success rate for the combined approach (with the majority being drained directly) is 86%.[63] The catheter is left in place until drainage ceases, the pseudocyst resolves, and there is no communication with the pancreatic duct.[63] The drainage period is generally longer than an uncomplicated abscess and closer to abscesses associated with fistula to the gastrointestinal tract.[63]

Endoscopic cystogastrostomy or duodenostomy is a recent alternative approach; however, it may be more time consuming than the radiologically-guided percutaneous approach.[65] If the above techniques are unavailable, if the anatomy precludes their usage, or if a pseudocyst is extensively multiloculated, a surgical decompression should be used.

Infected Pancreatic Lesions. The **uncircumscribed infected pancreatic focus** consists of entities that are not delimited by a wall, such as pancreatic necrosis, pancreatic fluid collections, and old pancreatic hemorrhage, which have been secondarily infected. Bacterial contamination of necrotic pancreatic tissue and fluid rises to a significant rate (71.4%) after 2 weeks of acute necrotic pancreatitis.[66] Sonographically, a sterile uncircumscribed focus cannot be distinguished from an infected one. Therefore a high index of suspicion is necessary to detect these lesions, and an ultrasound-guided (or CT-guided) needle aspiration with Gram's stain and culture of the aspirate should be performed to confirm the presence of infection. An uncircumscribed infected pancreatic focus is best treated by surgical debridement. Percutaneous catheter drainage is reserved for cases in which the patient is in refractory shock or cannot withstand immediate surgery.[67]

Sonographically, an **infected pancreatic pseudocyst** cannot be definitely distinguished from a sterile pseudocyst. Clinically, the patient may appear well with stable vital signs, except for an elevated temperature. Therefore a high index of suspicion is again necessary and a percutaneous ultrasound-guided aspiration with Gram's stain and culture should be employed whenever the question of infection arises. An infected pseudocyst is best treated (94% reported success) by percutaneous image-guided catheter drainage.[63,64]

A **pancreatic abscess** is distinguished from an infected pseudocyst by its greater risk for mortality (near 100% mortality if left untreated) and its need for surgical debridement (versus percutaneous catheter drainage).[68] The organisms obtained are usually gram-negative enteric bacteria and approximately half of the cultures are polymicrobial.[69] Pancreatic abscesses occur more frequently in postoperative patients than in those with alcohol or biliary pancreatitis.[70] Sonographically, one sees a thick-walled, mostly anechoic mass containing debris with bright echoes from gas bubbles. However, gas collections can also arise from noninfected fistulous communications with the gastrointestinal tract.[71] Whether ones sees gas bubbles, absence of gas, a cystic complex or solid structure, suspicious areas must be aspirated with a fine needle (22 gauge) under ultrasound or CT guidance to obtain specimens for Gram's stain, culture, and sensitivity tests. Pancreatic abscesses require surgical debridement. Also, the use of CT images may help to predict the success of draining a pancreatic abscess with a radiologic catheter.[72] Residual collections left after surgery can have a percutaneous catheter placed radiologically to help affect a complete cure.[72]

Pancreatic Ascites and Pleural Effusion. Pancreatic ascites results from slow leakage of pancreatic enzymes into the peritoneal cavity from a disruption of the main pancreatic duct or a poorly walled pseudocyst.[73] Anterior enzyme leakage enters the lesser sac and the peritoneal cavity, causing ascites. Posterior enzyme leakage moves cephaladly into the mediastinum and the pleural space, resulting in pancreatic pleural effusion (classically, left sided).[74] A "leaky" diaphragm or a pleural-subdiaphragmatic fistula may also allow ascites to become a pleural effusion. Pancreatic ascites is asymptomatic, causing an enlarging abdomen. ERCP can detect the location of pancreatic duct disruption.

Chronic Pancreatitis

Chronic pancreatitis is a progressive, irreversible destruction of the pancreas by repeated bouts of mild or subclinical pancreatitis resulting from high-alcohol intake or biliary tract disease. In chronic alcoholic pancreatitis, the chronic alcohol intake causes increased pancreatic protein secretion with subsequent obstruction of the ducts by the protein-rich plugs, resulting in the more common type, namely **chronic calcifying pancreatitis.**[20] The fibrous connective tissue proliferates around ducts and between parenchymal lobules causing interstitial scarring accompanied by loss of acini.[75] This process eventually leads to an irregular, nodular appearance of the surface of the pancreas and pancreatic calculi.[20,75] The less common type is **chronic obstructive pancreatitis** with a nonlobular distribution, less ductal epithelial damage, and rare calcified stones. This is usually due to stenosis of the sphincter of Oddi by cholelithiasis or pancreatic carcinoma.[20]

Sonographic findings of chronic pancreatitis consist of changes in the size and echotexture of the pancreas, focal mass lesions, calcifications, pancreatic duct dilation, and pseudocyst formation. Bile duct dilation and portal vein thrombosis are other associated findings.[15] The **echotexture** of the pancreas is usually mixed with patches of hypoechoic and hyperechoic foci. The hyperechoic foci are probably due to a combination of fibrosis and calcification. Hypoechoic areas are likely due to the associated inflammation.[15,76] The echotexture changes are relatively sensitive but nonspecific.[15] The

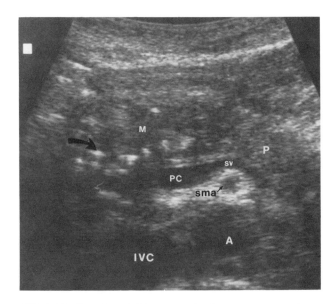

FIG 7-24. Chronic calcific pancreatis. Transverse scan shows focal hypoechoic enlargement *(M)* of head and proximal body of pancreas *(P)* with chronic calcific *(arrow)* pancreatitis. *A,* Aorta; *IVC,* inferior vena cava; *PC,* portal confluence; *sma,* superior mesenteric artery; *Sv,* splenic; *arrow,* calcification.

size of the pancreas depends on the degree of associated inflammation. In the absence of significant acute inflammation, the pancreas tends to be atrophied.

A **focal mass** or enlargement is found in approximately 40% of patients.[76,77] These changes result from progressive, mostly perilobular scarring in the interstitium accompanied by chronic edema and inflammatory infiltration. The presence of calcification helps to differentiate these focal enlargements from neoplasms (Fig. 7-24). However, in some cases differentiation is not possible (Fig. 7-13). Irregular **dilation of the pancreatic duct** occurs in chronic pancreatitis. In advanced cases the duct becomes very tortuous (Fig. 7-25). The differential diagnosis between chronic pancreatitis and pancreatic carcinoma in a patient with duct dilation can be difficult. However, as a general rule, chronic pancreatitis is more highly suspected when the duct contains calcification and no obstructing mass lesions is seen, whereas carcinoma is suggested when a parenchymal mass lesion is identified at the site of obstruction of the pancreatic duct.[78] In normal subjects, it has been shown that a variable degree of pancreatic duct dilation occurs following a standard meal or secretin stimulation.[15] Absent or diminished response has been shown in patients with chronic pancreatitis.[15]

Pancreatic calcifications are mostly intraductal in location and result from deposition of calcium carbonate on intraductal protein plugs (Fig. 7-26).[79] The presence of these calcifications has been used diagnostically and as a basis for treatment for chronic pancreatitis because they were thought to be associated with clinical pancreatic insufficiency. However, contrary to previous opinion, a recent study showed a poor correlation between exocrine function and pancreatic calcification.[80] Moreover, the degree and pattern of pancreatic calcification has been shown to change with time.[81] Three phases were identified: increasing calcification, stationary calcification, and decreasing calcification. The third phase, not previously recognized, occurred to a significant degree in one third of the patients studied; some of this loss resulted from drainage procedures, whereas others occurred spontaneously with continued loss of exocrine function.

Pancreatic pseudocysts are reported in 25% to 40% of patients with chronic pancreatitis.[15] They are better walled off in chronic pancreatitis as compared with the acute stage and tend not to resolve spontaneously.

Dilation of the common bile duct is present in 5% to 10% of the patients with chronic pancreatitis and characteristically causes smooth gradual tapering although abrupt tapering is rarely seen.[15]

Portosplenic vein thrombosis may occur as a complication of chronic pancreatitis and was recently reported as occurring in 5.1% of patients.[82] Because of the chronic nature of the disease, cavernous transformation may be present.

There is relatively good functional and morphologic correlation in advanced pancreatic disease, but poor correlation for mild to moderate disease. Bicarbonate secretion seems to correlate best with ductal imaging in chronic disease by ERCP, whereas enzyme secretion

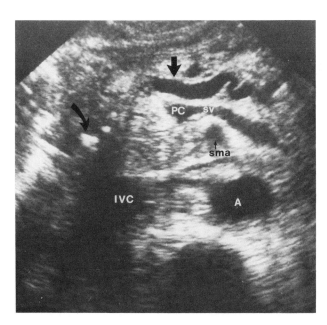

FIG 7-25. Chronic calcific pancreatitis. Transverse scan shows dilated tortuous pancreatic duct *(straight arrow)* and large head with calcification *(curved arrow)*. *A,* Aorta; *IVC,* inferior vena cava; *PC,* portal confluence; *sma,* superior mesenteric artery; *sv,* splenic vein.

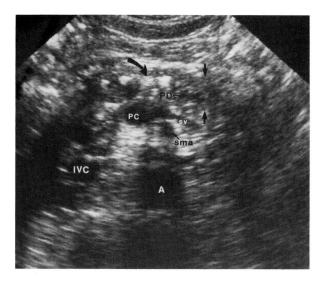

FIG 7-26. Pancreatic calculi *(curved arrow),* transverse scan. *PC,* Portal confluence; *sma,* superior mesenteric artery; *sv,* splenic vein; *PD,* pancreatic duct; *IVC,* inferior vena cava; *A,* aorta.

■ **TABLE 7-1**
Revised 'Cambridge' Classification of Chronic Pancreatitis

Class*		Ultrasound
1. Normal		Visualisation of entire gland and demonstration and measurement of main pancreatic duct
2. Equivocal	Less than 2 abnormal signs	Main duct enlarged (less than 4 mm)
		Gland enlarged (up to twice normal)
		Cavities (less than 10 mm)
		Irregular ducts
3. Mild		Focal reduction in parenchymal echogenicity
4. Moderate	2 or more abnormal signs	Echogenic foci in parenchyma
		Increased or irregular echogenicity of wall of main duct
		Irregular contour to gland, particularly focal enlargement
5. Marked		Large cavities (greater than 10 mm)
		Calculi
		Duct obstruction (greater than 4 mm)
		Major duct irregularity
		Gross enlargement (greater than 4 mm)
		Contiguous organ invasion

*If pathologic changes are limited to one third of the gland or less, they are classified as focal.
(Modified from Jones SN, Lees WR, Frost RA: Diagnosis and grading of chronic pancreatitis by morphological criteria derived by ultrasound and pancreatography. *Clin Radiol* 1988; 39:43-48. Reprinted with permission.)

correlates with gland imaging by ultrasound and CT.[83] However, recently, a revised "Cambridge" classification of chronic pancreatitis was proposed and preliminary studies indicate good correlations based on findings of ERCP and ultrasound (Table 7-1). Ductal abnormalities of more than three side branches are diagnostic of the early stages of chronic pancreatitis, while abnormality of the main duct indicates at least moderate disease.[84] The finding of intraductal calculi constitutes sufficient evidence for grading as advanced chronic pancreatitis.[85] Therefore, correlation of US findings with that of ERCP has recently become part of the basis of treatment of chronic pancreatitis.

NEOPLASMS
Adenocarcinoma

Pancreatic carcinoma is the fourth leading cause of death from cancer in the United States, preceded by cancer of the lung, colon, and breast. The incidence of this neoplasm has increased threefold in the past 40 years. Carcinoma of the pancreas is extremely rare before 40 years of age, and two thirds of patients present after age 60 years.[86] The prognosis is particularly poor, with a median survival time of 2 to 3 months and a 1-year survival of 8%. Clinical symptoms depend on the location. Tumors arising in the pancreatic head present earlier because of associated bile duct obstruction. A palpable, nontender gallbladder accompanied by jaundice (Courvoisier's sign) is present in about 25% of patients.[4] Tumors in the body and tail present later with less specific symptoms—most commonly weight loss, pain, jaundice, and vomiting when the gastrointestinal tract is invaded by the tumor. Diabetes and malabsorption are late findings.

Pathologically almost all adenocarcinomas originate in the ductal epithelium, with less than 1% arising in the acini. They may be either mucinous or nonmucinous secreting.[20] Approximately 70% of the pancreatic cancers arise in the region of the head, 15% to 20% in the body, and 5% in the tail. In 20% of cases the tumor is distributed diffusely throughout the gland.[20]

Because pancreatic head tumors present earlier, they can be fairly small and cause little or moderate expansion of the head. They may be inapparent on external examination and only create an impression of abnormal consistency or nodularity. On cut cross-section, they are poorly defined and present an irregular margin with few if any foci of hemorrhage.[20] Carcinoma of the body and tail of the pancreas are, on the average, larger than those of the head and tend to invade adjacent organs including the stomach, transverse colon, spleen, and adrenal gland. Carcinomas in the region of the body and tail are more likely to present with metastases, probably as a result of late presentation.[86] Massive hepatic metastases are characteristic. Metastases occur most frequently in the regional lymph nodes, liver, lungs, peritoneum, and adrenal glands. Peripancreatic, gastric, mesenteric, omental, and portohepatic nodes are frequent sites of spread.

Sonography

Direct Signs. The most common ultrasonographic finding in pancreatic carcinoma is a poorly defined, homogeneous or inhomogeneous hypoechoic mass in the pancreas or pancreatic fossa.[87] This may or may not be associated with expansion of the pancreas or compression of the adjacent structures. In patients whose pancreas shows increased echogenicity, the tumor will be better visualized as the contrast between the neoplasm and the normal pancreatic echotexture is accentuated. When an isoechoic mass is identified, attention should be given to the size of the pancreas and nodularity of its contour. In the uncinate process, the presence of a mass changes its pointed contour to a rounded appearance (Fig. 7-27). Necrosis, seen as a cystic area within the mass, is a rare manifestation of pancreatic carcinoma.[88] However, pseudocysts caused by associated pancreatitis may be seen adjacent to the carcinoma. The less common diffuse tumors can be mistaken for acute pancreatitis. At the time of diagnosis by ultrasonography, pancreatic carcinomas usually measure more than 2 cm. The tumor size is usually larger at surgery or autopsy than on the ultrasonograms. This may be due to the presence of microscopic infiltration of the tissues surrounding the tumor itself, which is undetected by ultrasound.

Indirect Signs. **Dilation of the pancreatic duct** proximal to a pancreatic mass is a common finding. A normal pancreatic duct usually measures less than 2 to 3 mm and has parallel walls and a straight course. When obstructed, it looses its parallel nature, becomes tortu-

ous, and ends or tapers abruptly. The pancreatic duct distends with aging, but it maintains its parallel straight course and can be followed to its entrance into the duodenum. Unfortunately, a similar appearance of the pancreatic duct may be seen in both pancreatic carcinoma and pancreatitis.

Bile duct dilation is commonly seen with lesions in the head of the pancreas. The gallbladder and cystic duct may or may not be dilated. The level of obstruction may be in the head, above the head, or in the porta hepatis, depending on the extent of the lesion or associated lymphadenopathy. Abrupt termination of the dilated bile duct is strongly suggestive of malignancy. Thick echogenic sludge in the common bile duct proximal to a tumor should not be mistaken for the tumor itself. These patients also often have thick sludge in the gallbladder. Uncommonly, the mass itself is seen inside the bile duct. Dilation of the common bile duct, pancreatic duct, or both may occasionally be the only ultrasonographic finding. Although the **double-duct sign** (combined dilation of the pancreatic and common bile duct) is also seen with chronic pancreatitis, it usually indicates the presence of pancreatic adenocarcinoma (Fig. 7-28).

Displacement and involvement of **adjacent vascular structures** may occur (Fig. 7-29). Compression of the inferior vena cava by the head of the pancreas is reported as an indication of a mass lesion.[89]

Associated **pancreatitis** proximal to the mass may obscure the underlying primary tumor because of the similar echogenicity. This is especially true when pseudocyst formation from pancreatitis distorts the gland and the underlying tumor. In these cases sonographic differentiation is difficult.

Atrophy of the gland proximal to an obstructing mass in the head may occur. In these patients, a disproportionate size of the head may be the only clue to the presence of a mass (Fig. 7-30).

Some patients presenting with carcinoma of the pancreas are very cachectic. In these circumstances, because the pancreas is situated anteriorly and close to the abdominal wall, a 7.5-MHz transducer or a transducer with a good near field should be used.

Occasionally, when there is occlusion of the pancreatic duct, the dilated duct may be the only structure left in the atrophied pancreas and the entire pathologic state can be overlooked if the duct is mistaken for a blood vessel. When dilation of the pancreatic duct or common bile duct or both are present, meticulous scanning should be performed in the region where one or both dilated ducts terminate.

Doppler Findings. Pancreatic carcinoma appears to have Doppler features similar to other malignant lesions (increased velocity and diminished flow impedance).[90] Taylor et al have shown a velocity greater than 3 KHz

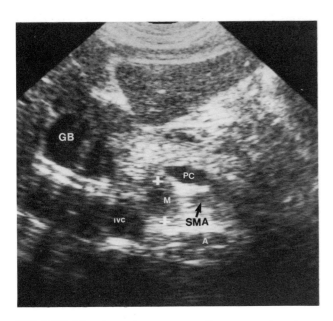

FIG 7-27. Mass in uncinate process. Transverse view shows hypoechoic mass *(M)* bulging contour of uncinate process. *A,* Aorta; *GB,* gallbladder; *IVC,* inferior vena cava; *PC,* portal confluence; *SMA,* superior mesenteric artery.

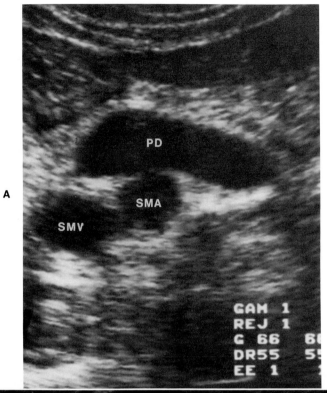

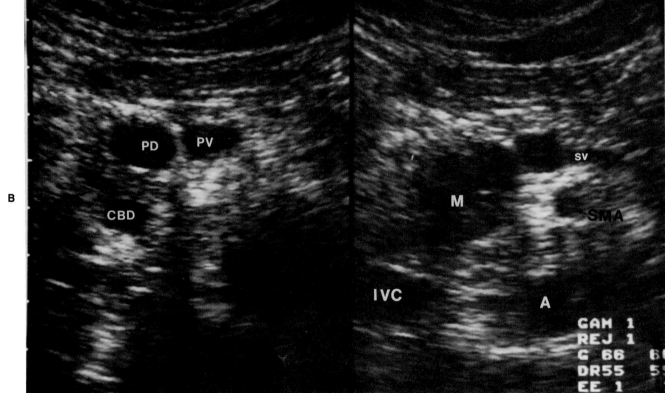

FIG 7-28. Double-duct sign, with adenocarcinoma of head of pancreas. **A,** Transverse view of body shows dilated pancreatic duct *(PD)*. **B,** Two adjacent cuts of head of pancreas show dilated common bile duct *(CBD)* and *PD*, leading to mass *(M)*. *A,* Aorta; *IVC,* inferior vena cava; *PV,* portal vein; *SMA,* superior mesenteric artery; *SMV,* superior mesenteric vein.

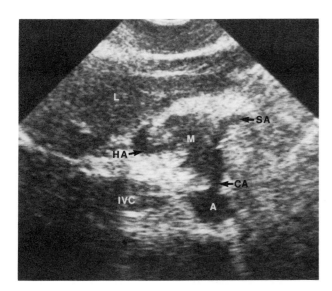

FIG 7-29. Pancreatic cancer, with encasement of celiac artery *(CA)*. Transverse view. *M,* Mass lesion; *A,* aorta; *HA,* hepatic artery; *IVC,* inferior vena cava; *L,* liver; *SA,* splenic artery.

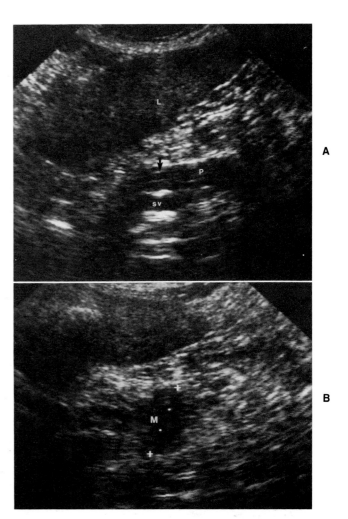

FIG 7-30. Atrophy of pancreas proximal to obstructing mass. **A,** Transverse view shows small atrophied pancreas *(P)* slightly dilated pancreatic duct *(arrow).* **B,** Head (caliper) is disproportionate in size, indicating presence of mass *(M). L,* Liver; *P,* pancreas; *sv,* splenic vein.

and a systolic/diastolic ratio of less than three in pancreatic carcinomas.[90] These results are similar to those reported for primary liver, kidney, and adrenal neoplasms. The increased velocity is attributed to arteriovenous shunting and the diminished impedance to vascular spaces that lack muscular walls.[90]

Pulsed Doppler can be used to evaluate venous and arterial structures for the presence or absence of encasement, occlusion, or thrombosis. The addition of color Doppler imagery makes the assessment of these structures easier and faster.

Staging of Pancreatic Carcinomas. The role of ultrasound is important not only in diagnosing pancreatic carcinomas but also in assessing the tumor's resectability. Surgery is still the treatment of choice in carcinomas that are considered resectable. However, it still carries a high mortality, morbidity, and poor results. Therefore every attempt should be made to preoperatively confirm the diagnosis and proper stage of the disease to prevent unnecessary surgery.

Extension of pancreatic carcinomas beyond the pancreatic parenchyma—including venous invasion, involvement of the retroperitoneal fat and adjacent organs, lymphadenopathy, and liver metastasis—precludes the feasibility of surgery. Some surgeons also consider arterial involvement a contraindication to surgery. It is generally difficult to differentiate between compression and invasion of the venous structures. Occlusion or thrombosis of the splenic vein is suggested with interruption of the vein, splenomegaly, and collateral formation in the peripancreatic and periportal region and along the stomach wall. Also, lack of visualization of the splenic vein should be regarded as suspicious for its invasion. The superior mesenteric and portal veins may also be affected with subsequent collateral formation in the mesentery. Cavernous transformation is rare because of the short duration of portal thrombosis in these patients. Encasement of the celiac axis or superior mesenteric artery as a result of lymphatic involvement is more easily recognizable and may be the only indication of the presence of the disease. Vascular structures should be evaluated with the help of the Doppler examination. Ascites is seen in more advanced cases.

Comparative Imaging. There is controversy concerning the role of ultrasound and CT in the detection of pancreatic carcinoma.[91-93] The superiority of ultrasound over CT for tissue characterization is generally accepted. Since sonography relies more on tissue characterization, which is a more objective sign than pancreatic enlargement for the diagnosis of pancreatic carcinoma, ultrasonography should be more accurate when the pancreas is optimally seen. Because CT relies more on indirect signs, such as enlargement of the pancreas, it has a lower specificity than ultrasound.[94] In one study 59% of the CT results falsely suggested a pancreatic mass solely on the basis of apparent localized enlargement of the pancreas without any other findings. All proved to be normal on the ultrasonographic examination.[94] Sensitivity of ultrasound for detection of pancreatic carcinoma is more operator dependent and is related to how much time is spent in visualizing the entire pancreas. Generally speaking, if the pancreas is optimally seen in its entirety and is normal, pancreatic carcinoma can be excluded with a high degree of certainty, considering the reported 98% sensitivity of US for detection of pancreatic carcinoma.[91] However, if the whole length of the pancreas is not seen, pancreatic carcinoma cannot be excluded. In one recent series comparing CT and ultrasound for the detection of pancreatic carcinoma, ultrasound showed the tumor itself in 86% as compared with 69% with CT. Ultrasound identified secondary signs but not the tumor in 11% compared with 25% for CT, and it was normal in 3% as compared to 6% for CT.[92]

CT should be performed following the ultrasonographic diagnosis of pancreatic carcinoma to assess resectability. CT appears to be more sensitive for assessment of local extension with regards to involvement of the adjacent retroperitoneal fat. However, if ultrasound confirms unresectability, no extra information is gained by performing CT.[91] Angiography is useful for the assessment of vascular invasion and resectability of the tumor. ERCP should be used in conjunction with ultrasound or CT, in which case it may be helpful to differentiate between malignant and inflammatory masses.[94]

Differential Diagnosis. The main differential diagnosis of pancreatic carcinoma is **focal pancreatitis** or a focal mass associated with chronic pancreatitis. If the findings are localized to the pancreas and limited to a hypoechoic area with or without mass effect, pancreatic carcinoma cannot be differentiated from focal pancreatitis unless the area has a calcification. With pancreatitis, CT scan may show more diffuse involvement of the pancreas or soft tissue changes in the adjacent fat. ERCP may show smooth tapering of the ducts at the site of the mass and associated changes of pancreatitis, especially distal to the mass.[94]

Peripancreatic lymphadenopathy can usually be differentiated from pancreatic cancer by the identification of echogenic septa between individual nodes. The absence of jaundice when a large pancreatic head mass is present close to the distal common bile duct favors lymphadenopathy.

Ampullary adenocarcinomas should be differentiated from pancreatic adenocarcinomas because they

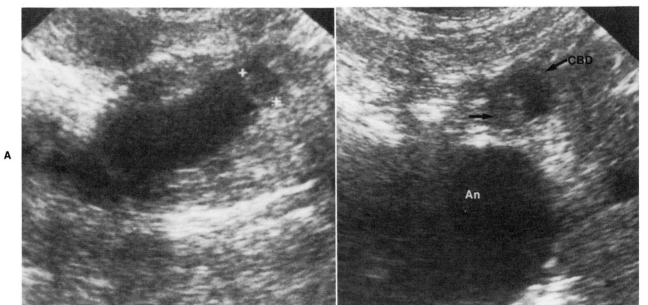

FIG 7-31. Intraluminal mass (*arrow* on **B**), with ampullary carcinoma. **A,** Sagittal and, **B,** transverse scan of dilated lower common bile duct *(CBD)*. *An,* Incidental aneurysm of abdominal aorta.

have a much better prognosis. For the three gross patterns of ampullary adenocarcinoma—intraampullary, periampullary, and mixed—the prognosis diminishes respectively. Masses larger than 2 cm have a similar prognosis to pancreatic carcinoma.[95] Most patients present with dilation of both the common bile duct and the pancreatic duct. However, the bile duct may be the only involved duct. Occasionally, an intraluminal mass is seen at the distal end of a dilated bile duct (Fig. 7-31).[96]

Cystic Neoplasms

Cystic neoplasms of the pancreas represent 10% to 15% of all pancreatic cysts and 1% of all pancreatic cancers. Both types of cystic neoplasms have a female to male preponderance of 3:2 for the microcystic and 6:1 for the macrocystic group.[97,98] Microcystic neoplasms are usually seen in patients past 60 years of age, whereas macrocystic tumors occur in both middle and old age.[98] Patients present with nonspecific abdominal symptoms, weight loss, abdominal mass, or jaundice. Tumors may be found incidentally at surgery or autopsy.[99] Microcystic neoplasms constitute a high percentage of cysts seen in patients with von Hippel-Lindau syndrome.[97]

Microcystic or serous cystadenoma is a moderately well-circumscribed, multilocular mass, often containing a central stellate scar with occasional calcification within this scar. Microcystic neoplasms are always benign and therefore do not require surgery, especially because they usually present in older patients. The cysts vary in size from less than 1 mm to 2 cm and are more numerous peripherally (Fig. 7-32). The cysts are lined with glycogen-containing cells.[97] In one study series, almost 30% of these cysts were located in the pancreatic head, with the rest distributed between the body and the tail. These tumors are often mistaken for lymphangiomas.[97]

Macrocystic or mucinous cystadenoma and cystadenocarcinoma are unilocular or multilocular smooth-surfaced cystic masses with occasional papillary projections or calcification. The cysts usually measure more than 2 cm and are lined with cells containing mucinous material.[98] These tumors are malignant or potentially malignant. Differentiation of benign and malignant forms is difficult even at surgery, and presumed benign tumors can present a few years later with metastasis. However, even the frankly malignant macrocystic tumors have a better prognosis than adenocarcinomas. Therefore these tumors should be surgically removed if possible.

Sonography. **Microcystic adenomas** are relatively well-defined tumors with external lobulation. They usually appear solid with mixed echogenicity because the smaller cysts are only depicted as interfaces. Occasionally, individual cysts may be visible, ranging in size from 1 to 20 mm. The scar that is present in some of these lesions is depicted on ultrasonographic examination as a central stellate-shaped echogenic area. Calcifications may be present within this scar (Fig. 7-33).[99] As a result of the small size of the cysts, meticulous scanning at a low-gain setting is required for their detection.

Macrocystic neoplasms commonly manifest sonographically as well-circumscribed, smooth-surfaced, thin- or thick-walled unilocular or multilocular cystic lesions of variable sizes, usually more than 2 cm.[99-101] The appearance of these cysts has been classified into four types[102]:
- Clear cysts
- Echogenic cysts containing debris
- Cysts with solid mural vegetations
- Completely filled or solid-looking cysts

The third type is the only one that can be correctly diagnosed with sonography, and the fourth can be mistaken for a solid mass. The first two types must be differentiated from a pseudocyst. The cysts may be septated or show peripheral or mural calcifications.[101] Although it is not possible to definitely differentiate between benign and malignant types, the lesions demonstrating more solid components or papillary projections are usually malignant.[99,101]

Ductectatic mucinous cystic neoplasm is a form of cystic neoplasm that has been recently reported.[103] They are seen in older age groups and are preponderant in males. The tumors are usually located in the uncinate process and result from cystic dilation of a branch of the pancreatic duct. They present as a multilocular cyst without nodularity, measuring less than 3 cm in diameter. ERCP shows a single or grapelike cluster of filling

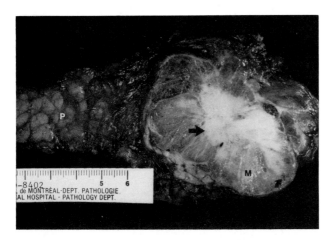

FIG 7-32. Microcystic neoplasm of pancreas. Pancreatectomy specimen. Mass *(M)* in pancreas *(P)* with multiple tiny cysts *(curved arrow)* peripherally and central radiating scar *(straight arrow)*.

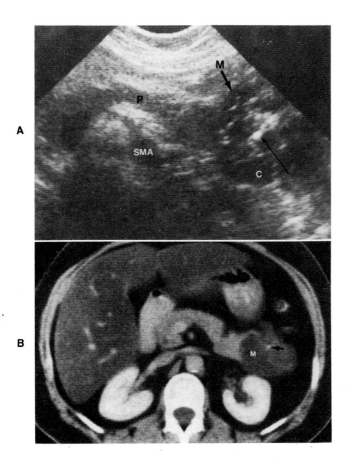

FIG 7-33. Cystic appearing microcystic neoplasm. **A,** Transverse ultrasound scan shows multicystic mass *(M)* in tail of pancreas *(P)* containing multiple small cysts *(C)* and central calcified scar *(arrow)*. **B,** Confirmatory CT scan shows hypodense mass *(M)* with central calcification *(arrow)*.

defects within the dilated ducts. Mucinous material may be seen exuding from the ampulla if the cysts are communicating with the pancreatic duct. Dilation of the pancreatic duct and intraluminal filling defects may be seen as a result of mucinous secretion.[103]

Comparative Imaging. Small cysts and mural nodules are better recognized on sonographic examinations than CT scans, whereas calcification is more evident on CT scan. Also, CT may show septal or mural enhancement.[99] Doppler imaging may prove useful in identifying microcystic neoplasms because they are known to be highly vascular. ERCP rarely shows communication with the pancreatic duct in macrocystic neoplasms.[104]

Differential Diagnosis. The microcystic type can only be differentiated from an **adenocarcinoma** if tiny cysts are visualized. Multilocularity and multiple septa are more in keeping with a cystic tumor than a pseudocyst. Communication with the pancreatic duct and parenchymal changes of pancreatitis on ERCP favor pseudocyst formation. Percutaneous fine needle aspiration can be used to differentiate between a pseudocyst (high amylase) and a mucinous tumor (mucinous material). **Choledochal cysts** may present as a cystic mass in the region of the head of the pancreas, but their communication with the common bile duct on cholangiography or direct opacification helps to differentiate them from the cystic neoplasms.[105]

Islet Cell Tumors

Islet cell tumors of the pancreas appear to arise from multipotential stem cells in ductal epithelium, referred to as the amine precursor uptake and decarboxylation (APUD) system. Islet cell tumors can be part of the multiple endocrine neoplasia (MEN) syndrome in which multiple tumors can secrete different polypeptides.[106] Although each specific tumor secretes multiple peptides, the clinical picture depends on the dominant hormone. Each of the syndromes may be caused by diffuse hyperplasia, benign adenoma, and malignant neoplasm.

Islet cell tumors are equally distributed through the gland.[20] Electron microscopy and immunoassay techniques are required for specific marking of the tumor.[20] Necrosis, hemorrhage, and calcification are more prominent in larger, malignant types, but malignancy cannot be differentiated microscopically and only dissemination provides indisputable evidence of malignancy. Even malignant tumors are slow growing, and spread beyond regional lymph nodes and liver is rare. Islet cell tumors are classified as functioning or nonfunctioning (silent). Silent tumors secrete a biologically inactive polypeptide hormone, or target cells are unresponsive or have blocked receptors.[107]

Functioning Tumors

B Cell Tumors (Insulinomas). Insulinomas are the most common islet cell tumors. they are usually benign, presenting in the fourth through six decades of life with hypoglycemic symptoms. B cell tumors are most commonly found in the body or tail of the pancreas.[88] They are usually well encapsulated and do not differ from normal islet cells on microscopic examination. Of these lesions, 70% are solitary adenomas, 10% are multiple adenomas and 10% are malignant. The remaining 10% are diffuse hyperplasia or extrapancreatic. Tumors range in size from minute lesions difficult to find on the dissecting table, to huge masses over 1500 gm (90% are less than 2 cm in diameter).[108] Ten to 27% of patients with biochemical and clinical indication of insulinomas have no tumor discovered at the time of the initial operation in which case a blind distal pancreatectomy may be performed.[109]

G Cell Tumors (Gastrinomas). Gastrinomas, producing the Zollinger-Ellison syndrome, are the second most common islet cell tumors after insulinomas. The presenting symptoms include diarrhea and peptic ulcer disease with a mean presentation at 50 years of age.[110]

Most gastrinomas are in the pancreas, with 10% to 15% arising in the duodenum.[20] Of those located in the pancreas, only 25% are solitary. Earlier reported malignancy rates were as high as 60% at presentation,[111] but recent studies confirm a decline in malignant cases, probably as a result of earlier detection because of radioimmunoassay tests for plasma gastrin levels.[112] However, it should be noted that all lesions are potentially malignant. Current management consists of medical treatment of the symptoms. Surgical intervention is limited to patients whose lesions are accurately localized.[112]

Rare Islet Cell Tumors. Glucagonoma, vipoma, somatostatinoma, and carcinoid and multihormonal tumors constitute rare functioning islet cell tumors. There is a high incidence of malignancy in glucagonomas and vipomas.[113] Vipomas are also associated with dilation of the gallbladder (caused by its paralysis as it fills with diluted bile), fluid-filled distended bowel loops (caused by inhibition of bowel motility) and excessive secretion of fluid and electrolytes. The gastric wall may also be thickened.[114]

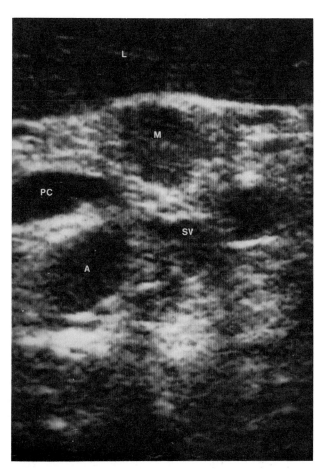

FIG 7-34. Islet cell tumor. Intraoperative scan shows hypoechoic mass *(M)* in body. *A,* Aorta; *L,* liver; *PC,* portal confluence; *SV,* splenic vein.

Nonfunctioning islet cell tumors constitute one third of all islet cell neoplasms and have a tendency to present as large tumors with a high incidence of malignancy. They are usually located in the head of the pancreas.[110]

Sonography. Preoperative ultrasonographic examination for detection of islet cell tumors is generally difficult, with identification varying from 25 to 60%.[115,116] This is due to the small size of these tumors in patients who are generally obese as a result of overeating because of fear of hypoglycemic episodes. Gastrinomas are even smaller, with an average accuracy of detection of 20%.[117] The usual small islet cell tumors are hypoechoic and well defined without calcifications or necrosis. However, these lesions can be isoechoic and only detectable by contour changes.[117] The larger tumors can be echogenic and irregular and may contain calcifications or areas of necrosis. The latter findings are usually associated with malignancy.[118] The metastatic lesions have a tendency to be echogenic.[118]

One of the most important contributions of **intraoperative ultrasound** (IOUS) is in the detection of the islet cell tumors (Fig. 7-34).[115,116] IOUS has improved the sensitivity of ultrasonographic detection from 61% to 84%,[115] and combined with palpation, it has a reported sensitivity of 100%.[115] In another study series, 86% of insulimonas and 83% of gastrinomas were detected by IOUS, and intrapancreatic lesions were identified in 100% of cases.[120] IOUS can also outline the relation of the neoplasm to the pancreatic or common bile duct.[115] Although more sensitive than both CT and preoperative ultrasonography, IOUS is less accurate for the detection of multiple adenomas, with a sensitivity of 36% because of the small size of the tumors.[115]

Comparative Imaging. Preoperative localization of islet cell tumors remains extremely difficult because of their small size and rare occurrence, which limits the experience of individual institutions.[119-122] Preoperative ultrasonographic, CT, and angiographic examinations appear to be comparable in the detection of islet cell tumors that are larger than 2 cm.

Rare Nonislet Cell Tumors

The rare nonislet cell tumors of the pancreas include: giant cell tumors, adenosquamous carcinomas, mucinous adenocarcinomas, anaplastic carcinomas, solid and papillary epithelial neoplasms, acinar cell carcinomas, pancreaticoblastomas, connective tissue tumors, metastases, lymphomas, and plasmocytomas.[123] There is no reported sonographic description for most of these tumors.

Solid and papillary tumors are usually seen in young females as large, well-defined, encapsulated tumors that may contain thick-walled cystic areas as a result of hemorrhage and necrosis. They have a predilection for the pancreatic tail and have a better prognosis and a tendency for long patient survival because of their local invasion and lack of metastases.[124]

Metastasis to the pancreas is not common and usually occurs as direct extensions from adjacent structures, such as the stomach, or contiguous lymphadenopathy. On autopsy, only 3% of all patients with a proven malignancy had metastasis to the pancreas.[125] Metastases to the pancreas occur in 8.4% of patients with lung cancer,[126] 19% of those with breast cancer,[127] and 37.5% with malignant melanomas.[128] Pancreatic metastasis[129] is usually hypoechoic and small, so the contour of the pancreas is not always affected. Larger lesions, especially from the ovary and melanoma, may show cystic changes. Single lesions may be mistaken for primary adenocarcinomas (Fig. 7-35) and multiple ones for acute pancreatitis, diffuse adenocarcinoma, or lymphoma.[129]

Non–Hodgkin's lymphomas, especially the histiocytic type, tend to involve the extra lymph node organs.

The extranodal involvement is usually associated with concomitant intraabdominal lymphadenopathy. Involvement of the pancreas may be either solitary or diffuse,[130] with multiple discrete nodules or diffuse involvement (Fig. 7-36).

ULTRASOUND-GUIDED PANCREATIC INTERVENTION
Biopsy

A percutaneous biopsy of pancreatic masses is performed to differentiate an inflammatory process from a pancreatic carcinoma. Although the sensitivity of percutaneous fine-needle aspiration biopsy (PFNA) for the diagnosis of pancreatic malignancy (50% to 86%)[131,132] is not as high as for diagnosis of liver malignancy, its reported specificity is as high as 100%.[131-133] Lower sensitivity results, both percutaneous and at surgery, are due to several factors:

- Presence of necrosis that is not visible on ultrasonograms
- Tendency for the neoplasm to produce significant desmoplastic fibrous reaction,[133] causing a negative biopsy result
- Associated pancreatitis that may complicate localization of the tumor
- Well-differentiated tumors that can be difficult to diagnose on cytologic examinations[133]

It is most efficacious to obtain biopsy specimens in the region where the pancreatic duct tapers. A positive biopsy result prevents unnecessary surgery when unresectability is confirmed by prior imaging.

The main complication of PFNA of the pancreas is the induction of pancreatitis, and a few deaths have

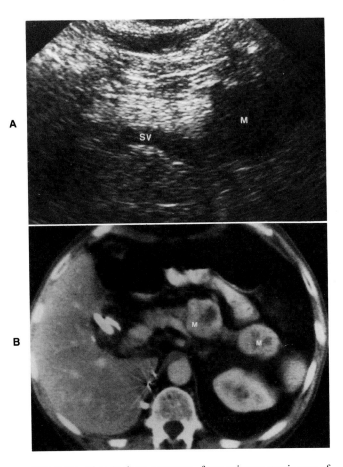

FIG 7-35. Metastasis to pancreas, from primary carcinoma of lung. **A,** Transverse ultrasound of pancreas shows well-defined solid mass *(M)* of tail of pancreas. **B,** CT scan shows two enhancing masses *(M)* of pancreas. *SV,* Splenic vein.

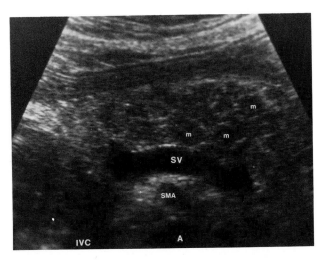

FIG 7-36. Non–Hodgkin's lymphoma, diffusely involving pancreas. Transverse scan of pancreas shows multiple, small, poorly defined hypoechoic solid masses *(m)* in body and tail of diffusely abnormal pancreas. *A,* Aorta; *IVC,* inferior vena cava; *SMA,* superior mesenteric artery; *SV,* splenic vein.

been reported from fulminant pancreatitis.[134,135] This usually occurs when a normal pancreas has undergone biopsy. There have also been isolated reports of seeding of pancreatic cancer along the path of the biopsy needle.[134,136]

Percutaneous Pancreatography

Although performing percutaneous pancreatography is feasible in a nondilated system (considering that the pancreatic duct is almost always seen under ultrasound guidance), the opacification of a nondilated pancreatic duct should be left to ERCP, except in cases in which ERCP is technically impossible. In patients with a dilated duct, a plain radiograph is obtained to document calcifications. The pancreatic duct is then punctured under ultrasound guidance using a 22-gauge needle. A small amount of pancreatic juice is aspirated for cytologic assessment, and water–soluble-contrast medium is injected at a low pressure using fluoroscopy.[137] The amount of contrast injected varies with visualization of the pancreatic duct or, in cases of occlusion, the amount of pressure needed to opacify and the patient's response to the injection. Excessive injection should be avoided, and at the end of the procedure, the contrast medium should be aspirated.[137] A success rate of 89% has been obtained in the largest study series reported.[137] No complications are reported, except for one case of bile leakage as a result of transgression of a dilated intrahepatic bile duct.[137]

Indications for percutaneous pancreatography include:

- Technical difficulty with ERCP, either as a result of failure of the procedure or modified anatomy from previous surgery (such as prior gastrecto-my, pancreaticojejunostomy, or a Whipple procedure)[137]
- Lack of ERCP visualization of the pancreatic duct in spite of opacification of the common bile duct
- Poor or nonopacification of the proximal pancreatic duct caused by significant narrowing or occlusion of the distal pancreatic duct
- Determination of the presence of stones and creation of a surgical map before pancreatic surgery
- A dilated pancreatic duct but no demonstrable mass on ultrasonographic or CT examinations (A pancreatogram can precisely localize a lesion for biopsy.) (Fig. 7-37)

PANCREATIC TRANSPLANTATION

Pancreatic transplants are complicated by ischemia, rejection, anastomotic leak, other arterial and venous anastomotic complications, and infection. Pancreatitis is the only complication unique to the pancreas.[138] There is no sensitive test for early detection of transplant rejection, and pancreatic biopsy is seldom performed because of the high risk of complications. However, when combined renal and pancreatic transplantations are performed, the two organs tend to be rejected at the same time.[138] The only established roles of ultrasound in pancreatic transplantation are to detect peripancreatic fluid collections and pancreatic enlargement[138,139] and to guide aspiration to characterize fluid.[140] Transplant rejection may cause an inhomogeneous echopattern,[138] but this is not specific.[138,140]

Recently, pulsed Doppler imaging has been used to diagnose early signs of transplant rejection, showing a resistance index of less than 0.7 in normal transplants and more than 0.7 in rejection with a sensitivity of 87.5%.[141] Pancreatic Doppler evaluation is more difficult technically than renal Doppler examination because of the lower vascularity of the pancreas.

ENDOSCOPIC ULTRASONOGRAPHY

Theoretically, endoscopic ultrasonography (EUS) overcomes the limiting factors of transabdominal pancreatic sonography (i.e., interfering gastrointestinal gas and attenuating fat). However, it is limited (in 24% of cases) by the endoscopic scanning arm, which is a rigid, oblique-viewing fiberoptic instrument.[142,143] A high-MHz sector scan transducer is mounted at the tip of the fibroscope and rotated by a motor, which provides a 360-degree scanning field.[143] The head of the pancreas, bile ducts, gallbladder, and portal vein are optimally seen with the transducer placed in the immediate postbulbar area or the second portion of the duodenum, whereas the body and the tail are best imaged through the posterior wall of the stomach (Fig. 7-38).[144]

EUS accurately discloses the presence or absence of disease in the pancreas[143] and has been shown to be

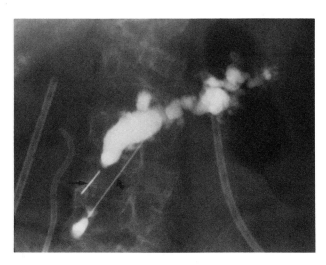

FIG 7-37. Percutaneous pancreatogram, performed under ultrasound guidance using 22-gauge needle *(curved arrow)*. Site of occlusion has been biopsied using 22-gauge needle *(straight arrow)* under fluoroscopic guidance.

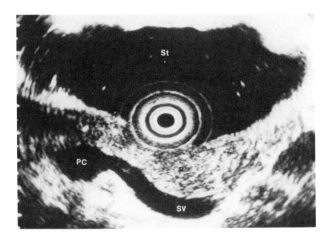

FIG 7-38. Transgastric endosonography, body and tail of normal pancreas *(P)*. *PC,* Portal confluence; *St,* stomach; *SV,* splenic vein.
(Courtesy Valette PJ, M.D., Hopital Edouard Herriot, Lion, France.)

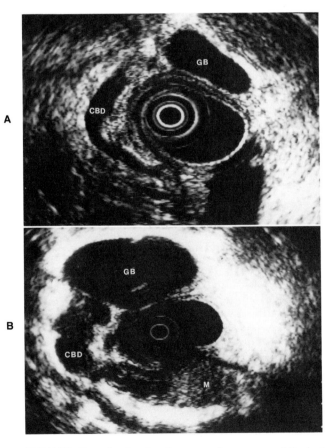

FIG 7-39. Transduodenal endosonography, common bile duct *(CBD)* and gallbladder *(GB)*. **A,** Normal common bile duct. **B,** Solid intraluminal mass *(M)* in distal dilated common bile duct is ampullary carcinoma. Gallbladder is distended.
(Courtesy Valette PJ, M.D., Hopital Edouard Herriot, Lion, France.)

more sensitive than transabdominal ultrasound, CT, and ERCP for the detection of pancreatic carcinoma.[144,145] Its major advantage is that it displays lesions of less than 20 mm[143,145] and those in the pancreatic head and tail.[145] EUS is superior to conventional ultrasound for the evaluation of vascular invasion[147] and other factors determining resectability.[146] EUS has also proved more accurate for the detection of ampullary carcinoma (Fig. 7-39), identification of stones in the lower common bile duct, and pancreatic ductal dilation.[147] Neuroendocrine tumors as small as 10 mm are detected with EUS.[148] Because of the technical difficulties and the invasive nature of this examination, the role of EUS is presently limited to specific cases rather than used for screening.

REFERENCES
Embryology

1. Clemente CD: The digestive system. In: *Gray's Anatomy.* 30th ed. Philadelphia: Lea & Febiger; 1985:1502-1507.
2. Berman LG, Prior JT, Abramow SM, et al: A study of the pancreatic duct system in man by the use of vinyl acetate casts of postmortem preparations. *Surg Gynecol Obstet* 1960;110:391-403.

Anatomy

3. Suramo I, Pèivènsalo M, Myllylè V: Cranio-caudal movements of the liver, pancreas and kidneys in respiration. *Acta Radiol* 1984;25(2):129-131.
4. Valenzvela JE: Pancreas. In: Gitnick G, Hollander D, Samloff IM, eds. *Principles and Practice of Gastroenterology and Hepatology.* New York: Elsvier Science Publishing; 1988:722-740.
5. Newman BM, Lebenthal E. In: Vay Liang WG, Gardner JD, Brooks FP et al, eds. Congenital anomalies of the exocrine pancreas, in the exocrine pancreas. New York: Raven Press; 1986:773-782.

Pancreatic Sonography

6. Bret PM, Reinhold C, Herba M, et al: Replaced or right accessory hepatic artery: can ultrasound replace angiography. *J Clin Ultrasound* 1988;16:245-249.
7. Bryan PJ: Appearance of normal pancreatic duct: a study using real-time ultrasound. *J Clin Ultrasound* 1982;10:63-66.
8. Hadidi A: Pancreatic duct diameter: sonographic measurement in normal subjects. *J Clin Ultrasound* 1983;11:17-22.
9. Didier D, Deschamps JP, Rohmer P, et al: Evaluation of the pancreatic duct: a reappraisal based on a retrospective correlative study by sonography and pancreatography in 117 normal and pathologic subjects. *Ultrasound Med Biol* 1983;9(5):509-518.
10. So CB, Cooperberg PL, Gibney RG, et al: Sonographic findings in pancreatic lipomatosis. *AJR* 1987;149:67-68.
11. Patel S, Bellon EM, Haaga J, et al: Fat replacement of the exocrine pancreas. *AJR* 1980;135:843-845.
12. Nakamura M, Katada N, Sakakibara, et al: Huge lipomatous pseudohypertrophy of the pancreas. *Am J Gastroenterol* 1979;72(2):171-174.
13. de Graaff CS, Taylor KJW, Simonds BD, et al: Gray-scale echography of he pancreas: re-evaluation of normal size. *Radiology* 1978;129:157-161.
14. Niederau C, Sonnenberg A, Muller JE, et al: Sonographic measurements of the normal liver, spleen, pancreas, and portal vein. *Radiology* 1983;149:537-540.

15. Bolondi L, Bassi, SL, Gaiani S: Sonography of chronic pancreatitis. *Radiol Clin North Am* 1989;27(4):815-833.

16. Tszékessy D, Pochhammer KF: Diurnal sonographic imaging of the pancreas. *Ultraschall Med* 1985;6:134-136.

17. Odo Op den Orth J: Tubeless hypotonic duodenography with water: a simple aid in sonography of the pancreatic head. *Radiology* 1985;154:826.

18. duCret RP, Jackson VP, Rees C, et al: Pancreatic sonography: enhancement by metoclopramide. *AJR* 1986;146:341-343.

19. Rauch RF, Bowie JD, Rosenberg ER, et al: Can ultrasonic examination of the pancreas and gallbladder follow a barium UGI series on the same day? *Invest Radiol* 1983;18(6):523-525.

Congenital Anomalies

20. Cotran RC, Kumar V, Robbins SL: *The Pancreas: Robins' Pathologic Basis of Disease*. 4th ed. Philadelphia: W B Saunders; 1989:981-1010.

21. Mares AJ, Hirsch M: Congenital cysts of the head of the pancreas. *J Pediatr Surg* 1977;12:547-552.

22. Oppenheimer EH, Esterly JR: Pathology of cystic fibrosis review of the literature and comparison with 146 autopsied cases. *Perspect Pediatr Pathol* 1975;2:241-278.

23. Swobodnik W, Wolf A, Wechsler JG, et al: Ultrasound characteristics of the pancreas in children with cystic fibrosis. *J Clin Ultrasound* 1985;13:469-474.

24. Dobson RL, Johnson MA, Henning RC, et al: sonography of the gallbladder, biliary tree, and pancreas in adults with cystic fibrosis. *J Can Assoc Radiol* 1988; 39:257-259.

25. Daneman A, Gaskin K, Martin DJ, et al: Pancreatic changes in cystic fibrosis: computed tomography and sonographic appearances. *AJR* 1983; 141:653-655.

26. Graham N, Manhire AR, Stead RJ, et al: Cystic fibrosis: ultrasonographic findings in the pancreas and hepatobiliary system correlated with clinical data and pathology. *Clin Radiol* 1985; 36(2):199-203.

27. Hernanz-Schulman M, Teele RL, Perez-Atayde A, et al: Pancreatic cytosis in cystic fibrosis. *Radiology* 1986;158:629-631.

28. Cooperman M, Ferrara JJ, Fromkes JJ, et al: Surgical management of pancreas divisum. *Am J Surg* 1982;143:107-112.

29. Cotton PB: Congenital anomaly of pancreas divisum as cause of obstructive pain and pancreatitis. *Gut* 1980;21:105-114.

30. Brinberg DE, Carr MF Jr, Premkumar A, et al: Isolated ventral pancreatitis in an alcoholic with pancreas divisum. *Gastrointest Radiol* 1988;13(4):323-326.

31. Jennings CM, Gaines PA: The abdominal manifestation of von Hippel-Lindau disease and a radiological screening protocol for an affected family. *Clin Radiol* 1988;39(4):363-367.

32. Levine E, Collins DL, Horton WA, et al: Computed tomography screening of the abdomen in von Hippel-Lindau disease. *AJR* 1982;139:505-510.

Inflammatory Processes

33. Ranson JHC, Ratkind KM, Turner JW: Prognostic signs and non-operative peritoneal lavage in acute pancreatitis. *Surg Gynecol Obstet* 1976;143:209-219.

34. Jeffrey RB, Laing FC, Wing VW: Ultrasound in acute pancreatic trauma. *Gastrointest Radiol* 1986;11:4448.

35. Jeffrey RB Jr, Federle MP, Crass RA: Computed tomography of pancreatic trauma. *Radiology* 1983;147:491-494.

36. Gyr KE, Singer MV, Sarles H: Pancreatitis: concepts and classification. International Congress Ser, vol 642, Feb, 1985.

37. Delhaye M, Engelholm L, Cremer M: Pancreas divisum: congenital anatomic variant or anomaly?—contribution of endoscopic retrograde dorsal pancreatography. *Gastroenterology* 1985;89:951-958.

38. Goekas MC: Etiology and pathogenesis of acute pancreatic inflammation: acute pancreatitis. *Ann Intern Med* 1985;103:86-100.

39. Jeffrey RB, Laing FC, Wing VW: Extrapancreatic spread of acute pancreatitis: new observations with real-time ultrasound. *Radiology* 1986;159:707-711.

40. Freeny PC: Classification of pancreatitis. *Radiol Clin North Am* 1989;27:1-3.

41. Neff CC, Simeone JF, Wittenberg J, et al: Inflammatory pancreatic masses: problems in differentiating focal pancreatitis from carcinoma. *Radiology* 1984;150:35-40.

42. Price J, Leung JWC: Ultrasound diagnosis of ascaris lumbricoides in the pancreatic duct: the "four-lines" sign. *Br J Radiol* 1988;61:411-413.

43. Warshaw AL: Inflammatory masses following acute pancreatitis. *Surg Clin North Am* 1974;54:621-636.

44. Bradley EL III, Clements JL Jr, Gonzalez AC: The natural history of pancreatic pseudocysts: a unified concept of management. *Am J Surg* 1979;137:135-141.

45. Donovan PJ, Sanders RC, Siegelman SS: Collections of fluid after pancreatitis: evaluation of computed tomography and ultrasonography. *Radiol Clin North Am* 1982;20:653-665.

46. Nyberg DA, Laing F: Ultrasonographic findings in peptic ulcer disease and pancreatitis that simulate primary gallbladder disease. *J Ultrasound Med* 1983;2:303-307.

47. Lee CM, Chang-Chien CS, Lim DY, et al: Real-time ultrasonography of pancreatic pseudocyst: comparison of infected and uninfected pseudocysts. *J Clin Ultrasound* 1988;16:393-397.

48. Bradley EL III: Pancreatic pseudocyst. In Bradley EL III, ed. *Complications of pancreatitis: Medical and Surgical*. Philadelphia: WB Saunders; 1982:124-153.

49. Rattner DW, Warshaw Al: Surgical intervention in acute pancreatitis. *Crit Care Med* 1988;16:8595.

50. Laing FC, Gooding GAW, Brown T, et al: Atypical pseudocysts of the pancreas: an ultrasonographic evaluation. *J Clin Ultrasound* 1979;7:27-33.

51. Maier W, Roscher R, Malfertheinar P, et al: Pancreatic pseudocyst of the mediastinum: evaluation by computed tomography. *Eur J Radiol* 1986;6:70-72.

52. Lye DJ, Stark RH, Cullen GM, et al: Ruptured pancreatic pseudocysts: extension into the thigh. *AJR* 1987;49:937-938.

53. Grace RR, Jordan PH Jr: Unresolved problems of pancreatic pseudocysts. *Ann Surg* 1976;184:16-21.

54. Rheingold OJ, Wilbar JA, Barkin JS: Gastric outlet obstruction due to pancreatic pseudocyst. a report of two cases. *Am J Gastroenterol* 1978;69:92-96.

55. Bellon EM, George CR, Schreiber H, et al: Pancreatic pseudocysts of the duodenum. *AJR* 1979;133:827-831.

56. Vick CW, Simeone JF, Ferrucci JT, et al: Pancreatitis associated fluid collection involving the spleen: sonographic and computed tomographic appearance. *Gastrointest Radiol* 1981;6:247-250.

57. Stanley JL, Frey CF, Miller TA, et al: Major arterial hemorrhage: a complication of pancreatic pseudocyst and chronic pancreatitis. *Arch Surg* 1976;111:435-440.

58. Frey CF, Lindenaver SM, Miller TA: Pancreatic abscess. *Surg Gynecol Obstet* 1979;149:722-726.

59. White AF, Barum S, Buranasiri S: Aneurysms secondary to pancreatitis. *AJR* 1976;127:393-396.

60. Falkoff GE, Taylor KJW, Morse SS: Hepatic artery pseudoaneurysm: diagnosis with real-time and pulsed doppler ultrasound. *Radiology* 1986;58:55-56.

61. Crass RA, Way LW. Acute and chronic pancreatic pseudocysts are different. *Am J Surg* 1981;142:660-663.

62. Sarti DA: Rapid development and spontaneous regression of

pancreatic pseudocysts documented by ultrasound. *Radiology* 1977; 125:789-793.

63. vanSonnenberg E, Wittich GR, Casola G, et al: Percutaneous drainage of infected and noninfected pancreatic pseudocysts: experience in 101 cases. *Radiology* 1989;170:757-761.

64. Matzinger FRK, Ho CS, Yee AC, et al: Pancreatic pseudocysts drained through a percutaneous transgastric approach: further experience. *Radiology* 1988;167:431-434.

65. Cremer M: Endoscopic cystoduodenostomy. *Endoscopy* 1981;2:29-30.

66. Beger HG, Bittner R, Block S, et al: Bacterial contamination of pancreatic necrosis: a prospective clinical study. *Gastroenterology* 1986;91:433-438.

67. van Sonnenberg E, Wittich GR, Casola G, et al: Complicated pancreatic inflammatory disease: diagnostic and therapeutic role of interventional radiology. *Radiology* 1985;155:340-355.

68. Banks PA: Clinical manifestations and treatment of pancreatitis. *Ann Intern Med* 1985;103:91-95.

69. Seiler JG, Polk HC: Factors contributing to fatal outcome after treatment of pancreatic abscess. *Ann Surg* 1986;203:605-612.

70. Ranson JHC, Spencer FC: Prevention, diagnosis and treatment of pancreatic abscess. *Surgery* 1977;82:99-105.

71. Federle MP, Jeffrey RB, Crass RA, et al: Computed tomography of pancreatic abscess. *AJR* 1981;136:879-882.

72. Vernacchia FS, Jeffrey RB Jr, Federle MP, et al: Pancreatic abscess: predictive value of early abdominal computed tomography. *Radiology* 1987;162:435-438.

73. Sankaran S, Walt A: Pancreatic ascites: recognition and management. *Arch Surg* 1976;(3):430-434.

74. Belfar HL, Radecki PD, Friedman AC, et al: Pancreatitis presenting as pleural effusions: computed tomography demonstration of pleural extension of pancreatic exudate. *CT* 1987; 11:184-186.

75. Howard JM, Nedurich A: Correlation of the histologic observations and operative findings in patients with chronic pancreatitis. *Surg Gynecol Obstet* 1971;132:387-395.

76. Alpern MB, Sandler MA, Kellman GM, et al: Chronic pancreatitis: ultrasonic features. *Radiology* 1985;155:215-219.

77. Ferrucci J Jr, Wittenberg J, Black EB, et al: Computed body tomography in chronic pancreatitis. *Radiology* 1979;130:175-182.

78. Fishman EK, Siegelman SS: Pancreatitis and its complications. In: Tavares JM, Ferrucci JT, eds. *Radiology: Diagnosis, Imaging, Intervention.* Philadelphia: JB Lippincott; 1986:1-12.

79. Weinstein BJ, Weinstein DP, Brodmeckel GJ Jr: Ultrasonography of pancreatic lithiasis. *Radiology* 1980;134:185-189.

80. Lankish PG, Otto J, Erkelenz I, et al: Pancreatic calcifications: no indicator of severe exocrine pancreatic insufficiency. *Gastroenterology* 1986;90:617-621.

81. Ammann RW, Meunch R, Otto R, et al: Evolution and regression of pancreatic calcification in chronic pancreatitis. *Gastroenterology* 1988;95:1018-1028.

82. Rosch N, Lux G, Rieman JF, et al: Chronic pancreatitis and the neighboring organs. *Fortschr Med* 1981;99:1118-1125.

83. Malfertheiner P, Buchler M: Correlation of imaging and function in chronic pancreatitis. *Radiol Clin North Am* 1989;27:51-64.

84. Ason ATA: Endoscopic retrograde cholangiopancreatography in chronic pancreatitis: Cambridge classification. *Radiol Clin North Am* 1989;27:39-50.

85. Jones SN, Lees WR, Frost RA: Diagnosis and grading of chronic pancreatitis by morphological criteria derived by ultrasound and pancreatography. *Clin Radiol* 1988;39:43-48.

Neoplasms

86. Kissane JM: *Anderson's Pathology.* 9th ed. St Louis: Mosby-Year Book; 1990;1347-1372.

87. Weinstein DP, Weinstein BJ: Pancreas. In: Goldberg BB, ed. *Clinics in Diagnostic Ultrasound: Ultrasound in cancer.* New York: Churchill Livingston; 1981:35-51.

88. Kaplan JO, Isikoff MB, Barkin J, et al: Necrotic carcinoma of the pancreas: "the pseudo-pseudocyst." *J Comput Assist Tomogr* 1980;4(2):166-167.

89. Walls WJ, Templeton AW: The ultrasonic demonstration of inferior vena caval compression: a guide to pancreatic head enlargement with emphasis on neoplasm. *Radiology* 1977; 123:165-167.

90. Taylor KJW, Ramos I, Carter D: Correlation of doppler US tumor signals with neovascular morphologic features. *Radiology* 1988;166:57-62.

91. Campbell JP, Wilson S: Pancreatic neoplasms: how useful is evaluation with ultrasound? *Radiology* 1988;167:341-344.

92. Pèivènsalo M, Lèhde S: Ultrasonography and computed tomography in pancreatic malignancy. *Acta Radiologica* 1988; 29(3):343-344.

93. Kamin PD, Bernardino ME, Wallace S, et al: Comparison of ultrasound and computed tomography in the detection of pancreatic malignancy. *Cancer* 1980;46:2410-2412.

94. Hildell J, Aspelin P, Wehlin L: Gray scale ultrasound and endoscopic ductography in the diagnosis of pancreatic disease. *Acta Chir Scand* 1979;145:239-245.

95. Cubilla AL, Fitzgerald PJ: Surgical pathology aspects of cancer of the ampulla-head-of-pancreas region. *Monogr Pathol* 1980;21:67-81.

96. Robledo R, Prieto ML, Pérez M, et al: Carcinoma of the hepaticopancreatic ampullar region: role of ultrasound. *Radiology* 1988;166:409-412.

97. Compagno J, Oertel JE: Microcystic adenomas of the pancreas (glycogen-rich cystadenomas): a clinicopathologic study of 34 cases. *Am J Clin Pathol* 1978;69(3):289-298.

98. Compagno J, Oertel JE: Mucinous cystic neoplasms of the pancreas with overt and latent malignancy (cystadenocarcinoma and cystadenoma): a clinicopathologic study of 41 cases. *Am J Clin Pathol* 1978;69(6):573-580.

99. Friedman AC, Lichtenstein JE, Dachman AH: Cystic neoplasms of the pancreas: radiological-pathological correlation. *Radiology* 1983;149:45-50.

100. Johnson CD, Stephens DH, Charboneau JW, et al: Cystic pancreatic tumors: computed tomography and sonographic assessment. *AJR* 1988;151:1133-1138.

101. Bastid C, Sahel J, Sastre B, et al: Mucinous cystadenocarcinoma of the pancreas: ultrasonographic findings in 5 cases. *Acta Radiologica* 1989;30(1):45-47.

102. Busilacchi P, Rizzatto G, Bazzocchi M, et al: Pancreatic cystadenocarcinoma: diagnostic problems. *Br J Radiol* 1982;55:558-561.

103. Itai Y, Ohhashi K, Nagai H, et al: "Ductectatic" mucinous cystadenoma and cystadenocarcinoma of the pancreas. *Radiology* 1986;161:697-700.

104. Herrera L, Glassman CI, Komins JI: Mucinous cystic neoplasm of the pancreas demonstrated by ultrasound and endoscopic retrograde pancreatography. *Am J Gastroenterol* 1980;73(6):512-515.

105. Markle BM, Friedman AC, Sachs L: Anomalies and congenital disorders. In: Friedman AC, ed. *Radiology of the liver, biliary tree, pancreas, and spleen.* Baltimore: Williams & Wilkins; 1987:351-385.

106. Friesen SR: Tumors of the endocrine pancreas. *N Engl J Med* 1982;306:580-590.

107. Toledo-Pereyra LH: *The Pancreas: Principles of Medical and Surgical Practice.* New York: Wiley Medical Publication; 1985.

108. van Heerden JA, Edis AJ, Service FJ: The surgical aspects of insulinomas. *Ann Surg* 1979;189:677-682.

109. Grant CS, van Heerden J, Charboneau JW, et al: Insulinoma: the value of intraoperative ultrasonography. *Arch Surg* 1988;123:843-848.

110. Rossi P, Allison DJ, Bezzi M, et al: Endocrine tumors of the pancreas. *Radiol Clin North Am* 1989;27(1):129-161.

111. Jensen RT, Gardner JD, Raufman JP, et al: Zollinger-Ellison syndrome: current concepts and management. *Ann Intern Med* 1983;98:59-75.

112. Stadil F: Gastrinomas: clinical syndromes. *Acta Oncologica* 1989;28(3):379-381.

113. Galiber AK, Reading CC, Charboneau JW, et al: Localization of pancreatic insulinoma: comparison of pre- and intraoperative ultrasound with computed tomography and angiography. *Radiology* 1988;166(2):405-408.

114. Gorman B, Charboneau JW, James EM, et al: Benign pancreatic insulinoma: preoperative and intraoperative sonographic localization. *AJR* 1986;147:929-934.

115. Kuhn FP, Gunther R, Ruckert K, et al: Ultrasonic demonstration of small pancreatic islet cell tumors. *J Clin Ultrasound* 1982;10:173-175.

116. Norton JA, Cromack DT, Shawker TH: Intraoperative ultrasonographic localization of islet cell tumors. *Ann Surg* 1988;207:160-168.

117. Katz LB, Aufses AH, Rayfield E, et al: Preoperative localization and intraoperative glucose monitoring in the management of patients with pancreatic insulinoma. *Surg Gynecol Obstet* 1986;163:509-512.

118. Rossi P, Baert A, Passariello R, et al: Computed tomography of functioning tumors of the pancreas. *AJR* 1985;144:57-60.

119. Roche A, Raisonnier A, Gillon-Savouret MC: Pancreatic venous sampling and arteriography in localizing insulinomas and gastrinomas: procedure and results in 55 cases. *Radiology* 1982;145:621-627.

120. Montenegro-Rodas F, Samaan NA: Glucagonoma tumors and syndrome. *Curr Prob Cancer* 1981;6(6):1-54.

121. Tjon A Tham RT, Jansen JB, Falke TH, et al: Magnetic resonance, computed tomography, and ultrasound findings of metastatic vipoma in pancreas. *J Comput Assist Tomogr* 1989;13(1):142-144.

122. Latshaw RF, Rohrer GV: Semierect and erect position in percutaneous transhepatic cholangiography. *AJR* 1978;131:171-172.

123. Rice NT, Woodring JH, Mostowycz L, et al: Pancreatic plasmacytoma: sonographic and computerized tomographic findings. *J Clin Ultrasound* 1981;9:46-48.

124. Lin JT, Wang TH, Wei TC, et al: Sonographic features of solid papillary neoplasm of the pancreas. *J Clin Ultrasound* 1985;13:339-342.

125. Willis RA: *The Spread of Tumors in the Human Body.* New York: Butterworths; 1975:216-220.

126. Budinger JM: Untreated bronchogenic carcinoma: a clinicopathological study of 250 autopsied cases. *Cancer* 1958;11:106-116.

127. de la Monte SM, Hutchins GM, Moore GW: Endocrine organ metastases from breast carcinoma. *Am J Pathol* 1984;114:131-136.

128. Patel JK, Didolkar MS, Pickren JW, et al: Metastatic pattern of malignant melanoma: a study of 216 autopsy cases. *Am J Surg* 1978;135:807-810.

129. Wernecke K, Peters PE, Galanski M: Pancreatic metastases: ultrasound evaluation. *Radiology* 1986;160:339-402.

130. Glazer HS, Lee JKT, Balfe DM, et al: non-Hodgkin lymphoma: computed tomographic demonstration of unusual extranodal involvement. *Radiology* 1983;149:211-217.

Ultrasound-Guided Pancreatic Intervention

131. Pilotti S, Rilke F, Claren R, et al: Conclusive diagnosis of hepatic and pancreatic malignancies by fine needle aspiration. *Acta Cytol* 1988;32(1):27-38.

132. Ekberg O, Bergenfeldt M, Aspelin P, et al: Reliability of ultrasound-guided fine-needle biopsy of pancreatic masses. *Acta Radiologica* 1988; 29(5):535-539.

133. Yamamoto R, Tatsuta M, Noguchi S, et al: Histocytologic diagnosis of pancreatic cancer by percutaneous aspiration biopsy under ultrasonic guidance. *Am J Clin Pathol* 1985;83(4):409-414.

134. Hancke S, Holm HH, Koch F: Ultrasonically guided puncture of solid pancreatic mass lesions. *Ultrasound Med Biol* 1984;10(5):613-615.

135. Evans WK, Ho CS, McLoughlin MJ, et al: Fatal necrotizing pancreatitis following fine-needle aspiration biopsy of the pancreas. *Radiology* 1981;141:61-62.

136. Caturelli E, Rapacci GL, Anti M, et al: Malignant seeding after fine-needle aspiration biopsy of the pancreas. *Diagn Imaging Clin Med* 1985;54(2):88-91.

137. Matter D, Bret PM, Bretagnolle M, et al: Pancreatic duct: ultrasound guided percutaneous opacification. *Radiology* 1987;163:635-636.

Pancreatic Transplantation

138. Patel B, Markivee C, Mahanta B, et al: Pancreatic transplantation: scintigraphy, ultrasound and computed tomography. *Radiology* 1988;167:685-687.

139. Yuh WTC, Wiese JA, Abu-Yousef MM, et al: Pancreatic transplant imaging. *Radiology* 1988;167:679-683.

140. Letourneau JG, Maile CW, Sutherland DER, et al: Ultrasound and computed tomography in the evaluation of pancreatic transplantation. *Radiol Clin North Am* 1987;25(2):345-355.

141. Patel B, Wolverson MK, Mahanta B: Pancreatic transplant rejection: assessment with duplex ultrasound. *Radiology* 1989;173(1):131-135.

Endoscopic Ultrasonography

142. Boyce GA, Sivak Jr MV: Endoscopic ultrasonography in the diagnosis of pancreatic tumors. *Gastrointest Endosc* 1990;36:S28-S32.

143. Kaufman AR, Sivak MV Jr: Endoscopic ultrasonography in the differential diagnosis of pancreatic disease. *Gastrointest Endosc* 1989;35(3):214-219.

144. Yasuda K, Tanaka Y, Fujimoto S, et al: Use of endoscopic ultrasonography in small pancreatic cancer. *Scand J Gastroenterol* 1984;19(102):9-17.

145. Yasuda K, Mukai H, Fujimoto S, et al: The diagnosis of pancreatic cancer by endoscopic ultrasonography. *Gastrointest Endosc* 1988;34(1):1-8.

146. Tio TL, Tytgat GNJ: Endoscopic ultrasonography in staging local resectability of pancreatic and periampullary malignancy. *Scand J Gastroenterol* 1986;21(123):135-142.

147. Strohm WD, Kurtz W, Hagenmuller F, et al: Diagnostic efficacy of endoscopic ultrasound tomography in pancreatic cancer and cholestasis. *Scand J Gastroenterol* 1984;19(102):18-23.

148. Dancygier H, Classen M: Endosonographic diagnosis of benign pancreatic and biliary lesions. *Scand J Gastroenterol* 1986;21(123):119-122.

CHAPTER 8

The Gastrointestinal Tract

- Stephanie R. Wilson, M.D.

BASIC PRINCIPLES

Gastrointestinal tract sonography is frequently frustrating and always challenging. Gas content within the gut lumen can make visibility difficult and even impossible, intraluminal fluid may mimic cystic masses, and fecal material may create a variety of artifacts and pseudotumors. Nevertheless, normal gut has a reproducible pattern or "gut signature," and a variety of gut pathologies create recognizable sonographic abnormalities. In addition, in a few conditions, such as acute appendicitis and acute diverticulitis, sonography may play a major primary investigative role. Further, endosonography, performed with high frequency transducers in the lumen of the gut, is an increasingly popular technique for assessing the esophagus, stomach, and rectum.

The Gut Signature

The gut is a continuous hollow tube with four concentric layers (Fig. 8-1). From the lumen outward, they are:

- Mucosa, which consists of an epithelial lining, loose connective tissue or lamina propria, and muscularis mucosa
- Submucosa
- Muscularis propria, with inner circular and outer longitudinal fibers
- Serosa or adventitia

These layers create a characteristic appearance or gut signature on sonography, where up to five layers may be visualized (Fig. 8-2). The correlation of the histologic layer with the sonographic appearance is depicted in Table 8-1.[1-3] The sonographic layers are alternately echogenic and hypoechoic: the first, third, and fifth layers are echogenic; and the second and fourth layers are hypoechoic. On routine sonograms, the gut signature (Fig. 8-3) may vary from a bull's eye in cross-section, with an echogenic central area and a hypoechoic rim, to full depiction of the five sonographic layers. The quality of the scan and the resolution of the transducer determine the degree of layer differentiation. The normal gut wall is uniform and compliant, with an average thickness of 3 mm if distended and 5 mm if not.[4]

The content and diameter of the gastrointestinal lumen and the motor activity of the gut are also assessed.

■ **TABLE 8-1**

Correlation of Sonographic and Histologic Layers
of the Gut Wall from the Lumen Outward

Sonography	Histology
Echogenic	Superficial mucosa
	+/− Luminal content/mucosal interface
Hypoechoic	Deep mucosa, including muscularis mucosa
Echogenic	Submucosa
	+ Submucosa/muscularis propria interface
Hypoechoic	Muscularis propria
Echogenic	Serosa
	+ Subserosal fat, + marginal interface

FIG 8-1. Schematic depiction of the histologic layers of the gut wall.

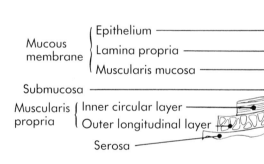

Mucous membrane { Epithelium
Lamina propria
Muscularis mucosa

Submucosa

Muscularis propria { Inner circular layer
Outer longitudinal layer

Serosa

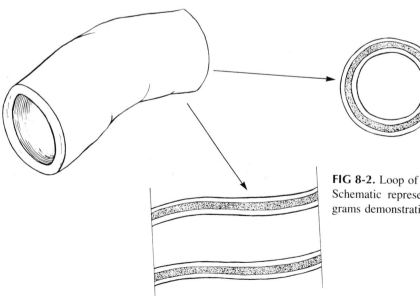

FIG 8-2. Loop of normal gut creating a normal gut signature. Schematic representation with sagittal and transverse sonograms demonstrating the five layers of the gut wall.

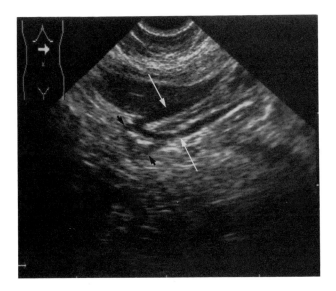

FIG 8-3. Normal gut signature. Transverse sonogram in epigastrium shows normal gastric antrum *(white arrows),* pylorus, and duodenal bulb *(black arrows)* with depiction of a normal gut signature with five sonographic layers. The submucosa is the thickest echogenic layer surrounded by the hypoechoic muscularis propria.

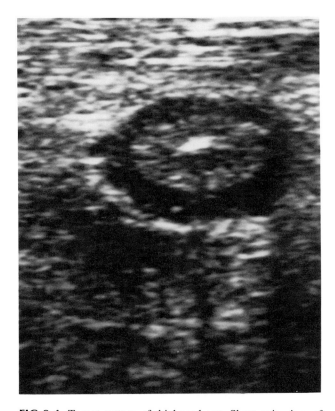

FIG 8-4. Target pattern of thickened gut. Short axis view of descending colon in a patient with Crohn's disease shows thickened gut wall creating a target pattern. The central echogenicity is the lumen. The low-level echoes are predominantly the submucosa. The hypoechoic external rim is the muscularis propria.

Hypersecretion, mechanical obstruction, and ileus are implicated when gut fluid is excessive. Peristalsis is normally seen in the small bowel and stomach. Activity may be increased with mechanical obstruction and with some inflammatory enteritides. Decreased activity is seen with paralytic ileus.

Gut Wall Pathology

Gut wall pathology creates characteristic sonographic patterns. The most familiar, the "target" pattern (Fig. 8-4), was first described by Lutz and Petzoldt in 1976[5] and later by Bluth et al[6] who referred to the pattern as a "pseudokidney" (Fig. 8-5), noting that a pathologically significant lesion was found in more than 90% of patients with this pattern. In both descriptions, the hypoechoic external rim corresponds to thickened gut wall whereas the echogenic center relates to residual gut lumen or mucosal ulceration (Fig. 8-6). The target and pseudokidney are the abnormal equivalents of the gut signature created by normal gut.

Gut pathology creating an exophytic mass (Fig. 8-7), with or without mucosal involvement or ulceration (Fig. 8-8), may form masses that are readily visualized but are difficult to assign to a gastrointestinal tract origin because typical gut signatures, targets, or pseudokidneys are not seen on sonography. Consequently, intraperitoneal masses of varying morphology, which do not clearly arise from the solid abdominal viscera or the lymph nodes, should be considered to have a potential gut origin (Fig. 8-9). Intraluminal gut masses and mu-

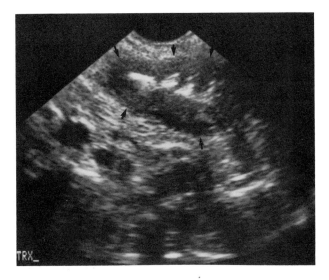

FIG 8-5. Pseudokidney pattern. Transverse sonogram in left upper quadrant shows pseudokidney *(arrows)* proven to be a large carcinoma of the gastric body. The central echogenicity represents the residual lumen. The hypoechoic rim is the tumor.

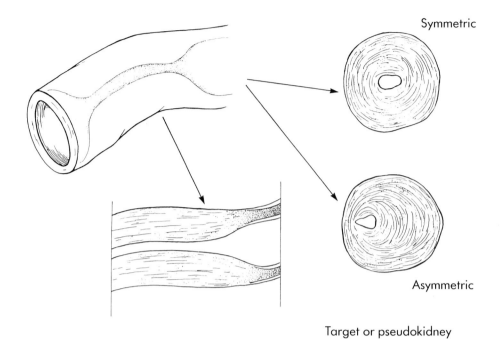

FIG 8-6. Gut wall thickening. Schematic of symmetric and asymmetric thickening, with corresponding sagittal and transverse sonograms creating target or pseudokidney appearance.

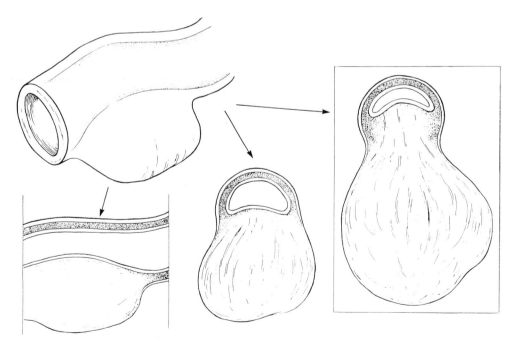

FIG 8-7. Exophytic gut mass. Schematic with corresponding sagittal and transverse sonographic appearances.

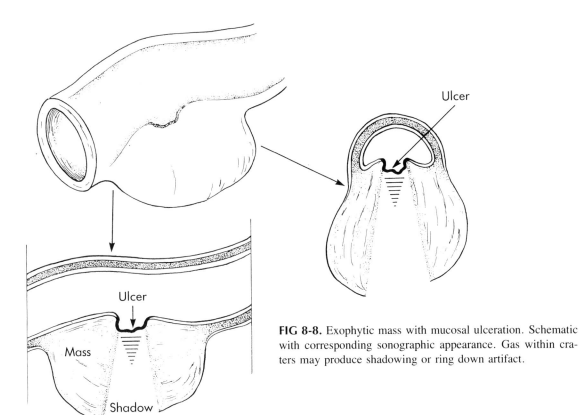

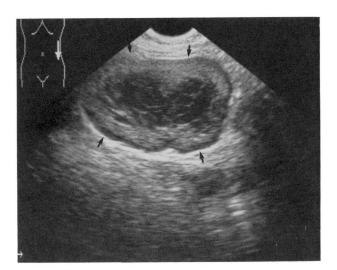

FIG 8-8. Exophytic mass with mucosal ulceration. Schematic with corresponding sonographic appearance. Gas within craters may produce shadowing or ring down artifact.

cosal masses may have a variable appearance and are frequently hidden by gas or luminal content.

Technique

Routine sonograms are best performed when the patient has fasted. A real-time survey of the entire abdomen is performed with a 3.5 and/or a 5 MHz transducer in which any obvious masses or gut signatures are ob-

FIG 8-9. Jejunal leiomyosarcoma. Left flank sagittal sonogram shows a well-defined mass *(arrows)* with solid rim and nonuniform cystic center consistent with necrosis. The gut origin of this mass was not definite on the sonogram.

served. The pelvis is scanned before and after the bladder is emptied because the full bladder facilitates visualization of pathologic conditions in some patients and displaces abdominal bowel loops in others. Areas of interest then receive detailed analysis, including *compression sonography*.[7] Although this technique was initially described utilizing high frequency linear probes, 5 MHz convex linear and some sector probes work extremely well. The critical factor is a transducer with a short focal zone allowing optimal resolution of structures close to the skin. Slow graded pressure is applied. Normal gut will be compressed, and gas pockets displaced away from the region of interest. In contrast, thickened abnormal loops of bowel and/or obstructed noncompressible loops will remain unchanged (Fig. 8-10). Patients with peritoneal irritation or local tenderness will usually tolerate the slow gentle increase in pressure of compression sonography, whereas they show a marked painful response if rapid uneven scanning is performed.

On occasion, oral fluid or a fluid enema may be helpful aids to sonography, particularly when one is attempting to determine the origin of a documented fluid collection or to confidently establish the gastric origin of intraluminal or intramural gastric masses.

GASTROINTESTINAL TRACT NEOPLASMS

The role of sonography in the evaluation of gastrointestinal tract neoplasms is similar to that of computed tomography (CT) scan. Visualization is rarely ob-

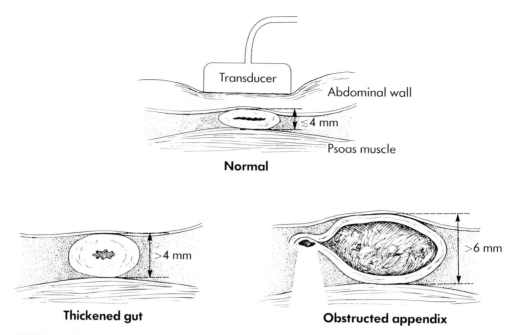

FIG 8-10. Compression sonography, schematic depiction. Normal gut is compressed. Abnormally thickened gut or an obstructed loop such as that seen in acute appendicitis will be noncompressible.
(Modified from Puylaert, JBCM; Acute appendicitis: Ultrasound evaluation using graded compression. *Radiology* 1986; 158:355-360.)

tained in early mucosal lesions or with small intramural nodules, whereas tumors growing to produce an exophytic mass, a thickened segment of gut with or without ulceration, or a sizable intraluminal mass may all be seen. Sonograms are frequently performed early in the diagnostic work up of patients with gastrointestinal tract tumors, often before their initial identification. Vague abdominal symptomatology, abdominal pain, a palpable abdominal mass, and anemia are common indications for these scans. Appreciation of the typical morphologies associated with gastrointestinal tract neoplasia may lead to accurate recognition, localization, and even staging of disease with the opportunity for directing appropriate further investigation, including sonographic-guided aspiration biopsy.

Adenocarcinoma

Pathology. Adenocarcinoma is the most common malignant tumor of the gastrointestinal tract. It accounts for 80% of all malignant gastric neoplasms. These tumors arise most commonly in the prepyloric region, the antrum and the lesser curve, which are the most optimally assessed portions of the stomach on sonography. Grossly their growth patterns are polypoid, fungating, ulcerated, and infiltrative. Infiltration may be superficial or transmural, the latter creating a linitis plastica or a "leather bottle" stomach.

Adenocarcinoma is much less frequent in the small bowel than in either the stomach or the large bowel. It accounts for approximately 50% of the tumors found in this region, 90% of them arising in either the proximal jejunum or the duodenum.[8] Crohn's disease is associated with a significantly increased incidence of adenocarcinoma that usually develops in the ileum. Small bowel adenocarcinomas are generally annular in gross morphology, frequently with ulceration.

Colon carcinoma is very common, its incidence surpassed only by lung and breast cancer. Colon carcinoma accounts for virtually all malignant colorectal neoplasms. Colorectal adenocarcinoma grows with two major gross morphologic patterns: polypoid intraluminal tumors, which are most prevalent in the cecum and ascending colon, and annular constricting lesions, which are most common in the descending and sigmoid colon.

Sonography of Adenocarcinoma. Most gastrointestinal tract mucosal cancers are not visualized on sonography; however, large masses, either intraluminal (Fig. 8-11) or exophytic, and annular tumors (Fig. 8-12) create sonographic abnormalities. Tumors of variable length may thicken the gut wall in either a concentric symmetric or an asymmetric pattern. A target (Fig. 8-13) or pseudokidney morphology may be created. Air in mucosal ulcerations typically produces linear echogenic foci, often with ring down artifact, within the bulk of the mass (Fig. 8-8). Tumors are usually, but not

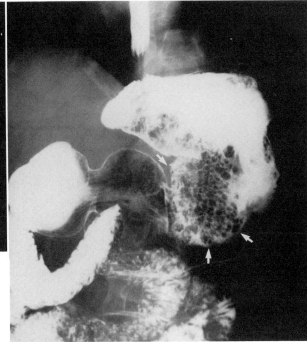

FIG 8-11. Intraluminal villous adenocarcinoma of the stomach. **A,** Transverse sonogram following oral fluid ingestion shows a relatively well-defined, nonhomogeneous, echogenic mass *(arrows)* within the body of the stomach. Fluid is in the stomach lumen *(S)*. **B,** Confirmatory barium swallow shows the villous tumor *(arrows)*.

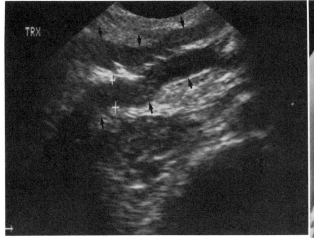

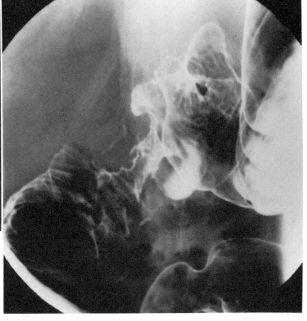

FIG 8-12. Annular carcinoma of the transverse colon. **A,** Transverse sonogram shows transverse colon *(arrows)* in long axis. The colon wall *(+)* is symmetrically thickened. The echogenic central area represents the narrowed lumen. **B,** Confirmatory barium enema.

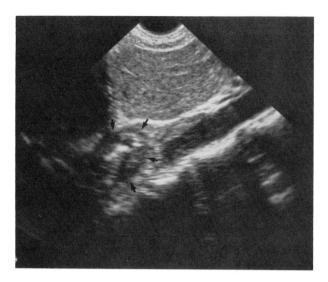

FIG 8-13. Carcinoma of the gastroesophageal junction. Sagittal sonogram in the left paramedian area shows target pattern *(arrows)*.

invariably, hypoechoic. Annular lesions may produce gut obstruction with dilatation, hyperperistalsis, and increased luminal fluid of the gut proximal to the tumor site. Evidence of direct invasion, regional lymph node enlargement, and liver metastases should be specifically sought in all cases.

Mesenchymal Tumors

Pathology. Of the mesenchymal tumors affecting the gut, those of smooth muscle are the most common and account for about 1% of all gastrointestinal tract neoplasms. Although they may be found as an incidental observation at surgery, sonography, or autopsy, these vascular tumors frequently become very large and may undergo ulceration, degeneration, necrosis, and hemorrhage.[9]

Sonography of Smooth Muscle Tumors. Smooth muscle tumors typically produce round mass lesions of varying size and echogenicity often with central cystic areas (Fig. 8-14).[10] Their gut origin is not always easily determined but if ulceration is present, pockets of gas in an ulcer crater may suggest the presence of tumors. Smooth muscle tumors of gut origin should be considered in the differential diagnosis of incidentally noted, indeterminate abdominal masses in asymptomatic patients. These tumors are very amenable to sonographic-guided aspiration biopsy.

Lymphoma

Pathology. The gut may be involved with lymphoma in two basic forms: as widespread dissemination in stage III or IV lymphoma of any cell type or, more commonly, as primary lymphoma of the gastrointestinal tract, which is virtually always a nonHodgkin's lym-

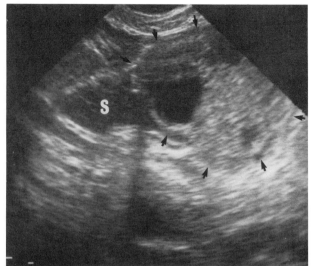

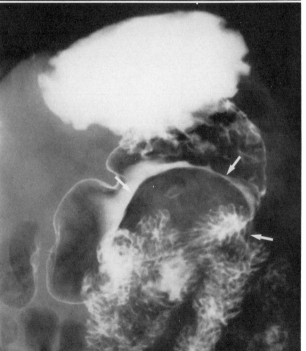

FIG 8-14. Gastric leiomyosarcoma. **A,** Transverse sonogram following oral ingestion of fluid shows a complex intramural mass *(arrows)* projecting into the fluid-filled stomach lumen *(S)*. **B,** Confirmatory barium swallow shows the intramural tumor *(arrows)*.

phoma. Primary tumors constitute only 2% to 4% of all gastrointestinal tract malignant tumors[11] but account for 20% of those found in the small bowel. Three predominant growth patterns are observed:

- Nodular or polypoid
- Carcinomalike ulcerative lesions
- Infiltrating tumor masses that frequently invade the adjacent mesentery and lymph nodes[8]

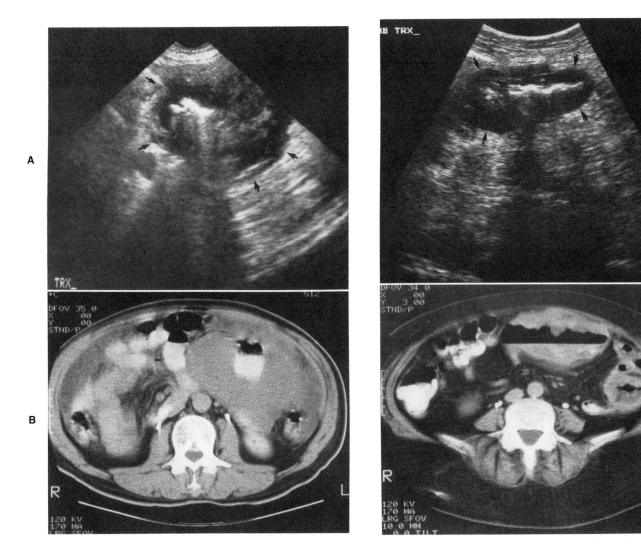

FIG 8-15. Small bowel lymphoma. **A,** Transverse left paramedian sonogram shows hypoechoic round mass lesion *(arrows)*. Central echogenicity with ring-down gas artifact suggests gut origin. **B,** Confirmatory CT scan shows large soft tissue mass with corresponding residual gut lumen.

FIG 8-16. Metastatic malignant melanoma to small bowel. **A,** Transverse paraumbilical sonogram shows well-defined, hypoechoic mass *(arrows)* with central irregular echogenicity with gas artifact suggesting gut origin. **B,** Confirmatory CT scan.

Sonography of Lymphoma. Although small submucosal nodules may be easily overlooked, many affected patients have large, very hypoechoic, ulcerated masses in the stomach or small bowel (Fig. 8-15).[12,13] Long, linear, high-amplitude echoes with ring down artifacts, indicating gas in the residual lumen or ulcerations, are frequently seen. Regional lymph node enlargement may be visualized, although generalized lymph node abnormality is uncommon.

Metastatic Tumors

Malignant melanoma and primary tumors of the lung and breast are the tumors most likely to have secondary involvement of the gastrointestinal tract.[14] In order of frequency, the stomach, small bowel, and colon are involved. Small submucosal nodules, with a tendency to ulcerate, are rarely seen on sonography. However, large diffusely infiltrative tumors with large ulcerations are common, particularly in the small bowel (Fig. 8-16), where they create hypoechoic well-defined masses that often have bright, specular echoes with ring down artifacts in areas of ulceration. Secondary neoplasm affecting the omentum and peritoneum may cause ascites, tiny superficial secondary nodules on the gut surface, or extensive omental cakes that virtually engulf the involved gut loops.[15,16]

INFLAMMATORY BOWEL DISEASE

Inflammatory bowel disease includes Crohn's disease and ulcerative colitis. Although barium study and endoscopy remain the major tools to evaluate mucosal and luminal abnormality, sonography, like CT, may offer valuable additional information about the gut wall, the lymph nodes, the mesentery, and the regional soft tissues.[17] The chronic nature of inflammatory bowel disease, characterized by multiple remissions and exacerbations, is well assessed by a noninvasive, sensitive modality such as sonography. The frequent association of extraluminal disease makes Crohn's disease the most optimally studied disorder. Baseline examination with follow-up predicts complications such as abscess, fistula, or obstruction; detects postoperative recurrence; and identifies patients who require more invasive imaging techniques.

Crohn's Disease

Pathology.   Crohn's disease, a chronic inflammatory disorder of the gastrointestinal tract of unknown pathogenesis and etiology, most commonly affects the terminal ileum and the colon although any portion of the gut may be involved. It is a transmural granulomatous inflammatory process affecting all layers of the gut wall. Grossly, the gut wall is typically very thick and rigid with secondary luminal narrowing. Discrete or continuous ulcers and deep fissures are characteristic, frequently leading to fistula formation. Mesenteric lymph node enlargement and matting of involved loops is common. The mesentery may be markedly thickened and fatty, creeping over the edges of the gut to the an-

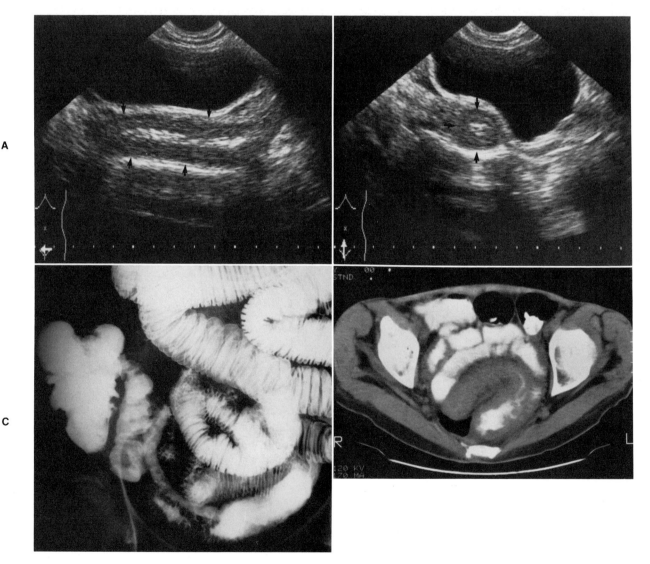

FIG 8-17. Crohn's disease of ileum. **A,** Long axis, and **B,** short axis sonograms of a diffusely thickened loop of gut *(arrows)* with narrowing of the central echogenic lumen. **C,** Confirmatory small bowel enema. **D,** Confirmatory CT scan.

timesenteric border. Recurrence after surgery, skip lesions, and perianal disease are classic features.

Sonography of Crohn's Disease. Sonography may be used in patients with Crohn's disease to:

- *Detect thickened loops of gut* (Fig. 8-17). This may be appropriate for initial detection, for detection of recurrence,[18] for determining the extent of disease, and in follow-up in the assessment of improvement. Gut wall thickening is most frequently concentric and may be quite marked.[19,20] Wall echogenicity varies depending on the degree of inflammatory infiltration and fibrosis. Stratification with retention of the gut layers may occur, or a target or pseudokidney appearance is possible. Involved gut appears rigid and fixed with no visible peristalsis. Skip areas are frequent. Involved segments vary in length from a few millimeters to several centimeters.

- *Assess strictures.* The caliber of the lumen and the length of involved segments are readily assessed; the lumen appears as a linear echogenic central area within a thickened gut loop. Peristaltic waves from the obstructed gut, proximal to a narrowed segment, may produce visible movement through the strictured segment. Incomplete mechanical obstruction is inferred if dilated hyperperistaltic segments are seen proximal to a stricture.

- *Characterize conglomerate masses.* These may have clumps of matted bowel, inflamed edematous mesentery, increased fat deposition in the mesentery, and uncommonly mesenteric lymphadenopathy. Involved loops may demonstrate angulation and fixation resulting from retraction of the thickened fibrotic mesentery. Mesenteric fat creeping onto the margins of the involved gut creates a uniform echogenic halo around the mesenteric border of the gut with a "thyroidlike" appearance in cross-section (Fig. 8-18).

- *Identify inflammatory masses or abscesses.* Abscesses are a frequent complication of Crohn's disease, producing complex or fluid-filled masses. Gas content within an abscess is a potential source of sonographic error, particularly if large quantities are present. Abscesses may be intraperitoneal or retroperitoneal or may be in remote locations such as the liver.

- *Assess fistula formation.* Although mucosal ulcerations are not well assessed on sonography, deep fissures in the gut wall appear as echogenic linear areas penetrating deeply into the wall beyond the margin of the gut lumen (Fig. 8-19). With fistula formation, linear bands of varying echogenicity can be seen extending from segments of abnormal

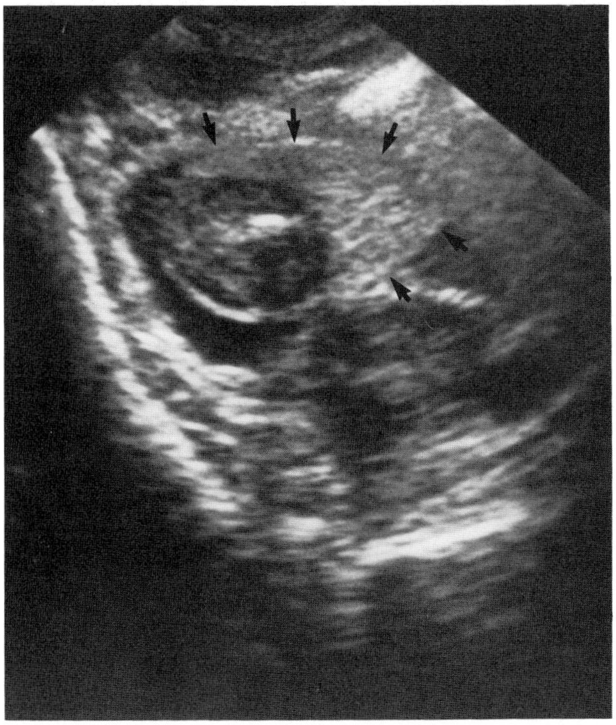

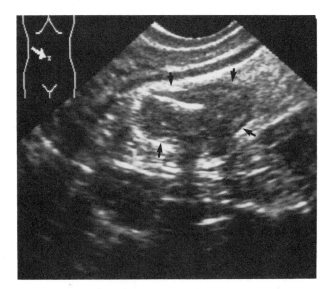

FIG 8-18. Crohn's disease—creeping fat. Transverse sonogram of thickened ascending colon shows fat *(arrows)* creeping onto the gut from the mesenteric margin. It produces a "thyroidlike" echogenic halo along the anteromedial aspect of the loop of gut.

FIG 8-19. Crohn's disease—deep fissure. Transverse sonogram of ascending colon *(arrows)* shows deep fissure, seen as an echogenic linear line, extending from the gut lumen to the serosa of the involved segment.

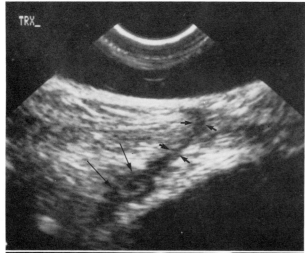

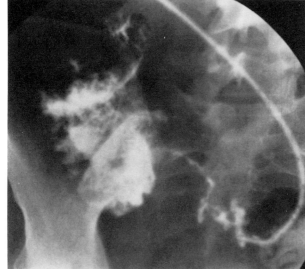

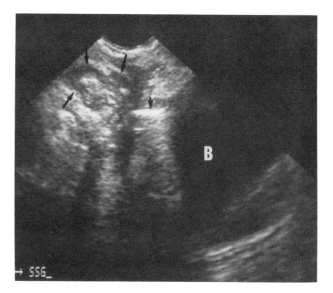

FIG 8-21. Crohn's disease—fistula from conglomerate mass of gut to bladder. Sagittal pelvic sonogram shows a clump of matted gut *(long arrows)*. A fistulous communication *(short arrow)*, seen as a linear echogenic line with air artifact, extends to the bladder *(B)*.

FIG 8-20. Crohn's disease—fistula to skin. **A,** Sonogram shows a mildly thickened loop of gut *(long arrows)* communicating with the skin by a faint linear hypoechoic fistulous tract *(short arrows)*. Image has been taken with a small standoff pad to place the fistula within the focal zone of the transducer. **B,** Confirmatory sinogram.

gut to the skin (Fig. 8-20), bladder (Fig. 8-21), or to other abnormal loops.

THE ACUTE ABDOMEN

Sonography is a valuable imaging tool in patients who may have specific gastrointestinal disease such as acute appendicitis or acute diverticulitis; however, its contribution to the assessment of patients with *possible* gastrointestinal tract disease is less certain. Seibert et al[21] emphasized its great value in assessing the patient with a distended and gasless abdomen, in detecting ascites, unsuspected masses, and abnormally dilated fluid-filled loops of small bowel. In my experience, sonography has

been helpful not only in the gasless abdomen but also in a wide variety of other situations. Sonography may add greatly to diagnostic acumen if used in conjunction with plain film radiography, CT, and other imaging modalities.

Several features should be specifically evaluated in assessing an acute abdomen. *Gas* within the abdomen should be assessed as to its intraluminal or extraluminal origin. Ring-down or comet tail artifact helps identify gas in a site where it is not normally found. Extraluminal gas may be intraperitoneal or retroperitoneal and its presence should raise the possibility of either hollow viscus perforation or infection with gas-forming organisms.[22] Nonluminal gas may be easily overlooked, particularly if the collection is large. Gas in the wall of the gastrointestinal tract, pneumatosis intestinalis, with or without gas in the portal veins raises the possibility of ischemic gut. Gas in the biliary ducts may be seen with spontaneous biliary enteric anastomosis.

Similarly, *fluid* should be assessed to determine whether it is luminal or extraluminal. Loculated fluid collections can mimic portions of the gastrointestinal tract. Left upper quadrant and pelvic collections suggestive of the stomach and rectum may be clarified by adding fluid orally and rectally. Assessing peristaltic activity and wall morphology also help in distinguishing luminal from extraluminal collections. Interloop and flank collections are aperistaltic and tend to correspond in contour to the adjacent abdominal wall or intestinal loops, frequently forming acute angles, which are rarely seen with intraluminal fluid.

Abnormal *masses* related to or causing gastrointestinal tract abnormality should also be sought. These are most commonly neoplastic or inflammatory in origin.

Acute Appendicitis

Acute appendicitis is the most common cause of the acute abdomen. Although many patients have a classic presentation, allowing prompt diagnosis and treatment, some patients have atypical and frequently confusing presentations, leading to misdiagnoses. This is especially problematic in females of child-bearing age.[23] Laparotomy resulting in removal of normal, noninflamed appendices is reported in 16% to 47% of cases, mean 26%.[24-26] Equally distressing, perforation may occur in up to 35%.[27]

Current medical practice recognizes the necessity of removing some normal appendices to minimize perforation rates. In 1986, Julien Puylaert described the value of graded compression sonography in the evaluation of 60 consecutive patients suspected of having acute appendicitis.[7] Since then, other investigators have improved the sonographic criteria for diagnosis, firmly establishing the value of sonography in assessing patients with equivocal evidence of this disease. The accuracy afforded by sonography should keep negative laparotomy rates at about 10%,[28] clearly an improvement over the rate achieved by instinct alone.

Pathology and Clinical Features. The underlying factor in the development of acute appendicitis is believed to be obstruction of the appendiceal lumen, 35% of cases demonstrating a fecalith.[29] Mucosal secretions continue, increasing the intraluminal pressure and compromising venous return. The mucosa becomes hypoxic and ulcerates. Bacterial infection ensues with ultimate gangrene and perforation. Walled-off abscess is more common than free peritoneal contamination.

Acute appendicitis begins with transient, visceral, or referred crampy pain in the periumbilical area associated with nausea and vomiting. Coincident with inflammation of the serosa of the appendix, the pain shifts to the right lower quadrant and may be associated with physical signs of peritoneal irritation.

Both clinical and experimental data support the belief that some patients have repeated attacks of appendicitis.[30,31] Surgical specimens have shown chronic inflammatory infiltrate in patients with recurrent attacks of right lower quadrant pain before appendectomy.

Sonography. Puylaert's[7] initial reports of success in diagnosing acute appendicitis with compression sonography depended solely on visualization of the appendix: a blind-ended, aperistaltic tube, arising from the tip of the cecum with a gut signature (Fig. 8-22). However, other investigators have reported seeing normal appendices on the sonogram.[32,33] Jeffrey[33] and his colleagues concluded that the size of an appendix can differentiate

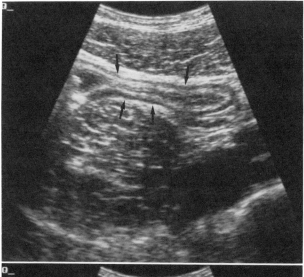

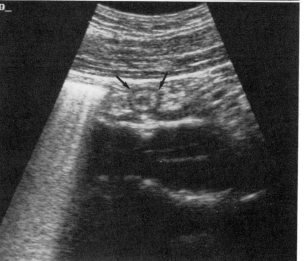

FIG 8-22. Normal appendix. **A,** Long axis, and **B,** short axis sonograms of a normal appendix *(arrows)* show a normal gut signature and a diameter less than 6 mm.

normal from acutely inflamed. Sonographic visualization of an appendix diameter greater than 6 mm (Fig. 8-23) in an adult patient with right lower quadrant pain is highly suggestive of acute appendicitis. Sonographic visualization of an appendix with an appendicolith, regardless of appendiceal diameter, should also be regarded as a positive test.

Although the sensitivity of sonography decreases with perforation, Borushok et al[34] describe three features statistically associated with its occurrence:

- Loculated pericecal fluid
- Prominent pericecal fat
- Circumferential loss of the submucosal layer of the appendix.

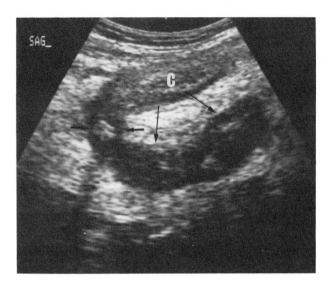

FIG 8-23. Acute appendicitis. The inflamed appendix *(long arrows)* is seen as a blind-ended, aperistaltic, noncompressible tubular structure, arising from the cecum *(C)*. A faintly shadowing appendicolith *(small arrows)* is seen.

Differential Diagnosis. False-positive diagnosis for acute appendicitis may occur if a normal appendix or a thickened terminal ileum is mistaken for an inflamed appendix. Awareness of the diagnostic criteria stated previously, particularly related to appendiceal diameter and morphology, should minimize these errors.

Clinical misdiagnosis occurs most frequently in young women with gynecologic conditions, especially acute pelvic inflammatory disease and rupture or torsion of ovarian cysts. Gastrointestinal illnesses clinically misdiagnosed as acute appendicitis include acute terminal ileitis with mesenteric adenitis,[35] acute typhlitis, acute diverticulitis, especially of a cecal tip diverticulum, and Crohn's disease in the ileocecal area or involving the appendix itself.[36] Urologic disease, especially stone-related, may also mimic acute appendicitis. The value of sonography in establishing an alternative diagnosis in patients with suspected acute appendicitis was addressed by Gaensler et al[37] who found that 70% of patients with another diagnosis had abnormalities visualized on the sonogram.

Acute Diverticulitis

Pathology and Clinical Features. Diverticula of the colon are acquired deformities and are found most frequently in western urban civilizations.[38] The incidence of diverticula increases with age,[39] affecting approximately half the population by the ninth decade. Muscular dysfunction and hypertrophy are constant associated features. Diverticula are usually multiple; their most common location is the sigmoid and left colon. They may be found singly and in the right colon, where no association with muscular hypertrophy and dysfunction has been established. Congenital or true diverticula with muscular walls are relatively rare. Acute diverticulitis and spastic diverticulosis may both be associated with a classical triad of presentation: left lower quadrant pain, fever, and leukocytosis.

Inspissated fecal material is believed to incite the initial inflammation in the apex of the diverticulum leading to acute diverticulitis.[40] Spread to the peridiverticular tissues and microperforation or macroperforation may follow. Localized abscess formation occurs more commonly than peritonitis. Fistula formation, with communication to the bladder, vagina, skin, or other bowel loops, is present in the minority of cases.

Surgical specimens demonstrate shortening and thickening of the involved segment of colon, which are associated with muscular hypertrophy. The peridiverticular inflammatory response may be minimal or very extensive.

Sonography. Sonography appears to be of value in early assessment of patients suspected of having acute diverticulitis[41,42] in which segments of thickened gut are detected and inflamed diverticula are identified. A negative scan combined with a low clinical suspicion is usually a good indication to stop investigation. However, a negative scan in a patient with a highly suggestive clinical picture justifies a CT scan. Similarly, demonstration of pericolonic inflammatory disease on the sonogram may be appropriately followed by CT scan to define the nature and extent of the pericolonic disease before surgery or other intervention.

Since diverticula and smooth muscle hypertrophy of the colon are so prevalent, it seems likely that they would be commonly seen on routine sonography but this is not the usual experience. However, with the development of acute diverticulitis, both the inflamed diverticulum and the thickened colon become evident. Presumably the impacted fecalith, with or without microabscess formation, accentuates the diverticulum, whereas smooth muscle spasm, inflammation, and edema accentuate the gut wall thickening. Diverticula on the sonogram strongly indicates diverticulitis.[41]

The diverticula are arranged in parallel rows along the margins of the teniae coli; therefore careful technique is required to make their identification. Following demonstration of a thickened loop of gut, the long axis of the loop should be determined. Slight tilting of the transducer to the margins of the loop will potentiate visualization of the diverticula because they may be on the lateral and medial edges of the loop rather than directly anterior or posterior. Cross-sectional views are then obtained running along the entire length of the thickened gut. Abnormalities must be confirmed on both views. Errors related to overlapping gut loops, in particular, can be virtually eliminated with this careful technique.

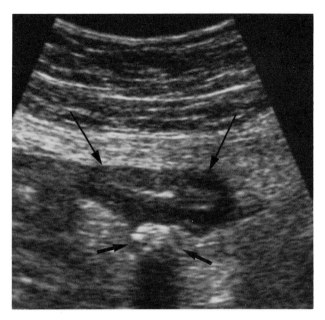

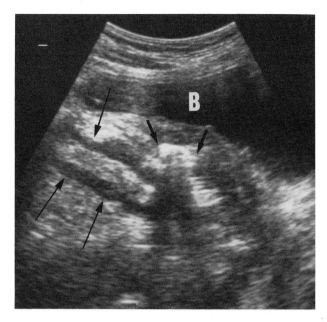

FIG 8-24. Acute diverticulitis. Cross-sectional sonogram of sigmoid colon shows a diffusely thickened loop of gut *(long arrows)*. An inflamed diverticulum *(short arrows)* is seen as an echogenic focus with acoustic shadowing located deep to the gut wall.

FIG 8-25. Acute diverticulitis—gas-containing abscess. This patient had recurring pelvic pain and cystitis. Sagittal pelvic sonogram shows a diffusely thickened loop of sigmoid colon *(long arrows)*, a large abscess containing a large focus of gas *(small arrows)*, and the urinary bladder *(B)*.

Gas-containing abscesses and interloop abscesses are the major potential sources of error when using sonography. The meticulous technique of following involved thickened segments of colon in long axis and transverse section will help detect even small amounts of extraluminal gas.

Sonographic features of diverticulitis include:

- Segmental concentric thickening of the gut wall that is frequently strikingly hypoechoic, reflecting the predominant thickening in the muscular layer.
- Inflamed diverticula, seen as bright echogenic foci, with acoustic shadowing or ring down artifact within or beyond the thickened gut wall (Fig. 8-24).
- Acute inflammatory changes in the pericolonic fat, seen as poorly defined hypoechoic zones without obvious gas or fluid content.
- Abscess formation, seen as loculated fluid collections in an intramural, pericolonic, or remote location (Fig. 8-25). With the development of extraluminal inflammatory masses, the diverticulum may no longer be identified on sonography, presumably being incorporated into the inflammatory process. Therefore, demonstration of a thickened segment of colon with an adjacent inflammatory mass may be consistent with diverticulitis but also with neoplastic or inflammatory disease.
- Intramural sinus tracts, seen as high amplitude lin-

ear echoes, often with ring down artifact, within the gut wall (Fig. 8-26). Typically they are deep, between the muscularis propria and the serosa.
- Fistulae, seen as linear tracts that extend from the involved segment of gut to the bladder, vagina, or adjacent loops. Their echogenicity depends on their content, usually gas or fluid.
- Thickening of the mesentery and the mesenteric fat in association with chronic inflammatory change.

Gastrointestinal Tract Obstruction

Occlusion of the gastrointestinal tract lumen producing obstruction may be mechanical, where an actual physical impediment to the progression of the luminal content exists, or may be functional, where paralysis of the intestinal musculature impedes progression (paralytic ileus).[43]

Mechanical Bowel Obstruction. Mechanical bowel obstruction is characterized by dilatation of the intestinal tract proximal to the site of luminal occlusion, accumulation of large quantities of fluid and/or gas, and hyperperistalsis as the gut attempts to pass the luminal content beyond the obstruction. If the process is prolonged, exhaustion and overdistention of the bowel loops may occur with secondary decrease in the peristaltic activity. There are three broad categories of mechanical obstruction: *obturation obstruction*, related to blockage of the lumen by material in the lumen; *intrinsic abnormalities* of the gut wall associated with lumi-

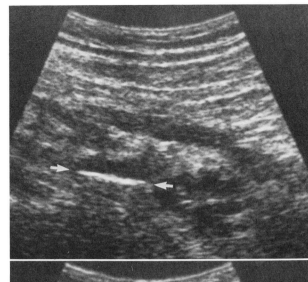

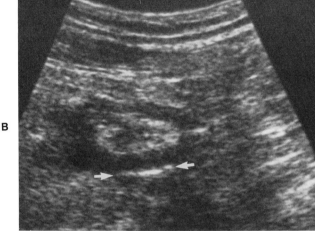

FIG 8-26. Acute diverticulitis—intramural sinus tract. **A,** Long axis, and **B,** short axis, sonograms of thickened sigmoid colon show linear echogenic tract *(arrows)* deep to the muscularis propria.

(Wilson SR, Toi A: The value of sonography in the diagnosis of acute diverticulitis of the colon. *AJR* 1990; 154:1199-1202.

nal narrowing; and *extrinsic bowel lesions,* including adhesions. Strangulation obstruction develops when the circulation of the obstructed intestinal loop becomes impaired.

Sonography in Suspected Mechanical Obstruction. In most patients with intestinal obstruction, sonography is not helpful. This is easily appreciated if one remembers that adhesions, the most common cause of intestinal obstruction, are not visible on the sonogram. Also, the presence of abundant gas in the intestinal tract, characteristic in most patients with obstruction, frequently produces sonograms of nondiagnostic quality. However, in the few patients with mechanical obstruction who do not have significant gaseous distention, sonography may be very helpful. In a prospective study of 48

patients, Meiser et al found that ultrasound was positive in 25% of the patients when the plain film was considered normal.[44] Ultrasound alone allowed complete diagnosis of the cause of obstruction in six patients.

Sonographic study should include assessment of:

- *Gastrointestinal tract caliber* from the stomach to the rectum, noting any point at which the caliber alters.
- *Content* of any dilated loops, with special attention to their fluid and/or gaseous nature.
- Peristaltic activity within the dilated loops, which is typically markedly exaggerated and abnormal, frequently producing a to and fro motion of the luminal content. With strangulation, peristalsis may decrease or cease.
- *Site* of obstruction for *luminal* (large gallstones, bezoars,[45] foreign bodies, intussusception, and occasional polypoid tumors); *intrinsic* (segmental gut wall thickening and stricture formation from Crohn's disease and annular carcinomas); and *extrinsic* (abscesses, endometriomas) abnormality as a cause of the obstruction.
- *Location of gut loops,* noting any abnormal position obstruction associated with external hernias are ideal for sonographic detection in that dilated loops of gut may be traced to a portion of the gut with normal caliber but abnormal location (Fig. 8-27). Spigelian and inguinal hernias are the disorders most commonly seen on sonograms.

Unique sonographic features are seen in the following:

- *Closed loop obstruction* occurs if the bowel lumen is occluded at two points along its length, a serious condition that facilitates strangulation and necrosis. As the obstructed loop is closed off from the more proximal portion of the gastrointestinal tract, little or no gas is present within the obstructed segments, which may become very dilated and fluid filled (Fig. 8-28). Consequently, the abdominal radiograph may be quite unremarkable and sonography may be most helpful.
- *Afferent loop obstruction* may occur by twisting at the anastomotic site, through internal hernias, or with anastomotic stricture. Again, a gasless dilated loop may be readily recognized on sonography.
- *Intussusception,* invagination of a bowel segment (the intussusceptum) into the next distal segment (the intussuscipiens), is a relatively infrequent cause of mechanical obstruction in the adult where it is usually associated with a tumor as a lead point. A sonographic appearance of multiple concentric rings, related to the invaginating layers of the telescoped bowel, seen in cross-section is virtually pathognomonic (Fig. 8-29).[46] Occasionally, only a target appearance may be seen.[47] The longi-

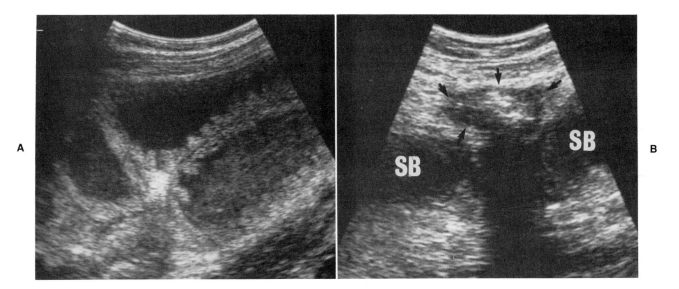

FIG 8-27. Mechanical small bowel obstruction—ventral hernia. **A,** Sonogram shows dilated fluid-filled loops of small bowel with edematous valvulae conniventes. **B,** Transverse paraumbilical sonogram shows normal caliber gut *(arrows)* lying in abnormal superficial location. Dilated loops of small bowel *(SB)* could be traced to this point.

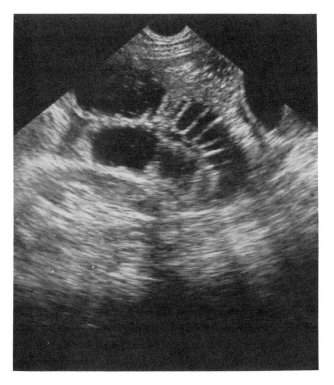

FIG 8-28. Closed loop obstruction. Representative sonogram shows markedly dilated, fluid-filled small bowel loop that was hyperperistaltic. Abdominal radiograph was normal.

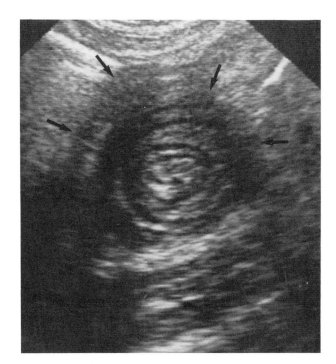

FIG 8-29. Intussusception—submucosal metastatic nodule as lead point. Sonogram shows multiple, concentric rings *(arrows)* representative of the invaginating intussuscipiens and the intussusceptum.

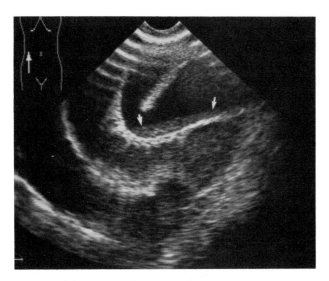

FIG 8-30. Paralytic ileus. Sagittal sonogram shows extensive small bowel dilatation. Loops are fluid-filled and quiet with fluid-fluid level *(arrows)*.

tudinal appearance suggesting a "hay fork"[48] is not as reliably detected.

- *Midgut malrotation* predisposes to bowel obstruction and infarction. It is infrequently encountered in adults. Sonographic abnormality related to the superior mesenteric vessels is suggestive of malrotation.[49] On transverse sonograms, the superior mesenteric vein is seen on the left ventral aspect of the superior mesenteric artery, a reversal of the normal relationship.

Paralytic Ileus. Paralysis of the intestinal musculature, in response to general or local insult, may impede the progression of luminal content. Although the lumen remains patent, no progression occurs. Sonography is usually of little value because these patients characteristically have poor quality sonograms resulting from large quantities of gas in the intestinal tract. However, on rare occasions, the sonogram may demonstrate dilated, fluid-filled, very quiet, or aperistaltic loops of intestine. A fluid-fluid level in a dilated loop is characteristic of paralytic ileus, reflecting lack of movement of the intestinal contents (Fig. 8-30).

GASTROINTESTINAL TRACT INFECTIONS

Although fluid-filled, actively peristaltic gut may be seen with infectious viral or bacterial gastroenteritis. Most affected patients do not demonstrate a sonographic abnormality. However, some pathogens, notably *Yersinia enterocolitica, Mycobacterium tuberculosis,* and *Campylobacter jejuni,* produce highly suggestive sonographic abnormalities in the ileocecal area. Also, certain high-risk populations, such as those with AIDS and neutropenia,[50] appear to be susceptible to

acute typhlitis and colitis, which also have a highly suggestive sonographic appearance.

Mesenteric Adenitis and Acute Ileitis

Mesenteric adenitis, in association with acute terminal ileitis, is the most frequent gastrointestinal cause of misdiagnosis of acute appendicitis. Patients typically have right lower quadrant pain and tenderness. During the sonographic examination, enlarged mesenteric lymph nodes and mural thickening of the terminal ileum are noted. *Yersinia enterocolitica* and *Campylobacter jejuni* are the most common causative agents.[51,52]

The AIDS Population

Sonography is frequently performed on AIDS patients; thus awareness of the gastrointestinal tract infections that produce sonographic abnormalities may lead to improved diagnosis and treatment. AIDS patients are at increased risk for development of both gastrointestinal tract neoplasia and unusual opportunistic infections, most commonly candidal esophagitis and cytomegalovirus (CMV) colitis.[53,54] The relative incidence of infection compared with neoplasia is about four or five to one. Acute abdominal catastrophe in patients with AIDS is usually a complication of CMV colitis and may result in hemorrhage, perforation, and peritonitis.[55]

Typhlitis and Colitis. Cytomegalovirus and *Mycobacterium tuberculosis* are the pathogens isolated most commonly in patients with typhlitis and colitis, although other organisms have been implicated. Sonographic study most commonly demonstrates striking concentric, uniform thickening of the colon wall, usually localized to the cecum and the adjacent ascending colon (Fig. 8-31). The colon wall may be several times normal in thickness, reflecting inflammatory infiltration throughout the gut wall. Cytomegalovirus is associated with deep ulcerations that may be complicated by perforation.

Tuberculous colitis is frequently associated with lymphadenopathy (particularly involving the mesenteric and omental nodes), splenomegaly, intrasplenic masses, ascites, and peritoneal masses, all of which may be assessed using sonography.

Pseudomembranous Colitis

Pseudomembranous colitis is a necrotizing inflammatory bowel condition that may occur as a response to a heterogeneous group of insults. Today, antibiotic therapy with effects from the toxin of *Clostridium difficile,* a normal inhabitant of the gastrointestinal tract, is most commonly implicated.[56] Watery diarrhea is the most common symptom and usually occurs during antibiotic therapy but may be quite remotely associated, occurring up to 6 weeks later. Endoscopic demonstration of pseudomembranous exudative plaques on the mu-

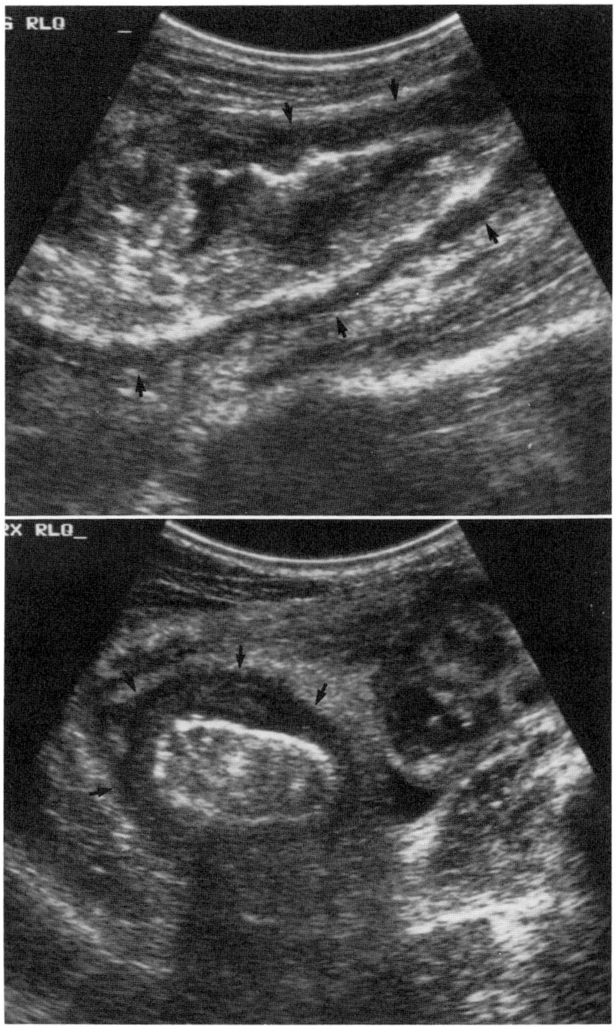

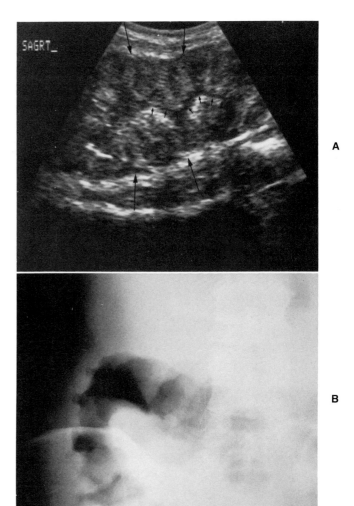

FIG 8-31. AIDS—acute typhlitis. **A,** Sagittal, and **B,** transverse sonograms of the cecum show diffuse concentric thickening of the cecal wall *(arrows)*. The cecal lumen is distended and partially fluid-filled.

FIG 8-32. Pseudomembranous colitis. **A,** Long axis scan of ascending colon shows grossly thickened gut *(long arrows)*, exaggerated haustral pattern, and virtual apposition of the mucosal surfaces of the gut wall *(short arrows)*. **B,** Plain abdominal radiograph shows thumb-printing.

cosal surface of the gut and culture of the enterotoxin of *C. difficile* is diagnostic. Superficial ulceration of the mucosa is associated with inflammatory infiltration of the lamina propria and the submucosa, which may be thickened to many times normal size.[57]

Sonography. Sonography is frequently performed before pseudomembranous colitis is diagnosed, often based on a history of fever, abdominal pain, and watery diarrhea. Sonographic features have only rarely been described[58,59] but are suggestive of pseudomembranous colitis. Usually the entire colon is involved in a process that may produce striking thickening of the colon wall. Exaggerated haustral markings and a nonhomogeneous thickened submucosa, with virtual apposition of the mucosal surfaces of the thickened walls, are character-

istic (Fig. 8-32). Pseudomembranous colitis should be suspected in any patient with diffuse colonic wall thickening without a previous history of inflammatory bowel disease. Since the history of concurrent or prior antibiotic therapy is not always given, direct questioning of the patient is frequently helpful.

MISCELLANEOUS GASTROINTESTINAL TRACT ABNORMALITIES
Congenital Abnormalities of the Gastrointestinal Tract

Duplication cysts, characterized by the presence of the normal layers of the gut wall, may occur in any portion of the gastrointestinal tract. These cysts may be visualized on the sonogram, either routine or endoscopic, and should be considered as diagnostic possibilities whenever unexplained abdominal cysts are seen.

Ischemic Bowel Disease

Ischemic bowel disease most commonly affects the colon and is most prevalent in elderly persons who have arteriosclerosis. In younger patients it may complicate cardiac arrhythmia, vasculitis, coagulopathy, embolism, shock, or sepsis.[60] Sonographic features have been poorly described, although gut wall thickening may be encountered. Pneumatosis intestinalis may complicate gut ischemia with a characteristic sonographic appearance.

Pneumatosis Intestinalis

Pneumatosis intestinalis is a relatively rare condition in which intramural pockets of gas are found throughout the gastrointestinal tract. It has been associated with a wide variety of underlying conditions including obstructive pulmonary disease, collagen vascular disease, inflammatory bowel disease, traumatic endoscopy, and postjejunoileal bypass. In many situations, affected patients are asymptomatic and the observation is incidental. However, its demonstration is of great clinical significance when necrotizing enterocolitis or ischemic bowel disease is present. Both conditions are associated with mucosal necrosis in which gas from the lumen passes to the gut wall.

Sonographic description is limited to isolated case

reports. High amplitude echoes may be demonstrated in the gut wall with typical air artifact or shadowing (Fig. 8-33).[61,62] Gut wall thickening may be noted if the pneumatosis is associated with underlying inflammatory bowel disease. If gut ischemia is suspect, careful evaluation of the liver is recommended to look for evidence of portal venous air.

Mucocele of the Appendix

Mucocele of the appendix is relatively uncommon, occurring in about 0.25% of 43,000 appendectomy specimens in one series.[63] Many patients with this condition are asymptomatic. A mass may be palpated in about 50% of cases. Both benign and malignant varieties occur in a ratio of approximately 10:1.[64] In the benign form, the appendiceal lumen is obstructed by either inflammatory scarring or fecaliths. The glandular mucosa in the isolated segment continues to secrete sterile mucus. The neoplastic variety of mucocele is associated with primary mucous cystadenoma or cystadenocarcinoma of the appendix. Although the gross morphology of the appendix may be similar in the benign and malignant varieties, the malignant form is often associated with pseudomyxoma peritonei if rupture occurs.

Mucoceles typically produce large, hypoechoic, well-defined right lower quadrant cystic masses with variable internal echogenicity, wall thickness, and wall calcification (Fig. 8-34). These masses are frequently retrocecal and may be mobile. Although their sonographic appearance is not always specific, this diagnostic possibility should be considered when an elongated oval cystic mass is found in the right lower quadrant in any patient with an appendix.[65]

Gut Edema

Hypoalbuminemia, congestive heart failure, and venous thrombosis may all be associated with diffuse edema of the gut wall. Prominent thickened hypoechoic valvulae conniventes (Fig. 8-35) and gastric rugae are relatively easy to recognize on the sonographic study.

Gastrointestinal Tract Hematoma

Blunt abdominal trauma, complicated by duodenal hematoma or rectal trauma, either sexual or iatrogenic following rectal biopsy, is the major cause of hematomas seen on sonography. Hematoma is usually localized to the submucosa. If large, diffuse gut wall thickening may be seen on sonograms.

Peptic Ulcer

Peptic ulcer, a defect in the epithelium to the depth of the submucosa, may be seen in either gastric or duodenal locations. Although rarely visualized, peptic ulcer has a fairly characteristic sonographic appearance. A

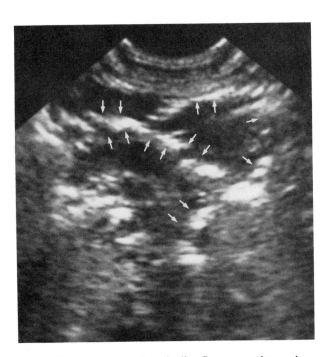

FIG 8-33. Pneumatosis intestinalis. Sonogram shows three loops of gut with bright, high amplitude echoes *(arrows)* originating within the gut wall.

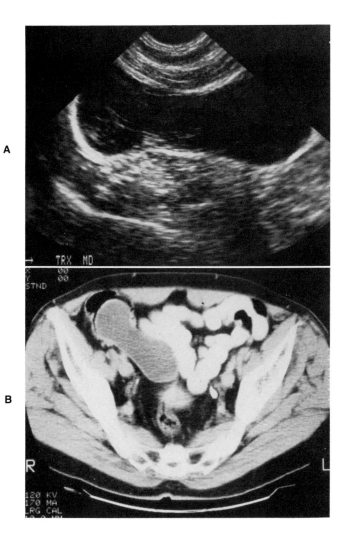

FIG 8-34. Mucocele of the appendix. **A,** Sonogram of right lower quadrant shows well-defined cystic mass with some low level echogenicity. **B,** Confirmatory CT scan.

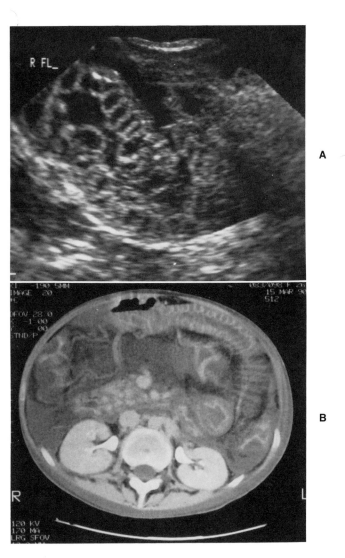

FIG 8-35. Grossly edematous small bowel wall in a patient with septic shock. **A,** Sonogram shows ascites and dilated grossly edematous small bowel characterized by strikingly edematous valvulae conniventes. **B,** Confirmatory CT scan.

gas-filled ulcer crater is seen as a bright echogenic focus with ring down artifact, either in a focal area of wall thickening or beyond the wall, depending on the depth of penetration. Edema in the acute phase and fibrosis in the chronic phase may produce localized wall thickening and deformity (Fig. 8-36).

Bezoars

Bezoars are masses of foreign material or food typically found in the stomach after surgery for peptic ulcer disease (phytobezoars) or after ingestion of indigestible organic substances such as hair (trichobezoars). These masses may produce shadowing intraluminal densities on the sonogram and have been documented as a rare cause of small bowel obstruction.[45]

Intraluminal Foreign Bodies

Large foreign bodies, including bottles, candles, sexual vibrators, contraband, tools, and food, may be identified, particularly in the rectum and sigmoid where they produce fairly sharp, distinct specular echoes with sharp acoustic shadows. Their recognition is enhanced by suspicion of their presence.

ENDOSONOGRAPHY

Endosonography that is performed with high frequency transducers in the lumen of the gut allows for detection of mucosal abnormality, delineation of the layers of the gut wall, and definition of the surrounding soft tissues to a depth of 8 to 10 cm from the transducer crystal. Thus tumors hidden below normal mucosa, tu-

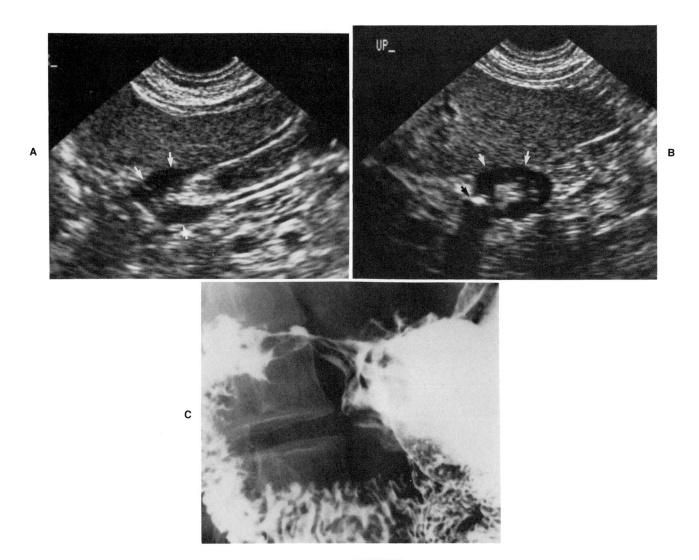

FIG 8-36. Peptic ulcer. **A,** Long axis, and **B,** short axis sonograms show focal hypoechoic thickening *(white arrows)* of the wall of the gut in the region of the pyloric channel. The ulcer crater *(black arrow)* is seen as an echogenic focus with acoustic shadowing. This focus projects beyond the lumen of the gut wall. **C,** Confirmatory barium swallow.

mor penetration into the layers of the gut wall, and tumor involvement of surrounding vital structures or lymph nodes may be well evaluated. Staging of previously identified mucosal tumors is one of the major applications of this technique.

Upper Gastrointestinal Tract Endosonography

Technique. Rotating high-frequency transducers, using 7.5 MHz crystals fitted into a fiberoptic endoscope, are most suitable for endosonography of the esophagus, stomach, and duodenum. Light sedation of the patient is usually required. The patient is placed in the left lateral decubitus position, and the endoscope is inserted to the desired location. Intraluminal gas is aspirated, and a balloon covering the transducer crystal is

inflated with deaerated water. Localization is determined from the distance of insertion from the teeth and identification of anatomic landmarks, such as the spleen, liver, pancreas, and gallbladder. Rotation and deflection of the transducer tip allow scanning of visualized lesions in different planes.[66]

Benign Lesions. Identification, localization, and characterization of benign masses are possible with endoscopic sonography. Varices are seen as compressible hypoechoic or cystic masses deep to the submucosa or in the outer layers of the esophagus, gastroesophageal junction, or gastric fundus.[67] Benign tumors, such as fibromas or leiomyomas, are well-defined solid masses without mucosal involvement that can be localized to the layer of the wall from which they arise, usually the submucosa and the muscularis propria respectively. Peptic ulcer typically produces marked thickening of all layers of the gastric wall with a demonstrated ulcer crater. Ménétrier's disease produces thickening of the mucosal folds.

Malignant Tumors. Staging of esophageal carcinoma involves assessment of depth of tumor invasion and evaluation of involvement of the local lymph nodes and adjacent vital structures.[68] Constricting lesions that do not allow passage of the endoscope may produce technically unsatisfactory or incomplete examinations.

Gastric lymphoma is typically very hypoechoic, its invasion is along the gastric wall or horizontal, and involvement of extramural structures and lymph nodes is less than with gastric carcinoma. Thus, localized mucosal ulceration with extensive infiltration of the deeper layers suggests lymphoma that may also grow with a polypoid pattern or as a diffuse infiltration without ulceration.[69] Gastric carcinoma, in contrast, arises from the gastric mucosa, is usually more echogenic, tends to invade vertically or through the gastric wall, and frequently involves the perigastric lymph nodes by the time of diagnosis.

Rectal Endosonography

Although a variety of pathologic conditions may be assessed with endorectal sonography, the staging of previously detected rectal carcinoma is its major role. Patients are scanned in the left lateral decubitus position following a cleansing enema. Both axial and sagittal images are obtained. A variety of rigid intrarectal

probes are now commercially available using a range of transducer technologies with phased array, mechanical sector, and rotating crystals. A sterile condom covers an inner balloon, which is inflated with 35 to 70 cc of deaerated water. The probe is moved to allow for visualization of the tumor within the focal zone of the transducer. Axial images demonstrate the rectum as a circle of layers (Fig. 8-37).

Tumors are staged according to the Astler-Coller modification of the Dukes classification[70] or more simply with the primary tumor (T) component of the "Union Internationale Contre le Cancer" (UICC) TNM classification[71] where T represents the primary tumor, N the nodal involvement, and M the distant metastases (box) (Figs. 8-38 to 8-40).

Rectal carcinoma arises from the mucosal surface of the gut. Tumors appear as relatively hypoechoic masses that may distort the rectal lumen. Invasion of the deeper layers, the submucosa, the muscularis propria, and the perirectal fat produces discontinuity of these layers on the sonogram. Superficial ulceration or crevices that allow small bubbles of gas to be trapped deep to the inflated balloon may demonstrate ring down artifact and shadowing, with loss of layer definition deep to the ulceration. Lymph nodes appear as round or oval hypoechoic masses in the perirectal fat. Sonographically, many visible nodes may be reactive rather than neoplastic, and normal-sized nodes may have microscopic invasion. Therefore, definitive staging requires pathological assessment of both the tumor and the regional nodes.

Wang and his associates[72] studied 6 normal and 16 neoplastic colorectal specimens in vitro with an 8.5 MHz ultrasound transducer. They accurately demonstrated invasion of the submucosa in 92.5% and invasion of the muscularis propria in 77%. Invasive tumors with extension beyond the muscularis propria were accurately predicted 90% of the time. In vivo studies support this excellent result.[73,74] Comparing preoperative transrectal ultrasound and CT staging in 102 consecutive patients, Rifkin et al found transrectal sonography superior to CT in assessment of tumor extent and in the detection of lymph node involvement.[75]

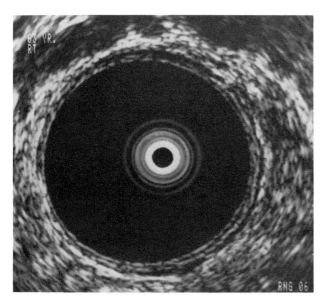

FIG 8-37. Normal rectal endosonogram. Axial view shows the probe centrally within the rectal lumen. The five layers of the gut wall are most optimally seen between the three o'clock and seven o'clock positions.

☐ **T COMPONENT FOR STAGING TUMORS—TNM UICC CLASSIFICATION**

T_1 Tumor confined to mucosa or submucosa
T_2 Invasion of the muscularis propria or serosa
T_3 Tumor invading the perirectal fat
T_4 Tumor involving an adjacent organ

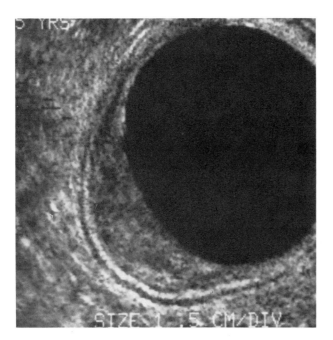

FIG 8-38. Rectal carcinoma—T$_1$. A hypoechoic mass between the six o'clock and eight o'clock positions is noted. The submucosa, the echogenic line, and the muscularis propria, the external hypoechoic line, are intact.

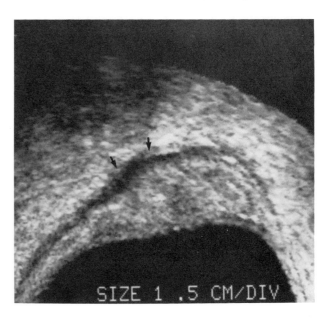

FIG 8-39. Rectal carcinoma—T$_2$. A tumor is seen anteriorly. The muscularis propria *(arrows)* is a hypoechoic line that is thickened and nodular consistent with tumor involvement.

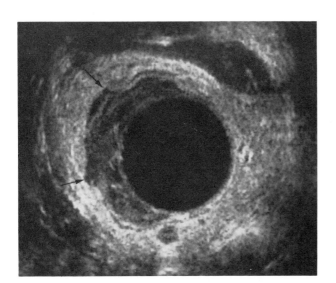

FIG 8-40. Rectal carcinoma—T$_3$. A large tumor involves the entire right lateral wall of the rectum. Invasion of the perirectal fat *(arrows)* is noted in several locations. A large node is seen at the six o'clock position; smaller nodes are seen at the five o'clock and eight o'clock positions.

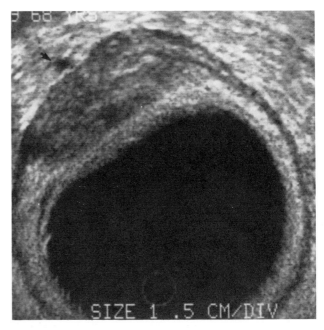

FIG 8-41. Metastatic carcinoma to rectal wall. A hypoechoic mass is seen between the ten o'clock and one o'clock positions. It involves the deep layers of the rectal wall and not the rectal mucosa. There is a small lymph node *(arrow)*.

Limitations of sonography include:

- Inability to identify microscopic tumor invasion
- Inability to image stenotic tumors
- Inability to image tumors greater than 15 cm from the anal verge
- Inability to distinguish nodes involved with tumor from those with reactive change
- Inability to identify normal-sized nodes with microscopic tumor invasion.

Despite these limitations, endorectal ultrasound appears to be an excellent imaging tool for preoperative staging of accessible rectal cancers.

Recurrent Rectal Carcinoma. Recurrent rectal cancer after local resection is usually extraluminal, involving the resection margin secondarily. Serial transrectal sonography may be used in conjunction with serum chorioembryonic antigen levels to detect these recurrences. A pericolic hypoechoic mass or local thickening of the rectal wall, in either deep or superficial layers, is taken as evidence of recurrence. Previous radiation treatment may produce a diffuse thickening of the entire rectal wall, usually of moderate or high echogenicity with an appearance that is usually easily differentiated from the focal hypoechoic appearance of recurrent cancer. Sonographic-guided biopsy of a detected abnormality facilitates histologic differentiation of recurrence from postoperative, inflammatory, or postradiation change.

Metastatic Rectal Carcinoma. Prostatic carcinoma may invade the rectum directly, or more remote tumors may involve the rectum, usually as a result of seeding to the posterior peritoneal pouch. Since these tumors initially involve the deeper layers of the rectal wall with mucosal involvement occurring as the disease progresses, their sonographic appearance is distinct from that of primary rectal carcinoma (Fig. 8-41).

Miscellaneous Rectal Abnormalities. Benign mesenchymal tumors, especially of smooth muscle origin, are uncommon in the rectum. When seen, their sonographic features are the same as elsewhere. Mucous retention cysts, caused by the obstruction of mucous glands, produce cystic masses of varying size that are located deep in the rectal wall.

Anal Endosonography

Preliminary anal endosonography, performed with addition of a hard cone attachment to a radial 7.5 MHz probe, allows accurate assessment of the anal canal, including the internal and external sphincters.[76]

REFERENCES
Basic principles

1. Heyder N, Kaarmann H, Giedl J: Experimental investigations into the possibility of differentiating early from invasive carcinoma of the stomach by means of ultrasound. *Endoscopy* 1987; 19:228-232.

2. Bolondi L, Caletti G, Casanova P, et al: Problems and variations in the interpretation of the ultrasound feature of the normal upper and lower gastrointestinal tract wall. *Scan J Gastroenterol* 1986; 21:16-26.

3. Kimmey MB, Martin RW, Haggitt RC, et al: Histologic correlates of gastrointestinal ultrasound images. *Gastroenterology* 1989; 96:433-441.

4. Fleischer AC, Muhletaler CA, James AE Jr: Sonographic assessment of the bowel wall. *AJR* 1981; 136:887-891.

5. Lutz H and Petzoldt R: Ultrasonic patterns of space occupying lesions of the stomach and the intestine. *Ultrasound Med Biol* 1976; 2:129-131.

6. Bluth EI, Merritt CRB, Sullivan MA: Ultrasonic evaluation of the stomach, small bowel, and colon. *Radiology* 1979; 133:677-680.

7. Puylaert JBCM: Acute appendicitis: Ultrasound evaluation using graded compression. *Radiology* 1986; 158:355-360.

Gastrointestinal tract neoplasms

8. Winawer SJ, Sherlock P: Malignant neoplasms of the small and large intestine. In: Sleisenger MH and Fordtran JS, editors. *Gastrointestinal Disease: Pathophysiology Diagnosis Management,* ed 3. Philadelphia: WB Saunders Co; 1983, 1220-1246.

9. Mesenchymal tumors. In: Fenoglio-Preiser CM, Lantz PE, Listrom MB, et al, editors. *Gastrointestinal Pathology: An Atlas and Text.* New York: Raven Press; 1989, 543-553.

10. Kaftori JK, Aharon M, Kleinhaus U: Sonographic features of gastrointestinal leiomyosarcoma. *J Clin Ultrasound* 1981; 9:11-15.

11. Primary lymphomas of the gastrointestinal tract. In: Fenoglio-Preiser CM, Lantz PE, Listrom MB, et al, editors. *Gastrointestinal Pathology: An Atlas and Text.* New York: Raven Press; 1989, 587-614.

12. Salem S, Hiltz CW: Ultrasonographic appearance of gastric lymphosarcoma. *J Clin Ultrasound* 1978; 6:429-430.

13. Derchi LE, Bandereali A, Bossi MC, et al: Sonographic appearance of gastric lymphoma. *J Ultrasound Med* 1984; 3:251-256.

14. Telerman A, Gerend B, Van der Heul B, et al: Gastrointestinal metastases from extra-abdominal tumors. *Endoscopy* 1985; 17:99.

15. Rubesin SE, Levine MS: Omental cakes: Colonic involvement by omental metastases. *Radiology* 1985; 54:593-596.

16. Yeh H-C: Ultrasonography of peritoneal tumors. *Radiology* 1979; 133:419-424.

Inflammatory bowel disease

17. Seitz K, Rettenmaier G: Inflammatory bowel disease. *Sonographic diagnostics.* Dr. Falk Pharma, West Germany, GmbH, 1988.

18. DiCandio G, Mosca F, Campatelli A, et al: Sonographic detection of postsurgical recurrence of Crohn's disease. *AJR* 1986; 146:523-526.

19. Worlicek H, Lutz H, Heyder N, et al: Ultrasound findings in Crohn's disease and ulcerative colitis: A prospective study. *J Clin Ultrasound* 1987; 15:153-163.

20. Dubbins PA: Ultrasound demonstration of bowel wall thickness in inflammatory bowel disease. *Clin Radiol* 1984; 35:227-231.

The acute abdomen

21. Seibert JJ, Williamson SL, Golladay ES, et al: The distended gasless abdomen: A fertile field for ultrasound. *J Ultrasound Med* 1986; 5:301-308.

22. Lee DH, Lim JH, Ko YT, et al: Sonographic detection of pneumoperitoneum in patients with acute abdomen. *AJR* 1990; 154:107-109.

23. Berry J Jr, Malt RA: Appendicitis near its centenary. *Ann Surg* 1984; 200(5):567-575.

24. Kazarian KK, Roeder W, Mersheiner WL: Decreasing mortality and increasing morbidity from acute appendicitis. *Am J Surg* 1970; 119:681-685.

25. Pieper R, Fonsell P, Kagen L: Perforating appendicitis: A nine year survey of treatment and results. *Acta Clin Scand* 1986; 530:51-57.

26. Go PMNYH, Luyendijk R, Murting JDK: Metnonidazo-protylaxe bij appendectomie. *Med Tijdschr Geneejk* 1986; 130:775-778.

27. Van Way CW III, Murphy JR, Dunn EL, et al: A feasibility study in computer-aided diagnosis in appendicitis. *Surg Gynecol Obstet* 1982; 155:685-688.

28. Jeffrey RB Jr, Laing FC, Lewis FR: Acute appendicitis: High-resolution real-time ultrasound findings. *Radiology* 1987; 163:11-14.

29. Shaw RE: Appendix calculi and acute appendicitis. *Br J Surg* 1965; 52:452-459.

30. Savrin RA, Clauren K, Martin EW Jr, et al: Chronic and recurrent appendicitis. *Am J Surg* 1979; 137:355-357.

31. Dachman AH, Nichols JB, Patrick DH, et al: Natural history of the obstructed rabbit appendix: Observations with radiography, sonography, and computed tomography. *AJR* 1987; 148:281-284.

32. Abu-Yousef MM, Bleicher JJ, Maher JW, et al: High-resolution sonography of acute appendicitis. *AJR* 1987; 149:53-58.

33. Jeffrey RB Jr, Laing FC, Townsend RR: Acute appendicitis: Sonographic criteria based on 250 cases. *Radiology* 1988; 67:327:329.

34. Borushok KF, Jeffrey RB Jr, Laing FC, et al: Sonographic diagnosis of perforation in patients with acute appendicitis. *AJR* 1990; 154:275-278.

35. Puylaert JBCM, Lalisang RI, van der Werf SDJ, et al: Campylobacter ileocolitis mimicking acute appendicitis: differentiation with graded-compression ultrasound. *Radiology* 1988; 166:737-740.

36. Agha FP, Ghahremani GG, Panella JS, et al: Appendicitis as the initial manifestation of Crohn's disease: Radiologic features and prognosis. *AJR* 1987; 149:515-518.

37. Gaensler EHL, Jeffrey RB Jr, Laing FC, et al: Sonography in patients with suspected acute appendicitis: Value in establishing alternative diagnoses. *AJR* 1989; 152:49.

38. Painter NS, Burkitt DP: Diverticular disease of the colon, a 20th century problem. *Clin Gastroenterol* 1975; 4:3.

39. Parks TG: Natural history of diverticular disease of the colon. *Clin Gastroenterol* 1975; 4:53.

40. Ming SC, Fleischner FG: Diverticulitis of the sigmoid colon: Reappraisal of pathology and pathogenesis. *Surgery* 1965; 58:627.

41. Wilson SR, Toi A: The value of sonography in the diagnosis of acute diverticulitis of the colon. *AJR* 1990; 154:1199-1202.

42. Parulekar SG: Sonography of colonic diverticulitis. *J Ultrasound Med* 1985;4:659-666.

43. Jones RS: Intestinal obstruction, pseudo-obstruction, and ileus. In: Sleisenger MH, Fordtran JS, editors. *Gastrointestinal Disease: Pathophysiology Diagnosis Management*. ed 4. Philadelphia: WB Saunders Co; 1988, 369-380.

44. Meiser G, Meissner K: Sonographic differential diagnosis of intestinal obstruction. Results of a prospective study of 48 patients. *Ultraschall Med* 1985; 6:39-45.

45. Tennenhouse JE, Wilson SR: Sonographic detection of a small bowel bezoar. *J Ultrasound Med* 1990; 9:603-605.

46. Parienty RA, Lepreux JF, Gruson B: Sonographic and computed tomography features of ileocolic intussusception. *AJR* 1981; 136:608-610.

47. Weissberg DL, Scheible W, Leopold GR: Ultrasonographic appearance of adult intussusception. *Radiology* 1977; 124:791-792.

48. Alessi V, Salerno G: The "hay-fork" sign in the ultrasonographic diagnosis of intussusception. *Gastrointest Radiol* 1985; 10:177-179.

49. Gaines PA, Saunders AJS, Drake D: Midgut malrotation diagnosed by ultrasound. *Clin Radiol* 1987; 38:51-53.

Gastrointestinal tract infections

50. Teefey SA, Montana MA, Goldfogel, et al: Sonographic diagnosis of neutropenic typhlitis. *AJR* 1987; 149:731-733.

51. Puylaert JBCM: Mesenteric adenitis and acute terminal ileitis: Sonographic evaluation using graded compression. *Radiology* 1986; 161:691-695.

52. Puylaert JBCM, Lalisang RI, van der Werf SDJ, et al: Campylobacter ileocolitis mimicking acute appendicitis: Differentiation with graded-compression ultrasound. *Radiology* 1988; 166:737-740.

53. Frager DH, Frager JD, Brandt LJ, et al: Gastrointestinal complications of AIDS: radiologic features. *Radiology* 1986; 158:597-603.

54. Balthazar EJ, Megibow AJ, Fazzini E, et al: Cytomegalovirus colitis in AIDS: Radiographic findings in 11 patients. *Radiology* 1985; 155:585-589.

55. Teixidor HS, Honig CL, Norsoph E, et al: Cytomegalovirus infection of the alimentary canal: Radiologic findings with pathologic correlation. *Radiology* 1987; 163:317-323.

56. Bartlett JG: The pseudomembranous enterocolitides. In: Sleisenger MH, Fordtran JS, editors. *Gastrointestinal Disease: Pathophysiology Diagnosis Management*, ed 4. Philadelphia: WB Saunders Co; 1988, 1307-1317.

57. Totten MA, Gregg JA, Fremont-Smith P, et al: Clinical and pathological spectrum of antibiotic associated colitis. *Am J of Gastroenterol* 1978; 69:311.

58. Bolondi L, Ferrentino M, Trevisani F, et al: Sonographic appearance of pseudomembranous colitis. *J Ultrasound Med* 1985; 4:489-492.

59. Downey DB, Wilson SR: The role of sonography in pseudomembranous colitis. *Radiology,* 1991; 180:61-64.

Miscellaneous gastrointestinal tract abnormalities

60. The Non-neoplastic Large Intestine. In: Fenoglio-Preiser CM, Lantz PE, Listrom MB, et al, editors.*Gastrointestinal Pathology: An Atlas and Text*. New York: Raven Press; 1989, 639-643.

61. Sigel B, Machi J, Ramos JR, et al: Ultrasonic features of pneumatosis intestinalis. *JCU* 1985; 13:675-678.

62. Vernacchia FS, Jeffrey RB, Laing FC, et al: Sonographic recognition of pneumatosis intestinalis. *AJR* 1985; 145:51-52.

63. Woodruff R, McDonald JR: Benign and malignant cystic tumors of the appendix. *Surg Gynecol Obstet* 1940; 71:750-755.

64. The gastrointestinal tract. In: Robbins SL, Cotran RS, Kumar V, editors. *Pathologic Basis of Disease*. ed 3. Philadelphia: WB Saunders Co; 1984, 874-877.

65. Horgan JG, Chow PP, Richter JO, et al: Computed tomography and sonography in the recognition of mucoceles of the appendix. *AJR* 1984; 143:959.

Endosonography

66. Shorvon PJ, Lees WR, Frost RA, et al: Upper gastrointestinal endoscopic ultrasonography in gastroenterology. *Br J Radiol* 1987; 60:429-438.

67. Strohm WD, Classen M: Benign lesions of the upper GI tract by means of endoscopic ultrasonography. *Scand J Gastroenterol* 1986; 21(123):41-46.

68. Takemoto T, Ito T, Aibe T, et al: Endoscopic ultrasonography in the diagnosis of esophageal carcinoma, with particular regard to staging it for operability. *Endoscopy* 1986; 18(3):22-25.

69. Bolondi L, Casanova P, Caletti GC, et al: Primary gastric lymphoma versus gastric carcinoma: Endoscopic ultrasound evaluation. *Radiology* 1987; 165:821-826.

70. Astler VB, Coller FA: The prognostic significance of direct extension of carcinoma of the colon and rectum. *Ann Surg* 1954; 139:816.

71. Spiessel B, Schiebe O, Wagner G: Union International Contre le cancer (UICC) TNM Atlas. New York: Springer Verlag; 1982.

72. Wang KY, Kimmey MB, Nyberg DA, et al: Colorectal neoplasms: Accuracy of ultrasound in demonstrating the depth of invasion. *Radiology* 1987;165:827-829.

73. Yamashita Y, Machi J, Shirouzu K, et al: Evaluation of endorectal ultrasound for the assessment of wall invasion of rectal cancer: Report of a case. *Dis Col & Rect* 1988; 31(8):617-623.

74. Hildebrandt U, Feifel G: Preoperative staging of rectal cancer by intrarectal ultrasound. *Dis Col & Rect* 1985; 28(1):42-46.

75. Rifkin MD, Ehrlich SM, Marks G: Staging of rectal carcinoma: Prospective comparison of endorectal ultrasound and computed tomography. *Radiology* 1989; 170:319-322.

76. Law PJ, Bartram CI: Anal endosonography: Technique and normal anatomy. *Gastrointest Radiol* 1989; 14:349-353.

CHAPTER 9

The Urinary Tract

- J. Scott Kriegshauser, M.D.
- Barbara A. Carroll, M.D.

The **urinary tract** consists of the kidneys, which produce urine; the ureters, which are long tubes that convey urine from the kidney; the urinary bladder, which acts as a temporary reservoir for urine; and the urethra, by which urine is discharged from the body. Normally, there are two kidneys located in the retroperitoneum on either side of the vertebrae. The position of the kidneys is variable: the right is slightly inferior in location to the left.[1-3] The right kidney is contiguous with the right adrenal gland in its superomedial extent, whereas the reminder of the superolateral aspect of the right kidney abuts the liver. The inferior aspect of the right kidney is adjacent to the right colic flexure and medially abuts the second portion of the duodenum and small bowel. The left kidney is bound by the left adrenal gland and the spleen superiorly. The tail of the pancreas comes into contact with the medial ventral surface of the left kidney, wheres the inferior aspect of the ventral surface of the left kidney abuts the left colic flexure. The dorsal aspects of both kidneys are embedded in fatty and areolar tissue and lie on the diaphragm, the psoas muscle, and the quadratus lumborum muscle.

Ultrasound evaluation of the urinary tract conveys morphologic information quickly, allows differentiation of cystic from solid lesions, and provides the ability to "see" urine-containing structures. As sonographic imaging is not dependent on renal function, it is often the first step in evaluating patients with renal failure. Renal artery Doppler imaging provides additional useful physiologic information and further solidifies the "front line" position of ultrasound in renal imaging.

NORMAL SONOGRAPHIC APPEARANCE

The normal adult kidney has a characteristic shape resembling a bean and ranges in size from 9 to 12 cm in length. The normal renal outline is smooth, and the cortical thickness between the capsule and cortical medullary junction is uniform with a slight prominence at the poles. Residual fetal lobulation can produce subtle indentations without significant cortical thinning. A **"dromedary hump"** (1.5 cm) appearance of lateral left cortical thickening is a common normal variant. The **junctional cortical defect** (Fig. 9-1),[4] a remnant of the junction of the reniculi, is most commonly seen in the right kidney but can occur on either side. A **column of Bertin** may create a renal "pseudomass" (Fig. 9-2).[5-7] However, several sonographic features help distinguish a column of Bertin from a pathologic mass:

- Isoechogenicity with the rest of the renal cortex
- Continuity with the renal cortex
- Lack of mass effect or splaying of central renal sinus fat

A duplication artifact caused by refraction of the sound beam at liver-fat, or spleen-fat interfaces is most common near the left upper pole. This can mimic an area of cortical thickening or a mass, either renal or suprarenal.[8] Changing the transducer position so that the liver or spleen are entirely interposed as an acoustic window over the kidney eliminates this artifact.

The normal **renal cortex** is classically described as less echogenic than the adjacent liver or spleen in adults (Fig. 9-3). However, Platt et al have shown that the renal cortex in patients with normal renal function is frequently isoechoic with liver (Fig. 9-4).[9,10] The neonatal renal cortex is normally isoechoic or hyperechoic when compared to the adjacent liver or spleen.[11] Furthermore, because the kidney is an anisotropic organ, renal echogenicity may vary as a function of the sonographic scan plane. For example, the kidney often appears more echogenic on transverse scans than on corresponding

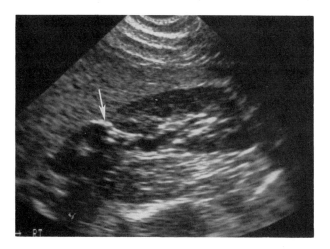

FIG 9-1. Junctional cortical defect *(arrow)*. This echogenic defect in cortex is due to fat extending from renal sinus to perirenal space (longitudinal view).

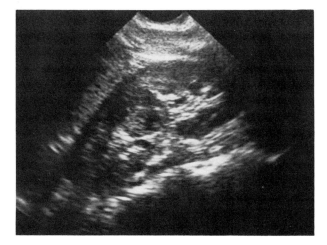

FIG 9-2. Column of Bertin on sagittal scan. Normal renal cortex is interposed between renal pyramids and extends into central sinus.

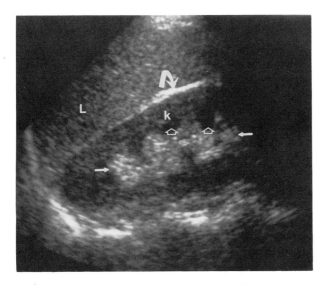

FIG 9-3. Normal renal echogenicity. Longitudinal sonogram shows normal kidney cortical echogenicity *(K)*, which is less than that of adjacent liver *(L)*, echogenic renal sinus *(arrows)*, and relatively hypoechoic medullary pyramids *(open arrows)*. Retroperitoneal fat stripe is shown *(curved arrow)*.

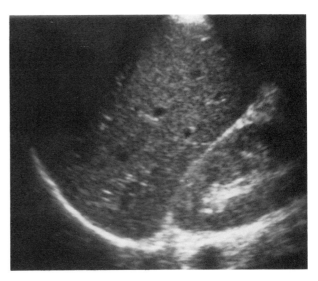

FIG 9-4. Normal variation of cortical echogenicity. Right longitudinal scan shows right renal cortex and liver parenchyma with similar echogenicity.

longitudinal images as a result of a relative difference in the number of the acoustic impedance-mismatch interfaces encountered. In addition, the use of electronically focused transducers has a tendency to increase the relative echogenicity in normal kidneys, vis-a-vis that seen using a fixed-focus transducer.[10]

Renal medullary pyramids are hypoechoic relative to the cortex and are more prominent in neonates.[11] However, the cortical medullary junction is usually identified in most normal adults. The **center of the kidney** contains sinus fat, calices, and infundibuli of the renal collecting system and the major vessels of the renal hilum, which enter the kidney medially. The normal central sinus is highly echogenic as a result of fat and multiple tissue interfaces. The renal pelvis may be intrarenal within the central sinus or extrarenal, in which case it may appear dilated (Fig. 9-5). Visualization of the collecting system depends on the degree of patient hydration and diuresis. Increased hydration also increases visualization of renal vessels.

Pulsed Doppler, color Doppler, or both virtually always identify flow in patent **renal hilar vessels;** however, identification of the proximal renal arteries and the renal veins as they enter the inferior vena cava (IVC) is more difficult. The right renal vein, which runs medially into the IVC, sometimes showing slight cephalic angulation, is more often seen in its entirety than the left renal vein, which normally courses over the aorta on its way to the IVC. The portion of the left renal vein between the hilum of the kidney and the point where it passes between the aorta and the superior

mesenteric artery is often quite prominent and may be mistaken for a pathologic structure (Fig. 9-6). Occasionally, the left renal vein takes a retroaortic course. The left renal artery has a shorter course than the right and is often difficult to image because of overlying bowel gas. The liver provides a better acoustic window on the right where the renal artery is frequently identified as it courses under the inferior vena cava (Fig. 9-7).

Portions of the normal proximal and distal **ureter** are often seen, but the midportion is rarely imaged for any

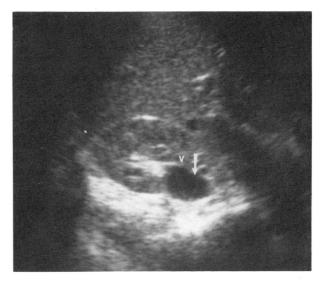

FIG 9-5. Extrarenal renal pelvis *(arrow)*. Transverse image of normal kidney. Renal vein is shown *(V)*.

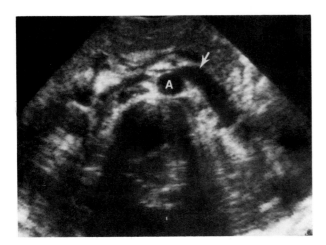

FIG 9-6. Normal left renal vein *(arrow)*. Transverse sonogram shows a prominent vein as it courses anterior to abdominal aorta *(A)*.

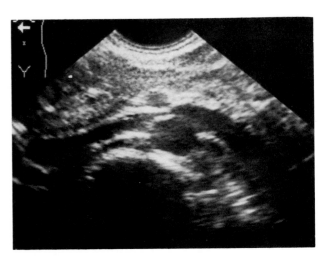

FIG 9-7. Normal right renal artery. Right renal artery *(arrows)* is shown on transverse scan as it courses posterior to IVC *(I)*. It almost never takes aberrant course.

significant length because of overlying bowel gas and because its small caliber causes it to blend in with retroperitoneal fat and adjacent structures. The proximal ureter emerges from the anteromedial renal pelvis posterior to the main renal vessels and runs caudally to insert into the bladder. The smoothly angled intramural portions of the ureters traversing the bladder wall can be seen in well-hydrated patients.[12] The ureteral orifices are associated with a focal elevation of surrounding mucosa at the base of the trigone along the posterior aspect of the bladder (Fig. 9-8).

Ureteric "jets," a normal phenomena, consist of an intermittent echogenic stream that traverses the urine-filled urinary bladder.[13] Experimental studies indicate that the "jet" is produced by fluid-fluid interfaces created by differences between the specific gravity of urine in ureters and the urinary bladder.[14] These "jets" are best appreciated in well-hydrated persons with partially filled bladders. Color Doppler ultrasound is particularly valuable in detecting ureteric "jets," which are invisible or poorly seen on a gray-scale image (Fig. 9-9).

The normal **bladder wall** thickness varies with the degree of bladder distention, measuring no more than 3 mm when fully distended and no more than 5 mm when nearly empty.[15,16] The bladder wall should have a uniform thickness with a smooth inner margin. With sufficient distension, the bladder may assume a somewhat square configuration on transverse images because of limitations of the bony pelvis. Ring-down artifacts frequently obscure the anterior wall of the bladder on transabdominal examinations and may create an appearance of echogenic debris within the bladder.

The **urethral opening** is located at the bladder base, inferiorly at the apex of the bladder trigone. The female

urethra can produce a characteristic soft tissue prominence at the bladder base, which should not be mistaken for a tumor (Fig. 9-10). The female urethra can be visualized on transabdominal ultrasound in 35% of patients and 100% of patients with catheters in place.[17,18] The female urethra can also be identified during endovaginal or translabial scanning. The proximal male urethra is identified as a hypoechoic tubular structure using endorectal ultrasound probes.[19,20]

SCANNING TECHNIQUES
Equipment and Machines

Transducer selection varies with availability and patient habitus (generally 3 to 5 MHz). The highest frequency possible should always be used. Gain, time gain compensation, and power output should be adjusted to optimize imaging, using the lowest exposure levels possible. Similarly, Doppler gain should be adjusted to obtain a satisfactory trace that minimizes background noise. The appropriate wall filter should be used to not hide important low-velocity information (Fig. 9-11). Color Doppler imaging can significantly shorten the examination time and add valuable information.[21]

Patient Preparation

Kidneys. Although no specific preparation is required for renal imaging, fasting optimizes visualization. Evaluation of renal vessels is augmented by adequate patient hydration. The bladder is best imaged when moderately full.

The kidneys should be thoroughly imaged in at least two orthogonal planes. This may require a change of patient position from supine to posterior oblique to decubitus, a variation in patient respiration, and use of an

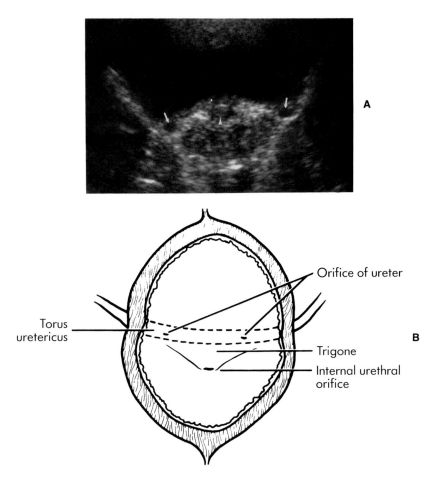

FIG 9-8. Normal bladder. **A,** Transverse image through base of trigone shows distal ureters *(arrows)* and periurethral musculature *(arrowhead)*. **B,** Diagram of same anatomy.

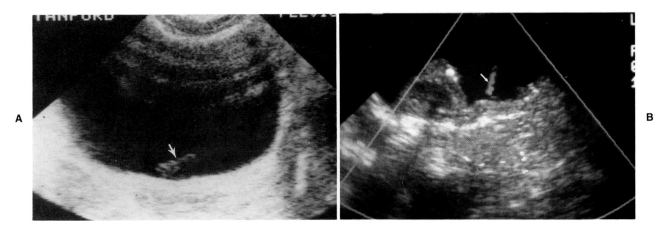

FIG 9-9. Ureteric jet from right ureteric orifice. **A,** Periodic low-level echo jets *(arrow)*, lasting several seconds, stream superomedially at roughly 45 degrees from ureteral orifices. **B,** Color Doppler image shows ureteral jet *(arrow)* adjacent to bladder wall mass in another patient.

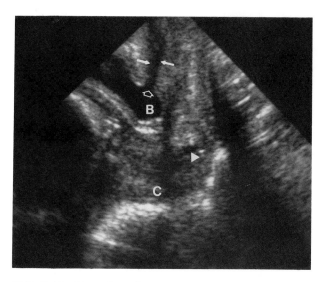

FIG 9-10. Normal urethra. Longitudinal translabial scan shows urethra *(arrows)* and internal urethral orifice *(open arrow)* at base of the trigone of the bladder *(B)*. *C* indicates cervix; *arrowhead*, nabothian cyst.

intercostal scanning technique. Rarely, the prone or upright position may be necessary to obtain a diagnostic image. Maximum renal-length measurements are obtained through the midlong axis of the kidney.

Any cystic structure in the renal sinus should be thoroughly evaluated to document connection with the pelvis or ureter (pyelocaliectasis) or lack of connection, as with peripelvic cysts. Doppler imaging may be used to distinguish prominent renal hilar vessels from a dilated pelvis (Fig. 9-12). If a dilated renal pelvis is confirmed, the examination should always include efforts to visualize the level and cause of obstruction.

Coronal views allow continuous real-time color Doppler evaluation of renal vessels during quiet respiration. Color Doppler imaging facilitates detection of intrarenal and renal hilar vessels; however, lack of color Doppler imaging does not preclude an adequate pulsed Doppler evaluation.

Ureters. The proximal ureter is best imaged in a coronal oblique view, using the kidney as a window. Transverse views can be used to locate the ureter for subsequent longitudinal imaging. The distal ureter can

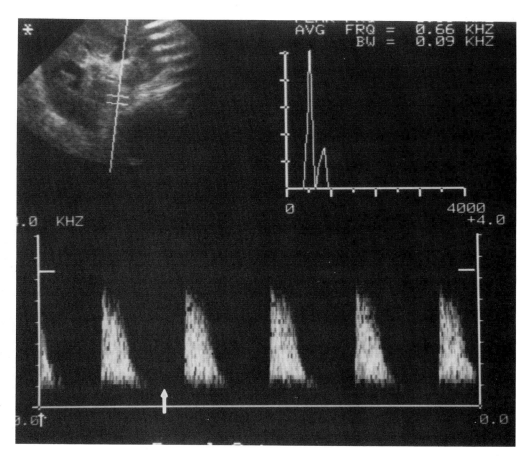

FIG 9-11. Wall-filter level *(arrow)* set too high. Wall filter *(dark band)* hides diastolic portion of waveform.

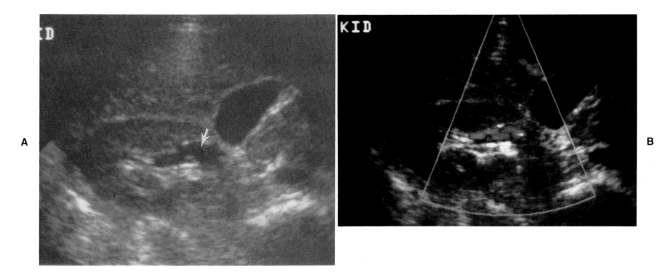

FIG 9-12. Normal hilar vessels mimicking hydronephrosis. **A,** Transverse sonogram shows possible mildly dilated right renal pelvis *(arrow).* **B,** Color Doppler image shows this is prominent renal vein.

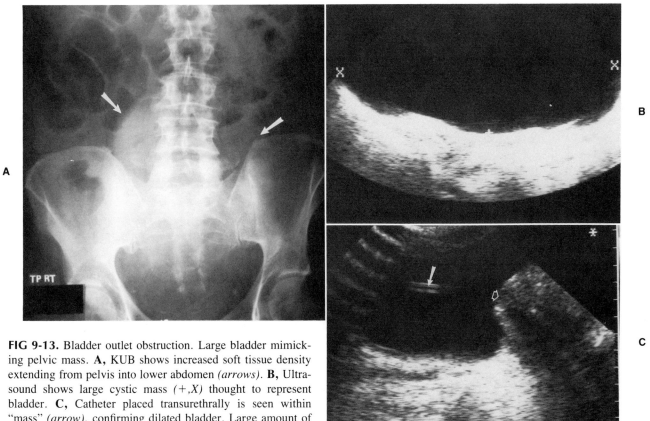

FIG 9-13. Bladder outlet obstruction. Large bladder mimicking pelvic mass. **A,** KUB shows increased soft tissue density extending from pelvis into lower abdomen *(arrows).* **B,** Ultrasound shows large cystic mass *(+,X)* thought to represent bladder. **C,** Catheter placed transurethrally is seen within "mass" *(arrow),* confirming dilated bladder. Large amount of fluid has been drained. Enlarged prostate *(open arrow)* was cause of bladder outlet obstruction.

(Courtesy J William Charboneau, M.D., Mayo Clinic, Rochester, MN.)

be visualized, particularly if it is dilated, using the urine-filled bladder as a window. Detection of ureteric "jets" is important because demonstration of this phenomenon excludes complete ureteric obstruction, showing some degree of renal function.

Bladder. The coronal view may be useful if standard views do not show the anterior wall. This can be obtained by placing the patient in the decubitus position and angling the transducer medially from the pelvic side wall. Additionally, standoff materials and high-frequency transducers are often necessary for optimal visualization of the anterior wall. If the nature of a large cystic pelvic structure is uncertain or if there are several cystic masses, voiding or insertion of a urethral catheter is useful to document which, if any, of the cystic structures represents the bladder (Fig. 9-13).

THE KIDNEY
Cystic Renal Disease

Simple Renal Cysts. Simple renal cysts occur in over 50% of people over age 50 years, and one study found simple renal cysts in 2% to 4% of autopsies performed on children.[22,23] **Ultrasound criteria** that diagnose a simple cyst include:

- Increased through transmission or enhancement
- Absence of internal echoes (anoechoic)
- Sharply defined far wall
- Nearly imperceptible cyst-wall thickness
- Round or ovoid shape (Fig. 9-14).

If a mass meets all of these criteria, no further evaluation is required except in the rare case in which a cyst is suspected to be the cause of symptoms, usually because of its large size.[24] In such instances cyst puncture may be performed to relieve symptoms.[22,25]

Atypical Renal Cysts. If one of the above-mentioned criteria is not met, a renal cyst is still the most likely diagnosis in many instances. For exmaple, cysts with a single thin septation, those with minimal wall calcification, those with internal echoes caused by artifact or hemorrhage, or those with lobulated shapes may all be benign cystic masses.[26] Evaluation using computed tomography (CT) is indicated in atypical cystic masses or if there is clinical suspicion of a neoplasm.[22] Cystic lesions that contain multiple thick septations, those with irregular walls, and those with large solid components should probably be removed surgically.

If a hyperdense cyst is seen on the CT scan, ultrasound is often required to differentiate a rare hyperdense renal cell carcinoma from a more common hemorrhagic cyst.[22,27] Such hemorrhagic cysts often meet all of the ultrasound criteria for a simple cyst, whereas hyperdense renal cell carcinomas are usually solid and highly echogenic on ultrasound. Low-level internal echoes (debris) may be seen in a hemorrhagic or infected cyst, but these usually vanish during serial imaging ex-

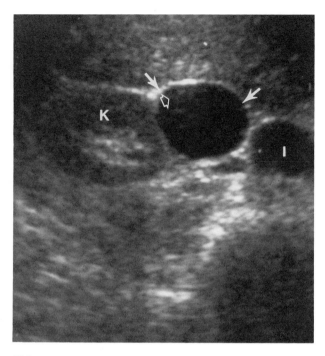

FIG 9-14. Exophytic simple renal cyst *(arrows)*. Right kidney, midportion *(K)* and inferior vena cava *(I)* Reverberations produce artifactual echoes in anterior aspect of cyst fluid *(open arrow)*.

aminations (Fig. 9-15). Rarely cyst aspiration or surgery may be required for definitive diagnosis.

Masses with equivocal densities on CT examination warrant ultrasound evaluation.[28] Both CT and ultrasound allow the diagnosis of simple cysts; however, the information gained from the two techniques is often complementary.[22,25,28] A mass that cannot be definitely diagnosed as a simple cyst after both CT (with intravenous contrast material if possible) and ultrasound have been performed should be removed surgically or followed very closely.

Most renal cysts are simple cortical cysts of the nephrogenic type and do not communicate with the collecting system. Pyelogenic cysts arise from the renal pelvis, infundibula, or calyces (calyceal diverticula) but have the ultrasound appearance of simple cysts.[29] Parapelvic cysts may be single or multiple, may cause symptoms, and can be mistaken on sonograms for hydronephrosis (Fig. 9-16).[30-32] Real-time ultrasound examination usually demonstrates communication between the renal pelvis and peripheral dilated cystic structures when hydronephrosis is present, or it documents lack of such commmunication with parapelvic cysts. When doubt remains, excretory urography is diagnostic.

A renal pseudoaneurysm may mimic a simple cyst.[33] In such instances there is usually a history of renal bi-

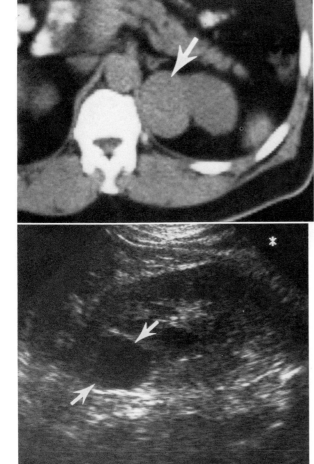

A

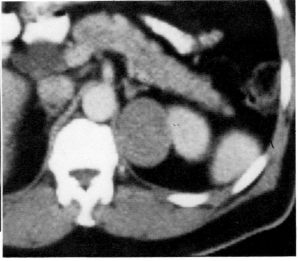

B

C

FIG 9-15. Hemorrhagic renal cyst. **A,** CT shows hyperdense left renal mass *(arrow).* **B,** Contrast-enhanced CT shows no enhancement. **C,** Ultrasound shows complicated cyst *(arrows)* with internal echoes. Cyst aspiration demonstrated amber fluid containing erythrocytes.

FIG 9-16. Parapelvic cysts. **A,** Longitudinal sonogram shows multiple cystic structures within renal hilum *(arrows),* which may mimic hydronephrosis. **B,** Excretory urogram shows distortion and compression of collecting system *(arrows)* by multiple cysts.

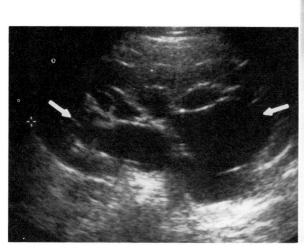

A

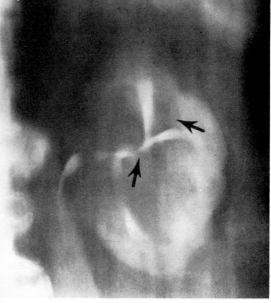

B

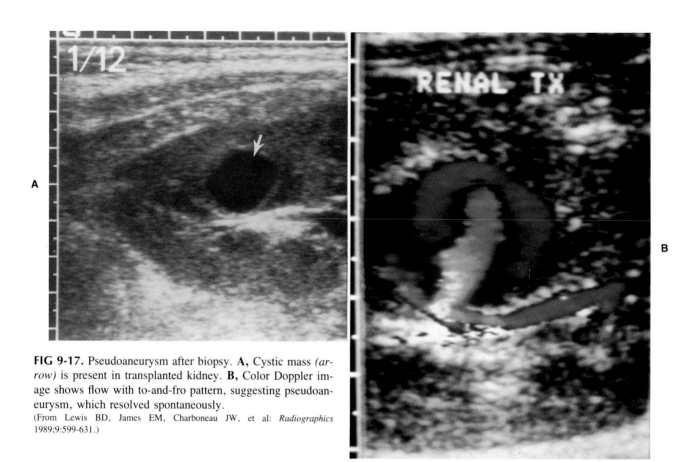

FIG 9-17. Pseudoaneurysm after biopsy. **A,** Cystic mass *(arrow)* is present in transplanted kidney. **B,** Color Doppler image shows flow with to-and-fro pattern, suggesting pseudoaneurysm, which resolved spontaneously.
(From Lewis BD, James EM, Charboneau JW, et al: *Radiographics* 1989;9:599-631.)

opsy, surgery, or trauma. Pulsed or color Doppler evaluation is diagnostic (Fig. 9-17). Splenorenal shunts in patients with severe portal hypertension may mimic exophytic renal cysts; Doppler evaluation is also diagnostic in these cases.[34]

Simple renal cysts are common in children and young adults with tuberous sclerosis, von Hippel-Lindau syndrome, and Turner's syndrome. The only significance of these benign cysts is that they may mask or draw attention away from the solid tumors that also occur in these patients. Increased risk of renal malignancy is well known in von Hippel-Lindau syndrome, but it has also been reported in polycystic kidney disease.[35]

Autosomal Dominant (Adult) Polycystic Kidney Disease. The diagnosis of autosomal dominant (adult) polycystic kidney disease (ADPKD) is made easily with ultrasound.[36] There is usually bilateral renal enlargement caused by numerous cysts of varying sizes (Fig. 9-18). The adjacent renal cortex frequently shows increased echogenicity. Other organs, such as the liver (30%), may be involved with multiple simple cysts, but symptomatic liver disease is not present.[29,30] Seventy-five percent of patients are hypertensive, and slowly progressive renal failure is common. However, acute renal failure may occur secondary to obstruction or in-

fection. Cerebral arterial (berry) aneurysms are present in 16% of patients with ADPKD, and 9% die from rupture of these.[29] When a patient presents with impaired renal function, enlarged kidneys, and cysts "too numerous to count," the diagnosis of ADPKD can be made with great confidence, even in the 20% who do not have a positive family history. Sonography is useful for family screening of ADPKD and genetic counseling in young patients in whom demonstration of even a few cysts makes the disease likely.[29,36] If no cysts are found on initial examination, follow-up is still necessary.[29,36]

Older patients often have multiple simple cysts that must be differentiated from ADPKD. As a rule, multiple simple cysts are less numerous and renal enlargement is not as marked as that in ADPKD. Furthermore, these patients with numerous renal cysts tend to be older at presentation than patients with ADPKD and have more normal renal function.

The cysts in ADPKD can cause pain, bleeding, or obstruction and may become infected. Such complications may require percutaneous drainage or nephrectomy. Frequently, one or more cysts in ADPKD will appear hyperdense on CT scans because of internal hemorrhage or proteinaceous material. On ultrasound examination, hemorrhagic cysts often contain echogenic

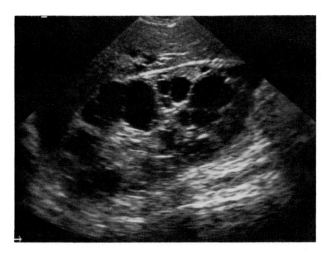

FIG 9-18. Autosomal dominant polycystic kidney disease (moderate involvement). Multiple cysts enlarge kidney.

debris, whereas simple cysts usually do not. However, it is often difficult to be certain that the same cysts are being imaged with both CT and ultrasound. If ultrasound demonstrates hemorrhagic debris within a cyst but no other abnormalities, follow-up with ultrasound is sufficient; hemorrhagic debris should clear over several months. However, if other atypical cyst features are present, follow-up with CT may be required because evidence suggests a higher incidence of renal cell carcinoma in ADPKD than in the general population.[35] An infected cyst may mimic a simple cyst, may contain internal debris, or may have a thick, indistinct wall. If cyst infection or abscess is suspected, percutaneous needle aspiration can be performed.

Autosomal Recessive Polycystic Kidney Disease. Infantile polycystic renal disease is associated with marked renal dysfunction and lung hypoplasia, incompatible with normal life. This disease may be detected in utero, often after suspected oligohydramnios prompts an ultrasound examination. Juvenile recessive polycystic kidney disease presents later with symptoms related to coexistent hepatobiliary dysfunction. **Sonographically,** the kidneys are bilaterally enlarged and echogenic with loss of cortical medullary distinction. Large macroscopic cysts are unusual.[29,30]

Multicystic Dysplastic Kidney. Multicystic dysplastic kidney (MCDK) is usually diagnosed in early childhood or in utero. In adults MCDK is implicated as a cause of renal agenesis, aplasia, and hypoplasia, but the natural history has only been reported in a small number of children and for only a few years after birth.[37,38]

Medullary Cystic Disease and Medullary Sponge Kidney. Medullary cystic disease, or nephronophthisis, is a rare disease of young adults (autosomal dominant form) and in children (autosomal recessive form).[39,40]

Clinical features include anemia, salt wasting, progressive azotemia, and polyuria. On **ultrasound,** the kidneys may demonstrate widening of the central sinus echoes because of multiple microscopic medullary cysts, which produce increased medullary echogenicity and cause the medullary pyramids to blend in with the sinus fat. Discrete cysts of up to 2 cm in size may be seen in the medulla or at the corticomedullary junction, but most cysts are only a few millimeters in size.[30] The kidneys are usually normal to slightly decreased in size; however, with advanced uremia, the entire kidney may be small and echogenic—findings consistent with an end-stage kidney disease from any cause.[39,40] Appropriate clinical features combined with the sonographic demonstration of discrete medullary cysts is diagnostic. However, as sonography does not always show cysts, biopsy may be necessary for diagnosis.[30,40]

Medullary sponge kidney is a common entity, usually of no clinical significance. Characteristic ectatic collecting tubules may be imaged with ultrasound but are best seen on excretory urography.[29] Calcium deposits and stones form in 10% to 15% of these dilated tubules. These deposits may result in echogenic medullary pyramids without posterior acoustic shadowing (Fig. 9-19); however, discrete shadowing may be seen behind stones within the affected medullary pyramids or collecting system. Stone formation and infection are the main concerns in these patients, but they rarely cause renal failure.[23,29] Papillary necrosis may produce cystic changes in the renal pyramids with medullary calcifications, which may mimic medullary cystic disease or medullary sponge kidney.

Acquired Cystic Kidney Disease. Up to 90% of patients on long-term hemodialysis develop cystic changes in their native kidneys.[41,42] These changes usually occur after 3 or more years of dialysis but may occur sooner.[42-45] **Sonographically,** the kidneys in acquired cystic kidney disease (ACKD) are normal to small in size and often show increased echogenicity with loss of corticomedullary distinction (Fig. 9-20). Cysts of varying sizes and number are seen throughout the kidney. Renal cortical irregularity may mimic solid masses, and CT correlation should be obtained if necessary in these cases. Coexistent solid masses (usually small) are reported in 7% to 40% of patients with ACKD.[41,44] These masses may be adenomas or renal cell carcinomas, and although the number of solid masses in these patients is worrisome, their clinical significance is controversial because only 0.33% of patients with ACKD develop metastatic renal cell carcinoma. This is the same incidence as in the general population.

It is not known if screening is necessary for detecting these cystic or solid masses in ACKD.[46,47] If patients are asymptomatic, the presence of these masses is of little significance to their medical management. CT

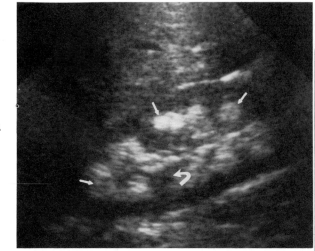
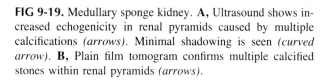
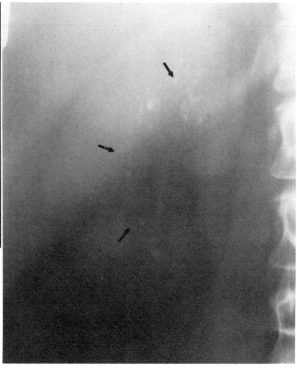

FIG 9-19. Medullary sponge kidney. **A,** Ultrasound shows increased echogenicity in renal pyramids caused by multiple calcifications *(arrows)*. Minimal shadowing is seen *(curved arrow)*. **B,** Plain film tomogram confirms multiple calcified stones within renal pyramids *(arrows)*.

is the preferred method for detecting cystic and solid masses in symptomatic ACKD. If hyperdense hemorrhagic cysts are present on CT, ultrasound can be used to confirm that these are cysts that contain echogenic debris, precluding further workup or allowing such cysts to be followed with either ultrasound or CT.[27,41] Mindell[41] states that sonography is the only practical, affordable method for screening such a large population. Further information is needed to determine the natural history of cystic and solid masses in patients with ACKD and to determine if any screening imaging test is warranted in all dialysis patients.

Multilocular Cystic Nephroma. Multilocular cystic nephroma (MCN) (multilocular renal cyst, benign cystic nephroma, fetal renal cystic hamartoma, or Pearlmann tumor)[48-50] is a rare, nonhereditary tumor with a bimodal distribution. Half of all cases occur in young children, predominately boys, and may contain elements of Wilms' tumor, whereas the other half occur predominantly in female adults.[30,48] Many cystic lymphangiomas, considered a separate entity, may also be MCNs because their radiographic appearance is identical.[48]

On **sonography,** MCN is a large (up to 10 cm or greater) cystic mass with a well-defined capsule and cysts separated by thick, echogenic septae.[30,48,49] Calcification in cartilaginous elements occurs in approximately 50% of these tumors and may produce posterior acoustic shadowing. The lower or midportion of the kidney, where they may distort or obstruct the collect-

ing system, is the most common location of these tumors. Occasionally CT or angiography may be helpful in distinguishing between malignant cystic masses and benign tumors, if tumor vascularity or an enhancing wall is seen on CT. In such cases nephrectomy or partial nephrectomy is indicated. However, failure to demonstrate these changes on CT or angiography may not indicate that the mass is definitively benign.[48,50] Many advocate resection of these masses in all cases for that reason.

Solid Renal Masses

Renal Cell Carcinoma. Renal cell carcinoma (RCC) is the most common solid renal mass in the adult.[51,52] These tumors are most frequently discovered in the sixth decade; however, they can occur at any age, including childhood. They tend to be large when discovered, but if discovered when small (less than 3 cm), the prognosis is very good.[52] Nephrectomy is recommended in most cases, even with small lesions.[53] There is a high incidence of RCC (10% to 25%), often bilateral or multifocal, in von Hippel-Lindau syndrome and patients with ACKD undergoing dialysis.[40] A slightly increased incidence of RCC is reported in autosomal dominant polycystic kidney disease, tuberous sclerosis, and other diseases and syndromes associated with multiple renal cysts.

On **Sonography,** RCC is usually a solid mass that is hypo- or isoechoic relative to normal adjacent renal pa-

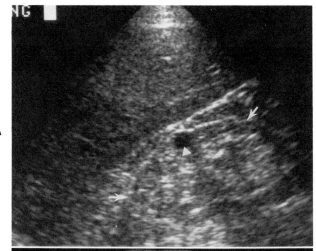

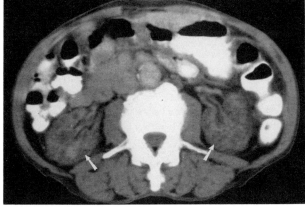

FIG 9-20. Acquired cystic disease in patient undergoing chronic dialysis. **A,** Longitudinal ultrasound shows small echogenic right kidney *(arrows)* with small cyst *(arrowhead)*. **B,** CT shows multiple cysts in small kidneys *(arrows)*.

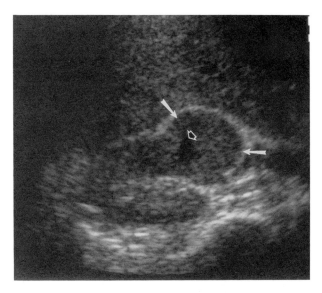

FIG 9-21. Renal cell carcinoma *(arrows)*. Transverse scan shows predominantly solid mass with cystic component *(open arrow)* arising from anteromedial cortex of upper pole of right kidney.

renchyma. Cystic areas of hemorrhage, necrosis, or tumor vascularity are present in about 40% (Fig. 9-21).[49] One to two percent of RCCs are predominantly cystic; rarely, these tumors may be entirely cystic or contain a single mural nodule of RCC in or contiguous with a simple cyst.[50,51]

Roughly 4% of RCCs have echogenicity equal to or greater than the renal sinus or perirenal fat (Fig. 9-22).[49] This may be due to diffuse fine calcification within the tumor but, sonographically, the appearance will resemble the echogenicity of fat in an angiomyolipoma. CT can easily separate high-density calcium from very low-density fat in angiomyolipoma. RCC calcifications may be focal or diffuse and clustered or stippled, and thus the type of calcifications cannot differentiate benign from malignant masses.

Tumor vascularity can be demonstrated in up to 92% of RCCs using color or pulsed Doppler ultrasound.[54,55] Doppler imaging features of RCC include high-systolic and high-diastolic arterial flow (arterio-venous shunt pattern) and high-velocity continuous flow, thought to represent flow within abnormal thin-walled venous structures.[55-57] A peak velocity of greater than 2.5 KHz with a 3-MHz transducer, detected in or along the edge of a renal mass, has been shown to be good evidence of RCC, although lesser peak velocities do not exclude malignancy.[58] In fact, any Doppler imaging evidence of abnormal vascularity in a mass suggests malignancy. No correlation has been found between tumor vascularity and tumor echogenicity.[59]

Solid, benign renal tumors cannot be unequivocally differentiated from RCC with ultrasound, and in fact, most solid masses should be considered malignant until proved otherwise because RCCs constitute 80% to 85% of adult renal neoplasms. One exception is that of a homogeneous highly echogenic mass, which is more likely to be an angiomylipoma. A poorly differentiated RCC may present as an infiltrative lesion, in which case the differential diagnosis includes transitional cell carcinoma, lymphoma, leukemia, metastases, and infection (Fig. 9-23).[60] Whenever a solid renal mass is detected, RCC should be suspected and the ipsilateral renal vein and inferior vena cava should be evaluated with ultrasound and Doppler imaging to exclude intraluminal tumor and determine the level of tumor thrombus (Fig. 9-24).[61,62] The ultrasound examination should include a thorough evaluation of the contralateral kidney, the renal vein, the retroperitoneum (searching for nodal disease), and the liver (for metastases) to determine tumor resectability and surgical approach. Although Doppler

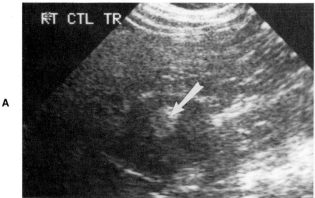

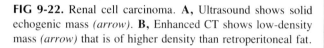

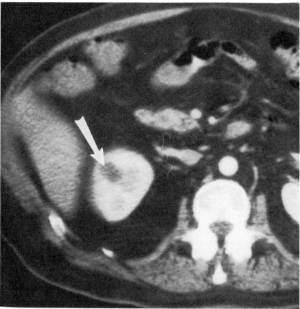

FIG 9-22. Renal cell carcinoma. **A,** Ultrasound shows solid echogenic mass *(arrow)*. **B,** Enhanced CT shows low-density mass *(arrow)* that is of higher density than retroperitoneal fat.

ultrasound is useful in the evaluation of venous extension, ultrasound imaging alone has been effective in detecting tumor thrombus in renal veins in the inferior vena cava. Tumor thrombus tends to be echogenic and more expansible than bland thrombus and is therefore easier to visualize. Occasionally RCC may hemorrhage into the subcapsular or perinephric space, producing an appearance indistinguishable from that associated with significant renal trauma.[51] The medical history, however, should differentiate between these entities. A CT examination is usually necessary for thorough staging and tumor characterization.

Angiomyolipoma. Multiple angiomyolipomas occur in up to 80% of patients with tuberous sclerosis (TS), but 50% of these tumors (usually solitary) arise in patients without this disease.[63,64] Isolated angiomyolipomas are most common in females aged 40 to 60 years. These tumors usually cause no symptoms, but occasionally tumor hemorrhage may result in pain or hematuria. Rarely, in TS, extensive bilateral involvement may produce renal failure.

The **classic ultrasound appearance** is of a homogeneous renal mass with echogenicity greater than or equal to renal sinus fat (Fig. 9-25). The mass may be

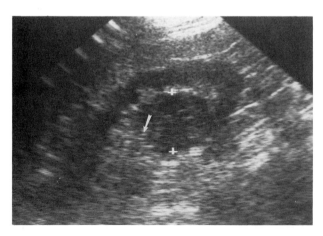

FIG 9-23. Renal cell carcinoma. Mass (+) infiltrating into central sinus fat *(arrow)* is isoechoic with renal cortex but is well separated from it.

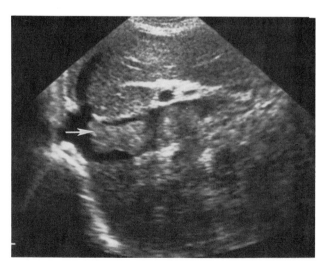

FIG 9-24. Tumor thrombus *(arrows)*. Extension of renal cell carcinoma from right renal vein into IVC.

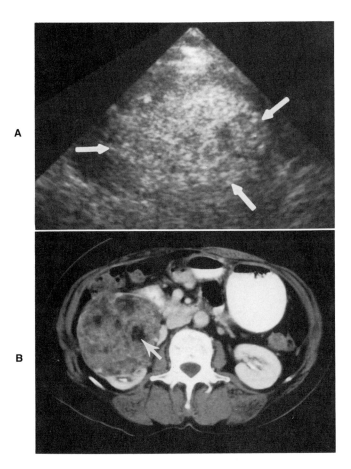

FIG 9-25. Angiomyolipoma. **A,** Large, central echogenic renal mass *(arrows)* is seen with ultrasound. **B,** CT confirms that mass contains fatty elements *(arrow).*

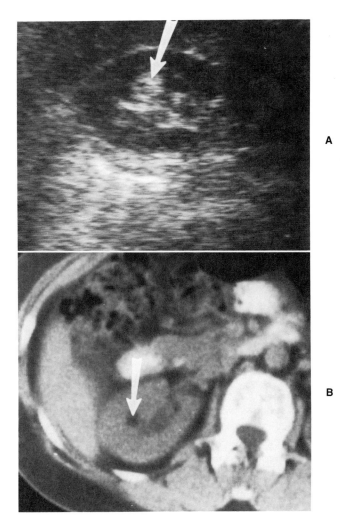

FIG 9-26. Angiomyolipoma. **A,** patient with small echogenic renal mass *(arrow)* found incidentally on ultrasound. **B,** CT shows fat density within mass *(arrow).*

less echogenic than sinus fat or have mixed echogenicity if there is hemorrhage or myomatous elements.[49,65] Apparent posterior displacement of structures behind these masses may be seen as a result of the slower acoustic velocity in these fatty tumors (speed propagation artifact). These masses are typically well circumscribed, but the borders can be indistinct. It is common to find incidental small (less than 2 cm) angiomyolipomas (Fig. 9-26). These tumors can be quite large (10 cm or greater) and exophytic. They can blend imperceptively into adjacent retroperitoneal fat, making it difficult to appreciate the true size of the tumor ("tip of the iceberg" effect). Pulsed and color Doppler imaging may demonstrate vascularity within these tumors but not the extremely high-velocity flow that is characteristic of RCC.[56,58]

CT confirmation of fat in an echogenic renal mass is considered diagnostic of angiomyolipoma.[65] Intratumoral fat in an oncocytoma or Wilms' tumor or a hemorrhagic lesion engulfing renal sinus fat may mimic an

angiomyolipoma.[66] Echogenic masses of less than 1 cm in diameter are usually too small for CT to definitively detect fat with CT. Such masses can be followed with serial imaging examinations.[67] If the mass enlarges, CT can be repeated with the knowledge that, if the mass is a RCC, the prognosis is still favorable when tumors are 3 cm or less in diameter.[52]

Adenomas. Renal adenomas have a histologic appearance identical to well-differentiated RCCs. An adenoma of greater than 3 cm should be considered malignant. By definition, adenomas lack invasive features and do not metastasize. These tumors are usually treated with total nephrectomy, although some surgeons may opt for partial nephrectomy in cases of small well-differentiated lesions.[44,68] Adenomas are usually asymptomatic, however, these tumors may cause recurrent painless hematuria.

Sonographically, adenomas are hypoechoic or iso-echoic relative to adjacent renal parenchyma. These tumors have well-defined margins and are homogeneous in composition. CT is more sensitive for detecting adenomas, but as with ultrasound, their appearance is nonspecific.

Oncocytoma. Benign oncocytomas are uncommon tumors that are usually seen in middle to old age. These tumors are thought to represent a type of adenoma, constituting 3% to 6% of renal neoplasms. Histologically, the central part of the tumor in 50% of cases shows a whitish, stellate scar, which is quite characteristic of a renal oncocytoma. These masses are usually incidental findings, but 30% are associated with a palpable flank mass or pain. Hematuria is uncommon.

Ultrasound shows a solid mass of variable size.[49,52,69] Oncocytomas of less than 5.5 cm in diameter tend to be well-circumscribed, homogeneous, and isoechoic with adjacent renal parenchyma. Larger tumors tend to be more inhomogeneous with less distinct margins. The characteristic stellate central scar is seen less commonly with ultrasound (7% to 25%) than CT (20% to 33%) and only in larger tumors.[69-71] Calcifications are rare. On angiography, a homogeneous blush and radiating vessels in a "spoke-wheel" configuration are characteristic but nonspecific.[71,72] Unfortunately, most oncocytomas are indistinguishable from RCC on ultrasonograms or CT scans.

Transitional Cell Carcinoma. Over 90% of malignancies that involve the renal pelvis and ureter are transitional cell carcinomas (TTCs). The majority of TCCs arise in the bladder and are associated with a 6% incidence of synchronous or metachronous TCC in the renal pelvis or ureter that may be bilateral (10%).[73-75] However, 32% of patients with renal TCC and 50% of patients with ureteral tumors will have synchronous or metachronous bladder involvement. Hematuria occurs early in these tumors, and thus TCCs usually present while they are relatively small in size and difficult to detect on sonography.

Sonographically, the typical appearance of a TCC is that of a hypoechoic mass within the collecting system (best seen when pelvocaliectasis is present) (Fig. 9-27).[73] TCCs may invade into adjacent renal parenchyma and form an infiltrating mass, which preserves the renal outline and contour but distorts internal renal architecture, displacing renal sinus fat, producing focal caliectasis, replacing central sinus echoes, and producing variable echogenicity of the renal parenchyma. Calcifications are rare. The epicenter of the TCC is typically located in the renal sinus, suggesting the diagnosis. As concurrent or subsequent involvement of the bladder and ureters is common, cystoscopy and bilateral retrograde pyelography should be performed to completely evaluate a suspected TCC within the kidney and

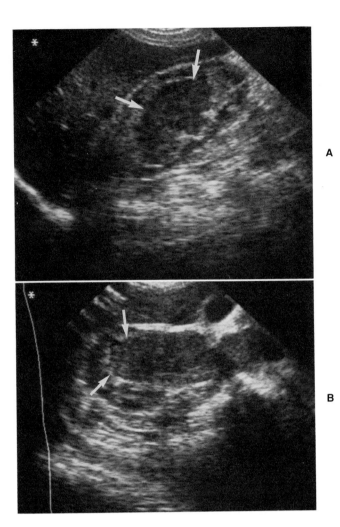

FIG 9-27. Transitional cell carcinoma. Mass *(arrows)* within central sinus is isoechoic with renal cortex. **A,** Longitudinal. **B,** Transverse.
(Courtesy of SR Wilson, M.D., Toronto General Hospital, Canada.)

to search for other tumors in the collecting system, ureter, or bladder.

Papillomas, the benign counterpart of TCC, tend to be smooth and more rounded than TCCs[75] but may have a higher risk of later developing into TCCs. Pathologic distinction from TCC may be difficult, and papillomas have been reported to recur. Other infiltrative processes, which may resemble TCC include lymphoma, metastatic disease, squamous cell carcinoma of the renal pelvis, infiltrative renal cell carcinoma, and acute bacterial nephritis.

Squamous cell carcinoma (SCC) of the renal pelvis is a rare neoplasm with imaging features similar to but more invasive than TCC. SCC often follows chronic irritation from chronic infection, leukoplakia, drug use (phenacetin), and urinary calculi. Leukoplakia or squamous metaplasia is considered a premalignant precursor of SCC. Both TCC and SCC are more commonly detected with intravenous urography or CT than with ultrasound.

Peripelvic Cysts and Central Sinus Lipomatosis. Ultrasound is frequently requested to define the cause of attenuation or compression of the renal pelvis or calyces seen on excretory urography. Renal sinus lipomatosis shows the increased echogenicity typical of fat and often apparent expansion of the central renal sinus echoes.[76] Tumor masses, which may distort the normal renal architecture, have an echogenicity between fluid and fat in most cases. When ultrasound is the initial imaging procedure, peripelvic cysts and central sinus lipomatosis can usually be diagnosed confidently. However, if questions remain or if tumor is suspected, excretory urography, CT, or both should be performed.

Renal Metastases. Autopsy findings show a 2% to 20% incidence of renal metastases (four times higher than the autopsy incidence of RCC). However, RCC is four and one half times more common than masslike metastases in patients with known metastatic disease.[77,78] Thus a new solitary renal mass is still likely to be a RCC, even if the patient has a known primary malignancy. Renal metastases tend to occur late in the course of disease and most commonly result from primary tumors in the lung, colon, skin (melanoma), head and neck, breast, and uterus. Metastases are usually small; approximately one third are bilateral, and over half are multifocal. Metastases can be large, solitary, and echogenic masses (particularly those from the colon). Infiltration of the perinephric space is particularly common in metastatic melanoma and lung carcinoma.

Sonographically, metastatic lesions usually present as multiple, poorly marginated, hypoechoic masses. Multiple metastases may produce an enlarged, inhomogeneous kidney without discrete masses. CT enhancement characteristics may be helpful in characterizing renal metastases.[77]

Renal Lymphoma. Primary renal lymphoma occurs rarely. Most renal lymphoma results from hematogenous spread or, less commonly, direct invasion from perinephric nodal disease.[79,80] The kidney is a common extranodal site of metastatic lymphoma, usually as a late manifestation of the disease. Non–Hodgkins' lymphoma involves the kidneys much more commonly than Hodgkins' disease. Lymphomatous renal involvement is seen in one third of patients at autopsy; however, this is usually not evident with ultrasonography or CT because the involvement is either microscopic disease, diffuse, or both. Bilateral renal involvement occurs in 75% of cases.

Sonographically, renal lymphoma usually demonstrates enlarged kidneys with multiple, bilateral, hypoechoic renal masses.[81,82] Occasionally lymphomatous

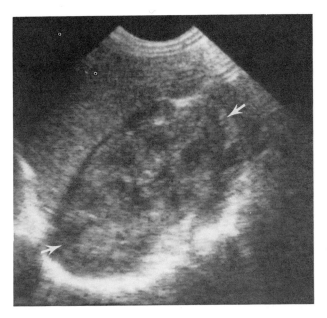

FIG 9-28. Lymphoma (diffuse). Most of right kidney *(arrows)* is involved with loss of normal hyperechoic central sinus.

masses may produce posterior acoustic enhancement. However, the margins of these masses are less discrete than those of cysts, and the degree of posterior enhancement is usually less than that anticipated posterior to a cyst of comparable size. Tumor invasion into the renal sinus may disrupt the echogenic central sinus (Fig. 9-28) but preserve the smooth renal contour.[78,81] CT is useful to study perirenal involvement or invasion.[79,81] Subcapsular lymphomatous invasion may be confused with hematoma or extramedullary hematopoiesis.[83,84]

Leukemia. Renal leukemia, similar to lymphoma, may cause diffuse enlargement of the kidney, although mild degrees of enlargement are seen in 15% to 30% of patients with leukemia without documented renal involvement. The cause of this enlargement is uncertain.[82] The kidney is frequently involved with leukemia during the active stages of the disease. Furthermore, the kidney may serve as a sanctuary site during hematologic remission. Although leukemia may present with diffuse enlargement of the kidney, leukemic infiltrates occasionally may present as focal, poorly marginated renal nodular masses that are hypoechoic to anechoic on ultrasound examination. Ultrasound can be used to monitor treatment in both lymphomatous or leukemic masses.[82,85]

Other Renal Neoplasms. Other rare renal neoplasms include sacromas, adult Wilms' tumor, juxtaglomerular tumors, carcinoid, renal sinus histiocytosis, hemangioma, lymphangioma, and malignant rhabdoid tumor.[86-94] The latter entity demonstrates a central mass, subcapsular nodules, and a large, subcapsular fluid collection, possibly from old hemorrhage. Juxtaglomerular tumors are a rare cause of hypertension (caused by excess renin production).[91,92] They have a variable echogenicity on ultrasound.[91] Hemangiomas also appear solid and echogenic on ultrasonograms.[94] A variety of other processes may mimic renal neoplasms, including inflammatory disease, infection, deposition diseases, and occasionally, vascular abnormalities such as aneurysms or pseudoaneurysms.

Renal Infection and Inflammatory Disease

Acute Pyelonephritis. Acute bacterial pyelonephritis usually results from ascending urinary tract infection. Ureteral reflux may play a positive role, as may urinary stasis or prior instrumentation. Gram-negative organisms, especially *Escherichia coli,* are responsible for approximately 85% of cases.[95,96] Females who are 15 to 35 years of age are most commonly affected.[95] Diabetes mellitus is an important predisposing medical condition and is often associated with fulminant bacterial pyelonephritis. Disease is usually unilateral but can be bilateral.[82,95] Imaging studies are often unnecessary because the diagnosis of pyelonephritis can be made clinically, but if there is no response to antibiotic treatment or if clinical symptoms progress, ultrasound examinations should be obtained to rule out obstruction or abscess.[97]

Sonographically, most kidneys with uncomplicated acute pyelonephritis demonstrate no abnormality.[95] However, renal enlargement with diffuse or focal decreased echogenicity caused by edema or acute lobar nephronia (focal bacterial nephritis) may occur.[96] Rarely, increased cortical echogenicity is present. Renal sinus echogenicity may be accentuated if the inflammatory process involves only the parenchyma, with discordant decrease in parenchymal echogenicity. Conversely, selective involvement of the renal sinus with central edema or purulent collections can decrease or obliterate the distinct boundaries between renal sinus fat and the renal parenchyma.[95] Differential diagnostic considerations in the acute clinical setting include acute renal vein thrombosis and renal infarction.

Acute "lobar nephronia" (focal bacterial nephritis) presents sonographically as a focal area of decreased echogenicity involving a renal lobe (Fig. 9-29). Typically, these abnormalities span the corticomedullary junction, but they do not demonstrate evidence of liquefaction or frank abscess formation. A characteristic wedge shape, suggesting a lobar infectious process, may not be seen on all views as a result of distortion and swelling of the renal lobe. A similar sonographic appearance can be seen in focal ischemia and renal infarction. Inflammatory masses may also have an infiltrative appearance, indistinguishable from neoplasm; however, clinical signs and symptoms usually suggest

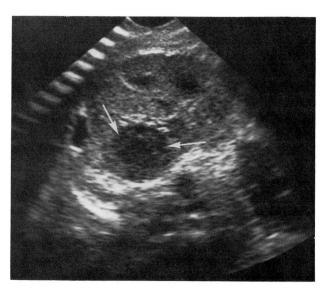

FIG 9-29. Lobar nephronia *(arrows).* Transverse sonogram shows poorly marginated hypoechoic area.
(Courtesy of SR Wilson, M.D., Toronto General Hospital, Canada.)

the correct diagnosis. Hemorrhagic acute bacterial nephritis may present as a wedge-shaped echogenic mass.[95,98] CT without contrast enhancement shows a hyperdense focal mass as opposed to the decreased density mass usually seen in focal bacterial nephritis. Acute bacterial nephritis may result in a renal cortical scar overlying a dilated calyx, similar to that seen with chronic atrophic pyelonephritis or reflux nephropathy.[95]

Focal bacterial nephritis may be difficult to distinguish from a renal abscess (Fig. 9-30). Abscesses tend to be larger, better defined, and frequently demonstrate increased through-sound transmission.[49,95,99] Suspicious hypoechoic renal lesions should be followed sonographically for the development of an abscess, which may require percutaneous ultrasound- or CT-guided aspiration and drainage for diagnosis, treatment, or both.[95]

Emphysematous pyelonephritis is most common in diabetics, immunosuppressed patients, or patients with urinary tract obstruction.[95,96] This fulminant necrotizing process, commonly associated with *E. coli* infection, is usually unilateral and may not respond to antibiotic treatment because of associated renal ischemia.[95] Nephrectomy is usually required to treat the infection—often urgently, because mortality has been reported to be as high as 33% to 35%. Ultrasound features of emphysematous pyelonephritis include shadowing echogenic foci located in the renal parenchyma, renal sinus, or both. The shadows produced by these echogenic collections of intrarenal gas tend to be less discrete than those seen posterior to renal calculi, and they frequently contain reverberations ("dirty shadowing").[95] In ex-

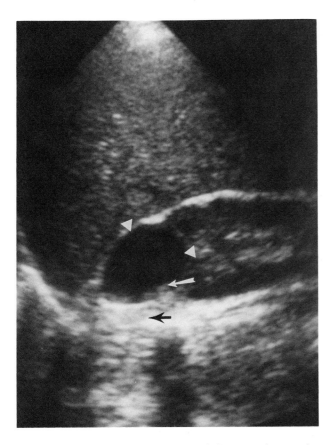

FIG 9-30. Abscess. Sagittal ultrasound shows cystic mass involving upper pole of right kidney *(arrowheads)* with dependent echoes or debris *(arrow)*. Note increased through transmission *(black arrow)*.

treme cases shadowing caused by intrarenal gas may obscure the entire renal bed and may be indistinguishable from bowel gas. Associated intestinal ileus may also hinder ultrasound evaluation.

Renal Abscess. Renal abscesses are usually the end result of acute bacterial nephritis.[95] *E. coli* is now the most common infecting organism. *Staphylococcus aureus* renal abscesses are usually caused by hematogenous seeding associated with immunocompromise, trauma, or IV-drug abuse.[95]

On ultrasound examination, renal abscesses are usually poorly marginated debris- and fluid-filled cystic masses with increased through transmission and peripheral sound-beam refraction (Fig. 9-30). Echogenic foci with posterior acoustic shadowing and a debris-fluid level in a cystic mass is very suggestive of an abscess.[95,99] Abscesses may mimic renal cysts, malignant tumors, or calyceal diverticuli. Rapid sequential changes in the appearance of a focal renal mass are the hallmark of infection and can usually exclude the presence of a cystic neoplasm.[98] Abscess invasion of the renal collecting system or perinephric space is best evalu-

ated with CT.[95] However, ultrasound can be used as an initial examination when a renal pathologic condition is highly suspected or known.[97]

Pyonephrosis. Pyonephrosis, which is purulent material in the collecting system, almost invariably occurs in patients with renal obstruction.[95,96,99,100] Percutaneous or surgical drainage is required for adequate treatment, and even in long-standing cases, some renal function can be recovered.

Ultrasound findings of echogenic debris or fluid-debris levels in a dilated renal collecting system are highly specific (97% to 100%) and should be considered diagnostic in the appropriate clinical setting.[95,96,100,101] Sonographic sensitivity for the diagnosis of pyonephrosis ranges from 62% to 90%. Failure to demonstrate echogenic debris within the collecting system does not exclude pyonephrosis. Percutaneous aspiration may be necessary for diagnosis.[95,96,100] Detection of gas within the urinary collecting system suggests infection, especially if there is no history of instrumentation.[95,100] It may difficult to differentiate gas from stones on ultrasonograms, and both may be present. Plain film radiographs or CT scans, however, can easily differentiate air and calcium if this is necessary.

Chronic Atrophic Pyelonephritis. Chronic vesicoureteral reflux is responsible for most cases of chronic atrophic pyelonephritis (CAP) (reflux nephropathy). Intrarenal reflux appears to be the main cause of damage, but controversy centers around whether concomitant infection is necessary to develop CAP.

The **sonographic features** of reflux nephropathy include a focal cortical scar overlying a dilated and blunted calyx (Fig. 9-31).[102] Focal increased echogenicity may be present in the region of the scar or where the renal sinus extends into the area of the scar. Involvement may be multicentric and bilateral. Upper and lower poles are more commonly affected than the midportion of the kidney. Discrete scars may be difficult to detect when cortical loss is diffuse, and chronically involved kidneys may be extremely small.[102] Postobstructive renal damage usually demonstrates more diffuse abnormalities, which involve the entire kidney. Treated, acute bacterial nephritis, renal tuberculosis, and papillary necrosis with cortical scarring may appear similar to CAP.[95] The cortical scarring in papillary necrosis does not necessarily occur directly over the calyces. Calyceal deformity and filling defects in the collecting system caused by sloughed papilla may help distinguish papillary necrosis from CAP.

Xanthogranulomatous Pyelonephritis. Xanthogranulomatous pyelonephritis (XGP) is an uncommon, severe, chronic renal parenchymal infection, usually affecting middle-aged females and diabetics.[82,95,103] Involvement is diffuse or segmental and extrarenal extension of infection is common.[95] Most patients give a history of re-

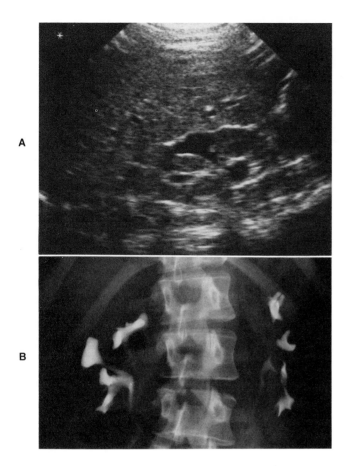

FIG 9-31. Chronic atrophic pyelonephritis. **A,** Longitudinal scan shows focal cortical scar overlying blunted dilated calyx. **B,** Confirmatory excretory urogram. Echogenic debris forms fluid-fluid level *(arrowhead)* within collecting system and is diagnostic of pyelonephrosis in this patient with symptoms of infection.

(Courtesy of SR Wilson, M.D., Toronto General Hospital, Canada.)

current urinary tract infections persisting in spite of antibiotic therapy. Up to 70% of patients have renal stones, especially staghorn calculi,[95,103] which obstruct a calyx or the ureteropelvic junction and contribute to the infectious process.

Sonographic features include a complex mass with cystic and solid components and renal stones or calcification.[95] Diffuse XGP presents with renal enlargement, loss of corticomedullary distinction, multiple hypoechoic areas (which mimic renal neoplasms), and frequently pelvocaliectasis.[95]

CT is the preferred imaging modality for determining the full extent of XGP into perirenal and pararenal areas. When contrast material is used, the degree of residual renal function can also be evaluated.[95,96] Combined ultrasound or CT findings and clinical history usually allow for the correct preoperative diagnosis.[95,103,104] However, if XGP presents as an intrarenal

mass without extrarenal extension or distinct renal calculi, preoperative differentiation from renal neoplasm or tuberculosis is difficult.

Renal Tuberculosis. Renal tuberculosis (TB) is acquired by hematogenous spread, usually associated with concurrent lung involvement. Although renal TB is usually a bilateral process, the clinical manifestations are often unilateral.[82,95,102] Cortical infection results in abscess and granuloma formation with caseation necrosis, fibrosis, and cortical destruction. Cortical lesions extend into the medullary pyramids and may eventually ulcerate into the collecting system with subsequent granuloma and stricture formation involving the renal pelvis and the ureters.[82] Ureteric granulomas caused by TB infection may produce a mass effect or ureteral strictures. Although these abnormalities may be difficult to identify directly with ultrasound, the resultant hydronephrosis is easily detected. Bladder involvement with TB usually follows renal infection, but unlike in the kidney, calcification is rare in the bladder.[105] Tuberculous granulomas may produce irregular thickening of the bladder wall, mimicking transitional cell carcinoma, but the most common sonographic findings are those of a small, spastic bladder. Bladder strictures may form, and the small bladder capacity may lead to vesicoureteral reflux.

On sonography, the kidney involved in renal TB may appear normal, even if it is nonfunctioning. Loss of corticomedullary distinction is common,[82,105] and distortion and dilation of the collecting system is frequent. Calcifications (10% of which are diffuse) are seen in 25% to 50% of cases; in fact, TB is the most common cause of diffuse calcification in a nonfunctioning kidney. Advanced parenchymal destruction results in a small, calcified, nonfunctioning kidney, also known as an "putty kidney" or "autonephrectomy" (Fig. 9-32). Hypoechoic regions of caseous necrosis adjacent to the collecting system may be difficult to differentiate from clubbed calyces filled with debris.[82,95] Approximately 25% of patients with renal TB demonstrate tumefactive masses similar to those seen in XGP. Bacterial abscesses and neoplasms occasionally demonstrate a similar appearance. Calyceal abnormalities caused by clubbed calyces and scarring seen on ultrasonograms may mimic changes seen in CAP, papillary necrosis, or calyceal diverticula.[82]

Most cases of renal TB, particularly when severe, can be diagnosed using a combination of CT, ultrasound, and excretory urography.[105] Excretory urography best defines the collecting system damage, but retrograde examinations may be required when renal function is poor. Treatment consists of triple antibiotic therapy, and when started early enough in the disease process, the prognosis is good. In rare instances nephrectomy may be required. However, scarring and ob-

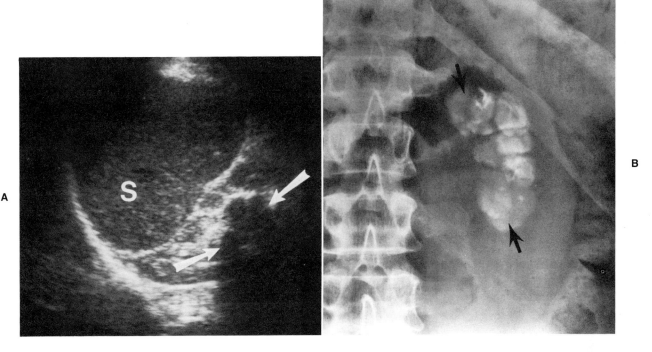

FIG 9-32. "Autonephrectomy" from TB. **A,** Sagittal sonogram shows spleen *(S)*. No left kidney is seen, but echoes with shadowing *(arrows)* are demonstrated in left renal bed. **B,** Plain film radiograph shows small, calcified left kidney *(arrows)*.

struction may progress even after successful treatment, and serial ultrasound examination is the preferred modality for long-term follow-up.

Renal Fungal Disease. Candidiasis is the most common renal fungal disease. Other fungal infections include aspergillosis, cryptococcosis, phycomycosis, and actinomycosis.[95] Most fungal infections result from hematogenous seeding; however, primary renal infections (probably caused by an ascending organism) also occur. Most patients wtih renal fungal infections are immunocompromised or have an underlying renal disease or a history of genitourinary surgery.[95,106] Renal fungal disease may be unilateral or bilateral.

On **sonography,** fungal infections may appear identical to acute bacterial nephritis or renal abscess.[95] Fungus balls, more echogenic than renal parenchyma, but without posterior acoustic shadowing may be seen in the collecting system[95,106] (Fig. 9-33). Renal tumors, blood clots, pyogenic debris, sloughed papilla, and nonshadowing renal stones can have a similar appearance. Rarely, a fungus ball will be hypoechoic or even anechoic internally. Fungus balls may produce obstruction, resulting in acute renal failure and anuria.[95]

Renal Parenchymal Malakoplakia. Malakoplakia is an uncommon inflammatory process, usually involving the bladder and collecting system; however, 16% to 33% of cases have renal parenchymal involvement.[49,95] Mala-

koplakia is associated with gram-negative urinary tract infection, usually *E. coli,* and is thought to result from impaired intracellular bacterial killing. Up to 40% of patients with malakoplakia are immunosuppressed; the process is more common in females by a 4:1 ratio, is

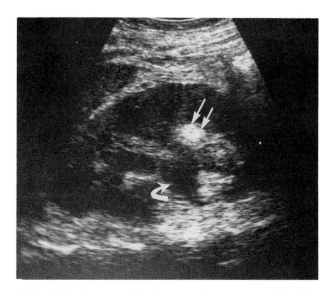

FIG 9-33. Fungus ball. Fungus ball *(arrows)* within obstructed midpole collecting system *(curved arrow)* is very echogenic.

bilateral in 50% of cases, and is multifocal in 74%.[95] On **sonography,** malakoplakia usually presents as a nonspecific hypoechoic mass or masses. However, sometimes the masses may have a cystic or complex appearance, or diffuse renal enlargement and disorganization of the central renal sinus complex may be noted.[49,107] Associated collecting system abnormalities are often present, as is renal obstruction.[95]

Renal Involvement in AIDS. Over 50% of AIDS patients in one study series demonstrated renal cortical echogenicity equal to or greater than the liver.[49] The kidneys may be normal in size or enlarged when involved in AIDS.[108,109] Enlarged echogenic kidneys may also be seen with many other disease processes, including acute tubular necrosis caused by drug administration, myoglobinuria, glomerulonephritis, amyloidosis, and diabetes.

Pathologic findings in AIDS include focal segmental glomerulosclerosis and tubular abnormalities.[108] The severity of the tubular abnormalities appears to correlate with the degree of renal echogenicity, suggesting that tubular abnormalities are the main factor contributing to increased renal echogenicity. However, Shaffer et al[109] reported no tubular abnormalities in 10 patients, most of whom had abnormally increased echogenicity and focal segmental glomerulosclerosis. Diffuse infection and renal calcification caused by *Pneumocystis carinii* (Fig. 9-34) and one case of diffuse parenchymal calcifications caused by *Mycobacterium avium* and *M. intracellulare* infections have been reported.[110,111]

Renal Congenital Abnormalities

Most congenital abnormalities are diagnosed in childhood or in utero. However, it is important to recognize congenital abnormalities in adults that may have escaped detection and that may have significant therapeutic implications. Documenting renal agenesis or excluding an ectopic kidney is important when a single functioning kidney is noted on excretion urography, in the evaluation of pelvic masses, in cases of trauma to a potential solitary kidney, or in considering a patient as a potential renal donor. Congenital renal abnormalities may also mimic other diseases. For example, a horseshoe kidney may present as a retroperitoneal mass (Fig. 9-35). Abnormal renal orientation and the ability to demonstrate continuity of renal parenchyma across the midline may suggest the correct diagnosis.

Renal Trauma

The role of ultrasound in evaluating renal trauma is controversial.[112,113] The initial evaluation of abdominal trauma is usually done using contrast-enhanced CT, provided the patient is stable. Ultrasound cannot provide information about renal function, does not readily image the entire abdomen, and provides only limited imaging of bowel. Nevertheless, in some countries, ultrasound is the procedure of choice in suspected renal injury, sometimes supplemented with excretory urography, and excellent results have been reported.[112,113] When ultrasound evaluation of the kidneys, including Doppler imaging, yields normal findings and hematuria is minimal, significant renal injury is unlikely. Ultrasound may also be used in conjunction with CT for follow-up of perirenal fluid collections, renal contusion, or fracture. Pulsed and color Doppler techniques may be helpful to document the integrity of the renal blood supply, but more experience is needed before Doppler imaging supplants CT or angiography in cases of suspected vascular injury.

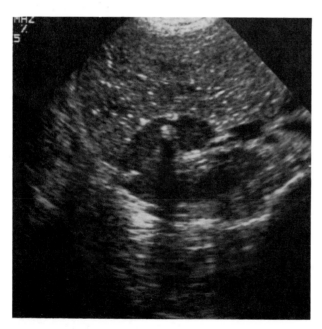

FIG 9-34. Disseminated *Pneumocystis carinii.* Transverse sonogram shows multiple, tiny, bright echogenic foci in liver and several larger echogenic foci, some with shadowing, in kidney.
(From Spouge AR, Wilson SR, et al: *AJR* 1990;155:176-78.

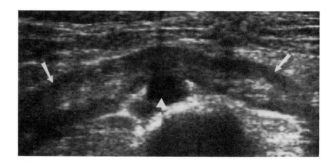

FIG 9-35. Horseshoe kidney. Transverse view shows right and left renal cortices *(arrows)*, connecting anterior to aorta *(arrowhead).*

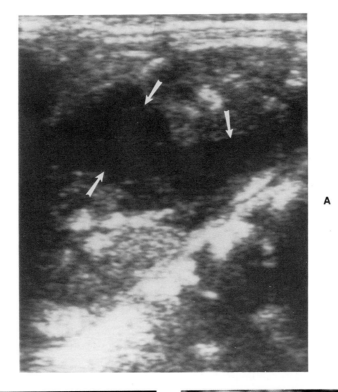

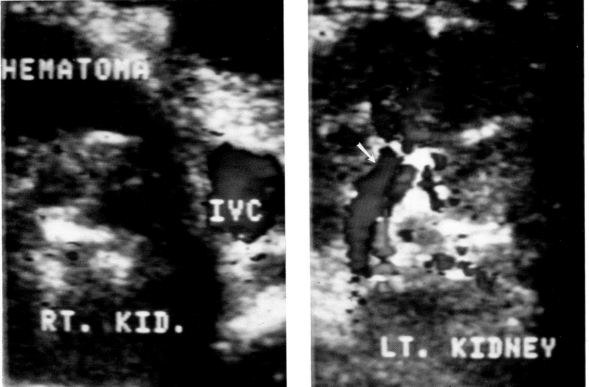

FIG 9-36. Fractured kidney, with hematoma. **A,** Sagittal scan shows linear hypoechoic defect *(arrows)* in midright kidney following trauma. **B,** Transverse color Doppler ultrasonogram of right kidney shows hematoma, no flow in renal parenchyma, and normal flow in adjacent IVC. **C,** Left kidney of same patient for comparison shows flow in left kidney *(arrow)*.
(From Lewis BD, James EM, Charboneau JW, et al: *Radiographics* 1989;9:599-631.)

Acute hemorrhage cannot usually be distinguished from other fluid collections (e.g., urinoma) with ultrasound. With time, hematomas generally become more echogenic and may contain fluid-debris levels. Subcapsular fluid collections can usually be distinguished from extrarenal fluid collections by the concave indentation of renal parenchyma produced by subcapsular processes. Renal parenchymal contusions, when visible, are hypoechoic and may appear masslike. Because hemorrhagic tumors may resemble a contusion with associated subcapsular or perinephric hemorrhage, renal neoplasm should be considered if significant trauma is not documented. Renal fractures may be diagnosed by demonstrating a linear defect (Fig. 9-36). Fragments of a shattered kidney may be visible within or surrounded by large collections of fluid. Echogenic blood clots may produce filling defects in the renal collecting system (Fig. 9-37) following trauma or renal biopsy.

Magnetic resonance imaging (MR) has shown changes in and around the kidney following extracorporeal shockwave lithotripsy (ESWL) in as many as 63% of patients, but ultrasound visualization of such abnormalities is less common.[114-117] Subcapsular hematomas occur in up to 15% of patients, but symptomatic hemorrhage is rare (less than 1%).[114,116-120] Perirenal and pararenal hematomas, as well as intraparenchymal hemorrhage, also occur. Hydronephrosis may be seen in up to 29% of patients following ESWL.[115,118]

Renal Vascular Ultrasound

Duplex and color Doppler ultrasound (CDU) are useful for identifying renal blood flow in normal renal arteries and veins and for characterizing intrarenal abnormalities.[21,55-58] Color Doppler imaging significantly shortens the examination time by providing a more global overview of renal blood flow, and it quickly identifies vessels for selective pulsed Doppler spectral analysis.[21,121] Segmental differences in organ blood flow, which are difficult to assess with pulsed Doppler and flow detection in small vessels, may be more readily appreciated with color Doppler ultrasound.[121]

A variety of measures, including the pulsatility index (PI = [peak systolic frequency (A) minus end-diastolic frequency (B)]/mean frequency) and the resistive index (RI = [peak systolic frequency (A) minus end-diastolic frequency (B)]/peak systolic frequency (A) are used to assess arterial resistance (Fig. 9-38). It should be noted, however, that these measurements are affected by significant variations in heart rate and blood pressure.[122] These indices are commonly used to evaluate renal allografts, to screen for renal artery stenosis, to assess suspected hydronephrosis, to evaluate medical renal disease, and to evaluate suspected renal neoplasms.

Renal Arterial Perfusion. The normal renal artery demonstrates continuous forward flow during diastole, typical of low-impedance (resistance) perfusion. Renal dysfunction caused by a variety of causes can result in increased renal arterial impedance.[123-129] Platt et al[129] report high sensitivity and specificity in differentiating obstructive versus nonobstructive nephropathy in the appropriate clinical setting using a threshold RI value of greater than 0.70 to define obstruction. They have also shown relatively similar RIs in bilateral native kidneys, with a RI difference of greater than 0.1, suggesting unilateral renal pathologic conditions in the kidney with the higher RI. Severe tubulointerstitial processes more often demonstrated markedly elevated resistivity indices than did purely glomerular processes.[130]

Renal Artery Occlusion. Kidneys with complete acute arterial occlusion may appear normal or may show mild renal enlargement initially.[131] Focal or seg-

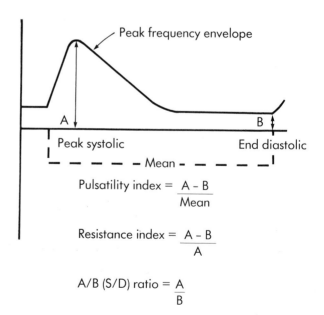

FIG 9-38. Doppler flow indices. Schematic representation of arterial waveform to demonstrate how flow indices are obtained.

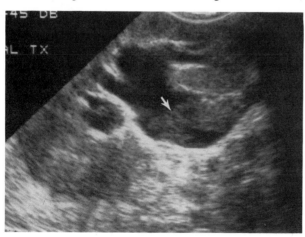

FIG 9-37. Blood clots. Echogenic mass *(arrow)* within obstructed upper collecting system is clot-producing obstruction in this transplant kidney following biopsy.

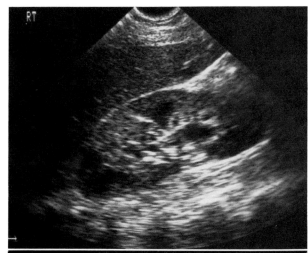

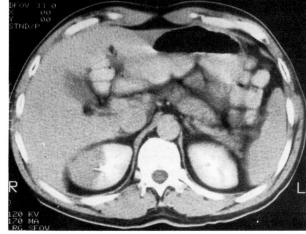

FIG 9-39. Segmental renal infarct. **A,** Sagittal scan of right kidney, 10 days after episode of right flank pain, shows wedge-shaped echogenic defect in anterior cortex of kidney. **B,** Confirmatory CT scan.
(Courtesy of SR Wilson, M.D., Toronto General Hospital, Canada.)

mental infarction (Fig. 9-39)[132] may produce a hypoechoic mass within the initial 24-hour period. Over several weeks, this mass often consolidates into an echogenic scar, which may mimic a solid mass. Chronic, complete, arterial occlusion or extensive multiple infarcts result in a shrunken, echogenic end-stage kidney. Although Doppler detection of flow rules out complete renal artery occlusion, failure to detect flow in patent renal arteries has been reported.[124]

Arteriovenous Fistulas. The arterial side of any arteriovenous fistula (AVF) typically shows an abnormally low-resistance arterial flow pattern with increased "turbulent" diastolic flow in the arterial limb.[33,133,134] Since renal arteries already demonstrate low resistance, this finding is most evident very close to the AFV and may be difficult to appreciate in a more distant location. Color or pulsed Doppler imaging typically demonstrates flow jets with high-systolic and high-diastolic velocity and marked spectral broadening (Fig. 9-40). A soft tissue "thrill" or bruit with random speckles of pulsatile

color may be seen adjacent to an AVF.[135] This finding is most pronounced in peripheral AVFs and can also occasionally be seen with severe arterial stenosis or in aneurysms. Arterial flow distal to an AVF may be damped. Venous flow demonstrates arterialization, particularly near the AVF, with increased velocity, pulsatility, and spectral broadening.

Renal AVFs are usually complications of a renal biopsy, but other etiologic factors include ruptured aneurysms and congenital malformations. Arteriovenous shunting is often seen in tumors such as renal cell carcinoma in which high-systolic and high-diastolic frequency shifts are suggestive of malignancy.[55-58]

Pseudoaneurysms. Renal pseudoaneurysms can be differentiated from other cystic masses by demonstrating pulsatile flow with a characteristic internal swirling color pattern and a to-and-fro pulsed Doppler signal at the neck of the mass (Fig. 9-17). Color Doppler imaging best demonstrates the connection between pseudoaneurysms and the adjacent artery.[136] Avascular cystic areas may show splashes of color during color Doppler ultrasound evaluation. This artifactual "flow" can be differentiated from true flow in a pseudoaneurysm by its random and homogeneous nature, lack of a characteristic pulsed Doppler waveform, and the ability to eliminate this artifact in many cases by changing color threshold and gain settings.

Renal pseudoaneurysms and AVFs may coexist after rupture of a pseudoaneurysm into an adjacent venous structure, which produces an arteriovenous communication. Renal pseudoaneurysm rupture may produce a subcapsular hematoma, which may lead to renal dysfunction or hypertension because of renal compression. Severe hemorrhage may require surgical repair.

Renal Artery Stenosis. Hypertension caused by renal vascular disease occurs in only 1% to 5% of patients with high blood pressure, but when diagnosed, it can often be definitively treated.[137] Renal vascular hypertension results when renal artery stenosis is severe enough to decrease renal blood flow and glomerular filtration, instigating a release of renin—which in turn starts a chain of conversions leading to increased amounts of angiotensin II in the blood stream. Angiotensin II, a potent vasoconstrictor, causes increased release of aldosterone, which further contributes to increased blood pressure. Approximately two thirds of renal artery stenoses are due to atherosclerosis, with most remaining cases caused by fibromuscular dysplasia.[137] Renal artery aneurysms, vasculitides, neurofibromatosis, unilateral renal parenchymal disease, infarction, and renal constriction (Page kidney) may also produce hypertension.[138]

Severe unilateral renal artery stenosis may produce renal size asymmetry, with the involved kidney being much smaller than the unaffected kidney (often less than 9 cm in length).[139] However, many cases of renal

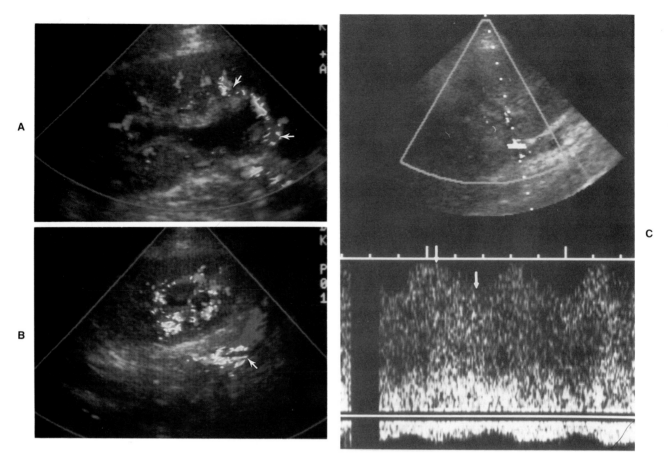

FIG 9-40. Arteriovenous fistula. **A,** Longitudinal color Doppler image shows focal areas of color heterogeneity and desaturation (increased velocity) *(arrows)* in lower pole of transplant kidney. **B,** Transverse scan confirms these flow abnormalities and shows high-velocity flow in adjacent internal iliac vein *(arrow)*. **C,** Pulsed Doppler signals *(arrows)* are characteristic of arteriovenous communication with disturbed, high-velocity flow, spectral broadening, and increased end diastolic flow.

artery stenosis do not produce marked renal asymmetry, making direct detection of renal artery stenosis essential for diagnosis.

Pulsed Doppler ultrasound screening for detection of renal artery stenosis in native kidneys is controversial.[137] The reported Doppler visualization rate for proximal native renal arteries ranges from 58% to 88%.[140-142] Recently, Handa et al[143] reported visualization of distal or hilar renal arteries in 98% of kidneys using a translumbar approach. Pulsed Doppler evaluation of the renal arteries is tedious, and the examination time is often a limiting factor in our experience. In addition, pulsed Doppler imaging has proved an unreliable method for detecting multiple renal arteries present in approximately 20% of cases. Two recently published studies[143,144] have not shown a significant improvement in the ability to detect renal artery stenosis using color Doppler ultrasound. Of particular disappointment was the failure of color Doppler ultrasound to improve detection of multiple renal arteries.

When renal arteries are adequately imaged, a variety of **Doppler imaging criteria** have been employed to determine if a significant stenosis is present. Sensitivities range from 0% to 100%, and specificities range from 37% to 100% in reported series. The lowest end of these ranges were obtained by Berland et al[143] using a peak angle-corrected velocity of more than 100 cm/sec or a ratio of peak renal artery to peak aortic velocity of more than 3.5 to 1 to determine if significant stenosis was present. It should be emphasized that this study intentionally kept the examination time to a minimum (average examination time was 17.5 minutes). Nevertheless, similar results were obtained by Desberg et al.[144] These relatively pessimistic results contradict earlier reports[139-141] which showed that a ratio of renal artery peak-systolic frequency shift to the peak-systolic frequency shift in the aorta of greater than 3.5 to 1 was highly sensitive for detecting renal artery stenosis. "Turbulent" flow combined with high peak-systolic frequencies (ranging from 4 KHz to 7.5 KHz in various studies) in stenotic renal arteries has also been reported to yield high sensitivities and specificities (Fig. 9-

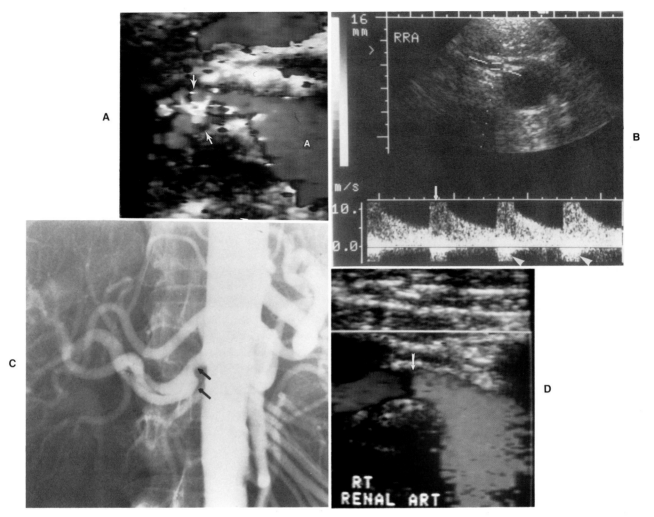

FIG 9-41. Renal artery stenosis. **A,** Transverse color Doppler image shows disturbed flow *(arrows)* in narrowed proximal right renal artery indicated by inhomogeneous color and intensity. *A* indicates aorta. **B,** Pulsed Doppler image shows high velocity through stenosis (velocity in excess of 10 m/s), "turbulence" (filling in of waveform), and aliasing *(arrowheads).* **C,** Arteriogram confirms right renal artery stenosis and poststenotic dilation *(arrows).* **D,** Normal right renal artery. Transverse color flow Doppler image shows proximal right renal artery *(arrow).* Homogeneous color indicates no turbulence. Note change of color in right renal artery caused by change in blood flow direction, vis-a-vis Doppler transducer.
(From Lewis BD, James EM, Charboneau JW, et al: *Radiographics* 1989;9:599-631.)

41).[139-141] **False-positive** and **false-negative examination results** are attributed to multiple renal arteries, branching arteries,[141] and distal fibromuscular dysplasia.[145] One prospective study demonstrated a negative predictive value of 94%, and several reports conclude that, if the renal artery is well seen and normal flow parameters are demonstrated, no further studies are required.[139,141] These series suggest that, when an abnormality is seen with pulsed Doppler imaging, angiographic evaluation is indicated. Some suggest that increased renal arterial resistance patterns within the kidney distal to a stenosis may predict a poor response to

surgery or angioplasty.[146] However, increased renal arterial resistance is a nonspecific finding, and further study of these observations is required.

The highest sensitivities for diagnosing renal artery stenosis have been reported using a translumbar ultrasound imaging approach. Only renal hilar artery waveforms were evaluated; an acceleration index was calculated and compared with values derived from normal controls.[142] Proximal stenosis results in a prolonged upslope decrease in the slope of the systolic waveform (delayed peak), the degree of which suggests significant stenoses (Fig. 9-42). Larger study series are needed to

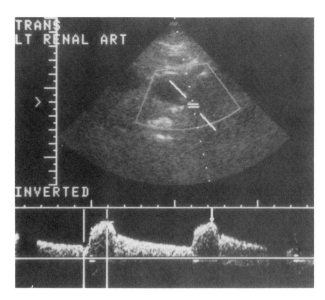

FIG 9-42. Renal artery stenosis. Waveform shows rounded and delayed systolic peak *(arrow)* distal to significant stenosis at origin of left renal artery.

further assess the accuracy of the translumbar approach in a Western population. Our initial experience indicates that renal hilar waveforms can be obtained in a high percentage of patients in a Western population, and findings of a delayed, rounded peak are suggestive of renal artery stenosis (Fig. 9-42). However, the measurements are technically complicated, and appropriate criteria to optimize renal artery stenosis detection and their accuracy are not yet established.

Currently, it appears that renal artery stenosis is most conclusively evaluated by arteriography (when stenosis is found, angioplasty can be performed with the hope of correcting hypertension).[137] However, not all renal artery stenoses are the cause of hypertension; currently, there is no way to predict which patients will respond to angioplasty by becoming normotensive.[146]

Renal Artery Aneurysm. Renal artery aneurysms (RAAs) are relatively rare in the general population but are more frequent in hypertensive patients.[147] Most are due to atherosclerotic disease; however, vasculitides and fibromuscular dysplasia are also important causes.[147,148] Congenital RAAs at vessel bifurcations may be mistaken for cysts. Pulsed or color Doppler imaging demonstration of arterial flow can readily identify the cystic mass as an aneurysm. The presence of hypertension and absence of a history of renal trauma or biopsy help differentiate true aneurysms from pseudoaneurysms, which rupture spontaneously more frequently than do true aneurysms.

RENAL FAILURE

Sonography plays a valuable role in the clinical evaluation and management of patients with renal failure.[82]

Renal failure can be categorized as:
- Prerenal (hypoperfusion caused by shock, sepsis, embolization, or renal artery or vein thrombosis)
- Renal (parenchymal disease including glomerulonephritides, autoimmune disease, acute tubular necrosis, and other interstitial diseases)
- Post-renal (obstruction of the collecting system)[82,97]

Sonography plays a major triage role in the initial evaluation and management of patients with renal failure by identifying postrenal obstructive abnormalities. Although only 5% to 10% of patients wtih acute renal failure have bilateral obstruction, this critical distinction can facilitate percutaneous nephrostomy tube placement or other interventional procedures to relieve the obstruction.

Prerenal Failure

Renal artery thrombosis is usually an acute event, presenting as acute flank pain and hematuria. Arterial thrombosis may be diagnosed sonographically by demonstration of absent arterial flow using either color Doppler or pulsed Doppler imaging, as well as identification of echogenic material within the renal arterial lumen.[82,97,149] The appearance of the kidney may be unremarkable in acute renal artery thrombosis. However, focal areas of infarction may present as hypoechoic wedge-shaped masses within the kidney. Areas of prior infarction may also appear as wedge-shaped atrophic scars or echogenic foci within the renal cortex, produced by fibrosis, fatty infiltration, or both.[132]

Renal Vein Thrombosis. Renal vein thrombosis may present as an acute or chronic event. When acute, symptoms include flank pain, hematuria, and (occasionally) fever and leukocytosis. The clinical differential diagnosis includes pyelonephritis and renal infarction. Incomplete or chronic renal vein thrombosis may escape detection because of a lack of significant signs or symptoms, possibly resulting from the presence of collateral venous flow. Patients at high risk of developing renal vein thrombosis include those with renal cell carcinoma, retroperitoneal malignancy, dehydration, nephrotic syndrome, renal transplants, amyloidosis, inferior vena cava thrombosis, and membranous glomerulonephritis and infants of diabetic mothers.

Sonographic features of acute renal vein thrombosis (RVT) are an enlarged, edematous, hypoechoic kidney with an indistinct corticomedullary junction.[150,151] Occasionally, areas of increased echogenicity caused by focal hemorrhage may be seen within the enlarged kidney. Thrombus may be visualized within a distended renal vein (Fig. 9-43), which may be dilated proximal to the area of occlusion. Although some studies report that tumor thrombus is more echogenic and expansible in nature than are bland thrombus,[61,62] the sonographic features of these two entities may be indistinguishable.

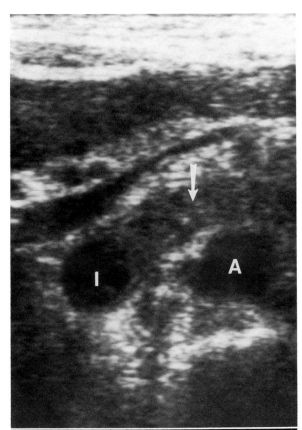

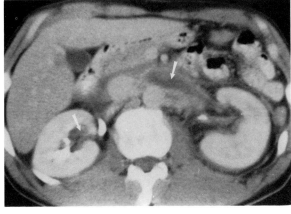

FIG 9-43. Bilateral renal vein thrombosis in patient with membranous glomerulonephritis. **A,** Transverse sonogram shows echogenic thrombus in left renal vein *(arrow)* as it crosses over aorta *(A)* to IVC *(I)*. **B,** CT shows filling defects *(arrows)* in dilated thrombosed renal veins.
(Courtesy of J. William Charboneau, M.D., Mayo Clinic, Rochester, MN.)

The use of Doppler, color Doppler, or both imaging modalities improves the ability to recognize thrombus within renal veins.[61,62,150,151]

In incomplete or partial RVT, the kidneys may appear normal or may exhibit decreased echogenicity as a result of edema. As the renal vein thrombosis progresses (10 days to 3 weeks after the acute event), renal cortical echogenicity may increase as a result of

cellular infiltration. Chronic RVT usually results in a shrunken, echogenic kidney with loss of corticomedullary definition caused by parenchymal fibrosis.

Recent studies report high-resistance renal artery flow waveforms (increased RI) secondary to RVT.[152] Although most such cases have been reported in patients with transplant kidneys in whom a lack of capsular venous anastomoses probably accents renal arterial changes, high impedance has also been reported in native kidneys with tumor thrombus involving the renal veins.[57,124,125] Increased arterial resistance is a nonspecific finding, however, when combined with absent renal vein flow, an increased RI is very suggestive of renal vein thrombosis even when no visible thrombus is detected. Color Doppler imaging, particularly when using low-flow detection levels, may facilitate evaluation of RVT, but the failure of Doppler imaging to detect flow in a patent renal vein has been reported.[124]

Medical Renal Disease

The normal adult kidney should be greater than 9 cm and less than 12 cm in length.[82] Normal or enlarged kidneys in patients with suspected medical renal disease usually require biopsy for definitive diagnosis of the underlying abnormality. In general, patients with renal lengths of less than 9 cm are considered to have abnormally small, end-stage kidneys, and biopsy is usually not required because the underlying renal disease is probably irreversible as this process is irreversible by any medical therapy, short of dialysis or renal transplant (Fig. 9-44). Although renal cortical thickness and length provide rough estimates of residual renal function, these measurements are relatively unreliable. Image assessment of renal function is better obtained with radionuclide or contrast-enhanced studies.

Common sonographic features of acute medical renal disease include: increased renal cortical echogenicity (echogenicity greater than that of the adjacent liver or spleen or echogenicity equal to or greater than that of the renal sinus) (Fig. 9-45), accentuated corticomedullary definition, and increased renal size.[153] Acute medical renal disease caused by infiltrative processes such as amyloidosis or leukemia frequently result in an enlarged kidney with either increased or decreased echogenicity.[82] Other causes of medical renal disease usually result in lesser degrees of renal enlargement or normal-sized kidneys with increased or decreased echogenicity. Any acute medical renal disease may progress to an "end-stage" shrunken echogenic kidney.

Acute Tubular Necrosis

Acute tubular necrosis (ATN) is the most common cause of acute renal failure.[82,87] ATN may result from a variety of processes, including toxic and ischemic insults leading to widespread tubular epithelial-cell damage. Toxins responsible for ATN include heavy metals,

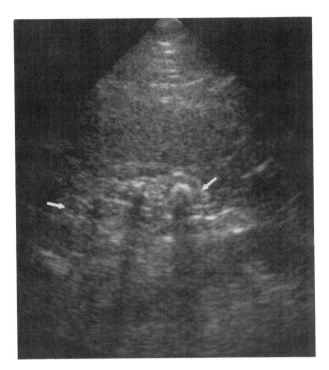

FIG 9-44. End-stage left kidney *(arrow)*. Small echogenic kidney measures 6 cm in length and contains two shadowing stones.

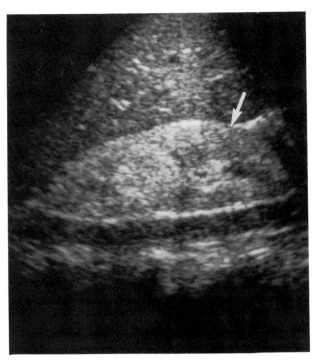

FIG 9-45. Glycogen storage disease (renal involvement). Right kidney *(arrow)* is more echogenic than adjacent liver.

antibiotics, anesthetics, and solvents. The renal insufficiency that occurs in ATN is often abrupt and severe; however, the process can be reversible. Histologically, there is tubular cell necrosis with cellular casts in the collecting tubules.

ATN caused by hypotensive ischemic episodes usually produces no sonographic abnormalities, although kidneys occasionally may develop increased cortical echogenicity and enlargement. Conversely, ATN caused by toxic effects of drugs or heavy metal exposure frequently demonstrates renal enlargement, increased cortical echogenicity,[82,154,155] and hypoechoic medullary pyramids with accentuated corticomedullary junction. Platt et al[156] have demonstrated increased RIs, which are most marked in active tubular interstitial processes, ATN, and severe vasculitis, but not with diseases limited to the glomeruli.

Myoglobulinuria is the cause of 5% to 7% of cases of ATN.[155] Even patients with small amounts of myoglobin in their blood over a period of time may develop chronic renal failure.[82,155] Myoglobinemia resulting from rhabdomyolysis with release of myoglobin into the bloodstream may follow alcohol or drug addiction,

crush injuries, strokes, toxins, fever, myositis, or significant ischemic muscle damage. Sonographically, kidneys with ATN secondary to myoglobulinuria demonstrate the same enlargement, increased cortical echogenicity, prominent medullary pyramids and elevated RIs seen with other causes of acute tubular necrosis (Fig. 9-46). Tamm-Horsfall protein precipitation in renal tubules in dehydrated infants can produce ATN and may have increased echogenicity of medullary pyramids that may mimic medullary nephrocalcinosis sonographically.[154]

Acute Cortical Necrosis

Acute cortical necrosis (ACN) is a rare cause of acute renal failure, which develops after renal injury caused by shock, hemorrhage, sepsis, burns, renal vein thrombosis, or severe dehydration.[82,157,158] The mechanism of injury is thought to be ischemic necrosis secondary to hypoperfusion, vasospasm, capillary damage, or intravascular thrombosis. Histologically, there is necrosis of the cortex and tubular cells with an interstitial cellular infiltrate. The renal medulla and a thin rim of subcapsular tissue supplied by capsular vessels remain intact. **Sonographically,** the renal cortex may be hypoechoic initially, and edema may produce slight renal enlargement.[82,158] However, increased cortical echogenicity caused by calcific and collagenous renal cortical deposits is usually seen in chronic stages of the disease.

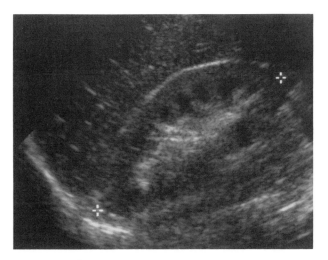

FIG 9-46. ATN from rhabdomyolysis. Kidney (+) is enlarged (14 cm) with increased cortical echogenicity. Medullary pyramids are prominent.

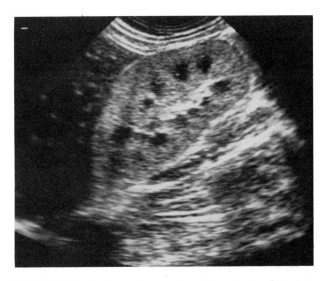

FIG 9-47. Acute glomerulonephritis; enlarged echogenic right kidney. Prominent medullary pyramids are seen on longitudinal scan.
(Courtesy of SR Wilson, M.D., Toronto General Hospital, Canada.)

Calcifications may appear as early as 24 hours following the ischemic insult, either at the junction between viable and necrotic tissue or diffusely throughout the cortex.[158] Calcification and increased echogenicity may become so great that both the kidney and the renal bed are obscured by posterior acoustic shadowing. Chronic glomerulonephritis and oxalosis may have a similar sonographic appearance. However, clinical features and radiographic confirmation of diffuse cortical calcifications should suggest the diagnosis of ACN.

Acute Glomerulonephritis

Glomerulonephritidies—including collagen vascular diseases such as lupus nephritis, poststreptococcal glomerulonephritis (GN), Goodpasture's syndrome, and rapidly progressive GN—represent autoimmune-induced renal inflammatory responses that produce glomerular damage. Patients typically present with hematuria, hypertension, azotemia, and red blood cell casts in the urine.[82]

Early in the disease, the kidneys may appear normal, but diffuse renal enlargement soon develops. Increased cortical echogenicity with medullary sparing may become quite prominent (Fig. 9-47). Hypoechoic cortical foci of ischemia or infarction caused by vasculitis may occur.[159] With time, renal size usually decreases. If treatment improves renal function, the kidneys may revert to a more normal appearance. The histologic cause for the increased echogenicity in acute GN has not been determined. In chronic GN, the kidneys may become small and echogenic, as in any sort of end-stage medical renal disease.[82]

Other Interstitial Nephritidies

Interstitial nephritis caused by infectious organisms is referred to as "pyelonephritis," which is usually a unilateral process and rarely a cause of renal failure. However, interstitial nephritis caused by systemic infections, drug hypersensitivity, or analgesic abuse may demonstrate interstitial white blood cell infiltration, which may result in echogenic kidneys associated with medical renal disease.[82]

Nephrocalcinosis

Some medical renal diseases that result in renal failure are associated with nephrocalcinosis—a broad term that denotes calcium deposits in the renal parenchyma.[160-163] Although ultrasound is more sensitive than plain film radiography, it is less sensitive than CT for detecting such calcific deposits. Sonographic findings of echogenic foci with posterior shadowing are nearly pathognomonic for renal stones or calcifications; however, shadows are not always present. When discrete shadowing is present, calcification is usually visible on plain radiographs. There are three broad categories of calcium distribution that should be considered, although there is often some overlap: intrarenal calculi, cortical nephrocalcinosis, and medullary calcification.[160-163]

Renal Stones. Renal stones usually arise in the collecting system. Most causes of nephrocalcinosis, whether cortical or medullary, are associated with stone formation, either from direct extrusion of a calcific focus into a calyx or from increased calcium or other metabolites in the urine that precipitate and act as a nidus for stone formation.[163] Focal renal calculi are usually

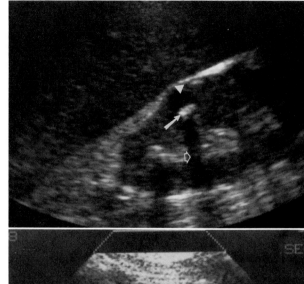

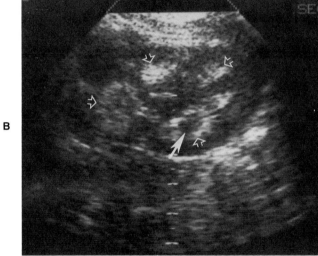

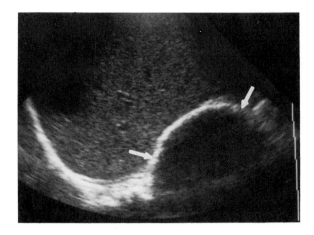

FIG 9-49. Primary oxalosis. Right kidney shows only echogenic rim *(arrows)* with shadowing caused by diffuse dense calcification.

FIG 9-48. Renal stone *(arrow)*. **A,** Sagittal sonogram shows upper pole with right renal stone, which casts discrete posterior shadow *(open arrow)*. Note obstructed calyx *(arrowhead)* caused by stone. **B,** Medullary nephrocalcinosis. Transverse scan shows highly echogenic pyramids *(open arrows)* but no shadowing. Relatively hypoechoic central areas within pyramids *(arrow)* exemplify Anderson-Carr progression.

easily distinguished from more diffuse forms of nephrocalcinosis (Fig. 9-48). Isolated renal stones are rarely a cause of renal failure unless there is only a single functioning kidney obstructed by a stone.

Cortical nephrocalcinosis. Cortical nephrocalcinosis is usually diffuse and bilateral. Unilateral or focal cortical calcifications are usually due to infection or tumor, although infection may also produce diffuse calcification. The most common causes of diffuse bilateral cortical calcifications are hypercalcemic states such as hyperparathyroidism, vitamin D intoxication or treatment, hypercalcemia associated with malignancies, acute cortical necrosis (ACN), and oxalosis.[164-167] ACN and ox-

alosis usually demonstrate predominantly cortical calcium deposits, whereas medullary involvement predominates in hypercalcemic states.

Primary oxalosis is a rare hereditary disorder in which renal calcification begins at the corticomedullary junction and can involve both the cortex and medullary pyramids (Fig. 9-49). Acquired oxalosis is associated with small bowel disease or bypass or a diet rich in oxalates. Sonographic findings of increased cortical echogenicity caused by calcium deposits may be impossible to distinguish from other causes of increased cortical echogenicity, unless calcification produces posterior shadowing or calcification is seen in a plain radiograph. Extensive calcification may obscure visualization of the kidney and renal bed in advanced cases.

Medullary Calcinosis. The most common causes of adult medullary nephrocalcinosis are hypercalcemic states and medullary sponge kidney.[159-169] In addition, patients with distal tubular acidosis may develop medullary nephrocalcinosis. Although the sonographic findings of echogenic medullary pyramids in adults (even without shadowing) are felt to indicate medullary nephrocalcinosis, there is some speculation that hyperuricemia and hyperkalemia in gout or primary aldosteronism may produce similar increased medullary echogenicity without calcification. However, this is currently being debated. Furthermore, there is some speculation that the multiple interfaces produced by the ectatic tubules in medullary sponge kidney may result in increased echogenicity without significant calcific deposits.

Sonographically, medullary nephrocalcinosis presents as highly echogenic pyramids with or without posterior acoustic shadowing. This is the reverse of the normal, in which pyramids are less echogenic than the renal cortex. The echogenic pyramids are readily identified by their shape, relation to the central sinus and columns of Bertin, and by visualization of arcuate vessels at their base.[82] The Anderson-Carr progression (Fig. 9-48, *B*) suggests that calcification initially develops at the peripheral interstitium around the collecting ducts as a result of a lymphatic calcium overload.[163] These collections of calcium act as a nidus for subsequent calcific deposits and stone growth, with stones ultimately extruding into the collecting system.

Renal Amyloidosis

Primary amyloidosis, which is present in 0.2% to 5% of routine autopsies, is a disease of uncertain etiologic factors that is unrelated to other underlying disease processes.[170] The most common clinical manifestation of primary amyloidosis is nephrotic syndrome, which occurs in 35% to 44% of patients. Histologic abnormalities include extensive amyloid deposits in glomeruli, arteries, and the renal interstitium. Although the nephrotic syndrome is a complication of primary and secondary amyloidosis, the amount of amyloid deposition does not appear to correlate with the degree of urinary protein loss, which is thought to be related to breaks in the tubular epithelium and damage to the podocytes.[170-172]

Secondary amyloidosis is associated with numerous chronic processes, especially inflammatory or rheumatoid disease. At postmortem, 14% to 26% of patients with rheumatoid arthritis have pathologic evidence of amyloidosis. In both juvenile and adult rheumatoid arthritis, the degree of amyloid involvement is directly related to the chronicity and severity of the underlying disease. Other immunologic diseases associated with secondary amyloidosis include ankylosing spondylitis, Reiter's syndrome, scleroderma, rheumatic heart disease, dermatomyositis, and systemic lupus erythematosus. Tuberculosis is the most common chronic infectious process associated with secondary amyloidosis; however, syphilis, colitis, or osteomyelitis may also underly this process. Tumors, including renal cell carcinoma, Hodgkins' disease, and multiple myeloma are associated with secondary amyloidosis, as are Waldenstrom's macroglobulinemia and chronic dialysis.

Sonographic findings are similar in primary and secondary amyloidosis and include renal enlargement and increased echogenicity. However, the kidneys may be large, normal, or small in size, depending on the stage of the disease.[82,171] Renal enlargement occurs predominantly in the acute stages of amyloidosis, with a progressive decrease in renal size as the disease advances. Increased cortical echogenicity and accentuated corticomedullary definition become more pronounced in the chronic stages of the disease. Eventually, a nonspecific end-stage shrunken kidney results. Although the findings of amyloidosis are nonspecific, clinical manifestations and a history of predisposing diseases, such as autoimmune processes or chronic infection, should raise the possibility of amyloidosis.

POSTRENAL FAILURE
Obstruction

Urinary obstruction causes roughly 5% of all cases of renal failure—usually in cases of bilateral obstruction or obstruction of a solitary kidney. Bilateral obstruction can also be encountered in patients with chronic renal failure. Patients at **high risk** for postrenal failure caused by obstruction include:

- Those with known pelvic malignancies or recent pelvic surgery
- Those with bladder outlet obstruction (of which benign prostatic hypertrophy is the most common cause)
- Those with known palpable masses or renal calculus disease
- Those with suspected renal sepsis

Although studies have shown that azotemic patients who are not in the high-risk category are unlikely to demonstrate obstruction and therefore will not require emergency intervention,[173] the ultrasound examination still provides valuable information with respect to the size and appearance of the kidney even when obstruction is not present. Thus ultrasound emergency procedures are of value in the triage of azotemic patients.

The normal renal sinus is a central echogenic area composed of peripelvic fat and numerous vascular and uroepithelial structures. Hydronephrosis produces separation of normal sinus echogenicity by an anechoic urine collection.[82] The **extent of hydronephrosis** can be graded as mild (minimal separation of sinus echoes [2mm]), moderate (anechoic separation of the entire central sinus), or marked (extensive separation of the central sinus and calyces with parenchymal thinning) (Fig. 9-50). Real-time sonography can demonstrate peristaltic waves that sweep through the renal pelvis at rates of two to four contractions per minute. The rate of renal pelvic contraction is directly related to the amount of urine the kidney produces. If urine-flow rates increase, as with increased hydration or diuretics, renal pelvic and ureteric peristalsis increases. With acute obstruction, the peristaltic rate becomes irregular. There are bursts of repeated incomplete contractions followed by aperistaltic periods. With chronic obstruction, renal pelvic contractions usually cease. Detection of these normal peristaltic waves and imaging of their direction and frequency may be helpful in distinguishing obstruction from renal pelvic distension secondary to diuresis.

False-Positive Diagnosis of Obstruction

Sonography readily detects pelvocaliectasis (sensitivity 93% to 100%); however, pelvocaliectasis does not equal obstruction. False-positive diagnoses of obstruction result from numerous causes: overhydration, overly full bladder, diuretics, large extrarenal pelvis, prominent hilar vessels, and peripelvic cysts.[175,176] Most false-positive study results occur with mild dilation or grade 1 hydronephrosis; however, in high-risk groups, findings of minimal dilation may be significant.[174-176] False-positive examination results occur in 10% to 26% of all ultrasound examinations, but 50% or more of cases diagnosed as grade-1 hydronephrosis may be normal.

Overdistention of the bladder from any cause may produce dilation of the ureters in the upper collecting system. Reevaluation of the collecting system following voiding or catheter drainage usually shows resolution of such pelvicaliectasis and ureterectasis. Evaluation of the kidneys at our institution includes imaging of the pelvis and urinary bladder if possible. If hydronephrosis is detected and the urinary bladder is full, reevaluation of the kidneys is routinely performed following voiding or bladder drainage.

Parapelvic cysts may mimic high-grade obstruction, but in most cases sonography distinguishes parapelvic cysts from obstruction by revealing a connection between all the cystic structures and the central renal pelvis when obstruction is present and a lack of this connection with parapelvic cysts (Fig. 9-16).[30-32] In equivocal cases excretory or retrograde urography should be performed.

Congenital Megacalices

Congenital megacalices develop as a result of an abnormality in the number and timing of divisions in the ureteral bed.[29] Calices are increased in size and number, and medullary thickness is decreased, whereas cortical thickness is normal. Renal function is usually normal, except for a mild reduction in concentrating ability. However, patients may develop stones and infection as a result of stasis. Excretory urography classically demonstrates polygonal or faceted calices, which are enlarged and increased in number. The sonographic appearance of large, clubbed calices extending into the medullary region may mimic hydronephrosis or renal papillary necrosis.[183] Contrast-enhanced studies and clinical findings will help differentiate between these entities.[177]

False-Negative Diagnosis of Obstruction

Sonographic false-negative diagnoses of obstruction occur in less than 1% of cases—most frequently in the setting of minimal dilation and interpreter error.[174-178] False-negative diagnoses also occur with staghorn calculi when posterior acoustic shadowing obscures the dilated collecting system (Fig. 9-51). Other causes of false-negative diagnoses include acute obstruction that has not yet produced dilation and decompression of

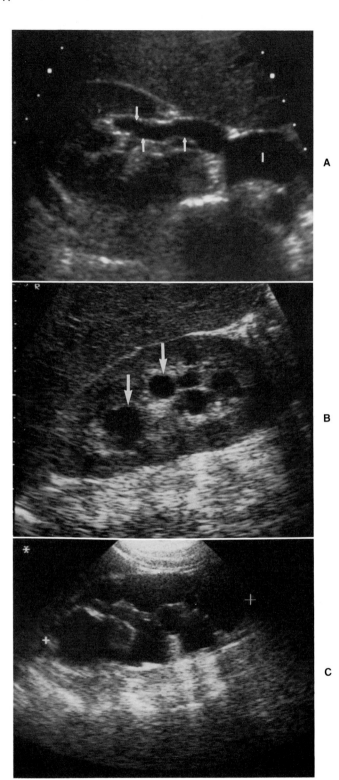

FIG 9-50. Degrees of hydronephrosis. **A,** Mild hydronephrosis *(arrows)* is seen on right transverse renal image. *I* indicates inferior vena cava. **B,** Moderate left hydronephrosis *(arrows)* seen on left coronal sonogram. **C,** Severe right renal obstruction caused by UPJ obstruction. Patient with nonvisualizing right kidney on excretory urogram shows total replacement of normal parenchyma by dilated fluid-filled calyces, indicating long-standing severe postobstructive atrophy with marked cortical thinning.

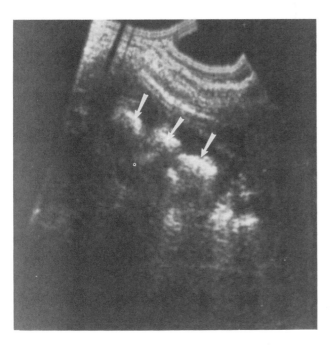

FIG 9-51. Staghorn calculus. Prone, longitudinal sonogram shows highly echogenic calyces with shadowing *(arrows)* caused by large staghorn calculus.

the obstructed system by tubular back flow or caliceal rupture. False-negative diagnoses may also arise if there is significant vascular insufficiency or when renal obstruction is associated with long-standing renal failure.[174-178] Obstruction may be difficult to diagnose in severely dehydrated patients or those with partial or intermittent obstruction. Retroperitoneal fibrosis or neoplastic encasement of the ureters may produce minimal dilation nephropathy, even with significant renal obstruction.[177-179] In cases in which nondilated obstructive uropathy is suspected, diuretic scintigraphy or retrograde studies are required before intervention.[178-179]

Platt et al have demonstrated a high sensitivity and specificity in differentiating obstructive versus nonobstructive nephropathy in the appropriate clinical setting, using a threshold resistivity index (RI) of greater than 0.7 to define obstruction.[129] Furthermore, they have shown relatively similar RIs in bilateral native kidneys so that a difference of greater than 0.1 in RI suggests unilateral renal pathologic conditions in the kidney with the higher RI. Although it appears that renal arterial RI values may help distinguish renal pelvic dilatation from acute renal obstruction, it is not clear that the same high degree of sensitivity and specificity exists in cases of long-standing chronic obstruction.

OBSTRUCTION WITHOUT RENAL FAILURE
Hydronephrosis of Pregnancy

Hydronephrosis occurs in 65% to 85% of pregnancies and is usually more marked on the right side.[180]

Such hydronephrosis is due to mechanical pressure on the ureters by the enlarged uterus. Other possible etiologic factors include muscular relaxation of the ureters resulting from hormonal factors.[179] Dilatation is often seen by 10 to 20 weeks of gestation and usually peaks at 24 to 28 weeks. In most cases this is a normal finding and dilatation usually resolves within several weeks postpartum. However, if a patient is symptomatic, pathologic renal obstruction must be considered.

In one study, measurements of the renal pelvis in the AP diameter in controls and during pregnancy were recorded in several hundred women.[180] Maximum measurements for first-trimester and second-trimester pregnant controls were 1.1 cm, 1.8 cm, and 2.8 cm on the right and 0.9 cm, 1.5 cm, and 1.8 cm on the left, respectively. These values provide useful guidelines for evaluating the pregnant patient with symptoms thought to be related to acute urinary obstruction.

A renal artery RI has yet to be evaluated in a large series of pregnant women. However, it is possible that some threshold value may be established for differentiating obstruction from the normal dilatation of pregnancy analogous to that reported for nonpregnant native kidneys.

Ureteropelvic Junction Obstruction

Ureteropelvic junction (UPJ) obstruction is a common congenital anomaly that rarely results in renal failure, unless it is severe and bilateral. In many cases UPJ obstruction may go undiagnosed until adulthood. Even if discovered late, surgical repair may preserve renal function. Other genitourinary tract anomlies are frequently associated with UPJ obstruction, particularly a contralateral multicystic dysplastic kidney.

Sonographic findings early in life show pelvocaliectasis with an abrupt cut off of the pelvic dilation at the UPJ. Long-standing cases detected in adults may present as a cystic mass without discernable renal parenchyma. In some cases differentiation of severe longstanding UPJ obstruction from multicystic dysplastic kidney may be impossible. In fact, some authors believe that these two entities are part of the disease continuum.[181,182]

Acute Flank Pain

Excretory urography is usually the procedure of choice to evaluate patients with acute flank pain.[183] However, ultrasound can be used as an alternative modality when a contrast-enhanced study is contraindicated, in patients with recurrent stone formation, or in obstetric patients. Although the obstructing stone or point of obstruction may not be visualized as often with ultrasound as with excretory urography (IVU), the observation of hydronephrosis localized to the symptomatic side suggests obstruction caused by a stone. In fact, Erwin et al demonstrated the presence of an obstructing

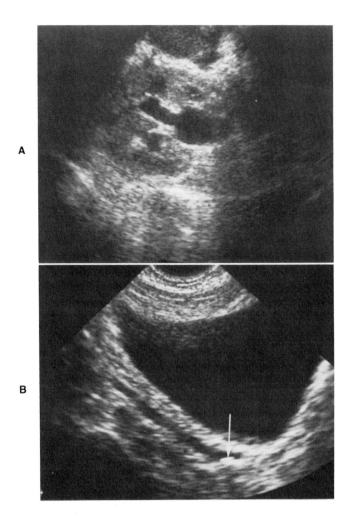

FIG 9-52. Ureteric stone. **A,** Transverse right renal sonogram shows moderate pelvocaliectasis in patient with acute right flank pain and hematuria. **B,** Partial obstructing stone. Sagittal scan shows dilated distal ureter with stone *(arrow)* just proximal to ureterovesical junction.

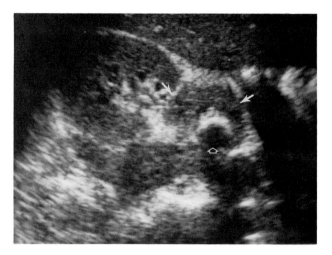

FIG 9-53. Ureteric calculi. Right transverse scan shows marked right ureteric thickening *(arrows)* caused by edema surrounding large calculus *(open arrow)*, which obstructs ureter. Surprisingly little right pelvocaliectasis is seen.

stone, hydronephrosis on the symptomatic side, or both in 100% of well-hydrated patients with acute renal colic.[184] Providing adequate hydration allows for visualization of the ureterovesicle junction (Fig. 9-52) and accentuates early pelvocaliectasis caused by acute obstruction. The ureterovesicle junction is the most common site for obstruction from renal calculi; the second most common site is the ureteropelvic junction; and the third most common level of ureteric obstruction is at the level of the pelvic inlet. Although ultrasound rarely detects stones in the midureter, coronal views allow for visualization of stones within the kidney, the region of the ureteropelvic junction, and proximal ureter (Fig. 9-53). With a well-distended bladder, distal ureteral stones are often visualized, as well as periureteric edema. In such cases visualization of ureteral jets indi-

cates partial rather than complete obstruction by the stone (Fig. 9-52, *B*).[185] Although pelvic tumors, trauma, or infection may produce obstruction, renal calculi are the most common cause of obstruction in patients with acute flank pain.

INTRALUMINAL-FILLING DEFECTS
Calculi

Renal stones are the most common intraluminal-filling defect. On ultrasound examination, they are echogenic foci that cast posterior acoustic shadows (Fig. 9-48). Stone shadowing is usually more discrete than that produced by gas, which is often poorly marginated and contains low-level echoes. Stone and shadow detection depends on stone size, transducer frequency, and transducer focal zone. Stones as small as 1.5 mm in diameter can be visualized.[186-188] There is no correlation between stone composition and the sonographic appearance.[187] Although renal artery calcification may mimic nephrolithiasis[189], the location serves to identify its source.

Sonography is equal to or slightly better than plain film radiography for the detection of calcified renal stones.[186] Plain film tomography improves stone detection, but CT is the most sensitive means for detecting calcified renal stones. Ultrasound can visualize noncalcified calculi such as uric acid stones, which are not visualized with plain film tomography.

Although ultrasound in conjunction with plain film radiographs is sufficiently accurate to guide extracorporeal renal shock-wave lithotripsy (ESWL), detection of stones in the ureters is suboptimal, and ultrasound does not accurately determine stone size or differentiate a single stone from a clump of several smaller stones.[114]

Other Intraluminal-Filling Defects

Echogenic, nonshadowing intraluminal masses include blood clots, pyogenic debris, sloughed papillae in cases of papillary necrosis, fungus balls, tumor, or very small stones (Fig. 9-48). Obviously, the clinical history is helpful in differentiating these entities. Hematuria suggests that filling defects are related to blood clots, tumor, or sloughed papillae. Conversely, fungus balls are rarely associated with hematuria and usually occur in the immunocompromised patient.[100,106] Pyogenic debris is usually associated with obstruction and symptoms of infection. An intravenous or retrograde contrast-enhanced study should be performed when the cause of an intraluminal mass is unclear, especially when the presence of a tumor is a possibility.

Papillary Necrosis

Papillary necrosis is most commonly caused by analgesic abuse.[190] Other causes include sickle cell anemia, obstruction, pyelonephritis, diabetes mellitis, ATN, renal vein thrombosis, and chronic alcohol abuse.[190] The clinical diagnosis is made by identifying sloughed papilla within the urine. IV or retrograde contrast-enhanced studies demonstrate characteristic irregular calices and sloughed papillae, which may cause obstruction. Contrast collections within the medulla may indicate necrosis before a papillae is sloughed.

Sonographic findings[191] include cystic collections in the medullary pyramids or triangular cystic collections replacing pyramids. When a papillae is sloughed, clubbed calices fill in where the pyramid was previously located; demonstration of the arcuate artery along the margin of the clubbed calyx may help confirm the diagnosis. Extensive changes of papillary necrosis with clubbed calices may occasionally mimic obstruction.

Sloughed papillae can be seen as echogenic nonshad-owing structures within the collection system; occasionally, they may calcify and mimic stones. Fulminant candidiasis may also produce papillary necrosis, making the differentiation between sloughed papillae and the fungus ball difficult.[190] Congenital megacalices or postobstructive atrophy may appear identical to papillary necrosis, with diffuse clubbed calices, but the clinical picture helps distinguish these entities. Prominent, normal papillae may be seen in a collecting system that is dilated or obstructed, but these appear smooth, and a connection with renal parenchyma can be demonstrated sonographically, distinguishing these from abnormal sloughed papillae (Fig. 9-54).[192]

URETERS

Coronal projections to image the proximal ureter and bladder filling to image the distal ureterovesical junction are essential in the evaluation of suspected ureteric pathologic conditions (Fig. 9-55). Furthermore, graded compression techniques similar to those used for the examination of the appendix may be useful, by compressing bowel gas out of overlying viscera and allowing visualization of the midportion of the ureters in some cases.

Ureteroceles

Simple ureteroceles are found more often in adults than in children. Most of these are round cystic structures that project into the bladder lumen at the ureterovesical junction, producing a "cyst within a cyst" appearance. The distal one third of the ureter may be dilated, but simple ureteroceles are usually asymptomatic and do not produce pelvocaliectasis. Characteristic sonographic demonstration of alternating filling and

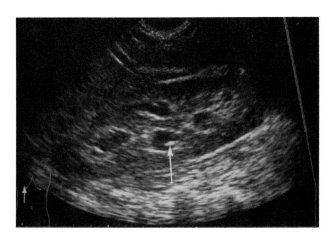

FIG 9-54. Normal papilla. Central echogenic focus *(arrow)* surrounded by fluid is normal papilla within dilated calyx. This appearance may mimic papillary necrosis.

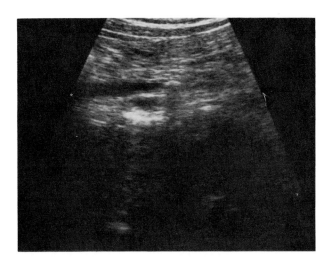

FIG 9-55. Dilated ureter. Right coronal sonogram shows dilated ureter to level of shadowing stone.
(Courtesy of SR Wilson, M.D., Toronto General Hospital, Canada.)

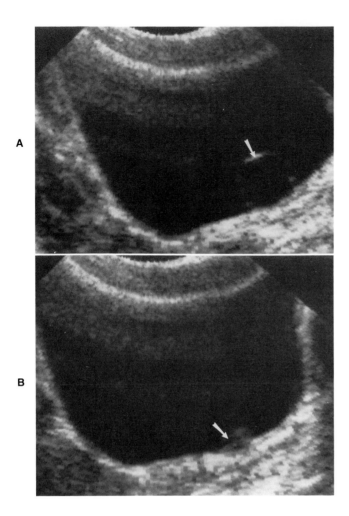

FIG 9-56. Ureterocele *(arrow),* showing "cyst within a cyst" appearance, with changing size. **A,** Filled. **B,** Empty ureterocele.

emptying of the ureterocele as a result of peristalsis can be seen on real-time ultrasonograms (Fig. 9-56). Ureteroceles within or outside the bladder wall may be difficult to distinguish from bladder diverticula, congenital cysts, or abscesses.

An **ectopic ureterocele** and its associated dilated ureter may mimic a multiseptated cystic mass within the pelvis.[193-195] Such ectopic ureteroceles are usually associated with partial or complete ureteral duplication, are frequently symptomatic, and thus are most commonly discovered in children. However, these duplicated systems may remain relatively asymptomatic until adulthood; in which case the obstructed upper pole moiety may present as a renal mass on intravenous urography (Fig. 9-57). Reflux into the lower pole moiety can be suggested by ultrasound when reflux is pronounced. However, voiding cystography is more sensitive for detecting reflux.[196]

Primary Megaureter

Primary megaureter caused by an aperistaltic distal ureteral segment can cause functional obstruction. Primary megaureter is thought to be related to abnormal muscle development around the ureteral bud, possibly caused by extrinsic compression by fetal vessels in utero.[29] It is more common on the left side and in males. In 25% of cases it is bilateral. Up to 42% of cases of primary megaureter are associated with additional GU anomalies, the most common of which is UPJ obstruction.

Typically, the lower ureter is dilated, but ureteric dilation can extend all the way to the renal calyces. Most patients are asymptomatic, and thus many of these lesions may not be discovered until adulthood. However, some patients may develop infection or stones. Progressive dilation is unusual, but when it occurs, it warrants resection of the aperistaltic segment. A dilated lower ureter without associated pelvocaliectasis is the most common sonographic appearance. Using the bladder as a window, the aperistaltic segment can sometimes be documented sonographically. Sequential ultrasound studies can document stability versus progressive dilation, and associated anomalies can be diagnosed.

Intramural and Extrinsic Ureteral Defects

Extrinsic ureteric compression at any level may cause complete or partial obstruction. Vascular compression may cause intermittent obstruction.[197] These vascular compressions usually occur at the junction of the upper ureter and the renal pelvis. Compression of the middle to lower portion of a retrocaval right ureter is seen where it courses behind the inferior vena cava. Whenever a pelvic mass is demonstrated, the kidneys should be imaged to evaluate potential ureteral obstruction. Bladder diverticula or ureteroceles may cause ipsilateral or contralateral ureteral obstruction. An ectopic ureterocele involving the upper pole ureter in a duplicated system can obstruct that moiety and produce reflux in the lower pole ureter.

Ultrasound is rarely used to image **ureteric masses;** however, when a ureteric mass is seen on ultrasonograms, it can be characterized as cystic or solid. Ureteric lesions in the region of the UVJ, such as ureteroceles and bladder diverticula, are the most commonly diagnosed.[193-195] Intramural ureteral lesions are particularly difficult to evaluate with ultrasound. Furthermore, most intramural lesions—such as tumor, edema, infection, or granulomas—have a similar appearance (Fig. 9-53). Periureteric edema and obstruction may persist after passage of a previously obstructing stone. Tuberculosis tends to form strictures or granulomatous lesions in the ureter, but in almost all cases there are changes in the ipsilateral kidney.[105]

Fibroepithelial polyps usually arise in the upper one

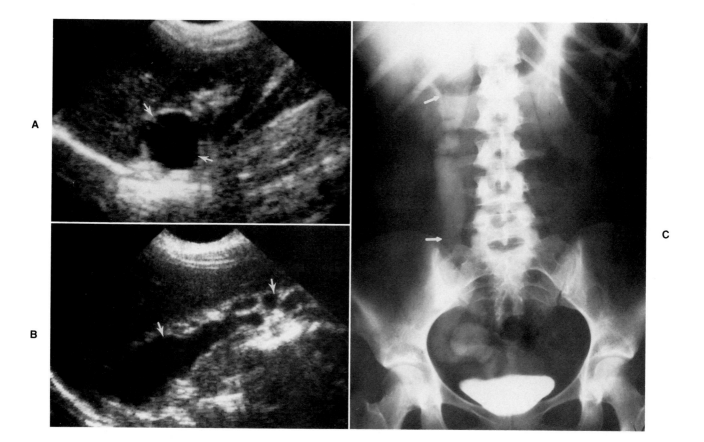

FIG 9-57. Obstructed upper pole moiety of duplex collecting system mimicking cyst. **A,** Longitudinal sonogram shows upper pole cystic mass *(arrows)* with single septation. **B,** More medial longitudinal scan demonstrates continuity between upper pole "cyst" and tortuous tubular dilated upper pole ureter *(arrows).* **C,** Delayed radiographic film from excretory urogram confirms poorly functioning obstructed upper pole moiety *(arrows).*

third of the ureters in young adults and are the most common benign primary neoplasm of the ureter or renal pelvis. The ultrasound appearance of these lesions has not been described. Radiographic contrast-enhanced studies may be normal or show hydronephrosis with a "cork-screw"-filling defect, which is classically described but not often seen.[198]

As ureteric masses have a relatively nonspecific appearance, biopsy or surgery is usually required for diagnosis. In many cases of ureteric pathologic conditions, resultant hydronephrosis is the only sonographically detected abnormality.

THE URINARY BLADDER
Bladder Neoplasms

Although cystoscopy and cystography are usually the initial imaging techniques for suspected bladder neoplasms, studies have shown that ultrasound is an accurate method for the detection, follow-up and staging of tumors.[199,200] Relatively large tumors may be missed

on transabdominal ultrasound as a result of technical factors and patient obesity. Optimal bladder distension is important.

Transitional Cell Carcinoma

Transitional cell carcinoma (TCC) is the most common primary bladder neoplasm (Fig. 9-58). Any mass or focal thickening of the bladder wall should raise the suspicion of the presence of TCC; however, the differential diagnosis of such masses is large, including invasive prostate carcinoma, cystitis, trabeculation, and wall thickening following long-standing bladder outlet obstruction, adherent blood clot, pyogenic debris, and postoperative changes or complications.[199-202] Other causes of bladder masses include endometriosis and neurofibromatosis.[203-205] The ultrasound appearance of a relatively hypoechoic mass—but one which is more echogenic than bladder mucosa and submucosa, although typical of TCC—is nonspecific. Thus cystoscopy and biopsy are necessary for definitive diagnosis

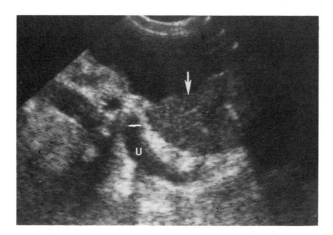

FIG 9-58. Transitional cell carcinoma of bladder. Longitudinal pelvic sonogram shows TCC *(arrows)* obstructing right ureter *(U)*.

when such bladder masses are identified. TCC may be a solitary mass or a multifocal process.

Benign **bladder papillomas,** which are forerunners of TCC, have a sonographic appearance identical to early TCC. Frequent cystoscopic evaluation and IV or retrograde contrast-enhanced urography should also be performed with these premalignant tumors.

Squamous cell carcinoma (SCC) accounts for approximately 3% of primary bladder neoplasms and is associated with chronic infection, stones, or strictures. There is a high incidence of SCC following schistosomiasis (estimated to be up to 27%).[206] SCC tends to be very aggressive and invasive but cannot be differentiated sonographically from TCC. SCC often arises in bladder diverticula, possibly as a result of the effects of chronic stasis or infection (Fig. 9-59). Leukoplakia of the bladder or squamous metaplasia are also associated with chronic infection and stones but are rarely imaged.

Neoplasms may develop in a **urachal remnant,** near the dome of the bladder, or between the bladder and the umbilicus. The vast majority of these neoplasms are mucinous adenocarcinomas and occur most commonly in males between the ages of 50 to 60 years.[207]

Prostate carcinoma often causes a large, irregular bladder-base mass, which may produce bladder outlet obstruction and invade the bladder wall.

Cystitis

Cystitis is more common in females than in males. Acutely, there is diffuse or focal bladder wall thickening.[202] In later stages the bladder may become small and contracted as a result of fibrosis or spasm. Focal bladder wall thickening mimicking carcinoma may be seen with most types of cystitis.[205] Fistula formation may occur with severe forms of cystitis, but it is most commonly a complication of radiation cystitis. **Bullous**

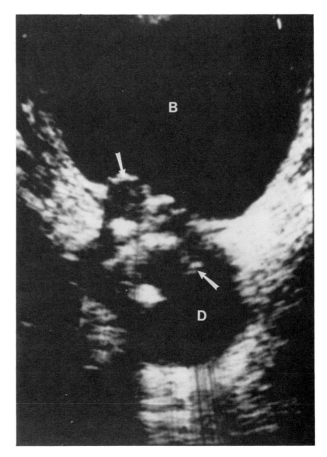

FIG 9-59. Squamous cell carcinoma *(arrows)* within bladder diverticulum *(D)* on transverse scan. *B* indicates bladder.

cystitis usually occurs after infection or catheterization.[208] Wall thickening may be focal, often occurring along the posterior bladder wall, and a polypoid appearance that may mimic carcinoma may develop as a result of redundant mucosa. With chronic catheterization, bladder wall thickening becomes more diffuse. **Hemorrhagic cystitis** may be caused by prolonged Cytoxan therapy. Ultrasound findings include intraluminal echogenic debris caused by blood clots, wall thickening, and even focal calcification. Cystitis glandularis may develop as a result of chronic infection and predisposes the patient to adenocarcinoma of the bladder.

Emphysematous cystitis may be diagnosed sonographically by demonstrating echogenic shadowing foci within the bladder wall.[209] The echogenic foci cause "dirty shadowing" posterior to gas collections. If the entire bladder wall is filled with gas, the bladder may mimic gas-containing bowel. Approximately half of patients with emphysematous cystitis have diabetes mellitus; infection is usually caused by *E. coli.*[209]

Schistosomiasis from *Schistosoma haematobium* in-

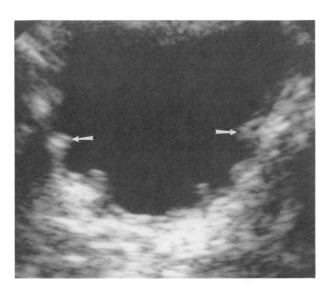

FIG 9-60. Bladder outlet obstruction. Transverse bladder sonogram shows marked trabeculation *(arrows)* caused by bladder outlet obstruction.

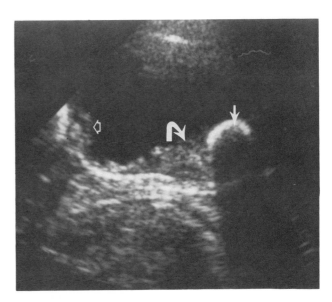

FIG 9-61. Bladder stone. Transverse scan shows left-sided bladder stone *(arrow)*, blood clot *(curved arrow)*, and bladder wall thickening *(open arrow)* in patient with severe cystitis.

fection causes polypoid bladder wall thickening as a result of granuloma formation. Later, fibrosis produces a small-capacity bladder, and bladder carcinoma may occur.[206,210] Vesicoureteral reflux may also develop. Bladder wall calcifications are common and produce discrete shadowing.

Bladder Outlet Obstruction

Bladder wall thickening and trabeculation occur with any type of bladder outlet obstruction (Fig. 9-60). The bladder is usually markedly distended, but in neurogenic dysfunction, the bladder lumen may be small[211,212] with striking muscular hypertrophy and trabeculation.

Spinal cord injury or spinal dysraphism may cause **neurogenic bladder dysfunction.** The internal sphincter cannot relax, and the bladder remains distended unless intermittent catheterization is performed. Vesicoureteral reflux may occur.[211] Sonographic voiding cystoureterography—performed using endorectal sonography to visualize the bladder, urethra, and sphincter—can demonstrate hyperreflexia produced by catheters in cases of spinal cord injury and can provide insights into the dynamic physiology of voiding in these patients.[212]

Tumors, especially prostatic carcinoma or TCC, may obstruct the bladder. Malignant bladder-base masses are usually asymmetric or eccentric (as opposed to BPH, which tends to be midline and symmetric). CT or MRI are generally required to evaluate the pelvic tumor extent in such cases.

Ectopic ureteroceles that are located medial and inferior to the normal ureteral insertion site may produce

bladder outlet obstruction, ureteral obstruction, and reflux.

Bladder stones may develop as a result of local stasis or may be passed down from the upper collecting system. These stones rarely cause bladder outlet obstruction, but they may serve as a nidus for infection. Ultrasound readily demonstrates bladder stones as mobile, echogenic intraluminal structures with acoustic shadowing (Fig. 9-61). Occasionally, stones may become adherent because of inflammation, infection, and hemorrhage. In such cases they may be indistinguishable from dystrophic calcification within adherent blood clots or tumors. **Blood clots** within the bladder typically do not demonstrate shadows, are echogenic, and are adherent to the bladder wall. In addition, fluid-fluid levels caused by extensive intracystic hemorrhage may be seen.

Extrinsic Bladder Compression

Endometriosis may produce focal masses outside and within the bladder lumen.[203,204] **Neurofibromatosis** may produce diffuse or focal bladder wall thickening.[205] Adherent bowel loops may indent the bladder and mimic masses; however, they can usually be identified by peristalsis. A water enema, confirming fluid-filled bowel loops with changing configuration, may be helpful.[202]

Colon cancer or **diverticulitis** may invade the bladder, resulting in bladder perforation or formation of an enterovesical fistula. Bladder wall irregularity, or a mass, is all that is usually demonstrated on ultrasound (Fig. 9-62). However, debris in the bladder can be

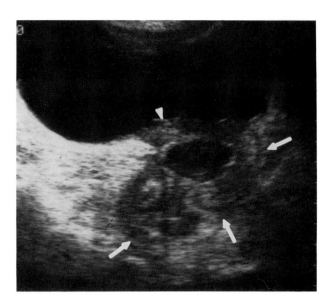

FIG 9-62. Crohn's disease, with enterovesical fistula. Thickened loops of small bowel with associated inflammatory mass *(arrows)* lie adjacent to left bladder base on this transverse scan. Bladder wall is thick and irregular in this region *(arrowhead)*.

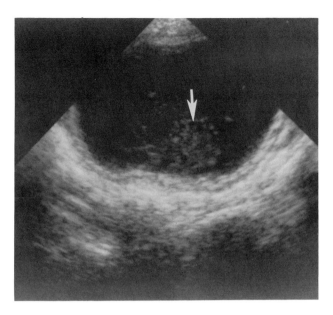

FIG 9-63. Mucous pseudomass after augmentation cystoplasty. Echogenic mass *(arrow)* is seen in bladder on this transverse image.
(Courtesy Barbara S. Hertzberg, M.D., Duke University Medical Center, Durham, NC.)

seen, suggesting infection and/or fistula. In the absence of instrumentation, air in the bladder suggests a fistula or infection by a gas-forming organism.

Cystic pelvic masses that frequently indent the bladder include urinomas, lymphoceles, abscesses, hematomas, ovarian or retroperitoneal cysts, vascular aneurysms, and fluid-filled bowel loops. **Solid pelvic masses** that may produce bladder indentation include organized hematomas, nonliquefactive abscesses, retroperitoneal neoplasms, uterine fibroids, and pelvic lipomatosis. Scarring and fibrosis after AP resection may also distort the bladder shape and contour.

Trauma

Extraperitoneal urinoma can be identified with ultrasound, but it may be difficult to distinguish from the bladder itself.[213] Differentiation of urinoma from a hematoma is not always possible, acutely; however, hematomas tend to become more echogenic and heterogeneous in appearance with time. Intraperitoneal leak produces urine ascites, which is sonographically indistinguishable from hemorrhage or ascites caused by other causes. Spontaneous postoperative bladder rupture from overdistention may occur at sites of previous suprapubic catheterization in children.

Postoperative Changes

Augmentation and replacement cystoplasty creates a variety of findings, including a thick or irregular bladder wall in 96% of cases, a pseudomass in the lumen in 89%, and fine debris or linear strands in 47%.[15]

Pseudomasses caused by folds of incorporated bowel, intraluminal mucous collections, or bowel intussucepted into the bladder to prevent reflux are potentially confusing findings (Fig. 9-63). Pancreas transplants are becoming more common, and the connecting fluid-filled duodenal segment can be identified at its attachment to the bladder. Segmental peristalsis can often be identified during real-time sonographic examination.

Instrumentation and catheterization of the bladder can introduce air, which fills the nondependent bladder lumen with echogenic foci. Irregular shadowing with reverberations is common, and extensive intracystic gas may obscure the bladder lumen. Differentiation of gas from stones is usually simple because stones are located in dependent portions of the lumen and produce discrete, well-defined posterior acoustic shadows. Fluid collections or masses behind the bladder can undergo biopsy or can be aspirated with a transcystic approach. In one report the only complication was a single case of transient hematuria.[214] This approach should be avoided if infection is suspected or if loops of bowel will be traversed during the biopsy. In our experience, the transcystic approach can be difficult as a result of bladder spasm and patient discomfort.

Congenital Anomalies

Bladder diverticula may be acquired or congenital and represent external herniation of mucosa through the muscularis. Occasionally, bladder diverticula may develop intraluminally or intramurally.[202] A **hutch diverticulum** may be difficult to differentiate from a uretero-

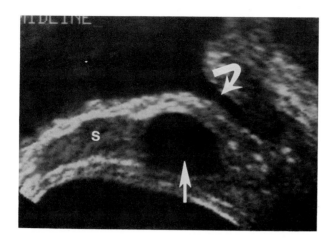

FIG 9-64. Urethra after previous transurethral resection. Transrectal ultrasound showing simple cyst *(arrow)* at base of prostate (probably within seminal vesicle *[S]*) separate from proximal urethra *(curved arrow)*. Proximal urethra is well seen because of previous TURP.

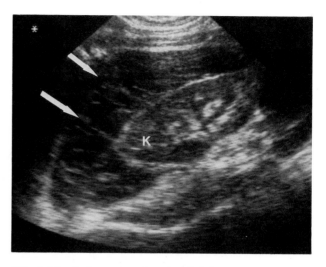

FIG 9-65. Peritransplant lymphocele. Large septated fluid collection *(arrows)* is seen adjacent to transplant kidney *(K)*. Minimal pelviectasis present.

cele with ultrasound, but the demonstration of peristaltic activity with real-time sonographic evaluation indicates a ureterocele. Urachal cysts or remnants occur between the dome of the bladder and the umbilicus. Ultrasound may demonstrate a cystic mass in this region or a diverticular outpouching from the dome of the bladder.[215,216] Infection, abscess, and occasionally an externally draining sinus may develop through the umbilicus.[215] Mucinous adenocarcinoma can develop in the urachal remnants.[207] Duplication of the bladder is very rare and is usually diagnosed in childhood.[217]

THE URETHRA

Abnormalities are uncommon in the adult urethra, and relatively few reports have dealt with ultrasound evaluation of the urethra.[17-20,218,219] Urethral diverticula in females may rarely be demonstrated with transabdominal ultrasound.[219] They appear as cystic structures below the base of the bladder along the anterior aspect of the vagina. One report showed that ultrasound better estimated the size of the diverticulum containing debris than occlusive urethrography. Although the proximal urethra can be visualized transrectally and the distal urethra is easily identified during penile artery evaluation, the ultrasound evaluations of urethral injuries are not well described. Translabial, transrectal, and transvaginal approaches hold promise for ultrasound evaluation of the urethra (Fig. 9-64).[212]

RENAL TRANSPLANT EVALUATION
Perinephric Fluid Collections

Perinephric fluid collections are reported in as many as 50% of renal transplantations[123,220] as complications

of surgery or biopsy or manifestations of rejection or infection.

The most common peritransplant fluid collections are **lymphoceles,** which usually arise 1 to 3 weeks after transplantation, although they may arise several months after surgery.[220] These fluid collections usually develop medially or inferiorally to the lower pole of the kidney and may become quite large. Sonographically, they frequently contain septations, and may contain debris (Fig. 9-65). Although lymphoceles are usually asymptomatic, when large they may cause obstruction, allograft dysfunction, or both. Secondary infection of lymphoceles should be suspected if significant amounts of internal debris are detected. Aspiration and drainage may provide adequate treatment of lymphoceles; however, they frequently recur after drainage, necessitating surgical excision to preserve renal function or relieve symptoms.

Urinomas are often early postoperative complications developing within the first 1 to 2 weeks after transplantation. These may be related to surgical complications and anastomotic leaks. They may also be related to vascular injuries of the transplant collecting system with subsequent infarction and necrosis leading to rupture and urine extravasation. Urinomas may also follow severe renal transplant obstruction. These fluid collections commonly arise near the lower pole of the transplant or in the region of the bladder and may be associated with ascites (Fig. 9-66). Contrast-enhanced CT, retrograde contrast-enhanced studies, radionuclide studies, or aspiration of the fluid collection may be needed to characterize the fluid.

Subcapsular or extracapsular **hematomas** are less common peritransplant fluid collections that usually arise soon after surgery or biopsy. Allograft pseudoan-

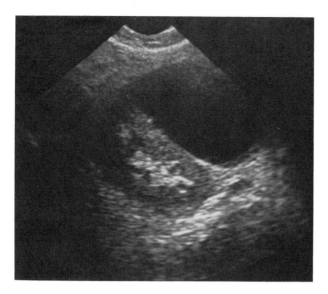

FIG 9-66. Urinoma. Transverse sonogram of renal transplant shows perinephric fluid collection without debris or septations.

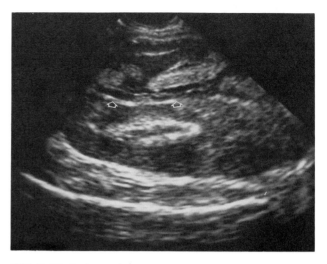

FIG 9-67. Peritransplant postbiopsy subcapsular hematoma. Longitudinal sonogram of renal allograft shows large, relatively complex collection *(open arrows)* anterior to kidney. (Courtesy of SR Wilson, M.D., Toronto General Hospital, Canada.)

eurysms, particularly peripheral ones, may rupture producing hematomas. **Sonographically,** hematomas may have a variety of appearances, depending on their age. Often they are complex masses that may contain debris or septations (Fig. 9-67). Subcapsular fluid collections may also indent the renal parenchyma, suggesting a subcapsular process.

Peritransplant **abscesses** rarely develop de novo, but rather they result from infection of a preexisting fluid collection, most commonly at 4 to 5 weeks after transplantation. Debris in a previously anechoic cystic mass should suggest superinfection in the appropriate clinical setting. Echogenic nondependent foci with "dirty shadowing" in a cystic mass is highly suggestive of an abscess.

Obstruction

Early postoperative edema at the ureteroneocystostomy site frequently causes mild, self-limited obstruction of the renal allograft. Once the edema has subsided, some degree of mild pelvic dilation may remain, although the obstruction has resolved and renal function is normal. **True obstruction** can result from a number of causes including extrinsic masses, ureteric stricture formation caused by vascular compromise or rejection, blood clots, sloughed papillae, or renal calculi (Fig. 9-68).[221] An overly distended urinary bladder may produce **functional obstruction** with a resultant sonogram demonstrating hydronephrosis, which frequently resolves following voiding. An increased RI may be seen with many complications of renal transplantation and cannot be used to distinguish a dilated system from other causes of renal transplant dysfunction.

Rejection

Renal transplant rejection can be hyperacute, accelerated acute, acute, or chronic.[222] The more severe and acute the rejection process, the more marked the **sonographic abnormalities** tend to be. Severe hyperacute or accelerated acute rejection may produce a markedly enlarged allograft with obscured corticomedullary definition and markedly abnormal Doppler flow velocity wave forms. The renal cortex is usually hypoechoic; however, in cases of severe rejection, marked hemorrhage in the parenchyma may result in scattered heterogeneous areas of increased echogenicity. Other features of less severe acute rejection include allograft enlargement, prominent hypoechoic medullary pyramids, increased or decreased renal cortical echogenicity, relative loss of corticomedullary definition, decreased renal sinus echogenicity, and thickening of the uroepithelium of the renal allograft, which can also be seen in infection, obstruction, and autoimmune disease (Fig. 9-69).[223] Papillary necrosis[152] or peritransplant fluid collections may also be present. Although the presence of several of these findings is highly suggestive of acute rejection, all of these abnormalities can be seen with other medical complications of transplantation.

Numerous recent studies have evaluated **pulsed Doppler imaging** assessment of renal allograft arterial flow in acute rejection.[123-127,224-229] The interlobar or segmental artery traces are the most reliable for analy-

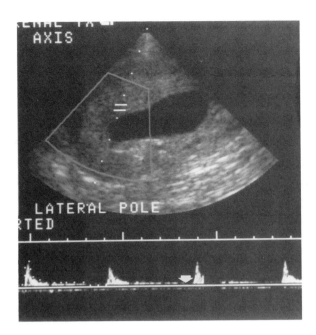

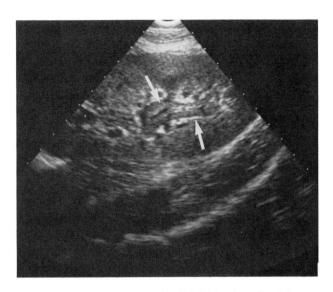

FIG 9-68. Obstructed renal transplant caused by ureteric stone shows markedly elevated RI with absent end diastolic flow *(arrow)*. RI returned to normal after obstruction was relieved.

FIG 9-69. Nonspecific uroepithelial thickening of pelvis *(arrows)* is seen in this patient with severe lupus nephritis. (Courtesy of SR Wilson, M.D., Toronto General Hospital, Canada.)

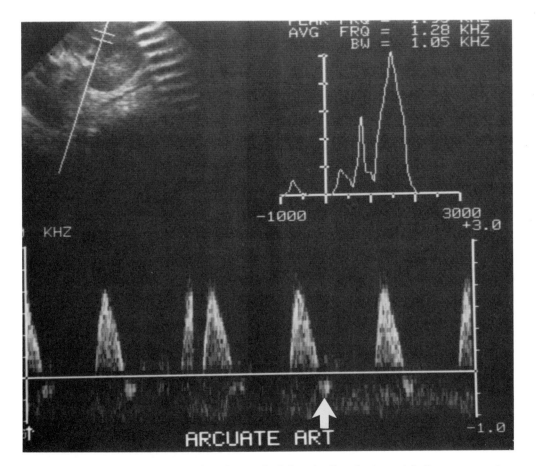

FIG 9-70. Acute transplant rejection. Reversal of flow in diastole *(arrow)* indicates extremely high resistance.

sis.[227] High-impedance flow waveforms with decreased, absent, or reversed end diastolic flow have been reported in acute rejection (Fig. 9-70). Color flow Doppler ultrasound demonstrates analogus qualitative changes with flashes of arterial flow noted during systole but little or no flow during diastole.[121] Color Doppler imaging has proved useful in rapid localization of arteries for pulsed Doppler spectral analysis, reducing examination time. Furthermore, it provides a more global appreciation of focal variation in organ perfusion.

Although initial studies indicated very high specificities using a RI threshold of 0.90 and a pulsatility index threshold of 1.80, sensitivities were low using these numbers.[130,226-228] When lower thresholds for the RI and pulsatility index were used (RI of 0.70, PI of 1.50), sensitivity increased, but specificity decreased significantly.

RI values greater than 0.90 are also reported in severe ATN, renal vein obstruction, pyelonephritis, extrarenal compression, ureteric obstruction, chronic rejection, Cyclosporin toxicity, and hemolytic-uremic syndrome.[125-127,230] Doppler waveforms, which demonstrate increased impedance or resistance in the renal arterial system, whether in an allograft or a native kidney, suggest renal dysfunction but are very nonspecific. Thus, unless clinical findings or image abnormalities are diagnostic of a likely cause of these abnormal waveforms, renal biopsy is usually required to diagnose the cause of transplant dysfunction.

Acute Tubular Necrosis

Acute tubular necrosis (ATN) usually presents soon after transplantation in the same clinical time frame as hyperacute or accelerated acute rejection. There are no sonographic features that reliably differentiate ATN from acute rejection.[127-129] Recent preliminary work using MRI suggests that this imaging modality may be more useful in making this distinction.[231]

Cyclosporin Toxicity

It is important to distinguish cyclosporin toxicity from rejection clinically because the appropriate treatment for this entity is diametrically different from that for rejection. Although in most cases cyclosporin toxicity is less likely to cause changes in the appearance of the allograft or to produce increased RIs, cyclosporin may produce an enlarged kidney with increased cortical echogenicity and prominent medullary pyramids (Fig. 9-71).[229] In addition, there are reports of significantly increased RIs associated with biopsy-proven cyclosporin toxicity.[126] Biopsy is frequently necessary for diagnosis.

Vascular Complications

The frequency of renal artery stenosis in renal allografts ranges from 1.6% to 16%.[232] Renal artery stenosis can result in decreased allograft function and hypertension and is divided into two major types.[133] Focal anastomotic site stenoses are probably caused by a reaction to suture material and occur most often with end-to-end anastomoses. **Long segment** stenoses distal to the anastomoses are related to scarring, possibly as a result of rejection, and are more common with end-to-side anastomoses.

Renal artery stenosis in an allograft demonstrates Doppler imaging abnormalities identical to those seen in the native kidney. Focal high-velocity disturbed flow is detected at and immediately distal to a stenosis. Velocity measurements exceeding 180 cm/sec are suggestive of stenosis. Intrarenal Doppler sampling distal to a stenosis may show a normal waveform, but overall flow may be damped and the initial systolic upslope may be prolonged (Fig. 9-41). Color Doppler imaging may be particularly useful in tracing the entire course of the main renal artery from the iliac vessels to the renal hi-

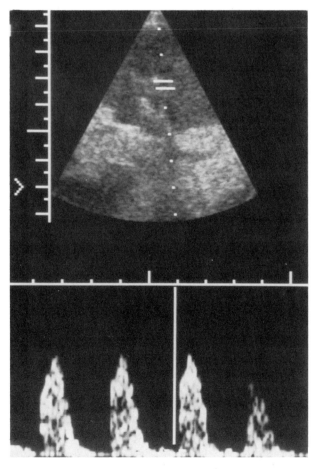

FIG 9-71. Cyclosporin toxicity. Decreased diastolic flow velocities indicating high resistance are seen; however, this is nonspecific finding.

lum. It also allows for detection of the appropriate Doppler angle, which facilitates calculation of renal artery velocities. Furthermore, color Doppler imaging may clearly demonstrate areas of luminal narrowing and disturbed flow. A perivascular color Doppler artifact caused by significant soft tissue vibrations surrounding severe stenoses may also be present.

Complete **arterial occlusion** and renal allograft infarction can be demonstrated with pulsed and color Doppler imaging. Severe acute vascular rejection is a common cause of allograft infarction and may result in complete occlusion of the renal arterial system.[133,227] Postoperative renal stenoses may also progress to total occlusion. There is controversy regarding whether further imaging is necessary if Doppler ultrasound indicates complete arterial occlusion in an allograft. Taylor et al[133] suggest it is appropriate to operate immediately on a patient if Doppler imaging indicates allograft arterial obstruction. Reuther et al[124] reported at least two cases in which Doppler imaging demonstrated no renal arterial or venous flow, but digital subtraction angiography showed flow was present. Nishioka et al[233] showed a correlation between color Doppler ultrasound visualization of renal allograft vasculature and serum creatinine, which implies that, if function is poor enough, blood flow in patent vessels may not be detected. Thus it would appear that the detection of renal arterial flow is useful, but failure to detect flow may not indicate complete obstruction.

Renal vein thrombosis (RVT) is a rare, serious complication of transplantation, usually occurring within the first postoperative days.[124] Absent capsular collaterals in the renal allografts produces considerable increased renal artery resistance in renal vein thrombosis. Markedly elevated RI or PI values indicative of high resistance are nonspecific in nature, but detection of reversed diastolic flow in the renal arterial system associated with absent renal vein flow is highly suggestive of acute renal vein thrombosis. Such markedly abnormal end-diastolic flow reversal may also be seen in acute rejection, acute tubular necrosis, severe obstruction, and in cases of transplant compression by extrarenal fluid collections (Fig. 9-67).[230] Sonography may also directly visualize thrombus in a distended vein.

Complications of renal biopsies, such as AVFs and pseudoaneurysms, can be readily evaluated with Doppler ultrasound, color Doppler ultrasound, or both. The sonographic features of these allograft vascular complications are similar to those seen in native kidneys. However, the superficial location of the allograft enhances their detection rate by color Doppler imaging.[233]

Transplant-Related Masses

When posttransplant patients demonstrate masses in the region of the transplant or in other portions of the body, the possibility of a **transplant-related malignancy** should be considered.[234] The Epstein-Barr virus has been implicated as a causative factor in the development of lymphomas in the posttransplant population, which may be augmented by use of cyclosporin A and OKT3 immunosuppression. Lymphomas and lymphoproliferative disorders often develop within 6 months following transplantation. Other malignancies that may develop include squamous cell carcinomas of the skin.

REFERENCES

1. Goss CM: *Gray's Anatomy.* Philadelphia: Lea & Febiger; 1969:1275-1287.
2. Dodds WJ, Darweesh RMA, Lawson TL, et al: The retroperitoneal spaces revisited. *AJR* 1986;147:1155-1161.
3. Chesbrough RM, Burkhard TK, Martinez AT, et al: Gerota versus Zuckerkandl: the renal fascia revisited. *Radiology* 1989;173:845-846.

Normal sonographic appearance

4. Carter AR, Horgan JG, Hennings TA, et al: The junctional parenchymal defect: a sonographic variant of renal anatomy. *Radiology* 1985;154:499–502.
5. Mahony BS, Jeffrey RB, Laing FC: Septa of Bertin: a sonographic pseudotumor. *J Clin Ultrasound* 1983;11:317-319.
6. Lafortune M, Constantin A, Breton G, et al: Sonography of the hypertrophied column of Bertin. *AJR* 1986;146:53-56.
7. Amendola MA, Bree RL, Pollack HM, et al: Small renal cell carcinomas: resolving a diagnostic dilemma. *Radiology* 1988;166:637-641
8. Middleton WD, Melson GL: Renal duplication artifact in ultrasound imaging. *Radiology* 1989;173:427-429.
9. Platt JF, Rubin JM, Bowerman RA, et al: The inability to detect kidney disease on the basis of echogenicity. *AJR* 1988;151:317-319.
10. Britt AR, Platt J, Rubin JM, et al: Reassessment of renal echogenicity: effect of electronically-focused vs fixed-focus transducers. *J Ultrasound Med* 1990;9:S20.
11. Hircak H, Slovis TL, Callen PW, et al: Neonatal kidneys: sonographic anatomic correlation. *Radiology* 1983;147:699-702.
12. Marchal GJ, Baert AL, Eeckels R, et al: Sonographic evaluation of normal ureteral submucosal tunnel in infancy and childhood. *Pediatr Radiol* 1983;13:125-129.
13. Elejalde BR, deElejalde MM: Ureteral ejaculation of urine visualized by ultrasound. *J Clin Ultrasound* 1983;11:475-476.
14. Kremer H, Dobrinski W, Mikyska M, et al: Ultrasonic in vivo and in vitro studies on the nature of the ureteral jet phenomenon. *Radiology* 1982;142:175-177.
15. Hertzberg BS, Bowie JD, King LR, et al: Augmentation and replacement cystoplasty: sonographic findings. *Radiology* 1987;3-856.
16. Jequier S, Rousseau O: Sonographic measurements of the normal bladder wall in children. *AJR* 1987;3:566.
17. Hennigan HW, DuBose TJ: Sonography of the normal fetal urethra. *AJR* 1985;145:839-841.
18. White RD, McQuown D, McCarthy TA, et al: Real-time ultrasonography in the evaluation of urinary stress incontinence. *Am J Obstet Gynecol* 1980;5:237.
19. Rifkin MD: Sonourethrography: technique of evaluation of the prostatic urethra. *Radiology* 1984;153:791-792.
20. Shapero LG, Friedland GW, Perkash I: Transrectal sonographic

voiding cystourethrography: studies in neuromuscular bladder dysfunction. *AJR* 1983;141:83-90.

Scanning techniques

21. Kriegshauser JS, Carroll BS: Doppler ultrasound in the genitourinary tract. *Radiology Report* 1990;2:250-262.

The kidney

22. Bosniak MA: The current radiological approach to renal cysts. *Radiology* 1986;158:1-10.
23. Hayden CK, Swischuk LE, Smith TH, et al: Renal cystic disease in childhood. *Radiographics* 1986;6:97-116.
24. Pollack HM, Banner MP, Arter PH, et al: The accuracy of gray-scale renal ultrasonography in differentiating cystic neoplasms from benign cysts. *Radiology* 1982;143:741-745.
25. Amis ES, Cronan JJ, Pfister RC: Needle puncture of cystic renal masses: a survey of the Society of Uroradiology. *AJR* 1987;148:297-299.
26. Rosenberg ER, Korobkin M, Foster W, et al: The significance of septations in a renal cyst. *AJR* 1985;144:593-595.
27. Zirinsky K, Auh YH, Rubenstein WA, et al: Computed tomography of the hyperdense renal cyst: sonographic correlation. *AJR* 1984;143:151-156.
28. Foster WL Jr, Roberts L Jr, Halvorsen RA Jr, et al: Sonography of small renal masses with indeterminant density characteristics on computed tomography. *Urol Radiol* 1988;10:59-67.
29. Mellins HZ: Cystic dilatation of the upper urinary tract: a radiologist's developmental model. *Radiology* 1984;153:291-301.
30. Grossman H, Rosenberg ER, Bowie JD, et al: Sonographic diagnosis of renal cystic diseases. *AJR* 1983;140:81-85.
31. Cronan JJ, Amis ES, Yoder IC, et al: Peripelvic cysts: an imposter of sonographic hydronephrosis. *J Ultrasound Med* 1982;1:229-236.
32. Hidalgo H, Dunnick MR, Rosenberg ER, et al: Parapelvic cysts: appearance on CT and sonography. *AJR* 1982;138:667-671.
33. Morton MJ, Charboneau JW: Arteriovenous fistula after biopsy of renal transplant: detection and monitoring with color flow and duplex ultrasonography. *Mayo Clin Proc* 1989;64:531-534.
34. Testa S, LiBassi S, Barbara L: Cyst of the kidney or spontaneous splenorenal shunt?: differentiation by pulsed Doppler sonography. *AJR* 1989;153:431.
35. Bernstein J, Evan AP, Gardner KD: Epithelial hyperplasia in human polycystic kidney diseases: its role in pathogenesis and risk of neoplasia. *Am J Pathol* 1987;129:92-101.
36. Rosenfield AT, Lipson MH, Wolf B, et al: Ultrasonography and nephrotomography in the presymptomatic diagnosis of dominantly inherited (adult-onset) polycystic kidney disease. *Radiology* 1980;135:423-427.
37. Pedicelli G, Jequier S, Bowen A, et al: Multicystic dysplastic kidneys: spontaneous regression demonstrated with ultrasound. *Radiology* 1986;160:23-26.
38. Avni EF, Thoua Y, Lalmand B, et al: Multicystic dysplastic kidney: natural history from in utero diagnosis and postnatal follow-up. *J Urol* 1987;138:1420-1424.
39. Garel LA, Habib R, Pariente D, et al: Juvenile nephronophthisis: sonography appearance in children with severe uremia. *Radiology* 1984;151:93-95.
40. Rego JD, Laing FC, Jeffrey RB: Ultrasonographic diagnosis of medullary cystic disease. *J Ultrasound Med* 1983;2:433-436.
41. Mindell HJ: Imaging studies for screening native kidneys in long-term dialysis patients. *AJR* 1989;153:768-769.
42. Jabour BA, Ralls PW, Tang WW, et al: Acquired cystic disease of the kidneys: computed tomography and ultrasonography appraisal in patients on peritoneal and hemodialysis. *Invest Radiol* 1987;22:728-732.
43. Andersen BL, Curry NS, Gobien RP: Sonography of evolving renal cystic transformation associated with hemodialysis. *AJR* 1983;141:1003-1004.
44. Bretan PN, Busch MP, Hricak H, et al: Chronic renal failure: a significant risk factor in the development of acquired renal cysts and renal cell carcinoma: case reports and review of the literature. *Cancer* 1986;57:1871-1879.
45. Boileau M, Foley R, Flechner S, et al: Renal adenocarcinoma and end stage kidney disease. *J Urol* 1987;138:603-606.
46. Taylor AJ, Cohen EP, Erickson SJ, et al: Renal imaging in long-term dialysis patients: a comparison of computed tomography and sonography. *AJR* 1989;153:765-767.
47. Kutcher R, Amodio JB, Rosenblatt R: Uremic renal cystic disease: value of sonographic screening. *Radiology* 1983;147:833-835.
48. Banner MP, Pollack HM, Chatten J, et al: Multilocular renal cysts: radiologic-pathologic correlation. *AJR* 1981;136:239-247.
49. Charboneau JW, Hattery RR, Ernst EC, et al: Spectrum of sonographic findings in 125 renal masses other than benign simple cysts. *AJR* 1983;140:87-94.
50. Feldberg MAM, vanWaes PFGM: Multilocular cystic renal cell carcinoma. *AJR* 1982;138:953-955.
51. Foster WL, Halvorsen RA, Dunnick NR: The clandestine renal cell carcinoma: atypical appearances and presentations. *Radiographics* 1985;5:175-192.
52. Levine E, Huntrakoon M, Wetzel LH: Small renal neoplasms: clinical, pathologic, and imaging features. *AJR* 1989;153:69-73.
53. Makamel E, Konichezky M, Engelstein D, et al: Incidental small renal tumors accompanying clinically overt renal cell carcinoma. *J Urol* 1988;140:22-24.
54. Shiamato K, Sadayuke S, Ishigaki T, et al: Intratumoral blood flow: evaluation with color Doppler echography. *Radiology* 1987;165:683-685.
55. Taylor KJW, Ramos I, Carter D, et al: Correlation of Doppler US tumor signals with neovascular morphologic features. *Radiology* 1988;166:57-62.
56. Kuijpers D, Jaspers R: Renal masses: differential diagnosis with pulsed Doppler ultrasound. *Radiology* 1989;170:59-60.
57. Dubbins PA, Wells I: Renal carcinoma: duplex Doppler evaluation. *Br J Radiol* 1986;59:231-236.
58. Kier R, Taylor KJW, Feyock AL, et al: Renal masses: characterization with Doppler ultrasound. *Radiology* 1990;176:703-707.
59. Pamilo M, Suramo I, Paivansalo M: Characteristics of hypernephromas as seen with ultrasound and computed tomography. *J Clin Ultrasound* 1983;11:254-259.
60. Hartman DS, Davidson AJ, Davis CJ, et al: Infiltrative renal lesions: computed tomographic-sonographic-pathologic correlation. *AJR* 1988;150:1061-1064.
61. Schwerk WB, Schwerk WN, Rodeck G: Venous renal tumor extension: a prospective ultrasound evaluation. *Radiology* 1985;156:491-495.
62. Hietala SO, Ekelund L, Ljungberg B: Venous invasion in renal cell carcinoma: a correlative clinical and radiologic study. *Urol Radiol* 1988;9:210-216.
63. Chonko AM, Weiss SM, Stein JH, et al: Renal involvement in tuberous sclerosis. *Am J Med* 1974;56:124.
64. McCullough DL, Scott R, Seybold HM: Renal angiomyolipoma (hamartoma): review of the literature and report of 7 cases. *J Urol* 1971;105:32.
65. Hartman DS, Goldman SM, Friedman AC, et al: Angiomyolipoma: ultrasonic-pathologic correlation. *Radiology* 1981;139:451-458.
66. Curry NS, Schabel SI, Garvin AJ, et al: Intratumoral fat in a renal oncocytoma mimicking angiomyolipoma. *AJR* 1990;154:307-308.

67. Zappasodi F, Sanna G, Fiorentini G, et al: Small hyperechoic nodules of the renal parenchyma. *J Clin Ultrasound* 1985;13:321-324.

68. Bennington JL, Beckwith JB: Tumors of the kidney, renal pelvis, and ureter. In: *Atlas of Tumor Pathology: Second Series.* Fascicle 12. Washington, DC: Armed Forces Institute of Pathology; 1975:94-99.

69. Goiney RC, Goldenberg L, Cooperberg PL, et al: Renal oncocytoma: sonographic analysis of 14 cases. *AJR* 1984;143:1001-1004.

70. Ball DS, Friedman AC, Hartman DS, et al: Scar sign of renal oncocytoma: magnetic resonance imaging appearance and lack of specificity. *Urol Radiol* 1986;8:46-48.

71. Quinn MJ, Hartman DS, Friedman AC, et al: Renal oncocytoma: new observations. *Radiology* 1984;153:49-53.

72. Lieber MM: Renal oncocytoma. In: Kaufman JJ, ed. *Current Urologic Therapy.* Philadelphia: WB Saunders; 1986:89-92.

73. Grant DC, Dee GJ, Yoder IC, et al: Sonography in transitional cell carcinoma of the renal pelvis. *Urol Radiol* 1986;8:1-5.

74. Yousem DM, Gatewood OMB, Goldman SM, et al: Synchronous and metachronous transitional cell carcinoma of the urinary tract: prevalence, incidence, and radiographic detection. *Radiology* 1988;167:613-618.

75. Winalski CS, Lipman JC, Tumch SS: Ureteral neoplasms. *RadioGraphics* 1990;10:271-283.

76. Cronan JJ, Yoder IC, Amis ES, et al: The myth of anechoic renal sinus fat. *Radiology* 1982;144:149-152.

77. Choyke PL, White EM, Zeman RK, et al: Renal metastases: clinicopathologic and radiologic correlation. *Radiology* 1987;162:359-363.

78. Pagani JJ: Solid renal mass in the cancer patient: second primary renal cell carcinoma versus renal metastasis. *J Comput Assist Tomogr* 1983;7:444-448.

79. Charnsangarej C: Lymphoma of the genitourinary tract. *Radiol Clin North Am* 1990;28-877, 1990.

80. Richmond JJ, Sherman RS, Diamond HD, et al: Renal lesions associated with malignant lymphomas. *Am J Med* 1962;32:184-207.

81. Hartman DS, Davis Jr CJ, Goldman SM, et al: Renal lymphoma: radiologic-pathologic correlation in 21 cases. *Radiology* 1982;144:759-766.

82. Green D, Carroll BA: Ultrasound of renal failure. In: Hricak H, ed: *Clinics in Ultrasound.* Vol 18. New York: Churchill Livingstone;1986:55-58.

83. Cadman PJ, Lindsell DRM, Golding SJ: An unsuual appearance of renal lymphoma. *Clin Radiol* 1988;39:452-453.

84. Deuskar K, Martin LFW, Leung W: Renal lymphoma: an unusual example. *J Can Assoc Radiol* 1987;38:133-135.

85. Gore RM, Shkolnik A: Abdominal manifestations of pediatric leukemias: sonographic assessment. *Radiology* 1982;142:207-210.

86. McKeown DK, Nguyen G, Rudrick B, et al: Carcinoid of the kidney: radiologic findings. *AJR* 1988;150:143-144.

87. Sisler CL, Siegel MJ: Malignant rhabdoid tumor of the kidney: radiologic features. *Radiology* 1989;172:211-212.

88. Bechtold RE, Wolfman NT, Karstaedt N, et al: Renal sinns histiocytosis. *Radiology* 1987;162:689-690.

89. Jacobs JE, Sussman SK, Glickstein MF: Renal lymphangiomyoma: a rare cause of a multiloculated mass. *AJR* 1989;152:307-308.

90. Pollack HM, Banner MP, Amendola MA: Other malignant neoplasms of the renal parenchyma. *Semin Roentgenol* 1987;22:260-274.

91. Harrison RB, Dyer R: Benign space-occupying conditions of the kidneys. *Semin Roentgenol* 1987;22:275-283.

92. Dunnick NR, Hartman DS, Ford KK, et al: The radiology of juxtaglomerular tumors. *Radiology* 1983;147:321-326.

93. Mucci B, Lewi HJE, Fleming S: The radiology of sarcomas and sarcomatoid carcinomas of the kidney. *Clin Radiol* 1987;38:249-254.

94. Goldman SM, Bohlman ME, Gatewood OMB: Neoplasms of the renal collecting system. *Semin Roentgenol* 1987;22:284-291.

95. Piccirillo M, Rigsby CM, Rosenfield AT: Sonography of renal inflammatory disease. *Urol Radiol* 1987;9:66-78.

96. Morehouse HT, Weiner SN, Hoffman-Tretin JC: Inflammatory disease of the kidney. *Semin Ultrasound CT MR* 1986;7:246-258.

97. Jeffrey RB, Federle MP: Computed tomography and ultrasonography of acute renal abnormalities. *Radiol Clin North Am* 1983;21:515-525.

98. Rigsby CM, Rosenfield AT, Glickman MG, et al: Hemorrhagic focal bacterial nephritis: findings on gray-scale sonography and computed tomography. *AJR* 1986;146:1173-1177.

99. Kuligowska E, Newman B, White SJ, et al: Interventional ultrasound in detection and treatment of renal inflammatory disease. *Radiology* 1983;147:521-526.

100. Jeffrey RB, Laing FC, Wing VW, et al: Sensitivity of sonography in pyonephrosis: a re-evaluation. *AJR* 1985;144:71-73.

101. Subramanyam BR, Raghavendra BN, Bosniak MA, et al: Sonography of pyonephrosis: a prospective study. *AJR* 1983;140:991-993.

102. Kay CJ, Rosenfield AT, Taylor KJW, et al: Ultrasonic characteristics of chronic atrophic pyelonephritis. *AJR* 1979;132:47-49.

103. Golomb J, Solomon A, Peer G, et al: Bilateral metachronous xanthogranulomatous pyelonephritis and end-stage renal failure. *Urol Radiol* 1986;8:95-97.

104. Subramanyam BR, Megibow AJ, Raghavendra N, et al: Diffuse xanthogranulomatous pyelonephritis: analysis by computed tomography and sonography. *Urol Radiol* 1982;4:5-9.

105. Premkumar A, Lattimer J, Newhouse JH: Computed tomography and sonography of advanced urinary tract tuberculosis. *AJR* 1987;148:65-69.

106. Stuck KJ, Silver TM, Jaffee MH, et al: Sonographic demonstration of renal fungus balls. *Radiology* 1981;142:473-474.

107. Charboneau JW, Hattery RR, Williamson Jr B, et al: Malacoplakia of the urinary tract and renal parenchymal involvement. *Urol Radiol* 1980;2:89-93.

108. Hamper UM, Goldblum LE, Hutchins GM, et al: Renal involvement in AIDS: sonographic-pathologic correlation. *AJR* 1988;150:1321-1325.

109. Schaffer RM, Schwartz GE, Becker JA, et al: Renal ultrasound in acquired immune deficiency syndrome. *Radiology* 1984;153:511-513.

110. Falkoff GE, Rigsby CM, Rosenfield AT: Partial, combined cortical and medullary nephrocalcinosis: ultrasound and computed tomography patterns in AIDS-associated MAI infection. *Radiology* 1987;162:343-344.

111. Spouge AR, Wilson SR, Gopinath N, et al: Extrapulmonary *Pneumocystis carinii* in a patient with AIDS: sonographic findings. *AJR* 1990;155:76-78.

112. Pollack HM, Wein AJ: Imaging of renal trauma. *Radiology* 1989;172:297-308.

113. Furtschegger A, Egender G, Jakse G: The value of sonography in the diagnosis and follow-up of patients with blunt renal trauma. *Br J Urol* 1988;62:110-116.

114. Baumgartner BR, Steinberg HV, Ambrose SS, et al: Sonographic evaluation of renal stones treated by extracorporeal shock-wave lithotripsy. *AJR* 1987;149:131-135.

115. Kaude JV, Williams CM, Millner MR, et al: Renal morphology and function immediately after extracorporeal shock-wave lithotripsy. *AJR* 1985;145:305-313.

116. Choyke PL, Pahira JH, Davros WJ, et al: Renal calculi after shock-wave lithotripsy: ultrasound evaluation with an in vitro phantom. *Radiology* 1989;170:39-44.

117. Papanicolaou N, Stafford SA, Pfister RC, et al: Significant renal hemorrhage following extracorporeal shock wave lithotripsy: imaging and clinical features. *Radiology* 1987;163:661-664.

118. Kaude JV, Williams JL, Wright PG, et al: Sonographic evaluation of the kidney following extracorporeal shock wave lithotripsy: induced perirenal hematomas. *J Urol* 1988;1139:700-703.

119. Rubin JI, Arger PH, Pollack HM, et al: Kidney changes after extracorporeal shock wave lithotripsy: computed tomography evaluation. *Radiology* 1987;162:21-24.

120. Knapp PM, Kulm TB, Lingeman JE, et al: Extracorporeal shock wave lithotripsy: induced perirenal hematomas. *J Urol* 1988;139:700-703.

121. Lewis BD, James EM, Charboneau JW, et al: Current applications of color Doppler imaging in the abdomen and extremities. *Radiographics* 1989;9:599-631.

122. Mostbeck GH, Gossinger HD, Mallek R, et al: Effect of heart rate on Doppler measurements of resistive index in renal arteries. *Radiology* 1990;175:511-513.

123. Letourneau JG, Day DL, Ascher NL, et al: Imaging of renal transplants. *AJR* 1988;150:833-838.

124. Reuther G, Wanjura D, Bauer H: Acute renal vein thrombosis in renal allografts: detection with duplex Doppler ultrasound. *Radiology* 1989;170:557-558.

125. Warshauer DM, Taylor KJW, Bia MJ, et al: Unusual causes of increased vascular impedance in renal transplants: duplex Doppler evaluation. *Radiology* 1988;169:367-370.

126. Genkins SM, Sanfilippo FP, Carroll BA: Duplex Doppler sonography of renal transplants: lack of sensitivity and specificity in establishing pathologic diagnosis. *AJR* 1989;152:535-539.

127. Don S, Kopecky KK, Filo RS et al: Duplex Doppler ultrasound of renal allografts: causes of elevated resistive index. *Radiology* 1989;171:709-712.

128. Wong SN: Renal blood flow pattern by noninvasive Doppler ultrasound in normal children and acute renal failure patients. *J Ultrasound Med* 1989;8:135-141.

129. Platt JF, Rubin JM, Ellis JH, et al: Duplex Doppler ultrasound of the kidney: differentiation of obstructive from nonobstructive dilatation. *Radiology* 1989;171:515-517.

130. Platt JF, Ellis JH, Rubin JM, et al: Intrarenal arterial Doppler sonography in patients with nonobstructive renal disease: correlation of resistive index with biopsy findings. *AJR* 1990;154:1223-1228.

131. Spies JB, Hricak H, Slemmer TM, et al: Sonographic evaluation of experimental acute renal arterial occlusion in dogs. *AJR* 1984;142:341-346.

132. Erwin BC, Carroll BA, Walter J, et al: Renal infarction appearing as an echogenic mass. *AJR* 1982;138:759-761.

133. Taylor KJW, Morse SS, Rigsby CM, et al: Vascular complications in renal allografts: detection with duplex Doppler ultrasound. *Radiology* 1987;162:31-38.

134. Middleton WD, Kellman GM, Melson GL, et al: Postbiopsy renal transplant arteriovenous fistulas: color Doppler ultrasound characteristics. *Radiology* 1989;171:253-257.

135. Middleton WD, Erickson S, Melson GL: Perivascular color artifact: pathologic significance and appearance on color Doppler ultrasound images. *Radiology* 1989;7-652.

136. Mitchell DG, Needleman L, Bezzi M, et al: Femoral artery pseudoaneurysm: diagnosis with conventional duplex and color Doppler ultrasound. *Radiology* 1987;165:687-690.

137. Hillman BJ: Imaging advances in the diagnosis of renovascular hypertension. *AJR* 1989;15:4-14.

138. Page I: The production of persistent arterial hypertension by cellophane nephritis. *JAMA* 1939;113:2046-2048.

139. Greene ER, Avasthi PS, Hodges JW: Noninvasive Doppler assessment of renal artery stenosis and hemodynamics. *J Clin Ultrasound* 1987;15:653-659.

140. Robertson R, Murphy A, Dubbins PA: Renal artery stenosis: the use of duplex ultrasound as a screening technique. *Br J Radiol* 1988;61:196-201.

141. Taylor DC, Kettler MD, Moneta GL, et al: Duplex ultrasound scanning in the diagnosis of renal artery stenosis: a prospective evaluation. *J Vasc Surg* 1988;7:363-369.

142. Handa N, Fukunaga R, Etani H, et al: Efficacy of echo-Doppler examination for the evaluation of renovascular disease. *Ultrasound Med Biol* 1988;14:1-5.

143. Berland LL, Koslin BD, Routh WD, et al: Renal artery stenosis: prospective evaluation of diagnosis with color Doppler ultrasound compared with angiography. *Radiology* 1990;174:421-423.

144. Desberg AL, Paushter DM, Lammert GK, et al: Renal artery stenosis: evaluation with color Doppler flow imaging. *Radiology* 1990;177:749-753.

145. Coughlin BF, Paushter DM: Peripheral pseudoaneurysms: evaluation with duplex ultrasound. *Radiology* 1988;168:339-342.

146. Martin LG, Casarella WJ, Gaylord GM: Azotemia caused by renal artery stenosis: treatment by percutaneous angioplasty. *AJR* 1988;150:839-944.

147. Vaughan TJ, Barry WF, Jeffords DL, et al: Renal artery aneurysms and hypertension. *Radiology* 1971;99:287-293.

148. VonRonnen JR: The roentgen diagnosis of calcified aneurysms of the splenic and renal arteries. *Acta Radiologica* 1953;39:385-400.

Renal failure

149. Rifkin MD, Pasto ME, Goldberg BB: Duplex Doppler examination in renal disease: evaluation of vascular involvement. *Ultrasound Med Biol* 1985;11:341-346.

150. Rosenfield AT, Zeman RK, Cronan JJ, et al: Ultrasound in experimental and clinical renal vein thrombosis. *Radiology* 1980;137:735-741.

151. Braun B, Weilemann LS, Weigand W: Ultrasonographic demonstration of renal vein thrombosis. *Radiology* 1981;138:157-158.

152. Reuther G, Wanjura D, Bauer H: Acute renal vein thrombosis in renal allografts: detection with duplex Doppler ultrasound. *Radiology* 1989;170:557-558.

153. Hricak H, Cruz C, Romanski R, et al: Renal parenchymal disease: sonographic/Histologic correlation. *Radiology* 1982;144:141-147.

154. Rosenfield AT, Zeman RK, Cicchetti DV, et al: Experimental acute tubular necrosis: ultrasound appearance. *Radiology* 1985;157:771-774.

155. Pardes JG, Auh YH, Kazam E: Sonographic findings in myoglobinuric renal failure and their clinical implications. *J Ultrasound Med* 1983;2:391-394.

156. Platt JF, Ellis JH, Rubin JM, et al: Intrarenal arterial Doppler sonography in patients with nonobstructive renal disease: correlation of restrictive index with biopsy findings. *AJR* 1990;154:1223-1227.

157. Sefzcek RJ, Beckman I, Lupetin AR, et al: Sonography of acute renal cortical necrosis. *AJR* 1984;142:553-554.

158. Sty JR, Starshak RJ, Hubbard AM: Acute renal cortical necrosis in hemolytic uremic syndrome. *J Clin Ultrasound* 1983;11:175-178.

159. Longmaid HE, Rider E, Tymkiw J: Lupus nephritis: new sonographic findings. *J Ultrasound Med* 1987;6:75-79.

160. Matsumoto J, Han BK, Restrepo de Rovetto C, et al: Hypercalciuric Bartter syndrome: resolution of nephrocalcinosis with Indomethacin. *AJR* 1989;152:1251-1253.

161. Glazer GM, Callen PW, Filly RA: Medullary nephrocalcinosis: sonographic evaluation. *AJR* 1982;138:55-57.

162. Afschrift M, Nachtegaele P, Van Rattinghe R, et al: Nephrocalcinosis demonstrated by ultrasound and computed tomography. *Pediatr Radiol* 1983;13:42-43.

163. Patriquin HB, Robitaille P: Renal calcium deposition in children: sonographic demonstration of the Anderson-Carr progression. *AJR* 1986;146:1253-1256.

164. Brennan JN, DiWan RV, Makker SP, et al: Ultrasonic diagnosis of primary hyperoxaluria in infancy. *Radiology* 1982;145:147-148.

165. Villimora PE, Fabian TM, Schulz EE, et al: Acquired renal oxalosis. *J Can Assoc Radiol* 1983;7:158-160.

166. Rosenfield AT: Letter re: ultrasonic diagnosis of primary hyperoxaluria in infancy. *Radiology* 1983;148:578.

167. Shuman WP, Mack LA, Rogers JV: Diffuse nephrocalcinosis: hyperechoic sonographic appearance. *AJR* 1981;136:830-832.

168. Toyoda K, Miyamoto Y, Ida M, et al: Hyperechoic medulla of the kidneys. *Radiology* 1989;173:431-434.

169. Patriquin HB, O'Regan S: Medullary sponge kidney in childhood. *AJR* 1985;145:315-319.

170. Gertz MA, Kyle RA: Primary systemic amyloidosis: a diagnostic primer. *Mayo Clin Proc* 1989;64:1505-1519.

171. Subramanyam BR: Renal amyloidosis in juvenile rheumatoid arthritis: sonographic features. *AJR* 1981;136:411-412.

172. Kyle RA, Greipp PR: Amyloidosis (AL): clinical and laboratory features in 229 cases. *Mayo Clin Proc* 1983;58:665-683.

Postrenal failure

173. Ritchie WW, Vick CW, Glocheski SK, et al: Evaluation of azotemic patients: diagnostic yield of ultrasound examination. *Radiology* 1988;167:145-247.

174. Kamholtz RG, Cronan JJ, Dorfman GS: Obstruction and the minimally dilated renal collecting system: ultrasound evaluation. *Radiology* 1989;170:51-53.

175. Ellenbogen PH, Scheible FW, Talner LB, et al: Sensitivity of gray scale ultrasound in detecting urinary tract obstruction. *AJR* 1978;130:731-733.

176. Stuck KJ, White GM, Granke DS, et al: Urinary obstruction in azotemic patients: detection by sonography. *AJR* 1987;149:1191-1193.

177. Garcia CJ, Taylor KJW, Weiss RM: Congenital megalyces: ultrasound appearance. *J Ultrasound Med* 1987;6:163-165.

178. Naidich JB, Rackson ME, Mossey RT, et al: Nondilated obstructive uropathy: percutaneous nephrostomy performed to reverse renal failure. *Radiology* 1986;160:653-657.

179. Goldford CR, Ongseng F, Chokski V: Nondilated obstructive uropathy. *Radiology* 1987;162:879.

180. Fried AM, Woodring JH, Thompson OJ: Hydronephrosis of pregnancy: a prospective sequential study of the course of dilatation. *J Ultrasound Med* 1983;2:244.

181. Stuck KJ, Koff SA, Silver TM: Ultrasonic features of multicystic dysplastic kidney: expanded diagnostic criteria. *Radiology* 1982;143:217-221.

182. Sanders RC, Nussbaum AR, Solez K: Renal dysplasia: sonographic findings. *Radiology* 1988;167:623-626.

Obstruction without renal failure

183. Laing FC, Jeffrey RB, Wing VW: Ultrasound versus excretory urography in evaluating acute flank pain. *Radiology* 1985;154:613-616.

184. Erwin BC, Carroll BA, Sommer FG: Renal colic: the role of ultrasound in initial evaluation. *Radiology* 1984;152:147-150.

185. Dubbins PA, Kurtz AB, Darby J, et al: Ureteric jet effect: the echographic appearance of urine entering the bladder. *Radiology* 1981;140:513-515.

Intraluminal filling defects

186. Middleton WD, Dodds WJ, Lawson TL, et al: Renal calculi: sensitivity for detection with ultrasound. *Radiology* 1988;167:239-244.

187. King W, Kimme-Smith C, Winder J: Renal stone shadowing: investigation of contributing factors. *Radiology* 1985;154:191-196.

188. Stafford SJ, Jenkins JM, Staab EV, et al: Ultrasonic detection of renal calculae: accuracy tested in an in vitro porcine kidney model. *J Clin Ultrasound* 1981;9:359-363.

189. Kane RA, Manco LG: Renal arterial calcification simulating nephrolithiasis sonography. *AJR* 1983;140:101-104.

190. Puvaneswary M, Segasothy M: Analgesic nephropathy: ultrasonic features. *Aust Radiol* 1988;32:247-250.

191. Hoffman JC, Schnur MJ, Koenigsburg M: Demonstration of renal papillary necrosis by sonography. *Radiology* 1982;145:785-787.

192. Dillard JP, Talner LB, Pinckney L: Normal renal papillae simulating caliceal filling defects on sonography. *AJR* 1987;148:895-896.

Ureters

193. Share JC, Lebowitz RL: Ectopic ureterocele without ureteral and calyceal dilatation (ureterocele disproportion): findings on urography and sonography. *AJR* 1989;152:567-571.

194. Athey PA, Carpenter RJ, Hadlock FP, et al: Ultrasonic demonstration of ectopic ureterocele. *Pediatrics* 1983;71:568-571.

195. Nussbaum AR, Dorst JP, Jeffs RD, et al: Ectopic ureter and ureterocele: their varied sonographic manifestations. *Radiology* 1986;159:227-235.

196. Kessler RM, Altman DH: Real time sonographic detection of vesicoureteral reflux in children. *AJR* 1982;138:1033-1036.

197. Hoffer FA, Lebowitz RL: Intermittent hydronephrosis: a unique feature of ureteropelvic junction obstruction caused by a crossing renal vessel. *Radiology* 1985;156:655-658.

198. Williams PR, Feggetter J, Miller RA, et al: The diagnosis and management of benign fibrous uretric polyps. *Br J Urol* 1980;52:253-256.

The urinary bladder

199. Abu-Yousef MM, Narayana AS, Franken EA, et al: Urinary bladder tumors studied by cystosonography, I: detection. *Radiology* 1984;153:223-226.

200. Abu-Yousef MM, Narayana AS, Franken EA, et al: Urinary bladder tumors studied by cystosonography, II: staging. *Radiology* 1984;153:227-231.

201. Dershaw DD, Scher HI: Serial transabdominal sonography of bladder cancer. *AJR* 1988;150:1055-1059.

202. Friedman AP, Haller JO, Schulze G, et al: Sonography of vesical and perivesical abnormalities in children. *J Ultrasound Med* 1983;2:385-390.

203. Goodman JD, Macchia RJ, Macasaet MA, et al: Endometriosis of the urinary bladder: sonographic findings. *AJR* 1980;135:625-626.

204. Kumar R, Haque AK, Cohen MS: Endometriosis of the urinary bladder: demonstration by sonography. *J Clin Ultrasound* 1984;12:363-365.

205. Miller WB, Boal DK, Teele R: Neurofibromatosis of the bladder: sonographic findings. *J Clin Ultrasound* 1983;11:460-462.

206. Jorulf H, Lindstedt E: Urogenital schistosomiasis: computed tomography evaluation. *Radiology* 1985;745-749, 1985.

207. Han SY, Witten DM: Carcinoma of the urachus. *AJR* 1976;127:351-353.

208. Abu-Yousef MM, Narayana AS, Brown RC: Catheter-induced cystitis: evaluation by cystosonography. *Radiology* 1984;151:471-473.

209. Kauzlauric D, Barmeir E: Sonography of emphysematous cystitis. *J Ultrasound Med* 1985;4:319-320.

210. Bessette PL, Abell MR, Herwig KR: A clinicopathologic study of squamous cell carcinoma of the bladder. *J Urol* 1974;112:66-67.

211. Brandt TD, Neiman HL, Calenoff L, et al: Ultrasound evaluation of the urinary system in spinal cord injury patients. *Radiology* 1981;141:473-477.

212. Perkash I, Friedland GW: Catheter induced hyperreflexia in spinal cord injury patients: diagnosis by sonographic voiding cystoureterography. *Radiology* 1986;159:453.

213. Zerin JM, Lebowitz RL: Spontaneous extraperitoneal rupture of the urinary baldder in children. *Radiology* 1989;170:487-488.

214. Steiner E, Mueller PR, Simeone JF, et al: Transcystic biopsy: a new approach to posterior pelvic lesions. *AJR* 1987;149:93-95.

215. Williams BD, Fisk JD: Sonographic diagnosis of giant urachal cyst in the adult. *AJR* 1981;136:417-418.

216. Bovier JF, Pascaud E, Mailhes F, et al: Urachal cyst in the adult: ultrasound diagnosis. *J Clin Ultrasound* 1984;12:48-50.

217. Richman TS, Taylor KJW: Sonographic demonstration of bladder duplication. *AJR* 1982;139:604-605.

218. McAlister WH: Demonstration of the dilated prostatic urethra in posterior urethral valve patients. *J Ultrasound Med* 1984;3:189-190.

The urethra

219. Wexler JS, McGovern TP: Ultrasonography of female urethral diverticula. *AJR* 1980;134:737-740.

Renal transplant evaluation

220. Silver TM, Campbell D, Wicks JD, et al: Peritransplant fluid collections. *Radiology* 1981;138:145-151.

221. Shapeero LG, Vordemark JS: Papillary necrosis causing hydronephrosis in the renal allograft: sonographic findings. *J Ultrasound Med* 1989;8:579-581.

222. Becker JA, Kutcher R: The renal transplant: rejection and acute tubular necrosis. *Semin Roentgenol* 1978;13:352-362.

223. Nicolet V, Carignan L, Dubuc G, et al: Thickening of the renal collecting system: a nonspecific finding at ultrasound. *Radiology* 1988;168:411-413.

224. Berland LL, Lawson TL, Adams MB, et al: Evaluation of renal transplants with pulsed Doppler sonography. *J Ultrasound Med* 1982;1:215-222.

225. Steinberg HV, Nelson RC, Murphy FB, et al: Renal allograft rejection: evaluation by Doppler ultrasound and magnetic resonance imaging. *Radiology* 1987;162:337-342.

226. Rifkin MD, Needleman L, Pasto ME, et al: Evaluation of renal transplant rejection by duplex Doppler examination: value of the resistive index. *AJR* 1987;148:759-762.

227. Rigsby CM, Burns PN, Weltin GG, et al: Doppler signal quantitation in renal allografts: comparison in normal and rejecting transplants with pathologic correlation. *Radiology* 1987;162:39-42.

228. Allen KS, Jorkasky DK, Arger PH, et al: Renal allografts: prospective analysis of Doppler sonography. *Radiology* 1987;169:371-376.

229. Buckely AR, Cooperberg PL, Reeve CE, et al: The distinction between acute renal transplant rejection and cyclosporine nephrotoxicity: value of duplex sonography. *AJR* 1987;1:525.

230. Kaveggia LP, Perrella RR, Grant EG, et al: Duplex Doppler sonography in renal allografts: the significance of reversed flow in diastole. *AJR* 1990;155:295-298.

231. Grist TM, Charles HC, Sostman HD: Renal transplant rejection: diagnosis with ^{31}P MR spectroscopy. *AJR* 1991;156:105-112.

232. Grenier N, Douws C, Morel D, et al: Detection of vascular complications in renal allografts with color Doppler flow imaging. *Radiology* 1991;178:217-223.

233. Nishioka T, Ikegami M, Imanishi M, et al: Renal transplant blood flow evaluation by color Doppler echography. *Transplant Proc* 1990;21:1919-1922.

234. Tubman DE, Frick MP, Hanto DW: Lymphoma after organ transplantation: radiologic manifestations in the central nervous system, thorax and abdomen. *Radiology* 1983;149:625-631.

CHAPTER 10

The Prostate

- Robert L. Bree, M.D.

The use of transrectal ultrasound of the prostate is an issue embroiled in controversy. Its current use in the diagnosis, staging, and screening of prostate cancer has been the subject of many studies and debates. Recently, a multiinstitutional cooperative clinical trial sponsored by the National Cancer Institute reported relatively poor results for sonographic identification and staging of prostate cancer.[1] This study, however, did not assess accuracy of detection since all patients had known cancer. There is significant published information highlighting the uses and abuses of this procedure, generally indicating favorable results.[2-6] A recent diagnostic and therapeutic technology assessment concluded that the technique is safe, although effectiveness in staging, screening, and even detection of prostate cancer remains unclear.[7]

HISTORY OF PROSTATE ULTRASOUND

The prostate is located deep in the pelvis and, when enlarged, is sonographically accessible from a transabdominal, transvesicle approach. Correlative studies have shown that volumetric evaluation of the prostate with suprapubic ultrasound is accurate and that a gram of prostate tissue is equivalent to one cubic centimeter. Most of the current interest in prostatic imaging relates to transrectal techniques. In 1974 the Japanese[8] were the first to publish their experience with a radial scanner situated on a chair. The technique has evolved slowly since that time, with significant advances occurring with the development of gray scale, real-time imaging, improved transducer crystal design, and most recently, biplane probes that allow for prostatic assessment in both axial and longitudinal planes.[9-12] The usefulness of the transvesicle examination for detection of prostate tumors is limited because most prostate cancers occur posteriorly and their small size makes identification difficult.

Many early investigators enthusiastically undertook studies to evaluate the role of transrectal ultrasound in patients with prostate cancer. Their reports suggested that even small cancers produced areas of hyperechogenicity.[13-15] Further studies suggested that prostate cancer was difficult to detect, particularly in its early stages.[16,17] With the evolution of higher frequency probes, larger study series of cases of prostate cancer were reported. Authors have sparked a continuing debate concerning the sonographic appearance of prostate cancer, with some series describing small hypoechoic lesions[18] and others describing large hyperechoic cancers.[19]

ANATOMY

Original textbook anatomic descriptions of the prostate use **lobar anatomy,** describing anterior, posterior, and median lobes. Although the concept of a median lobe may be useful in the evaluation of patients with benign prostatic hypertrophy, this lobar anatomy has not been useful in identification of carcinoma of the prostate.[20] Detailed anatomic dissections of the prostate reveal **zonal anatomy,** whereby the prostate is divided into four glandular zones surrounding the prostatic urethra: the peripheral zone, transition zone, central zone, and the periurethral glandular area (Figs. 10-1 to 10-5). In the normal gland, however, sonography can rarely identify these zones unless a pathologic condition is present. Therefore, on sonography, it is more useful to separate the prostate into a peripheral zone and the inner gland, which encompasses the transition and central zones and the periurethral glandular area. A nonglandular region on the anterior surface of the prostate is termed the anterior fibromuscular stroma. Other fibromuscular structures in the prostate include the preprostatic sphincter, postprostatic sphincter, and longitudinal smooth muscle of the proximal urethra.[21,22]

The **peripheral zone,** the largest of the glandular zones, contains approximately 70% of the prostatic glandular tissue and is the source of most prostate can-

cer. It surrounds the distal urethral segment and is separated from the transition zone and central zone by the surgical capsule, which is often hyperechoic as a result of corpora amylacea or calcification. The peripheral zone occupies the posterior, lateral, and apical regions of the prostate, extending somewhat anteriorly (Figs. 10-1 to 10-5). The ducts of the peripheral zone enter the distal urethra.

The **transition zone** in the normal patient contains approximately 5% of the prostatic glandular tissue. It is seen as two small glandular areas located adjacent to the proximal urethral segment. It is the site of origin of benign prostatic hyperplasia. The ducts of the transition zone end in the proximal urethra at the level of the verumontanum, which bounds the transition zone caudally (Figs. 10-1 to 10-5).

The **central zone** constitutes approximately 25% of the glandular tissue. It is located at the prostatic base.

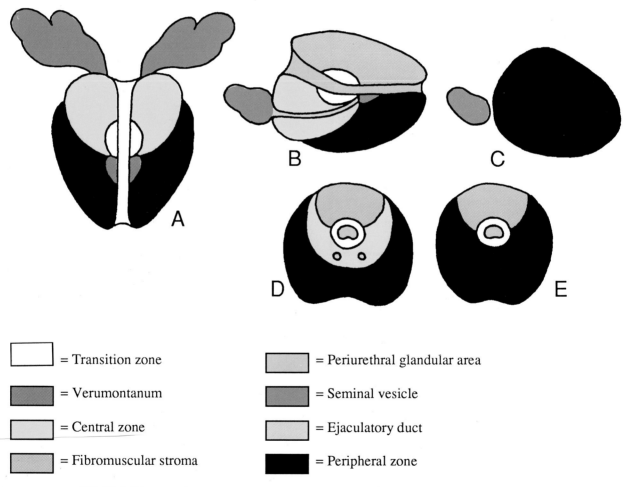

⬜ = Transition zone	▨ = Periurethral glandular area
⬛ = Verumontanum	▨ = Seminal vesicle
⬜ = Central zone	⬜ = Ejaculatory duct
▨ = Fibromuscular stroma	⬛ = Peripheral zone

FIG 10-1. Diagram of prostate zonal anatomy. **A,** Coronal section, mid prostate. **B,** Sagittal midline section. **C,** Sagittal section, lateral prostate and seminal vesicle. **D,** Axial section, prostatic base. Paired ejaculatory ducts are seen posterior to urethra and periurethral glandular area. Peripheral zone encompasses most of posterior and lateral aspect of gland. **E,** Axial section, apex of gland showing mostly peripheral zone, and urethral and periurethral glandular area.

The ducts of the vas deferens and seminal vesicles enter the central zone, and the ejaculatory ducts pass through it (Figs. 10-1 to 10-5). The central zone is relatively resistant to disease processes and is the site of origin of only 5% of prostate cancers. Central zone ducts terminate in the proximal urethra near the verumontanum. The **periurethral glands** form about 1% of the glandular volume. They are embedded in the longi-tudinal smooth muscle of the proximal urethra, also known as the internal prostatic sphincter (Figs. 10-1 to 10-5).[20-22]

Scan Orientation

Using a transrectal approach, various scanning orientations have been proposed. The most commonly used convention illustrated is similar to that for transabdom-

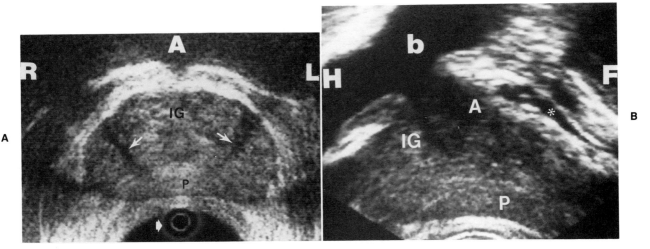

FIG 10-2. Normal prostate anatomy. **A,** Axial image, midprostate gland. Peripheral zone *(p)* and inner gland *(IG)* are of same echogenicity. Lateral edges of surgical capsule are seen as hypo-echoic linear bands *(thin arrows)*. Patient's left *(L)* and right *(R)* and anterior abdominal wall *(A)* indicated. Probe *(fat arrow)* is near anterior rectal wall, allowing for excellent resolution of entire prostate gland. **B,** Midline (true) parasagittal scan. Inner gland *(IG)* and peripheral zone *(P)* are isoechoic. Anterior fibromuscular stroma *(A)* is hypoechoic. Periurethral glandular area and anterior urethra lie between anterior fibromuscular stroma and inner gland. Large periprostatic vessel is noted in periprostatic fat *(*)*. *H,* Patient's head; *F,* patient's feet; *b,* bladder.

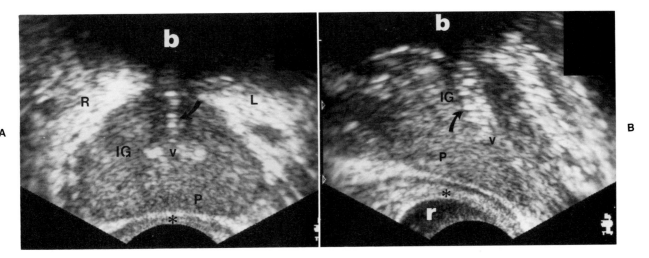

FIG 10-3. Normal prostate with corpora amylacea. **A,** Oblique coronal view. **B,** Oblique sagittal view. Images show that corpora amylacea in periurethral glandular tissue produce multiple bright echoes ("Eiffel tower"), surrounding urethra *(arrows)* extending down to verumontanum *(V)*. *R,* Right; *L,* left; *b,* bladder; *IG,* inner gland; *P,* peripheral zone; *r,* rectum; *(*)* rectal wall.

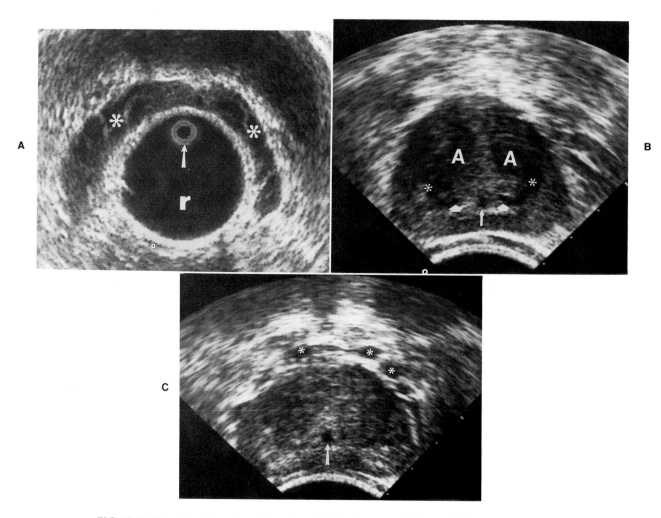

FIG 10-4. Normal axial anatomy in patient with benign prostatic hyperplasia (BPH). **A,** Seminal vesicles (*) are seen as paired hypoechoic multiseptated structures surrounding rectum *(r)*. *Arrow,* Rotating radial probe. **B,** Base of prostate gland. *A,* Adenoma; *, surgical capsule; *short arrows,* ejaculatory ducts; *long arrow,* urethra. **C,** Caudal to verumontanum, urethra *(arrow)* is seen posteriorly as a result of BPH. *, Prominent periprostatic vessels.

inal sonography (Fig. 10-1). As if standing at the foot of a supine patient, looking up, the rectum is displayed at the bottom of the screen with the ultrasound beam emanating from within the rectum. On transverse imaging, the anterior abdominal wall is at the top the screen with the right side of the patient on the left side of the image. In a sagittal plane, the anterior abdominal wall is again located at the top of the screen and the head of the patient is on the left side of the image (Fig. 10-2).

Several manufacturers have developed probes that fire from the end and can be used for both transrectal and transvaginal imaging; longitudinal and axial scans are obtained by rotating the probe through a 180-degree axis. The sagittal and axial images are relatively more oblique than those obtained with side-firing probes. Therefore axial images near the base of the gland are

considered semicoronal in orientation. In addition, the prostate appears more elongated when imaged with a end-firing probe than when a true axial orientation is presented (Figs. 10-1, *A* and 10-3). With end-firing probes, the top of the image is in an oblique direction toward the head and the bottom of the image is in an oblique direction toward the feet. Because of these differences in probe design, the anatomy that is depicted may vary from machine to machine.

Axial and Coronal Anatomy

The seminal vesicles are seen as paired, relatively hypoechoic, multiseptated structures surrounding the rectum cephalad to the base of the prostate gland (Figs. 10-1, 10-4, *A* and 10-5, *B,C*). In the axial plane, the anterior urethra and its surrounding smooth muscle and

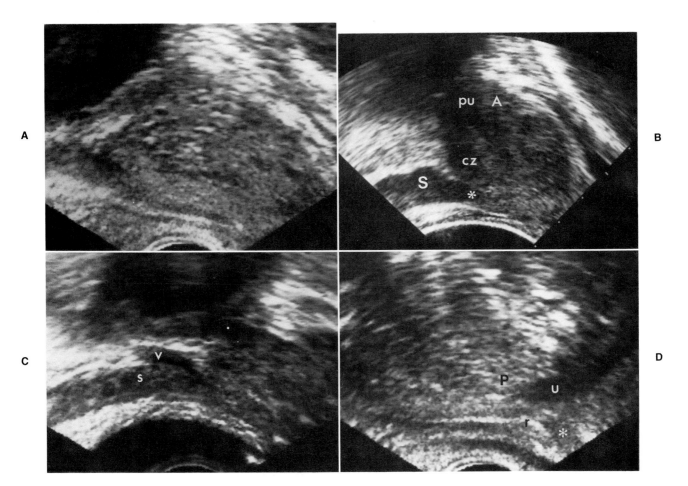

FIG 10-5. Normal sagittal anatomy. **A,** Lateral scan of mildly enlarged gland with sector side-firing probe. Peripheral zone is isoechogenic. Linear inhomogeneities seen in central gland represent cystic dilation of ducts, a normal variant. **B,** Midline sagittal image. Seminal vesicle *(S)* extends into prostate, creating beak (*). *cz,* Central zone; *pu,* periurethral glandular area; *A,* anterior fibromuscular stroma. **C,** Lateral scan through junction of prostate gland and seminal vesicle shows vas deferens *(v)* entering seminal vesicle *(s)* as it joins with prostate. **D,** Apex of prostate centers around trapezoid area. Boundaries are membranous urethra *(u),* peripheral zone *(P),* rectum *(r)* and rectourethralis muscle (*).

glandular area appear relatively hypoechoic (Fig. 10-4, *B* and 10-13, *B*). When corpora amylacea fill the periurethral glands, they may form a linear hyperechoic configuration, which has been termed the eiffel tower (Fig. 10-2, *B* and 10-3, *A*).[20] The inner gland is separated from the peripheral zone by the surgical capsule. This can be seen occasionally in the normal gland (Fig. 10-2, *A*). More often corpora amylacea, seen as echogenic foci, develop at the level of the surgical capsule (Figs. 10-11, 10-12, and 10-13). Frequently, the separation between the zones on transverse imaging is only positional, and no distinct structures will be present to clarify the anatomy (Fig. 10-4, *B* and *C*).

With hyperplasia in the transition zone, the urethra may be displaced posteriorly. Near the base of the gland the ejaculatory ducts may be seen on either side of the

urethra. At the verumontanum, the ducts are no longer identified (Fig. 10-4). As the probe is withdrawn toward the apex of the gland, most of the tissue is of the peripheral zone and should be uniform in echogenicity.

Sagittal Anatomy

The most lateral images of the gland in the sagittal plane show peripheral zone tissue with uniform echogenicity. With glandular hyperplasia, the transition zone may extend laterally, compressing the peripheral zone posteriorly (Fig. 10-5, *A*). At the base of the gland, the seminal vesicles immediately adjoin the central and peripheral zone (Fig. 10-5, *B*). The entrance of the seminal vesicles and vas deferens into the central zone produces an invaginated extraprostatic space, which is a pathway for a neoplasm to extend from the prostate gland into the seminal vesicle. A hypoechoic beak like configuration is formed by the entrance of the seminal vesicles and vas deferens into the central zone (Fig. 10-5, *B* and *C*). The ejaculatory ducts can occasionally be seen coursing through the central zone from the seminal vesicles and joining the urethra at the verumontanum as it extends from an anterior to more posterior position. The urethra and surrounding glands and smooth muscle are most often hypoechoic (Figs. 10-2, *B,* and 10-5, *B*) but when corpora amylacea are present, may be hyperechoic (Fig. 10-3, *B*). The anterior fibromuscular stroma can be seen well on sagittal imaging anterior to the urethra (Figs. 10-2, *B,* and 10-5, *B*).

Prostate Capsule

On transverse and sagittal imaging, the border of the prostate with the periprostatic fat may be sharply defined or, occasionally, less sharply defined, particularly in areas far from the transducer or on the edge of the imaging field. Histologically, the prostatic capsule is not well defined, and vessels and nerves course through the periprostatic tissue, which includes smooth muscle, skeletal muscle, and loose connective tissue. Posteriorly, the periprostatic tissue is fibroadipose, and no true surrounding capsule exists (Figs. 10-2, *A* and 10-3, *A*).[23] In addition to the absence of a well-defined capsule, the presence of prominent vessels in the periprostatic soft tissues may make assessment of capsular integrity difficult in patients with prostate cancer (Figs. 10-2, *B* and 10-4, *C*). At the apex of the gland, a trapezoid area is formed by the rectourethralis muscle, the rectum, the urethra, and the prostate gland. This area of potential weakness is a site of extraprostatic spread of cancer (Fig. 10-5, *D*).[21]

Normal Prostatic Echo Patterns

Three echo levels are seen on prostatic sonographic examinations:

- Isoechoic
- Hyperechoic
- Hypoechoic

An isoechoic structure contains middle-range echoes and is most characteristic of the peripheral, transition, and central zones in the normal patient. Smooth muscle produces a hypoechoic appearance, although an enlarged transition zone is also able to produce such echogenicity. Hyperechoic structures are most characteristic of fat, corpora amylacea, or calculi.

EQUIPMENT AND TECHNIQUES

Most modern ultrasound machines have transrectal probes, which have been developed to perform ultrasound of the prostate and rectum. Probe design and biopsy attachments vary. Probes are at least 5 MHz, and most are as high as 7 or 8 MHz.

Transducer Design

Following the initial development of linear array and rotating radial probe designs, manufacturers have now developed probes for biplane transrectal prostate scanning with either a single probe or multiple probes on the same machine.[24] A convenient probe design is an **end-viewing transducer,** which allows for multiplanar imaging in semicoronal and axial projections (Fig. 10-6). The limitations of these probes include problems with patient discomfort as a result of the size and frequent necessity to include a water path and the difference in anatomic presentation between true transverse, axial, and oblique image planes. Other probe designs include **biplane sector scanners,** a combination of a sector transverse and linear sagittal scanner; also in a biplane probe is a rotating sector scanner with a symmetric axis and a rotating scanner with an asymmetric axis.[4-6,20] In addition, some manufacturers have produced separate probes for transverse and sagittal imaging. The advantages of biplane probe designs include patient convenience and ease of use. It probably makes little difference to the patient, however, if a single probe is in

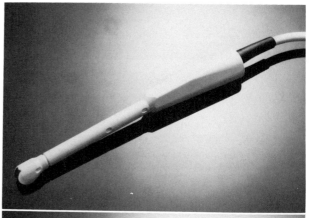

A

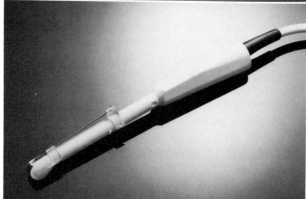

B

FIG 10-6. Transrectal probe. **A,** Curved linear end-firing design. **B,** Probe fitted with biopsy guide, which snaps onto probe handle.
(Courtesy General Electric Medical System, Milwaukee, WI).

place for the same length of time as two individual probes. The only difference is the discomfort of insertion.

Probes must be covered during the examination. Condoms, which have been developed to fit individual probes, are often made of latex. It was recently suggested that some patients may have latex allergies. Therefore patients should be quizzed to determine if this condition exists, in which case alternate covers should be used. Between usages, the probes should be soaked in an antiseptic solution such as glutaraldehyde. Recommendations from the manufacturer should be followed, particularly concerning the depth of insertion of the probe into the solution.

Many probes require a water path between the crystal and the rectal mucosa. This decreases the near-field artifact and allows for better visualization of the peripheral zone which may be very close to the rectal wall (Figs. 10-2 and 10-3). The amount of water necessary depends on the focal zone of the probe and the probe frequency. Careful attention should be paid to correctly positioning the probe to take advantage of the focal zone. A disadvantage of the water-path design is the occasional inadvertent introduction of air into the water path, creating an artifact (Fig. 10-7, A). Occasionally, pressure on the balloon can force the air bubble more laterally, but often it is necessary to remove the fluid and eliminate the air bubble from the system with a series of flushes after removing the probe from the rectum. In addition, when a water path is used, a "ringdown" artifact may be seen from the interface between the water and the rectal wall. This may be positioned in the prostate so that it creates annoying echoes (Fig. 10-7, B). This can be overcome by placing the probe as close to the rectal wall as possible.

Scanning Technique

Most clinicians who perform prostate ultrasound prefer that the patient lie in a left lateral decubitus position for the scan. Others prefer a lithotomy position, particularly if the examination is done in conjunction with other urologic procedures. A self-administered enema is routinely used before scanning. It is advantageous to perform a rectal examination before probe insertion to correlate the imaging with any abnormalities on physical examination and to ensure that there are no rectal abnormalities that could interfere with the scan. Following adequate lubrication, the probe is gently inserted into the rectum and the balloon inflated with water if necessary. Insertion is often painless, particularly in older men with decreased rectal sphincter tone. Hard-copy images are obtained on a multiimage camera at multiple levels throughout the prostate gland. An image-labeling technique has been developed to enable localization of the scan plane. This involves placement of a cursor in a rela-

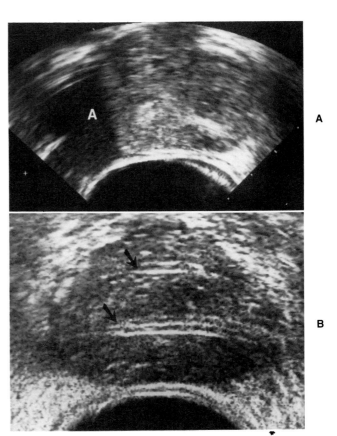

FIG 10-7. Artifacts. **A,** Transverse image. Large air bubble, inadvertently placed in water-filled balloon, gravitates to superior (right side) of balloon, causing reflective artifact *(A)*, and shadowing much of right side of prostate gland. **B,** Reverberation (ring down) artifacts *(arrows)* arise from strong interface between water path and rectal wall.

tive position between right and left on the sagittal plane and base and the apex in the axial plane (Fig. 10-14).

When examining the prostate gland, a systematic approach is necessary. If one begins in the transverse or semicoronal plane, the seminal vesicles are seen at the cephalad portion of the prostate gland above the prostatic base. These paired structures have different sizes and shapes, depending on age and sexual activity. They are generally hypoechoic and irregular and usually symmetrical bilaterally (Fig. 10-4, A). Continuing in the transverse or semicoronal plane, the base of the prostate is then examined with demonstration of the central zone, transition zone, and periurethral glandular area. The anterior fibromuscular stroma is hypoechoic. In a semicoronal plane, the periurethral area may be very hypoechoic and simulate a transurethral resection defect. The urethra and the ejaculatory ducts may be identified. At the level of the verumontanum, the ejaculatory ducts and urethra merge. Near the apex of the gland, most of the tissue seen is of the peripheral zone.

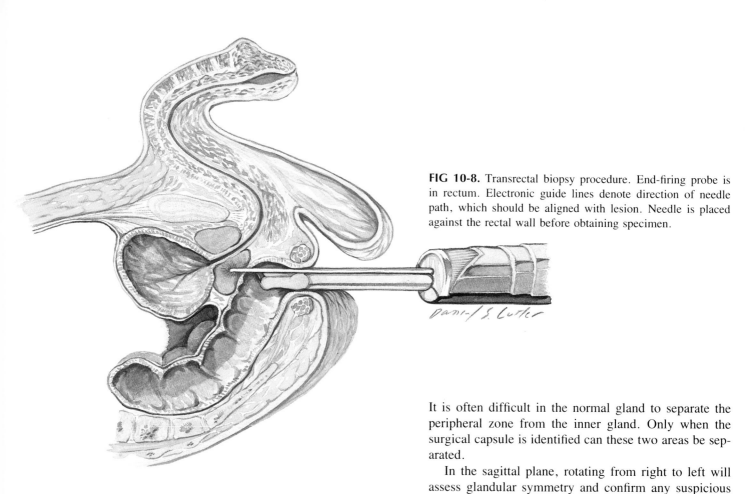

FIG 10-8. Transrectal biopsy procedure. End-firing probe is in rectum. Electronic guide lines denote direction of needle path, which should be aligned with lesion. Needle is placed against the rectal wall before obtaining specimen.

It is often difficult in the normal gland to separate the peripheral zone from the inner gland. Only when the surgical capsule is identified can these two areas be separated.

In the sagittal plane, rotating from right to left will assess glandular symmetry and confirm any suspicious abnormalities seen on axial or coronal imaging. The seminal vesicles and periurethral area are better evaluated in the sagittal plane.

Biopsy Techniques

The addition of ultrasound-guided biopsy procedures to the diagnostic examination adds a significant dimension to prostate ultrasound. Conventional prostate biopsy uses the examining finger in the rectum and transperineal or transrectal needle placement. The use of transrectal ultrasound for biopsy guidance was first performed with a transperineal approach using an axial rotating scanner.[25] Many investigators have described their experiences with transrectal and transperineal ultrasound-guided biopsy techniques.[4,10,20,26-28]

Currently, ultrasound-guided prostate biopsy is most often performed with a transrectal approach. Needle-guidance systems that clamp onto the side of the probe, are available for end-firing and side-firing probes (Figs. 10-6, *B*, and 10-8). Electronic guide lines show the needle path (Fig. 10-9), facilitating the procedure. Some of the newer probes allow the needle to pass through the probe shaft, permitting side-firing probes to use water paths for better visualization of the prostate during biopsy. Both systems allow for precise needle localization throughout the procedure.

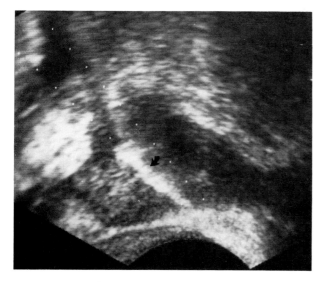

FIG 10-9. Prostate biopsy 1-cm dots. Guidelines denote path that needle will traverse. Needle echo *(arrow)* obscures lesion.

A common device now used for transrectal prostate biopsies is an automatic biopsy gun with 18-gauge needles. Thus a type of core biopsy specimen is obtained with minimal manipulation and with remarkable safety as a result of the speed at which the biopsy is performed.[20,26] The needle advances approximately 2 to 3 cm with the push of a button. The inner needle advances, and the outer needle cuts the tissue core and fixes it into the beveled chamber of the inner needle (Fig. 10-10). There are some who advocate the use of cytologic examinations in the prostate, although the ease of obtaining histologic cores has made cytologic techniques less popular.

Prostate biopsy may be performed in an ambulatory setting with little or no patient preparation. Patients on anticoagulants or aspirin should not undergo biopsy until these drugs have been discontinued for several days. It has become standard practice to administer a rapidly absorbed antibiotic such as ciprofloxacin in one dose just before and in several doses following the biopsy.[29-31] Informed consent should be obtained as with other biopsy procedures.

Transrectal biopsy is often performed immediately following the diagnostic examination. The patient remains in the left lateral decubitus position and the biopsy attachment is placed on the probe using a sterile

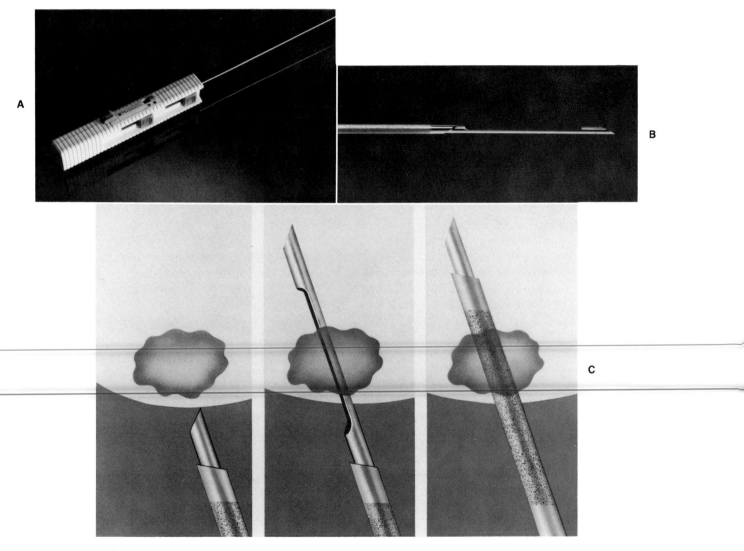

Fig 10-10. Tru-cut automatic biopsy needle. **A,** Needle is cocked with two buttons on side and fired with button on top. **B,** Side view of needle shows beveled chamber of inner needle and outer needle, which cuts tissue. **C,** Tru-cut technique with automatic needle. Inner needle traverses lesion and outer needle cuts biopsy core into beveled chamber.
(Courtesy Microvasive, Watertown, MA).

technique (Fig. 10-6). Although no great attempt is made to provide a sterile field, some have advocated the use of antiseptic enemas before performing the biopsy. The lesion is localized, and the needle is placed into the guidance system and moved to a position so that the needle tip is approximately 1 cm proximal to the lesion. The lesion can then be sampled one or more times. It may be useful to perform a biopsy of the opposite lobe in an area where no sonographic abnormality is noted.[27,31] Others have suggested that a higher yield of cancer can be obtained by using random systematic biopsies throughout the prostate gland.[31]

Significant **complications** from prostate biopsy—regardless of the mode of guidance, needle size, or approach—have been relatively low. Minor complications, primarily related to bleeding, are common and may seen in at least 30% to 40% of patients undergoing transrectal biopsy. Major complications include sepsis, large hematomas, and tumor seeding. With the use of prophylactic antibiotics, the incidence of septic complications requiring therapy should be less than 1%.[28,29,32]

Ultrasound guided *biopsy results* depend directly on the index of suspicion of the lesion that is biopsied. If all palpable and nonpalpable abnormalities are sampled with ultrasound guidance, higher positive results for cancer will be found than if only nonpalpable lesions undergo ultrasound-guided biopsy and the remainder undergo conventional biopsy techniques. In a large study series, 52% of lesions that were biopsied were adenocarcinoma. An additional 11% were diagnosed as prostatic intraepithelial neoplasia, a premalignant disorder.[28] In general, positive biopsy result rates, when using ultrasound criteria for selection, range from 40% to 60%.[33] Controversy exists over whether ultrasound guidance is necessary in the biopsy of palpable prostatic nodules. Some believe that a ultrasound-guided biopsy has no advantage as compared with a digitally directed prostatic biopsy. Some palpable lesions may be better sampled with digital guidance because they may not be seen at all with ultrasound. When a palpable abnormality is not discovered sonographically, it should undergo biopsy with conventional digital techniques.[34-36] Conversely, when a digitally guided biopsy yields negative results in a suspicious gland, repeat biopsy with ultrasound guidance is important.[36]

BENIGN ABNORMALITIES OF THE PROSTATE AND SEMINAL VESICLES
Benign Prostatic Hyperplasia

Enlargement of the prostate gland is common in older men. The gland size, however, does not always correlate with symptoms of prostatism, although there appears to be correlation between symptoms and growth of the gland as it relates to the anterior urethra. Glandular volumes can be determined accurately by volumetric

techniques performed sonographically.[37,38] Volumes can be measured by using a stepping device, whereby areas of the prostate are cumulatively added to create a volume, or by using volume formulas, depending on the prostatic shape. Most often the prostate is elliptical in shape, and using the formula for a prolate ellipse (L × W × H × 0.523) gives an accurate volume measurement. For a sphere, use $4/3 \pi r^3$, and for a cylinder, use πr^2 × height (r = radius). These formulas can also be used to calculate the volume of tumor in the gland. Volume can be converted to weight because 1 cc of prostate tissue is equivalent to 1 g. Glandular weight and volume is age related. The weight of the gland in a younger patient is approximately 20 g. Beginning at age 50 years, the doubling time of the weight of the prostate is approximately 10 years. Prostate glands weighing more than 40 g are generally considered enlarged in older men.[39]

The **sonographic appearance** of benign prostatic hyperplasia (BPH) is varied and depends on the histopathologic changes. Distinct nodules or diffuse enlargement can be present in the transition zone, the periurethral glandular tissue or both.[20,22] The typical sonographic feature of BPH is enlargement of the inner gland, which remains relatively hypoechoic to the peripheral zone (Fig. 10-11). The echo pattern depends on the admixture of glandular and stromal elements because nodules may be fibroblastic, fibromuscular, muscular, hyperadenomatous, and fibroadenomatous.[5,20] This combination may allow for a hyperechoic appearance (Fig. 10-12).

Other sonographic features of BPH include calcifications and rounded hyperechoic nodules (Fig. 10-13). The occasional hypoechoic nodule that simulates carci-

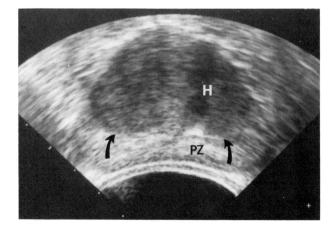

FIG 10-11. Benign prostatic hyperplasia, typical appearance. Transverse image shows echogenic peripheral zone *(PZ)* is separated from hypoechoic hyperplastic inner gland *(H)* by surgical capsule *(arrows)*, which contains calcification in corpora amylacea.

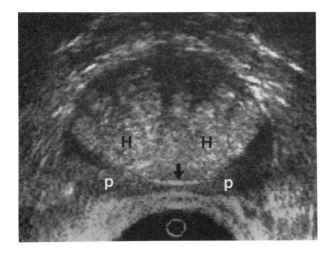

FIG 10-12. Benign prostatic hyperplasia (BPH), atypical appearance. Transverse image shows isoechoic peripheral zone *(p)*, hyperechoic inner gland with transition zone hyperplasia *(H)* and surgical capsule *(arrow)*.

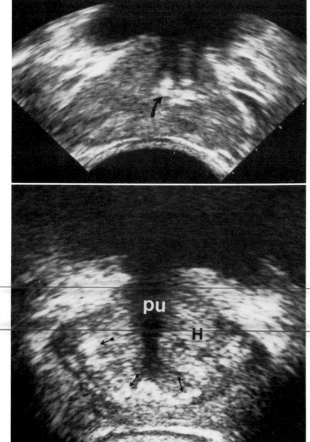

FIG 10-13. Benign prostatic hyperplasia. **A,** Prostatic calcifications, common feature in hyperplasia, are seen in transition zone *(arrow)*. Acoustic shadowing is anterior because probe is in rectum. **B,** Hyperplastic echogenic nodule *(H)* and corpora amylacea *(arrows)* are seen in this oblique coronal image. Elongated periurethral glandular area *(pu)* is hypoechoic because of glandular and smooth muscular tissue.

noma and that histologically represents hyperplasia may also be seen (Fig. 10-14). Because of the distortion of the gland in patients with BPH, these nodules may appear to be in the peripheral zone, when they actually lie in the transition zone. The surgical capsule can be a distinct demarcation between the inner gland and peripheral zone. When in the transition zone, hypoechoic nodules will be hyperplastic in approximately 80% to 90%.[20,40,41] When asymmetry of the gland occurs in BPH, this can be indicative of carcinoma, and biopsy may be necessary (Fig. 10-15).

In the patient with symptoms of prostatism, ultrasound can be useful to determine prostatic volume. Many surgeons prefer to perform an open prostatectomy in glands that are larger than 60 to 80 g. Because the growth of the gland is primarily anterior, particularly in patients with symptoms, the volume or weight cannot be estimated well by digital palpation. In addition, preoperative sonographic evaluation of the bladder and kidneys can be performed.[42,43] Ultrasound can analyze the effect of the hyperplasia on the anterior urethra and assess "median lobe" enlargement (Fig. 10-16). Often, very large glands may be seen in asymptomatic patients, whereas patients with severe symptoms of prostatism have only enlargement anteriorly and centrally.

In patients who have had transurethral resections, ultrasound is useful in evaluating the anterior urethra, extending from the bladder to the verumontanum. It is interesting to note that, although urologic surgeons may believe they have removed a large amount of the prostate, scans done relatively soon after transurethral resection show small- to moderate-sized defects in the periurethral glandular tissue and transition zone. There may

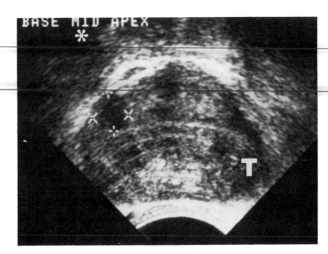

FIG 10-14. Tumor and hyperplasia. Transverse image shows large tumor on left side of gland *(T)*. Well-defined hypoechoic nodule of hyperplasia is seen in right transition zone *(cursor marks)*.

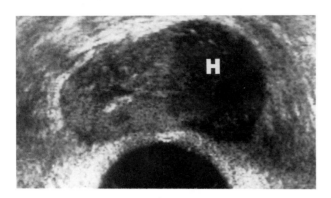

FIG 10-15. Large hyperplastic nodule (biopsy proven). Large hypoechoic mass *(H)* on left side of gland cannot be distinguished from carcinoma sonographically.

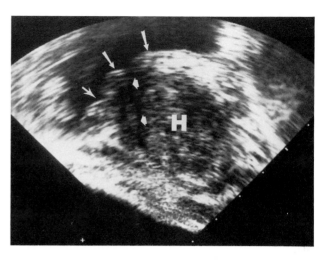

FIG 10-16. Median lobe hypertrophy. Midline sagittal scan shows hyperplasia *(H)* of periurethral glandular tissue, displacement of urethra *(short arrows)*, and nodular extension into bladder *(long arrows)*.

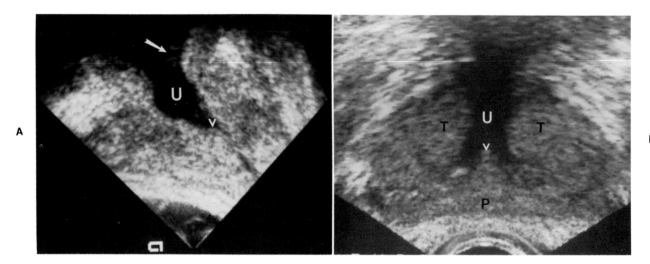

FIG 10-17. Posttransurethral prostatectomy (TURP). **A,** Sagittal midline image shows small nodule of tissue *(arrow)* that commonly protrudes into urethral lumen following resection. Anterior urethra is dilated to verumontanum *(v)* allowing posterior urethra and prostate to act as sphincter. **B,** Oblique coronal scan through base of gland shows dilated urethra *(U)* and verumontanum *(v)*. Some hyperplasia is seen in transition zone *(T)* on either side of urethra. Peripheral zone *(P)* is isoechoic.

be some redistribution of prostatic tissue to account for the large amount of prostate mass remaining. Patients, however, are uniformly symptom free following these procedures, suggesting that the amount of prostatic tissue removed does not necessarily correlate with the success of the procedure (Fig. 10-17).

Recently, techniques of transurethral dilation of the prostate have been developed, particularly for symptomatic patients with only mild enlargement of the periurethral glandular tissue. Ultrasound may play a role in monitoring the balloon dilation procedure (Fig. 10-18).[44]

Patients with benign prostatic hypertrophy often have glands that are abnormal to palpation. The role of ultrasound in these patients is to separate benign from malignant lesions and to guide biopsies when this distinction cannot be made sonographically. A patient with a hard nodule that is felt by digital rectal examination

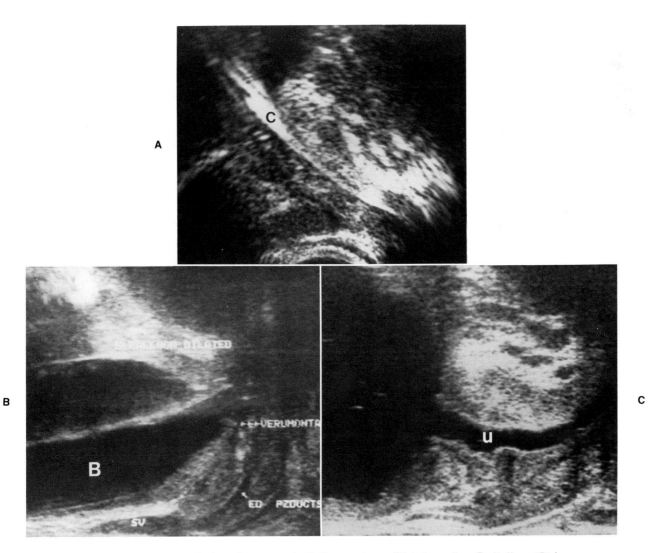

FIG 10-18. Balloon dilation of prostate. **A,** Balloon catheter *(C)* is in urethra. **B,** Balloon *(B)* is distended above verumontanum. **C,** Following removal of balloon urethra *(u)* is dilated without significant angulation at bladder neck.
(Courtesy F. Lee, M.D.)

and that contains calcification with shadowing can be spared an unnecessary biopsy if the palpable lesion corresponds to that seen with ultrasound.

Hyperplastic nodules are the most common cause of false-positive prostate ultrasound examination results. However, a small number of patients with BPH may harbor prostatic intraepithelial neoplasia (atypical hyperplasia), which is a premalignant lesion. When follow-up biopsies are done, these lesions may develop into prostatic carcinoma. Also, prostate cancer may coexist adjacent to or within the same gland as prostatic intraepithelial neoplasia (PIN). Close follow-up, subsequent biopsies, and correlation with prostate specific antigen is helpful when evaluating these patients further. Care must be taken to avoid overdiagnosis of carcinoma (Fig. 10-19).[5,45,46]

Inflammation of the Prostate and Seminal Vesicles

With the major emphasis of transrectal ultrasound on carcinoma of the prostate, there have been few studies analyzing its usefulness in inflammatory diseases. There is a significant incidence of acute and chronic prostatitis with varied symptoms. **Chronic prostatitis** may be associated with specific pathogens such as *Chlamydia* or *Mycoplasma* Organisms. If no known etiologic factor can be found, the condition is then termed *prostatodynia*.[47,48] Sonographic findings that can be seen with chronic prostatitis include focal masses of different degrees of echogenicity, ejaculatory duct calcifications, capsular thickening or irregularity, and periurethral glandular irregularity. Dilation of periprostatic veins and distended seminal vesicles have been described

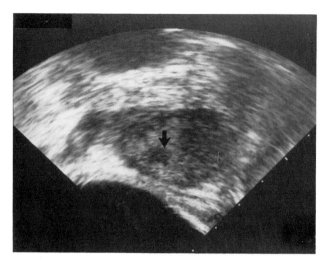

FIG 10-19. Prostatic intraepithelial neoplasia. Sagittal scan shows small hypoechoic lesion (biopsy proven) *(arrow)* in peripheral zone.

with chronic prostatitis or prostatodynia.[48] Sonographic-guided biopsy has been used to identify chronic prostatitis and to confirm the presence of bacteria.[49] Chronic prostatitis or seminal vesiculitis can lead to hemospermia. Transrectal ultrasound may be useful to rule out neoplasm and also to guide aspiration and injection of steroids and antibiotics to treat the infection.[50,51] Chronic granulomatous prostatitis has been described and can mimic the sonographic features of prostatic carcinoma. Diffuse large and small hypoechoic zones or a solitary hypoechoic lesion may be seen. Patients undergoing bacillus Calmette-Guerin (BCG) therapy for bladder cancer are at risk of development of granulomatous prostatitis (Fig. 10-20).[52]

In patients with **acute prostatitis,** the role of ultrasound is somewhat limited. Physical examination and placing a probe in the rectum is often difficult because of pain, and ultrasound may demonstrate significant abnormality, mimicking carcinoma. In general, the glands are hypoechoic (Fig. 10-21). Ultrasound can lead to an early diagnosis of a prostatic abscess. In a patient with acute prostatitis refractory to treatment, the development of an anechoic mass with or without internal echoes suggests the presence of an abscess (Fig. 10-22). Sonography-guided aspiration and installation of antibiotic into the abscess may be performed using a transrectal or transperineal approach.[53,54]

Prostatic and Seminal Vesicle Cysts

Most patients with cystic lesions in the prostate and seminal vesicle will be asymptomatic. Occasionally, these cysts can cause symptoms or become infected, particularly if they are large.

Congenital abnormalities are common in and around

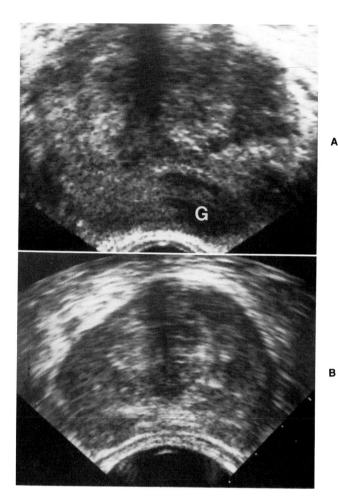

FIG 10-20. Granulomatous prostatitis *(G),* biopsy proven. **A,** Focal pattern. Patient with benign prostatic hyperplasia has large hypoechoic mass on left side of peripheral zone. **B,** Diffuse pattern. Inhomogeneity throughout gland and large and small hypoechoic and hyperechoic nodules are seen.

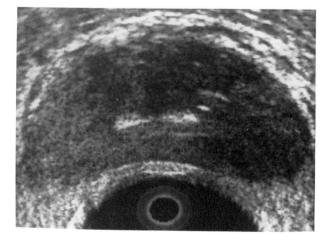

FIG 10-21. Acute prostatitis. Transverse scan shows large hypoechoic area on left side of gland, which could mimic carcinoma. Follow-up examination was normal.

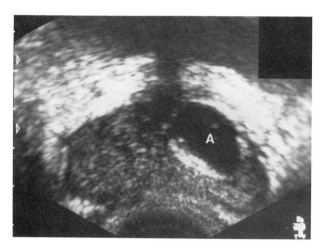

FIG 10-22. Prostate abscess *(A)*, aspirate proven, in patient with incompletely treated urinary tract infection. Cystic mass with internal echoes is present in transition zone. Aspiration of mass yielded purulent material.

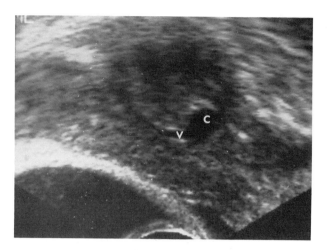

FIG 10-23. Utricle cyst, an isolated congenital anomaly. Sagittal scan shows small midline cyst *(c)* extending from verumontanum *(v)*.

the prostate and seminal vesicles. The müllerian tubercle gives rise to the prostatic utricle, a midline, small, blind-ending pouch that is situated near the summit of the colliculus seminalis, which is a mound on the posterior wall of the prostatic urethra. **Prostatic utricle cysts** are due to dilation of the prostatic utricle. Utricle cysts can be associated with unilateral renal agenesis and rarely contain spermatozoa. Utricle cysts are always in the midline and are usually small (Fig. 10-23). **Müllerian duct cysts** may arise from remnants of the müllerian duct. Müllerian duct cysts may extend lateral to the midline and can be large. They have no other associations and never contain spermatozoa.[55,56] **Ejaculatory duct cysts** are usually small and probably represent cystic dilation of the ejaculatory duct possibly as a result of obstruction (Fig.

10-24). These cysts do contain spermatozoa when aspirated. They may cause perineal pain.[55,57] Cysts occurring within the prostate gland may be caused by benign prostatic hyperplasia or may be **retention cysts. Seminal vesicle cysts,** when large and solitary, may be associated with ipsilateral renal agenesis. This is the result of a wolffian duct anomaly (Fig. 10-25). Affected patients may also benefit from aspiration when cysts are large and symptomatic.[56,57]

PROSTATE CANCER
Clinical Aspects

In the United States, among all cancers that are seen in men, prostate cancer is the third leading cause of death, and it is the highest cause of death in men older

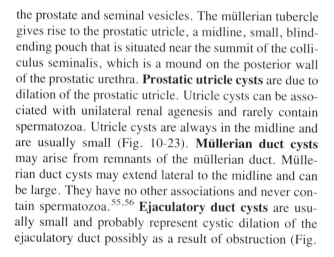

FIG 10-24. Ejaculatory duct cyst. A 1.5-cm cystic mass *(C)* extends into central zone from region of seminal vesicle. Aspiration revealed spermatozoa.

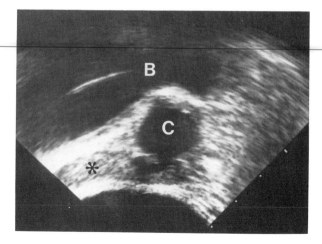

FIG 10-25. Seminal vesicle cyst. Transverse scan shows large cyst *(C)* extending anteriorly from left seminal vesicle and indenting bladder *(B)*. Normal right seminal vesicle (*).

A1

A2

B1

B2

C

D

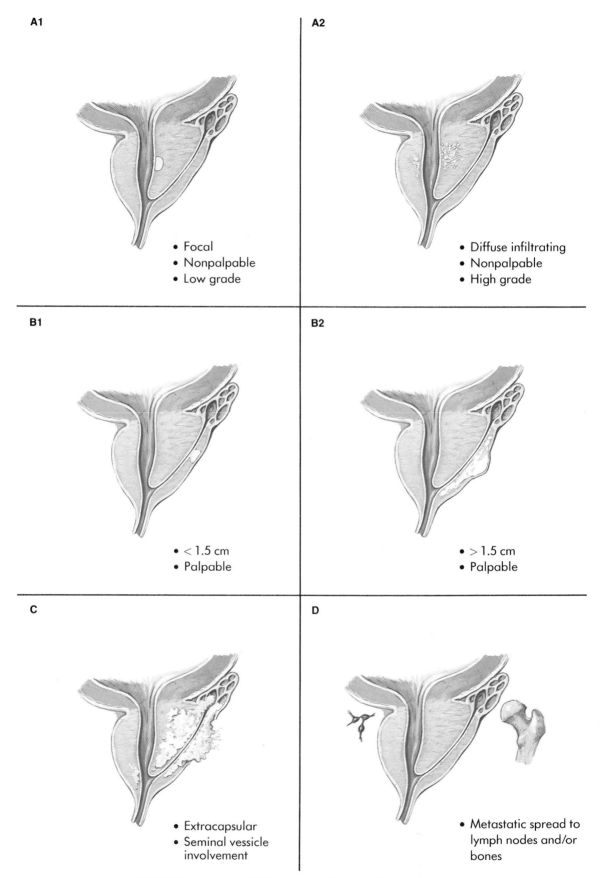

- Focal
- Nonpalpable
- Low grade

- Diffuse infiltrating
- Nonpalpable
- High grade

- < 1.5 cm
- Palpable

- > 1.5 cm
- Palpable

- Extracapsular
- Seminal vessicle involvement

- Metastatic spread to lymph nodes and/or bones

FIG 10-26. Jewett and Whitmore classification of prostatic tumors.

than 75 years of age. Approximately 10% of men who are age 50 years will develop clinical prostate cancer during their lifetime.[58] Annually, there are approximately 100,000 new cases with 30,000 deaths from prostate cancer in the United States.[7]

A number of surgical and autopsy reports suggest that prostate cancer may be divided into two major prognostic groups: latent and overt. Latent carcinoma may be seen in as many as 50% of men over 75 years of age and represents prostate cancer with low-histologic grades and no biological aggressiveness.[59] This is particularly important when considering the number of patients who will have incidental cancer found during transurethral resection of the prostate. There is considerable debate in the literature as to whether incidental cancer found at the time of transurethral resection is indeed distinct from cancer in the peripheral zone discovered at the time of rectal sonographic examination. It is probable that virulent cancer can be discovered anywhere in the prostate gland and that there is no reliable way to predict clinical activity. The degree of differentiation and tumor volume can be used to help determine further treatment modalities, particularly in patients whose cancers are discovered incidentally at the time of transurethral resection.[60,61]

Clinical Stage and Grade

Prostate cancer is most commonly staged by the Jewett and Whitmore classification (Fig. 10-26 and Table 10-1).[62] In addition to clinical staging, the Gleason histologic grading system analyzes the degree of glandular differentiation and dedifferentiation microscopically; grade 1 is well differentiated and 5 is poorly differentiated. The cancers are graded by evaluating the most representative histologic pattern and a less representative area and adding the grades of the two areas together to obtain a number between 2 and 10.[63] Most urologists accept the Jewett stage and Gleason grading systems to define the tumor and assign prognosis.

Stage A tumors are nonpalpable clinically. The tumors are typically located in the inner gland, having developed in the transition zone or periurethral glandular tissue (A1). If a stage A tumor is extensive (A2), it may extend into the peripheral zone from the inner gland or it may be diffuse in the peripheral zone and extend into the inner gland so that it is not detectable by digital rectal examination. **Stage B and C tumors** are palpable by digital rectal examination and represent local cancer, typically in the peripheral zone. Stage C tumors extend into the seminal vesicles or periprostatic soft tissue. **Stage D tumors** represents cancer that, at the time of presentation, is present either in lymph nodes or distant organs or bones. When initially discovered, most prostate cancers are stages A or D, with the minority of patients being discovered with stages B or C. With the increasing use of prostate ultrasound, this data may change as local cancers are discovered at an earlier stage.

Indications for Transrectal Ultrasound of the Prostate

The indications for transrectal ultrasound of the prostate in patients with known or suspected prostate cancer are:

- Evaluation of the patient with a palpably abnormal digital rectal examination
- Evaluation of the patient with abnormal laboratory test results indicative of prostate cancer, including prostate specific antigen, acid phosphatase, or other evidence of metastatic disease
- Guidance for directed sonographic biopsy
- Staging of known prostate cancer
- Screening for prostate cancer
- Monitoring response following treatment for prostate cancer[3,4,6,7,20,64]

Sonographic Appearance

The sonographic appearance of prostate cancer has been the subject of much debate. Early investigators felt that most prostate cancers were hyperechoic.[19] With the development of higher frequency transducers, the concept of the hypoechoic and mixed appearance of prostate cancer evolved.[18,40,65]

With currently available high-frequency transrectal probes, prostate cancer may have varied appearances, depending on the size and background of the prostate in which it is growing. Small prostate cancers are generally hypoechoic because of the nodular cellular appearance of the carcinoma against the background of normal peripheral zone glandular tissue (Fig. 10-27).[46] When

■ **TABLE 10-1**
Jewett and Whitmore Classification of Prostatic Tumors

Stage	Definition
A	Nonpalpable cancers
A1	<5% of tissue and Gleason grade <7
A2	>5% of tissue or Gleason grade >7
B	Palpable nodule
B1	Palpable nodule <1.5 cm in diameter
B2	Palpable nodule >1.5 cm in diameter, confined within the prostatic capsule
C	Extension beyond the prostatic capsule without distant metastases
D	Metastases
D1	Metastases to regional lymph nodes
D2	Metastases to bone or viscera

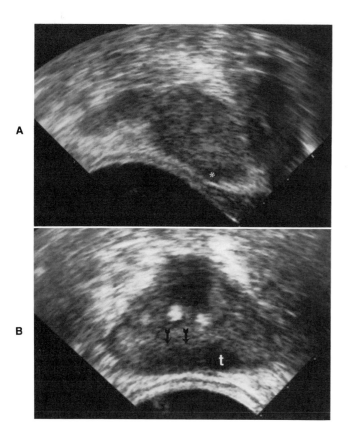

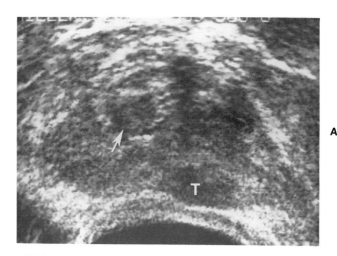

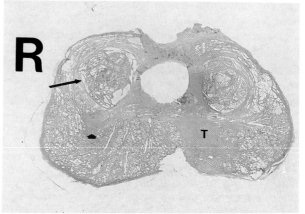

FIG 10-27. Small, typical, palpable hypoechoic prostate cancer. **A,** Sagittal image shows 8-mm, nonpalpable oval-shaped hypoechoic mass (*) in peripheral zone near apex of gland. **B,** Solid anechoic portion of tumor *(t)* is located on left with infiltration into peripheral zone toward midline *(arrows).*

FIG 10-28. Sonographic pathologic correlation of prostate cancer. **A,** Preoperative sonogram in axial plane shows palpable hypoechoic lesion *(T)* in left peripheral zone and second hypoechoic area *(arrow)* in right transition zone. **B,** Whole mount specimen following radical prostatectomy shows peripheral zone tumor *(T)* as solid area surrounded by glandular tissue. Second focus of tumor *(thick arrow)* in anterior peripheral zone (less than 5 mm) could not be appreciated on preoperative sonogram. Second hypoechoic area in transition zone *(thin arrow)* is area of nodular hyperplasia.

attempting to correlate the echogenicity of neoplasms with the amount of stromal fibrosis, it was found that hypoechoic lesions had less stromal fibrosis than did their more echogenic counterparts (Fig. 10-28). In addition, the hypoechoic lesions tended to be better differentiated with lower Gleason grades.[66] Another report, however, found the opposite information in a correlative study with pathologic states, suggesting that the hypoechoic tumors were poorly differentiated and that the poorly differentiated tumors were better seen with ultrasound.[67] The validity of these analyses needs further study.

Hyperechoic cancer, although seen infrequently, has been identified. With large cancers, the appearance may be caused by a desmoplastic response of the surrounding glandular tissue to the presence of the tumor or to infiltration of neoplasm into a background of benign prostatic hyperplasia[3,4,65,66,68,69] (Fig. 10-29). Other histologic types of cancer, including the cribriform pattern and comedonecrosis, also correlate with echogenic can-

cer (Fig. 10-30). Rarely are prostate cancers associated with deposits of intraluminal crystalloid material, which also can produce increased echogenicity[70] (Fig. 10-31). At times, these lesions may not be large enough and can mimic areas of hyperplasia. It has been our experience that a few extensive large cancers have a hyperechoic appearance, probably as a result of the infiltration of the neoplasm into a background of benign prostatic hyperplasia. Biopsy of hyperechoic lesions with sonographic guidance is the only way in which one can prove that the lesion seen represents a neoplasm (Figs. 10-29, 10-30, and 10-31).

A significant number of prostate cancers are difficult or impossible to detect with transrectal ultrasound be-

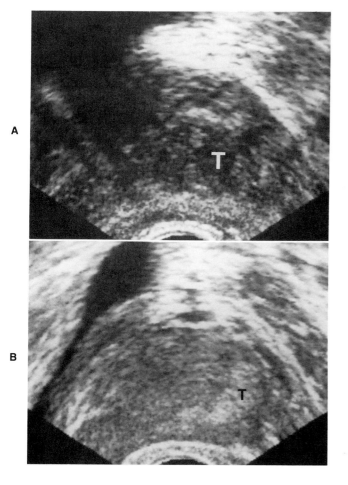

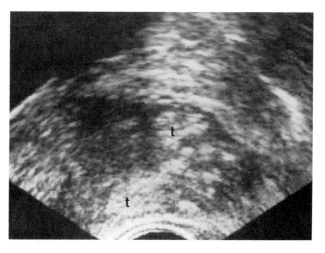

FIG 10-30. Hyperechoic cancer; Cribriform and comedocarcinoma, biopsy proven. Diffuse cancer through gland with foci of hyperechoic tumor *(t).*

FIG 10-29. Hyperechoic cancers. **A,** Sagittal image shows large hyperechoic tumor *(T)* with multiple hyperechoic foci. Histologically, there was significant desmoplasia with tumor intermixed with hyperplasia. **B,** Sagittal scan in lateral aspect of this gland shows small hyperechoic focus of tumor *(T)* in peripheral zone. Biopsy demonstrated significant desmoplastic response to this high-grade neoplasm.

cause they are isoechoic with the surrounding prostate gland. When an isoechoic lesion is present, it can be detected only if secondary signs are appreciated, including glandular asymmetry (Fig. 10-32), capsular bulging, and areas of attenuation (Fig. 10-33).[3,71] When isoechoic tumors are subjected to histopathologic correlation, it can be seen grossly that they are larger and tend to blend into the background of hyperplasia (Fig. 10-34). If there is strong clinical suspicion of prostate cancer and a palpable nodule is present, a biopsy should be performed.[65]

The ability to define prostate cancer both with the digital rectal examination and with ultrasound is determined by the ability to differentiate the cancer from the background of normal or hyperplastic tissue. When the cancer totally replaces an entire zone or the entire gland, this distinction becomes more difficult. This

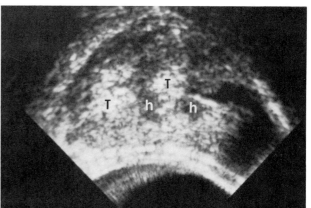

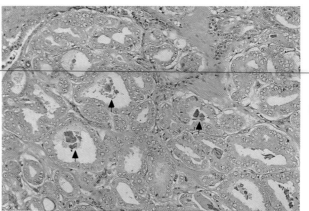

FIG 10-31. Hyperechoic cancer with crystals. **A,** Transverse scan shows transurethral resection defect and extensive stage A2 cancer with multiple hyperechoic foci *(T)* intermixed with hypoechoic foci *(h)* in inner gland. **B,** Histologic specimen demonstrates multiple intraluminal crystalloid deposits in tumor acini *(arrows).*

diffuse type of cancer must be identified based on the expected echogenicity of the area examined rather than its relation to surrounding structures. When the tumor replaces the entire peripheral zone, it will often be less echogenic than the inner gland, which is a reversal of the normal sonographic relation (Fig. 10-35). When the entire gland is replaced with tumor, on a background of hyperplasia, the gland may be diffusely inhomogeneous (Fig. 10-36). A very hypoechoic appearance is expected when the gland is not enlarged and the hyperplastic background is totally replaced (Fig. 10-37).

Prostate cancer is often multifocal, but the sonographer may not appreciate the multiple foci when encountering a well-defined hypoechoic lesion (Figs. 10-28 and 10-38).[1] In a recent study, 66% of biopsies yielded positive results from a hypoechoic lesion palpable by digital examination; random biopsies of the contralateral lobes were also found to yield positive results in a high percentage of cases, despite apparent sonographically normal isoechoic features.[36] These sonographic false-negative results support the opinion of some that reliance on prostate ultrasound for screening is inappropriate.[58]

Ancillary techniques for determining the significance of abnormalities seen with prostate ultrasound include prostate specific antigen (PSA) and Doppler imaging. The prostate specific antigen, a serum marker, was felt to be primarily useful to determine recurrence of prostate cancer following treatment.[72] More recently, it has been used for screening for prostate cancer. When combined with digital rectal examination and prostate ultra-

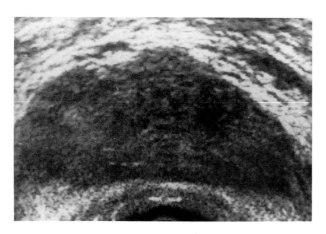

FIG 10-32. Isoechoic cancer. Transverse scan with palpably abnormal gland on right side shows asymmetry with bulging of right side caused by extensive tumor in peripheral zone and inner gland.

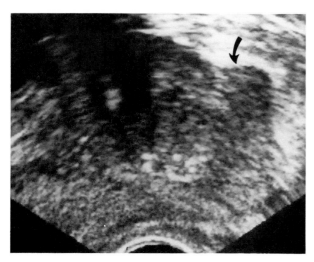

FIG 10-33. Isoechoic cancer with focal bulge *(arrow)*. This gland had extensive cancer throughout.

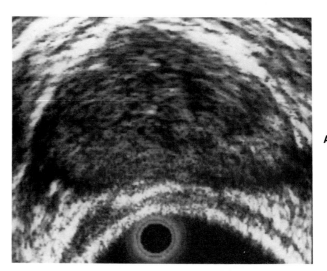

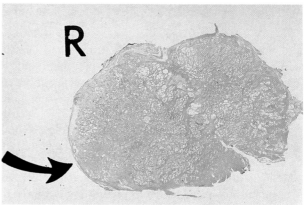

FIG 10-34. Isoechoic cancer, sonographic and histologic correlation. **A,** Transverse scan shows subtle asymmetry of gland with enlarged right side. Biopsy proved palpable carcinoma. **B,** Radical prostatectomy specimen shows diffuse glandular hyperplasia throughout both lobes. Tumor *(arrow)* infiltrating glandular hyperplasia cannot be identified at this magnification and was only seen microscopically.

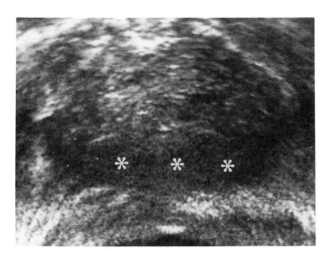

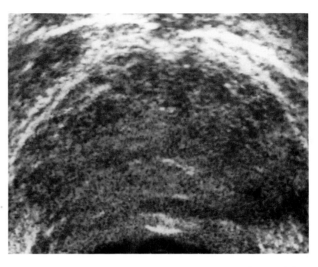

FIG 10-35. Diffuse, peripheral zone, high-grade cancer in patient with palpably normal prostate and markedly elevated prostate specific antigen. Ultrasonogram shows diffusely hypoechoic peripheral zone (*) with isoechoic inner gland.

FIG 10-36. Diffuse cancer. Axial scan shows diffusely inhomogeneous gland with loss of definition of peripheral and central zones.

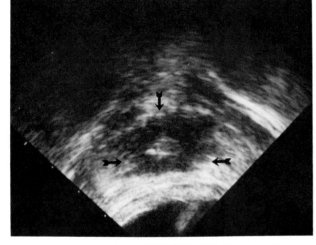

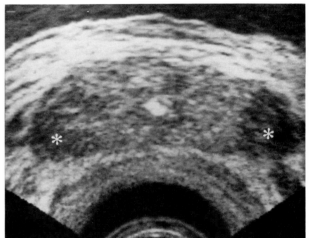

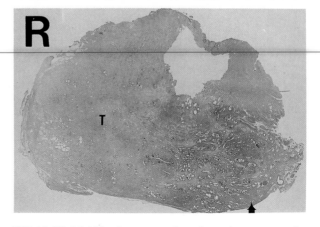

FIG 10-37. Diffuse carcinoma with atrophy. **A,** Transverse sonogram shows very small hypoechoic gland *(arrows)* with irregular borders. Central echogenic focus is corpora amylacea. **B,** Whole mount specimen shows complete replacement of gland with tumor and extensive infiltration beyond capsule.

FIG 10-38. Multifocal cancer underestimated on sonography. **A,** Transverse sonogram shows bilateral hypoechoic masses (*). **B,** Photograph of whole-mount specimen shows tumor on right side is much more extensive than appreciated on preoperative sonogram because of its isoechoic nature medially. Tumor *(T)* extends into left side of gland *(arrow).*

sound, PSA may be useful to determine which patients should undergo biopsies of suspicious lesions. Using a monoclonal assay, the normal is up to 1.3 ng/mL, and with the polyclonal assay, the normal is up to 2.6 ng/mL.[32,72,73] Benign prostatic hyperplasia elevates the level of PSA but at a much lower rate than carcinoma. Using volume-adjusted valves of PSA determined by Littrup et al can further define patients at high risk of cancer.[74] Using a cut off of 10 ng/mL (polyclonal assay) can be useful in deciding which patients will benefit from biopsy. A normal PSA does not exclude the presence of cancer.

Doppler ultrasound has the potential to separate benign from malignant lesions by evaluating flow patterns of vessels in and around mass lesions. Doppler imaging can also distinguish vessels from tumor, particularly at the periphery of the gland. Early anecdotal studies suggest carcinomas have increased flow with low resistance.

Location of Prostate Cancer

About 70% of prostate cancers arise in the peripheral zone, 20% in the transition zone, and 10% in the central zone.[75] With ultrasound, peripheral zone cancers are the most commonly detected, and one must have a high incidence of suspicion to identify and biopsy lesions outside of the peripheral zone (Fig. 10-39). Prostate cancer that begins in the peripheral zone often grows longitudinally along the peripheral zone before extending into the inner gland. The surgical capsule acts as an anatomic barrier to inner gland spread. When using ultrasound in conjunction with PSA, higher positive biopsy result rates can be expected in all inner gland lesions (Figs. 10-28 and 10-39). In a large study series of patients undergoing ultrasound and ultrasound-guided biopsy, 13% of lesions in the transition zone were malignant as opposed to 41% in the peripheral zone. In this study series, however, only hypoechoic lesions underwent biopsy.[73]

Results of Prostate Ultrasound in Cancer Detection

Because there is no gold standard by which to measure the accuracy of prostate ultrasound in the detection of prostate cancer, there is uniform lack of agreement on the accuracy of this technique. Only those studies that correlate sonographic findings with ultrasound-guided biopsy or radical prostatectomy can be used to determine the sensitivity of the procedure. In the recent NIH trial, lesion detection was poor, but detection of cancer in individual patients was not assessed because all patients had known cancer.[1] Positive biopsy result rates range from as low as 20% for small hypoechoic masses to as high as 65% for all suspected masses in different study series of patients (Fig. 10-40).[30-33,36,73,76,77] If sonographic abnormalities are correlated with tumor size, digital rectal examination, and prostate specific antigen, it has been shown that normal PSA and digital rectal examination can obviate the need for biopsy, particularly when lesions are 1 cm or smaller. When lesions that are 1.5 cm or larger are detected and when biopsy is performed, up to 70% of these lesions may represent cancer.[73] The majority of tumors of less than 3 cc in volume have not spread beyond the capsule.[32] Unfortunately, sonographic studies have shown than ultrasound tends to underestimate the size and volume of individual lesions, making size a less accurate factor in determining the significance of a lesion.[78]

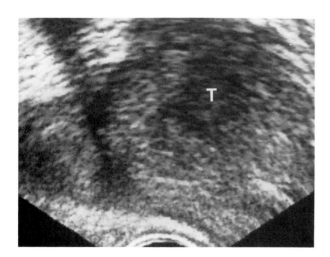

FIG 10-39. Transition zone cancer. Sagittal scan shows hypoechoic area *(T)* in transition zone in patient with carcinoma in another section in peripheral zone.

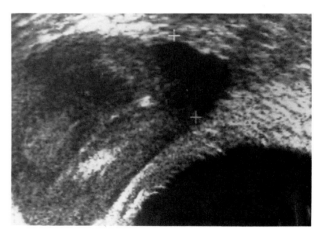

FIG 10-40. Benign hypoechoic mass that is biopsy-proven hyperplasia. Axial scan shows large anechoic mass in left peripheral zone (between *cursor marks*).

Screening for Prostate Cancer

Several screening studies have been published in the literature, and some are ongoing. A study of 784 self-referred men revealed 22 cancers, of which 20 were detected with transrectal ultrasound and 10 by digital examination. This suggested that ultrasound was twice as effective as digital examination for detection of unsuspected prostate cancer.[79] It was found that there was a cost of $6500 per diagnosed cancer with the use of transrectal ultrasound with a slightly higher cost for diagnosing early cancer. This is less than the cost of diagnosing breast cancer with screening mammography programs.[80] More recently, studies using prostate specific antigen and transrectal ultrasound have been reported. Two hundred and twenty-five men with negative rectal examination results were followed in a urology office. Because of suspicious prostate ultrasonograms, an elevated prostate specific antigen level, or both, biopsies were performed. Thirty percent of the biopsies were positive for carcinoma. As with other screening studies, no proof of negative examination findings was obtained.[81] Additional screening studies have shown a small but significant yield of carcinoma in patients without clinical suspicion.[82-84] In other screening studies, only 7% to 15% of the hypoechoic masses defined in an asymptomatic patient population represented carcinoma, which limits the value of detecting cancer in a massive screening program. Sonography is complementary to the digital rectal examination but cannot stand alone as a screening tool.[85,86]

Based on the studies comparing digital rectal examination with prostate ultrasound with the screening studies of asymptomatic patients, it could be concluded that all men in the high-risk age group should have routine PSA, *sonographic*, and digital rectal examinations. This would detect prostate cancer in 5.3% of men over 50 years of age who will contract prostate cancer sometime in their lifetime.[20] Unfortunately, early detection of cancer may not add to patient survival. Also, patients with the best prognosis may be the ones identified with screening. Therefore the possibility of overdetection with screening is raised. Considering the operative mortality and morbidity and the lack of evidence that detecting nonpalpable cancer affects the morbidity and mortality of the disease, there is currently no good data to support screening with ultrasound. A long-term randomized clinical trial is necessary to prove that screening is beneficial.[7,30,58,87]

Staging of Prostate Cancer

Following the diagnosis of prostate cancer, definitive therapeutic decisions cannot be made unless adequate knowledge of the stage of prostate cancer is determined. In general, incidental prostate cancer found on transurethral prostatectomy (TURP) (A1) only needs follow-up examinations without further therapy. Prostate sonography with ultrasound-guided biopsy has been suggested to evaluate these patients in addition to or instead of a repeat transurethral resection or blind needle biopsy. For example, if a minimal amount of cancer were found on a transurethral resection as the result of resection sampling of the edge of a large cancer, ultrasound could properly assess and determine the stage of these patients.[88]

Clinical stages A2, B1, and B2 can be treated with radical prostatectomy or radiation therapy. Controversy exists concerning the best therapy for locally invasive prostate cancer (Stage C). If microscopic invasion is

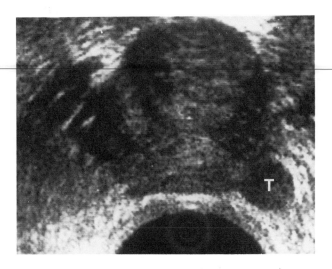

FIG 10-41. Macroscopic local extension. Axial scan shows large extraprostatic nodular extension of tumor *(T)* on left side of the gland in the region of the neurovascular bundle.

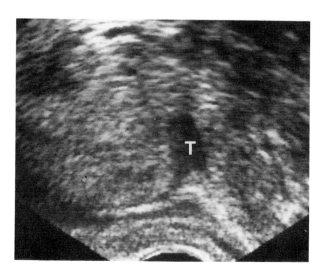

FIG 10-42. Apical cancer with local extension. Sagittal scan shows tumor *(T)* in trapezoid area.

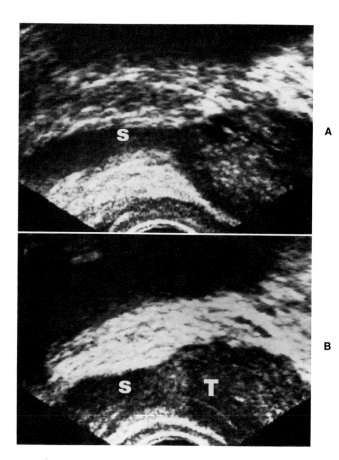

FIG 10-43. Seminal vesicle invasion. **A,** Right sagittal scan shows normal right seminal vesicle *(S)*. **B,** Left sagittal scan shows large tumor *(T)* with extension into large left seminal vesicle *(S)* with loss of seminal vesicle beak.

found, surgery followed by radiation seems to be an acceptable approach. With macroscopic invasion, there appears to be no advantage to surgery, and radiation therapy is recommended. Sonographic staging allows for separation of those patients with macroscopic local extension into the periprostatic fat, seminal vesicles, or local lymph nodes from those with disease confined to the prostate gland. The neurovascular bundle has been identified on sonography in as many as 70% of patients. Involvement would alert the urologist to not attempt a nerve-sparing procedure on that side. Sexual potency can be maintained if one bundle is left intact. Evaluation of the neurovascular bundle has not been used extensively, and its accuracy is poor (Fig. 10-41).[89,90]

The role of ultrasound in local staging has been assessed. Investigators have found sensitivities for local extension into the capsule or seminal vesicles to be as high as 90% and as low as 40% to 60%. More importantly, specificities for invasion ranged from 46% to 90%, depending on the size of the primary tumor.[1,91,92] Large tumors can be easily seen to extend outside of the capsule as a result of the loss of symmetry and capsular irregularity (Figs. 10-32, 10-33, 10-37, 10-38, and 10-41). Anatomically, however, the prostate does not contain a true capsule but a fibromuscular band. This creates a dilemma for the pathologist and urologist in determining the exact significance of the depth of invasion outside this band and into the periprostatic soft tissues.[23]

A point of weakness through the trapezoid area at the prostatic apex has been described (Fig. 10-42).[69] Another potential pathway through the prostate, the invaginated extraprostatic space, allows the tumor to extend through the central zone into the seminal vesicle region (Fig. 10-45).[69] Seminal vesicle extension can be

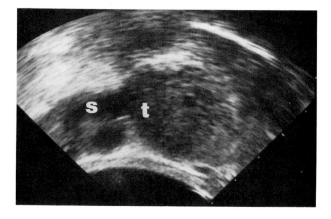

FIG 10-44. Seminal vesicle obstruction. Right sagittal scan shows seminal vesicle *(s)* is dilated because of obstruction by extensive prostatic tumor *(t)* at base. This cannot be separated from direct seminal vesicle tumor extension or hemorrhage following biopsy.

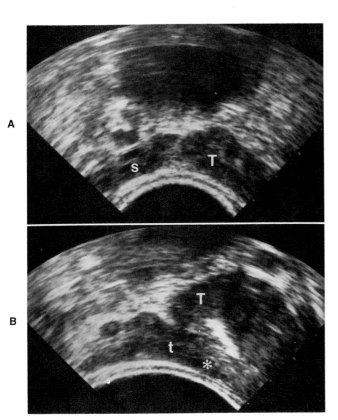

FIG 10-45. Seminal vesicle extension of carcinoma. **A,** Axial image shows normal right seminal vesicle *(s)* and tumor invasion of left seminal vesicle *(T)*. **B,** Sagittal scan shows extensive prostate tumor *(T)* with tumor extension into seminal vesicle *(t)*. Invaginated extraprostatic space (*) is route by which tumor extends into seminal vesicle. Ultrasound-guided biopsy of the seminal vesicle revealed carcinoma.

defined sonographically by enlargement, cystic dilation, asymmetry, anterior displacement, hyperechogenicity, and loss of the seminal vesicle beak (Fig. 10-43).[21,93] This phenomenon is best appreciated when comparing the normal with the abnormal side.[93] Tumors that extend into the seminal vesicle can also obstruct the seminal vesicle, causing diffuse enlargement (Fig. 10-44). Hemorrhage into the seminal vesicle following biopsy can simulate obstruction.

Both seminal vesicle invasion and local periprostatic invasion have been studied with computed tomography and magnetic resonance imaging and compared with ultrasound. Computed tomography is a poor staging technique, for involvement of both local periprostatic structures and lymph nodes.[94,95] Magnetic resonance imaging is slightly more advantageous than ultrasound in detecting local invasion and involvement of the seminal vesicles.[1] The recent introduction of endorectal surface coils may further enhance the ability of magnetic resonance imaging of the prostate.[96]

Transrectal ultrasound used for preoperative staging must be combined with ultrasound-guided biopsy. Selective biopsy of the region of the prostatic capsule and seminal vesicle is essential if local invasion is suspected (Fig. 10-45).[21]

Monitoring for Treatment and Response to Therapy

Ultrasound has been used as a guidance technique for placement of ^{125}I seed implantations for interstitial therapy of prostate cancer. Follow-up examinations have shown significant volume reduction, although biopsy of lesions in these patients revealed residual cancer in 50% (Fig. 10-46).[97-100] Research is now underway to study intraprostatic implantation of iridium and catheters for hyperthermia therapy with ultrasound guidance. In advanced cancer, volume decrease in patients following orchiectomy of at least 50% was a good

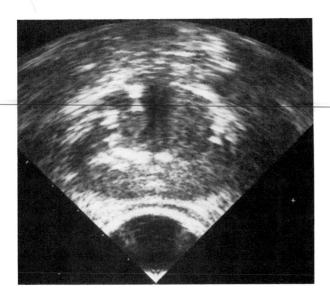

FIG 10-46. I-125 seeds in patient treated previously for prostate cancer. Axial scan shows multiple very bright echoes with reverberation artifacts beyond. No abnormal masses are seen in this gland.

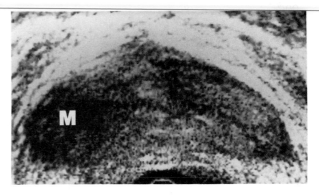

FIG 10-47. Radiation fibrosis (biopsy proven) in patient previously treated with external beam radiation. Palpable and sonographically identifiably mass *(M)* suggestive of carcinoma is seen in right lobe.

prognostic sign.[101] Patients with sonographic abnormalities following radiation therapy for prostate cancer had positive biopsy findings in a high percentage of hypoechoic lesions, particularly when the prostate specific antigen was elevated (Fig. 10-47). As with the preradiation prostate, a significant number of patients underwent random biopsies, which also yielded positive results for cancer, particularly when there was a high suspicion of recurrence.[102,103] A newly developing technique for treating prostate cancer using ultrasound guidance is cryosurgery.[104]

REFERENCES

1. Rifkin MD, Zerhouni EA, Gastsonis CA: Comparison of magnetic resonance imaging and ultrasound in staging early prostate cancer. *N Engl J Med* 1990;323(10):621-626.
2. Griffiths GJ, Clements R, Peeling WB: The current status of transrectal ultrasonography in the diagnosis and management of prostatic cancer. *Clin Radiol* 1989;40:337-340.
3. Resnick MI: Transrectal ultrasonography in the detection and staging of prostate cancer. *World J Urol* 1989;7:2-6.
4. Rifkin MD, Dahnert W, Kurtz AB: State of the art: endorectal sonography of the prostate gland *AJR* 1990;154:691-700.
5. Shinohara K, Scardino PT, Carter S, et al: Pathologic basis of the sonographic appearance of the normal and malignant prostate. *Urol Clin North Am* 1989;16:675-691.
6. Waterhouse RL, Resnick MI: The use of transrectal prostatic ultrasonography in the evaluation of patients with prostatic carcinoma. *J Urol* 1989;141:233-239.
7. Transrectal ultrasonography: Reassessment. *JAMA* 1990;263:1563-1568.

History of prostate ultrasound

8. Watanabe H, Igari D, Tanahasi Y, et al: Development and application of new equipment for transrectal ultrasonography. *J Clin Ultrasound* 1974;2:91-98.
9. Gammelgaard J, Holm HH: Transurethral and transrectal ultrasonic scanning in urology. *J Urol* 1980; 124:863-868.
10. Rifkin MD, Kurtz AB, Goldberg BB: Prostate biopsy utilizing transrectal ultrasound guidance. *J Ultrasound Med* 1983;2:165-167.
11. Rifkin MD, Kurtz AB, Goldberg BB: Sonographically guided transperineal prostatic biopsy: preliminary experience with a longitudinal linear-array transducer. *AJR* 1983;140:745-747.
12. Sekine H, Oka K, Takehara Y. Transrectal longitudinal ultrasonotomography of the prostate by electronic linear scanning. *J Urol* 1982;127:62.
13. Boyce WH, McKinney WM, Resnick MI, et al: Ultrasonography as an aid in the diagnosis and management of surgical diseases of the pelvis. *Ann Surg* 1976;184:477-489.
14. King WW, Wilkiemeyer RM, Boyce WH, et al: Current status of prostatic echography. *JAMA* 1973;226:444-447.
15. Watanabe H: History and applications of transrectal sonography of the prostate. *Urol Clin North Am* 1989;16:617-622.
16. Fritzsche PJ, Axford PD, Ching VC, et al: Correlation of transrectal sonographic findings in patients with suspected and unsuspected prostatic disease. *J Urol* 1983;130:272-274.
17. Spirnak JP, Resnick MI: Transrectal ultrasonography. *Urology* 1983;23:461-467.
18. Lee F, Gray JM, McLeary RD, et al: Prostatic evaluation by transrectal sonography: criteria for diagnosis of early carcinoma. *Radiology* 1986;158:91-95.
19. Rifkin MD, Friedland GW, Shortliffe L: Prostatic evaluation by transrectal endosonography: detection of carcinoma. *Radiology* 1986;158:85-90.

Anatomy

20. Lee F, Torp-Pedersen ST, Siders DB, et al: Transrectal ultrasound in the diagnosis and staging of prostatic carcinoma. *Radiology* 1989;170:609-615.
21. Kaye KW, Richter L: Ultrasonographic anatomy of normal prostate gland: reconstruction by computer graphics. *Urology* 1990;35:12-17.
22. McNeal JE: The zonal anatomy of the prostate. *Prostate* 1981;2:35-49.
23. Ayala AG, Ro JY, Babaian R, et al: The prostatic capsule: does it exist? *Am J Surg Pathol* 1989;13:21-27.

Equipment and scanning techniques

24. Rifkin MD: Endorectal sonography of the prostate: clinical implications. *AJR* 1987;148:1137-1142.
25. Holm HH, Gammelgaard J: Ultrasonically guided precise needle placement in the prostate and seminal vesicles. *J Urol* 1981;125:385-387.
26. Parker SH, Hopper KD, Yakes WF, et al: Image-directed percutaneous biopsies with a biopsy gun. *Radiology* 1989;171:663-669.
27. Torp-Pedersen ST, Lee F: Transrectal biopsy of the prostate guided by transrectal ultrasound. *Urol Clin North Am* 1989;16(4):703.
28. Torp-Pedersen S, Lee F, Littrup PJ, et al: Transrectal biopsy of the prostate guided with transrectal ultrasound: longitudinal and multiplanar scanning. *Radiology* 1989;170:23-27.
29. Bree RL: Prostate and other transrectally guided biopsies. In: McGahan JP, ed. *Interventional Ultrasound.* Baltimore: Williams & Wilkins; 1990:221-237.
30. Hodge KK, McNeal JE, Terris MK, et al: Random systematic versus directed ultrasound guided transrectal core biopsies of the prostate. *J Urol* 1989;142:71-75.
31. Dyke CH, Toi A, Sweet JM: Value of random ultrasound-guided transrectal prostate biopsy. *Radiology* 1990;176:345-349.
32. Cooner WH, Mosley BR, Rutherford CL Jr, et al: Prostate cancer detection in a clinical urological practice by ultrasonography, digital rectal examination and prostate specific antigen. *J Urol* 1990;143:1146-1154.
33. Lee F, Littrup PJ, McLeary RD, et al: Needle aspiration and core biopsy of prostate cancer: comparative evaluation with biplanar transrectal ultrasound guidance. *Radiology* 1987;163:515-520.
34. Resnick MI: Transrectal ultrasound guided versus digitally directed prostatic biopsy: a comparative study. *J Urol* 1987;139:754-757.
35. Ajzen SA, Goldenberg SL, Allen GJ, et al: Palpable prostatic nodules: comparison of ultrasound and digital guidance for fine-needle aspiration biopsy. *Radiology* 1989;171:521-523.
36. Hodge KK, McNeal JE, Stamey TA: Ultrasound guided transrectal core biopsies of the palpably abnormal prostate. *J Urol* 1988;142:66-70.

Benign abnormalities of the prostate and seminal vesicles

37. Berry SJ, Coffey DS, Walsh PC, et al: The development of human benign prostatic hyperplasia with age. *J Urol* 1984;132:474-479.
38. Hendrikx AJ, van Helvoort, van Dommelen CA, et al: Ultrasonic determination of prostatic volume: a cadaver study. *Urology* 1989;34(3):123-125.

39. Jakobsen H, Torp-Pedersen S, Juul N: Ultrasonic evaluation of age-related human prostatic growth and development of benign prostatic hyperplasia. *Scand J Urol Nephrol* 1988;107(suppl):26-31.

40. Burks DD, Drolshagen LF, Fleischer AC, et al: Transrectal sonography of benign and malignant prostatic lesions. *AJR* 1986;146:1187-1191.

41. Lee F, Torp-Pedersen ST, McLeary RD: Diagnosis of prostate cancer by transrectal ultrasound. *Urol Clin North Am* 1989;16:663-673.

42. Hendrikx AJ, Doesburg WH, Reintjes AG, et al: Determination of prostatic volume by ultrasonography. *Urology* 1989;33(4):336-339

43. Hendrikx AJ, Doesburg WH, Reintjes AG, et al: Effectiveness of ultrasound in the preoperative evaluation of patients with prostatism. *Prostate* 1988;13:199-208.

44. Castaneda F, Reddy P, Wasserman N, et al: Benign prostatic hypertrophy: retrograde transurethral dilation of the prostatic urethra in humans. *Radiology* 1987;163:649-653.

45. Brawer MK, Rennels MA, Nagle RB, et al: Prostatic intraepithelial neoplasia: A lesion that may be confused with cancer on prostatic ultrasound. *J Urol* 1989;142:1510-1512.

46. Lee F, Torp-Pedersen S, Carroll JT, et al: Use of transrectal ultrasound and prostate-specific antigen in diagnosis of prostatic intraepithelial neoplasia. *Urology* 1989;34(suppl):4-8.

47. Doble A, Carter S: Ultrasonographic findings in prostatitis. *Urol Clin North Am* 1989;16(4):763-772.

48. Di Trapani D, Pavone C, Serretta V, et al: Chronic prostatitis and prostatodynia: ultrasonographic alterations of the prostate, bladder neck, seminal vesicles and periprostatic venous plexus. *Eur Urol* 1988;15:230-234.

49. Doble A, Thomas BJ, Furr PM, et al: A search for infectious agents in chronic abacterial prostatitis using ultrasound guided biopsy. *Br J Urol* 1989;64:297-301.

50. Fuse H, Sumiya H, Ishii H, et al: Treatment of hemospermia caused by dilated seminal vesicles by direct drug injection guided by ultrasonography. *J Urol* 1988; 140:991-992.

51. Tzai T, Chang C, Yang C, et al: Transrectal sonography of the prostate and seminal vesicles on patients with hemospermia. *J Formosan Med Assoc* 1989; 88:232-235.

52. Bude R, Bree RL, Adler RS, et al: Transrectal ultrasound appearance of granulomatous prostatitis. *J Ultrasound Med* 1990;9:677-680.

53. Cytron S, Weinberger M, Pitlik S, et al: Value of transrectal ultrasonography for diagnosis and treatment of prostatic abscess. *Urology* 1988;32(5):454-458.

54. Papanicolaou N, Pfister R, Stafford S, et al: Prostatic abscess: imaging with transrectal sonography and magnetic resonance. *AJR* 1987;149:981-982.

55. Nghiem HT, Kellman GM, Sandberg SA, et al: Cystic lesions of the prostate. *Radiographics* 1990;10:635-650.

56. Shabsigh R, Lerner S, Fishman IJ, et al: The role of transrectal ultrasonography in the diagnosis and management of prostatic and seminal vesicle cysts. *J Urol* 1989;141:1206-1209.

57. Littrup PJ, Lee F, McLeary RD, et al: Transrectal ultrasound of the seminal vesicles and ejaculatory ducts: clinical correlation. *Radiology* 1988;168:625-628.

Prostate Cancer

58. McClennan BL: Transrectal ultrasound of the prostate: Is the technology leading the science? *Radiology* 1988; 168:571-575.

59. Dhom G: Incipient prostate cancer: definition, histology and clinical consequences. *Recent Results Cancer Res* 1988;106:86-93.

60. Baran GW, Golin AL, Bergsma CJ, et al: Biologic aggressiveness of palpable and nonpalpable prostate cancer: assessment with endosonography. *Radiology* 1991;178:201-206.

61. McNeal JE, Price HM, Redwine EA, et al: Stage A versus stage B adenocarcinoma of the prostate: morphological comparison and biological significance. *J Urol* 1988;139:61-65.

62. Whitmore WF Jr: Natural history staging of prostate cancer. *Urol Clin North Am* 1984; 11:205-220.

63. Gleason DF, Veterans Administration Cooperative Urological Research Group. *Histologic Grading and Clinical Staging of Prostatic Carcinoma*. Philadelphia: Lea & Febiger; 1977.

64. Muldoon L, Resnick MI: Results of ultrasonography of the prostate. *Urol Clin North Am* 1989;16:693-702.

65. Dahnert WF, Hamper UM, Eggleston JC, et al: Prostatic evaluation by transrectal sonography with histopathologic correlation: the echogenic appearance of early carcinoma. *Radiology*; 1986;158:97-102.

66. Rifkin MD, McGlynn ET, Choi H: Echogenicity of prostatic cancer correlated with histologic grade and stromal fibrosis: endorectal ultrasound studies. *J Urol* 1989;170:549-552.

67. Shinohara K, Wheeler TM, Scardino PT: The appearance of prostate cancer on transrectal ultrasonography: correlation of imaging and pathological examinations. *J Urol* 1989;142:76-82.

68. Dahnert WF, Hamper UM, Walsh PC, et al: The echogenic focus in prostatic sonograms, with xeroradiographic and histopathologic correlation. *Radiology* 1986;159:95-100.

69. Lee F. Transrectal ultrasound: diagnosis and staging of prostatic carcinoma. *Urology* 1989;33(suppl):5-10.

70. Hamper UM, Sheth S, Walsh PC, et al: Bright echogenic foci in early prostatic carcinoma: sonographic and pathologic correlation. *Radiology* 1990;176:339-343.

71. Dahnert WF: Ultrasonography of carcinoma of the prostate: a critical review. *Appl Radiol* 1988;17:39-44.

72. Stamey TA, Yang N, Hay AR, et al: Prostate-specific antigen as a serum marker for adenocarcinoma of the prostate. *N Engl J Med* 1987; 317:909-955.

73. Lee F, Torp-Pedersen S, Littrup PJ, et al: Hypoechoic lesions of the prostate: clinical relevance of tumor size, digital rectal examination, and prostate-specific antigen. *Radiology* 1989; 170:29-32.

74. Littrup PJ, Kane RA, Williams CR, et al: Determination of prostate volume with transrectal ultrasound for cancer screening. *Radiology* 1991;178:537-542.

75. McNeal JE, Redwine EA, Freiha FS, et al: Zonal distribution of prostatic adenocarcinoma. *Am J Surg Pathol* 1988;12:897-906.

76. Hunter PT, Butler SA, Hodge GB, et al: Detection of prostatic cancer using transrectal ultrasound and sonographically guided biopsy in 1410 symptomatic patients. *J Endourol* 1989; 3:167-175.

77. Rifkin MD, Choi H: Implications of small, peripheral hypoechoic lesions in endorectal ultrasound of the prostate. *Radiology* 1988;166:619-622.

78. Palken M, Cobb OE, Warren BH, et al: Prostate cancer: correlation of digital rectal examination, transrectal ultrasound and prostate specific antigen levels with tumor volumes in radical prostatectomy specimens. *J Urol* 1990;143:115-162.

79. Lee F, Littrup PJ, Torp-Pedersen S, et al: Prostate cancer: comparison of transrectal ultrasound and digital rectal examination. *Radiology* 1988;168:389-394.

80. Torp-Pedersen S, Littrup PJ, Lee F, et al: Early prostate cancer: diagnostic costs of screening transrectal ultrasound and digital rectal examination. *Radiology* 1988;169:351-354.

81. Cooner WH, Mosley BR, Rutherford CL, et al: Clinical application of transrectal ultrasonography and prostate specific antigen in the search for prostate cancer. *J Urol* 1988;139:758-761.

82. Nesbitt JA, Drago JR, Badalament RA: Transrectal ultrasonography. *Urology* 1989;34(3):120-122.

83. Drago JR, Nesbitt JA, Badalament RA: Use of transrectal ultrasound in detection of prostatic carcinoma: a preliminary report. *J Surg Oncol* 1989;41:274-277.

84. Imai K, Zinbo S, Shimizu K, et al: Clinical characteristics of prostatic cancer detected by mass screening. *Prostate* 1988; 12:199-207.

85. Carter HB, Hamper UM, Sheth S, et al: Evaluation of transrectal ultrasound in the early detection of prostate cancer. *J Urol* 1989;142:1008-1010.

86. Perrin P, Mouriquand P, Monsallier M, et al: Hypothetical place of transrectal ultrasound in the diagnosis of prostatic cancer at an early stage. *J Endourol* 1989;3:109-113.

87. Chodak GW: Screening for prostate cancer. *Urol Clin North Am* 1989;16:657-661.

88. Parra RO, Gregory JG: Transrectal ultrasound in stage A1 prostate cancer. *Urology* 1989;34:344-346.

89. Hamper UM, Sheth S, Holtz PM, et al: Evaluation of the periprostatic neurovascular bundle: a sonographic surgical pathological correlation. *J Ultrasound Med* 1900;9:545.

90. Hamper UM, Sheth S, Walsh PC, et al: Carcinoma of the prostate: value of transrectal sonography in detecting extension into the neurovascular bundle. *AJR* 1990;155:1015-1019.

91. Andriole GL, Coplen DE, Mikkelsen DJ, et al: Sonographic and pathological staging of patients with clinically localized prostate cancer. *J Urol* 1989;142:1259-1261.

92. Hardeman SW, Causey JQ, Hickey DP, et al: Transrectal ultrasound for staging prior to radical prostatectomy. *Urology* 1989;34:175-180.

93. Terris MK, McNeal JE, Stamey TA: Invasion of the seminal vesicles by prostatic cancer: detection with transrectal sonography. *AJR* 1990; 155:811-815.

94. Platt J, Bree RL, Schwab RE: Accuracy of computed tomography in the staging of carcinoma of the prostate. *AJR* 1987;149:315-318.

95. Salo JO, Kivisaari L, Rannikko S, et al: Computerized tomography and transrectal ultrasound in the assessment of local extension of prostatic cancer before radical retropubic prostatectomy. *J Urol* 1987;137:435-438.

96. Schnall MD, Lenkinski RE, Pollack HM, et al: Prostate: magnetic resonance imaging with an endorectal surface coil. *Radiology* 1989; 172:570-574.

97. Iversen P, Bak M, Juul N, et al: Ultrasonically guided 125 iodine seed implantation with external radiation in management of localized prostatic carcinoma. *Urology* 1989;34:181-186.

98. Broseta E, Boronat F, Domimguez C, et al: Modification del patron ecografico del carcinoma de prostata tratado mediante agonistas Lh-rh. *Arch Esp de Urol* 1989;42:125-128.

99. Clements R, Griffiths GJ, Peeling WB, et al: Transrectal ultrasound in monitoring response to treatment of prostate disease. *Urol Clin North Am* 1989;16:735-740.

100. Egender G, Pirker E, Rapf C, et al: Transrectal ultrasonography as follow-up method in prostatic carcinoma after external beam and interstitial radiotherapy. *Eur J Radiol* 1988;8:37-43.

101. Carpentier P, Schroeder FH, Schmitz PIM: Transrectal ultrasonometry of the prostate: the prognostic relevance of volume changes under endocrine management. *World J Urol* 1986;4:159-162.

102. Egawa S, Carter SSC, Wheeler Tm, et al: Ultrasonographic changes in the normal and malignant prostate after definitive radiotherapy. *Urol Clin North Am* 1989;16:741-749.

103. Kabalin JN, Hodge KK, McNeal JE, et al: Identification of residual cancer in the prostate following radiation therapy: role of transrectal ultrasound guided biopsy and prostate specific antigen. *J Urol* 1989;142:326-33.

104. Onik G, Cobb C, Cohen J, et al: Ultrasound characteristics of frozen prostate. *Radiology* 1988;168:629-631.

CHAPTER 11

The Adrenal Glands and Retroperitoneum

- J. Scott Kriegshauser, M.D.
- Barbara A. Carroll, M.D.

Although computed tomography (CT) is generally superior to sonography for imaging the retroperitoneum and adrenal glands in adults, ultrasound frequently detects retroperitoneal abnormalities.[1,2] It is particularly useful in the evaluation of slender adults and in those with pulsatile, palpable abdominal masses. A wide range of retroperitoneal pathology will be imaged initially with ultrasound, and in many instances, sonographic demonstration of a retroperitoneal abnormality may obviate the need for additional imaging studies. Thus a thorough appreciation of the sonographic features of the normal retroperitoneum, including the adrenal glands, and the pathology that arises in this space is crucial.

TECHNIQUE

Fasting for 6 to 8 hours before the exam usually decreases the bowel gas that can greatly interfere with visualization of the adrenals and retroperitoneum. If the left adrenal gland is difficult to see because of bowel gas, having the patient drink water and fill the stomach with fluid may be useful to provide a sonographic window for imaging.

In most adults, a 3 to 3.5 MHz transducer will provide adequate penetration for evaluation of the adrenals and retroperitoneum. In larger patients, in patients with fatty infiltration of the liver, or when evaluating very deep structures, a 2 to 2.5 MHz transducer may be required. Conversely, slender patients may be evaluated with a 5 Mhz transducer. Sector transducers provide access through the intercostal spaces better than linear array transducers. When large masses are being evaluated, a linear transducer may be valuable because of the wide near field of view.

It is important to identify the echogenic retroperitoneal fat of the anterior pararenal and perirenal spaces on a longitudinal scan and to assess any displacement of this structure. Anterior displacement of the retroperitoneal fat echoes denotes a retroperitoneal process (Fig. 11-1), while masses arising in the liver or subhepatic space displace the fat echoes posteriorly or inferiorly.[3] Furthermore, a wedge-shaped anterior displacement suggests an adrenal or suprarenal mass (Fig. 11-1) rather than one of renal origin.

Evaluation of the adrenal glands and retroperitoneum should be done in both the transverse and longitudinal planes, in the supine and lateral decubitus positions. Some studies suggest that the transverse plane is better for visualizing the adrenal glands themselves, but other studies favor longitudinal scans for evaluation of the adrenal gland and the adrenal bed.[4,5] An intercostal approach through the liver at the middle or anterior axillary line is usually best for evaluation of the right adrenal gland. Scanning in the left lateral decubitus position or anteriorly through the liver with the patient supine may also be useful. The left adrenal gland is best eval-

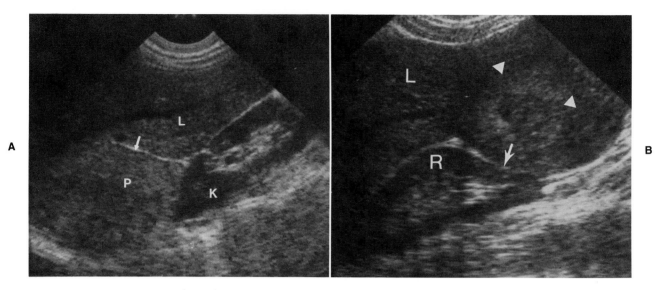

FIG 11-1. Retroperitoneal fat stripe displacement. **A,** Longitudinal sonogram shows a wedge-shaped anterior displacement of the right retroperitoneal fat stripe *(arrow)* caused by a right adrenal pheochromocytoma *(P)*. **B,** Longitudinal scan shows postero-inferior displacement of the right retroperitoneal fat stripe *(arrow)* by a bulging Liver metastasis *(arrowheads)*. *L,* Liver; *R,* right kidney.

(Courtesy Stephanie R. Wilson, M.D., Toronto General Hospital, Canada.)

uated from an intercostal approach along the posterior axillary line or even farther posteriorly using the spleen as a window. The right posterior oblique position relative to the table, a right lateral decubitus position, or scanning anteriorly using the fluid-filled stomach as a window may also be helpful. Scanning from a posterior approach rarely offers any advantage, possibly because of the large number of interfaces in the fat and muscle tissues in the back as well as the low position of the posterior lung.[4,6]

Initial sonographic evaluation of the retroperitoneum is performed with the subject in a supine position. The great vessels are identified in the midline, and the paraaortic and paracaval regions are examined from the level of the diaphragm to, and including, the iliac vessels when possible. Generally the aorta enters the abdominal cavity far posterior but becomes progressively more anterior as it travels caudally. The inferior vena cava (IVC), in contrast, maintains a more horizontal course throughout the retroperitoneum. Overlying bowel gas obscures more of the structures in the retroperitoneum as one moves lower in the abdomen and within the pelvis. Coronal or near-coronal scans, using the kidneys and posterior musculature as an acoustic window, can give excellent images of retroperitoneal structures in some patients, even if bowel gas obscures the region on supine scans (Fig. 11-2).[7]

Renal morphology and movement should be assessed. Normal respiratory excursion may be absent or decreased when a perinephric process is present. The retroperitoneal muscles should be evaluated for morphology and symmetry. An attempt should be made to identify both diaphragmatic crura and exclude pathology around these structures. The transverse plane is most helpful, often with the patient in the lateral decu-

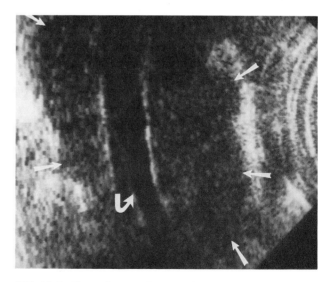

FIG 11-2. Coronal scan of retroperitoneal adenopathy. Massive retroperitoneal adenopathy *(arrows)* surrounding the abdominal aorta down to the bifurcation *(curved arrow)* is demonstrated on this coronal scan through the left flank.

bitus position. Longitudinal or coronal planes may be helpful for the right crus but usually are not rewarding for evaluating the left crus.[8]

ADRENAL GLANDS
Normal Appearance

The adrenal glands consist of an anteromedial ridge and lateral and medial wings. They measure 4 to 6 cm in length and 2 to 3 cm in width, but only 3 to 6 mm in thickness.[4] The adrenal glands lie within the perirenal space, anteromedial to the kidneys, and are connected to Gerota's fascia (Fig. 11-3). The distance from the kidney to the adrenal is somewhat variable because of this attachment, whereas the relationship of the adrenal to the great vessels and more anterior structures is relatively more constant (Fig. 11-4).[6] Typically, the lateral wing is more horizontal and superior, while the medial wing is directed more longitudinally and inferiorly.

The medial wing of the right adrenal lies posterior to the IVC. Some of the right adrenal extends superior to the upper pole of the kidney. However, the medial wing is usually located more inferiorly, adjacent to the upper pole of the kidney when viewed in a transverse plane. The liver lies laterally and anterolaterally. The crus of the diaphragm lies medial and posterior to the right adrenal gland (Fig. 11-5).

The left adrenal gland lies anteromedial to the upper pole of the left kidney. In 10% of patients it extends inferiorly to the level of the renal hilum.[4,9] As on the right, portions of the left adrenal may extend superior to the upper pole of the kidney. The aorta and crus of the diaphragm are located medial to the left adrenal. The tail of the pancreas and splenic vein are anterior to the left adrenal gland at one level; at a higher level, the lesser sac and posterior portions of the stomach form the anterior border. Portions of the spleen occasionally

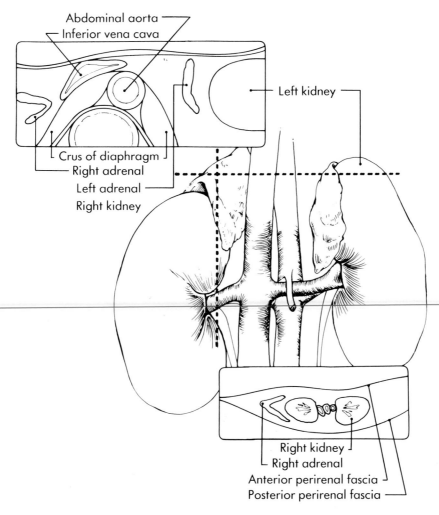

FIG 11-3. Normal anatomy. Schematic representation of the relationship of the adrenal glands to the kidney, great vessels, and perirenal fascia. *Upper insert,* transverse plane, *lower insert,* sagittal plane.

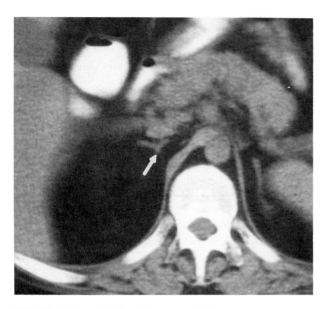

FIG 11-4. Normal adrenals, congenitally atrophic right kidney. CT shows the right adrenal *(arrow)* remains very close to the IVC because of its attachment to Gerota's fascia.

extend more medially and can lie adjacent to the left adrenal.

Real-time sonographic visualization of the normal adrenal gland has been reported to be as high as 92% on the right and 71% on the left.[5] However, Gunther et al[6] reported visualization of the adrenal glands in only 1 of 60 normal volunteers. Yeh[4,9,10] reported visualization of the adrenal gland on the right in 78% and on the left in 44% of normal subjects using manual static scanning techniques. Visualization is higher in the neonate and the adult with a hypertrophic gland.[10]

Sonographically, the adrenal gland is usually slightly less echogenic than the surrounding retroperitoneal fat. The medulla may be seen as an echogenic central linear structure within the adrenal gland. This is especially prominent in neonates and is a distinguishing feature between adrenal hyperplasia and an infiltrative process enlarging the adrenal gland, which obliterates this structure (Fig. 11-6).

Adrenal Masses

Ultrasound can detect approximately 90% of known adrenal masses, which are better studied first by CT.[6,11] Obesity and overlying bowel gas are the most common reasons for failure to visualize adrenal masses; this oc-

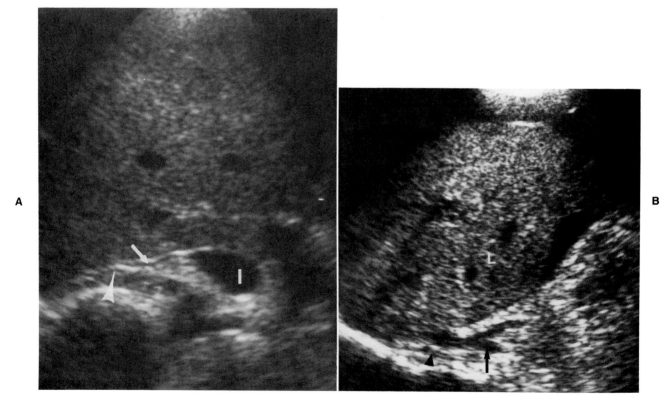

FIG 11-5. Normal right adrenal. **A,** Transverse image shows a portion of the right adrenal *(arrow)* between liver and the diaphragmatic crus *(arrowhead). I,* IVC. **B,** Longitudinal sonogram shows the normal right adrenal *(arrow)* in a patient with cirrhosis and ascites. *I,* IVC; *L,* liver.

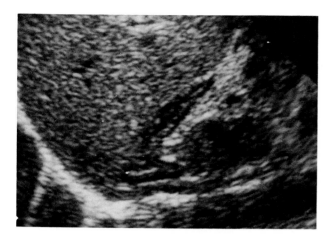

FIG 11-6. Newborn right adrenal gland seen on a longitudinal image shows the echogenic central adrenal medulla *(arrow)*.

curs more often on the left.[5] False-positive examinations are also more common on the left. Fluid-filled bowel and periadrenal fat may suggest a mass when one is not present. Peristalsis in the "suspected" mass confirms its bowel origin. An accessory spleen also may mimic a left adrenal mass, but these are usually located lateral to the adrenal bed, have a characteristic round or oval shape, and are isoechoic with the spleen.[12] Occasionally a splenic lobule will project into the renal bed, and in some planes, resemble an adrenal mass. In this situation, scanning in other planes will usually demonstrate a connection with the rest of the spleen and identical echotexture.

Ultrasound may be useful for:

- Characterizing a known adrenal mass as cystic or solid (particularly when CT numbers are low, as occurs in the cysts and masses with a high lipid content)
- Evaluating the position and patency of the IVC and draining veins
- Evaluating tumor invasion into adjacent structures
- Determining the origin of a large retroperitoneal mass
- Follow-up of an adrenal mass that is not surgically removed[2]

The ability to use multiple scanning planes gives ultrasound and magnetic resonance imaging (MR) an advantage over CT in determining the organ of origin of a suspected adrenal mass or invasion of adjacent structures. A wedge- or triangular-shaped anterior or superior displacement of the echogenic retroperitoneal fat stripe is good evidence for a retroperitoneal mass of adrenal origin, whereas posterior (and inferior) displacement suggests a hepatic or subhepatic process (Fig. 11-1).[3] Invagination of the liver capsule is good evidence for an extrahepatic mass, whereas external bulging of

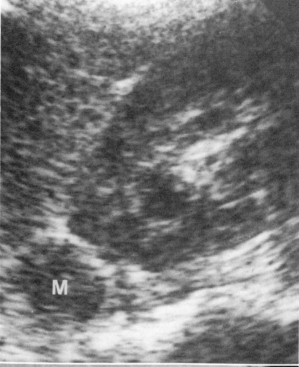

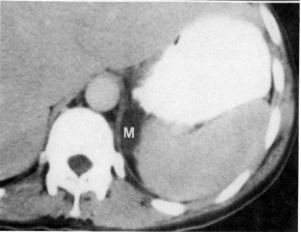

FIG 11-7. Adrenal adenoma. **A,** Longitudinal ultrasound shows a solid mass in the left adrenal bed *(M)*. **B,** CT shows low-density left adrenal mass *(M)*.
(Courtesy J. William Charboneau, M.D., Mayo Clinic, Rochester, Minn.)

the capsule suggests an intrahepatic mass.[13] Calcification within an adrenal mass is entirely nonspecific and may be seen in almost any benign or malignant processes.

Neoplasms of the Adrenal Cortex

Adenomas. Adrenal nodules less than 2.5 cm in diameter are commonly found at autopsy (2% to 9% incidence), and most are nonfunctioning adenomas.[14,15] However, clinical imaging of these lesions is less frequent and usually incidental. One report found adrenal masses incidentally with CT in 0.6% of their patients.[16] Incidentally detected masses of the adrenal gland are most commonly nonfunctioning adenomas, however a significant percentage of these may be malignant.[15,17] The decision to resect such an adrenal mass is usually based on size when endocrine studies are negative. Reports of the maximum size of an incidental adrenal mass that can be safely watched instead of resected vary from 3 to 6 cm.[15,17] In patients with a known primary malignancy, percutaneous biopsy is often performed even on small adrenal masses to exclude metastatic disease. Clinical or biochemical evidence of Cushing's syndrome or hyperaldosteronism is usually an indication for resection of an adrenal mass, even if it is small.

Cushing's syndrome is most commonly caused by pituitary adenomas (80%). Therefore, when a pituitary adenoma is demonstrated, there is no need to image the adrenals even though up to 50% may show adrenal hyperplasia. Adrenal adenomas are the cause of Cushing's syndrome in 18% of patients. These are usually small (2 to 5 cm in diameter). CT is the study of choice for their identification, but ultrasound may help if a low-density mass seen on CT needs to be differentiated from a cyst (Fig. 11-7).[2,18]

Approximately half of patients with hyperaldosteronism have a single unilateral adenoma. These most commonly measure between 0.5 cm and 3 cm in diameter. One half of cases are due to bilateral hyperplasia, and this is an important differentiation since surgery is more helpful for adenomas but often not indicated with hyperplasia.[2]

When adrenal masses are small, differentiation of a solitary mass, such as an adenoma, from a hyperplastic nodule may be difficult or impossible. Hyperplastic nodules may be multiple and are often associated with bilateral hyperplasia, whereas a functioning adenoma is typically associated with contralateral adrenal atrophy.[10]

Adrenal Cortical Carcinoma. Adrenal cortical carcinomas are highly malignant tumors with a very poor prognosis.[2,19] They occur in both children and adults and are more common in females. Approximately half are hormonally active. There is a wide variation in size, ranging from 3 to 22 cm in one study.[19] Smaller tumors (less than 6 cm) are hormonally active more often than larger tumors. Differentiation from benign adenoma is sometimes difficult, even histologically, but most authors recommend removal of a tumor (or biopsy) based on size (threshold ranges from 3 to 6 cm).[15,17]

The sonographic appearance is typically that of a well-defined homogenous mass when the tumor is small (less than 2 to 6 cm), whereas larger tumors tend to have necrosis and hemorrhage centrally, and they more often calcify (Fig. 11-8).[19] Calcifications are seen in up to 19%. Tumor may invade into the adrenal or renal

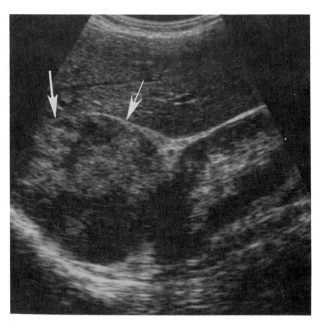

FIG 11-8. Adrenal carcinoma. Longitudinal scan shows a large inhomogeneous mass *(arrows)*.
(Courtesy Stephanie R. Wilson, M.D., Toronto General Hospital, Canada.)

veins, as well as the IVC, hepatic veins, and even the right atrium.[2,20] Ultrasound and Doppler are often useful for evaluation of such venous involvement.[2,20]

Neoplasms of the Adrenal Medulla

Pheochromocytoma. Pheochromocytoma originates in the adrenal medulla in 90% of cases. This rare tumor occurs most commonly in adults between the fourth and sixth decades but can be seen in children.[1] Tumors are multicentric in 10% and bilateral in 5% with a higher incidence of multiple tumors during childhood. Secretion of epinephrine and norepinephrine can lead to hypertension. Evaluation of urinary metanephrines is the preferred screening procedure. In one study this was positive in 102 out of 104 cases.[1] Pheochromocytoma is associated with neuroectodermal disorders such as von Hippel-Lindau disease, tuberous sclerosis, and neurofibromatosis, and is also seen in multiple endocrine neoplasm (MEN) syndromes (Fig. 11-9). Patients with these syndromes tend to have more frequent occurrence of pheochromocytoma in childhood, more frequent multiple tumors, but a lower incidence of malignancy.[1,14] The overall incidence of malignancy in pheochromocytomas is 5% to 13%. Invasion of adjacent structures is not by itself an indicator of malignancy, and metastatic disease is the only reliable indicator of malignancy, according to some reports.[1,14]

Ultrasound is reported to have a sensitivity of between 89% and 97% for detection of adrenal

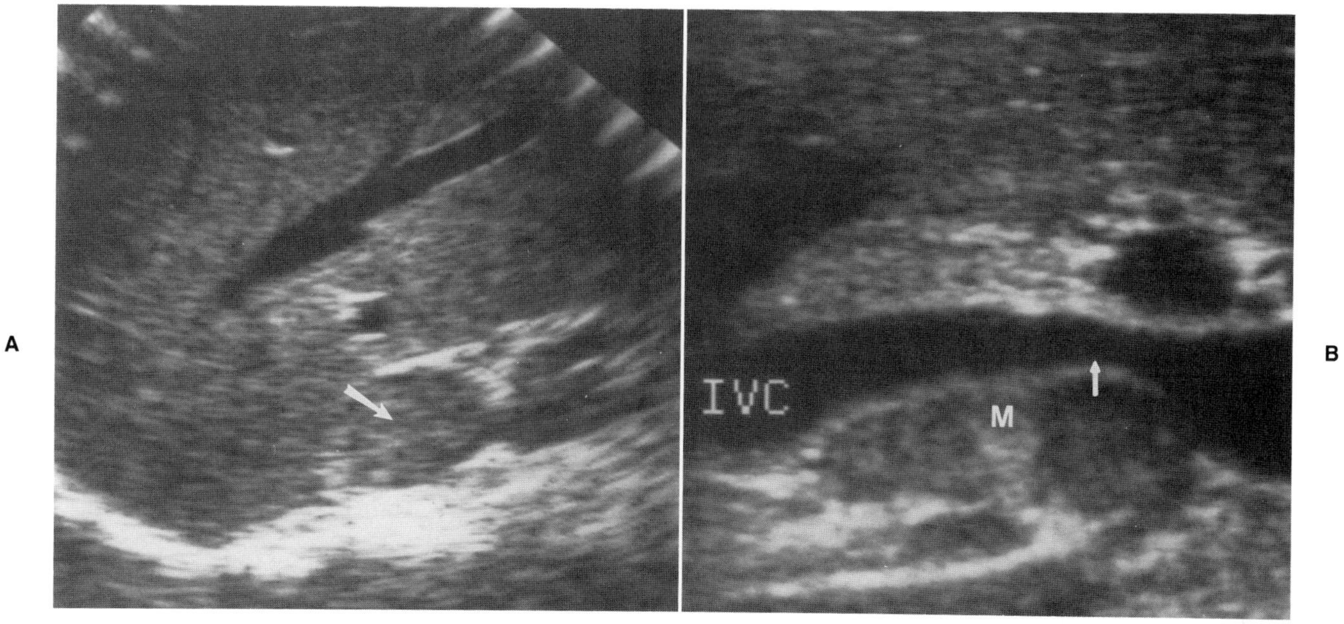

FIG 11-9. Pheochromocytoma. **A,** Von Hippel-Lindau disease. Longitudinal sonogram shows a solid right adrenal mass *(arrow)*. Patient also had an islet cell tumor of the pancreas (not shown). **B,** Multiple endocrine tumor syndrome II. Longitudinal sonogram shows pheochromocytoma (inhomogeneous mass) *(M)* that displaces the IVC anteriorly *(arrow)*.
(Courtesy J. William Charboneau, M.D., Mayo Clinic, Rochester, Minn.)

pheochromocytoma, whereas CT sensitivity approaches 100%.[1,21] These tumors tend to be large (average 5 to 6 cm) and sharply marginated, and have a significant solid component. Central hemorrhagic and necrotic changes are common and may produce a cystic component (Fig. 11-10) or focal echogenic abnormalities.[22] There are reports of pheochromocytomas that are almost entirely cystic in appearance, and a fluid-fluid level was identified in one tumor.[21,23]

Other Medullary Neoplasms. Other tumors originating from the adrenal medulla, including neuroblastoma, ganglioneuroblastoma, and ganglioneuroma, occur most commonly in childhood (see Chapter 60).

Myelolipoma. Adrenal myelolipomas are rare, benign, nonfunctioning hamartomas that contain both fatty and bone marrow elements.[14,24] These tumors range in size from microscopic to 30 cm, but most are 2 to 9 cm.[24,25] They have been reported to be bilateral, but most are unilateral;[14] most occur between the fourth and sixth decades. Patients are usually asymptomatic; however, hemorrhage may cause flank pain.[14,24] Some reports associate myelolipomas with concurrent chronic illness.[25,26]

Ultrasound most commonly shows an echogenic or predominantly echogenic mass in the adrenal bed.

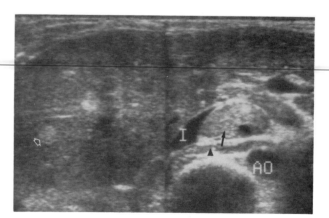

FIG 11-10. Adrenal pheochromocytoma *(arrow),* with a small cystic component, is seen displacing the IVC *(I)* laterally and anteriorly. The diaphragmatic crus *(arrowhead)* is well seen along the spine between the right adrenal mass and the aorta *(AO).* Hepatic metastases *(open arrow)* are present.
(Courtesy J. William Charboneau, M.D., Mayo Clinic, Rochester, Minn.)

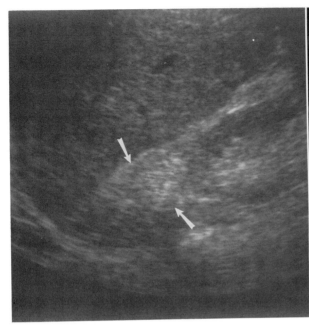

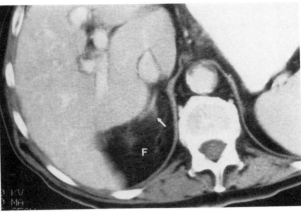

FIG 11-11. Pseudomass from prominent fat. **A,** Longitudinal sonogram suggests an echogenic "mass" *(arrows)* in the right adrenal bed. **B,** CT shows a normal right adrenal gland *(arrow)* and prominent perirenal fat *(F)*.

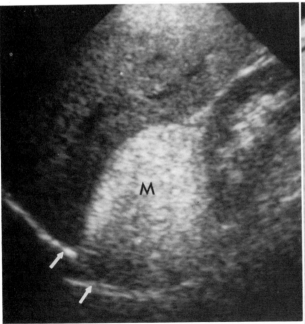

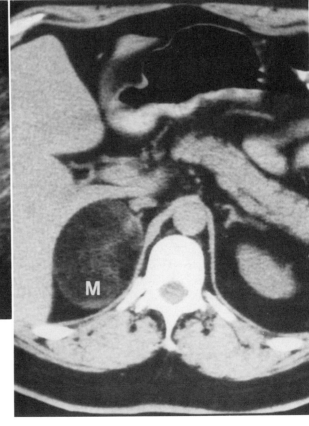

FIG 11-12. Myelolipoma with speed propagation artifact. **A,** Longitudinal sonogram shows an echogenic right adrenal mass *(M)*. Break in the diaphragm echoes *(arrows)* displaced posteriorly behind the adrenal mass resulting from speed propagation artifact caused by fat within the mass. **B,** CT shows the predominantly fatty right adrenal mass *(M)*.

Roughly half of these tumors have a homogeneous echo texture. Hypoechoic regions correlate pathologically with myeloid elements, with a tendency to enhance on CT.[24] CT will confirm a fatty component in the majority of myelolipomas, even those containing predominantly myeloid elements. If a fatty component is not definitely demonstrated with CT, biopsy may be necessary for diagnosis. A small fatty tumor may be masked by the surrounding periadrenal fat on both CT and with ultrasound. Conversely, normal periadrenal fat may mimic a mass on ultrasound, suggesting a myelolipoma (Fig. 11-11). Diffuse or scattered calcifications may cause posterior acoustic shadowing.[24,25]

Propagation speed artifact was originally described in a case of myelolipoma, and the presence of this artifact is excellent evidence of a fat-containing mass (Fig. 11-12).[24,27] The slower speed of sound within fat or lipid elements, as in a myelolipoma, is not compensated for by the ultrasound machine's computer, which maps the echoes in and behind the tumor as farther away from the transducer than they really are. This will make the adrenal mass appear larger and may produce artifactual discontinuities in structures behind the mass, such as the diaphragm.

The differential diagnosis of a hyperechoic adrenal mass includes any adrenal mass with diffuse calcifica-tion, such as hematoma, as well as any mass containing fat, including a renal angiomyelolipoma, retroperitoneal lipomas and liposarcomas, and teratomas.[24,25] However, when ultrasound and CT confirm the adrenal origin of a fat-containing mass, myelolipoma can be comfortably diagnosed.

Adrenal Cysts. Adrenal cysts are rare, usually asymptomatic, and most often found incidentally. They are usually unilateral and occur equally on the right and left sides (Fig. 11-13). They occur at any age but are most commonly seen between the third and sixth decades in females.[28,29] Lymphangiomatous cysts are most common pathologically (41%). Pseudocysts, while less common pathologically (39%), are more often discovered clinically because of their larger size. Pseudocysts are thought to result from previous hemorrhage, with organization of the clot and subsequent cyst formation. Calcification, which is usually peripheral and curvilinear, is seen in approximately 15% of pseudocysts.[23,28,29] Most cysts are not large enough to cause clinical manifestations, but if they attain a very large size, these can cause symptoms resulting from pressure on adjacent structures.

On ultrasound, increased through transmission, posterior enhancement, and well-defined walls are generally necessary to confidently diagnose a cyst sonograph-

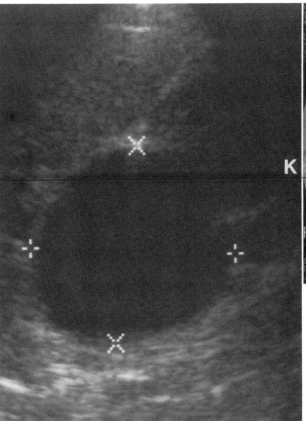

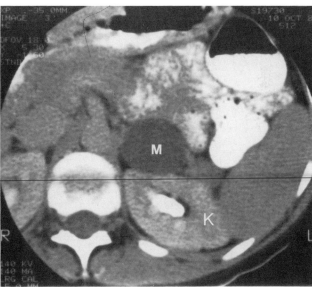

FIG 11-13. Adrenal cyst. **A,** Transverse ultrasound shows a simple cyst (×,+) in the left adrenal bed. **B,** CT scan shows a low-density mass *(M)* anterior to the left kidney. *K,* Left kidney.

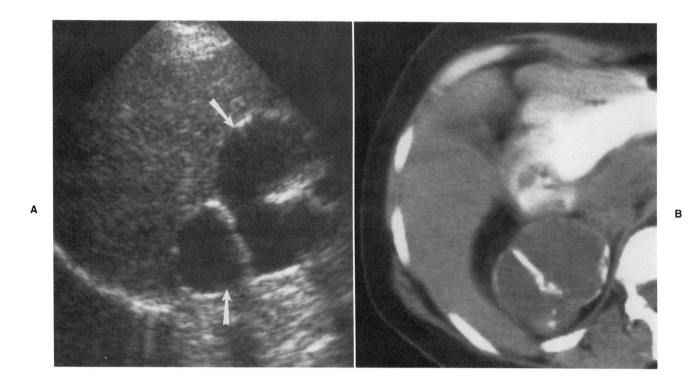

FIG 11-14. Adrenal pseudocyst. **A,** Sonogram demonstrates a cystic right adrenal mass *(arrows)* with echogenic walls and septations. Acoustic shadowing indicates wall calcification. **B,** CT confirms the calcifications and septations.

ically. Adrenal pseudocysts demonstrate thin, smooth walls. They may be septated and contain calcifications or occasional scattered internal echoes (Fig. 11-14). When the diagnosis is in doubt or the mass is large, aspiration may be helpful for diagnosis.[14,28] Differential diagnosis includes cystic degeneration of a malignant adrenal mass, abscess, and occasionally a very hypoechoic lymphoma.

Hemangiomas. Adrenal hemangiomas have been reported, but the ultrasound and CT findings are nonspecific. Ultrasound may show a large heterogeneous mass, and CT may demonstrate a mass with a hypodense central region and thick, irregular, high-density tissue peripherally.[22] Calcifications may occur.

Lymphoma. Adrenal involvement with lymphoma is common and frequently bilateral. Non-Hodgkin's lymphoma is reported to involve the adrenal in up to 4% of patients on radiographic studies and 24% of patients at autopsy.[30] Involvement may be diffuse, resembling hyperplasia, or masslike. Lymphadenopathy is usually present. Unilateral adrenal lymphoma as a primary manifestation of disease is rare.[30,31]

Adrenal lymphoma is usually hypoechoic and may even resemble a cystic mass. Central necrosis and hemorrhage in a patient who has not had chemotherapy are rare. Lymphomatous adrenal masses may also appear echogenic and when bilateral the sonographic appearance on one side may be completely different from that on the other side.[32] One report claims a histologic diagnosis of large-cell lymphoma in the adrenal gland should be suggested when a solid mass containing nodular sonolucent components is seen in conjunction with adenopathy (Fig. 11-15).[31]

Adrenal Metastases. Metastatic disease to the adrenal glands is common, especially from primary lung and renal cell carcinomas.[9,11] Bilateral involvement was seen in slightly more than half of the patients in one study,[11] the masses ranging from 1 to 10 cm in size with a mean of 3.5 cm. Differentiation of a common benign adenoma from a metastatic lesion is sometimes difficult when there is no other evidence of metastatic disease and the adrenal mass is unilateral. Often, needle aspiration/biopsy is necessary for diagnosis, and this is usually done with CT guidance.[17]

Sonographically, metastatic lesions have a nonspecific appearance (Fig. 11-16). Larger masses may contain central areas of necrosis or hemorrhage. There has been one report in the literature of IVC invasion from a metastatic adrenal mass.[33]

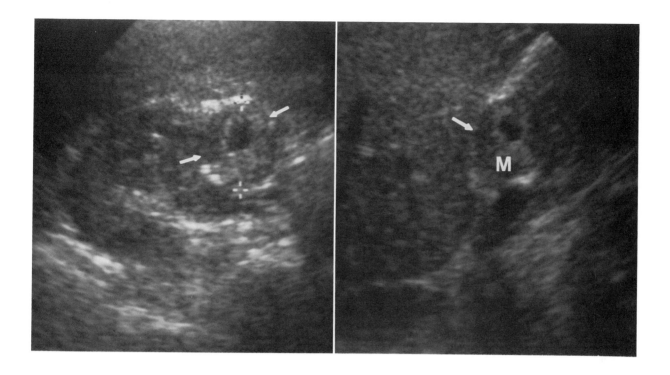

FIG 11-15. Adrenal lymphoma. **A,** A mixed echogenicity mass *(arrows)* is seen medial to the right kidney on a transverse image. **B,** Longitudinal scan confirms anterior retroperitoneal fat stripe displacement *(arrow)* by the right suprarenal mass *(M)*.

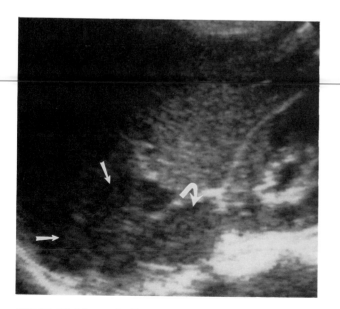

FIG 11-16. Metastatic disease to the right adrenal *(curved arrow)* and liver *(arrows)*.

Hemorrhage

Adrenal hemorrhage is most common in the neonate, caused by the large size of the adrenals and their high degree of vascularity, which make them vulnerable to peripartum trauma and asphyxial injuries.[9,34,35] Hemorrhage can also occur with infection, especially meningococcemia (Waterhouse-Friderichsen syndrome). Trauma is the most common cause of adrenal hemorrhage in the adult, with hemorrhage occurring in up to 25% of severely traumatized patients. In contrast to neonatal adrenal hemorrhage, which is usually bilateral, posttraumatic bleeding is more common on the right side (85%), with approximately 20% occurring bilaterally.[36]

Ultrasound initially shows an echogenic adrenal mass that may contain a bright central region. Later the mass will become hypoechoic or anechoic centrally (Fig. 11-17) and, with time, may shrink. With progressive decrease in size the mass may again become more echogenic and calcifications often develop. Alternatively, a pseudocyst with all the ultrasound characteris-

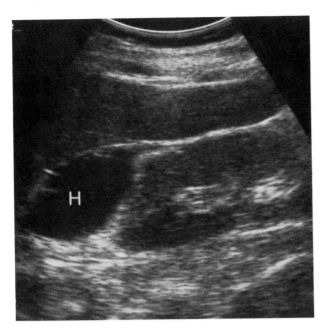

FIG 11-17. Adrenal hemorrhage *(H)* in a patient with meningococcemia. The right adrenal is large and hypoechoic.

tics of a simple cyst may be left behind.[36,37] Acute adrenal hemorrhage is more commonly seen with CT, which shows a soft tissue (or higher) density mass with adjacent stranding in the retroperitoneal fat and occasionally enlargement of the adjacent diaphragmatic crus.[36,37]

Infection

Tuberculosis and histoplasmosis are the most common infections involving the adrenal glands.[14] Both organisms can cause enlargement of the adrenal to several times its normal size and granuloma formation. Calcification is common, and this may remain even after resolution of the acute infectious process. Tuberculosis used to be the leading cause of Addison's disease, but with the advent of triple antibiotic treatment, autoimmune disease is now a more common cause. Tuberculosis and fungal and viral infections can involve the adrenals in AIDS patients.[18] These infections may produce adrenal masses, which are usually hypoechoic on ultrasound.[9] Pyogenic infections in or around the adrenal gland may produce cystic masses, which have an ultrasound appearance indistinguishable from necrotic malignancy or, occasionally, cysts. Aspiration biopsy is sometimes necessary for diagnosis. Excess steroids (endogenous or exogenous) cause an increased incidence of infection in many locations, including the adrenal glands. Most common of such steroid-related infections are histoplasmosis and cytomegalovirus.[18]

Adrenal Hyperplasia

Hyperplasia of the adrenal glands can occur:
- From any cause of Cushing's syndrome
- In approximately 50% of patients with hyperaldosteronism
- In various other syndromes
- As a primary process

Differentiation of an adenoma from a hyperplastic enlargement in patients with hyperaldosteronism is important since surgery is indicated for an adenoma.[2,14] Bilateral adrenal enlargement is seen with hyperplasia, whereas a functioning adenoma often produces contralateral adrenal atrophy.[10]

Adrenal hyperplasia may present as multiple bilateral nodules or as diffuse bilateral enlargement of the adrenal glands.[38] The differential diagnosis of diffuse enlargement includes lymphoma, metastatic disease, and infection.[4] Nodular hyperplasia is generally distinguishable from other causes of bilateral adrenal masses, such as metastatic disease and lymphoma, because the nodules tend to be 1 cm or less in size and are often seen in conjunction with generalized bilateral enlargement. Sonographically, the hypoechoic cortical portion of the gland is enlarged in adrenal hyperplasia, with sparing of the hyperechoic medulla. Nodularity can distort the contour and shape of the adrenal gland.[4,9]

RETROPERITONEUM
Normal Anatomy

Compartmental division of the retroperitoneum is somewhat controversial, although generally it is divided into the perirenal, anterior pararenal, and posterior pararenal spaces. The kidneys and adrenals lie within the perirenal space and are separated from the pararenal spaces by the renal fascia, often called Gerota's fascia or Toldt's fascia anteriorly and Zuckerkandl's fascia posteriorly (Fig. 11-18).[39-41] The right anterior pararenal space contains the IVC and portions of the duodenum and pancreas; the left anterior pararenal space contains the splenic vein and the pancreatic tail. The aorta and the diaphragm crura are located in the midline. Retroperitoneal portions of the colon lie within the lateral confines of the anterior pararenal space on each side. Occasionally, peritoneal recesses extend posterolaterally to the renal fascia.[40] The anterior pararenal and perirenal spaces contain abundant amounts of fatty and fibrous connective tissues, which produce an echogenic anterior border for the superior extent of the retroperitoneum (Fig. 11-19). Usually, it is not possible to distinguish echogenic fat in the perirenal space from that in the anterior pararenal space, but occasionally Gerota's fascia can be visualized.

The posterior pararenal space is of variable size and contains mostly fat. Retroperitoneal muscles are sepa-

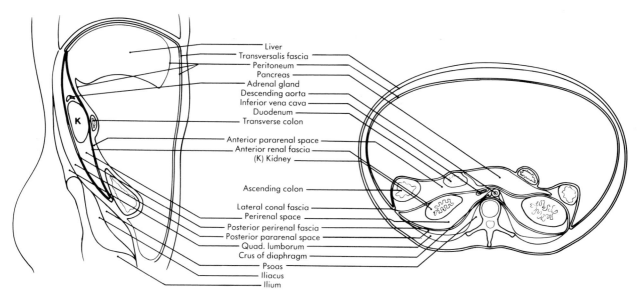

FIG 11-18. Normal anatomy. Transverse and right sagittal diagrams of retroperitoneal anatomy.

rated from this space by their own fascia. The quadratus lumborum muscle appears as a hypoechoic structure posterior to the kidneys (Fig. 11-20). In large patients or with improper settings, this muscle may give the appearance of a mass or a fluid collection, but no through enhancement should be seen, and it is a bilaterally symmetric structure with a characteristic appearance on coronal scans.[42] The psoas muscle lies in the paraspinal region, posterior and medial to the kidneys. It extends into the iliac fossa, combining with the iliacus muscle and paralleling the common iliac vessels. Symmetry is

important when evaluating the muscles of the retroperitoneum, as pathologic processes affecting these muscles, either directly or indirectly, may produce enlargement or atrophy.

The diaphragmatic crura are useful sonographic anatomic landmarks, but may be misinterpreted as an abnormality, especially when they are thickened. Transverse scans identify the right crus in approximately 90% of patients and the left in approximately 50%. Longitudinally, the right crus is identified in only 50% of patients, and the left crus is almost never seen in this

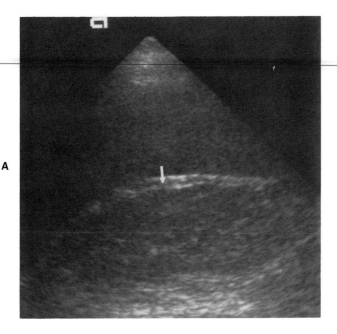

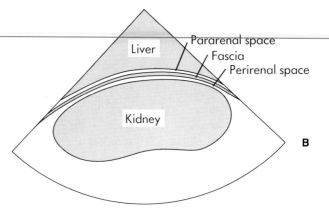

FIG 11-19. Fascia surrounded by echogenic fat. **A,** Longitudinal right-sided scan shows the separation of the echogenic fat in the perirenal and anterior pararenal space by Gerota's fascia *(arrow).* **B,** Diagram of the same normal anatomy.

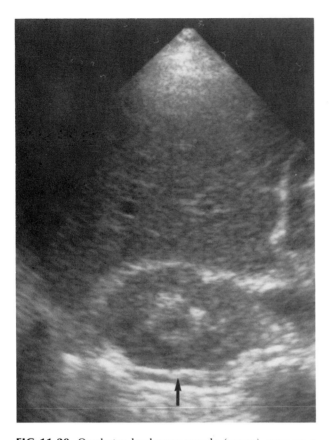

FIG 11-20. Quadratus lumborum muscle *(arrow)*, seen on a transverse right upper quadrant scan through the liver and right kidney.

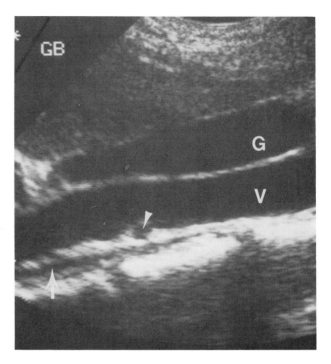

FIG 11-21. Right diaphragmatic crus. Longitudinal right sonogram shows the relationship of the diaphragmatic crus *(arrow)* to the right renal artery *(arrowhead)* and IVC *(V)*. *G,* Gallbladder.

plane.[8] The right crus extends to the L3 transverse process and is longer, larger, and more lobular than the left crus. The right renal artery travels anterior to the crus and posterior to the IVC (Fig. 11-21). The adrenal gland and right lobe of the liver lie lateral and anterior to the right crus. The left crus lies medial and posterior to the left adrenal gland, the gastroesophageal junction, the celiac plexus, and the splenic vasculature. Superior to the celiac artery, a portion of the right crus extends anterior to the aorta along the left aspect of the esophagus, joining with the left crus (Fig. 11-22).[8]

The retroperitoneum extends into the pelvis. Other structures contained in the retroperitoneum include lymph nodes and lymphatics, the ureters, portions of the colon, the major vessels of the abdomen and pelvis, and variable amounts of fat.

Lymphadenopathy and Lymphoma

Ultrasound has been reported to be 80% to 90% accurate in the detection of retroperitoneal nodal lymphoma, and can also evaluate extranodal involvement.[43-45] Ultrasound accuracy compares favorably with that of CT for detection of abdominal lymphoma

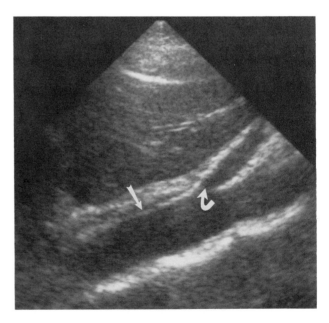

FIG 11-22. Diaphragmatic crus. A portion of the crus *(straight arrow)* is seen anterior to the aorta, just superior to the origin of the celiac artery *(curved arrow)* on this left-sided sagittal image.

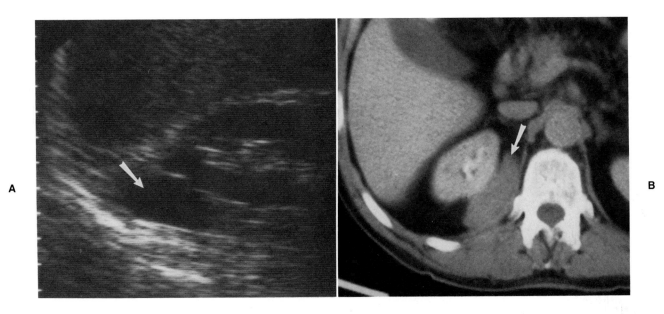

FIG 11-23. Perirenal lymphoma. **A,** Longitudinal sonogram shows an anechoic, well-circumscribed perirenal mass *(arrow)* without the amount of posterior through-transmission anticipated behind a cyst of this size. **B,** CT shows a low-density mass *(arrow)*.

in some series, but patient preparation is necessary for optimal ultrasound visualization of the retroperitoneum. In addition, ultrasound imaging is operator dependent, and scan planes are difficult to reproduce from one exam to the next. Thus, although ultrasound can potentially visualize abdominal lymphoma, CT is the preferred imaging technique, except when there is insufficient retroperitoneal fat. In such cases, ultrasound can be superior to CT for the detection of retroperitoneal adenopathy.[43] Neither CT nor ultrasound will detect disease in normal-size nodes, present in roughly 10% of patients, unless prior lymphography has opacified normal-size nodes, allowing CT demonstration of focal filling defects. Retroperitoneal nodal involvement is seen in both Hodgkin's and non-Hodgkin's lymphoma, but is more common in non-Hodgkin's disease. Paraaortic nodal involvement is present in roughly 25% of newly diagnosed Hodgkin's disease patients and 40% of patients with non-Hodgkin's lymphoma. More than 12% of patients with Hodgkin's disease with normal paraaortic nodes will have lymphomatous involvement of celiac, mesenteric, or perisplenic nodes, and more than 40% of non-Hodgkin's disease patients will show similar distribution of disease. If lymphangiography demonstrates paraaortic nodal disease, more than 76% of non-Hodgkin's lymphoma patients will have mesenteric nodal disease.[43-47]

On ultrasound, lymphoma typically produces hypoechoic or even anechoic lymph node masses (Fig. 11-23). However, echogenicity is variable and nonspecific. Nodes with lymphoma demonstrate a spectrum of sonographic appearances related to internal histology, surrounding retroperitoneal fat, and ultrasound technical factors, such as the time gain compensation curve or transducer focal zone. There is no correlation between node appearance and lymphoma histology.[48] Retroperitoneal involvement may appear as a platelike mass extending from the vertebral bodies anteriorly, surrounding the aorta and IVC. It may also present as multiple, separate, lobulated lymph nodes (greater than 1-2 cm) (Fig. 11-24) or as a bulky conglomerate mass of enlarged lymph nodes (Fig. 11-25). Paraaortic lymph nodes frequently obscure the echogenic anterior aortic border, producing a "sonographic silhouette," which helps distinguish paraaortic disease from mesenteric nodes (Fig. 11-26). Such distinction is important as the demonstration of mesenteric nodal disease in non-Hodgkin's patients may obviate a staging laparotomy or change radiation ports.[43,46] When the mesentery is involved with lymphoma one may see a characteristic appearance that has been called the "sandwich sign," produced by entrapment of mesenteric vessels and fat between hypoechoic lymphomatous nodes invading the space between the mesenteric leaves.[49] Mesenteric

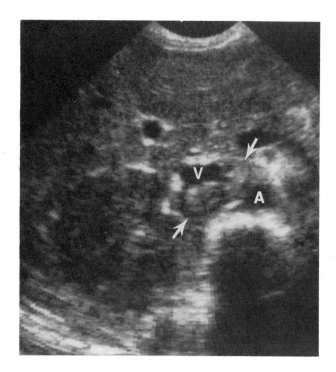

FIG 11-24. Lymphoma. Several lymphomatous nodes *(arrows)* extend anteriorly from the vertebral body to encase the IVC *(V)* and aorta *(A)*.

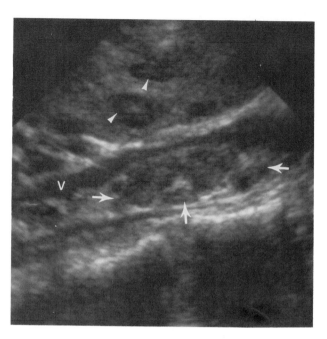

FIG 11-25. Lymphoma. Longitudinal image of a conglomerate of retrocaval nodes *(arrows)* in non-Hodgkin's lymphoma. Note also multiple hypoechoic liver metastases *(arrowheads)*. *V,* IVC.

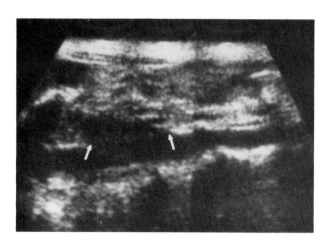

FIG 11-26. Paraaortic adenopathy *(arrows)*. A mass of retroperitoneal lymphomatous nodes silhouette a segment of the anterior echogenic border of the abdominal aorta.

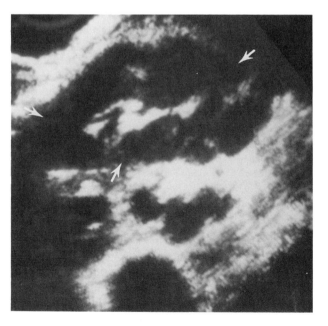

FIG 11-27. Mesenteric adenopathy *(arrows)*. A transverse scan shows the "sandwich" or "pseudokidney" sign.

lymphadenopathy may also create a "pseudokidney" appearance produced by the same distribution of disease (Fig. 11-27). Lymphomatous masses involving the perinephric space or retroperitoneal muscles tend to be hyechoic or even anechoic, occasionally with through transmission, which mimics a cystic mass (Fig. 11-23).[49]

Besides lymphoma, the differential diagnosis of retroperitoneal lymphadenopathy includes nodal metastases, infection of any kind, and AIDS and AIDS-related diseases (including lymphoma). The ultrasound findings are nonspecific and identical to lymphoma.

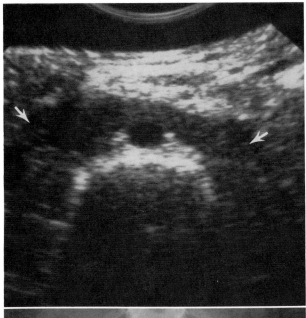

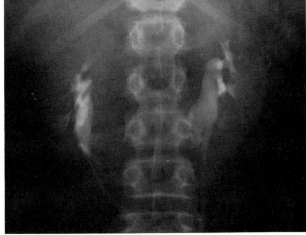

FIG 11-28. Horseshoe kidney. **A,** Transverse sonogram. The horseshoe kidney *(arrows)* may be confused with platelike lymphadenopathy, retroperitoneal fibrosis, or renal vein thrombosis. Often the connection with the renal cortices can be demonstrated with ultrasound. **B,** Excretory urogram shows the horseshoe kidney.

Retroperitoneal fibrosis and lymphoma may be indistinguishable, although retroperitoneal fibrosis often has smoother, less lobulated borders and involves the anterolateral aspects of the retroperitoneal vessels more extensively than the posterior region. This is especially true with perianeurysmal fibrosis due to inflammatory changes caused by leaking inflammatory aneurysms of the abdominal aorta. However, such characteristics are nonspecific. A thrombosed left renal vein crossing the aorta, as well as the midline portion of a horseshoe kidney, may also mimic lymphoma or lymphadenopathy (Fig. 11-28). Dilated vascular structures, such as with varices, may at first glance mimic lymphadenopathy. Demonstration of flow with Doppler, as well as demonstration of a tubular appearance in different planes, distinguishes these as vascular structures.[50] Rarely, a dilated lymphatic vessel may present as a mass, but this should also appear tubular.[51]

Retroperitoneal lymphomatous nodal disease can encase or invade adjacent organs and produce significant organ displacement. It is curious that massive retroperitoneal adenopathy often produces disproportionately little renal obstruction relative to other bulky retroperitoneal diseases. Lymphadenopathy resulting from metastatic disease may also appear hypoechoic and be indistinguishable from lymphoma. However, in a considerable number of cases, metastatic adenopathy is more echogenic than lymphoma (Fig. 11-29). Metastatic involvement in the retroperitoneum may produce a fibrotic reaction indistinguishable from benign causes of retroperitoneal fibrosis and give the impression of more extensive retroperitoneal involvement than is actually present pathologically.

Primary Neoplasms of the Retroperitoneum

Primary malignant neoplasms are more common than benign retroperitoneal neoplasms, but both are

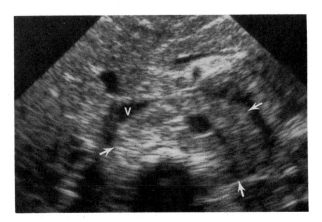

FIG 11-29. Metastatic neuroblastoma. Very echogenic retroperitoneal adenopathy *(arrows)* is seen surrounding the aorta and displacing the IVC *(V)* anteriorly.

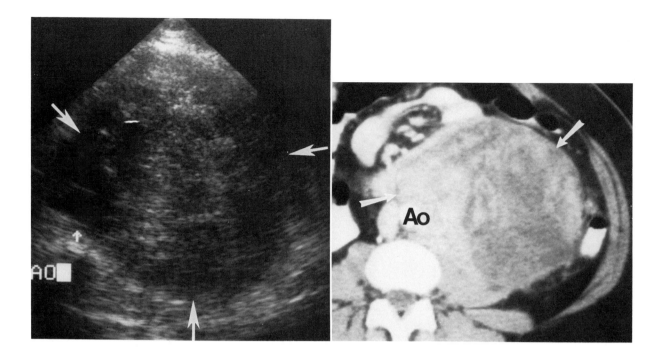

FIG 11-30. Retroperitoneal leiomyosarcoma. **A,** Transverse sonogram shows an inhomogeneous retroperitoneal mass *(arrows)* with partial encasement of the aorta *(Ao).* **B,** CT after injection of IV contrast material confirms and defines the edges of the mass *(arrows)* and aortic encasement.

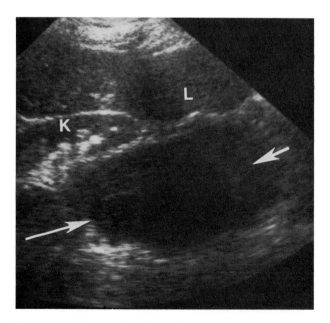

FIG 11-31. Retroperitoneal malignant fibrous histiocytoma. The hypoechoic mass *(arrows)* is only slightly inhomogeneous. The kidney *(K)* is displaced, but the kidney and liver *(L)* are clearly separate from the mass.

rare.[52] The relative number of cases of primary retroperitoneal tumors versus lymphomas that are detected varies with the referral base of various institutions.[52,53] In our experience, lymphoma is many times more common than other malignant retroperitoneal tumors. Leiomyosarcoma, liposarcoma, and malignant fibrous histiocytoma (MFH) account for the vast majority of retroperitoneal malignancies (93% in one study).[52,54,55]

Retroperitoneal primary malignancies show a strong male predominance (2:1 or 3:1); these tumors may be found at any age. The 5-year survival ranges from 22% to 50%.[54,55] Fixation of the tumor and involvement of adjacent organs are the most important prognostic indicators and, when present, indicate poor 5-year survival and a high risk of recurrence.

On sonography and CT, primary retroperitoneal malignancies tend to be more heterogeneous than lymphomas (Fig. 11-30).[53,56] Increased echogenicity may be related to fat content (liposarcomas), calcification, vascularity (hemangiopericytoma)[57] or hemorrhage.[58] Hypoechogenicity or cystic portions may be due to necrosis or hemorrhage, and septations may be seen.[59] Although CT usually visualizes the extent of tumor better, ultrasound may be useful in some instances to help evaluate the extent of involvement and invasion of adjacent organs (Figure 11-31). This helps in planning surgical resection, which is the treatment of choice. The ultrasound appearance of all these tumors is nonspecific, although extreme invasiveness is more suggestive of fibrosarcoma or rhabdomyosarcoma.

Tumors of Mesenchymal Origin. Mesenchymal cells found within the connective tissues of the retroperitoneum are capable of differentiating into various mesenchymal cell types, such as lipoblasts and fibroblasts. Tumors formed of well-differentiated cells tend to be benign or of low-grade malignancy and are more easily classified by the primary cell type. Poorly differentiated tumors are more difficult to characterize and may contain more than one derivative. Special immunohistochemical stains may be required to characterize the cell of origin.

Benign lipomas consist almost entirely of fat, whereas liposarcomas have variable amounts of detectable fat. Most fat-containing tumors in the retroperitoneum are liposarcomas. The echogenicity of fat in a liposarcoma may be similar to that of the normal retroperitoneal fat, causing the tumor to blend in with the normal fat, rendering the tumor imperceptible with ultrasound. The sonographic appearance of these tumors is nonspecific. Focal echogenicity within a mass is not specific for fat and may represent areas of hemorrhage or necrosis; conversely, liposarcoma may not contain detectable fat.

Other primary tumors of mesenchymal origin include malignant fibrous histiocytomas,[59] fibrosarcomas, fibromas, and desmoid tumors.[52,60] All are nonspecific sonographically. Desmoid tumors are benign histologically but are locally invasive. They occur sporadically and in association with Gardner's syndrome.

Neurogenic Tumors. Neurogenic tumors are usually located in the paravertebral region and may be benign or malignant. They may extend into the retroperitoneum or arise from peripheral nerves within the retroperitoneum. Larger tumors may contain central areas of necrosis, and those with invasion of adjacent structures are often malignant. However, ultrasound features are not specific for malignant versus benign tumors. Pheochromocytomas may occur anywhere along the sympathetic chain.

Tumors of Muscle Origin. Leiomyosarcomas may originate from smooth muscle of small blood vessels or develop from previously undifferentiated mesenchymal cells and may occur anywhere within the retroperitoneum. They also may develop within stomach or bowel walls and extend exophytically into the retroperitoneum. Large size and echogenic or cystic areas of central necrosis favor leiomyosarcoma over leiomyoma.

Tumors of Vascular Origin. Hemangiopericytomas (which are most often benign) and hemangiomas tend to be diffusely echogenic because of their vascular nature.[58] Extrahepatic hemangiomas may also have a fatty component. These tumors, like lipomas, may be difficult to evaluate with ultrasound if they occur within echogenic retroperitoneal fat. Hemangioendotheliomas occur most often in childhood.[57]

Germ Cell Tumors. Both malignant and benign germ cell tumors occur in the retroperitoneum.[52,60] Teratomas are rare and most commonly found in the pediatric age group.[61] Fat within these tumors may produce increased tumor echogenicity. However, this fat is not reliably distinguished from other causes of increased echogenicity with ultrasound. A fat-fluid level or chunky calcifications may suggest the diagnosis.

Retroperitoneal Cysts. Ultrasound may be helpful in characterizing cystic retroperitoneal structures. Primary retroperitoneal cysts can be quite large (up to 15 cm) and have the ultrasound characteristics of a simple cyst.[62] Differential diagnosis includes urinoma, lymphocele, and exophytic renal cysts. Abscesses, hematomas, dermoids, and hydatid cysts are usually more complex with septations and debris.[62] Lymphangiomas may be unilocular or multilocular cysts with thick septations. Approximately 44% contain debris.[63] An elongated appearance suggests the diagnosis of lymphangioma (Fig. 11-32). Retroperitoneal cystic hamartoma is very rare and seems to occur most often in the presacral or precoccygeal space.[64]

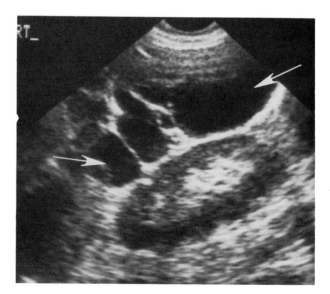

FIG 11-32. Lymphangioma. Longitudinal sonogram shows elongated cystic mass *(arrows)* with multiple septations adjacent to the kidney.

(Courtesy Stephanie R. Wilson, M.D., Toronto General Hospital, Canada.)

Other Tumors. Castleman's disease is an extremely rare benign lymphoid tumor.[65] Ultrasound characteristics have not been well described.

Retroperitoneal Metastatic Disease

Metastatic disease may occur anywhere in the retroperitoneum secondary to hematogenous spread, within lymph nodes resulting from lymphatic spread, or by direct extension. Ultrasound characteristics are nonspecific. Metastatic nodules within the perirenal space were most commonly caused by melanoma in one study.[66] Renal cell carcinomas may also metastasize to the contralateral perirenal space. The most common disease processes involving the perirenal space are primary renal tumors, inflammatory conditions, lymphoma, and metastases (Fig. 11-29). Retroperitoneal hemorrhage may occur with metastatic disease or primary tumors.[67]

Hemorrhage

Hemorrhage can occur anywhere in the retroperitoneum and may occur spontaneously or result from a bleeding diathesis, tumor, anticoagulation therapy, trauma, or catheterization.[68-70] Common sites of hemorrhage include the perinephric space and the psoas muscle (Figs. 11-33 and 11-34). Persistent bleeding from a femoral arterial puncture site or from a ruptured femoral pseudoaneurysm may track superiorly within the retroperitoneal musculature. Lithotripsy of renal stones rarely can cause extrarenal hemorrhage.[71]

Ultrasound findings are nonspecific, and CT is the most sensitive and specific modality for evaluating the presence and extent of these hemorrhages.[67] The sonographic appearance of hemorrhage is quite variable, and the extent is difficult to assess.[67] In the perinephric space, there may be fluid surrounding the kidney, which may contain internal debris. Occasionally hemorrhage may be uniformly echogenic and blend in with the retroperitoneal fat. Totally anechoic hemorrhage can appear similar to an abscess or urinoma. Homogeneous tumors such as lymphoma may also mimic a hematoma, but usually lymphomas do not display the same degree of increased posterior sound transmission as that routinely seen posterior to large hematomas. Furthermore, the clinical history and a drop in hemoglobin will confirm the diagnosis of hematoma. Cellular debris may be seen layered dependently, also suggesting the diagnosis. Hemorrhage into the psoas muscles often causes diffuse enlargement, which may produce diffusely hypoechoic muscles or anechoic pockets within the musculature (Fig. 11-34).

Bladder flap hematomas can be identified with ultrasound as solid- or mixed-echogenicity masses between the uterus and the bladder after low transverse cesarean section.[72] They may be associated with significant blood loss, fever, and infection. A subfascial hematoma

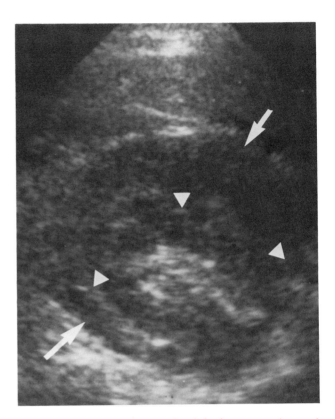

FIG 11-33. Posttraumatic perinephric hematoma *(arrows)* surrounding the right kidney *(arrowheads)* seen on a transverse scan.

may also be identified postoperatively and is also associated with potentially significant blood loss or infection.[73] These occur anterior to the bladder, and high-frequency transducers or sufficient stand-offs may be required for diagnosis. Superficial hematomas are not commonly associated with significant bleeding and can be differentiated by their location anterior to the rectus muscles, as opposed to the subfascial hematoma, which is located posterior to the rectus muscles.

Lymphoceles, Urinomas, and Pseudocysts

Lymphoceles are common complications of surgical procedures. They occur in 10% to 27% of patients after staging lymphadenectomy.[74] Most arise lateral to the bladder and within 3 cm of the anterior abdominal wall, but they can occur anywhere in the pelvis and may be found within the abdomen.[74,75] After renal transplantation, they are found near or adjacent to the transplanted kidney (Fig. 11-35).

Most often lymphoceles are anechoic and appear similar to simple cysts.[74,76] However, in 20% to 25% of patients they may be complex masses. Septations are probably of no significance, but internal debris may indicate infection. Localized symptoms and enlarging size

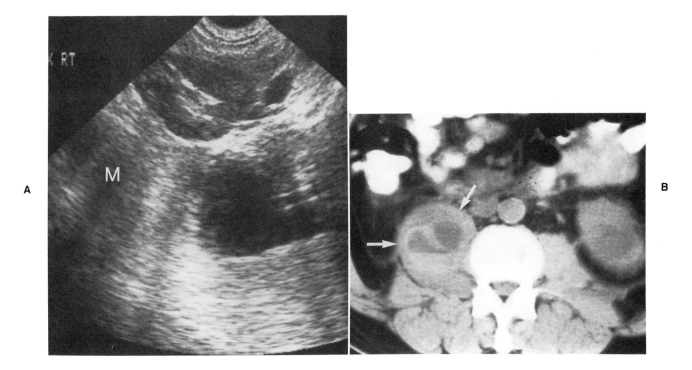

FIG 11-34. Psoas hematoma. **A,** Transverse sonogram shows enlargement of the right psoas muscle *(M)* and the anterior displacement of the right kidney caused by a psoas hematoma. **B,** CT scan below the kidney confirms the psoas hematoma *(arrows)* with focal inhomogeneity.

are other indicators of infection in a known lymphocele.

Differentiation from abscess, hematoma, or urinoma cannot usually be made sonographically, especially when internal debris is present. Abnormal fluid-filled loops of bowel and, rarely, postoperative lymphatic duct dilation are also in the differential diagnosis.[51,76] Most lymphoceles develop within 10-21 days of surgery.[74] Psoas hematoma may be particularly difficult to differentiate from lymphoceles in the early postoperative state.

Small echo-free lymphoceles are most likely to resolve spontaneously and are indistinguishable from "seromas." Lymphoceles that are larger or contain echoes are more likely to require surgery. Percutaneous drainage, often combined with sclerosing therapy, is most frequently indicated to evaluate for potential infection or to relieve symptoms. However, surgical treatment may be required eventually to prevent recurrence of lymphoceles.

Urinomas usually occur after trauma, interventional procedures, or high-grade acute ureteral obstruction. As urine within the retroperitoneal spaces may incite a fibrotic reaction, percutaneous or surgical drainage is indicated if a urinoma persists. Furthermore, urinomas may become infected if not drained. A urinoma will often resolve after decompression of the collecting system in patients with obstruction.[77]

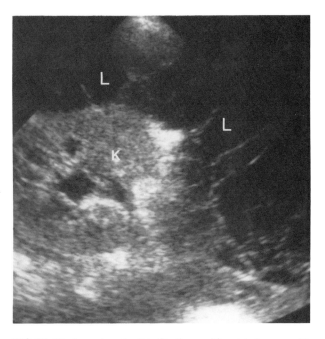

FIG 11-35. Lymphocele *(L)*. Cystic, multiseptated mass with internal debris surrounds the anteromedial aspect of a transplant kidney *(K)*.

Pancreatitis may cause fluid collections within the pararenal space. It may also involve the perirenal space either through inferior connections with the pararenal space or from disruption of Gerota's fascia caused by the enzymatic action of pancreatic fluid.[39,40] The clinical situation and the radiographic appearance of the pancreas are usually suggestive. Pseudocysts are well-circumscribed fluid collections that develop within the inflamed pancreas or peripancreatic tissue as a complication of pancreatitis. Occasionally it may be difficult to differentiate pseudocysts from lymphoceles or urinomas, especially in a postoperative or posttraumatic patient. Analysis of aspirated fluid is usually diagnostic.

Infection

Primary retroperitoneal abscesses may occur, but most often retroperitoneal abscesses result from direct extension of a renal inflammatory process or secondarily within an existing fluid collection, such as a lymphocele, hematoma, urinoma, or pseudocyst. Paraspinal abscesses may occur from vertebral or disk-space infections, e.g., tuberculosis, or as a complication of spinal surgery. Predisposing factors include diabetes mellitus, ureteral obstruction, trauma or recent surgery, alcohol or drug abuse, and AIDS.[78,79] Percutaneous drainage is the treatment of choice initially and is the only treatment necessary in the majority of cases.[80] When surgery is required, prior percutaneous drainage will decrease morbidity in most cases.

Sonographically, abscesses often have variable echogenicity related to internal content. Generally, there is increased sound transmission through abscesses indicating their underlying cystic nature. Air within an abscess may obscure parts of the mass and produce bright echoes and shadowing. A debris-fluid level may be present. Ultrasound may be useful for characterization of a retroperitoneal abscess, however, an abscess may be sonographically indistinguishable from a hematoma. Percutaneous drainage can be guided by either ultrasound or CT.

Some inflammatory processes may cause masses within the retroperitoneum,[81-84] and most have a nonspecific appearance. Xanthogranulomatous pyelonephritis commonly extends into the perirenal and pararenal spaces.[85] Typically the mass is complex sonographically and associated with renal calculi. The connection of the retroperitoneal process with the kidney can be demonstrated with ultrasound.

Retroperitoneal Fibrosis

Retroperitoneal fibrosis may be an idiopathic condition or may be associated with infiltrating neoplasms or acute immune diseases such as Crohn's disease, ulcerative colitis, sclerosing cholangitis, or Riedel's struma.[86-89] When seen around an abdominal aortic an-

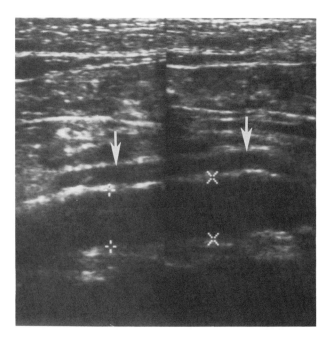

FIG 11-36. Inflammatory aneurysm. Longitudinal composite sonogram shows hypoechoic tissue *(arrows)* along the anterior aspect of the abdominal aorta $(+,\times)$.

eurysm, it is sometimes termed an inflammatory aneurysm and may be related to previous or recurrent leak from the aneurysm (Fig. 11-36). Whether this is a distinct type of retroperitoneal fibrosis, caused by the leaking aneurysm, or just idiopathic retroperitoneal fibrosis in a patient who incidentally has an aneurysm, is controversial. Methysergide treatment and urine extravasation have also been implicated as causes of retroperitoneal fibrosis. Medial displacement and obstruction of the ureters are on excretory urography. CT is the primary radiographic modality for evaluating retroperitoneal fibrosis, and MR may prove to be helpful in determining whether malignancy is present.[82,83] Malignancy may be implied in patients with known metastatic disease or lymphoma, but in other patients, surgically obtained tissue is often required to exclude malignancy. Pathologically, benign retroperitoneal fibrosis is characterized by ill-defined fibrous masses with an associated inflammatory infiltrate.

Sonographically abnormal hypoechoic tissue is seen surrounding the anterolateral aspect of the aorta and/or IVC (Fig. 11-37).[84,88,89] Generally this is smoothly marginated and homogeneous, whereas lymphadenopathy tends to be more lobulated or nodular appearing and completely encompasses the major vessels. The midline portion of a horseshoe kidney may be difficult to differentiate from retroperitoneal fibrosis, especially if overlying bowel gas prevents connection of the abnormal mass with the kidneys. Ultrasound may be useful for serial evaluation of the kidneys for hydronephro-

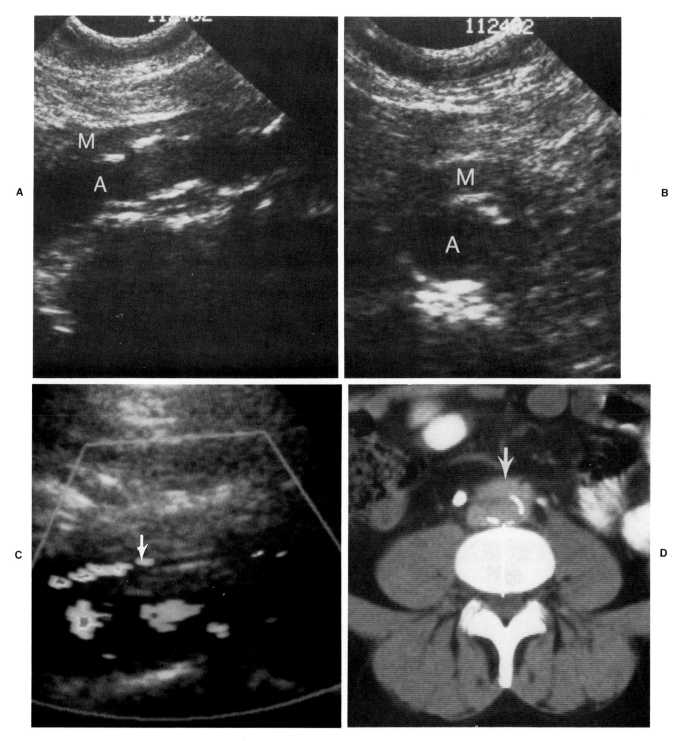

FIG 11-37. Retroperitoneal fibrosis. **A,** Transverse sonogram shows hypoechoic mass *(M)* anterior to the distal abdominal aorta *(A)*. **B,** Longitudinal sonogram confirms a homogeneous, smoothly bordered mass. **C,** Color Doppler shows the inferior mesenteric artery *(arrow)* is entrapped by this fibrotic process. **D,** CT confirms the mass *(arrow)*.

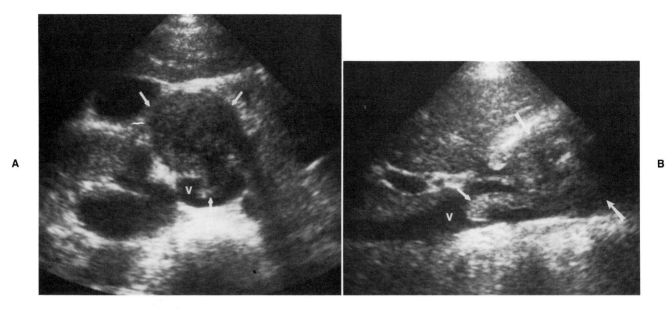

FIG 11-38. Ovarian vein thrombosis. A tubular hypoechoic, inhomogeneous mass was seen arising out of the pelvis in a patient after cesarean delivery. **A,** Transverse and **B,** longitudinal sonograms show the superior extent of this large thrombus *(arrows)* which extends into the IVC *(V)* from its anterior aspect.

sis as well as evaluation of fibrosis regression in response to steroid therapy.

Vascular Structures

Occasionally, large varices may mimic adenopathy or fluid collections.[50,76] Doppler ultrasound can clarify the vascular nature of these structures. Ovarian vein thrombosis (Fig. 11-38) may produce massive enlargement of the ovarian vein and may mimic a retroperitoneal neoplasm, especially when overlying bowel gas prevents visualization of the entire process extending from the pelvis to the IVC in the midabdomen. CT and MR may be helpful in this situation.[90,91] Ovarian vein thrombosis most often occurs postpartum and is associated with surgery or endometritis. Renal vein thrombosis may mimic other disease processes, such as retroperitoneal fibrosis or lymphadenopathy, and may have an appearance similar to a horseshoe kidney. Demonstration of extension into the IVC helps confirm the diagnosis of venous thrombosis in these situations (Fig. 11-38). Extension of tumor into renal veins or the IVC may also be confirmed with ultrasound, and CT or MR may again be helpful for clarification. Generally, tumor thrombus tends to be more echogenic and expansible than bland thrombus, but this is not always the case.

REFERENCES

1. Johnson CM, Welch TJ, Hattery RR, et al: Computed tomography of the adrenal medulla. *Semin Ultrasound, CT, MR* 1985;6:219-240.

2. Johnson CM, Sheedy PF, Welch TJ, et al: Computed tomography of the adrenal cortex. *Semin Ultrasound, CT, MR* 1985; 6:241-260.

Technique

3. Gore RM, Callen PW, Filly RA: Displaced retroperitoneal fat: sonographic guide to right upper quadrant mass localization. *Radiology* 1982;142:701-705.

4. Yeh H: Ultrasonography of the adrenals. *Semin Roentgenol* 1988;23:250-258.

5. Marchal G, Gelin J, Verbeken E, et al: High-resolution real-time sonography of the adrenal glands: a routine examination? *J Ultrasound Med* 1986;5:65-68.

6. Gunther RW, Kelbel C, Lenner V: Real-time ultrasound of normal adrenal glands and small tumors. *J Clin Ultrasound* 1984;12:211-217.

7. Magill HL, Tonkin ILD, Bada H, et al: Advantages of coronal ultrasonography in evaluating the neonatal retroperitoneum. *J Ultrasound Med* 1983;2:289-295.

8. Callen PW, Filly RA, Sarti DA, et al: Ultrasonography of the diaphragmatic crura. *Radiology* 1979;130:721-724.

The Adrenal Glands

9. Yeh H: Adrenal and retroperitoneal sonography. In Leopold GR, ed: *Ultrasound in Breast and Endocrine Disease.* New York: Churchill Livingstone; 1984.

10. Yeh H: Adrenal gland and nonrenal retroperitoneum. *Urol Radiol* 1987;9:127-140.

11. Paivansalo M, Merikanto J, Kallioinen M, et al: Ultrasound in the detection of adrenal tumors. *Eur J Radiol* 1988; 8:183-187.

12. Subramanyam BR, Balthazar EJ, Horii SC: Sonography of the accessory spleen. *AJR* 1984;143:47-49.

13. Graif M, Manor A, Itzchak Y: Sonographic differentiation of extra- and intrahepatic masses. *AJR* 1983;141:553-556.

14. Silverman ML, Lee AK: Anatomy and pathology of the adrenal glands. *Urol Clin North Am* 1989;16:417-432.

15. Hubbard MM, Husami TW, Abumrad NN: Nonfunctioning adrenal tumors: dilemmas in management. *Am J Surg* 1989;5:516-522.

16. Glazer HS, Weyman PJ, Sagel SS, et al: Nonfunctioning adrenal masses: incidental discovery on computed tomography. *AJR* 1982;139:81-85.

17. Bitter DA, Ross DS: Incidentally discovered adrenal masses. *Am J Surg* 1989;158:159-161.

18. Grizzle WE: Pathology of the adrenal gland. *Semin Roentgenol* 1988;23:323-331.

19. Hamper UM, Fishman EK, Hartma DS, et al: Primary adrenocortical carcinoma: sonographic evaluation with clinical and pathologic correlation in 26 patients. *AJR* 1987;148:915-919.

20. Davies RP, Lam AH: Adrenocortical neoplasm in children: ultrasound appearance. *J Ultrasound Med* 1987;6:325-328.

21. Bowerman RA, Silver TM, Jaffe MH, et al: Sonography of adrenal pheochromocytomas. *AJR* 1981;137:1227-1231.

22. Derchi LE, Rapaccini GL, Banderali A, et al: Ultrasound and computed tomography findings in two cases of hemangioma of the adrenal gland. *J Comput Assist Tomogr* 1989;13:659-661.

23. Barki Y, Eilig I, Moses M, et al: Sonographic diagnosis of a large hemorrhagic adrenal cyst in an adult. *J Clin Ultrasound* 1987;15:194-197.

24. Musante F, Derchi LE, Zappasodi F, et al: Myelolipoma of the adrenal gland: sonographic and computed tomography features. *AJR* 1988;151:961-964.

25. Vick CW, Zeman RK, Mannes E, et al: Adrenal myelolipoma: computed tomography and ultrasound findings. *Urol Radiol* 1984;6:7-13.

26. Gould JD, Mitty HA, Pertsemlidis D, et al: Adrenal myelolipoma: Diagnosis by fine-needle aspiration. *AJR* 1987;148:921-922.

27. Richman TS, Taylor KJW, Kremkau FW: Propagation speed artifact in a fatty tumor (myelolipoma): significance for tissue differential diagnosis. *J Ultrasound Med* 1983;2:45-47.

28. Tung GA, Pfister RC, Papanicolaou N, et al: Adrenal cysts: imaging and percutaneous aspiration. *Radiology* 1989;173:107-110.

29. Foster DG: Adrenal cysts. *Arch Surg* 1966;92:131-143.

30. Vicks BS, Perusek M, Johnson J, et al: Primary adrenal lymphoma: computed tomography and sonographic appearances. *J Clin Ultrasound* 1987;15:135-139.

31. Cunningham JJ: Ultrasonic findings in "primary" lymphoma of the adrenal area. *J Ultrasound Med* 1983;2:467-469.

32. Antoniou A, Spetseropoulos J, Vlahos L, et al: The sonographic appearance of adrenal involvement in non-Hodgkin's lymphoma. *J Ultrasound Med* 1983;2:235-236.

33. Ritchey ML, Kinard R, Novicki DE: Adrenal tumors: Involvement of the inferior vena cava. *J Urol* 1987;138:1134-1136.

34. Wu C: Sonographic spectrum of neonatal adrenal hemorrhage: report of a case simulating solid tumor. *J Clin Ultrasound* 1989;17:45-49.

35. Sarnakl AP, Sanfilippo DJ, Slovis TL: Ultrasound diagnosis of adrenal hemorrhage in meningococcemia. *Pediatr Radiol* 1988;18:427-428.

36. Wilms G, Marchal G, Baert A, et al: Computed tomography and ultrasound features of post-traumatic adrenal hemorrhage. *J Comput Assist Tomogr* 1987;11:112-115.

37. Murphy BJ, Casillas J, Yrizarry JM: Traumatic adrenal hemorrhage: radiologic findings. *Radiology* 1988;169:701-703.

38. Bryan PJ, Caldamone AA, Morrison SC, et al: Ultrasound findings in the adreno-genital syndrome (congenital adrenal hyperplasia). *J Ultrasound Med* 1988;7:675-679.

The Retroperitoneum

39. Dodds WJ, Darweesh RMA, Lawson TL, et al: The retroperitoneal spaces revisited. *AJR* 147:1155-1161.

40. Rubenstein WA, Whalen JP: Extraperitoneal spaces. *AJR* 1986;147:1162-1164.

41. Chesbrough RM, Burkhard TK, Martinez AT, et al: Gerota versus Zuckerkandl: the renal fascia revisited. *Radiology* 1989;173:845-846.

42. Callen PW, Filly RA, Marks WM: The quadratus lumborum muscle: a possible source of confusion in sonographic evaluation of the retroperitoneum. *J Clin Ultrasound* 1979;7:349-352.

43. Jing B: Diagnostic imaging of abdominal and pelvic lymph nodes in lymphoma. In Libshitz HI, ed: *Imaging the Lymphomas*. Radiol Clin North Am 1990, pp 801-803.

44. Carroll BA: Ultrasound of lymphoma. *Semin Ultrasound* 1982;3:114-122.

45. Carroll BA, Ta HN: The ultrasonic appearance of extranodal abdominal lymphoma. *Radiology* 1990;136:419-425.

46. Brascho DL, Durant JR, Green LE: The accuracy of retroperitoneal ultrasonography in Hodgkin's disease and non-Hodgkin' lymphoma. *Radiology* 1977;125:485-487.

47. Rochester D, Bowie JD, Kunzmann A, et al: Ultrasound in the staging of lymphoma. *Radiology* 1977;124:483-487.

48. Hillman BJ, Haber K: Echographic characteristics of malignant lymph nodes. *J Clin Ultrasound* 1980;8:213-215.

49. Mueller PR, Ferrucci JT, Harbin WP, et al: Appearance of lymphomatous involvement of the mesentery by ultrasonography and body computed tomography: the "sandwich sign". *Radiology* 1980;134:467-473.

50. Creed L, Reger K, Pond GD, et al: Potential pitfall in computed tomography and sonographic evaluation of suspected lymphoma. *AJR* 1982;139:606-607.

51. Verbanck JJ, Vermeulen JT, Rutgeerts LJ, et al: Dilated abdominal paraaortic lymphatic duct: a possible pitfall in retroperitoneal ultrasound. *Radiology* 1988;167:701-702.

52. Pinson CW, ReMine SG, Fletcher WS, et al: Long-term results with primary retroperitoneal tumors. *Arch Surg* 1989;124:1168-1173.

53. Cohan RC, Baker ME, Cooper C, et al: Computed tomography of primary retroperitoneal malignancies. *J Comput Assist Tomogr* 1988;12:804-810.

54. Dalton RR, Donohue JH, Mucha P, et al: Management of retroperitoneal sarcomas. *Surgery* 1989;106:725-733.

55. Solla JA, Reed K: Primary retroperitoneal sarcomas. *Am J Surg* 1986;152:496-498.

56. Bahnson RR, Zaontz MR, Maizels M, et al: Ultrasonography and diagnosis of pediatric genitourinary rhabdomyosarcoma. *Urology* 1989;33:64-68.

57. Koci TM, Worthen NJ, Phillips JJ, et al: Perirenal hemangioendothelioma in a newborn: sonography and magnetic resonance findings. *J Comput Assist Tomogr* 1989; 13:145-147.

58. Goldman SM, Davidson AJ, Neal J: Retroperitoneal and pelvic hemangiopericytomas: clinical, radiologic, and pathologic correlation. *Radiology* 1988;168:13-17.

59. Schut JM, van Imhoff WL: Retroperitoneal malignant fibrosis histiocytoma: an unusual echographic presentation. *J Clin Ultrasound* 1987;15:145-149.

60. Lane RH, Stephens DH, Reiman HM: Primary retroperitoneal neoplasms: computed tomography findings in 90 cases with clinical and pathologic correlation. *AJR* 1989;152:83-89.

61. Davidson AJ, Hartman DS, Goldman SM: Mature teratoma of the retroperitoneum: radiologic, pathologic, and clinical correlation. *Radiology* 1989;172:421-425.

62. Derchi LE, Rizzatto G, Banderali A, et al: Sonographic appearance of primary retroperitoneal cysts. *J Ultrasound Med* 1989;8:381-384.

63. Davidson AJ, Hartman DS: Lymphangioma of the retroperitoneum: computed tomography and sonographic characteristics. *Radiology* 1990;175:507-510.

64. DeLange EE, Black WC, Mills SE: Radiologic features of retroperitoneal cystic hamartoma. *Gastrointest Radiol* 1988;13:266-270.

65. Ebisuno S, Yamauchi T, Fukatani T, et al: Retroperitoneal Castleman's disease: a case report and brief review of tumors of the pararenal area. *Urol Int* 1989;44:169-172.

66. Shirkhoda A: Computed tomography of perirenal metastases. *J Comput Assist Tomogr* 1986;10:435-438.

67. Belville JS, Morgentaler A, Loughlin KR, et al: Spontaneous perinephric and subcapsular renal hemorrhage: evaluation with computed tomography, ultrasound and angiography. *Radiology* 1989;172:733:738.

68. Shirkhoda A, Mann MA, Staab EV, et al: Soft-tissue hemorrhage in hemophiliac patients: computed tomography and ultrasound study. *Radiology* 1983;147:811-814.

69. Graif M, Martinovitz U, Strauss S, et al: Sonographic localization of hematomas in hemophilic patients with positive iliopsoas sign. *AJR* 1987;148:121-123.

70. Kaufman RA, Towbin R, Babcock DS, et al: Upper abdominal trauma in children: imaging evaluation. *AJR* 1984;142:449-460.

71. Papanicolaou N, Stafford SA, Pfister RC, et al: Significant renal hemorrhage following extracorporeal shock wave lithotripsy: imaging and clinical features. *Radiology* 1987; 163:661-664.

72. Baker ME, Bowie JD, Killam AP: Sonography of post-cesarean-section bladder flap hematoma. *AJR* 1985;144:757-759.

73. Wiener MD, Bowie JD, Baker ME, et al: Sonography of subfascial hematoma after caesarean delivery. *AJR* 1987;148:907-910.

74. Spring DB, Schroeder D, Babu S, et al: Ultrasonic evaluation of lymphocele formation after staging lymphadenectomy for prostatic carcinoma. *Radiology* 1981;141:479-483.

75. Fried AM, Williams CB, Litvak AS: High retroperitoneal lymphocele: unusual clinical presentation and diagnosis by ultrasonography. *J Urol* 1980;123:583-584.

76. Rifkin MD, Needleman L, Kurtz AB, et al: Sonography of nongynecologic cystic masses of the pelvis. *AJR* 1984; 142:1169-1174.

77. McAninch JW: Complications of renal, vesical, and urethral trauma. In Marshall FF, ed: *Urologic Complications. Medical and Surgical, Adult and Pediatric*. Chicago: Year Book Medical Publishers, Inc; 1986.

78. Sacks D, Banner MP, Meranze SG, et al: Renal and related retroperitoneal abscesses: percutaneous drainage. *Radiology* 1988;167:447-451.

79. Soffer M, Abecassis J, Bonnin A: Percutaneous drainage of retroperitoneal abscesses. *Radiology* 1989;170:280-281.

80. Lang EK: Renal, perirenal, and pararenal abscesses: percutaneous drainage. *Radiology* 1990;174:109-113.

81. Piccirillo M, Rigsby CM, Rosenfield AT: Sonography of renal inflammatory disease. *Urol Radiol* 1987;9:66-78.

82. Morehouse HT, Weiner SN, Hoffman-Treatin JC: Inflammatory disease of the kidney. *Semin Ultrasound, CT, MR* 1986;7:246-258.

83. Suesada Y, Nakao N, Miura K, et al: Pseudolymphoma of the retroperitoneum. *Eur J Radiol* 1987;6:144-146.

84. Glynn TP, Kreipke DL, Irons JM: Amyloidosis: Diffuse involvement of the retroperitoneum. *Radiology* 1989;170:726.

85. Merine D, Fishman EK, Siegelman SS: Renal xanthogranulomatosis: radiological, clinical, and pathologic features in two cases. *J Comput Assist Tomogr* 1987;11:785-789.

86. Degesys GE, Dunnick NR, Silverman PM, et al: Retroperitoneal fibrosis: use of computed tomography in distinguishing among possible causes. *AJR* 1986;146:57-60.

87. Baker LRI, Mallinson WJW, Gregory MC, et al: Idiopathic retroperitoneal fibrosis: a retrospective analysis of 60 cases. *Br J Urol* 1988;160:497-503.

88. Sanders RC, Duff T, McLoughlin MG, et al: Sonography in the diagnosis of retroperitoneal fibrosis. *J Urol* 1977;118:944-946.

89. Fagan CJ, Amparo EG, Davis M: Retroperitoneal fibrosis. *Semin Ultrasound* 1982;3:123-138.

90. Savader SJ, Otero RR, Savader BL: Puerperal ovarian vein thrombosis: evaluation with computed tomography, ultrasound and magnetic resonance. *Radiology* 1988;167:637-639.

91. Baran GW, Frisch KM: Duplex Doppler evaluation of puerperal ovarian vein thrombosis. *AJR* 1987;149:321-322.

CHAPTER 12

Doppler Assessment of the Abdomen

- Christopher R.B. Merritt, M.D.

The traditional approach to abdominal ultrasound has emphasized two dimensional real-time imaging with the display of morphologic changes in organ size, shape, position, contour, and parenchymal patterns. With B-mode gray scale ultrasound, large vessels such as the aorta and the inferior vena cava (IVC) and smaller vessels such as the mesenteric, portal, splenic, hepatic, and renal vessels are readily identified. Although the vessel wall and lumen are seen, real-time imaging provides little if any information about flow; and significant pathologic conditions related to vascular thrombosis, narrow-

ing, or changes in flow direction or dynamics may be overlooked. With Doppler ultrasound, details of flow are provided and rapid determination of the presence and direction of flow is possible along with more subtle information related to flow velocity and organ perfusion. The addition of information related to organ blood supply and organ perfusion, which is available with Doppler instrumentation, may have a profound impact on the sonographic evaluation of the abdomen, increasing the role and range of applications of this modality. Abdominal duplex Doppler imaging or color Doppler imaging (CDI) combines anatomic and flow information most optimally. To properly use these tools in abdominal diagnosis, an understanding of the elementary principles of Doppler ultrasound is essential. Because the specific use of Doppler ultrasound in abdominal evaluation is discussed in individual chapters, this chapter provides an overview with an emphasis on the principles, instrumentation, and diagnostic techniques of Doppler examination, using duplex and color flow instruments.

Quality Doppler ultrasonography demands special operational skills. The operator must monitor the quality of the data generated in the examination and differentiate real and clinically important from artifactual findings. This is particularly true in the abdomen where greater examination depths result in the potential for artifacts and technical errors, which usually are not encountered in peripheral vascular applications. Interpretation of the results requires training and experience, including an understanding of the basic principles and the unique nature of the Doppler information, as well as knowledge of the techniques and instrumentation necessary to ensure the generation of high-quality data. Also needed is a knowledge of the patterns of normal and abnormal flow necessary to establish a diagnosis. Serious pitfalls await the careless or poorly trained sonographer—no matter how sophisticated the machine being used. Ultimately, the success or failure of the investigation is determined by clinical, technical, and interpretative skill and not the machine.[1]

PRINCIPLES OF DOPPLER ULTRASONOGRAPHY

Conventional B-mode ultrasound imaging uses pulse-echo transmission, detection, and display techniques. Brief pulses of ultrasound energy emitted by the transducer are reflected from acoustic interfaces within the body. Precise timing allows for determination of the depth from which the echo originates. When pulsed ul-

trasound is reflected from an interface, the backscattered (reflected) signal contains amplitude, phase, and frequency information. This information permits inference of the position, nature, and motion of the interface, reflecting the pulse.[2] B-mode ultrasound imaging uses only the amplitude information in the backscattered signal to generate the image, with differences in the strength of reflectors displayed in the image in vary-

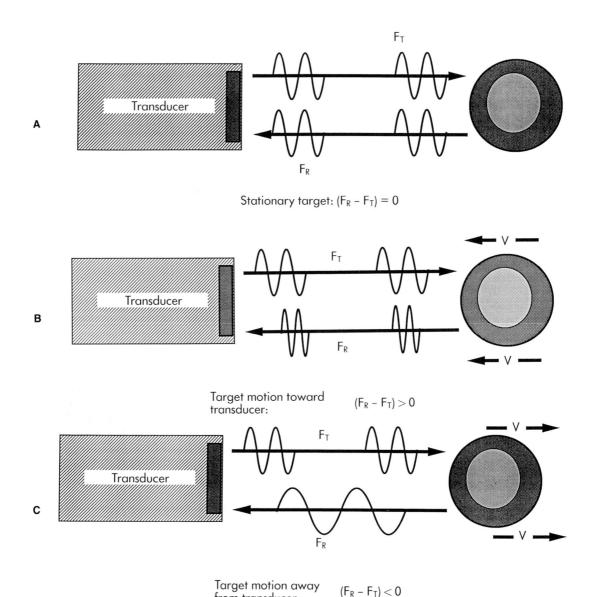

FIG 12-1. Doppler principles, effect of target movement. **A,** If the reflecting interface is stationary, the frequency of the reflected ultrasound (F_R) is essentially the same as the frequency of the transmitted sound, (F_T). **B,** If the reflecting interface is moving with respect to the sound beam emitted from the transducer, there is a change in the frequency of the sound scattered by the moving object. If the interface moves toward the transducer, the difference in reflected and transmitted frequencies is greater than 0. **C,** If the target is moving away from the transducer, this difference is less than 0. The Doppler equation is used to relate this change in frequency to the velocity of the moving object.

(From Merritt CRB: Doppler principles: the basics. *Radiographics;* 1991;11:109-119. Used with permission.)

ing shades of gray. Rapidly moving targets, such as red blood cells within the bloodstream, produce echoes of low amplitude that are not commonly displayed, resulting in a relatively anechoic pattern within the lumens of large vessels. Although gray scale display relies on the amplitude of the backscattered ultrasound signal, additional information is present in the returning echoes, which can be used to evaluate the motion of moving targets. When high-frequency sound impinges on a stationary interface, the reflected ultrasound has essentially the same frequency or wavelength as the transmitted sound (Fig. 12-1, *A*). However, if the reflecting interface is moving with respect to the sound beam emitted from the transducer, there is a change in the frequency of the sound that is scattered by moving object (Fig. 12-1, *B* and *C*). This change in frequency is directly proportional to the velocity of the reflecting interface, relative to the transducer, and is a result of the Doppler ef-

fect. The relation of the returning ultrasound frequency to the velocity of the reflector is described by the Doppler equation:

$$\Delta = (F_R - F_T) = 2F_T \, v/c$$

The Doppler frequency shift is $\mathbf{\Delta F}$; $\mathbf{F_R}$ is the frequency of sound reflected from the moving target; $\mathbf{F_T}$ is the frequency of sound emitted from the transducer; v is the velocity of the target toward the transducer; and c is the velocity of sound in the medium. The Doppler frequency shift $\mathbf{\Delta F}$ applies only if the target is moving directly toward or away from the transducer (Fig. 12-2, *A*). In the clinical setting, the direction of the ultrasound beam is seldom directly toward or away from the direction of flow. The ultrasound beam usually approaches the moving target at an angle designated as θ, the Doppler angle (Fig. 12-2, *B*). In this case the frequency shift $\mathbf{\Delta F}$ is reduced in proportion to the cosine

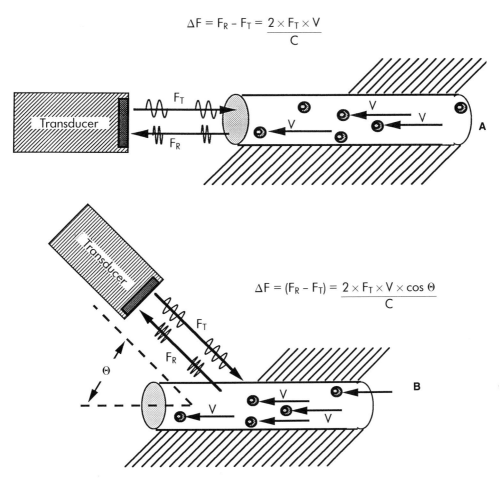

FIG 12-2. The Doppler equation describes the relationship of the Doppler frequency shift to target velocity. **A,** In its simplest form, it is assumed that the direction of the ultrasound beam is parallel to the direction of movement of the target. **B,** This situation is unusual in clinical practice and requires that the equation take into account the angle of the Doppler beam to the direction of flow.
(From Merritt CRB: Doppler principles: the basics. *Radiographics;* 1991;11:109-119. Used with permission.)

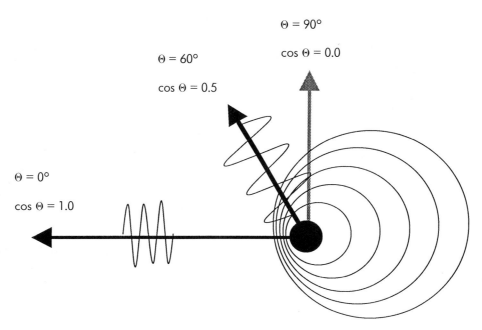

FIG 12-3. Effect of the Doppler angle on detected Doppler frequency shift. At an angle of 60 degrees, the detected frequency shift is only 50% of the shift detected at an angle of 0 degrees. At 90 degrees there is no relative movement of the target toward or away from the transducer, and therefore no frequency shift is detected. The detected Doppler frequency shift is reduced in proportion to the cosine of the Doppler angle. Because the cosine of the angle changes rapidly at angles above 60 degrees, the use of Doppler angles of less than 60 degrees is recommended in making velocity estimates.
(From Merritt CRB: Doppler principles: the basics. *Radiographics* 1991;11:109-119. Used with permission.)

of this angle and

$$\Delta F = (F_R - F_T) = (2F_T \, v/c) \cos \theta$$

where θ is the angle between the axis of flow and the incident ultrasound beam. If the Doppler angle can be measured, estimation of flow velocity is possible. Accurate estimation of target velocity requires precise measurements of both the Doppler frequency shift and the angle of insonation to the direction of target movement. As the Doppler angle θ approaches 90 degrees, the cosine of θ approaches 0 degrees. At an angle of 90 degrees, there is no relative movement of the target toward or away from the transducer, and no Doppler frequency shift is detected (Fig. 12-3). Because the cosine of the Doppler angle changes rapidly for angles of more than 60 degrees, accurate angle correction requires that Doppler measurements be made at angles of less than 60 degrees. Above 60 degrees, relatively small errors in estimation of the Doppler angle may result in a large error in the estimation of velocity. These considerations are important in using both duplex and color flow instruments because optimal imaging of the vessel wall is obtained when the axis of transducer is perpendicular to the wall, whereas maximal Doppler frequency differences are obtained when the transducer axis and the di-

rection of flow are at a relatively small angle. In peripheral vascular applications, it is highly desirable that measured Doppler frequencies be corrected for the Doppler angle to provide velocity measurement. This provides data from systems using different Doppler frequencies to be compared and eliminates errors in the interpretation of frequency data obtained at different Doppler angles. For abdominal applications, angle-corrected velocity measurements are encouraged, although qualitative assessments of flow are often made, using only the Doppler frequency shift data. The interrelation of transducer frequency $\mathbf{F_T}$ and the Doppler angle θ to the Doppler frequency shift and target velocity, which are described by the Doppler equation, are of great importance in the proper clinical use of Doppler equipment.

Doppler Signal Processing and Display

Several options exist for the processing of $\Delta \mathbf{F}$, the Doppler frequency shift, to provide useful information regarding the direction and velocity of blood. Doppler frequency shifts encountered clinically fall in the audible range. This audible signal may be analyzed by ear, and with training, many flow characteristics may be identified. More commonly, the Doppler shift data are

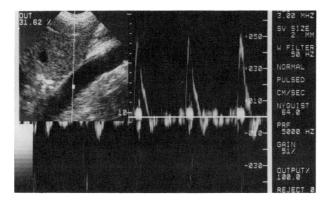

FIG 12-4. Doppler frequency spectrum of flow in proximal abdominal aorta. Changes in flow velocity and direction are indicated by vertical deflections of waveform above and below baseline. Width of spectral waveform is determined by range of frequencies present at any instant in time. Brightness (gray) scale is used to indicate relative amplitudes of each frequency component.

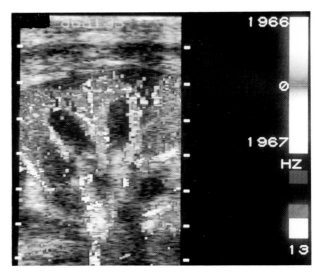

FIG 12-5. Doppler color imaging (DCI). With DCI, amplitude data from stationary targets provide basis for B-mode image. Signal phase provides information about presence and direction of motion, and changes in frequency relate to velocity of target. Backscattered signals from red blood cells are displayed in color as function of their motion toward or away from transducer. Degree of saturation of color is used to indicate relative velocity of moving red blood cells. Image of renal transplant and flow toward transducer in interlobar renal arteries is shown in red; flow away from transducer in veins is shown in blue. Less saturated colors indicate higher mean velocities.
(From Merritt CRB: Real-time Doppler color flow imaging: other applications. In: Bernstein EF, ed. *Non-Invasive Diagnostic Techniques in Vascular Disease.* St Louis: Mosby-Year Book; 1990: 42-56; with permission.)

displayed in graphic form as a time-varying plot of the frequency spectrum of the returning signal. A fast Fourier transformation is used to perform the frequency analysis. The resulting Doppler frequency spectrum displays the variation with time of the Doppler frequencies present in the volume sampled, with the envelope of the spectrum representing the maximum frequencies at any given point in time and the width of the spectrum at any point indicating the range of frequencies present (Fig. 12-4). In many instruments the amplitude of each frequency component is displayed in gray scale. The presence of a large number of different frequencies at a given point in the cardiac cycle results in so-called spectral broadening.

In Doppler color imaging systems, velocity information determined from Doppler measurements is displayed as a feature of the image itself (Fig. 12-5).[3] In addition to the detection of Doppler frequency shift data from each pixel in the image, these systems may also provide range-gated pulsed Doppler with spectral analysis for display of Doppler data.

Doppler Instrumentation

In contrast to A-mode, M-mode, and B-mode gray scale ultrasonography, which display the information from tissue interfaces, Doppler ultrasound instruments are optimized to display flow information. The simplest Doppler devices use continuous rather than pulsed ultrasound, employing two transducers that transmit and receive ultrasound continuously (continuous wave [CW] Doppler). The transmit and receive beams overlap in a sensitive volume at some distance from the transducer face (Fig. 12-6, *A*). Although direction of flow can be determined with CW Doppler imaging, these devices do

not allow for discrimination of motion coming from various depths, and the source of the signal being detected is difficult if not impossible to ascertain with certainty. Inexpensive and portable CW Doppler instruments are used primarily at the bedside or during surgery to confirm the presence of flow in superficial vessels.

Because of the limitation of CW systems, most abdominal applications employ range-gated pulsed Doppler. Rather than a continuous wave of ultrasound emission, pulsed Doppler devices emit brief pulses of ultrasound energy (Fig. 12-6, *B*). Using pulses of sound permits use of the time interval between the transmission of a pulse and the return of the echo as a means of determining the depth from which the Doppler shift arises. In a pulsed Doppler system the sensitive volume from which flow data are sampled can be controlled in terms of shape, depth, and position. When combined with a two-dimensional real-time B-mode image in the form of a duplex scanner, the position of the Doppler sample can be precisely controlled and monitored.

The most recent form of Doppler ultrasound used for abdominal applications is DCI. In color flow imaging

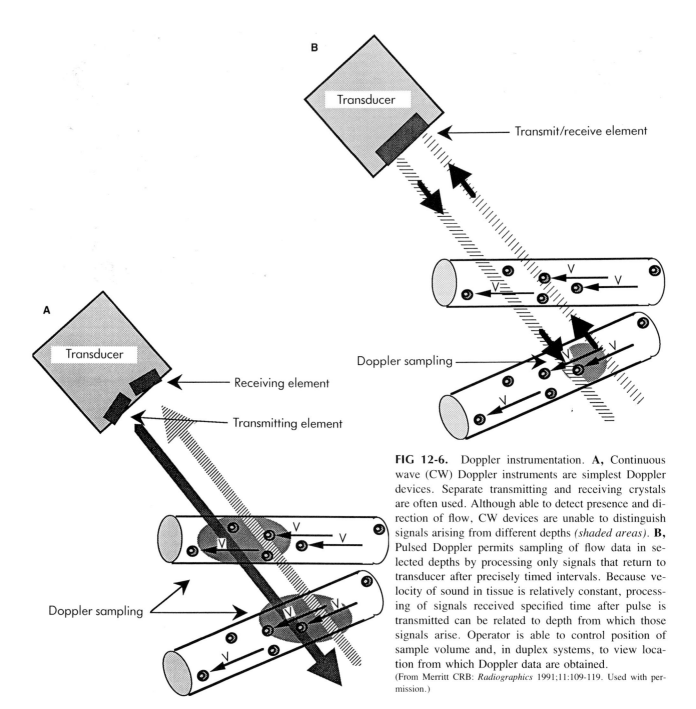

FIG 12-6. Doppler instrumentation. **A,** Continuous wave (CW) Doppler instruments are simplest Doppler devices. Separate transmitting and receiving crystals are often used. Although able to detect presence and direction of flow, CW devices are unable to distinguish signals arising from different depths *(shaded areas).* **B,** Pulsed Doppler permits sampling of flow data in selected depths by processing only signals that return to transducer after precisely timed intervals. Because velocity of sound in tissue is relatively constant, processing of signals received specified time after pulse is transmitted can be related to depth from which those signals arise. Operator is able to control position of sample volume and, in duplex systems, to view location from which Doppler data are obtained.
(From Merritt CRB: *Radiographics* 1991;11:109-119. Used with permission.)

systems, flow information that is determined from Doppler measurements is displayed as a feature of the image itself. Stationary or slowly moving targets provide the basis for the B-mode image (Fig. 12-5).[3] Signal phase provides information about the presence and direction of motion and changes in echo signal frequency, relative to the velocity of the target. Backscattered signals from red blood cells are displayed in color as a function of their motion toward or away from the transducer. The degree of the saturation of the color is used to indicate the relative velocity of the moving red blood

cells. Doppler color imaging expands conventional duplex sonography by providing additional capabilities. The use of color saturation to display variations in Doppler shift frequency allows for a semiquantative estimate of flow to be made from the image alone, provided that variations in the Doppler angle are noted. The display of flow throughout the image field allows the position and orientation of the vessel of interest to be observed at all times. The display of spatial information with respect to velocity is ideal for the display of small localized areas of turbulence within a vessel, which provides clues to stenosis or irregularity of the vessel wall caused by atheroma, trauma, or other disease. Flow within the vessel is observed at all points, and stenotic jets and focal areas of turbulence, which might be overlooked with duplex instrumentation, are displayed. The contrast of flow within the vessel lumen permits small vessels, which are invisible to conventional imagers, to be seen and enhances the visibility of wall irregularity. DCI aids in precise determination of the direction of flow and measurement of the Doppler angle. Limitations of DCI include the inability to display the entire Doppler spectrum in the image, the limited sensitivity of some instruments and artifacts as a result of high-amplitude low-frequency targets and phase shifts from intestinal gas.

Interpretation of the Doppler Signal

Components of the Doppler data, which must be evaluated both in spectral display and color flow imaging, include the Doppler shift frequency and amplitude, the Doppler angle, the spatial distribution of frequencies across the vessel, and the temporal variation of the signal. Because the Doppler signal itself has no anatomic significance, the examiner must interpret the Doppler signal and then determine its relevance in the context of the image.

The detection of a **Doppler frequency shift** indicates movement of the target, which in most applications is related to the presence of flow. The sign of frequency shift (positive or negative) indicates the direction of flow relative to the transducer. Vessel stenosis is typically associated with large Doppler frequency shifts in both systole and diastole at the site of greatest narrowing, with turbulent flow in poststenotic regions. In peripheral vessels, analysis of the Doppler changes allows for accurate prediction of the degree of vessel narrowing. In addition, information related to the resistance to flow in the distal vascular tree can be obtained by analysis of changes of blood velocity with time shown in the Doppler spectral display. Figure 12-7 provides a graphic example of the changes in the Doppler spectral waveform, resulting from physiologic changes in the resistance of the vascular bed, supplied by the brachial artery of a normal individual. In Figure 12-7, *A*, the waveform shows the typical high-resistance pattern associated with arteries supplying a muscular vascular bed. In Figure 12-7, *B*, a blood pressure cuff has been inflated to above systolic pressure to occlude the distal branches supplied by the brachial artery. This causes a profound drop in systolic amplitude and cessation of diastolic flow, resulting in a quite different waveform than that found in the normal resting state (Fig. 12-7, *A*). Figure 12-7, *C* shows the waveform in the brachial artery immediately after release after 3 minutes of occluding pressure. During the period of

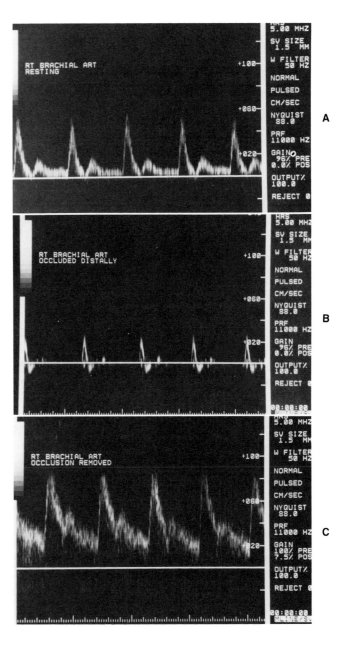

FIG 12-7. Physiologic changes in resistance of vascular bed. Changes in Doppler spectral waveform of brachial artery were recorded under identical measurement conditions, with no changes in velocity scale. **A,** Waveform shows typical high-resistance pattern of peripheral artery supplying muscular vascular bed. **B,** Blood pressure cuff has been inflated to above systolic pressure. Resulting occlusion of distal branches supplied by brachial artery causes profound drop in systolic amplitude and cessation of diastolic flow, resulting in quite different waveform than found in normal resting state **(A). C,** Shows waveform in brachial artery immediately after release of 3 minutes of occluding pressure. During period of ischemia induced by pressure cuff occlusion of the forearm vessels, vasodilation has occurred, resulting in significantly diminished peripheral vascular resistance. Doppler waveform now reflects low-resistance peripheral vascular bed with increased systolic amplitude and continuous rapid flow throughout diastole.

ischemia induced by pressure cuff occlusion of the forearm vessels, vasodilation has occurred. The Doppler waveform now reflects a low-resistance peripheral vascular bed with increased systolic amplitude and rapid flow throughout diastole. Doppler indices, such as the systolic-diastolic ratio, resistive index and pulsatility index, which compare the flow in systole and diastole, provide an indication of the resistance in the peripheral vascular bed, and are used to aid in the evaluation of the placenta and uterus and perfusion of renal transplants. With Doppler ultrasound, it is therefore possible to identify vessels, determine the direction of blood flow, evaluate narrowing or occlusion, and characterize flow to organs and tumors.

Analysis of the Doppler shift frequency with time can be used to infer both proximal stenosis and changes in distal vascular impedance. Most research using pulsed Doppler has emphasized the detection of stenosis, thrombosis, and flow disturbance in major peripheral arteries and veins. In these applications, measurements of peak systolic and end diastolic frequency or velocity, analysis of the Doppler spectrum, and calculation of certain frequency or velocity ratios have been the basis of analysis (Fig 12-8, *A*). Changes in the spectral waveform, which are measured by indices comparing flow in systole and diastole, provide insight into the

resistance of the vascular bed supplied by the vessel and indicate changes caused by a variety of pathologic states (Fig. 12-8, *B*). Changes of these indices from normal may be important in the early indication of rejection of transplanted organs, parenchymal dysfunction, and malignancy. Although these indices are useful, it is important to keep in mind that these measurements are influenced not only by the resistance to flow in peripheral vessels but by many other factors, including heart rate, blood pressure, vessel wall length and elasticity, and extrinsic organ compression. Interpretation must therefore always take into account all of these variables.

Although the more graphic presentation of color Doppler imaging makes interpretation easier, the complexity of the color Doppler image actually yields an image that is more demanding to evaluate than the simple Doppler spectrum. Nevertheless, DCI has important advantages over pulsed duplex Doppler images because flow data are obtained only from a small portion of the area being imaged. To be confident that a conventional Doppler study has achieved reasonable sensitivity and specificity in detection of flow disturbances, a methodical search and sampling of multiple sites within the field of interest must be performed. Doppler color flow imaging devices permit simultaneous sampling of multiple sites and are less susceptible to this error.

FIG 12-8. A, Dop-pler imaging is capable of providing information about flow in large vessels and may detect stenosis, thromboses, and flow disturbances. **B,** Doppler flow indices reflecting impedance or resistance of small vessels distal to site of measurement include systolic-diastolic ratio (S/D ratio), resistive index (RI), and pulsatility index (PI). In calculation of PI, minimum diastolic velocity or frequency is used; calculation of S/D ratio and RI use end diastolic value. These indices are influenced by heart rate, blood pressure, vessel length, vessel wall elasticity, and compression of vessels.
(**A,** From Merritt CRB: *Radiographics* 1991;11:109-119.)

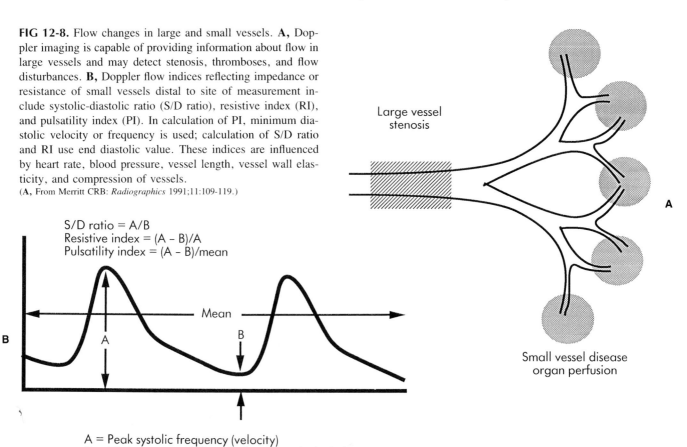

S/D ratio = A/B
Resistive index = (A − B)/A
Pulsatility index = (A − B)/mean

A = Peak systolic frequency (velocity)
B = Minimum or end diastolic frequency (velocity)

Other Technical Considerations

Although many of the problems and artifacts associated with B-mode imaging, such as shadowing, are encountered with Doppler ultrasonography, the detection and display of frequency information related to moving targets adds a group of special technical considerations that are not found with other forms of ultrasonography. An understanding of the source of these artifacts and their influence on the interpretation of the flow measurements obtained in clinical practice is important. Major sources of Doppler inaccuracy or artifacts include the following.

Doppler Frequency. A primary objective of the Doppler examination is the accurate measurement of characteristics of flow within a vascular structure. The moving red blood cells that serve as the primary source of the Doppler signal act as point scatterers of ultrasound rather than specular reflectors. This interaction results in variations of the intensity of the scattered sound in proportion to the fourth power of the frequency to be used for a given examination. As the transducer frequency increases, Doppler sensitivity improves, but attenuation by tissue also increases, resulting in diminished penetration. Careful balancing of the requirements for sensitivity and penetration are an important responsibility of the operator during a Doppler examination. Because many abdominal vessels lie several centimeters beneath the surface, Doppler frequencies in the range of 3 to 3.5 MHz are usually required to permit adequate penetration.

Wall Filters. Doppler instruments detect motion not only from blood flow but from adjacent structures. To eliminate these low-frequency signals from the display, most instruments employ high-pass filters, or "wall" filters, which remove signals that fall below a given frequency limit. Although effective in eliminating low-frequency noise, these filters may also remove signal from low-velocity blood flow. In certain clinical situations, the measurement of these slower flow velocities is of clinical importance and the improper selection of the wall filter may result in serious errors of interpretation. For example, low-velocity venous flow may not be detected if an improper filter is used, and low-velocity diastolic flow (in certain arteries) may not be eliminated from the display, resulting in errors in calculation of Doppler indices, such as the systolic-diastolic ratio or resistive index. In general, the filter should be kept at the lowest practical level (usually in the range of 50 to 100 Hz).

Spectral Broadening. Spectral broadening refers to the presence of a large range of flow velocities at a given point in the pulse cycle and is an important criterion of high-grade vessel narrowing (Fig. 12-9). Excessive system gain or changes in the dynamic range of the gray scale display of the Doppler spectrum may suggest

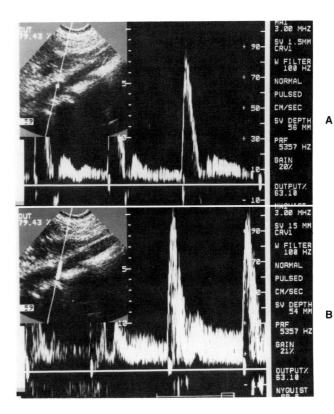

FIG 12-9. Spectral broadening describes range of velocities present at any given time in pulse cycle **A,** Doppler waveform is defined by narrow band of frequencies throughout pulse cycle. This indicates that, at any given instance, most of red blood cells in sample volume are flowing at approximately same velocity. **B,** Sample volume contains number of different frequencies at each instant in time. Shape of Doppler waveform or envelope is defined by maximum frequencies or velocities in sample volume. Signal within envelope indicates presence of lower frequencies and is referred to as spectral broadening. Spectral broadening may indicate presence of turbulent flow but may also be caused by use of excessively large Doppler sample volume, improper placement of Doppler sample, or excessive Doppler gain.

spectral broadening, whereas opposite settings may mask broadening of the Doppler spectrum, causing diagnostic inaccuracy. Spectral broadening may also be produced by selection of an excessively large sample volume or by the placement of the sample volume too near the vessel wall where slower velocities are present.

Aliasing. Aliasing is an artifact arising from ambiguity in the measurement of high-Doppler frequency shifts. To ensure that samples originate only from selected depths when using a pulsed Doppler system, it is necessary to wait for the echo from the area of interest before transmitting the next pulse. This limits the rate with which pulses can be generated—it provides for a lower pulse repetition frequency (PRF) required for

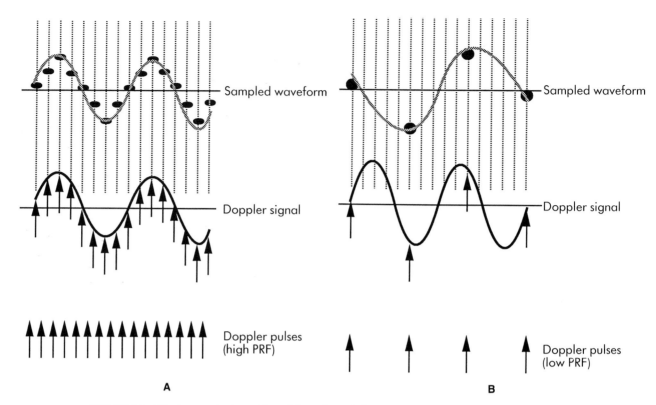

FIG 12-10. Aliasing results in artifactual lowering of displayed Doppler frequency shift because of inadequate sampling. If pulse repetition frequency (PRF) is sufficiently high, sampled waveform resembles original waveform **(A)**. If sampling frequency is too low as result of low PRF, sampled waveform will have lower frequency than original **(B)**.
(From Merritt CRB: *Radiographics* 1991;11:109-119. Used with permission.)

greater depth. The PRF also determines the maximum depth from which unambiguous data can be obtained. If the PRF is less than twice the maximum frequency shift produced by movement of the target (the Nyquist limit), an artifact called aliasing results (Fig. 12-10). If the PRF is less than twice the frequency shift being detected, lower frequency shifts than are actually present are displayed. Because of the need for lower PRFs to reach deep vessels, signals from deep abdominal arteries are prone to aliasing if high velocities are present. In practice, aliasing is usually readily recognized. Aliasing can be reduced by increasing the pulse repetition frequency by increasing the Doppler angle (thereby decreasing the frequency shift) or by using a lower frequency Doppler transducer (Fig. 12-11) (Table 12-1).

Doppler Angle. When making Doppler measurements, it is desirable to correct the Doppler angle and display the measurements in terms of velocity. These measurements are independent of the Doppler frequency. The accuracy of a velocity estimate obtained with Doppler is only as great as the accuracy of the measurement of the Doppler angle. This is particularly true as the Doppler angle exceeds 60 degrees. In general, the Doppler angle is best kept at 60 degrees or less because small changes in the Doppler angle above 60 degrees result in significant changes in the calculated velocity. Therefore measurement inaccuracies result in much greater errors in velocity estimates than similar errors at lower Doppler angles.

Sample Volume Size. With pulsed Doppler systems, the length of the Doppler sample volume can be controlled by the sonographer, whereas the width is determined by the beam profile. Analysis of Doppler signals requires that the sample volume be adjusted to exclude as much of the unwanted clutter from near the vessel walls as possible.

ABDOMINAL APPLICATIONS

Currently, the most important abdominal applications of Doppler are:

- To aid in the identification of vessels
- To determine the direction of blood flow
- To evaluate vessel narrowing or occlusion
- To aid in the characterization of flow to organs and tumors

Although most of the research using pulsed Doppler has

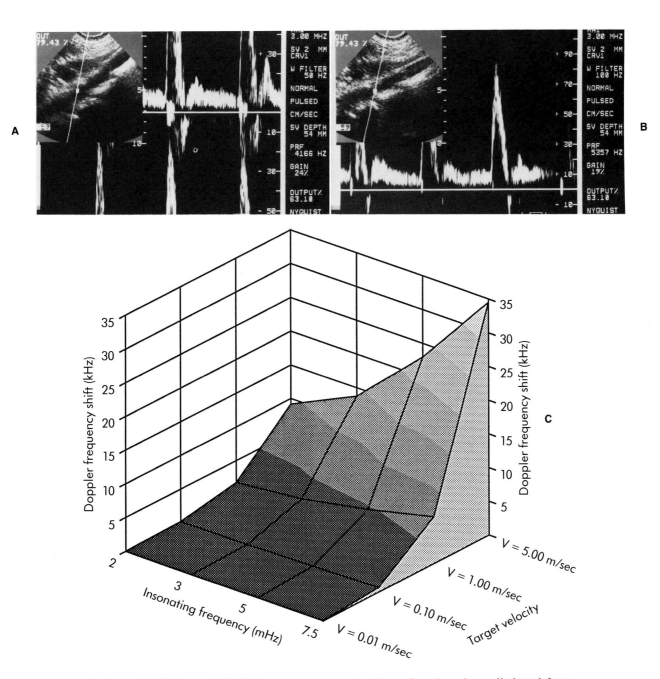

FIG 12-11. Aliasing. **A,** High-frequency components of waveform have been eliminated from their normal display location and are shown, instead, at bottom of image as lower frequency components. **B,** PRF has been increased to permit adequate sampling of high-frequency components of signal, and appearance of waveform has returned to normal. **C,** Relationship between insonating Doppler frequency and Doppler frequency shift, which is associated with given velocity. Higher Doppler frequencies result in higher Doppler shifts for given velocity and therefore are more prone to aliasing. When aliasing is a problem, the use of lower frequency Doppler transducer may eliminate difficulty.

■ **TABLE 12-1**
Relationship of Doppler frequency shift associated with a target moving at a given velocity to the Doppler angle and transmitted frequency.

F_T(mHz)	$\theta = 0°$	$\theta = 45°$	$\theta = 60°$	$\theta = 80°$
2.0	2.6	1.8	1.3	0.5
2.5	3.2	2.3	1.6	0.6
3.0	3.9	2.8	1.9	0.7
5.0	6.5	4.6	3.2	1.1
7.5	9.7	6.8	4.9	1.6

Doppler shift frequencies (kHz) for a target moving 1.00 m/sec

(From Merritt CRB: *Radiographics* 1991;11:109-119. Used with permission.)
*F_T, Transmitted frequency.

emphasized the detection of occlusions, stenoses, and flow disturbances in major vessels, Doppler information is of growing importance in the inference of abnormalities in the peripheral vascular bed of organs or tissue. Changes in the spectral waveform—or in the case of DCI in the appearance of flow in diastole—provide insight into the resistance of the vascular bed supplied by the vessel and (although not specific) indicate changes caused by a variety of pathologic states.

In abdominal applications, semiquantitative analysis of the Doppler shift frequency obtained from both large and small vessels may be used to infer both proximal stenosis and changes in distal vascular impedance.[4] For example, large vessel changes such as flow reversal in the portal vein, the presence of portosystemic collaterals, the occlusion of portal, splenic, or renal veins, and mesenteric or renal artery stenosis are all identifiable by Doppler ultrasonographic methods. Doppler changes, which reflect abnormal impedance of the vascular bed, may also be important in the early identification of transplant organ rejection and may aid in the differentiation of benign from malignant masses. It is well accepted that changes in tissue function are often associated with changes in blood flow, and duplex Doppler ultrasound and DCI, with their abilities to display such changes, are leading closer to the long sought after goal of noninvasive tissue characterization.[5-7] In the following section, an overview of the major implications of Doppler methods in the abdomen is given.

The Liver

Doppler methods permit the evaluation of flow within normal and abnormal hepatic and portal veins and the hepatic artery. Doppler and imaging frequencies of 3 to 5 MHz are used, depending on patient size and the depth of the vessel to be examined. Normal vascular anatomy and anatomic variations, involving vessels in the porta hepatis, can be rapidly evaluated using Doppler to differentiate vascular structures. Doppler color imaging promptly identifies the major hepatic vessels, confirms their patency, and evaluates flow direction and dynamics.

Hepatic Veins

Normal. The inferior vena cava (IVC) and the main left, middle, and right hepatic veins are normally visible with two-dimensional real-time imaging. The Doppler spectral waveforms in the hepatic veins and IVC are among the more complex venous waveforms encountered in the abdomen. Doppler spectral images obtained from normal hepatic veins are similar to those of the IVC with a forward phasic pattern (Fig. 12-12). Because of the lack of a competent valve between the IVC, the hepatic veins, and the right atrium, variations in flow related to cardiac pulsation are transmitted directly to these vessels. Flow varies with changes in respiration, abdominal pressure, and right atrial pressure. During atrial systole, a rapid reversal of flow caused by regurgitation of blood from the right atrium is noted with antegrade flow in diastole. Flow velocity in the hepatic veins and IVC is also affected by respiration with diminished flow or cessation of flow, accompanying increased intrathoracic pressure or reduced intraabdominal pressure (at the end of inspiration or during a Valsalva maneuver), and increased flow when intrathoracic pressure is reduced and abdominal pressures are increased. During inspiration intrathoracic pressure decreases and intraabdominal pressure increases, causing increased flow toward the heart. These dynamics are reversed in expiration. In most individuals, at the end of inspiration (which is when most patients are requested to suspend respiration for scanning), there is an increase in thoracic pressure (a Valsalva maneuver) and flow diminishes or stops. This makes the collection of more than a few cardiac cycles of Doppler information from the hepatic veins difficult in many patients.

Hepatic Vein Abnormalities. The major abnormalities affecting the IVC and hepatic veins are thrombosis and compression or occlusion as a result of space-occupying disease. In the **Budd-Chiari syndrome,** hepatic venous outflow obstruction may result from obstruction of the hepatic vein from the level of the hepatic lobule to the IVC. Duplex Doppler is valuable in the evaluation of patients with Budd-Chiari syndrome and, generally, correlates well with therapeutic results and angiographic findings. Pulsed Doppler sonography in Budd-Chiari syndrome may reveal absent blood flow in the IVC and hepatic veins or reversed, turbulent, or continuous flow patterns.[8] Pulsed Doppler images may also show communicating vessels between hepatic veins or between occluded veins and the retrohepatic IVC.[9] When compared with computed tomography (CT) and

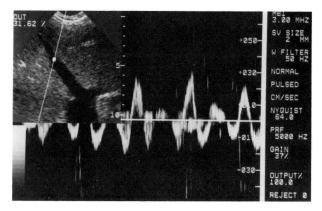

FIG 12-12. Doppler spectrum from middle hepatic vein exhibits complex pattern. Although overall flow direction is away from the transducer or toward heart, transient reversals of flow are present as a result of right atrial contraction. This is indicated by presence of signals both above and below baseline.

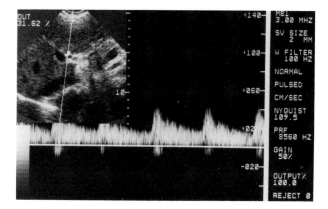

FIG 12-13. Normal hepatic artery spectral waveform reveals pattern of flow typically associated with low-vascular resistance. Forward flow is maintained throughout diastole.

technetium 99m–liver scanning in patients with the Budd-Chiari syndrome, Doppler sonography has been shown to demonstrate intrahepatic venous abnormalities better and to have the unique benefit of showing the direction of blood flow.[10] Color flow Doppler also permits the excellent delineation of intrahepatic, portal, and IVC circulatory dynamics and intrahepatic flow abnormalities, including flow reversal and abnormal hepatic venous connections decompressing obstructed segments of the hepatic venous circulation. DCI frequently permits identification of flow in small or compressed hepatic veins that is not visible with gray scale imaging alone, and it overcomes the difficulty of visualizing the hepatic veins, which may occur with duplex sonography.[11] Because of its ease of use and high sensitivity, color flow is now recommended in the initial appraisal of patients suspected of having Budd-Chiari syndrome.

In addition to evaluation of suspected Budd-Chiari syndrome, both duplex Doppler and DCI are useful in the evaluation of mesoatrial shunts and mesocaval shunts performed to treat hepatic vein occlusion and provide rapid noninvasive confirmation of shunt patency and flow direction. Doppler sampling directly from mesocaval and mesoatrial shunts should show evidence of flow toward the IVC or heart if the shunt is patent and functioning properly. As an adjunct to imaging, Doppler imaging, particularly color imaging, aids in the identification of hepatic vein invasion and tumor thrombus by hepatocellular carcinoma and metastatic tumors involving the liver.

Hepatic Artery

Normal. The normal hepatic artery can be evaluated at multiple sites along its course. Axial or sagittal imaging planes in the epigastrium and subxiphoid region permit interrogation of the origin of the hepatic artery from the celiac axis or, in the case of anomaly, from the superior mesenteric artery. There is considerable variation in the relation of the intrahepatic branches of the hepatic artery relative to the portal vein and bile duct. Most often, the main hepatic artery lies anterior and to the left of the portal vein and next to the bile duct. At the level of the hepatoduodenal ligament, the hepatic artery usually lies between the portal vein and bile duct, although in about 15% of patients it lies anterior to the bile duct. Within the liver the usual location is also between the portal vein and bile duct; however, in 10% to 15% of patients, it will be anterior to and, in 5% to 10%, posterior to the portal vein.[12] The intrahepatic portions of the hepatic artery along the portal vein are usually best evaluated using intercostal or subcostal acoustic windows to scan through the liver. We prefer to use a small sample volume when measuring hepatic arterial waveforms with Doppler imaging, although a somewhat larger sample window is sometimes necessary when searching for the vessel. Once the vessel is located, the sample volume size should be reduced. DCI has proved to be particularly helpful in identifying the presence and location of the hepatic artery for Doppler sampling, especially in hepatic transplant patients. The normal hepatic artery has a low impedance Doppler waveform with continuous diastolic flow (Fig. 12-13).

Because anatomic variants in the portahepatis are relatively common, perhaps the most frequent and useful application of Doppler ultrasonography is in quickly differentiating tubular structures in the porta hepatis. Frequently, the hepatic artery is as large as or larger than the bile duct, giving rise to possible confusion and misdiagnoses, which are easily resolved with the use of Doppler imaging.[13] We have found DCI to be singularly helpful in providing rapid differentiation of vascular from nonvascular structures. For example, quick and accurate differentiation of an enlarged hepatic artery from the bile duct is sometimes useful. DCI has also allowed for identification of flow redistribution between the portal venous and hepatic arterial systems in patients with portal hypertension.[14]

Hepatic Transplantation. Doppler ultrasound is of critical importance in both the pre- and postoperative assessment of hepatic transplant recipients. Before transplantation, the anatomy and patency of the IVC, hepatic, and portal veins must be confirmed. In children with biliary atresia, identification of common anatomic variants of the IVC and hepatic vessels is facilitated with Doppler imaging, especially with the use of color instruments. After transplantation, Doppler methods are essential to confirm hepatic arterial and portal venous patency in the early postoperative period when the risk of thrombosis is greatest. Regular Doppler evaluation of the major hepatic vessels, using both spectral duplex and color flow Doppler is indicated. The use of portable scanners for frequent examinations performed at the patient's bedside obviates the need for angiography. Hepatic artery thrombosis after liver transplantation is difficult to detect clinically in its early stages but is a devastating event requiring emergency retransplantation in most patients. Loss of hepatic arterial flow in the early posttransplant period indicates possible arterial thrombosis. With early identification by Doppler imaging of this complication, thrombectomy rather than retransplantation may be successful. Duplex sonography is highly sensitive in detecting hepatic artery thrombosis after liver transplantation, and Doppler imaging of the hepatic artery combined with real-time sonography of the liver parenchyma is regarded as the optimal procedure for selecting patients who require hepatic angiography after liver transplantation. Doppler ultrasonography has also been found to be useful in monitoring the response to intraarterial thrombolytic treatment for hepatic artery thrombosis following liver transplantation.[15] The role of Doppler in the diagnosis of hepatic transplant rejection is less well established. Although changes in the hepatic arterial resistive index have been suggested as indicating graft dysfunction in some studies, this index is generally not considered to contribute to the diagnosis of hepatic rejection.[16,17] It should be noted that rejection in the absence of Doppler waveform abnormalities may also occur.

Hepatic Tumors. Characteristic signal patterns from malignant tumors, using both continuous wave and pulsed Doppler images, have been reported.[18] The patterns generally described involve the periphery of the tumor and include a characteristic Doppler spectrum with relatively high-peak systolic velocities and a predominance of high-power, low-frequency elements. In

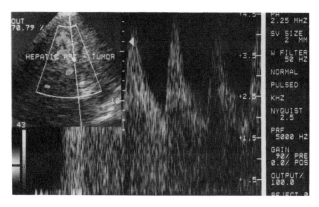

FIG 12-14. Tumor neovascularity. Characteristic Doppler waveform is shown in this patient with hepatocellular carcinoma. Maximum frequency shifts exceed 4.5 KHz (3 MHz, transmitted frequency) and are well above frequencies normally encountered.

the liver, Doppler signals from small hepatic arterial branches may aid in the characterization of hepatic masses.[19] The presence of high-frequency (5 KHz or greater) shifts attributed to arterioportal shunting has been described in hepatomas and some metastatic tumors; these appear relatively specific for highly vascular tumors (Fig. 12-14).[20] Abnormal patterns associated with highly vascular hepatic lesions have also been described using DCI.[7] In contrast to malignant tumors, which have high-velocity arteriovenous shunts, hemangiomas have slow flow velocities and thus are not associated with abnormal Doppler signals.

Portal Vein Doppler

Normal. Subcostal and transhepatic approaches using 3- to 3.5-MHz Doppler imaging are usually required to evaluate the intrahepatic and extrahepatic portions of the portal vein. Because the left portal vein ascends vertically, it is customarily possible to easily obtain a small Doppler angle from this vessel by scanning in the subxiphoid region. The horizontal portion of the main right portal vein is best sampled by scanning in the intercostal spaces laterally. Attention to the Doppler angles is particularly important in obtaining measurements from the right portal vein, because the use of a large (>60 degrees) angle may make it difficult to detect flow and can also result in an ambiguous display of flow direction.

Doppler imaging of the main portal vein reveals a continuous flow pattern with variations in velocity induced by respiration (Fig. 12-15). On inspiration, there is mechanical compression of the liver, resulting in increased pressure in the portal vein with diminished flow velocity; on expiration, the situation is reversed, and flow increases. Normal portal venous flow is hepatope-

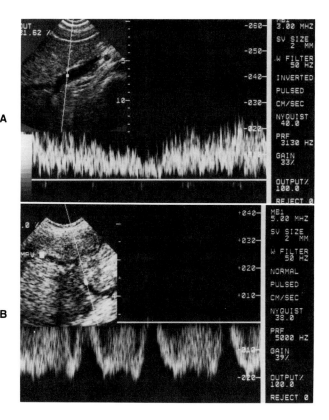

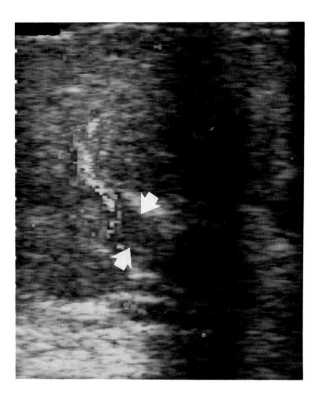

FIG 12-15. A, Normal portal vein flow is toward liver (hepatopedal) and exhibits slight variations in velocity related to respiration. **B,** Reversal of portal vein flow may occur with intrahepatic obstruction of portal vein due to cirrhosis. This is readily demonstrated with duplex of color Doppler with appearance of flow below baseline.

FIG 12-16. Partial portal vein thrombosis. DCI is particularly valuable. Echogenic thrombus *(arrows)* totally occludes proximal right portal vein. More distally, anterior segmental branch is reconstituted by collaterals and shows hepatopedal flow (blue signals).

dal (toward the liver). In some individuals, DCI shows complex helical patterns of hepatopedal flow. Recognition of this is important because sampling with pulsed spectral Doppler images may indicate reversed flow if the vessel is not completely examined.

Portal Vein Thrombosis. Noninvasive diagnosis of portal vein thrombosis, using ultrasound imaging, dynamic CT, and duplex Doppler ultrasound has been reported.[21,22] Although quite accurate, the differentiation of a complete from a partial portal vein occlusion is difficult with these techniques. With duplex sonography, a sensitivity and specificity for main portal vein disorders of 83% and 93%, respectively, have been reported.[23] Duplex ultrasound is accurate in prospectively assessing the direction of flow and the presence of total thrombosis in the portal vein, but partial thrombosis may not be detected. DCI gives a rapid evaluation of the portal vein and is very effective in revealing flow in the residual lumen if partial thrombosis is present (Fig. 12-16). Detection of the presence of collaterals (cavernous transformation), which frequently form following portal vein

occlusion, is another application for which DCI is especially well suited. Typical findings of cavernous transformation include numerous tubular structures that exhibit low-velocity venous flow patterns in the region of the porta hepatis. DCI also demonstrates increased hepatic artery size and flow, which accompany this pathologic condition.

Portal Hypertension. In patients with portal hypertension, Doppler ultrasound allows for the rapid determination of the **direction** of portal blood flow. This information is important in planning surgical treatment because the presence of hepatofugal flow indicates the need for a portocaval or mesocaval (rather than a splenorenal) shunt. It has been suggested that measurement of portal vein flow velocity is of value in establishing the prognosis in patients with portal hypertension with lower flow velocities, indicating more advanced disease. Studies in Europe have indicated that patients with large varices have significantly lower portal blood velocity and portal blood flow than do patients without varices, suggesting that, in patients with cirrhosis, circulatory alterations in the portal vascular bed may be—at least in part—an indicator of the stage of liver disease.[24] In children with biliary atresia, a decline in portal vein flow velocity has been indicated to be useful in predicting deterioration of liver function.[25] Interobserver variation in the measurement of portal vein velocity may be quite high, however, casting some doubt on the reliability of these measurements, except in carefully controlled clinical settings.[26] **Portosystemic collateral vessels** in patients with portal hypertension are detected readily using Doppler ultrasonography—again with DCI proving to be especially valuable. Parumbilical, gastroesophageal, pancreaticoduodenal, retroperitoneal, splenorenal, and gastrorenal collaterals have all been described with duplex or DCI methods. In all patients with chronic liver disease or portal hypertension, any unusual tubular structure in the abdomen should be evaluated with Doppler imaging because many of these will turn out to be collateral veins that decompress the obstructed portal venous system. DCI often indicates the presence of more extensive collaterals than does gray scale imaging alone.

When portal hypertension is treated by portocaval, mesocaval, mesoatrial, or splenorenal shunting, shunt patency may be evaluated with duplex or DCI. Portacaval shunts are more amenable to study by duplex ultrasound than are more peripheral shunts because the liver can be used as an acoustic window.[27] In patients with distal splenorenal (Warren) shunts, scanning through the spleen usually allows for good visualization of the vessels of interest. Color Doppler imaging has been shown to have a high sensitivity and high specificity in evaluating shunt patency. Comparison of duplex and DCI has shown that, although the two techniques are almost equally effective in establishing patency in portacaval, mesocaval, and mesoatrial shunts, DCI was far more helpful in the assessment of splenorenal shunts.[28] In the evaluation of portocaval shunts, it is essential that both the portal vein and IVC be imaged. Duplex Doppler or DCI will show flow from the shunt into the IVC if the shunt is patent. In functioning splenorenal shunts Doppler imaging shows the flow within the portal vein, as well as in the splenic and renal segments of the shunt, with flow directed toward the renal vein and IVC.

Other Portal Vein Changes. In the proper clinical setting, portal vein Doppler ultrasonography is capable of showing manifestations of hepatic venoocclusive disease, demonstrating decreased or reversed flow in the portal vein.[29] In patients with right ventricular failure and tricuspid regurgitation, variations in the Doppler waveforms may be seen in portal veins. Normal portal flow is not pulsatile and is characterized by relatively little variation in velocity, except for changes related to respiration. In the presence of elevated right atrial pressure, flow within the portal vein becomes more pulsatile, with reversal of flow during each cardiac cycle. A similar pattern of pulsatile portal vein flow has been de-

scribed in association with tricuspid regurgitation. Thus the identification of pulsatile portal vein waveforms that are similar to those in hepatic veins may aid in the diagnosis and treatment of patients with right ventricular failure.[30-32]

Splenic and Mesenteric Vessels

Measurements of flow in the splenic artery have been reported but currently are of limited clinical value.[33] In approximately 25% of subjects, Doppler examination is limited because of patient size, debility, distorted vascular anatomy, and excessive gas in the stomach. The measurement of flow in the superior mesenteric artery is potentially of greater clinical relevance, particularly in the workup of patients with intestinal angina. In the past diagnosis of mesenteric arterial occlusive disease has required arteriography, but a growing role for duplex sonography is likely. Mesenteric duplex scanning has been used successfully to measure postprandial changes in celiac and superior mesenteric arterial blood flow, as well as changes in visceral flow produced by other pharmacologic stimuli.[34] The spectral waveform obtained from the proximal superior mesenteric artery varies with intestinal activity. During fasting, a high-resistance waveform with little diastolic flow is present (Fig. 12-17). After eating, increased intestinal blood flow is accompanied by increased diastolic flow and a low-resistance waveform. Studies of neonates have shown alterations in the resistance of the vascular bed of the superior mesenteric artery in small for gestational age infants and in full-term neonates with cardiovascular abnormalities, which may help in the evaluation of intestinal abnormalities related to perfusion disturbance.[35] Intraoperative CW Doppler probes are helpful in assessing intestinal viability during intestinal surgery. Criteria used in the assessment of in-

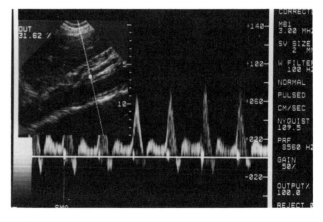

FIG 12-17. Superior mesenteric artery (normal spectrum). Lack of early diastolic flow is indicative of high resistance in distal vascular bed. This pattern is seen in fasting patients. After eating, low-resistance waveform is present.

testinal viability include the presence of flow within the vessel of interest and measurements of velocity.

A major difficulty in the Doppler assessment of the splenic and mesenteric vessels is limited visualization, resulting from superimposed intestinal gas. If the patient is thin and gas is minimal, the ability of DCI to image the splenic and mesenteric arteries and veins is excellent, permitting the potential diagnosis and characterization of stenosis and occlusion.

The Native Kidney

Currently, Doppler evaluation of the native kidney has proved to be of somewhat limited value. The location of the renal arteries, the common occurrence of multiple arteries, and superimposed bowel and bone have increased the difficulty of obtaining consistent results. Confirmation of arterial and venous patency in the kidney is possible using pulsed Doppler and DCI and may be particularly useful in infants and children when renal arterial occlusion or renal vein thrombosis is suspected. The use of renal artery Doppler as a screening method for renovascular hypertension has yet to be universally accepted. In the evaluation of the transplanted kidney, Doppler imaging provides an indispensable adjunct to the imaging examination, allowing for rapid confirmation of arterial and venous flow. The role of Doppler imaging in the evaluation of transplant rejection has been the subject of much controversy; however, carefully performed measurements that are interpreted in the proper clinical context are useful in the management of transplant dysfunction.

Normal Renal Artery and Vein

In the native kidney, Doppler measurement of renal arterial flow can be made along the extrarenal course of the vessel, provided that a suitable acoustical window also is found for the segmental, interlobar, and arcuate arteries. Both supine transabdominal and prone translumbar approaches are possible. Usually, the renal arteries are imaged in the axial plane at the level of the superior mesenteric artery and left renal vein. In sagittal scan planes, identification of the right renal artery as it passes posterior to the IVC may be helpful. The acoustical window provided by the liver and IVC makes evaluation of the right renal vessels easier to perform than evaluation of the left. Doppler frequencies of 3 to 3.5 MHz are used. DCI aids in identifying the renal vessels and is a useful adjunct to duplex scanning. With duplex Doppler imaging, the segmental, interlobar, and arcuate vessels are not visible. Samples are obtained by blind sampling between the medullary pyramids at the corticomedullary junction. DCI permits visualization of these small vessels and aids in precise sampling. The spectral waveform obtained from the main renal artery and its branches shows a pattern typical of a low-resis-

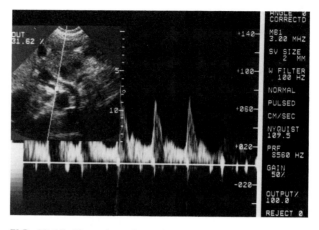

FIG. 12-18. Normal renal arterial spectrum, similar to hepatic arterial, shows flow throughout diastole, indicating low resistance.

tance vessel with high-flow velocity, persisting throughout diastole (Fig. 12-18). Velocity measurements in the main renal artery are normally less than 100 cm/sec. With duplex and DCI instruments, venous flow can be measured from within both the kidney and the main renal veins. The identification of normal and symmetric venous waveforms from the kidney may be useful in excluding main renal vein thrombosis.

Renal Artery Stenosis. Duplex Doppler imaging has been shown (with varying degrees of success) to permit diagnosis of renal artery stenosis and occlusion. Criteria for the diagnosis of significant (>50%) stenosis in the main renal artery include:

- The presence of a systolic velocity of greater than 100 cm/sec[36]
- A ratio of peak renal artery velocity to peak aortic velocity of 3.5 or greater[37]
- Spectral broadening
- Absence of diastolic flow
- Lack of flow, indicating occlusion

Using these criteria, sensitivities of 89% to 91% and specificities of 73% to 95% have been obtained in the detection of significant stenosis. Using similar criteria, other investigators have reported much less encouraging results, noting a specificity for Doppler imaging of only 37%.[38] Because accurate evaluation demands that the entire course of each renal artery be examined, the study may be compromised in many patients because of superimposed bowel gas, bone, or fat. The accuracy of renal artery Doppler imaging is impaired by the difficulty of obtaining adequate samples from both renal arteries,[39] and the occurrence of multiple renal arteries is more than 20% of patients. With DCI, normal renal arteries and veins are regularly imaged in thin patients and children but are less consistently imaged in adults. Criteria for the diagnosis of stenosis using DCI include not only the spectral changes described with duplex Doppler imaging but the direct visualization of vessel narrowing and the stenotic jet. Currently, however, Doppler methods, including color flow Doppler imaging, are not generally regarded as suitable for use in the initial screening for renal artery stenosis in hypertensive patients. The need for a simple, accurate, and noninvasive screening technique for renovascular disease undoubtedly will stimulate continued interest in the improvement of Doppler criteria and techniques for renal artery evaluation.

Renal Carcinoma. As with liver tumors, vascular changes associated with malignant renal tumors may be demonstrated by Doppler ultrasound. Using a Doppler frequency shift in excess of 2.5 KHz (for 3-MHz insonating frequency) as the criterion for diagnosis, tumor signals have been reported in up to 83% of untreated renal cell carcinomas, 75% of Wilms' tumors, and in patients with metastases to the kidney not associated with benign renal masses.[40] DCI has also been reported to show changes associated with renal carcinoma.[41] The sensitivity of Doppler imaging in identifying malignant tumors of the kidney is reported to be 70%, with a specificity of 94%.[42] Doppler ultrasound adds useful information to the study of renal masses, and the detection of high-velocity signals can aid in the differential diagnosis of renal masses.[43]

Other Conditions. Renal obstruction has been shown to increase renal vascular resistance in animals, and there is now evidence that this also may occur in humans. Resistive index (RI) measurements have been reported to show a significant difference between obstructed and nonobstructed kidneys. In normal kidneys, the RI measured in the interlobar arteries is usually less than 0.70%.[44] With obstruction, higher values are encountered. An RI of 0.7 or greater appears to correlate well with obstruction, resulting in a sensitivity of 92%, a specificity of 88%, and an accuracy of 90%.[45] Doppler measurements therefore are quite promising in aiding the differentiation of obstructive from nonobstructive calyectasis.

Experience with Doppler ultrasonography in **renal vein thrombosis** is limited, but our experience is encouraging in patients in whom size and gas levels do not prevent assessment. The demonstration of a distended renal vein without evidence of flow has correlated well with other studies, indicating renal vein thrombosis in a small number of patients. Doppler imaging, particularly DCI, is also useful in confirming tumor invasion of the renal veins when imaging findings are equivocal. With DCI, intrarenal vessels—including segmental, interlobar, and arcuate vessels—are visible in many patients, and we have noted diminished patterns of flow in these vessels in patients with advanced renal parenchymal disease. The future role of DCI in the evaluation of renal perfusion remains to be defined,

but the capabilities provided by new imaging methods are promising and deserve further study.

Renal Transplants

Transplant dysfunction may result from vessel stenosis, occlusion, or parenchymal changes caused by rejection, tubular necrosis, or drug toxicity. The ability of Doppler ultrasonography to assess major vessels for primary abnormalities and to document dynamics of flow that reflect changes in smaller vessels has encouraged the routine postoperative use of ultrasound in the evaluation of renal transplants. Because of the superficial location of the transplanted kidney and the lack of superimposed gas, high-quality Doppler studies are possible in essentially all patients. DCI can be performed at 5 to 7.5 MHz, permitting excellent detail of intrarenal and extrarenal vessels (Fig. 12-5). Duplex or DCI examinations provide rapid and accurate diagnosis of stenosis or thrombosis of the main renal artery and vein. In the normal renal transplant, flow in the segmental, interlobar, and arcuate vessels continues throughout both systole and diastole; RI values range from 0.5 to 0.7 in the segmental and interlobar arteries. With duplex Doppler imaging, significant differences in perfusion patterns from the norm have been observed, with elevation of RI values in patients with rejection and acute tubular necrosis (Fig. 12-19).[46] Although high-RIs have been associated with acute rejection, other causes of RI elevation, including acute tubular necrosis, renal vein thrombosis, renal compression, pyelonephritis, and obstruction have been described.[47-50] Lack of RI elevation in significant numbers of patients with pathologic evidence of acute transplant rejection has also been reported.[51,52] It is clear that more recent studies have not shown the degree of sensitivity and specificity for Doppler ultrasound in the identification of rejection that was initially reported. Despite these shortcomings, an abnormal Doppler imaging finding warrants clinical correlation and additional workup to establish the cause of the abnormality.[53]

DCI has been used following biopsy of renal transplants to identify complications, including arteriovenous fistula and pseudoaneurysm. With color Doppler, arteriovenous fistulas may be directly visualized. Often, an associated tissue vibration (bruit) is present and is imaged with DCI. Color and spectral Doppler images demonstrate higher than normal arterial and venous velocities, and a pulsatile venous waveform, resulting from the arteriovenous shunting, is present. Pseudoaneurysms may vary from several millimeters to several centimeters in diameter. Imaging alone may suggest a cystic mass, but the use of duplex or color Doppler permits the identification of flow within the mass, confirming its vascular nature. Color Doppler imaging is particularly helpful in permitting rapid identification both of the turbulent flow within the pseudoaneurysm and the connection from the feeding vessel. The ease and speed of diagnosis make DCI superior to duplex ultrasound in the identification of these complications. DCI is the method of choice for noninvasive detection of vascular lesions caused by percutaneous biopsy.[54]

Other Applications

Currently, the major role of abdominal Doppler and DCI has been to evaluate the presence and direction of flow in large vessels to abdominal viscera and to assist in the evaluation of renal and hepatic transplant perfusion. In addition to these applications, Doppler sonography is also used in the assessment of blood flow to the transplanted pancreas, permitting early identification of mechanical problems with arterial and venous anastomoses.

Tumor vascularity has also been evaluated in a number of abdominal organs, in addition to the liver and kidney. A high sensitivity is required to detect the low-amplitude signals present in tumor vessels, and the highest Doppler frequency available should be used. Careful Doppler interrogation of the margin of the tumor is required to identify the vessels of interest. Because arteriovenous shunting in tumor vessels results in high-velocity flow, aliasing may occur. In the pancreas, signals of much higher frequency than normally encountered have been described with Doppler imaging having a sensitivity of 83% and a specificity of 94% in differentiating benign from malignant tumors.[55] In the future, the use of DCI with ultrasound contrast agents may further enhance the role of ultrasonography in tumor analysis.

REFERENCES

1. Merritt CRB: Ultrasound safety: what are the Issues? Editorial. *Radiology* 1989;173:304-306

Principles of Doppler ultrasonography

2. Merritt CRB: Doppler principles: the basics. *Radiographics* 1991; 11: 109-119.
3. Merritt CRB: Real time Doppler Color flow imaging: other applications. In: Bernstein EF: *Non-Invasive Diagnostic Techniques in Vascular Disease.* St Louis: Mosby-Year Book; 1990:42-56.

Abdominal applications

4. Taylor KJW, Burns PN: Duplex Doppler scanning in the pelvis and abdomen. *Ultrasound Med Bio* 1985;11:643-658.
5. Wells PNT, Halliwell M, Skidmore R, et al: Tumor detection by ultrasonic Doppler blood-flow signals. *Ultrasonics* 1977;5:231-232.
6. Dubbins PA, Wells I: Renal carcinoma: duplex Doppler evaluation. *Br J Radiol* 1986;59:231-236.
7. Merritt CRB: Doppler color flow imaging. *J Clin Ultrasound* 1987;15:591-597.
8. Hosoki T, Kuroda C, Tokunaga K, et al: Hepatic venous outflow obstruction: evaluation with pulsed duplex sonography. *Radiology* 1989;170:733-737.
9. Ohnishi K, Terabayashi H, Tsunoda T, et al: Budd-Chiari syndrome: diagnosis with duplex sonography. *Am J Gastroenterol* 1990;85:165-169.

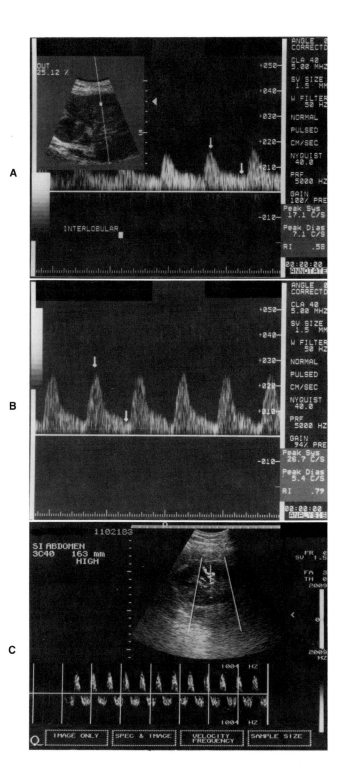

FIG 12-19. Renal transplants. Changes in renal arterial resistive index may aid in evaluation of transplant dysfunction. **A,** Normal transplant with resistive index (RI) of 0.58. **B,** RI is abnormal (0.79); biopsy indicated rejection. **C,** There is reversal of diastolic flow; highly abnormal pattern is associated in this case with acute rejection. RI changes are not specific.

10. Gupta S, Barter S, Phillips GW, et al: Comparison of ultrasonography, computed tomography and 99m Tc liver scan in diagnosis of Budd-Chiari syndrome. *Gut* 1987;28:242-247.

11. Grant EG, Perrella R, Tessler FN, et al: Budd-Chiari syndrome: the results of duplex and color Doppler imaging. *AJR* 1989;152:377-381.

12. Ralls PW, Quinn MF, Rogers W, et al: Sonographic anatomy of the hepatic artery. *AJR* 1981;136:1059-1063.

13. Berland LL, Lawson TL, Foley WD: Porta hepatis: sonographic discrimination of bile ducts from arteries with pulsed Doppler with new anatomic criteria. *AJR* 1982;138:833-840.

14. Ralls PW: Color Doppler sonography of the hepatic artery and portal venous system. *AJR* 1990;155:517-525.

15. Hidalgo EG, Abad J, Cantarero JM, et al: High-dose intraarterial urokinase for the treatment of hepatic artery thrombosis in liver transplantation. *Hepatogastroenterology* 1989;36:529-532.

16. Zonderland HM, Lameris JS, Terpstra OT, et al: Auxiliary partial liver transplantation: imaging evaluation in 10 patients. *AJR* 1989;153:981-985.

17. Taylor KJ, Morse SS, Weltin GG, et al: Liver transplant recipients: portable duplex ultrasound with correlative angiography. *Radiology*. 1986;159:357-363.

18. Taylor KJ, Ramos I, Carter D, et al: Correlation of Doppler ultrasound tumor signals with neovascular morphologic features. *Radiology* 1988;166:57-62.

19. Taylor KJ, Ramos I, Morses SS, et al: Focal liver masses: Differential diagnosis with pulsed Doppler ultrasound. *Radiology* 1988;166:57-62.

20. Scoutt LM, Zawin ML, Taylor KJW: Doppler ultrasound, II; clinical applications. *Radiology* 1990;174:309-319.

21. Merritt CRB: Ultrasound demonstration of portal vein thrombosis. *Radiology* 1979;133:425-442.

22. Miller VE, Berland LL: Pulsed Doppler duplex sonography and computed tomography of portal vein thrombosis. *AJR* 1985;145:73-76.

23. Alpern MV, Rubin JM, Williams DM, et al: Porta hepatis: duplex Doppler ultrasound with angiographic correlation. *Radiology* 1987;162:53-56.

24. Ljubicic N, Duvnjak M, Rotkvic K, et al: Influence of the degree of liver failure on portal blood flow in patients with liver cirrhosis. *Scand J Gastroenterol* 1990;25:395-400.

25. Wanek EA, Horgan JG, Karrer FM, et al: Portal venous velocity in biliary atresia. *J Pediatr Surg* 1990;25:146-148.

26. Sabba C, Weltin GG, Cicchetti DV, et al: Observer variability in echo-Doppler measurements of portal flow in cirrhotic patients and normal volunteers. *Gastroenterology* 1990;9:1603-1611.

27. Finn JP, Gibson RN, Dunn GD: Duplex ultrasound in the evaluation of portacaval shunts. *Clin Radiol* 1987;38:87-89.

28. Grant EG, Tessler FN, Gomes AS, et al: Color Doppler imaging of portosystemic shunts. *AJR* 1990;154(2):393-397.

29. Brown BP, Abu-Yousel M, Farner R, et al: Doppler sonography: a non-invasive method for evaluation of hepatic venoocclusive disease. *AJR* 1990;154:721-724.

30. Alvarez G. Sanchez la Fuente J, Lopez J, et al: Flow changes in hepatic veins in congestive cardiac insufficiency: a study of pulsed Doppler ultrasound. *Eur J Radiol* 1989;9:163-166.

31. Duerinckx AJ, Grant EG, Perrella RR, et al: The pulsatile portal vein in cases of congestive heart failure: correlation of duplex Doppler findings with right atrial pressures. *Radiology* 1990;176:655-658.

32. Abu-Yousef MM, Milam SG, Farner RM: Pulsatile portal vein flow: a sign of tricuspid regurgitation on duplex Doppler sonography. *AJR* 1990;155:785-788.

33. Manoharan A, Gill RW, Griffiths KA: Splenic blood flow measurements by Doppler ultrasound: a preliminary report. *Cardiovasc Res* 1987;21:779-782.

34. Flinn WR, Rizzo RJ, Park JS, et al: Duplex scanning for assessment of mesenteric ischemia. *Surg Clin North Am* 1990;70:99-107.

35. Van Bel F, Van Zwieten PHT, Guit GL, et al: Superior mesenteric artery blood flow velocity and estimated volume flow: duplex Doppler ultrasound study of preterm and term neonates. *Radiology* 1990;174:165-169.

36. Avasthi PS, Voyles WF, Greene ER: Non-invasive diagnosis of renal artery stenosis by echo-Doppler velocimetry. *Kidney Int* 1984;25:824-829.

37. Kohler Tr, Zierler RE, Martin RL, et al: Non-invasive diagnosis of renal artery stenosis by ultrasonic duplex scanning. *J Vasc Surg* 1986;4:450-456.

38. Berland LL, Koslin DB, Routh WD, et al: Renal artery stenosis: prospective evaluation of diagnosis with color duplex ultrasound compared with angiography: work in progress. *Radiology* 1990;174:421-423.

39. Dubbins PA: Renal artery stenosis: duplex Doppler evaluation. *Br J Radiol* 1986;59:225-229.

40. Ramos IM, Taylor KJW, Kier R, et al: Tumor vascular signals in renal masses: detection with Doppler ultrasound. *Radiology* 1988;168:633-637.

41. Shimamoto K, Sakuma S, Ishigaki T, et al: Intratumoral blood flow: evaluation with color Doppler echography. Radiology 1987;165:683-685.

42. Kier R, Taylor KJW, Feycock AL, et al: Renal masses: characterization with Doppler ultrasound. *Radiology* 1990;176:703-707.

43. Dubbins PA, Wells P: Renal carcinoma: duplex Doppler evaluation. *Br J Radiol* 1986;50:231-236.

44. Gottlieb RH, Luhmann K IV, Oates RP: Duplex ultrasound evaluation of normal native kidneys and native kidneys with urinary tract obstruction. *J Ultrasound Med* 1989;8:609-611.

45. Platt JF, Rubin JM, Ellis JH: Distinction between obstructive and nonobstructive pyelocaliectasis with duplex Doppler sonography. *AJR* 1989;153:997-1000.

46. Rigsby CM, Taylor KJW, Weltin GG, et al: Renal allografts in acute rejection: evaluation using duplex sonography. *Radiology* 19867;1548:375-378.

47. Rifkin MD, Needleman L, Pasto ME, et al: Evaluation of renal transplant rejection by duplex Doppler examination: value of the resistive index. *AJR* 1987;148:759-762.

48. Buckley AR, Cooperberg PL, Reeve CE, et al: The distinction between acute renal transplant rejection and cyclosporine nephrotoxicity: value of duplex sonography. *AJR* 1987;149:521-525.

49. Warshauer DM, Taylor KJW, Bia MJ, et al: Unusual causes in increased vascular impedance in renal transplants: duplex Doppler evaluation. *Radiology* 1988;169:367-370.

50. Allen KS, Jorkasky DK, Arger PH, et al: Renal allografts: prospective analysis of Doppler sonography. *Radiology* 1988; 169:371-376.

51. Genkins SM, Sanfilippo FP, Carroll BA: Duplex Doppler sonography of renal transplants: lack of sensitivity and specificity in establishing pathologic diagnosis. *AJR* 1989;152:535-539.

52. Keicz F, Pozniak MA, Pirsh JD, et al: Pyramidal appearance and resistive index: insensitive and nonspecific sonographic indicators of renal transplants rejection. *AJR* 1990;155:531-535.

53. Taylor KJW, Marks WH: Commentary: use of Doppler imaging for evaluation of dysfunction in renal allografts. *AJR* 1990;155:536-537.

54. Hubsch PJ, Mostbeck G, Barton PP, et al: Evaluation of arteriovenous fistulas and pseudoaneurysms in renal allografts following percutaneous needle biopsy: color coded Doppler sonography versus duplex Doppler sonography. *J Ultrasound Med* 1990;9:95-100.

55. Orr NM, Taylor KJW: Doppler detection of tumor vascularity. In: Taylor KJW, Strandness DE, eds. *Clinic in Diagnostic Ultrasound*. New York: Churchill Livingstone; 1990:149-163.

CHAPTER 13

The Abdominal Great Vessels

- Gretchen A.W. Gooding, M.D.

AORTA

The abdominal aorta enters the abdomen through the aortic hiatus of the diaphragm and descends a little to the left of midline, bifurcating at the level of the umbilicus into the left and right common iliac arteries. The aorta has three ventral or anterior branches: the celiac artery, the superior mesenteric artery, and the inferior mesenteric artery. These branches supply blood to the gastrointestinal tract, liver, spleen, and pancreas. The renal arteries are the largest lateral branches of the aorta and are the only lateral branches of significance to sonographers.

Abdominal aortic blood flow is characterized as plug flow, with the red blood cells all moving at the same velocity.[1] This contrasts with the parabolic flow seen in smaller vessels, in which the red blood cells move faster in the central portion of the vessel and slower at the periphery. Color-coded Doppler imaging enables the examiner to visualize the slower peripheral flow as a different color from the central faster flow—that is, red (slow) versus white (fast). During diastole, no flow may be demonstrated by color along the periphery of the vessel, although newer methods now incorporate a program in the ultrasonic instrumentation to facilitate detection of slow flow.[1]

The abdominal aorta is the major supplier of the peripheral musculature. As such, the duplex Doppler examination reveals a triphasic high-resistance waveform on spectral analysis.

Examination

No preparation is required for sonographic examination of the aorta. Overlying bowel gas may obscure portions of the vessel, but changes in patient position, coronal imaging, and return to the region after other parts of the abdomen have been examined may yield better results.[2] A large panniculus may be pushed to the side in obese patients to gain an acoustic window closer to the aorta.

The abdominal aorta should be examined from the diaphragm to the iliac bifurcation at the umbilicus in parasagittal and transverse planes. The standard transducer frequency for the aortic examination is 3.5 MHz. If the patient is thin, 5 MHz will suffice. A long linear transducer shows a longer viewing segment than does a sector transducer. The normal aorta is a long tubular structure that lies just anterior to the vertebral bodies (Fig. 13-1). It is positioned more anteriorly at the level of the bifurcation than at the diaphragmatic hiatus. Normally, the diameter of the aorta is less than 3 cm in an anteroposterior dimension.

The **sonographic aortic examination** is performed:
- To define aortic size
- To determine the extent of atherosclerosis
- To detect aortic dissection
- To assess the periaortic soft tissues

Limitations of aortic sonography are related to suboptimal visualization caused by overlying bowel gas, obesity, or both. The origins of the renal arteries are obscured in many patients.[3] Inter- and intraobserver er-

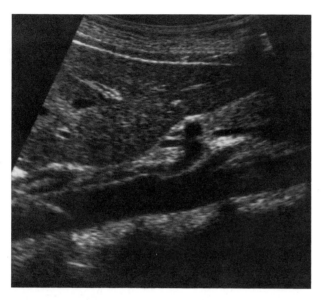

FIG 13-1. Normal aorta. Sagittal scan shows aorta as long tubular structure lying just anterior to lumbar spine. Large anterior branches, celiac axis, and superior mesenteric artery, are seen.

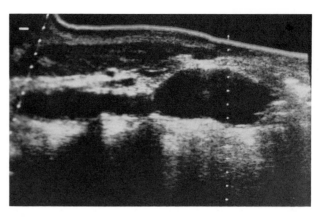

FIG 13-2. Bifurcation abdominal aortic aneurysm. Sagittal scan shows focal fusiform expansion of the distal abdominal aorta.
(Courtesy Dr. Stephanie Wilson, Toronto General Hospital, Canada.)

rors in abdominal aortic aneurysm measurement may also limit the accuracy of sonography.[4]

Abdominal Aortic Aneurysm

An abdominal aortic aneurysm is defined as a focal enlargement of the aorta of 3 cm or greater in the anteroposterior diameter. The majority of abdominal aortic aneurysms are atherosclerotic and infrarenal. Trauma, syphilis, and mycotic etiologic factors should be considered for those with a suprarenal location. Morphologically, abdominal aneurysms are usually fusiform or saccular (Fig. 13-2).

Aneurysms of the aorta are common in elderly men. Early diagnosis and surgical treatment with graft replacement offers long-term survival rates for patients who are low-operative risks and who have aneurysms that are greater than 4 cm in diameter.[5] A population-based sonographic study notes a risk of rupture of 3% at 10 years after graft replacement in aneurysms of less than 5 cm; the risk increases to 25% at 5 years in aneurysms 5 cm or greater.[6] This is distinctly less than an older autopsy study series that reported a 9.5% risk of rupture for aneurysms of less than 4 cm, a 23.5% risk for those of 4.1 to 5 cm, and a 60.5% risk for those of more than 10 cm.[7] Abdominal aortic aneurysms increase in diameter an average of of about 0.2 cm per year.[6] Because recent surgical mortality in elective cases is less than 2%, many aneurysms are now resected.[8]

Features of aortic aneurysms that favor surgery include:

- Size, particularly those of 6 cm or greater in diameter
- Associated pain or tenderness
- Documented enlargement (Fig. 13-3)
- Associated distal emboli
- Renal obstruction or gastrointestinal bleeding
- Suspected rupture

In experienced hands, the sonographic diagnosis of an abdominal aortic aneurysm is extremely accurate, approaching 100%. Duplex Doppler imaging adds the new dimension of actual flow characterization.

Objectives of the sonographic examination of an aortic aneurysm are:

- To determine the location, length, and breadth of the aneurysm
- To assess the extent of mural thrombus and calcification
- To define the patent channel and the flow characteristics by duplex Doppler imaging
- To determine whether the iliac arteries or the proximal aorta are involved
- To detect dissection
- To evaluate the periaortic region for masses, hemorrhage, or adenopathy

The patient who is a surgical candidate should also undergo a renal sonogram to exclude unsuspected hydronephrosis because this will affect the surgical risk.

An abdominal aorta may develop tortuosity throughout its length. Sonographically, a tortuous aneurysmal aorta requires special attention to define actual size. Overestimation of size results when oblique views rather than true anterior to posterior dimensions are taken on transverse scans. To avoid this pitfall, the aorta should be noted in a longitudinal plane, and the transducer then rotated 90 degrees to a true transverse section. This plane may not be a true transverse of the

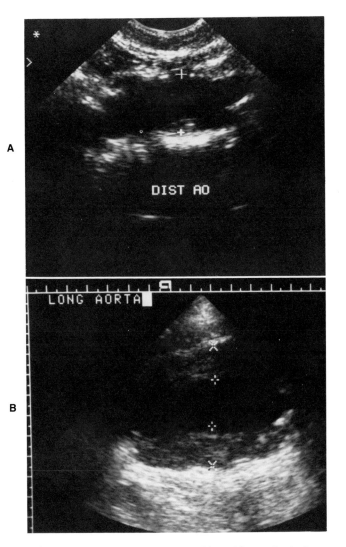

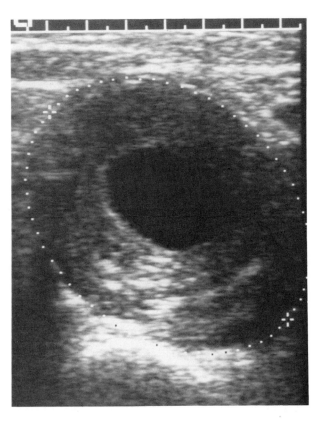

FIG 13-3. Distal aortic aneurysm with rapid growth. **A,** Longitudinal scan shows aneurysm of 3.2 cm in diameter. **B,** One year later, aneurysm has grown to 5.8 cm in diameter. This rapid expansion is distinctly unusual.

FIG 13-4. Aortic aneurysm. Transverse image shows large distal abdominal aortic aneurysm with circumferential intraluminal thrombus.

abdomen. The transducer should be moved along the length of the vessel to include the common iliac arteries.

Intraluminal thrombus, which is usually anterior and often eccentric, occurs in the majority of abdominal aortic aneurysms. Color flow Doppler imaging has shown that an aneurysm with a flow that jets against a wall is associated with less thrombus at that site. Thrombus may also be circumferential along the walls, leaving a central or eccentric lumen (Fig. 13-4). The thrombus or the intimal surface may calcify. This thrombus is a source of peripheral embolism and may eventually result in peripheral vessel occlusion. Complete thrombosis of an aneurysm is much less likely to occur in the aorta than in the peripheral arteries.

With aneurysmal dilation, **duplex sonographic evaluation** reveals a holosystolic waveform. Systolic flow is seen both above and below the baseline, reflecting turbulence. Using color flow Doppler sonography, the turbulent flow in aneurysms is recognized by red, white, and blue pixels of color, which rapidly change in a swirling configuration.

An isolated **suprarenal aneurysm** of the aorta is uncommon and more likely occurs as a result of trauma or infection than of atherosclerosis. In contrast, an aortic aneurysm at the level of the diaphragm suggests extension of a thoracic aneurysm (Fig. 13-5). Although ultrasound is the primary screening study to detect an aneurysm and to determine its size, the relation of the aorta to the origins of the renal arteries is more often inferred from its position rather than actual visualization. Positional clues suggesting renal artery involvement include visualization of the aneurysm on transverse scans at the level of the left renal vein or on parasagittal scans at the level of the right renal artery.

Rupture of the aorta is a life-threatening event. The larger the aneurysm, the greater the likelihood of rupture (Fig. 13-6). Although small (less than 4 cm) aortic aneurysms can rupture, they are much less likely to do so than are larger ones. Risk factors for rupture in

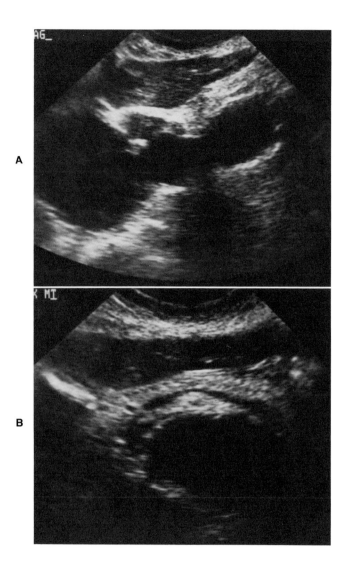

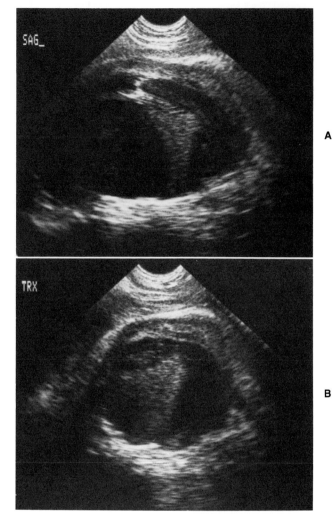

FIG 13-5. Suprarenal abdominal aortic aneurysm. **A,** Sagittal scan shows continuation of large thoracic aortic aneurysm into abdomen. **B,** Transverse scan shows abdominal aortic aneurysm at level of pancreas.

(Courtesy Dr. Stephanie Wilson, Toronto General Hospital, Canada.)

FIG 13-6. Large abdominal aortic aneurysm with high risk of rupture. **A,** Sagittal and, **B,** transverse scans show large (8 cm in diameter) aneurysm with nonuniform laminated thrombus and irregular external contour.

(Courtesy Dr. Stephanie Wilson, Toronto Hospital, Canada.)

these small aneurysms appear to be diastolic hypertension and chronic obstructive pulmonary disease.[9] Mortality from aortic rupture is greater than 80% if the patient is in shock. Sonographically, a large retroperitoneal hematoma is the rule, especially around the left psoas muscle (Fig. 13-7).[10] A rapid change in aneurysm size is a warning of impending rupture.

Postoperative **complications of aneurysmectomy** include hemorrhage, shock, renal failure, ureteral injury, paraplegia, infection, occlusion of the aortic prosthesis, anastomotic aneurysm, and aortoenteric fistula. An unusual complication of aneurysmectomy, is the development of a fistula with an adjacent vein (1%). The most common communication is between the aorta and the inferior vena cava. Duplex Doppler imaging can confirm an aortic aneurysm–left renal vein fistula, showing high-velocity turbulent flow at the confluence. This condition is almost always associated with the variant retroaortic left renal vein (92%).[11]

Rarely, aneurysms of the aorta develop a dense perianeurysmal fibrosis. These are called **inflammatory aneurysms.** The etiologic factors of this process are obscure (Fig. 13-8).[12]

Atherosclerosis in the absence of an aortic aneurysm results in vessel tortuosity. The intima appears irregular as a result of plaque, which often contains focal calcifi-

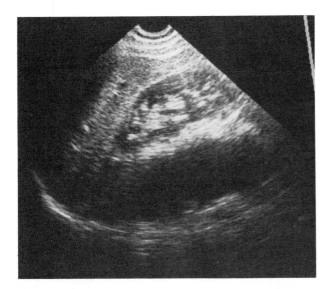

FIG 13-7. Retroperitoneal hematoma caused by ruptured abdominal aortic aneurysm. Sagittal scan shows hypoechoic fluid collection posterior to left kidney.
(Courtesy Dr. Stephanie Wilson, Toronto General Hospital, Canada.)

cation. Another atherosclerotic phenomenon is diffuse aortic enlargement, which may affect not only the abdominal aorta but also the distal iliac, femoral, and popliteal arteries. This condition is called **"arteria magna"** and is caused by atheromatous disease or a degenerative process of the elastic media.

Aortic Dissection

Aortic dissection occurs when an intimal tear allows passage of blood into the layers of the aortic wall. Both an entry and exit point exist, creating both a true and false lumen. Isolated abdominal aortic dissections represent only about 4% of the total cases of aortic dissection. More commonly, the abdominal aorta is involved as a distal extension of a thoracic dissection (especially of type 3), which originates distal to the origin of the left subclavian artery. When the false lumen dissects down the aortic wall, a renal artery may be narrowed or occluded from the aortic dissection. Dissection occurs most often in elderly men with atherosclerosis, but it also occurs in Marfan's disease, pregnancy, bicuspid aortic valve, coarctation, trauma, aortic stenosis, and hypertension.[13]

Sonographically, the intima-media disruption from the media-adventitia may cause a mobile flap in a zig-zag configuration noted along the length of the dissection (Fig. 13-9). In acute dissection, flow can be demonstrated in both the true and false lumina. Chronic dissection is difficult to diagnose because the false lumen may be filled with a clot, and thus motion of the intimal flap will not be appreciated. Occasionally during interventional procedures, a local dissection will result. This

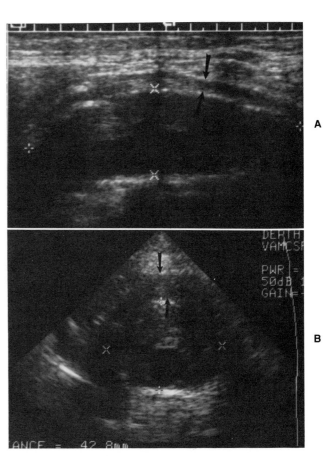

FIG 13-8. Inflammatory abdominal aortic aneurysm. **A,** Longitudinal and, **B,** transverse scans show aneurysm with thin layer *(arrows)* of fibrous tissue, anterior and adjacent to aortic wall.

is usually confined to a small area and is not associated with the flapping motion of the classic abdominal aortic dissection. Dissection may be simulated sonographically when layers of thrombus have different echogenicities and an anechoic crescent of thrombus is seen peripheral to the more hyperechoic thrombus, which is adjacent to the lumen (Fig. 13-10).[14]

Coarctation of the Aorta

Coarctation of the aorta typically occurs at the level of the ductus arteriosus. Atypically, coarctations occur in the distal abdominal aorta and are classified as infrarenal, suprarenal, and interrenal.[13] The etiologic factors are unknown although there is an association with Takayasu's arteritis.

Aortic Thrombosis

Just as atherosclerotic aortic aneurysms are below the renal arteries in 95% to 98%, **arteriosclerotic occlusive disease** is also commonly an infrarenal process. Before the development of duplex Doppler imaging, the

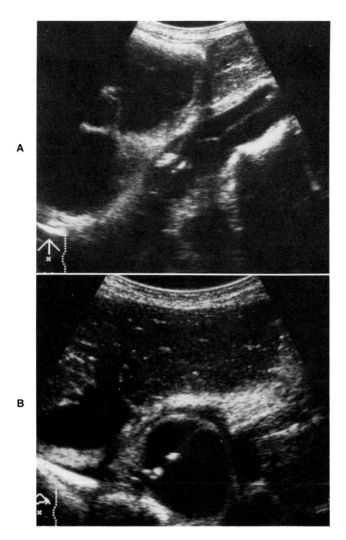

FIG 13-9. Aortic dissection. **A,** Sagittal and, **B,** transverse scans show irregular echogenic line, which represents intimal flap, separating true and false lumens.
(Courtesy Dr. C Withers, Sunnybrook Medical Center, Toronto.)

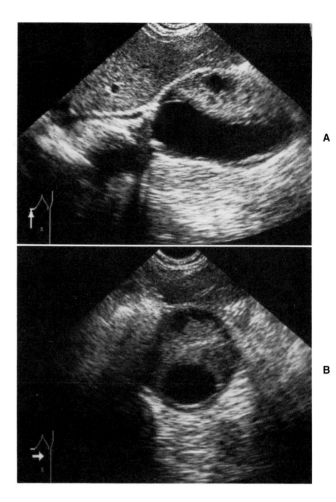

FIG 13-10. Hypoechoic thrombus mimicking dissection. **A,** Sagittal and, **B,** transverse sonograms show hypoechoic zone near outer margin of laminated thrombus. Clot in this area is recent, as compared with more echogenic laminated thrombus closer to lumen.
(Courtesy Dr. Stephanie Wilson, Toronto General Hospital, Canada.)

abdominal aorta could appear perfectly normal sonographically, yet it could be occluded. Ultrasound was not sensitive to the detection of thrombosis.[15,16] As resolution and sensitivity in sonographic instrumentation have increased and greater experience has evolved, it has become clear that there is an evolutionary continuum in the sonographic appearance of a thrombus, which ranges from anechoic to hyperechoic (Fig. 13-11).

The development of duplex Doppler imaging allows the sonographer to determine not only the presence and absence of flow but also the actual flow velocity. Because a thrombus may be anechoic, routine Doppler interrogation will diagnose an unsuspected aortic occlusion, a condition that may occur in the absence of aortic

aneurysm. Color-coded examination has the advantage of flow visualization, in addition to allowing spectral analysis.

Aortic Grafts

Surgery is the only definitive treatment for aortic aneurysms. The walls of the aneurysm are incised and wrapped around the prosthetic graft (Fig. 13-12). With concomitant iliac disease, an aortoiliac or aortofemoral graft is implanted. The proximal anastomosis may be end-to-end or end-to-side—that is, the end of the graft is sewn to the end or to the anterior side of the distal aorta, respectively.

Aortoiliac disease is progressive, atherosclerotic, and multifocal. The treatment of this occlusive disease

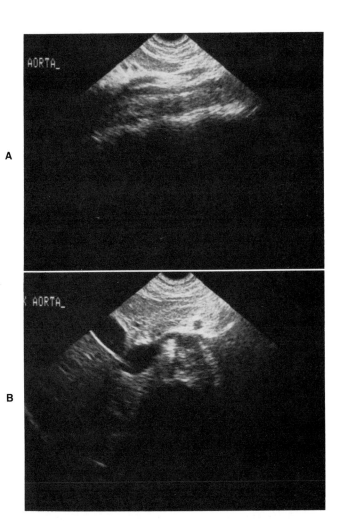

FIG 13-11. Aortic thrombosis. **A,** Sagittal and, **B,** transverse sonograms show echogenic thrombus filling aortic lumen. (Courtesy Dr. Stephanie Wilson, Toronto General Hospital, Canada.)

is also aortofemoral, axillofemoral, femorofemoral, or iliofemoral bypass. **Sonography after graft implantation** is used to:

- Verify patency
- Measure velocity of flow
- Localize stenosis
- Define complications, such as arteriovenous shunting, occlusion, or anastomotic aneurysm

Intraoperative ultrasound, which was initially confined to Doppler velocitometers, now allows the surgeon to check visually for vascular integrity before closing the incision, thereby excluding mechanical problems of stenosis or intimal flap.[17]

The **sonographic appearance** of a graft is that of a tube with discrete echogenic walls. The end-to-side aortic anastomosis appears as two adjacent tubes, with one on top of the other.[18] The aortoiliac or aortofemoral graft lies anterior to the distal aorta and native external iliac artery.[19] The aortofemoral graft is placed end-to-side—that is, the end of the distal graft connects to the anterior side of the common femoral artery (Fig. 13-13). The scanning plane for the best visualization of the iliofemoral region is along an imaginary line from the umbilicus to the common femoral artery just below the inguinal ligament.

An axillofemoral bypass is placed to salvage a limb when an abdominal approach is not feasible. Sonographically, the graft is seen just beneath the skin, extending from the axilla along the midaxillary line to the common femoral artery. A femorofemoral bypass may be placed for unilateral iliac disease. This short superficial graft ends in bilateral anastomosis to the common femoral arteries. It is visualized in transverse and longi-

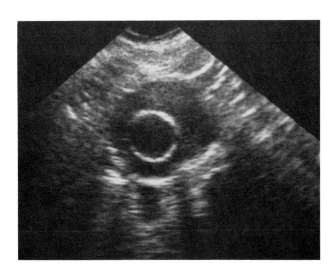

FIG 13-12. "Wrap-around" appearance following graft for aortic aneurysm repair. (Courtesy Dr. Stephanie Wilson, Toronto General Hospital, Canada.)

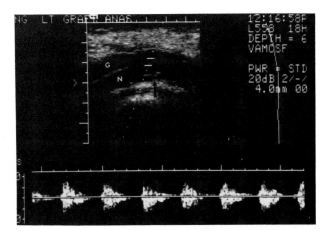

FIG 13-13. Anastomosis of aortofemoral graft to common femoral artery. Spectral analysis shows holosystolic flow from turbulence, which becomes accentuated with development of pseudoaneurysms at that site. Some atherosclerotic plaque is noted in posterior common femoral artery *(arrow)*. *G,* indicates graft; *N,* native artery.

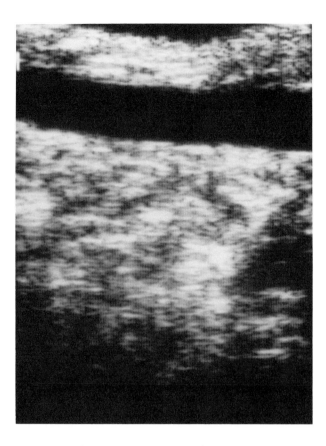

FIG 13-14. Normal bifemoral graft just beneath skin surface of pubis *(longitudinal scan)*.

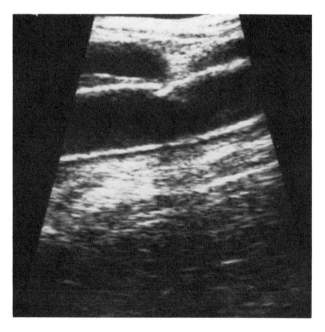

FIG 13-15. Pseudoaneurysm with graft leak: femorofemoral graft. Longitudinal scan shows break in graft and anterior perigraft fluid collection. Positive arterial Doppler signal could be obtained within this collection.
(Courtesy Dr. Stephanie Wilson, Toronto General Hospital, Canada.)

tudinal planes in the soft tissues anterior to the pubis (Fig. 13-14).

The principal **postoperative complications** of any graft implantation include:

- False aneurysm (anastomotic aneurysm) (Fig. 13-15)
- Stenosis
- Infection
- Hematoma
- Seroma

Patients who have an aortic graft are at risk of developing an **anastomotic aneurysm.** These are false aneurysms, which are confined in a fibrous sac and communicate with the lumen of the affected artery. They do not have layers of intima, media, and adventitia. Anastomotic aneurysms may occur after an aortofemoral graft. They usually develop in the groin and are proba-

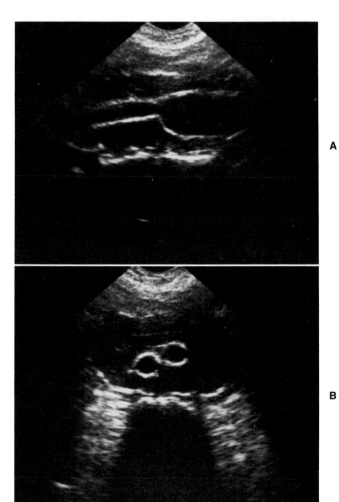

A

B

FIG 13-16. Perigraft fluid. **A,** Sagittal and, **B,** transverse sonograms show aortobifemoral graft surrounded by hypoechoic fluid collection. On aspiration, this was seroma.
(Courtesy Dr. Stephanie Wilson, Toronto General Hospital, Canada.)

bly related to motion, the surgical repair, and perigraft hematoma or infection. False aneurysms constitute less than 2% of all anastomoses. Intraabdominal proximal anastomotic aneurysms are less common and tend to be silent, although they may erode into the adjacent bowel with subsequent hemorrhage. Anastomotic aneurysms are a source of distal emboli. They may thrombose or continue to expand and if untreated are prone to rupture. The typical sonographic appearance is that of a focal circumscribed collection at the site of the anastomosis, which, upon insonation, has a holosystolic flow of marked turbulence.

Fluid around a graft anastomosis in the immediate postoperative period is the rule rather than the exception (Fig. 13-16). After 3 months, however, periaortic fluid is abnormal and most often related to hemorrhage, seroma, or infection.[20] Aspiration of a perigraft fluid collection is easily performed if infection is suspected.

Extrinsic Masses

Retroperitoneal masses may be detected on the basis of their morphologic characteristics or as a result of compression (especially venous) or displacement of the regional vessels. Both the aorta and inferior vena cava normally lie immediately adjacent to the vertebral bodies. Anterior displacement should raise the possibility of a retroaortic or retrocaval mass (Figs. 13-17 and 13-18).

A **horseshoe kidney** is a fusion anomaly. The fused lower renal poles appear as a soft tissue mass anterior to the aorta at the level of the fourth lumbar vertebra. If

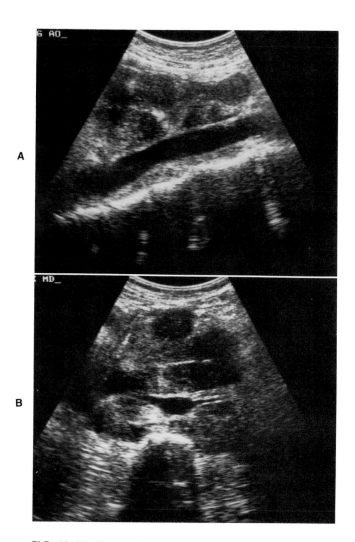

FIG 13-17. Para-aortic lymph nodes. Multiple hypoechoic masses surround aorta and aortic branches. Aorta is displaced slightly anteriorly from spine by retroaortic nodes. **A,** Sagittal and, **B,** transverse scans.
(Courtesy Dr. Stephanie Wilson, Toronto General Hospital, Canada.)

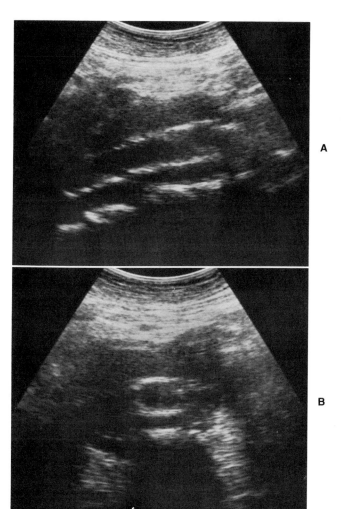

FIG 13-18. Pseudoabdominal aortic aneurysm caused by para-aortic lymph node mantle. Confluent lymphadenopathy may be mistaken for abdominal aortic aneurysm if lymph nodes are mistaken for circumferential thrombus. **A,** Sagittal and, **B,** transverse scans.
(Courtesy Dr. Stephanie Wilson, Toronto General Hospital, Canada.)

not recognized, this normal variant may be confused with adenopathy, primary mass, or retroperitoneal fibrosis. Aortic aneurysms are rarely associated with horseshoe kidney.[21]

Retroperitoneal fibrosis is characterized by dense fibrous masses, which envelop the distal aorta and iliac vessels. The majority of cases are idiopathic (68%), although the disease has been linked with methysergide maleate administration (12%) and malignancy (8%).[22] On ultrasound examination, retroperitoneal fibrosis appears as a hypoechoic, often circumferential irregular mass that may be associated with concomitant hydronephrosis.[23]

Adenopathy, primary retroperitoneal tumors, and **hemorrhage** may all give rise to hypoechoic para-aortic masses.

PRINCIPAL AORTIC BRANCHES
The Celiac Artery

The first major branch of the abdominal aorta is the celiac artery, which immediately bifurcates into the common hepatic, left gastric, and splenic arteries. On

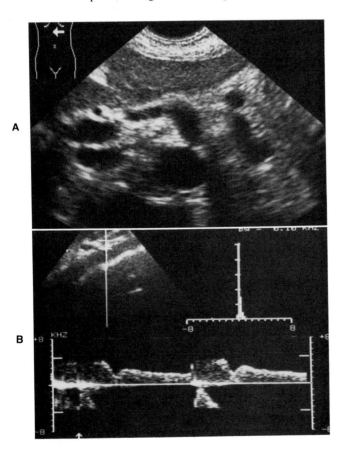

sonography, the celiac artery is noted just inferior to the caudate lobe of the liver and just superior to the superior mesenteric artery and pancreas. It is usually quite perpendicular or angled cephaladly from the aorta, and its characteristic branching produces a Y or T configuration on transverse scans.

The waveform of the celiac artery on spectral analysis is one of low resistance with forward flow in both systole and diastole. It has more spectral broadening than the aorta because of its small size.[1,24] The diagnosis of abdominal angina caused by celiac and superior mesenteric artery stenosis can be made by the delineation of a high-velocity jet at the vessel origins (Fig. 13-19).

Superior Mesenteric Artery

The superior mesenteric artery (SMA), which originates approximately 1 cm below the origin of the celiac artery, is the second major anterior branch of the abdominal aorta. It has a triphasic waveform of a peripheral artery with forward velocities throughout the diastolic phase. After a meal, the waveform converts to a low-impedance profile and forward diastolic flow increases markedly.[25]

Malrotation of the intestine associated with polysplenia alters the position of the SMA so that it appears to the right of the superior mesenteric vein and anterior to the inferior vena cava rather than the aorta. As malrotation is associated with hepatic vascular anomalies, it may represent a contraindication for liver transplantation.[26]

Splanchnic Aneurysms

Aneurysms may be congenital, atherosclerotic, traumatic, mycotic, or inflammatory. About 10% of the patients with chronic pancreatitis will develop aneurysms

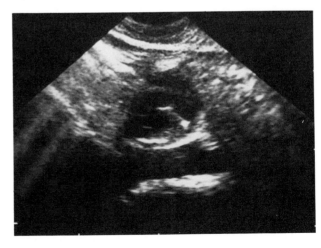

FIG 13-19. Celiac axis stenosis. **A,** Transverse sonogram shows tight narrowing of celiac axis at its origin from aorta. **B,** Duplex Doppler image shows aliasing at 8 kHz, consistent with high-velocity jet.
(Courtesy Dr. Stephanie Wilson, Toronto General Hospital, Canada.)

FIG 13-20. Celiac artery aneurysm. Sagittal scan shows cystic mass with laminated thrombus anterior to aorta.
(Courtesy Dr. Stephanie Wilson, Toronto General Hospital, Canada.)

of the hepatic, superior mesenteric, splenic, or gastroduodenal arteries.[27-29] Splanchnic aneurysms are fusiform or saccular (Fig. 13-20) and typically have a holosystolic waveform. Turbulence can be detected with color-coded Doppler imaging unless thrombus has filled all the lumen but a narrow channel. Turbulence with color Doppler imaging is manifested by breakup of the uniform color into a disorganized pattern with both forward and reversed flow patterns.

Renal Arteries

Of patients with renal disorders, 20% to 30% have more than one renal artery supplying a kidney; 22% have two, and 1% to 2% have more than two.[30] This complicates the evaluation of renal artery stenosis because all renal vessels must be examined from their origins at the aorta to the renal hilum. The renal artery origins can be seen by ultrasound (86%),[31] nonvisualization occurs particularly on the left as a result of overlying bowel gas. The right renal artery is usually seen crossing behind the inferior vena cava. Placing the patient in a left lateral decubitus position may aid visualization.

Renal Artery Stenosis. Renal artery stenosis may result from atherosclerosis (the most common cause), fibrodysplasia, or trauma. Atherosclerosis of the renal arteries is progressive and usually asymmetric. It may occur from primary involvement of the renal arteries or from extension of aortic disease. Abdominal aortic aneurysms may occlude or narrow the origins of the renal arteries because of thrombosis or compression. Poststenotic dilation may occur. Fibrodysplasia is a disease of younger patients, particularly females. Traumatic renal artery stenosis may result from blunt trauma or interventional and surgical procedures. Other causes of renal artery stenosis include developmental entrapment of the right by the crura of the diaphragm,[32] syphilitic arteritis, vasculitis, and neoplasm.

The normal renal artery has a low-impedance signal on spectral analysis. The peak systolic velocity is below 100 cm/sec, and diastolic flow is prominent. With the increased resistance of stenosis, peak systolic flow rises to above 125 cm/sec.[33] As resistance increases the diastolic component decreases. A peak systolic velocity in the area of stenosis in the renal artery, divided by the peak systolic velocity in the distal aorta, results in a ratio of greater than 3.5 in patients with renal artery stenosis.[34] Doppler interrogation is time consuming, and visualization of all renal arteries from their aortic origin to the kidney is not always possible.[34]

Although ultrasound has potential in the followup of patients after percutaneous transluminal angioplasty for renal artery stenosis, there is no large body of work to show that it is, indeed, effective.

Renal Artery Aneurysms. **Renal artery aneurysms**

commonly develop as a complication of large-bore renal biopsy, as do arteriovenous fistulae. Isolated renal artery aneurysms may cause hypertension. Renal artery aneurysms noted by sonography are hypoechoic fluid-filled lesions contiguous with the renal artery.

Arteriovenous Fistula. The majority of renal arteriovenous fistulae are acquired; a quarter are congenital; and a few spontaneously develop as a result of malignancy.[13] Arteriovenous fistulae are recognized sonographically as focal areas of both forward and reversed flow.

Iliac Arteries

The common and the external iliac artery are well seen by sonography.[35] The common iliac artery is approximately 1.5 cm in anteroposterior diameter and the external iliac artery approximately 1 cm. The internal iliac artery is not identified routinely. The scanning plane is along an imaginary line from the umbilicus to the femoral artery at the inguinal ligament. The iliac vessels are better visualized with a full bladder because they traverse the lateral bladder walls. The use of transvaginal sonography enables the sonographer to identify the iliac artery and vein along the lateral aspect of the pelvis.[36] The waveform of the iliac artery is triphasic because, as a peripheral artery, the impedance is high.

Iliac artery aneurysms occur predominantly in older men and are usually asymptomatic. They are atherosclerotic, progressive, and subject to erosion or rupture into the iliac vein, the rectosigmoid colon, or the ureter.[37] Because the ureter crosses the iliac artery, hydronephrosis may result from aneurysmal compression.

INFERIOR VENA CAVA

The inferior vena cava (IVC) is a large vein that returns blood from the lower extremities and the entire abdomen to the right ventricle. Sonographically, it is examined in sagittal, coronal, and transverse planes in either the supine or left lateral decubitus positions. Views from the diaphragm to the bifurcation are attempted, although the IVC is frequently not visualized beyond the inferior margin of the liver. Usually examined with a 3.5-MHz transducer, the vein in thin patients is well seen with the shorter penetration of a 5-MHz transducer (Fig. 13-21). When the vessel is relatively superficial, a linear transducer defines the vein in a longer segment of view than does a sector transducer. In the long axis, the vessel is often visibly pulsatile, responding to both breathing and cardiac pulsations. On transverse scan, the IVC is often more elliptical than round, with a smaller anteroposterior than transverse diameter.

Duplex Doppler interrogation of the IVC shows a characteristic waveform on spectral analysis. Transmission of the adjacent right atrial pulsation to the vein re-

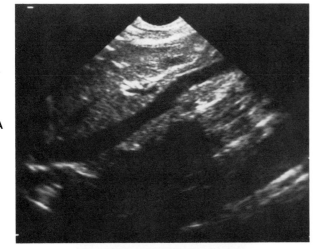

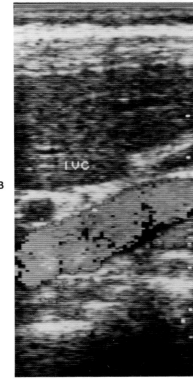

FIG 13-21. Normal inferior vena cava. **A,** Sagittal scan shows inferior vena cava as long tubular structure entering right atrium at its upper end. **B,** Longitudinal color-coded Doppler image.

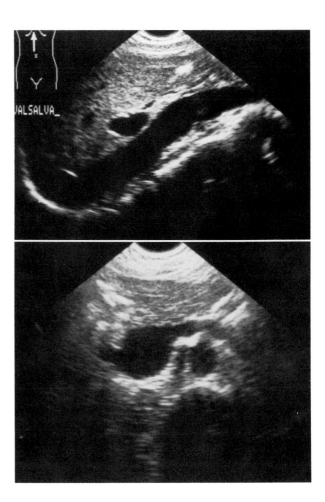

FIG 13-22. Congestive heart failure. Inferior vena cava is dilated and has decreased respiratory variation on real-time scan.

(Courtesy Dr. Stephanie Wilson, Toronto General Hospital, Canada.)

sults in a kind of zigzag pattern above and below the baseline, reminiscent of rick-rack. This is also the waveform of the hepatic veins. With portal vein occlusion, the IVC and the hepatic veins lose this typical waveform. In this situation, the waveform converts to one more typical of the portal vein—a low-velocity continuous venous signal hovering around the baseline.

The sonographic hallmark of venous patency is collapse of the vessel with compression. The IVC, lying deep in the abdomen, is not as accessible to compression as is the peripheral veins. Respiratory maneuvers are also difficult to define precisely because the vessel tends to move out of the field of view with a Valsalva maneuver.[38] Therefore duplex Doppler imaging offers a real advantage in defining actual flow velocity, while depicting the normal rhythmic response to respiration.

Although the IVC is not always identified in the normal patient distal to the acoustic window of the liver, when cardiac failure is present, the cava enlarges and is noted sonographically throughout its length (Fig. 13-22). Cardiac failure may also contribute to slow flow. Blood flow in the cava is usually anechoic. With cardiac failure, layers of increased echogenicity may be apparent within the caval lumen, simulating thrombus (Fig. 13-23). The echoes produced by flowing blood occur from Rayleigh scattering of the individual red blood cells. As flow slows significantly, it becomes more echogenic. This has been explained on the basis

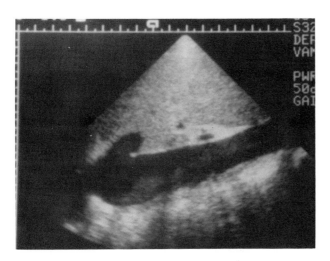

FIG 13-23. Congestive heart failure. Longitudinal sonogram shows enlarged inferior vena cava with large hepatic vein and very slow flow, causing flow-level echoes in inferior vena cava. These findings disappeared with aggressive treatment for congestion.

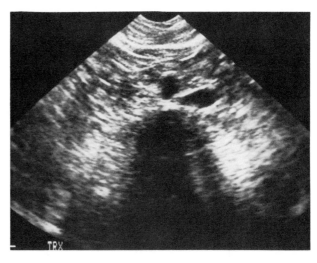

FIG 13-24. Persistent left inferior vena cava. Transverse scan just above umbilicus shows normal round aorta on right and more flattened inferior vena cava on left.

(Courtesy Dr. Stephanie Wilson, Toronto General Hospital, Canada.)

of shear forces and red blood cell aggregation.[17] A lower shear rate of flow is associated with greater blood echogenicity and erythrocyte aggregation. As blood flow and shear rate increase, blood becomes less echogenic.[39] Others have postulated that echogenicity of blood is related to cavitation effects from the abrupt drop in pressure caused by changes in fluid dynamics in situations of turbulent or sluggish flow.[40]

With congestive heart failure, the hepatic veins and the peripheral veins of the lower extremity also engorge. The peripheral veins have an increased capacitance, which diminishes their normal ability to be easily compressed. Obstruction of the IVC may also cause engorgement of the peripheral veins and an increase in peripheral venous diameter.

Congenital Anomalies

In the embryo, the paired posterior cardinal veins are joined to paired subcardinal veins. The IVC develops from segmental portions of this venous complex. Anomalies are a result of incomplete or aberrant regression or failure of regression of these channels. Anomalies of the IVC are readily detected with CT. Ultrasound is not the primary tool to detect these abnormalities, but it can be used to recognize anomalies that are usually unsuspected. The **anomalies of the IVC** include:

- Infrahepatic **interruption of the IVC:** In these rare cases, the IVC is not identified in the abdomen proximal to the renal arteries. This is due to failure of the precursor right subcardinal vein to fuse with the hepatic veins.

- A **single left-sided IVC** (.2%): This results from a persistent left supracardinal vein that persists when the right supracardinal vein regresses (Fig. 13-24). It arises from the left common iliac vein and usually joins the left renal vein.

- A **double IVC** (.3% to 2.8%): This results from failure of regression of the subdiaphragmatic supracardinal veins (Fig. 13-25).[41] On transverse

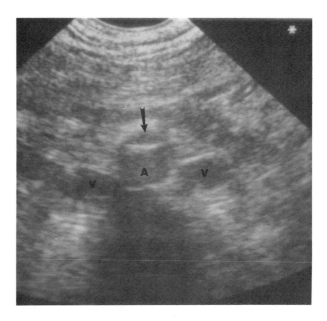

FIG 13-25. Double inferior vena cava. Transverse sonogram shows vein (V) on either side of aorta (A), which incidentally shows chronic dissection anteriorly (arrow).

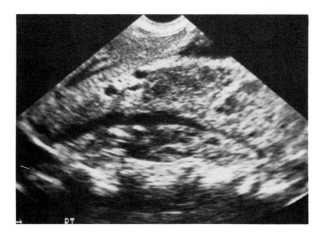

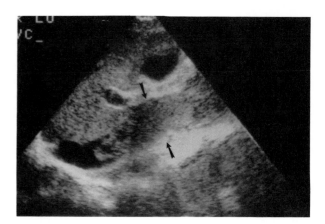

FIG 13-26. Retrocaval adenopathy. Sagittal scan shows multiple hypoechoic nodes, which displace inferior vena cava anteriorly from spine.
(Courtesy Dr. Stephanie Wilson, Toronto General Hospital, Canada.)

FIG 13-27. Leiomyosarcoma of inferior vena cava. Longitudinal sonogram shows large solid intracaval mass *(arrows)*.

sonograms, the left-sided IVC may be confused with adenopathy.

Hydronephrosis may be the presenting sign of a **retrocaval ureter,** which usually occurs on the right side. Patients generally present in the third or fourth decade of life. In this condition the ureter descends posteromedially to the IVC and then abruptly turns anterolaterally to cross it. At this point, ureteral obstruction may occur. The incidence of this anomaly is .9 of 1000 cases.[41,42]

Extrinsic Masses

The IVC may be compressed or deviated by peritoneal or retroperitoneal masses (Fig. 13-26), including primary retroperitoneal tumors, adenopathy, retroperitoneal hematoma, abdominal aortic aneurysm, hepatomegaly or liver mass, adrenal neoplasm, and adjacent inflammatory conditions such as retroperitoneal fibrosis.

Intrinsic Masses

Neoplasms, which extend into the IVC, include renal cell carcinoma (2% to 5%), Wilms' tumor, adrenal cancer, hepatoma, lymphoma, renal angiomyolipoma, and atrial myxoma.[43] The most common primary neoplasm of the IVC, although rare, is leiomyosarcoma (Fig. 13-27).

Sonography is highly effective in the detection of intraluminal caval masses. Intrinsic tumor can produce an intraluminal mass and can completely occlude and even expand the lumen of the inferior vena cava. Color Doppler imaging is particularly effective in demonstrating a partially patent lumen when the standard gray scale examination suggests total occlusion. Ultrasound may be used to detect extension of tumor into the right atrium. Recognition of atrial extension allows the surgeon to

prepare for a cardiac bypass procedure so that the atrial extension may be removed at the time of primary tumor resection.[44-46]

Intrinsic obstruction of the IVC may also be related to **thrombosis,** either partial or complete.[47] Most thrombi ascends from the peripheral veins. Renal vein thrombosis may also result from this ascension. Partial thrombosis produces some signal on duplex Doppler imaging analogous to partial deep venous thrombosis in the extremity. Focal thrombi in the IVC occasionally calcify, which may cause acoustic shadowing on ultrasound.

Greenfield filters placed in the IVC prevent the propagation of thrombi to the lungs in 98% of patients, without occluding the vein itself. Generally, the filters maintain a stable position and are biologically inert, although they have the potential to migrate or perforate the vessel.

Sonographically, filters are seen as local, bright hyperechoic foci in the IVC. Sonographic evaluation of veins at the placement site for Greenfield filters, usually from femoral or jugular approaches, has shown that site complications are low. Venous thrombosis at the site (14% to 19%) is usually transient and tends to occur most commonly in the left common femoral vein.[48,49] Early indicators suggest that insertion of Greenfield filters, using balloon angioplasty catheterization techniques, has the potential to reduce site complications.[49]

Traumatic rupture of the IVC may produce occlusion by compression from hematoma or from mural injury analogous to plaque causing stenosis. Once IVC occlusion has occurred, nephrotic syndrome and malignant hypertension are associated complications.[43]

Occasionally, a dilated, right, ascending lumbar vein is visualized posterior to and midway between the IVC and aorta on a transverse scan. This finding may be an important sonographic sign of congenital absence, compression or obstruction of the inferior vena cava. Blood is diverted through the prevertebral venous system and ascends into the thorax through the azygous or hemizygous veins.[50]

PRINCIPAL INFERIOR VENA CAVAL BRANCHES AND TRIBUTARIES
Renal Veins

The right renal vein has a short course from the right kidney directly to the IVC. The left renal vein, in contrast, has a longer course traversing between the aorta and the SMA to enter the IVC. Sonographic visualization of the right renal vein is more common than the left because of the hepatic acoustic window. The left renal vein is often well seen on transverse scans at the level of the pancreas. Circumaortic renal veins are rare. The retroaortic left renal vein variant, which occurs in 1.8% to 3.4% of patients, is of importance to the surgeon contemplating retroperitoneal surgery or aortic aneurysm repair because injury and subsequent hemorrhage may inadvertently result from failure to recognize this position.[51]

Decompression of the portal venous system in patients with portal hypertension may involve collaterals, including the left renal vein. Retrograde flow may be detected with duplex Doppler imaging. Color-coded Doppler imaging is particularly effective in the detection of the direction of flow.

The renal veins may be compressed from **extrinsic disease** or affected by **intrinsic processes.** Retroperitoneal hemorrhage, aortic aneurysm, tumors, or aberrant vessels may cause compression and thrombosis. Malignant extension into the renal veins may occur from renal cell carcinoma, renal lymphoma, transitional cell carcinoma, Wilms' tumor, and adrenal carcinoma. The left gonadal vein drains directly into the left renal vein, and thus tumor may extend through this route. The right gonadal vein empties directly into the IVC below the level of the right renal vein.

Causes of **renal vein thrombosis** include renal diseases such as glomerulonephritis, lupus, amyloidosis, hypercoagulable states, sepsis, trauma, or dehydration.[52] Renal vein thrombosis as a complication of renal transplantation occurs in less than 1% of patients. On sonographic examination, there may be dilation of the vein proximal to the obstruction.[53] Acute thrombosis of the renal veins causes the kidneys to enlarge with decreased echogenicity from edema.[54] In neonates, renal vein thrombosis may be a cause of intrarenal calcification.[55] Before the advent of duplex Doppler imaging, absence of venous pulsations was used to suggest renal vein occlusion.[56] Color flow imaging allows for direct visual confirmation of flow.

Hepatic Veins

Three main hepatic veins drain the liver: the left, the middle, and the right hepatic veins. The hepatic veins have Doppler appearance similar to the IVC, showing flow above and below the baseline on spectral analysis secondary to transmitted atrial contractions. These veins on color Doppler images are predominantly blue, in contrast to the main portal vein, which is red.

The hepatic veins enlarge with congestive heart failure and become compressed with hepatomegaly. **Budd-Chiari syndrome,**[57] which may involve both the IVC and the hepatic veins, has been associated with thrombosis, congenital webs or bands, neoplasms, hypercoagulable states, trauma, pregnancy, polycythemia vera, and oral contraceptives (Fig. 13-28).[58-60] Hepatomegaly, ascites, and portal hypertension are the rule. Because an enlarged liver tends to compress hepatic veins,

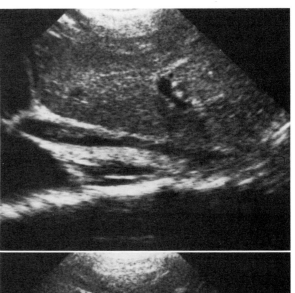

A

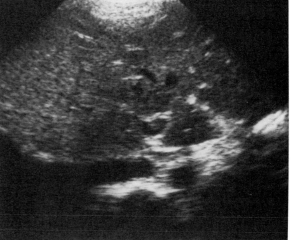

B

FIG 13-28. Inferior vena cava thrombus. **A,** Sagittal and, **B,** transverse scans show small echogenic intraluminal mass in patient with Budd-Chiari syndrome.

(Courtesy Dr. Stephanie Wilson, Toronto General Hospital, Canada.)

color Doppler imaging offers an advantage to detect the compressed venous flow that rushes through the narrowed vessels. With color Doppler imaging, unusual tiny venous hepatic collaterals to peripheral hepatic or retroperitoneal veins may be noted. It is difficult, however, to differentiate collateral hepatic venous flow caused by hepatic vein thrombosis from residual patent hepatic veins compressed by hepatomegaly. A typical finding is the inability to detect the hepatic veins at all. Thrombolytic therapy may be effective in the acute phase of hepatic venoocclusive disease. Later treatment consists of portosystemic shunting, ablation of a web, or thrombectomy. Vessel patency can be assessed with sonography.[61,62]

Inferior Mesenteric Vein

The inferior mesenteric vein is not routinely noted in adults. In children it is best noted in a parasagittal plane through the left flank anterior and lateral to the aorta.[63] It may dilate in portal hypertension.

Iliac Veins

In the supine or decubitus position, the common iliac veins are seen adjacent to the common iliac arteries. The external iliac veins extend from a superficial position at the inguinal ligament to a deep one in the pelvis, lateral to the bladder, where they join with the deeper internal iliac veins to form the common iliac veins.

The veins have respiratory phasicity. They can be compressed by adjacent masses such as lymphoceles, abscess, iliac aneurysm, neoplasm, or hematoma. Because of their intraabdominal position, they will collapse with a Valsalva maneuver because of increased intraabdominal pressure, and they respond to augmentation, which can be produced by squeezing the thigh.

CONTRAST AGENTS

Perfluorooctylbromide injection enhances the visualization of the color-coded Doppler signals.[64] Experimental research with animals suggests that air-filled albumin microspheres also transiently enhance arterial and venous Doppler signals when injected.[65] Although these studies are preliminary in nature, contrast agents potentially will provide advantages to visualization of color-coded Doppler images.

REFERENCES
Aorta

1. Taylor KJW, Holland S: Doppler ultrasound, I; basic principles, instrumentation and pitfalls. *Radiology* 1990;174:297-307.
2. Elam EA, Hunter TB, Hunt KR: The lack of sonographic image degradation after barium upper gastrointestinal examination. *AJR* 1989;153:993-994.
3. Gomes MN, Choyke PL: Pre-operative evaluation of abdominal aortic aneurysms: ultrasound or computed tomography? *J Cardiovasc Surg* 1987;28:159-166.
4. Graeve AH, Carpenter CM, Wicks JD, et al: Discordance in the sizing of abdominal aortic aneurysm and its significance. *Am J Surg* 1982;144:627-634.
5. Crawford ES, Hess KR: Abdominal aortic aneurysm. *N Engl J Med* 1989;321:1040-1042.
6. Nevitt MP, Ballard DJ, Hallett JW Jr: Prognosis of abdominal aortic aneurysms: a population-based study. *N Engl J Med* 1989;321:1009-1014.
7. Darling RC, Messina CR, Brewster DC, et al: Autopsy study of unoperated abdominal aortic aneurysms: the case for early resection. *Circulation* 1977;56(3/11):161-164.
8. Crawford ES, Saleh SA, Babb JW III, et al: Infrarenal abdominal aortic aneurysm: factors influencing survival after operation performed over a 25-year period. *Ann Surg* 1981;193:699-709.
9. Cronenwett JL, Murphy TF, Zelenock GB, et al: Actuarial analysis of variables associated with rupture of small abdominal aorta aneurysms. *Surgery* 1985;98:472-483.
10. Gooding GAW: Ruptured abdominal aorta: postoperative ultrasound appearance. *Radiology* 1982;145:781-783.
11. Mansour MA, Russ PD, Subber SW, et al: Aorto-left renal vein fistula: diagnosis by duplex sonography. *AJR* 1989;152:1107-1108.
12. Sterpetti AV, Hunter WJ, Feldhaus RJ, et al: Inflammatory aneurysm of abdominal aorta: incidence of pathologic and etiologic considerations. *J Vasc Surg* 1989;9:643-650.
13. Hillman BJ: Disorders of the renal arterial circulation and renal vascular hypertension. In: Pollack HM, ed. *Clinical Urography.* Philadelphia: WB Saunders; 1990:2127-2185.
14. King PS, Cooperberg PL, Madigan SM: The anechoic crescent in abdominal aortic aneurysms: not a sign of dissection. *AJR* 1986;146:345-348.
15. Anderson JC, Baltaxe MA, Wolf GL, et al: Inability to show clot: one limitation of ultrasonography of the abdominal aorta. *Radiology* 1979;132:693-696.
16. Gooding GAW, Effeney DJ: Static and real-time B-mode sonography of arterial occlusions. *AJR* 1982;139:949-952.
17. Sigel B, Machi J, Beitler JC, et al: Red cell aggregation as a cause of blood flow echogenicity. *Radiology* 1983;148:799-802.
18. Gooding GAW, Herzog KA, Hedgcock MW, et al: B-mode ultrasonography of prosthetic vascular grafts. *Radiology* 1978;127:763-766.
19. Gooding GAW, Effeney DJ, Goldstone J: The aortofemoral graft: detection and identification of healing complications by ultrasonography. *Surgery* 1981;8:94-101.
20. Aufferman W, Olofsson PA, Rabahie GN, et al: Incorporation versus infection of retroperitoneal aortic grafts: MR imaging features. *Radiology* 1989;172:359-362.
21. Killen DA, Scott HW Jr, Rhamy RK: Aneurysm and arterial occlusive disease of the abdominal aorta and its major branches associated with horseshoe kidney. *Am J Surg* 1968;116:920-924.
22. Witten DM: Retroperitoneal fibrosis. In: Pollack HM, ed. *Clinical Urography.* Philadelphia: WB Saunders; 1990:2469-2483.
23. Fagan CJ, Larrieu AJ, Amparo EG: Retroperitoneal fibrosis: ultrasound and CT features. *AJR* 1979;133:239-243.

Principal aortic branches

24. Taylor KJW, Burns PN, Woodcock JP, et al: Blood flow in deep abdominal and pelvic vessels: ultrasonic pulsed-Doppler analysis. *Radiology* 1985;154:487-495.
25. Sata S, Ohnishi K, Sujita S, et al: Splenic artery and superior mesenteric artery blood flow: non-surgical Doppler ultrasound measurement in healthy subjects and patients with chronic liver disease. *Radiology* 1987;164:347-352.
26. Chandra RS: Biliary atresia and other structural anomalies in the congenital polysplenia syndrome. *J Pediatrics* 1974;85:649-655.
27. Gooding GAW: Ultrasound of a superior mesenteric artery aneurysm secondary to pancreatitis: a plea for real-time ultrasound of

sonolucent masses in pancreatitis. *J Clin Ultrasound* 1981;9:255-256.

28. Derchi LE, Biggi E, Cicio GR, et al: Aneurysm of splenic artery: noninvasive diagnosis by pulsed Doppler sonography. *J Ultrasound Med* 1984;3:41-44.

29. Athey PA, Sox SL, Lamki N, et al: Sonography of diagnosis of hepatic artery aneurysms. *AJR* 1986;147:725-727.

30. Boijsen E: Angiographic studies of the anatomy of single and multiple renal arteries. *Acta Radio* 1959;183:1-135.

31. Avasthi PS, Voyles WF, Greene ER: Noninvasive diagnosis of renal artery stenosis by echo-Doppler velocimetry. *Kidney Int* 1984;25:824-829.

32. Spies JB, Lequire MH, Robinson JG, et al: Renovascular hypertension caused by compression of the renal artery by the diaphragmatic crus. *AJR* 1987;149:1195-1196.

33. Berland LL, Koslin DB, Routh WD, et al: Renal artery stenosis: prospective evaluation of diagnosis with color duplex ultrasound compared with angiography. *Radiology* 1990;174:421-423.

34. Kohler TR, Zierler RE, Martin RL, et al: Noninvasive diagnosis of renal artery stenosis by ultrasonic duplex scanning. *J Vasc Surg* 1986;4:450-456.

35. Gooding GAW: Ultrasonography of the iliac arteries. *Radiology* 1980;135:161-163.

36. Timor-Tritsch IE, Rotten S, Thaler I: Review of transvaginal ultrasonography: a description with clinical application. *Ultrasound Q* 1988;6:1-34.

37. Richardson JW, Greenfield LJ: Natural history and management of iliac aneurysms. *J Vasc Surg* 1988;8:165-171.

Inferior vena cava

38. Grant E, Rendano F, Sevinc E, et al: Normal inferior vena cava caliber changes observed by dynamic ultrasound. *AJR* 1980;135:335-338.

39. Kalio T, Alanen A: A new ultrasonic technique for quantifying blood echogenicity. *Invest Radiol* 1988;23:832-835.

40. Yousefzadeh DK, Ben-Ami T: Impact of flow dynamics of echogenicity of body fluids. *Radiology* 1989;173(P):181.

41. Mellins HZ: Anomalies of the inferior vena cava. In: Pollack HM, ed. *Clinical Urography*. Philadelphia: WB Saunders; 1990:2097-2104.

42. Schaffer RM, Sunshine AG, Becker JA, et al: Retrocaval ureter: sonographic appearance. *J Ultrasound Med* 1985;4:199-201.

43. Mellins HZ: Inferior vena cava obstruction. In: Pollack HM, ed. *Clinical Urography*. Philadelphia: WB Saunders; 1990:2105-2111.

44. Clayman RV Jr, Gonzalez R, Fraley EE: Renal cell cancer invading the inferior vena cava: clinical review and anatomical approach. *J Urol* 1980;123:157-163.

45. Sonnenfeld M, Finberg HJ: Ultrasonographic diagnosis of incomplete inferior vena caval thrombosis secondary to periphlebitis: the importance of a complete survey examination. *Radiology* 1980;137:743-744.

46. Dal Bianco M, Breda G, Artobani W, et al: Echography in vena cava invasion from renal tumors. *Eur Urol* 1985;11:95-99.

47. Goiney R: Ultrasound imaging of inferior vena cava thrombosis. *J Ultrasound Med* 1985; 4:387-389.

48. Dorfman GS, Cronan JJ, Paolella LP, et al: Iatrogenic changes at the venotomy site after percutaneous placement of the Greenfield filter. *Radiology* 1989;173:159-162.

49. Mewissen MW, Erickson SJ, Foley WD, et al: Thrombosis at venous insertion sites after inferior vena caval filter placement. *Radiology* 1989;173:155-157.

50. Manor A, Itzchak Y, Strauss S, et al: Sonographic demonstration of the right ascending lumbar vein. *AJR* 1982;138:339-341.

Principal inferior vena caval branches and tributaries

51. Beckman CF, Abrams HL: Renal venography: anatomy, technique, applications, analysis of 132 venograms, and a review of the literature. *Cardiovasc Interv Radiol* 1980;3:45-70.

52. Mellins HZ: Renal vein obstruction. In: Pollack HM, ed. *Clinical Urography*. Philadelphia: WB Saunders; 1990:2119-2126.

53. Braun B, Weilemann LS, Weigand W: Ultrasonographic demonstration of renal vein thrombosis. *Radiology* 1981;138:157-158.

54. Rosenberg ER, Trought WS, Kirks DR, et al: Ultrasonic diagnosis of renal vein thrombosis in neonates. *AJR* 1980;134:35-38.

55. Brill PW, Mitty HA, Strauss L: Renal vein thrombosis: a cause of intrarenal calcification in the newborn. *Pediatr Radiol* 1977;6:172-175.

56. Rosenfield AT, Zeman RK, Cronan JJ, et al: Ultrasound in experimental and clinical renal vein thrombosis. *Radiology* 1980;137:735-741.

57. Mori H Maeda H, Fukuda T, et al: Acute thrombosis of the inferior vena cava and hepatic veins in patients with Budd-Chiari syndrome: CT demonstration. *AJR* 1989;153:987-991.

58. Becker CD, Scheidegger J, Marinek B: Hepatic vein occlusion: morphologic features on computed tomography and ultrasonography. *Gastrointest Radiol* 1986;4:305-311.

59. Grant EG, Evela R, Tessler FN, et al: Budd-Chiari syndrome: the results of duplex and color Doppler imaging. *AJR* 1989;152:377-381.

60. Hosoki T, Kuroda C, Tokunaga K, et al: Hepatic venous outflow obstruction evaluation with pulsed duplex sonography. *Radiology* 1989;170:733-737.

61. LaFortune M, Patriquin HB, Pomier G, et al: Hemodynamic changes of portal circulation following porto-systemic shunts: a study of 45 patients using duplex ultrasonography. *AJR* 1987;147:701-706.

62. LaFortune M, Pomier G, Dery R, et al: Ultrasonographic and Doppler observations in patients with the Budd-Chiari syndrome. *J Ultrasound Med* 1988;7:62-63.

63. Patriquin HB, Babcock DS, Paltiel H: Color Doppler: applications in children. *Ultrasound Quarterly* 1989;7:243-269.

Contrast agents

64. Huet PM, Villeneuve JP, Pomier-Layrargues G, et al: Hepatic circulation in cirrhosis. *Clin Gastroenerol* 1985;14:155-168.

65. Hilpert Pl, Mattrey RF, Mitten RM, et al: IV injection of air-filled human albumin microspheres to enhance arterial Doppler signal: a preliminary study in rabbits. *AJR* 1989;153:613-616.

CHAPTER 14

The Abdominal Wall

- Khanh T. Nguyen, M.D.
- Eric E. Sauerbrei, M.D.
- Bernard J. Lewandowski, M.D.
- Robert L. Nolan, M.D.

A common indication for scanning the abdominal wall is the presence of a palpable mass. Is the mass in the wall or inside the abdominal cavity? Is it cystic or solid? Sonography can readily give the answer to these questions. Occasionally, an abnormality is found in the abdominal wall during routine scanning of the intraabdominal organs.

SCANNING TECHNIQUES

Because the skin is "out of focus" with even the highest frequency transducers, scanning the skin requires various stand-off techniques to obtain the best resolution and to avoid the "bang effect" of direct transducer placement on the skin. Flotation pads that are liquid-filled micro cell sponges,* synthetic polymer

---

*Reston flotation pad, 3M Company, Minneapolis, Minn.

†Kitecko, 3M Company, St. Paul, Minn.

‡Echomould, AHS/Belgium, Steenweg op Zellick 30, B-1080, Brussels, Belgium.

blocks,† and silicone elastomer blocks‡ are commercially available. These substances are dense enough to stand unsupported and have a uniform consistency to minimize artifacts.

Scanning the abdominal wall requires no special patient preparation. The examination can be performed over surgical wounds by applying an adhesive plastic membrane* over the wound after removing the dressing.[1] The adhesive is sterile and prevents both contamination of the wound by the transducer and contamination of the transducer by an infected wound or draining sinus. Gentle pressure with the transducer is applied, but one should avoid excessive pressure over wounds and other tender areas. One should use the highest frequency possible that allows penetration to the area of interest; this is usually a high-frequency linear array probe.

ANATOMY

The abdominal wall is divided into anterior, anterolateral, and posterior parts, best appreciated on a transverse CT scan (Fig. 14-1) or in schematic form (Fig. 14-2, *A* and *B*). The anterior abdominal wall is a laminated structure. From the outermost layer working in, the wall includes the skin, the superficial fascia, the subcutaneous fat, the muscle layers, the transversalis fascia, and a layer of extraperitoneal fat. The anterior muscle layer is composed of the paired midline rectus muscles and the anterolaterally situated external oblique, the internal oblique, and transversus abdominis muscles. The rectus abdominis muscles insert superiorly into the fifth, sixth, and seventh ribs and extend inferiorly to the pubic crest. They are enclosed anteriorly and posteriorly by the rectus sheath, which is formed by the aponeuroses of the internal oblique, external oblique, and transversus muscles. The posterior caudal aspect of the sheath ends at the arcuate line, which is situated usually midway between the umbilicus and the

---

*Op-site, Smith and Nephew, Welwyn Garden City, Hertfordshire, England.

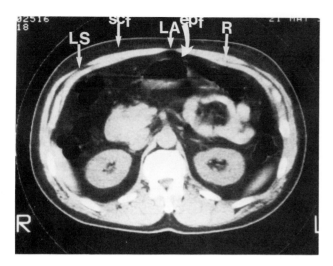

FIG 14-1. CT of abdomen showing the normal anatomy of anterior abdominal wall. *LA*, linea alba; *LS*, linea semilunaris; *R*, rectus muscle; *scf*, subcutaneous fat; *epf*, extraperioneal fat.

symphysis pubis. Distal to the arcuate line, the aponeuroses of all three muscles pass in front of the rectus muscle, which is then separated posteriorly from the peritoneum only by the transversalis fascia.[2] At the medial border of the rectus, the aponeuroses fuse to form the linea alba, which separates the rectus muscles in the midline.

The normal epidermis is a highly reflective layer measuring 1 to 4 millimeters in thickness.[3] The subcu-

taneous fat layer is of variable thickness. A significant amount of work has been done to determine the usefulness of this sonographic measurement to predict total body density and to compare the ability of ultrasound assessment with traditional caliper techniques in measuring subcutaneous fat. Real time sonography has proven as effective as caliper techniques in cadaver experiments,[4] as well as in young male and obese subjects, whereas A mode is less effective but probably more convenient than CT scanning.[5-8] One report, however, concluded that total abdominal circumference provides a better estimate of body fat in obese women than does ultrasound measurement of subcutaneous fat, because ultrasound did not measure the deep fat. Nonetheless, these measurements are important in sports medicine and in obesity clinics.

Over the years there have been conflicting reports concerning the echogenicity of fat. Some fatty tissues—for example, breast lipomas—are relatively anechoic, and subcutaneous fat is relatively hypoechoic; however, fat in the liver is echogenic.[9] The spectrum of echogenicities displayed by fat and fatty tissues can be explained by the water content within the fat. In an in vitro experiment, margarine (containing 85% vegetable oil and 15% water), scanned in a water bath, was echogenic and attenuated sound, whereas when the margarine melted, floating echogenic globules were seen. When the margarine was heated until the water vaporized and then rescanned after cooling, the substance was anechoic.[9] The authors concluded that not only is pure fat anechoic, but that a mixture of fat and water is echogenic.

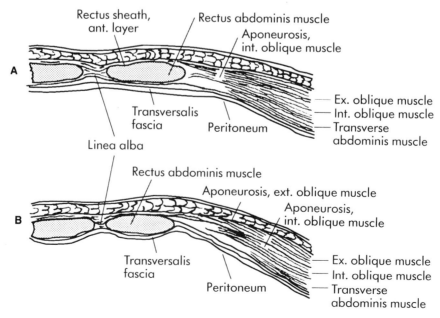

FIG 14-2. Schema of anterior abdominal wall, **A,** above arcuate line, and **B,** below arcuate line.

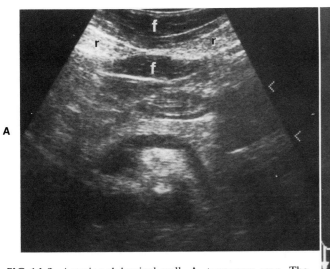

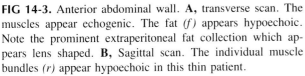

A

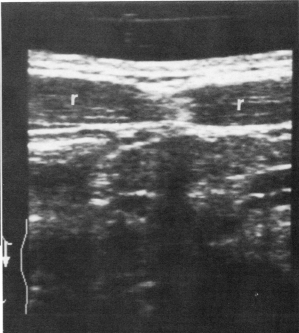

B

FIG 14-3. Anterior abdominal wall. **A,** transverse scan. The muscles appear echogenic. The fat (f) appears hypoechoic. Note the prominent extraperitoneal fat collection which appears lens shaped. **B,** Sagittal scan. The individual muscle bundles (r) appear hypoechoic in this thin patient.

Because water and fat are immiscible, there are multiple fat/water and water/fat interfaces, each with a significant acoustic impedance mismatch that causes the marked echogenicity.[10]

The musculofascial layer is usually more echogenic than the subcutaneous fat layer (Fig. 14-3, A). With high resolution probes, individual muscle bundles can be identified that show fairly uniform texture and orientation (Fig. 14-3, B). Because the muscles of the back are thicker, they are more difficult to visualize in detail than the muscles of the anterolateral walls.

The extraperitoneal fat collection posterior to the muscles appears quite thick in many people, particularly those who are obese, at the level of the linea alba and linea semilunaris (see Fig. 14-3, This A). This acts as the source of the split image artifact, which will be discussed later in this chapter. It should not be mistaken for a tumor.

PATHOLOGY
Cutaneous Lesions

Sonographic evaluation of the skin has been used to detect clinically occult foci of recurrent or metastatic melanoma and has been used to guide fine-needle aspiration biopsies of these lesions.[11,12] Pigmented nevi and malignant melanomas are clearly demarcated from normal skin (Fig. 14-4). Most melanomas are hypoechoic and demonstrate enhancement through transmission.

Although malignant melanoma is rarely found on the anterior abdominal wall, almost 75% of patients with melanoma develop cutaneous or subcutaneous metastases.[12] More importantly, the nodules may be found in unexpected locations.

Hernias

Ventral Hernia. *Ventral hernias* may be acquired or congenital. Acquired hernias are more frequently seen in patients who are obese or elderly or in those with previous trauma or surgery. The typical locations are at

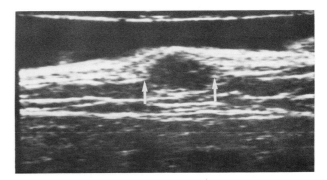

FIG 14-4. Subcutaneous metastatic melanoma. The nodule appears hypoechoic. Note disruption of the skin layer (arrows).

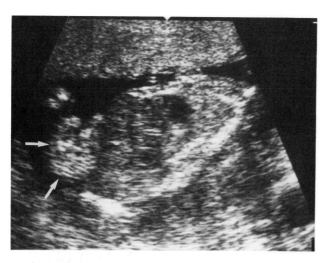

FIG 14-5. Gastroschisis seen in utero at 17 weeks' menstrual age. Note the mass of herniated bowel *(arrows)* in the parasagittal view of the fetus.

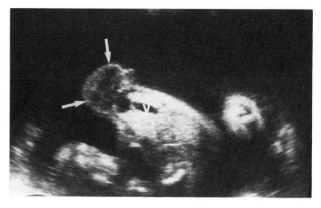

FIG 14-6. Omphalocele seen in utero at 18 weeks' menstrual age. Note the umbilical vein *(v)* running into the omphalocele *(arrows)*, which is covered by a membrane.

points of weakness where no muscle is present, along the linea alba in the midline or the linea semilunaris on each side (Spieghelian hernia), and in the inferior lumbar space.[13-15] The fascial defect and the herniated contents (omental fat or bowel) are usually identified by careful scanning with a 7.5 MHz linear array transducer. Seen in cross-section, herniated bowel loops appear as target lesions with strong reflective central echoes representing air in the lumen. When obstructed, they appear as tubular fluid-filled structures containing valvulae conniventes (small bowel) or fecal material (colon). Congenital ventral hernias consist of gastroschisis and omphalocele. Gastroschisis (Fig. 14-5) occurs in about 1 per 174,000 births and usually as an isolated anomaly. The abdominal wall defect is usually on the right side of the umbilical cord insertion, with herniation of small bowel not covered by a membrane. In contrast, omphalocele (Fig. 14-6) occurs directly at the site of the umbilical cord insertion. It is three times more common than gastroschisis and is associated with other organ malformations. The hernia sac usually contains liver and/or bowel. Both conditions may be detected by sonography in the fetus in utero as early as 18 weeks' menstrual age.[16]

Spieghelian Hernia. Spieghelian hernia, the only spontaneous hernia of the lateral abdominal wall, was first described in the year 1721.[17,18] It consists of a defect in the aponeurosis of the transversus abdominis muscle lateral to the rectus sheath. The most common location of Spieghelian hernias is at or near the junction of linea semilunaris and the arcuate line. Before the use of high-resolution sonography, the diagnosis of Spieghelian hernia was missed in 50% of cases preoperatively, because the classic findings are often miss-

ing.[19,20] The sonographic diagnosis of a Spieghelian hernia depends on the demonstration of a defect at any point in the linea semilunaris that represents the hernial orifice[21] (Fig. 14-7, *A* and *B*). If associated with protrusion of deep tissues, the hernia is usually bounded anteriorly by the external oblique aponeurosis. The external aponeurosis is so thick at this level that only 15 of 876 patients have been reported to have a subcutaneous hernial sac. More than 280 articles and 5 medical theses have been published on Spieghelian hernias, yet a review of the literature by Spangen revealed that only 876 patients had undergone surgery.[22] It should be noted that all patients with a Spieghelian hernia have tenderness over the orifice on palpation.

Lumbar Hernia. Lumbar hernias are uncommon and are most often acquired rather than congenital.[23,24] Spontaneous hernias occur in two areas of weakness in the flank: the inferior (Petit's hernia) and superior (Grynfeltt hernia) lumbar triangles. Acquired lumbar hernias are usually post-traumatic or iatrogenic.[25,26]

Lumbar hernias are usually asymptomatic. Since the neck of the hernia is wide, strangulation is uncommon, occurring in about 10% of cases. It is postulated that they are more common in females because of the wider pelvis.[27] The diagnosis depends on cross-sectional imaging, usually CT.[28-30] There has been, however, at least one case report in which the diagnosis was made sonographically.[31] In this case, sonography showed fluid-filled loops of small bowel extending from the peritoneal cavity into a mid-flank mass.

Incisional Hernia. Incisional hernias are delayed complications of abdominal surgery and occur in 0.5% to 14% of patients;[32-34] the current rate is about 4%. Since almost two million abdominal operations are performed in the United States every year, the problem is not a trivial one.[35,36] Enlargement of these hernias will

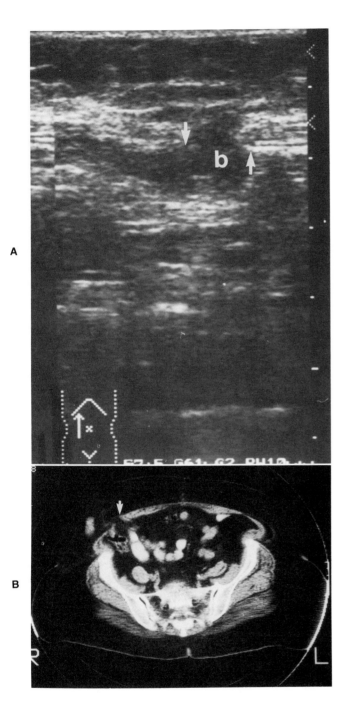

FIG 14-7. Spieghelian hernia. **A,** Ultrasound appearance. Bowel *(b)* is seen herniating through the fascial defect *(arrows).* **B,** CT appearance. Note the hernia orifice *(arrow).*

usually manifest within the first year; however, 5% to 10% will remain silent.[37] Clinically unsuspected incisional hernias are often detected by CT scanning.[38] Sonography may occasionally identify herniated bowel loop at the incision site.

Inguinal Hernia. The inguinal canal extends from the deep inguinal ring to the superficial inguinal ring.

The deep inguinal ring is a defect in the transversalis fascia anterior to the femoral vessels, above the inguinal ligament. The superficial inguinal ring is an opening in the aponeurosis of the external oblique muscle. Hesselbach's triangle is formed by the lateral border of the rectus sheath medially, the inferior epigastric artery laterally, and the inguinal ligament inferiorly. Direct inguinal hernias protrude through a weakened inguinal canal floor medial to the inferior epigastric artery, whereas an indirect hernia exits via the deep inguinal ring—that is, lateral to the inferior epigastric artery—and courses through the inguinal canal. Both direct and indirect inguinal hernias can extend into the scrotum.

Since both the superficial inguinal ring and the inferior epigastric artery are not easily seen sonographically, ultrasound has not been helpful in distinguishing direct from indirect inguinal hernias. However, sonography can distinguish hernias from other inguinal canal masses such as undescended testicles or varicoceles.[39] Inguinal sonography can be useful in delineating the superior aspects of a scrotal mass[40] and defining the presence of intestine and/or omentum in a hernial sac.

Sonography can detect complications of inguinal herniorrhaphy. The most common acute complication is hematoma extending from the inguinal canal into the scrotum. Less common complications include epididymitis and ischemic orchitis. Delayed scrotal swelling (several months after surgery) is usually secondary to a small hydrocele.[41] One theory is that inguinal herniorrhaphy aggravates an existing hydrocele by disturbing the lymphatic drainage.[42]

Femoral Hernia. Sonography is recommended in patients with groin pain and no palpable mass,[43] questionable palpable masses, and elderly obese patients with unexplained abdominal pain.[44] Up to 70% of nonobstructed femoral hernias are misdiagnosed by nonsurgical practitioners,[45] and 25% of femoral hernias are misdiagnosed surgically, because they can be incarcerated and yet be impalpable.[46] The boundaries of the femoral canal are the femoral vein laterally, the superior pubic ramus posteriorly, and the ileopubic tract anteromedially. The sonographic detection of a femoral hernia depends on the demonstration of a mass medial to the femoral vein (Fig. 14-8, *A* and *B*). The mass must then be differentiated from other masses found in the femoral triangle, which includes haematomas, pseudoaneurysms, A-V fistulae, lipomas, lymph nodes, hydroceles, saphenous varices, and inguinal hernias.

Rectus Sheath Hematoma

Rectus sheath hematomas are either post-traumatic or spontaneous. The traumatic causes include direct trauma, surgery, or sudden vigorous abdominal contractions that may occur with seizures, paroxysms of

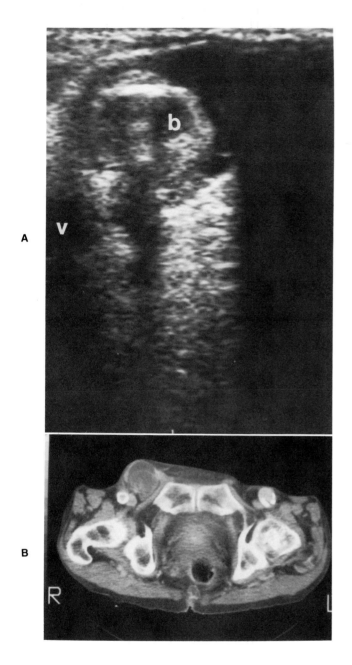

FIG 14-8. A, Strangulated femoral hernia—transverse scan. Note the target appearance typical of a dilated bowel loop *(b)* medial to the vessels *(v)*. **B,** CT scan. The mass in the right groin is indistinguishable from a vascular or nodal lesion.

coughing,[47] sneezing, defecation, urination, and intercourse.[48,49] Recently a single case of rectus sheath hematoma as a complication of tetanus has been reported.[50] Anticoagulant therapy is the most common cause of spontaneous rectus sheath hematoma. Other less common associations include collagen diseases, steroid therapy, pregnancy,[51] and bleeding disorders.[52] Bleeding is usually secondary to either the rupture of the epigastric artery or veins or a primary tear of the muscle

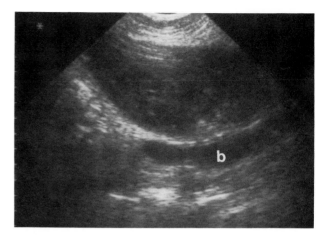

FIG 14-9. Sagittal scan of rectus sheath hematoma. Distal to the arcuate line, the echogenic mass dips down into the pelvis to compress the urinary bladder *(b)*.

fibers.[53] The bleeding is usually intramuscular but may be extramuscular and confined by the rectus sheath. The tamponade effect of the sheath usually limits the size of the hematomas; however, there is a case report of a massive hematoma, where the bleeding site was identified sonographically.[54] Clinical findings include abdominal pain, palpable mass, ecchymosis, and the Fothergill sign,[55,56,57] which involves palpating the suspected abdominal mass while the patient tenses the abdominal muscles. An abdominal wall mass will remain fixed, whereas an intraabdominal mass will become less apparent. The sonographic appearance depends on the location of bleed with respect to the arcuate line, its age, and the transducer frequency. Above the arcuate line, the linea alba prevents the spread of hematoma across the midline; thus the hematoma are ovoid transversely and biconcave in the long axis.[58,59] Below the arcuate line, blood can spread to the pelvis or cross the midline, forming a large mass that indents on the dome of the urinary bladder (Fig. 14-9).

Fluid Collections

Fluid collections are usually seromas, liquifying hematomas, or abscesses related to previous surgery or trauma. Occasionally, a urachal cyst may be seen extending from the umbilicus to the dome of the urinary bladder.[39] A urachal cyst may be complicated by hemorrhage or infection (urachal abscess).[59] Uncommonly, tumors may arise in the urachus in children or young adults.[60]

Sterile fluid collections are usually echofree. When complicated by hemorrhage or infection, they appear more complex, with septations and/or layering low-level echoes representing blood cells or debris (Fig. 14-10). Fluid collections may be aspirated percutaneously

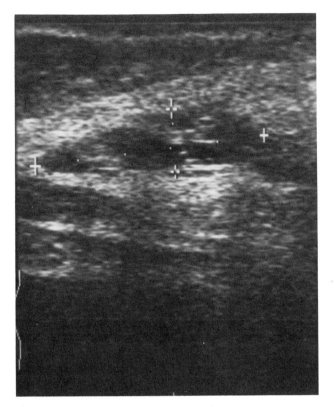

FIG 14-10. Infected seroma. Pus was obtained from this irregular septated collection beneath a recent surgical incision.

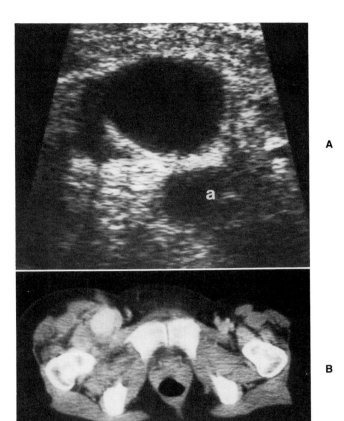

FIG 14-11. Pseudoaneurysm. **A,** Transverse scan of right groin shows a cystic pulsatile mass anterior to the femoral artery *(a)*. **B,** CT scan through the level of the right groin shows contrast material in the pseudoaneurysm.

under ultrasound guidance, with specimen sent for gram stain and culture and sensitivity.

Vascular Lesions

Subcutaneous Arterial Bypass Grafts. High resolution sonography is ideal in imaging subcutaneous axillofemoral and femorofemoral arterial bypass grafts[61,62,63,64] Postoperatively the grafts demonstrate transient small perigraft fluid collections at the level of the surgical tunnels, which disappear as the graft is incorporated into the subcutaneous tissues. Persistent perigraft fluid collections, or localized collections are abnormal, and are usually seromas, or abscesses.[65] Any abnormal perigraft fluid collection should be followed until it resolves, or a definitive diagnosis is made. Although loss of pulsatility within the graft may indicate thrombosis,[66] duplex Doppler and color flow Doppler makes the diagnosis easier. Other reported complications include graft aneurysms due to failure of the graft and pseudoaneurysms.

Pseudoaneurysms and Arteriovenous (AV) Fistulas. Most femoral artery pseudoaneurysms involve the common femoral artery and are secondary to vascular reconstruction.[67,68] Pseudoaneurysm is also a well known but uncommon complication of femoral artery catheterization, with an incidence of 0.1%.[69] Arteriovenous fis-

tulas are considerably rarer. A pseudoaneurysm is a pulsatile hematoma, secondary to bleeding into the soft tissue, with fibrous encapsulation and a persistent communication between the vessel and the fluid space. The vessel wall does not heal, and the blood flows back and forth between the two spaces during the cardiac cycle.[70-72] Most hematomas and pseudoaneurysms are within 2 cm of the arterial injury. The real-time criteria of pseudoaneurysm include echogenic swirls within a cystic cavity, expansile pulsatility, hypoechoic mass, and a visible tract.[73] When present, echogenic swirls are diagnostic of a pseudoaneurysm. Unfortunately, they are not often seen. Similarly, expansile pulsatility is difficult to evaluate and has not always been helpful.[74] A fistulous tract is the least observed sonographic finding (Fig. 14-11, *A* and *B*). Thus the ultrasound findings alone may not be sufficient to distinguish a hematoma from a pseudoaneurysm.[75] Duplex Doppler and color Doppler have increased our ability to distinguish these entities.[76] The Doppler characteristics of a

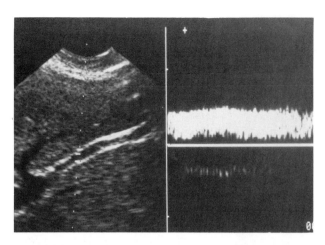

FIG 14-12. Recanalized paraumbilical vein (sagittal scan). Typical venous Doppler signal was obtained from this tubular structure running from the left portal vein to the umbilicus.

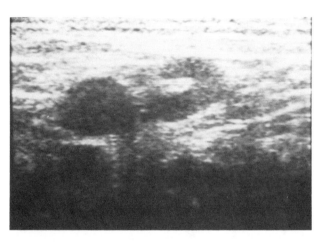

FIG 14-13. Lymphomatous nodes in the groin. The majority of lymphamatous nodes are hypoechoic or even anechoic. Biopsies are required to confirm the diagnosis.

pseudoaneurysm include arterial flow within a mass separate from the artery and to-and-fro flow between the artery and the mass. One author states that demonstration of to-and-fro flow at the neck of the pseudoaneurysm is not a necessary condition for the diagnosis of a pseudoaneurysm and reports sensitivities of 94% and specificities of 97%, with an accuracy of 96% using the first criterion alone.[77] With duplex Doppler one should be sure that the sample volume is interrogating the cavity and not an adjacent small vessel, whereas with color Doppler one should not interpret a perivascular color flow artifact as representing abnormal flow within a pseudoaneurysm.[78] A false positive diagnosis using color has been reported in a case of necrotizing lymphadenitis after an arteriography, where the mass was mistaken for a false aneurysms on the basis of a jet within the hilus of the inflamed inguinal lymph node.[79]

Varices. Recanalized umbilical vein seen in portal hypertension (Fig. 14-12), saphenous varices, and varicoceles found in the femoral triangle and inguinal area are easily identified since they are characteristically compressible and have typical venous Doppler characteristics.

Lymph Nodes

Ultrasound can be used to detect lymphadenopathy when there is no palpable mass, or it can be used to categorize a palpable groin mass as lymphadenopathy. Although it was originally thought that normal lymph nodes are not detected sonographically because they are indistinguishable from subcutaneous fat,[80] high-resolution sonography can detect pathologically normal superficial lymph nodes. Most nodes are ovoid in shape and are variable in size. Very few are homogeneous. They vary in echogenicity, depending on the degree of cen-

tral lipomatosis.[81] Thus the center of the node is echogenic, and the periphery is hypoechoic. With extensive lipomatosis, the node may become indistinguishable from the surrounding subcutaneous tissue. Ultrasound is more effective in demonstrating lymphadenopathy than is clinical palpation,[82-84] and it is useful for staging lymphoma and for monitoring therapy.[85] There is no criterion to distinguish malignant from inflammatory lymphadenopathy, and the metastatic inference must be confirmed by biopsy. Although not all enlarged nodes are malignant and not all malignant nodes are enlarged, there are some sonographic clues available to help distinguish malignant from inflamed nodes. Lymphomatous nodes are extremely hypoechoic (Fig. 14-13) and may even be anechoic, especially in non-Hodgkin's lymphoma.[86] A recent study of patients with palpable lymph nodes suggests that a 1-to-3 mm central artery can be seen centrally within enlarged lymphomatous nodes, whereas in lymph nodes with carcinomatous involvement the central artery is not seen sonographically, because it is infiltrated and destroyed on microscopy.[87] As discussed in the section on pseudoaneurysms, this central artery has been identified in one case of lymphadenitis.

Undescended Testicles

Cryptorchidism is the most common congenital anomaly of the male reproductive system, with an incidence of between 0.23% and 0.8% in the adult population.[88] It is bilateral in 10% to 25% of all cases.[89,90] Testicular descent can stop at any point between the hilus of the ipsilateral kidney to the external inguinal ring.[91,92] Of all undescended testicles, 80% are palpable and 20% are not palpable. Of those that are not palpable, 80% are in the inguinal canal and the remaining

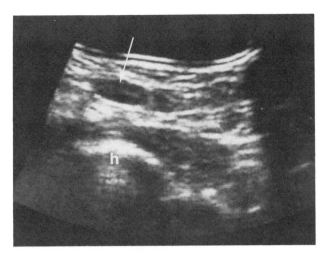

FIG 14-14. Undescended testicle. Sagittal scan of the right groin reveals an ovoid hypoechoic mass*(arrow)* anterior to the hip *(h)*.

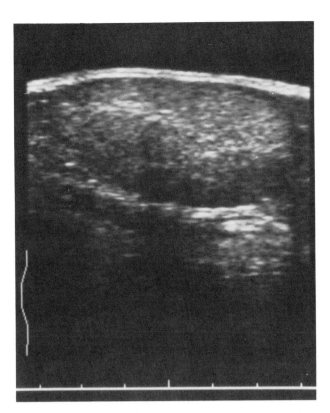

FIG 14-15. Lipoma of anterior abdominal wall. The lesion is well encapsulated and highly echogenic.

20% are intraabdominal;[93,94] the testicle is absent in 4% of cases when it is not palpable. Sonography is useful in the detection of undescended testicles (Fig. 14-14). The undescended testis often appears smaller than the normal testis. It usually appears ovoid, and its long axis is usually parallel to the inguinal canal. Visualization of the echogenic hilus of the lymph node should distinguish the structure from a testicle. Unfortunately, although sonography can often detect testicles that are in the inguinal canal, it is less successful in detecting intraabdominal testicles.[95,96,97]

Neoplasms

The abdominal wall is an uncommon site for neoplastic disease. The most common primary neoplasms are **desmoid tumors,** which arise from fascia or aponeurosis of muscles. The most common location is in the anterior abdominal wall. Desmoid tumors are usually seen in patients with previous abdominal surgery and often occur at the site of the previous laparotomy scar. They also occur in patients with familial polyposis and are often associated with pregnancy. Of patients with desmoid tumors, 70% are between 20 to 40 years of age. There is a three-to-one female preponderance.[98-103] Computed tomography and ultrasound are ideal methods to demonstrate both the site and extent of the mass.[104] Lipoma (Fig. 14-15), neuroma, and neurofibroma are occasionally seen.

The most frequent malignant subcutaneous nodules are **metastatic melanoma.** Secondaries from lymphoma or carcinoma of the lung, breast, ovary, and colon are less frequent.[39,59] The metastasis may occur as an isolated finding (Fig. 14-16), but more often it is seen in patients with widespread metastatic disease else-

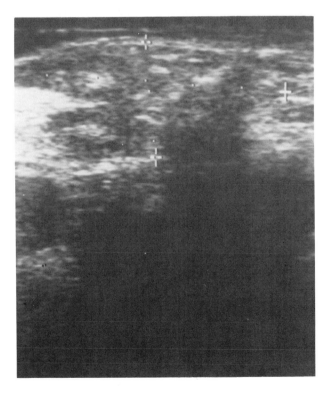

FIG 14-16. Metastasis in anterior abdominal wall. Note the large, irregular mass in the abdominal wall. Biopsy revealed metastasis from bronchogenic carcinoma.

where. The abdominal wall may also be locally invaded by malignancies arising from the pleura, peritoneum, diaphragm (mesothelioma, rhabdomyosarcoma, fibrosarcoma), or intraabdominal organs such as the colon.

ARTIFACTS

The anatomic arrangement of the lower abdominal wall has been implicated in an important artifact observed deep in the pelvis. It has been called a "ghost artifact," named after the "ghosting" seen in television images, or more appropriately the split-image artifact.[105,106,107]

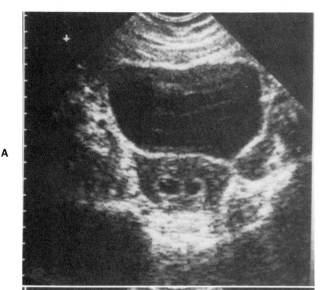

A

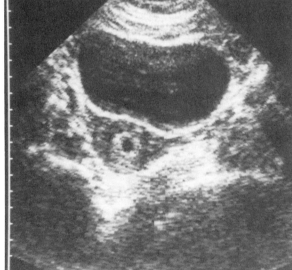

B

FIG 14-17. Split image artifact. **A,** Two gestational sacs were seen in this transverse scan of the pelvis. **B,** In fact, only one gestational sac was present. When the transducer is angled or the parasagittal plane is scanned, the artifact will disappear. In the upper abdomen, a double aorta or double superior mesenteric artery may be seen due to this artifact.

The split-image artifact arises because of the presence of extraperitoneal fat deep to the linea alba and rectus abdominis muscles. In transverse scan planes at the midline, sound rays are refracted at the muscle-fat interfaces in such a way that smaller structures in the abdomen or pelvis may be completely duplicated. For example, a small gestational sac may appear as two sacs, one small embryo may appear as two embryos, one aorta may appear as two aortas, and so on. The effect is usually seen only when the collection of fat beneath the linea alba is large (and thus the muscle-fat interfaces lie in an oblique orientation) and the structure of interest is deep below the abdominal wall.

Scanning in sagittal and oblique scan planes will fail to demonstrate the duplicated images seen in the transverse scans and thus resolve the ambiguity (Fig. 14-17).

REFERENCES
Scanning techniques

1. Fataar S, Goodman H, Tuft R, et al: Postoperative abdominal sonography using a transsonic sealing membrane. *AJR* 1983; 141:565-566.

Anatomy

2. The muscles of the abdomen. In: Warwick R, Williams PL (eds.), *Gray's Anatomy.* Edinburgh: Longman Group Ltd. 1978; 519-527.
3. Shafir R, Itzchak Y, Heymen Z, et al: Preoperative ultrasonic measurements of the thickness of cutaneous malignant melanoma. *J Ultrasound Med* 1984; 3:205-208.
4. Jones PR, Davies PS, Norgan NG: Ultrasonic measurements of subcutaneous adipose tissue in man. *Am J Phys Anthropology* 1986; 73:359-363.
5. Weits T, van der Beek EJ, Wedel M: Comparison of skinfold calliper measurements of subcutaneous fat tissue. *Int J Obesity* 1986; 10:161-168.
6. Kuczmarski RJ, Fanelli MT: Ultrasonic assessment of body composition in obese adults: overcoming the limitations of the skinfold calliper. *Am J Clin Nutrition* 1987; 45:717-724.
7. Chumlea WC, Roche AF: Ultrasonic and skinfold calliper measures of subcutaneous adipose tissue thickness in elderly men and women. *Am J Phys Anthropology* 1986; 71:351-357.
8. Black D, Vora J, Hayward M, et al: Measurement of subcutaneous fat thickness with high frequency pulsed ultrasound: comparison with a calliper and a radiographic technique. *Clin Phys & Physiol Measurement* 1988; 9:57-64.
9. Behan M, Kazam E: The echogenic characteristics of fatty tissues and tumors. *Radiology* 1978; 129:143-151.
10. Errabolu RL, Sehgal CM, Bahn RC, et al: Measurement of ultrasonic nonlinear parameter in excised fat tissue. *Ultrasound Med Biol* 1988; 14:137-146.

Pathology

11. Fornage BD: Fine-needle aspiration biopsy with a vacuum test tube. *Radiology* 1988; 169:553.
12. Fornage BD, Lorigan JG: Sonographic detection and fine-needle aspiration biopsy of nonpalpable recurrent or metastatic melanoma in subcutaneous tissues. *J Ultrasound Med* 1989; 8:421-424.
13. Thomas JL, Cunningham JJ: Ultrasonic evaluation of ventral hernias disguised as intra-abdominal neoplasms. *Arch Surg* 1978; 113:589-590.

14. Rubio PA, Del Castillo H, Alvaraz A: Ventral hernia in a massively obese patient: diagnosis by computed tomography. *Southern Med J* 1981; 10:1307-1308.

15. Spangen L: Ultrasound as a diagnostic aid in ventral abdominal hernia. *JCU* 1975; 3:211-213.

16. Sauerbrei EE, Nguyen TK, Nolan RL: The fetus. In: Sauerbrei EE (ed.) *A practical guide to ultrasound in obstetrics and gynecology.* New York: Raven Press; 1987: 111-159.

17. La Chausse BI. De hernia ventrali [1746], in Haller: Disputations chirurgicales. Bosquet (Lausanne) 1755; 3:181-211.

18. LeDran HF: Observation de Chirurgie. Paris: C. Osmont, 1771; p. 143.

19. Weiss Y, Lernau O, Nissan S: Spigelian hernia. *Ann Surg* 1974; 180:836-839.

20. Deitch EA, Engel JM: Spigelian hernia: an ultrasound diagnosis. *Arch Surg* 1980; 115:93.

21. Spangen L: Spigelian hernia. *Acta Chir Scand* (Suppl) 1976; 462.

22. Spangen L: Spigelian hernia. *World J Surg* 1989; 13:573-580.

23. Swartz WT: Lumbar hernia. In: Nyhus LM, Condon RE (eds.) *Hernia,* 2nd ed., Philadelphia: JB Lippincott Co; 1978:409-426.

24. Ponka JL: Lumbar hernia. In: Ponka JL. *Hernias of the abdominal wall.* Philadelphia: WB Saunders Co; 1980:465-477.

25. Quick CR: Traumatic lumbar hernia. *Br J Surg* 1982; 69:160-162.

26. Castelein RM, Sauter AJ: Lumbar hernia in an iliac bone graft. *Acta Orthop Scand* 1985; 56:2273-2274.

27. Light HG: Hernia of the inferior lumbar space: a cause of back pain. *Arch Surg* 1983; 118:1077-1080.

28. Lawdahl R, Moss CN, Van Dyke JA: Inferior lumbar (Petit's) hernia. *AJR* 1986; 147:744-745.

29. Baker ME, Weinerth JL, Andriani RT, et al: Lumbar hernia: diagnosis by CT. *AJR* 1987; 148:565-567.

30. Chenoweth J, Vas W: Computed tomography demonstration of inferior lumbar (Petit's) hernia. *Clin Imaging* 1989; 13:164-166.

31. Siffring PA, Forrest TS, Frick MP: Hernia of the inferior lumbar space: diagnosis with US. *Radiology* 1989; 170:190.

32. Fischer JD, Turner FW: Abdominal incisional hernias—a 10 year review. *Can J Surg* 1974; 17:202-204.

33. Bucknall TE, Cox PJ, Ellis H: Burst abdomen and incisional hernia: a prospective study of 1129 major laparotomies. *Br Med J* 1982; 284:931-933.

34. Baker RJ: Incisional hernia. In: Nyhus LM, Condon RE (eds.) *Hernia.* Philadelphia: JB Lippincott Co; 1978:329-341.

35. Larson GM, Vandertoll DJ: Approaches to repair of ventral hernia and full thickness losses of the abdominal wall. *Surg Clin North Am* 1984; 64:335-349.

36. Ghahremani GG, Meyers MA: Iatrogenic abdominal hernias. In: Meyers MA, Ghahremani GG. *Iatrogenic gastrointestinal complications.* New York: Springer-Verlag; 1981:269-278.

37. Ellis H, Gajraj H, George CD: Incisional hernias: when do they occur? *Br J Surg* 1983; 70:290-291.

38. Ghahremani GG, Jimenez MA, Rosenfeld M, et al: CT diagnosis of occult incisional hernias. *AJR* 1987; 148:139-142.

39. Engel JM, Deitch EE: Sonography of the anterior abdominal wall. *AJR* 1981; 137:73-77.

40. Subramanyam BR, Balthazar EJ, Raghavendra BN, et al: Sonographic diagnosis of scrotal hernia. *AJR* 1982; 139:535-538.

41. Archer A, Choyke PL, O'Brien W, et al: Scrotal enlargement following inguinal herniorrhaphy: ultrasound evaluation. *Urol Radiol* 1988; 9:249-252.

42. Wantz GE: Complications of inguinal hernia repair. *Surg Clin N Am* 1984; 64:287-298.

43. Ekberg O, Abrahamsson P, Kesek P: Inguinal hernia in urological patients: the value of herniography. *J Urol* 1988; 139:1253-1255.

44. Deitch EA, Soncrant M: The value of ultrasound in the diagnosis of nonpalpable femoral hernias. *Arch Surg* 1981; 116:185-187.

45. Waddington RT: Femoral hernia: a recent appraisal. *Br J Surg* 1971; 59:920-922.

46. Ponka PL, Brush BE: Problem of femoral hernia. *Arch Surg* 1971; 102:411-413.

47. Lee TM, Greenberger PA, Nahrwold DL, et al: Rectus sheath hematoma complicating an exacerbation of asthma. *J Allergy Clin Immunol* 1986; 78:290-292.

48. Lee PWR, Bark M, Macfie J, Pratt D: The ultrasound diagnosis of rectus sheath haematoma. *Br J Surg* 1977; 64:633-634.

49. Manier JW: Rectus sheath haematoma. Six case reports and a literature review. *Am J Gastroenterol* 1972; 54:433-435.

50. Suhr GM, Green AE: Rectus abdominis sheath hematoma as a complication of tetanus: diagnosis by computed tomography scanning. *Clinical Imaging* 1989; 13:82-86.

51. Torpin R, Coleman J, Handkins JR: Hematoma of the rectus abdominis muscle in pregnancy, labor, or puerperium: report of three cases. *J Med Assoc Ga* 1969; 58:158-159.

52. DeLaurentis DA, Rosemond GP: Hematoma of the rectus abdominis muscle complicated by anticoagulant therapy. *Am J Surg* 1966; 112:359.

53. Henzel JH, Pories WJ, Smith JL, et al: Pathogenesis and management of abdominal wall haematomas. *Arch Surg* 1966; 93:929-935.

54. Savage PE, Joseph AEA, Adam EJ: Massive abdominal wall hematoma: real-time ultrasound localization of bleeding. *J Ultrasound Med* 1985; 4:157-158.

55. Gocke JE, MacCarty RL, Faulk WT: Rectus sheath hematoma: diagnosis by computed tomography scanning. *Mayo Clin Proc* 1981; 56:757-761.

56. Fisch AE, Brodey PA: Computed tomography of the anterior abdominal wall: normal anatomy and pathology. *J Comput Assist Tomogr* 1981; 5:728-733.

57. Tromans A, Campbell N, Sykes P: Rectus sheath haematoma. Diagnosis by ultrasound. *Br J Surg* 1981; 68:518-519.

58. Kaftori JK, Rosenberger A, Pollack S, Fish JH: Rectus sheath hematoma: ultrasonographic diagnosis. *AJR* 1977; 128:283-285.

59. Diakoumakis EE, Weinberg B, Seife B: Unusual case studies of anterior wall mass as diagnosed by ultrasonography. *J Clin Ultrasound* 1984; 12:351-354.

60. Kwok-Liu JP, Zikman JM, Cockshott WP: Carcinoma of the urachus: the role of computed tomography. *Radiology* 1980; 137:731-734.

61. Gooding GAW, Herzog KA, Hedgecock NW, Eisenberg RL: B-mode ultrasonography of prosthetic vascular grafts. *Radiology* 1978; 127:763-766.

62. Gooding GAW, Effeney DJ, Goldstone J: The aortofemoral graft: detection and identification of healing complications by ultrasonography. *Surgery* 1981; 89:949-1001.

63. Clifford PC, Skidmore R, Bird DR, et al: Pulsed Doppler and real-time "duplex" imaging of Dacron arterial grafts. *Ultrasonic Imaging* 1980; 2:381-390.

64. Wolson AH, Kaupp HA, McDonald K: Ultrasound of arterial graft surgery complications. *AJR* 1979; 133:869-875.

65. Gooding GAW, Effeney DJ: Sonography of axillofemoral and femorofemoral subcutaneous arterial bypass grafts. *AJR* 1985; 144:1005-1008.

66. Gooding GAW, Effeney DJ: Static and real-time scanning B-mode sonography of arterial occlusions. *AJR* 1982; 139:949-952.

67. Lang EK: A survey of the complications of percutaneous retrograde arteriography: Seldinger technique. *Radiology* 1973; 81:257-263.

68. Szilagyi DE, Smith RE, Elliot JP, et al: Anastomotic aneurysms after vascular reconstruction: problems of incidence, etiology and treatment. *Surgery* 1975; 78:800-816.

69. Brener BJ, Couch NP: Peripheral arterial complications of left heart catheterization and their management. *Am J Surg* 1973; 125:521-525.

70. Rapoport S, Sniderman KW, Morse SS, et al: Pseudoaneurysm: complication of faulty technique in femoral arterial puncture. *Radiology* 1985; 154:529-530.

71. Quera LA, Flinn WR, Yao JST, Bergan JJ: Management of peripheral arterial aneurysms. *Surg Clin N Amer* 1979; 59:693-706.

72. Perl S, Wener L, Lyon WS: Pseudoaneurysms after angiography. *Med Ann DC* 1973; 42:173-175.

73. Abu-Yousef MM, Wiese JA, Shamma AR: Case report. The "to-and-fro" sign: duplex Doppler evidence of femoral artery pseudoaneurysm. *AJR* 1988; 150:632-634.

74. Mitchell DG, Needleman L, Bezzi M, et al: Femoral artery pseudoaneurysm: diagnosis with conventional duplex and color Doppler US. *Radiology* 1987; 164:687-690.

75. Sandler MA, Alpern MB, Madrazo BL, et al: Inflammatory lesions of the groin: ultrasonic evaluation. *Radiology* 1984; 151:747-750.

76. Sacks D, Robinson MD, Perlmutter GS: Femoral arterial injury following catheterization duplex evaluation. *J Ultrasound Med* 1989; 8:241-246.

77. Coughlin BF, Paushter DM: Peripheral pseudoaneurysms: evaluation with duplex US. *Radiology* 1988; 168:339-342.

78. Middleton WD, Erickson S, Melson GL: Perivascular color artifact: pathologic significance and appearance on color Doppler US images. *Radiology* 1989; 171:647-652.

79. Morton MJ, Charboneau JW, Banks PM: Inguinal lymphadenopathy simulating a false aneurysm on color-flow Doppler sonography. *AJR* 1988; 151:115-116.

80. Hillman BJ, Haber K: Echographic characteristics of malignant lymph nodes. *JCU* 1980; 8:213-215.

81. Marchal G, Oyen R, Verschakelen J, et al: Sonographic appearance of normal lymph nodes. *J Ultrasound Med* 1985; 4:417-419.

82. Bruneton JN, Roux P, Caramella E, et al: Ear, nose, and throat cancer: ultrasound diagnosis of metastasis to cervical lymph nodes. *Radiology* 1984; 142:771-773.

83. Bruneton JN, Normand F. Cervical lymph nodes: In: Bruneton JN (ed.) *Ultrasonography of the neck.* Berlin: Springer; 1987:81-92.

84. Bruneton JN, Caramella E, Hery M, et al: Axillary lymph node metastasis in breast cancer: preoperative detection with US. *Radiology* 1986; 158:325-326.

85. Bruneton JN, Normand F, Balu-Maestro C, et al: Lymphomatous superficial lymph nodes: US detection. *Radiology* 1987; 165:233-235.

86. Hillman BJ, Haber K: Echographic characteristics of malignant lymph nodes. *JCU* 1980; 8:213-215.

87. Majer MC, Hess CF, Kolbel G, Schmiedl U: Small arteries in peripheral lymph nodes: a specific sign of lymphomatous involvement. *Radiology* 1988; 168:241-243.

88. Martin DC: The undescended testis—evolving concepts in management. *J Cont Ed in Urol* 1977; 1:17-31.

89. Glickman MG, Weiss RM, Itzchak Y: Testicular venography for undescended testicles. *Am J Roentgenol* 1977; 129:67-70.

90. Pinch L, Aceto T, Meyer-Bahlburg HF: Cryptorchidism: a paediatric review. *Urol Clin North Am* 1974; 1:573-592.

91. Diamond AB, Meng CH, Kodroff M, et al: Testicular venography in the nonpalpable testis. *Am J Roentgenol* 1977; 129:71-75.

92. Levitt SB, Kogan SJ, Schneider KM, et al: Endocrine tests in phenotypic children with bilateral impalpable testes can reliably predict "congenital" anorchism. *Urology* 1978; 11:11-14.

93. Kogan SJ, Gill B, Bennett B, et al: Human monorchism: a clinicopathological study of unilateral absent testes in 65 boys. *J Urol* 1986; 135:758-761.

94. Madrazo BL, Klugo RC, Parks JA, et al: Ultrasonographic demonstration of undescended testes. *Radiology* 1979; 133:181-183.

95. Wolverson MK, Jagannadharao B, Sundaram M, et al: CT in localization of impalpable cryptorchid testes. *AJR* 1980; 134:725-729.

96. Wolverson KW, Houttuin E, Heiberg H, et al: Comparison of computed tomography with high-resolution real-time ultrasound in the localization of the impalpable undescended testis. *Radiology* 146:133-136.

97. Weiss RM, Carter AR, Rosenfield AT: High-resolution real-time ultrasonography in the location of the undescended testis. *J Urol* 1986; 135:936-938.

98. Pasciak RM, Kozlowski JM: Mesenteric desmoid tumor presenting as an abdominal mass following salvage cystectomy for invasive bladder cancer. *J Urol* 1987; 138:145-146.

99. McAdam WAF, Golinger JC: The occurrence of desmoids in patients with familial polyposis coli. *Br J Surg* 1970; 57:618.

100. Baron RL, Lee JK: Mesenteric desmoid tumours. *Radiology* 1981; 140:777-779.

101. Brasfield RD, Das Gupta TK: Desmoid tumours of the anterior abdominal wall. *Surgery* 1969; 65:241-246.

102. Mantello MT, Haller JO, Marquis JR: Sonography of abdominal desmoid tumors in adolescents. *J Ultrasound Med* 1989; 8:467-470.

103. Magid D, Fishman EK, Bronwyn J, et al: Desmoid tumors in Gardner's syndrome: use of computed tomography. *AJR* 1984; 142:1141-1145.

104. Baron RL, Lee JKT: Mesenteric desmoid tumour: sonographic and computed tomographic appearance. *Radiology* 1981; 140:777-779.

Artifacts

105. Buttery B, Davison G: The ghost artifact. *J Ultrasound Med* 1984; 3:49-52.

106. Muller N, Cooperberg PL, Rowley VA, et al: Ultrasonic refraction by the rectus abdominis muscles: the double image artifact. *J Ultrasound Med* 1984; 3:515-519.

107. Sauerbrei EE: The split image artifact in pelvic sonography: the anatomy and physics. *J Ultrasound Med* 1985; 4:29-34.

CHAPTER 15

The Peritoneum and the Diaphragm

- Khanh T. Nguyen, M.D.
- Eric E. Sauerbrei, M.D.
- R.L. Nolan, M.D.

The peritoneum is the largest serous membrane of the body. It consists of a single layer of flattened mesothelial cells covering a layer of loose connective tissue. The mesothelium forms a dialysing membrane across which substances in complete solution (solutes) are absorbed directly into the blood capillaries. Particulate matters in suspension pass into the lymphatic circulation probably with the aid of phagocytes. The parietal peritoneum is the membrane lining the inside of the abdominal wall; the visceral peritoneum is reflected over the intraabdominal organs to which it is firmly attached; it is an integral part of the organ that it covers. The peritoneal cavity is the potential space between the parietal and visceral membranes.

The diaphragm, in addition to its function as an active muscle of respiration, is a musculofibrous sheet separating the thoracic from the abdominal cavity. It is innervated by the phrenic and lower intercostal nerves; it is vascularized by the phrenic arteries, which are branches of the aorta.

SCANNING TECHNIQUES

No special patient preparation is required for scanning. Routinely, a 3.5 or 5 MHz sector probe is used. If a superficial lesion is detected, a higher frequency linear array probe may be used for better visualization.

The patient is usually scanned in the supine position. Decubitus or erect positions will help to determine whether a fluid collection is free or loculated. When scanning a collection with an air-fluid level, it is helpful to scan from a posterior approach, through the fluid-filled dependent portion. In this way, one avoids scanning through the air, which reflects all the sound.[1]

Scanning the diaphragm is performed with the patient in the supine or sitting positions, in quiet respiration. Coughing or sniffing tests may be used to evaluate diaphragmatic motion. Measurements for normal diaphragmatic excursion have been established for newborns.[2] On sagittal scans of neonates, the average normal excursion of the right hemidiaphragm measures 2.6 cm ($\pm$ 0.1) for the anterior third, 3.6 cm ($\pm$ 0.2) for the middle third, and 4.5 ($\pm$ 0.2) cm for the posterior third. Measurements for adults are not available.

Peritoneum

Multiple peritoneal ligaments and folds connect the viscera to each other and to the abdominal and pelvic walls. The lesser omentum is the fold connecting the liver to the stomach (hepatogastric ligament) and to the duodenum (hepatoduodenal ligament). The lesser omentum contains the portal vein, hepatic artery, and common bile duct at its free margin. The greater omentum is the largest fold, extending inferiorly from the greater curvature of the stomach to cover the anterior aspect of the transverse colon and hanging down like a curtain in front of the small bowel. The right border of the greater omentum extends as far as the proximal duodenum; its left border is continuous with the gastrosplenic ligament. In addition to functioning as a storehouse for fat, the greater omentum may limit the spread of disease in the peritoneal cavity. The mesenteries refer to peritoneal folds, which suspend the small bowel and colon from the posterior abdominal and pelvic wall. They include the mesentery of the small bowel, the mesoappendix, the transverse mesocolon, and the sigmoid mesocolon. The transverse mesocolon divides the peritoneal cavity into the supramesocolic and inframesocolic compartments.[3,4]

The *supramesocolic* compartment is in turn divided into two spaces by the falciform ligament, which runs in the midline from the umbilicus to the diaphragm and suspends the liver from the diaphragm and anterior abdominal wall. The two spaces are the *right* and *left* supramesocolic spaces (Figs. 15-1 to 15-3).

The *right* supramesocolic space consists of the *lesser sac* and the *right perihepatic space*. The lesser sac has a superior recess that lies on the right side adjacent to the caudate lobe of the liver and an inferior recess on the left side separating the stomach anteriorly from the pancreas posteriorly. It communicates with the greater peritoneal sac through the foramen of Winslow (Epiploic foramen), which is located inferior to the caudate lobe and posterior to the free edge of the lesser omentum.

The right perihepatic space consists of the *right subphrenic* and *right subhepatic* spaces. The subphrenic space is immediately inferior to the diaphragm; it is bounded posteromedially by the right superior coronary ligament. Medial to this ligament is the bare area of the liver not covered by the peritoneum and in direct contact with the retroperitoneal space. The right subhepatic space lies inferior to the liver. It has an anterior component adjacent to the gall bladder fossa and a posterior compartment that is the hepatorenal recess or Morison's pouch.

The *left* supramesocolic space consists of four compartments: the *left perihepatic* spaces (anterior and posterior) and the *left subphrenic* spaces (anterior perigastric and posterior perisplenic). The left anterior subphrenic space is separated from the lesser sac posteriorly by the left coronary ligament that suspends the left lobe of the liver from the diaphragm. It extends over the liver to the most superior left upper quadrant.

The oblique root of the mesentery extending from the duodenojejunal flexure (ligament of Treitz) to the ileocecal junction divides the *inframesocolic* compartment into the smaller *right* and a larger *left* space. The right space is bounded laterally by the ascending colon and inferiorly by the ileocecal junction; the left space is bounded laterally by the descending colon and inferiorly by the sigmoid colon. The two spaces open inferiorly to the pelvic cavity, which is the most dependent part of the peritoneal cavity in both the erect and recumbent positions. The pelvic recesses communicate freely with the right supramesocolic compartment via the right paracolic gutter lateral to the ascending colon; on the left side, the phrenocolic ligament at the ceph-

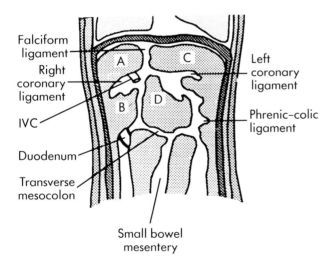

FIG 15-1. Frontal diagram of peritoneal compartments. *A,* Right subphrenic space; *B,* right subhephatic space, *C,* left subphrenic space; *D,* lesser sac; *IVC,* inferior vena cava.
(Adapted from Halvorsen RA, Jones MA, Rice RP, Thompson WM: *AJR* 1982; 139:233-289.)

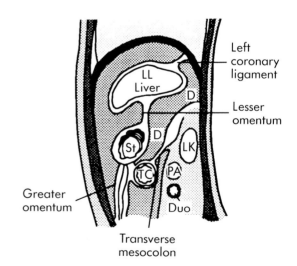

FIG 15-2. Parasagittal diagram of left subphrenic spaces. *D,* Lesser sac; *St,* stomach; *TC,* transverse colon; *PA,* pancreas; *LK,* left kidney; *Duo,* duodenum.
(Adapted from Halvorsen RA, Jones MA, Rice RP, Thompson WM: *AJR* 1982;139:233-289.)

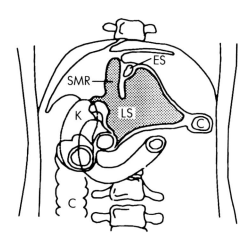

FIG 15-3. Frontal diagram of lesser sac. *SMR,* Superomedial recess; *LS,* lateral recess; *ES,* esophagus; *C,* colon; *K,* kidney. (Adapted from Halvorsen RA, Jones MA, Rice RP, Thompson WM: *AJR* 1982;139:233-289.)

alad end of the left paracolic gutter prevents communication with the left supramesocolic compartment.[3,4]

When the peritoneal spaces are filled with fluid or tumour or when the membranes are thickened by disease, they may be identified by using sonography. The normal small bowel mesentery, which usually contains fat and blood vessels, is better seen by CT than by ultrasound.

Diaphragm

The diaphragm consists of a central crescent-shaped tendinous plate connected by peripheral muscular bundles to the lower sternum and lower six ribs anteriorly and to the lumbar spine posteriorly. The anterior muscular fibers are shorter than the posterior ones. Because of this, the diaphragm has a dome-shaped configuration with convexity toward the thorax. The two crura anchoring the diaphragm to the spine join in the midline to form the arcuate ligament; posterior to this and in front of the spine at the level of the twelfth dorsal vertebra is the aortic hiatus. The esophageal hiatus is usually at the level of the tenth dorsal vertebra, slightly to the left of the midline, between the decussating mitral fibers of the right crus. The inferior vena cava passes through the right side of the central tendon, usually at the level of the eighth or ninth dorsal vertebra (Fig. 15-4).

Sonographically, the muscles of the diaphragm are seen as a thin hypoechoic band. The interface between diaphragm and liver (or spleen) appears as a thin echogenic line. The interface between diaphragm and lung appears as a stronger and thicker echogenic band. Occasionally, another thin echogenic line is present cephalad to the diaphragm–lung interface.[5] This is a mirror-image artifact of the diaphragm–liver interface (Figs. 15-5 and 15-6). The term "diaphragmatic slips" refers to normal prominent muscular insertions. In cross section, they may appear as focal echogenic masses of

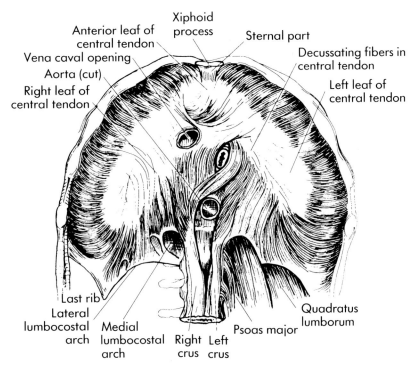

FIG 15-4. Abdominal aspect of diaphragm.
(Adapted from *Gray's Anatomy,* 35th ed. Edinburg: Longman Group Ltd; 1973: 516.)

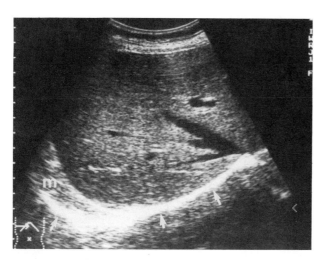

FIG 15-5. The right hemidiaphragm in transverse scan. The echogenic curved line *(arrows)* represents the diaphragm-lung interface. The triangular hypoechoic band *(m)* represents the peripheral muscular bundles.

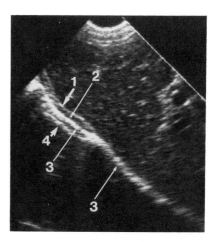

FIG 15-6. The right hemidiaphragm in parasagittal view. *1,* Diaphragm–liver interface; *2,* muscles of diaphragm; *3,* diaphragm–lung interface; *4,* mirror-image of diaphragm–liver interface.

various shapes (round, triangular, oval) that may be mistaken for focal liver or peritoneal lesions.[6] By rotating the transducer and scanning in their long axis, they appear elongated and become larger in inspiration (Figs. 15-7 and 15-8). The diaphragmatic crura may be seen as thin hypoechoic bands anterior to the upper abdominal aorta and posterior to the inferior vena cava. They also become thicker in deep inspiration.[6]

PERITONEAL PATHOLOGY
Ascites

Accumulation of fluid in the peritoneal cavity is termed *ascites.* The fluid may be a transudate or an ex-

udate; it may be blood, pancreatic juice, chyle, pus, or urine.

The anatomic compartmentalization, together with the action of gravity and variation in intraabdominal pressure during respiration, determine the distribution of fluid and its contents throughout the peritoneal cavity. Gravity causes fluid to flow along peritoneal reflections: the fluid tends to pool in the lower end of the mesenteric root at the ileocecal junction and in the sigmoid mesocolon (Fig. 15-9). From there, it spills into the pelvic cul-de-sac and paravesical recesses. In the recumbent position, fluid flows preferentially cephalad along the right paracolic gutter and collects in the right

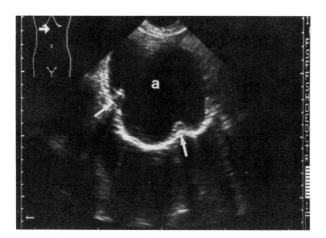

FIG 15-7. The diaphragmatic slips in cross section. Transverse scan. They appear as small hypoechoic masses *(arrows).* Note the large ascites *(a).*

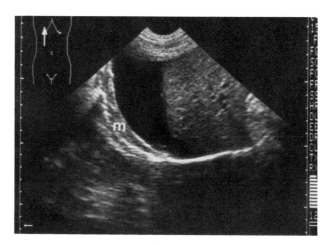

FIG 15-8. When scanned in their long axis, the diaphragmatic slips appear elongated *(m)* and also become thicker in deep inspiration.

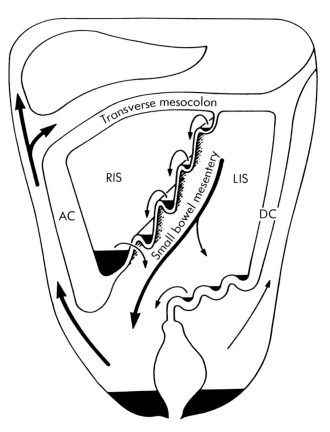

FIG 15-9. Diagram of ascitic fluid distribution. *RIS,* Right inframesocolic space; *LIS,* left inframescocolic space; *AC,* ascending colon; *DC,* descending colon.
(Reprinted with permission from Siegel MJ: Spleen and peritoneal cavity. In: Siegel MJ, ed. *Pediatric sonography.* New York: Raven Press, 1991: 173.)

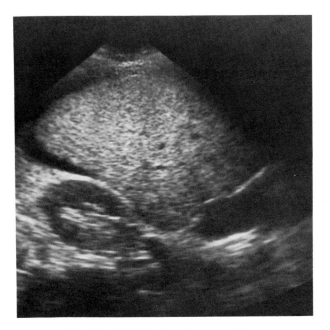

FIG 15-10. Minimal ascites around liver.

subphrenic and perihepatic spaces. On the left side, flow is weak and limited cephalad by the phrenocolic ligament.[7] Because of this, minimal ascites is most frequently found in the hepatorenal recess (Morison's pouch) and in the pelvic cul-de-sac, which are the most dependent spaces of the peritoneal cavity (Fig. 15-10). It is possible to detect with real-time sonography as little as a few milliliters of free fluid in these locations.[8,9,10] It is also apparent from the above discussion that the abdominal and pelvic cavity form an anatomic continuum. If fluid is seen in the abdomen, one should look for it in the pelvis and vice versa. This should be remembered when evaluating certain conditions such as blunt abdominal trauma, ruptured ectopic pregnancy, and intraperitoneal abscesses. A small amount of fluid in the pelvic cul-de-sac may be the only sign of injury to the upper abdominal viscera. Similarly, fluid in the hepatorenal recess may be seen in a ruptured ectopic pregnancy. A right subphrenic collection may originate from a pelvic source.

Ultrasound performs better than CT in localizing as-

citic fluid in relation to the peritoneal spaces, because it allows instant visualization in different planes. It is worthwhile to note that fluid in the bare area of the liver is not intraperitoneal; it is either pleural or subcapsular. A right subphrenic collection does not extend posterior to the inferior vena cava, as a right pleural effusion often does.[11] In massive ascites, the liver, spleen, and bowel are displaced medially and toward the center of the abdomen.[12] The bowel may appear as echogenic structures distributed around the periphery of the fan-shaped mesentery (Fig. 15-11). Loculated ascites as an isolated finding simulates mesenteric or omental cyst, lymphocele, abscess, or a cystic neoplasm (Fig. 15-12). Diagnosis often requires fine-needle percutaneous aspiration, which is frequently performed under ultrasound guidance.

The sonographic appearance of the fluid is variable. In general, simple ascites or a transudate is usually sonolucent. Fluid collections complicated by hemorrhage or infection or an exudate may contain septations or floating debris.[13]

Intraperitoneal Abscess

Intraperitoneal abscesses may develop following spillage of contaminated material from perforated bowel; or they may occur as the result of direct contamination during surgery; or they may be seen as a complication of trauma, pancreatitis, or in conditions associated with decreased immune response. The majority of intraperitoneal abscesses occur in the upper abdomen between the transverse colon and diaphragm: 60% per-

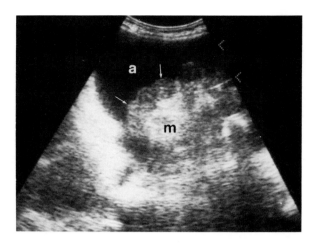

FIG 15-11. Bowel loops *(arrows)* are arranged around the periphery of the mesentery *(m)*. Ascites *(a)* surrounds the bowel.

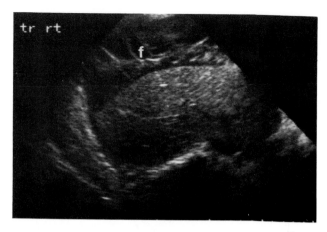

FIG 15-12. Loculated septated ascites *(f)* is seen around the liver in this transverse scan.

cent are found on the right side, 25% occur on the left, and about 15% are bilateral. The most common offending organisms are *Escherichia coli,* Streptococci, Staphylococci, and *Klebsiella.* Mixed infections are also common.[14] Clinical findings typically include fever, leukocytosis, abdominal pain, and tenderness.

It is generally accepted that sonography performs better than CT in the detection of subphrenic and perihepatic abscesses, although the left upper quadrant may present some difficulties.[15,16] Ultrasound is also the screening modality of choice for thin patients and for patients with vague clinical findings. CT performs better in detecting intraloop abscesses and those located in the lower abdomen and pelvis. CT is also the best imaging technique for obese patients and for patients with recent surgery.[15,16] Therefore, the choice of the initial imaging modality should be tailored to the patient's size and clinical status. Most often the best results are obtained with the appropriate use of more than one imaging technique (US, CT, nuclear medicine, and MRI).

An air-fluid collection in the mid upper abdomen may be in the lesser sac or in the left anterior subphrenic space. Both spaces may extend across the midline.[17] Most lesser sac abscesses usually originate from disease processes in contiguous organs, particularly the pancreas. They are seen posterior to the stomach and at a lower plane than the subphrenic abscesses, which are anterior to the stomach and may simulate abscesses in the left lobe of the liver (Figs. 15-13 and 15-14).

A loculated fluid collection containing gas bubbles is strongly suggestive of an abscess. This is not often seen. More frequently one finds a fluid collection ovoid or spherical or irregular in shape, which may or may not contain septations or debris. Occasionally a fluid-fluid level may be detected (Figs. 15-15 and 15-16). Some abscesses may simulate an echogenic solid mass or a simple cystic lesion. Others show a complex appearance, partly cystic, partly solid (Figs. 15-17 and 15-18). Diagnosis and drainage are established by using the percutaneous approach.[18] Ultrasound or CT guidance may be used depending on the location of the abscess.

A few authors claim an accuracy approaching 90 percent in the sonographic detection of intraabdominal abscesses.[15,16] This includes abscesses affecting the solid viscera. In practice, the results are probably in the range of 40% to 50%, as published by Lundstedt et al., for the sonographic detection of abscesses occurring in the peritoneal cavity.[19] The ultrasound examination is often severely limited by the presence of open wounds, drainage tubes, large dressings, and bowel gas.

Lymphoceles

Disruption of lymphatic vessels following surgery (lymphadenectomy, kidney transplant) or trauma results in the development of lymphoceles, which are lymph-containing collections that occur most commonly in the pelvis, in the abdominal peritoneal recesses, or in the retroperitoneum.[20]

Lymphoceles are usually small. However, some may attain considerable size, measuring many centimeters in diameter and causing pressure symptoms or hydronephrosis of the transplanted kidney. Small lymphoceles frequently resorb over time. Large and symptomatic lymphoceles (Fig. 15-19) are usually decompressed percutaneously or surgically.[21] Some success has been obtained with sclerotherapy using instillation of Tetracycline into the cyst.[22]

Uncomplicated lymphoceles appear as echo-free collections mimicking loculated ascites or mesenteric and

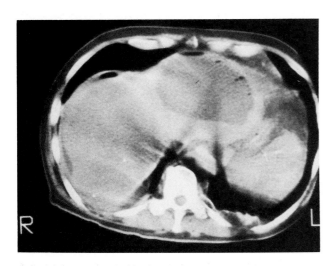

FIG 15-13. Left anterior subphrenic abscess. CT scan of upper abdomen. There is a well-defined fluid collection *(a)* in the mid abdomen, which may be in the left lobe of the liver.

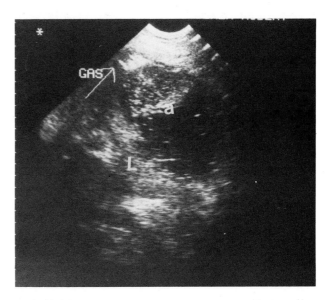

FIG 15-14. Left anterior subphrenic abscess. On the ultrasound scan, the left lobe of the liver *(L)* appears compressed and displaced posteriorly by the collection *(a)*. The midline location high under the diaphragm anterior to the liver suggests an anterior left subphrenic abscess. This was successfully drained via a percutaneous approach. Note the gas collection floating on the top of the abscess.

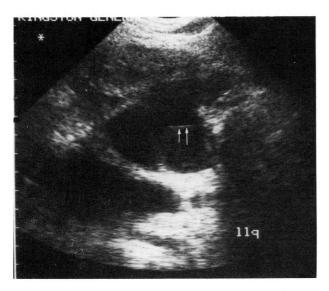

FIG 15-15. Abscess in left lower quadrant. Parasagittal scan reveals an fluid collection on the left side of the abdomen. A faint fluid-fluid level is seen *(arrows)*. It is not possible to say whether this is sterile or infected.

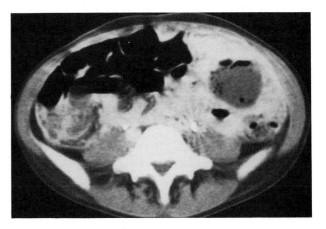

FIG 15-16. Abscess in left lower quadrant. CT scan shows the presence of gas bubbles in the abscess that is partially surrounded by bowel and is successfully drained via a percutaneous approach. CT performs better in detecting small gas bubbles. Sonography detects fluid levels and septation more easily.

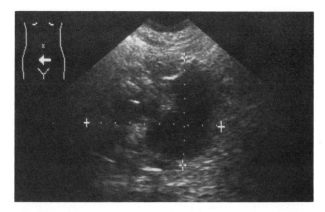

FIG 15-17. Diverticular abscess. Transverse scan of pelvis. A complex mass is partly cystic, partly solid on the left side of the pelvis.

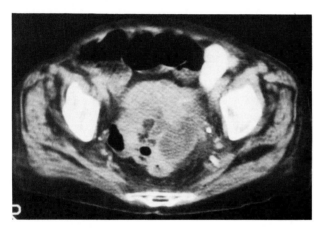

FIG 15-18. Diverticular abscess. CT scan of pelvis. There is a mass of inhomogenous density adjacent to bowel. This proved to be a diverticular abscess that was drained transrectally under ultrasound guidance.

omental cysts or pancreatic pseudocysts. Septation and floating debris are usually seen when they are complicated by hemorrhage or infection. Diagnosis requires percutaneous aspiration under ultrasound or CT guidance. Fat globules are found in the fluid.

Omental and Mesenteric Cysts

Omental and mesenteric cysts are lesions of obscure etiology. Some authors consider them to be hamartomas, part of lymphangiomatosis; others believe they are caused by congenital lymphatic obstruction.[23] Mesenteric cysts are usually found in the root of the mesentery; omental cysts occur adjacent to the bowel. The fluid they contain may be serous, bloody or mixed, or a "cheesy white" material thought to be inspissated chyle.[24] The majority of the patients present with a palpable abdominal mass.

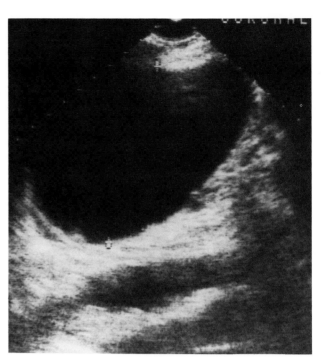

FIG 15-19. Lymphocele. This appears as a large simple fluid collection on the left side of the abdomen in this patient who had previous nodal dissection.

Sonographically, omental and mesenteric cysts often appear as unilocular cystic lesions (Figs. 15-20 and 15-21) that may be septated.[25,26] Rarely a fat-fluid level may be seen; this is thought to be because of the presence of chyle associated with an inflammatory exudate.[27] In contrast to bowel duplication cysts, they are not lined with a mucosal layer. Differentiation from other cystic lesions of the abdomen is often difficult without percutaneous needle aspiration. The rare cystic teratoma and lymphangioma of the mesentery have been reported.[28,29]

Meconium Peritonitis

Prenatal bowel perforation results in aseptic chemical inflammation of the peritoneum termed *meconium peritonitis*. Intestinal stenosis or atresia and meconium ileus (cystic fibrosis) are the most common causes, accounting for 65 percent of cases. Other causes include perforated Meckel's diverticulum or appendix, bowel perforation related to volvulus, internal hernia, and vascular thrombosis.[30]

Extravasated meconium causes an intense foreign body reaction. This results in a fibroadhesive peritonitis that may calcify over time. A fibrous wall may develop around the mass of spilled meconium, producing a pseudocyst that may appear echogenic (Figs. 15-22 and 15-23). Antenatal detection of meconium peritonitis has been made by showing a mass in the fetal abdomen that

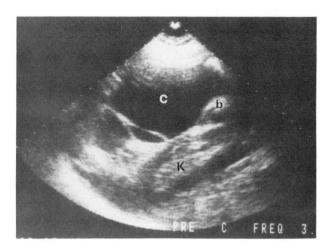

FIG 15-20. Mesenteric cyst. This left parasagittal scan reveals a cystic lesion *(c)* adjacent to bowel *(b)*. *K,* Kidney.

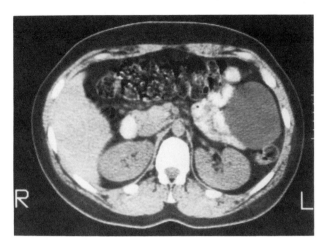

FIG 15-21. Mesenteric cyst. CT appearance. The lesion is closely adjacent to the small bowel.

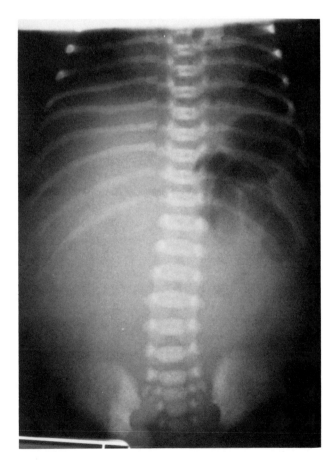

FIG 15-22. Meconium pseudocyst. A large soft tissue pelvo-abdominal mass is seen in this abdominal radiograph of a newborn.

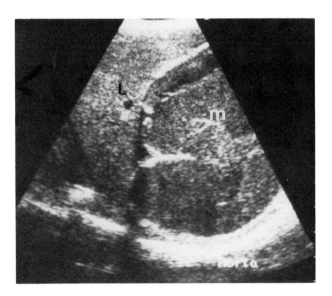

FIG 15-23. Meconium pseudocyst. Abdominal sonogram reveals an echogenic mass *(m)* filling the abdomen. *L,* Liver. At surgery, this proves to be a meconium pseudocyst resulting from ileal atresia.

may be complex or cystic with an echogenic wall.[30-33] Calcified peritoneal thickening may be seen as scattered linear echoes with or without acoustic shadowing. After birth, there may be a diffuse echogenicity throughout the abdomen described as a "snowstorm" appearance. Other findings include fetal ascites, dilated bowel loops, and polyhydraminos.[31-34]

Peritoneal Tuberculosis

Inflammation of the peritoneum caused by *Mycobacterium tuberculosis* is now a rare occurrence, particularly in the Western world. This is usually caused by direct spread from gastrointestinal tuberculosis or following hematogenous dissemination from a lung focus. Only a few reports exist in the sonographic literature, describing ascites, enlarged necrotic mesenteric nodes, and echogenic epigastric masses representing caseating granulomata.[35,36] The greater omentum may be thickened by granulomatous deposits and adhesions. This may appear on sonography as an "omental cake" indistinguishable from peritoneal carcinomatosis or mesothelioma,[37] which will be described later in this chapter. Diagnosis requires peritoneoscopy and biopsies.

Mesenteritis

Inflammation and thickening as well as fat necrosis of the mesentery may develop in a number of conditions including Crohn's disease, pancreatitis, trauma, surgery, or as part of retroperitoneal fibrosis. Occasionally, this may appear as a focal echo-poor mass simulating a neoplasm.[38,39] Diagnosis may be suspected in the appropriate clinical setting but may require percutaneous fine-needle biopsy.

Retained Surgical Sponges

Surgical sponges may be forgotten in the abdomen after surgery. Without opaque markers, they cannot be detected by radiography.

Surgical sponges may be seen in abdominal sonography and may cause diagnostic confusion if one is not aware of and familiar with their appearance. The ones surrounded by an abscess usually appear as infected collections or masses.[40] The ones not associated with abscess usually show a clean, clear-cut acoustic shadow in relation to a palpable mass.[41] The abdominal radiograph helps to exclude residual barium in the bowel or a calcified neoplasm.

Peritoneal Neoplasms

Mesenteric and omental neoplasms are rare. The most common benign primary mesenteric neoplasm is desmoid tumor. Common peritoneal malignancies include lymphoma, mesothelioma, and carcinomatosis.

Desmoid Tumors. Desmoid tumors arise from fascia and aponeuroses. They occur most commonly in the ab-

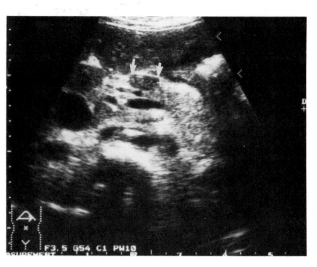

FIG 15-24. Isolated enlarged peripancreatic node *(arrows)*. This is seen in a patient with known non-Hodgkin's lymphoma.

dominal wall. Mesenteric desmoids usually appear as hypoechoic masses that may contain areas of acoustic shadowing thought to arise from fibrotic collagenous tissue and not from calcification.[42]

Lymphoma. The most common primary mesenteric malignancy is lymphoma. Fifty percent of patients with non-Hodgkin's lymphoma and only 5 percent of patients with Hodgkin's lymphoma have mesenteric involvement.[43]

Isolated enlarged lymph nodes measuring more than 1.5 centimeters in maximal diameter may be detected around the celiac axis, the superior mesenteric artery or in the porta hepatis. They are often hypoechoic, but they may be echogenic (Figs. 15-24). More frequently, mesenteric lymphoma appears as a lobulated mass encasing the mesenteric vessels that manifest as linear echoes within the mass (Figs. 15-25 and 15-26). This has been described as the "sandwich sign", more commonly seen in lymphoma than in metastatic disease.[44]

Mesothelioma. Mesothelioma is a sarcoma arising from a serous membrane. Closely related to asbestos exposure, it affects the pleura (65% of cases) more often than the peritoneum (33% of cases); both pleura and peritoneum are affected in 2% of cases.[45] Clinical signs and symptoms are usually vague. The latent period may be as long as 40 years following the initial exposure to asbestos.

The disease typically causes thickening of the omentum, which appears sonographically as sheetlike superficial masses described as "omental mantle or cake."[46,47] The anterior surface follows the contour of the abdominal cavity; the posterior surface is adjacent to bowel loops and is often outlined by a thin collection of fluid (Figs. 15-27 and 15-28). However, this appearance may

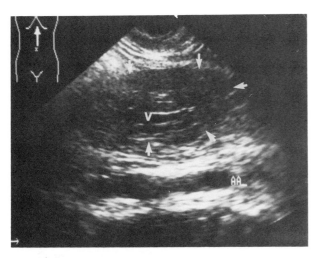

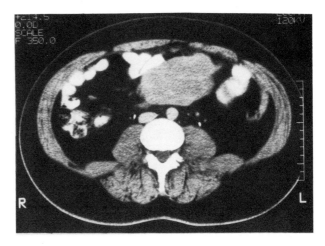

FIG 15-25. Mesenteric lymphoma. The mesenteric vessels *(v)* are surrounded by a hypoechoic mass *(arrows)*. The appearance has been described as the "sandwich" sign. This is also seen with metastatic disease. *AA,* Abdominal aorta.

FIG 15-26. Mesenteric lymphoma CT scan.

also be seen with peritoneal carcinomatosis and tuberculosis. The surrounding bowel may be invaded and become fixed, not changing location with different patient position. Ascites when present is usually minimal, although massive ascites may sometimes occur. Liver metastases, pleural plaques, and effusions are readily identified by sonography. CT scanning performs better than ultrasound in detecting small nodules attached to the peritoneal surface or buried in the mesenteric fat, focal peritoneal thickening, and calcified pleural plaques. Gallium uptake by pleural and peritoneal mesotheliomas has been reported.[48] Diagnosis may be made by fine-needle aspiration biopsies, which should be performed at different sites in order to obtain adequate samples.[49] In most cases peritoneoscopy or laparotomy is required. The extremely rare cystic mesothe-

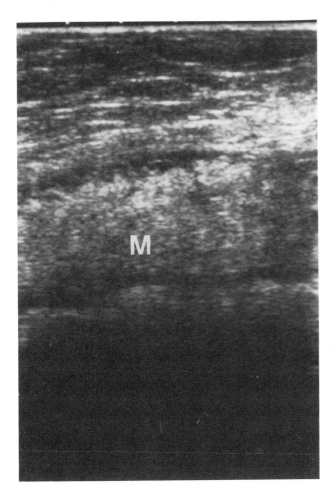

FIG 15-27. Peritoneal mesothelioma. Sonogram shows typical "omental cake" *(M)* resulting from thickening of the omentum. The lobulated posterior contour is due to adjacent bowel.

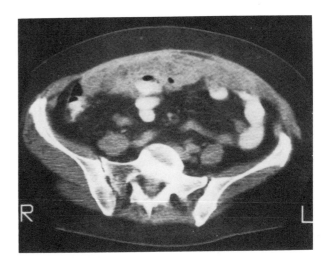

FIG 15-28. Peritoneal mesothelioma. CT appearance. Note absence of ascites.

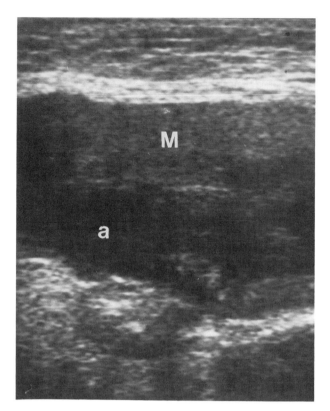

FIG 15-29. Peritoneal metastasis—Omental cake *(M)*. The omental thickening is indistinguishable from peritoneal mesothelioma or tuberculosis. Note significant ascites *(a)*. The patient had ovarian carcinoma.

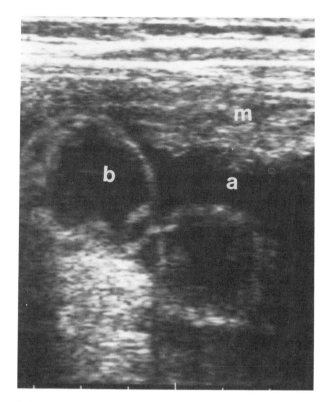

FIG 15-30. Peritoneal implants. The metastic deposits *(m)* are well seen because of surrounding ascites *(a)*. Note dilated fluid-filled bowel loops *(b)*.

lioma of the peritoneum is a separate entity that has no relation to previous exposure to asbestos.[50,51]

Carcinomatosis. Metastases to the peritoneum and mesentery arise from a variety of sources, the most common being carcinoma of the ovaries and of the gastrointestinal tract.[43] Four mechanisms determine the spread of metastatic disease in the abdomen: mesenteric pathways, intraperitoneal seeding, and lymphatic and hematogenous spread.

Gastrointestinal malignancies often invade surrounding viscera by growing along mesenteric and ligamentous attachments. This has been well illustrated by Meyers et al.[52] Carcinoma of the stomach spreads along the gastrocolic ligament to affect the transverse colon; conversely, carcinoma of the transverse colon may extend cephalad along the same ligament to affect the stomach. The transverse mesocolon may serve as a conduit for spread of pancreatic carcinoma, which tends to invade the posteroinferior border of the transverse colon.

The natural flow of ascitic fluid and its contents determine the intraperitoneal seeding of malignancies in the peritoneal cavity. Malignant cells that shed in the fluid grow at specific sites where fluid tends to collect.

These sites are the pelvic cul-de-sac, the root of the mesentery at the ileo-cecal junction, the sigmoid mesocolon, and the right paracolic gutter. They are locations where peritoneal metastases are commonly found and these can be detected by barium studies and sonography.[53] When the greater omentum is thickened by secondary infiltration, it may be detected by ultrasound or CT scanning as sheetlike masses described as "omental mantle or cake" seen in mesothelioma or tuberculosis (Fig. 15-29). When ascites is present, small nodules attached to the abdominal wall or peritoneal surface are easily identified. (Fig. 15-30).

Lymphatic spread results in enlarged mesenteric nodes that may be isolated or may appear as conglomerated lobulated hypoechoic masses indistinguishable from lymphoma.

Hematogenous dissemination occurs via the mesenteric arteries, which carry the metastatic emboli to the vasa recta on the antimesenteric border of the bowel, where they grow submucosally into large masses that can be detected by sonography. Melanoma and carcinoma of the breast and lung commonly disseminate this way.[54]

In the search for metastatic disease in the abdomen,

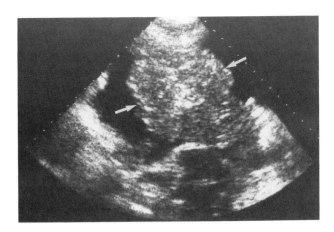

FIG 15-31. Pseudomyxoma peritoneii. Large calcified peritoneal mass *(arrows)* surrounded by ascites. A number of similar lesions are seen throughout the abdomen of this patient with ovarian cancer.

it should be stressed that a negative ultrasound scan does not preclude other imaging tests, including barium studies, CT, MRI, and intraperitoneal injection of I-131 labelled B72.3 antibody.[55] Ultrasound may also be used to guide percutaneous biopsy and to monitor response to treatment.

Pseudomyxoma Peritoneii. Pseudomyxoma peritoneii is characterized by mucinous peritoneal implants and gelatinous ascites. It is most often caused by secondaries from mucin-producing adenocarcinoma of the ovary, appendix, colon and rectum, although a few be-

nign neoplasms of the ovary and appendix may be responsible for the condition.[56] It is not frequently seen in ultrasound practice. A few reports describe nodular masses ranging from hypoechoic to strongly echogenic distributed throughout the peritoneal cavity[57,58,59] (Fig. 15-31). The masses correspond to calcified lesions seen on abdominal radiographs.

Leiomyomatosis Peritonealis Disseminata. Leiomyomatosis peritonealis disseminata is an extremely rare condition that should be included in the differential diagnosis of peritoneal mesothelioma and carcinomatosis. It affects pregnant women or women of childbearing age. It is characterized by the presence of peritoneal masses that are disseminated benign leiomyoma. Ascites is usually not present.[60]

Diffuse Infiltrative Lipomatosis. Diffuse infiltrative lipomatosis is a rare condition that usually affects young patients. It is characterized by extensive overgrowth of fatty tissue in the mesentery. Sonography shows a strongly echogenic mass; the fatty nature of the mass is apparent on CT scanning. Differentiation from a liposarcoma is difficult.[61]

DIAPHRAGMATIC PATHOLOGY
Paralysis

Sonography is increasingly used instead of fluoroscopy in the evaluation of the diaphragm. The technique offers several advantages:

- it is free of ionizing radiation, therefore more suitable for children and pregnant women
- it can be easily performed at the patient's bedside with portable equipment
- it can identify the diaphragm even when the latter is obscured by peridiaphragmatic abnormalities such as effusion or tumor (Figs. 15-32 and 15-33)

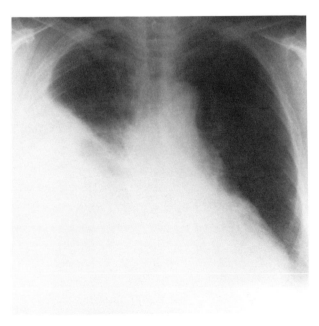

FIG 15-32. Chest (PA projection). Increased density is present in the right base obscuring the outline of the right hemidiaphragm.

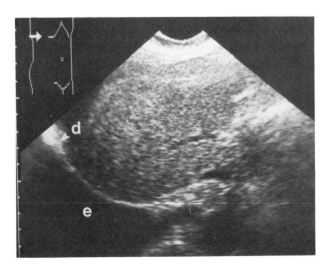

FIG 15-33. Transverse scan. Right pleural effusion *(e)*. The diaphragm *(d)* is seen in normal position.

■ for patients on a respirator, scanning may be done with the respirator disconnected for a few seconds in order to evaluate unassisted ventilation.

The examination is made in the parasagittal and transverse position in quiet respiration; scanning transversely over the xiphoid usually allows simultaneous visualization of both hemidiaphragms. Paradoxical motions may be elicited by the coughing and sniffing tests. Paralysis of one hemidiaphragm can be detected by showing absent or paradoxical motion on the affected side compared with the usual or exaggerated excursion on the opposite side.[62,63]

Eventration

This condition accounts for 5 percent of all diaphragmatic defects. Traditionally, it is considered a congenital malformation resulting from incomplete muscularization of the membranous diaphragm. Others suggest that it may be acquired, secondary to focal ischemia, infarct, or neuromuscular weakness.[6]

Eventration may be complete or partial. The complete form occurs more commonly on the left and in males. The partial form more commonly affects the anterior portion of the right hemidiaphragm. Eventration may be bilateral; in this case, it is frequently seen in Trisomies 13-15 and 18 and in Beckwith-Wiedemann syndrome.[64,65] Diaphragmatic eventration has been diagnosed prenatally.[66]

Partial eventration is usually of no clinical significance and should not be subject to multiple investigations. Complete eventration may cause respiratory distress in the newborn or in the obese and may require surgical plication.[64] Chest radiographs in partial eventration may suggest a mass in the lower thorax or in the liver. Ultrasound helps clarify the issue by showing absence of a mass and the typical diaphragmatic bulge filled by the liver.[6] Complete eventration has not been described in the ultrasound literature.

Inversion

Normally, the convexity of the diaphragmatic dome is toward the thorax. A large pleural effusion or neoplasm may push the diaphragm such that its convexity is toward the abdomen (Fig. 15-34). This is called diaphragmatic inversion and occurs more commonly on the left side. Only part or the entire hemidiaphragm may be affected.[6,67] The inverted hemidiaphragm shows little or asynchronous motion, resulting in paradoxical ventilation and air exchange between the two lungs thus causing respiratory distress. It may simulate a mass on CT scanning because of its inverted cone shape. Parasagittal and transverse sonographic scan planes help to clarify the situation.

Hernia

Acquired defects in the diaphragm are less common than congenital ones, which occur in about 1/2000 to 1/12,500 live births. Of congenital diaphragmatic hernias (CDH), 50% are associated with other malformations.[68] Two major types are recognized: the posterior Bochdalek hernia and the anterior Morgagni hernia.

Posterior Bochdalek hernias are the most common congenital diaphragmatic defect resulting from defective closure of the pleuroperitoneal canal during development. There is a left-sided preponderance ranging from 9/1 to 2/1. On the left side, there may be herniation of the stomach, spleen, or kidney into the lower thorax; on the right side, part of the liver or right kidney may herniate through the defect; most frequently,

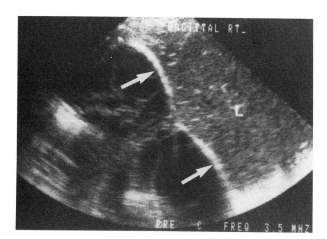

FIG 15-34. Parasagittal scan shows inversion of the right hemidiaphragm *(arrows)* by a septated pleural effusion. *L,* Liver.

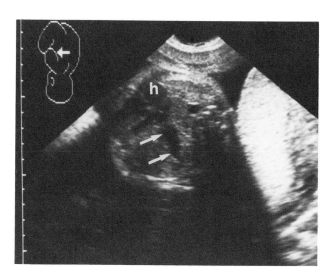

FIG 15-35. Congenital diaphragmatic hernia. Scan through the fetal thorax reveals herniated fluid-filled stomach *(arrows)* in the thorax adjacent to and displacing the heart *(h).*

however, omental fat is found above the diaphragm. Chest radiographs usually show in the diaphragmatic contour a focal posterior hump corresponding to the herniated organ.[69]

The rare anterior Morgagni hernias are due to maldevelopment of the septum transversum. It is often associated with a pericardial defect. There may be herniation of an abdominal organ or fat into the pericardial sac or herniation of the heart into the upper abdomen.[70] Morgagni hernia usually appears as a triangular mass in the right cardiophrenic angle anteriorly and medially, posterior to the sternum. Diaphragmatic hernias are best demonstrated by CT scanning.[68]

Antenatal detection of CDH by ultrasound has been reported.[71,72] The diagnosis should be suspected when the fetal heart is displaced either by an intrathoracic solid mass (liver, kidney) or by a fluid-filled structure (stomach, bowel) (Fig. 15-35). Pulmonary hypoplasia often results from compression of the fetal lung by the herniated viscera. Over 50 percent of infants with CDH die from respiratory failure.[73]

Rupture

Diaphragmatic rupture is usually caused from penetrating injury and blunt trauma and rarely occurs because of infection such as liver amebiasis. The left side is more commonly affected in blunt trauma.[74,75,76]

The diagnosis of diaphragmatic rupture is often difficult without using multiple imaging modalities, which include chest radiographs, contrast studies of the bowel, CT, and MRI scanning. Chest radiography may offer a clue to the diagnosis that is often obscured by life-threatening conditions associated with multiple injuries.[77] Ultrasound usually offers a limited contribution but may detect a large rent (over 10 cm long) showing disruption of diaphragmatic echoes and herniation of abdominal viscera into the thorax.[78,79]

Neoplasms

Diaphragmatic neoplasms, either primary or secondary, are rare. Primary tumours include various types of sarcomas. Secondary involvement is often due to local invasion by adjacent pleural, peritoneal, or thoracic and abdominal wall malignancies. Distant metastases from bronchogenic or ovarian carcinoma, Wilm's tumor, and osteogenic sarcoma are less common.[80]

The metastatic deposits usually cause disruption or interruption of the diaphragmatic echoes seen on sonography.[81] They may produce partial or complete inversion of the involved hemidiaphragm (Fig. 15-36).

ARTIFACTS
Disruption and Displacement of Diaphragmatic Echoes

A fatty mass in the liver or right adrenal or a cystic lesion in the liver may cause apparent interruption and displacement of the right diaphragmatic echoes (Fig. 15-37). This artifact has been referred to as the propagation speed artifact and has been used to suggest the tissue characteristic of the mass causing the artifact.[82,83] It is caused by the difference in velocity of the sound beam through the liver and through the fatty or cystic mass; Cooperberg et al. suggested that refraction at the edge of the lesion may also play a role in the production of the artifact.[84]

Mirror-Image Artifact

Mirror-image artifact is caused by scattered reflection of sound. The right lung–diaphragm interface acts as an acoustic mirror resulting from presence of air in

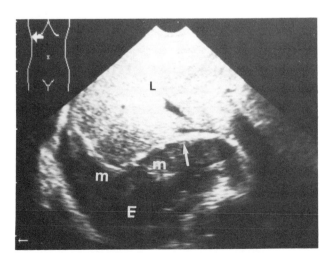

FIG 15-36. Diaphragmatic metastases. Transverse scan shows multiple solid masses, *(m)* causing segmental inversion and disruption of the right hemidiaphragm *(arrow)*. E, Pleural effusion. Metastases from bronchogenic carcinoma. *L,* Liver.

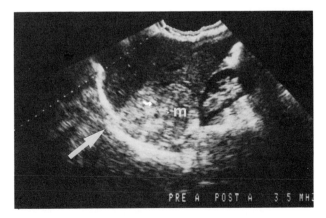

FIG 15-37. Propagation speed artifact. Note apparent disruption and posterior displacement of the right hemidiaphragm *(arrow)*. This is caused by the difference in velocity of the sound beam through the liver and the fatty mass *(m)* in the liver.

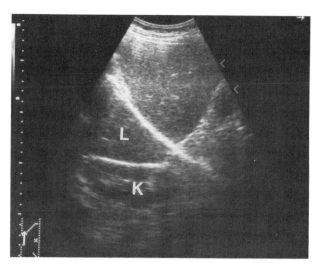

FIG 15-38. Mirror image artifact. Phantom images of liver *(L)* and kidney *(K)* at the base of the thorax caused by reflection of sound beam at the diaphragm.

the lung, which is a strong reflector of sound. When two or more reflectors are on the way of the sound beam, objects that are on one side of a strong reflector may be artificially reproduced on the other side (Fig. 15-38). The formation of this artifact can be explained as follows[85,86]: when the incident sound beam hits the diaphragm–lung interface, some of the beam is reflected away from the incident path into the abdomen. This reflected beam is in turn reflected back from various structures to the diaphragm and thence, back to the probe along the incident path. It takes longer for the reflected beam to reach the transducer. The longer time is translated into a printed signal that appears to originate from the other side of the diaphragm along the direction of the beam (Fig 15-39).

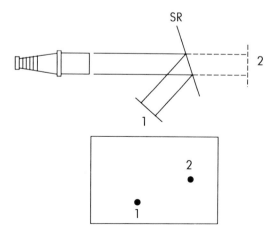

FIG 15-39. Mirror-image artifact. Schema of mechanism.
(From Kremkau FW: Imaging artifacts. In Kremkau FW, ed. Diagnostic ultrasound-principles, instruments and exercises. Philadelphia: WB Saunders Co, 1989: 147-176.)

REFERENCES

Scanning Techniques

1. Golding RH, Li DKB, Cooperberg PL: Sonographic demonstration of air-fluid levels in abdominal abscesses. *J Ultrasound Med* 1982; 1:151-155.
2. Laing IA, Teele RL, Stark AR: Diaphragmatic movements in newborn infants. *J Pediatr* 1988; 112:638-643.

Anatomy

3. Heiken JP: Abdominal wall and peritoneal cavity. In: Leek TL, Sagel SS, Stanley RJ (eds). *Computed tomography with MRI correlation.* New York: Raven Press; 1988:661-705.
4. Whalen JP: Anatomy and radiologic diagnosis of perihepatic abscesses. *Radiol Clin North Am* 1976; 14:406-428.
5. Lewandowski BJ, Winsberg F: Echographic appearance of the right hemidiaphragm. *J Ultrasound Med* 1983; 2:243-249.
6. Yeh H-C, Halton KP, Gray CE: Anatomic variations and abnormalities in the diaphragm seen with ultrasound. *Radiographics* 1990; 10:1019-1030.

Peritoneal Pathology

7. Myers MA (ed.): *Dynamic radiology of the abdomen: normal and pathologic anatomy,* 3rd ed. New York: Springer-Verlag; 1988.
8. Gooding GAW, Cummings SR: Sonographic detection of ascites in liver disease. *J Ultrasound Med* 1984; 3:169-172.
9. Proto AV, Lane EJ, Marangola JA: A new concept of ascitic fluid distribution. *AJR* 1976; 126:974.
10. Meyers MA: The spread and localization of acute intraperitoneal effusions. *Radiology* 1970; 95:547-554.
11. Halvorsen RA, Fedyshin PJ, Korobkin M, Thompson WM: CT differentiation of pleural effusion from ascites: an evaluation of four signs using blinded analysis of 52 cases. *Invest Radiol* 1986; 21:391-395.
12. Yeh H-C, Wolf BS: Ultrasonography in ascites. *Radiology* 1977; 124:783-790.
13. Edell SL, Geften WB: Ultrasonic differentiation of types of ascitic fluid. *AJR* 1979; 133:111-114.
14. Magilligan DJ Jr: Suprahepatic abscess. *Arch Surg* 1968; 96:14-19.
15. Taylor KJW, Wasson JFM, de Graaf C, et al: Accuracy of grey-scale ultrasound in the diagnosis of abdominal and pelvic abscesses in 220 patients. *Lancet* 1978; 1:83-84.
16. Mueller PR, Simeone JF: Intra-abdominal abscess: diagnosis by sonography and computed tomography. *Radiol Clin North Am* 1983; 21:425-443.
17. Halvorsen RA, Jones MA, Rice RP, Thompson WM: Anterior left subphrenic abscesses: characteristic plain film and CT appearance. *AJR* 1982; 139:283-289.
18. van Sonnenberg E, Müeller PR, Ferrucci JT: Percutaneous drainage of 250 abdominal abscesses and fluid collections. Part I: results, failures and complications. *Radiology* 1984; 151:337-341.
19. Lundstedt C, Hederström E, Holmin T, et al: Radiological diagnosis in proven intra-abdominal abscesses formation: a comparison between plain films of the abdomen, ultrasonography and computed tomography. *Gastroinest Radiol* 1983; 8:261-266.
20. Spring DB, Schroeder D, Babu S, et al: Ultrasonic evaluation of lymphocele formation after staging lymphadenectomy for prostatic cancer. *Radiology* 1981; 141:479-483.

21. Lessner AM, Lempert N, Pietrocola DM, et al: Diagnosis and treatment of pelvic lymphoceles in the renal transplant patient. *NY State J Med* 1984; 84:491-494.

22. White M, Mueller PR, Ferrucci JT Jr, et al: Percutaneous drainage of postoperative abdominal and pelvic lymphoceles. *AJR* 1985; 145:1065-1069.

23. Fragoyamis SG, Anagnostopoulos G: Hemangiolymphomatous hamartoma of the mesentery. *Am J Dis Child* 1974; 128:233-234.

24. Walker AR, Putnam TC: Omental, mesenteric and retroperitoneal cysts: a clinical study of 33 new cases. *Ann Surg* 1973; 178:13-19.

25. Geer LL, Mittelstaedt CA, Staab EV, Gaisier G: Mesenteric cyst: sonographic appearance with CT correlation. *Pediatr Radiol* 1984; 14:102-104.

26. Mittelstaedt C: Ultrasonic diagnosis of omental cysts. *Radiology* 1975; 114:673-676.

27. van Mil JBC, Laméris JS: Unusual appearance of a mesenteric cyst. *Diagn Imaging* 1983; 52:28-32.

28. Pricto ML, Casanova A, Delgado J, et al: Cystic teratoma of the mesentery. *Pediatr Radiol* 1989; 19:439.

29. Nicolet V, Gagnon A, Filiatrault D, Boisvert J: Sonographic appearance of an abdominal cystic lymphangioma. *J Ultrasound Med* 1984; 3:85-86.

30. Brugman SM, Bjelland JJ, Thomasson JE, et al: Sonographic findings with radiographic correlation in meconium peritonitis. *J Clin Ultrasound* 1979; 7:305-306.

31. Garb M, Riseborough J. Meconium peritonitis presenting as fetal ascites on ultrasound. *Br J Radiol* 1980; 53:602-604.

32. Blumenthal D, Rushorich AM, Williams RK, Rochester D: Prenatal sonographic findings of meconium peritonitis with pathologic correlation. *J Clin Ultrasound* 1982; 10:350-352.

33. Hartung RW, Kilcheski TS, Greaney RC, et al: Antenatal diagnosis of cystic meconium peritonitis. *J Ultrasound Med* 1983; 2:49-50.

34. Laver JD, Cradock TV: Meconium pseudocyst: prenatal sonographic and antenatal radiologic correlation. *J Ultrasound Med* 1982; 1:333-335.

35. Borgia G, Ciampi R, Nappa S, et al: Tuberculous mesenteric lymphadenitis clinically presenting as abdominal mass: CT and sonographic findings. *J Clin Ultrasound* 1985; 13:491-493.

36. Epstein BM, Mann JH: CT of abdominal tuberculosis. *AJR* 1982; 139:861-866.

37. Wu C-C, Chow K-S, Lü T-N, Huang F-T: Sonographic features of tuberculous omental cakes in peritoneal tuberculosis. *J Clin Ultrasound* 1988; 16:195-198.

38. Marshak RH, Lindner AE, Maklansky D, et al: Mesenteric fat necrosis simulating a carcinoma of the cecum. *Am J Gastroenterol* 1980; 5:459-462.

39. Kordan B, Payne SD. Fat necrosis simulating a primary tumor of the mesentery: sonographic diagnosis. *J Ultrasound Med* 1988; 7:345-347.

40. Sekiba K, Akamatsu N, Niwa K: Ultrasound characteristics of abdominal abscesses involving foreign bodies (gauze). *J Clin Ultrasound* 1979; 7:284-285.

41. Barriga P, Garcia C. Ultrasonography in the detection of intraabdominal retained surgical sponges. *J Ultrasound Med* 1984; 3:173-176.

42. Baron RL, Lee JK: Mesenteric desmoid tumours. *Radiology* 1981; 140:777-779.

43. Levitt RG, Koehler RE, Sagel SS, et al: Metastatic disease of the mesentery and omentum. *Radiol Clin North Am* 1982; 20:501-510.

44. Mueller PR, Ferrucci JT Jr, Harbin WP, et al: Appearance of lymphomatous involvement of the mesentery by ultrasonography and body computed tomography: the "sandwich sign". *Radiology* 1980; 134:467-473.

45. Moertel CG: Peritoneal mesothelioma. *Gastroenterol* 1972; 63:346-350.

46. Yeh H-C, Chahinian AP: Ultrasonography and computed tomography of peritoneal mesothelioma. *Radiology* 1980; 135:705-712.

47. Cooper C, Jeffrey RB, Silverman PM, et al: Computed tomography of omental pathology. *J Computer Assisted Tomography* 1986; 10:62-66.

48. Dach J, Patel N, Patel S, Petassnick J: Peritoneal mesothelioma: CT, sonography and gallium-67 scan. *AJR* 1980; 135:614-616.

49. Reuter K, Raptopoulos V, Reale F, et al: Diagnosis of peritoneal mesothelioma: computed tomography, sonography and fine needle aspiration biopsy. *AJR* 1983; 140:1189-1194.

50. O'Neil JD, Ros PR, Storm BL, et al: Cystic mesothelioma of the peritoneum. *Radiology* 1989; 170:333-337.

51. Schneider JA, Zelnick EJ: Benign cystic peritoneal mesothelioma. *J Clin Ultrasound* 1985; 13:190-192.

52. Meyers MA: Metastatic disease along the small bowel mesentery: roentgen features. *AJR* 1975; 123:67-73.

53. Meyers MA: Distribution of intra-abdominal malignant seeding: dependency on dynamics of flow and ascitic fluid. *AJR* 1973; 119:198-206.

54. Meyers MA, McSweeney J: Secondary neoplasms of the bowel. *Radiology* 1979; 133:419-424.

55. Carrasquillo JA, Sugarbaker P, Colcher D, et al: Peritoneal carcinomatosis: imaging with intraperitoneal injection of I-131 labelled B72.3 monoclonal antibody. *Radiology* 1988; 167:34-40.

56. Fernandez R, Daly JM: Pseudomyxoma peritoneii. *Arch Surg* 1980; 115:409-414.

57. Merritt CB, Williams SM: Ultrasound findings in a patient with pseudomyxoma peritoneii. *J Clin Ultrasound* 1978; 6:417-418.

58. Seshill MB, Coulam CM: Pseudomyxoma peritoneii: computed tomography and sonography. *AJR* 1981; 136:803-806.

59. Seale WB: Sonographic findings in a patient with pseudomyxoma peritoneii. *J Clin Ultrasound* 1982; 10:441-443.

60. Remigers SA, Michael AS, Bardawil WWA, et al: Sonographic findings in leiomyomatosis peritonealis disseminata. A case report and literature review. *J Ultrasound Med* 1985; 4:497-500.

61. Siegel MJ. Spleen and peritoneal cavity. In: Siegel MJ (ed.) *Pediatric Sonography*. New York: Raven Press; 1991; 6:161-178.

Diaphragmatic Pathology

62. Haber K, Asher WM, Freimann AK: Echographic evaluation of diaphragmatic motion in intra-abdominal disease. *Radiology* 1975; 114:141-144.

63. Diament MJ, Boerhat MI, Kangarloo H: Real-time sector ultrasound in the evaluation of suspected abnormalities of diaphragmatic motion. *J Clin Ultrasound* 1985; 13:539-543.

64. Symbas PN, Hatcher CR Jr, Waldo W: Diaphragmatic eventration in infancy and childhood. *Ann Thorac Surg* 1977; 24:113-119.,

65. Weller MH: Bilateral eventration of the diaphragm. *West J Med* 1976; 124:415-419.

66. Jurcak-Zaleski S, Comstock C, Kirk JS: Eventration of the diaphragm - prenatal diagnosis. *J Ultrasound Med* 1990; 9:351-354.

67. Subramanyam BR, Raghavendra BN, LeFleur RS: Sonography of the inverted right hemidiaphragm. *AJR* 1981; 136:1004-1006.

68. Panicek DM, Benson CB, Gottlieb RH, Heitzman ER: The diaphragm: anatomic, pathologic and radiologic considerations. *Radiographics* 1988; 8:385-424.

69. Gale ME: Bochdalek hernia: prevalence and CT characteristics. *Radiology* 1985; 156:449-452.

70. Gale ME: Anterior diaphragm: variations in the CT appearance. *Radiology* 1986; 161:635-639.

71. Chinn DH, Filly RA, Callen PW, et al: Congenital diaphragmatic hernia diagnosed prenatally by ultrasound. *Radiology* 1983; 148:119-123.

72. Comstock CH: The antenatal diagnosis of diaphragmatic anomalies. *J Ultrasound Med* 1986; 5:391-396.

73. Benaceraff BK, Adzick NS: Fetal diaphragmatic hernia: ultrasound diagnosis and clinical outcome in 19 cases. *Am J Obstet Gynecol* 1987; 156:573-575.

74. Landay MJ, Setiawan H, Hirsch G, et al: Hepatic and thoracic amebiasis. *AJR* 1980; 135:449-454.

75. Ball T, McCrory R, Smith JO, Clements JL Jr: Traumatic diaphragmatic hernia: errors in diagnosis. *AJR* 1988; 138:633-637.

76. Bergqvist D, Dahlgren S, Hedelin H: Rupture of the diaphragm in patients wearing seatbelts. *J Trauma* 1978; 18:781-783.

77. Gelman R, Mirris SE, Gens D: Diaphragmatic rupture due to blunt trauma: sensitivity on Plain Chest Radiographs. *AJR* 1991; 156:51-57.

78. Rao KG, Woodlief RM: Grey-scale ultrasonic documentation of ruptured right hemidiaphragm. *Br J Radiol* 1980; 53:812-814.

79. Ammann AM, Brewer WH, Mauhl KI, Walsh JW: Traumatic rupture of the diaphragm: real-time sonographic diagnosis. *AJR* 1983; 140:915-916.

80. Kangarloo H, Sukor R, Sample WF, et al: Ultrasonographic evaluation of juxtadiaphragmatic mass in children. *Radiology* 1977; 125:785-787.

81. Worthen NJ, Worthen WF II: Disruption of the diaphragmatic echoes: a sonographic sign of diaphragmatic disease. *J Clin Ultrasound* 1982; 10:43-45.

82. Pierce G, Golding RH, Cooperberg PL: The effects of tissue velocity on acoustical interfaces. *J Ultrasound Med* 1982; 1:185-187.

Artifacts

83. Richman TS, Taylor KJW, Kremkase FW: Propagation speed artifact in a fatty tumour (myelolipoma): significance for tissue differential diagnosis. *J Ultrasound Med* 1983; 2:45-47.

84. Mayo J, Cooperberg PL: Displacement of the diaphragmatic echo by hepatic cysts: a new explanation with computer simulation. *J Ultrasound Med* 1984; 3:337-340.

85. Kremkau FW. Imaging artifacts. In: Kremkau FW (ed.) *Diagnostic ultrasound - principles, instruments and exercises.* Philadelphia: WB Saunders Company; 1989;147-176.

86. Zagzebski JA: Images and artifacts. In: Hagen-Ansert SL (ed.) *Textbook of diagnostic sonography.* St. Louis: Mosby–Yearbook, Inc; 1983:44-60.

CHAPTER 16

The Uterus and Adnexa

- Shia Salem, M.D.

The development of high-frequency vaginal probes with excellent resolution has improved the detail and diagnostic accuracy in the demonstration of both normal pelvic anatomy and pathologic states. Sonography plays an extremely important role in the management of the infertility patient (see Chapter 52). It is considered the initial imaging modality in evaluating the patient with a pelvic mass and may be used in guidance of aspiration or biopsy procedures. Furthermore, Doppler imaging techniques, especially color Doppler, may prove to be of value in assessing the pelvic vascularity.

When a pelvic mass is found by sonographic examination, it may be characterized by its size, location (uterine or extrauterine), external contour (well-defined, ill-defined, or irregular borders), and internal consistency (cystic, complex predominantly cystic, complex predominantly solid, and solid). Generally, uterine masses are mainly solid, as opposed to ovarian masses, which are mainly cystic. Although a specific diagnosis cannot be made in many instances, a more limited differential diagnosis can be given based on this classification.

NORMAL PELVIC ANATOMY

The **uterus** is a hollow thick-walled muscular organ. Its internal structure consists of a muscular layer, or **myometrium,** which forms most of the substance of the uterus, and a mucous layer, the **endometrium,** which is firmly adherent to the myometrium. The **uterus** is located between the two layers of the broad ligament laterally, the bladder anteriorly, and the rectosigmoid colon posteriorly. It is divided into two major portions, the **body** and **cervix,** by a slight narrowing at the level of the internal os. The **fundus** is the superior area above the entrance of the fallopian tubes. The area of the body where the tubes enter the uterus is called the **cornua.** The cervix opens into the upper vagina through the external os. The **vagina** is a fibromuscular canal that lies in the midline and runs from the cervix to the vestibule of the external genitalia. The cervix projects into the proximal vagina, creating a space between the vaginal walls and surface of the cervix called the **vaginal fornix.** Although the space is continuous, it is divided into anterior, posterior, and two lateral fornices.[1]

The two **fallopian tubes** run laterally from the uterus in the upper free margin of the broad ligament. Each tube varies from 7 to 12 cm in length and is divided into intramural, isthmic, ampullary, and infundibular portions.[2] The **intramural** portion, which is approximately 1 cm long, is contained within the muscular wall of the uterus and is the narrowest part of the tube. The **isthmus,** constituting the medial third, is slightly wider, round, cordlike, and continuous with the **ampulla,** which is tortuous and forms approximately one half the length of the tube.[1] The ampulla terminates in the most distal portion, the **infundibulum,** or fimbriated end, which is funnel shaped and opens into the peritoneal cavity (Fig. 16-1).

The **ovaries** are elliptical in shape with the long axis usually oriented vertically. The surface of the ovary is not covered by peritoneum but by a single layer of cuboidal or columnar cells called the **germinal epithelium** that becomes continuous with the peritoneum at the hilum of the ovary. The internal structure of the ovary is divided into an outer cortex and inner medulla. The cortex consists of an interstitial framework, or stroma, which is composed of reticular fibers and spindle-shaped cells and which contains the ovarian follicles and corpus lutea. Beneath the germinal epithelium, the connective tissue of the cortex is condensed to form a fibrous capsule, the **tunica albuginea.** The medulla, which is smaller in volume than the cortex, is composed of fibrous tissue and blood vessels, especially veins. In the nulliparous female, the ovary is located in a depression on the lateral pelvic wall called the **ovarian fossa,** which is bound anteriorly by the obliterated umbilical artery, posteriorly by the ureter and the internal iliac artery, and superiorly by the external iliac vein.[1] The fimbriae of the fallopian tube lie superior and lateral to the ovary. The anterior surface of the ovary is attached to the posterior surface of the broad ligament by a short mesovarium. The lower pole of the ovary is attached to the uterus by the ovarian ligament, whereas the upper pole is attached to the lateral wall of the pelvis by the lateral extension of the broad ligament known as the suspensory (infundibulopelvic) ligament of the ovary. The suspensory ligament contains the ovarian vessels and nerves. These ligaments are not rigid, and therefore the ovary can be quite mobile, especially in women who have had pregnancies.

The **arterial blood supply** to the uterus comes primarily from the **uterine artery,** a major branch of the internal iliac artery. This artery ascends along the lateral margin of the uterus in the broad ligament and, at the level of the uterine cornua, runs laterally to anastomose with the ovarian artery. The uterine arteries anastomose extensively across the midline through the anterior and posterior arcuate arteries, which run within the broad ligament and then enter the myometrium.[1,2] The uterine plexus of veins accompany the arteries. The **ovarian artery** arises from the aorta slightly inferior to the renal arteries. It crosses the external iliac vessels and runs medially within the suspensory ligament of the ovary. After giving off branches to the ovary, it continues medially in the broad ligament to anastomose with the uterine artery. The **ovarian veins** leave the ovarian hilum and form a plexus of veins in the broad ligament that communicate with the uterine plexus of veins. The right ovarian vein drains into the inferior vena cava, whereas the left ovarian vein drains directly into left renal vein.[1]

TECHNIQUE

The standard **transabdominal sonogram** is performed with a distended urinary bladder, which provides an acoustic window to view the pelvic organs and serves as a reference standard for evaluating cystic structures. The distended bladder displaces the bowel

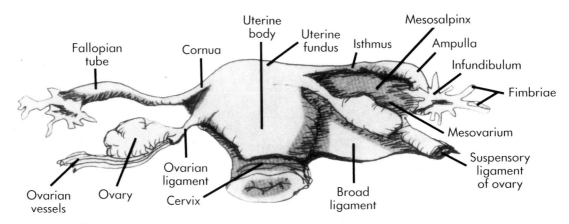

FIG 16-1. Normal gynecologic organs. Diagram of uterus, ovaries, tubes, and related structures. On left side, broad ligament has been removed.
(Courtesy of Jocelyne Salem.)

cephaladly out of the pelvis and displaces the pelvic organs 5 to 10 cm from the anterior abdominal wall. The pelvic organs lie within the focal zone of most 3.5-MHz transducers, which are usually adequate for evaluating the entire pelvis. A 5-MHz transducer may be necessary to identify an ovary that lies anteriorly and away from the uterus. Gentle pressure on the transducer may be necessary to bring the area of interest within the focal zone. The urinary bladder is considered ideally filled when it covers the entire fundus of the uterus. Overdistension may distort the anatomy by compression and may also push the pelvic organs beyond the focal zone

of the transducer, limiting detail. Imaging of the uterus and adnexa is performed in both sagittal and transverse planes. The long axis of the uterus is identified in the sagittal plane and a somewhat oblique angulation may be necessary to visualize the entire uterus and cervix. The adnexae may be imaged by scanning obliquely from the contralateral side, although in many instances visualization can be achieved by scanning directly over the adnexa, especially when an overdistended bladder pushes the adnexae beyond the focal zone of the transducer. The **limitations** of this technique include the examination of patients who are unable to fill their blad-

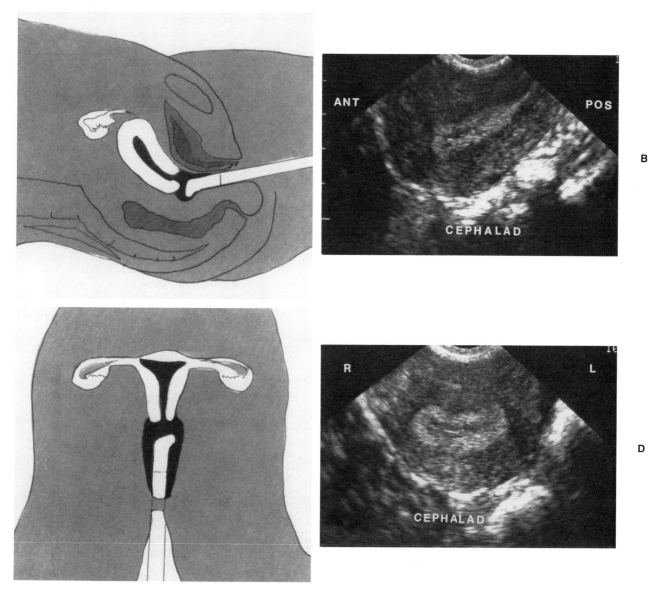

FIG 16-2. Transvaginal sonography orientation. **A,** Illustration of transvaginal scanning in sagittal plane. **B,** Corresponding sagittal sonogram of uterus. **C,** Illustration of transvaginal scanning in coronal plane. **D,** Corresponding coronal sonogram of uterus. *R* indicates right; *L*, left.
(**A** and **C** courtesy of Jocelyne Salem.)

ders, obese patients, and patients with a retroverted uterus in which the fundus may be located beyond the focal zone of the transducer.

For **transvaginal sonography,** the bladder must be empty to bring the pelvic organs into the focal zone of the transvaginal transducer. An empty bladder also provides patient comfort during the examination. Transvaginal transducers range in frequency from 5 to 7.5 MHz and have a focal zone from 1 to 5 cm. The transducer is prepared with ultrasound gel and then covered with a latex condom. An external lubricant is then applied to the outside of the condom. The transducer is inserted into the vagina with the patient in a supine position, with knees gently flexed and hips elevated slightly on a pillow. With gentle rotation and angulation of the transducer, both sagittal and coronal images are obtained. Slight anterior angulation will bring the fundus of an anteverted uterus into view. To visualize the cervix, the transducer must be pulled slightly outward away from the external os. Extreme angulation may be needed to visualize the entire adnexae and cul-de-sac. **Image orientation** may be confusing initially as the sagittal images are displayed 90 degrees counterclockwise from their actual orientation, whereas the coronal scans are similarly rotated in their craniocaudad direction but correctly displayed as to right-left orientation (Fig. 16-2). The main **disadvantage** of this technique is the limited field of view. Large masses may fill the entire field, making orientation difficult, and superiorly placed ovaries may not be visualized. Transvaginal sonography better distinguishes adnexal masses from bowel loops and provides greater detail of the internal characteristics of a pelvic mass because of its improved resolution. Although some authors suggest that transvaginal sonography should be the initial examination method for evaluating the nonpregnant female pelvis,[3] the more accepted current view is to use transvaginal sonography to supplement the transabdominal examination if necessary to establish a more accurate diagnosis.[4-7] The two methods are complimentary, and further experience will undoubtedly establish their individual roles.

UTERUS
Normal Sonographic Anatomy

The uterus lies between the bladder anteriorly and the rectosigmoid colon posteriorly (Fig. 16-3). Uterine position is variable and changes with varying degrees of bladder and rectal distention. The cervix usually lies in the midline, but the fundus may lie obliquely on either side of the midline. In an anteverted uterus, the fundus is usually more anterior in position than appreciated on transabdominal sonograms because the distended bladder displaces the fundus more posteriorly. The uterus may be retroflexed with the body tilted posteriorly (rel-

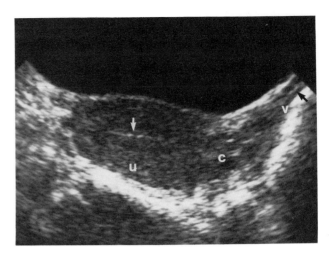

FIG 16-3. Normal uterus *(u)*, cervix *(c)*, and vagina *(v)* sagittal scan. Note thin echogenic menstrual phase endometrium *(white arrow)* and central linear echo, representing apposed surfaces of vaginal mucosa *(black arrow)*.

ative to the cervix) or retroverted when the entire uterus is tilted backwards (relative to the vagina). It is usually difficult to distinguish between these two conditions sonographically. The fundus of a retroverted or retroflexed uterus is frequently difficult to assess by transabdominal sonography. As this portion of the uterus is situated at a distance from the transducer, it may appear hypoechoic and simulate a fibroid. Transvaginal sonography has proved to be excellent for assessing the retroverted or retroflexed uterus because the transducer is in close proximity to the posteriorly located fundus.[8]

The **size** and **shape** of the normal uterus varies throughout life. The infantile uterus ranges from 2 to 3.3 cm in length, with the cervix accounting for two thirds of the total length, and 0.5 to 1 cm in anteroposterior (AP) diameter.[9] The infantile uterus has a tubular or inverse pear-shaped appearance, with the AP diameter of the cervix being greater than that of the fundus.[10] This infantile appearance persists until puberty. In the immediate neonatal period, because of residual maternal hormone stimulation, the neonatal uterus (Fig. 16-4) is approximately 0.6 to 0.9 cm longer and 0.7 to 0.8 cm greater in AP diameter than the infantile uterus.[11] As puberty approaches, the uterus gradually increases in size, with more pronounced growth in the body, to the eventual adult pear-shaped appearance, with the diameter and length of the body being approximately double that of the cervix.[10] The normal postpubertal uterus varies considerably in size. The maximum dimensions of the nulliparous uterus are approximately 8 cm in length by 5 cm in width by 4 cm in AP diameter.[12,13] Multiparity increases the normal size by more than 1 cm in each dimension.[13] The postmenopausal uterus at-

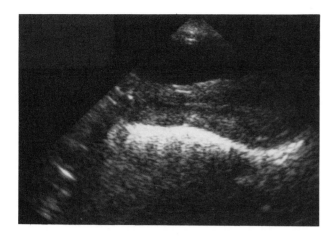

FIG 16-4. Normal neonatal uterus, sagittal scan. Note inverse pear shape with cervix having greater AP diameter and length than body.

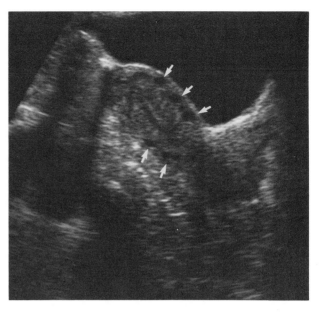

FIG 16-5. Uterine veins. Sagittal scan of normal uterus shows multiple small peripheral anechoic areas *(arrows)*.

rophies in the first 5 to 10 years following cessation of menstruation and ranges from 3.5 to 6.5 cm in length and 1.2 to 1.8 cm in AP diameter in patients over age 65 years.[13]

The normal **myometrium** has a uniformly homogeneous texture of low to moderate echogenicity. Uterine veins may be seen peripherally as small focal anechoic areas (Fig. 16-5) and can be confirmed by Doppler examination.[14,15]

The normal **endometrial cavity** is seen as a thin echogenic line as a result of specular reflection from the interface between the opposing surfaces of the endometrium.[16] The sonographic appearance of the **endome-**

trium varies during the menstrual cycle (Fig. 16-6) and has been correlated with histology.[17-19] The endometrium is composed of a functional and basal layer. The functional layer thickens throughout the menstrual cycle and is shed with each menses. The basal layer remains intact during the cycle and contains vessels that elongate to supply the functional layer as it thickens. The proliferative phase of the cycle before ovulation is under the influence of estrogen, whereas progesterone is mainly responsible for maintenance of the endometrium

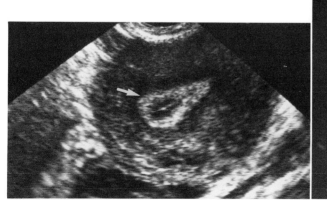

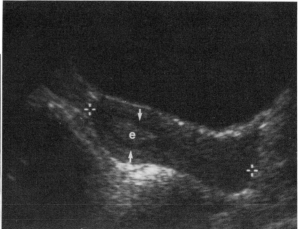

FIG 16-6. Normal endometrium. **A,** Sagittal transvaginal sonogram shows early secretory phase endometrium *(arrow)*. Note inner hypoechoic layer and outer thicker hyperechoic layer. **B,** Sagittal transabdominal scan of uterus (between *asterisks*) shows late secretory phase endometrium *(e)* and thin hypoechoic inner layer of myometrium *(arrows)*.

in the secretory phase following ovulation. The menstrual phase endometrium consists of a thin, broken echogenic line. During the proliferative phase, the endometrium thickens, reaching 2 to 4 mm. The endometrium is best measured on a midline sagittal scan of the uterus. The measurements are taken from the anterior myometrial-endometrial junction to the central cavity echo. If the latter is not seen, the total AP measurement of the endometrium is halved, as this represents two layers of endometrium. A relatively hypoechoic region that represents the functional layer can be seen around the central echogenic line. In the early proliferative phase, this hypoechoic area is thin but increases and becomes more clearly defined in the later proliferative phase, probably as a result of edema. The hypoechoic appearance of the proliferative endometrium has been related to the relatively homogeneous histologic structure because of the orderly arrangement of the glandular elements. Following ovulation, the functional layer of the endometrium changes from hypoechoic to hyperechoic as the endometrium progresses to the secretory phase.[17,18] The endometrium in this phase measures 5 to 6 mm in thickness. The hyperechoic texture in the secretory endometrium is related to increased mucus and glycogen within the glands, as well as the increased number of interfaces caused by the tortuosity of the glands. Acoustic enhancement may be seen posterior to the secretory endometrium; however, it is not specific because it has also been seen with proliferative endometrium, although not as frequently.[18] A thin hypoechoic layer surrounding the relatively echogenic endometrium has been noted and referred to as the subendometrial halo. This most likely represents the compact, relatively hypovascular, inner layer of myometrium.[19,20] The **postmenopausal endometrium** is thin (2 to 3 mm), undergoing atrophy following menopause. In postmenopausal patients an endometrium measuring more than 5 mm should be considered abnormal.[19]

Congenital Abnormalities

Congenital uterine abnormalities occur in approximately 0.5% of females and are associated with an increased incidence of abortion and other obstetric complications.[21] The fused caudal ends of the two müllerian (paramesonephric) ducts form the uterus, cervix and upper vagina, whereas the unfused cranial ends form the paired fallopian tubes. Fusion occurs in a cephalad direction, and the median septum formed by the medial walls of the müllerian ducts resorbs, leaving a single uterine cavity.[2]

Uterine malformations (Fig. 16-7) may be due to either:

- Arrested development of the müllerian ducts
- Failure of fusion of the müllerian ducts
- Failure of resorption of the median septum

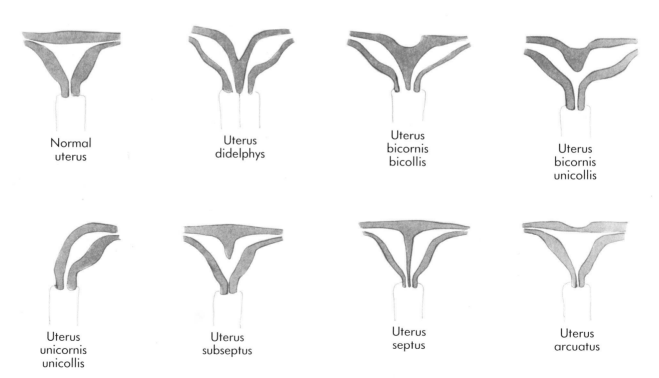

Normal uterus

Uterus didelphys

Uterus bicornis bicollis

Uterus bicornis unicollis

Uterus unicornis unicollis

Uterus subseptus

Uterus septus

Uterus arcuatus

FIG 16-7. Congenital uterine abnormalities. Diagram of common types. (Courtesy of Jocelyne Salem.)

Arrested development of the müllerian ducts may be either unilateral or bilateral. Arrested bilateral development is extremely rare resulting in uterine aplasia. Unilateral arrested development results in a uterus unicornis unicollis (one uterine horn, and one cervix). Hypoplasia of one müllerian duct may result in a rudimentary uterine horn. Most rudimentary horns are noncommunicating and connected to the opposite cornua by fibrous bands. If the endometrium in a rudimentary horn is nonfunctional, no clinical symptoms occur, but if functional endometrium is present, retention of menstrual blood in the rudimentary horn may occur.

Failure of fusion of the müllerian ducts may be complete, resulting in a uterus didelphys (two vaginas, two cervices, and two uteri) or partial, which may result in either a uterus bicornis bicollis (one vagina, two cervices, and two uterine horns) or a uterus bicornis unicollis (one vagina, one cervix, and two uterine horns). Uterus arcuatus is the mildest fusion anomaly, resulting in a partial indentation of the uterine fundus with a relatively normal endometrial cavity and is considered either a very mild form of the bicornuate uterus or a normal variant.

Failure of resorption of the median septum results in a septate or subseptate uterus, depending on whether the failure is complete or partial, respectively. This results in complete or partial duplication of the uterine cavities without duplication of the uterine horns and is the most common uterine abnormality. The septate or subseptate uterus can be distinguished from the bicornuate uterus only by seeing the external contour of the uterus.

There is a high association between uterine malformations and congenital renal abnormalities, especially renal agenesis and ectopia.[22] The most common anomaly associated with renal agenesis is the uterus bicornis bicollis with a partial vaginal septum in which one side has no outlet for menstrual blood, resulting in a unilateral hematometrocolpos.[23] In all patients with uterine malformations, the kidneys should be evaluated sonographically. Also, in females with an absent or ectopic kidney, the uterus should be scanned for malformations. The abnormalities are always on the same side.

Sonography may detect anomalies of the nongravid uterus.[24] Two endometrial echo complexes may be seen in the bicornuate or septate uterus (Fig. 16-8, *A*). Sonography can demonstrate the external contour of the uterus and, in combination with hysterosalpingography, has been shown to be useful in distinguishing between the septate and bicornuate uterus. It is important to differentiate these two conditions as the septated uterus can now be treated by outpatient laparoscopic surgery.[25] The unicornuate uterus is difficult to differentiate from the normal uterus by sonography. It may be suspected when the uterus appears small and laterally positioned. Hydrome-

tra in the opposite rudimentary horn may be seen. If the central endometrial echo complex is not seen in one horn, the bicornuate uterus may be confused with a uterine fibroid or adnexal mass. In many instances, the bicornuate uterus is first diagnosed incidentally in early pregnancy when a gestational sac is present in one horn and decidual reaction in the other (Fig. 16-8, *B*).

Abnormalities of the Myometrium

Leiomyoma (Fibroid). Leiomyomas (Fig. 16-9) are the most common neoplasms of the uterus, occurring in approximately 20% to 30% of females over the age of 30 years.[26] These tumors are more common in black women. They are usually multiple and are the commonest cause of enlargement of the nonpregnant uterus. Although frequently asymptomatic, pain and uterine bleeding may occur. Leiomyomas may be classified as:

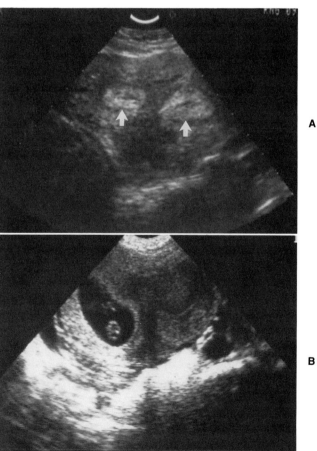

FIG 16-8. Bicornuate uterus. **A,** Transverse scan shows two prominent endometrial echo complexes *(arrows).* **B,** Transverse scan shows gestational sac and embryo in right horn and decidual reaction in left horn.

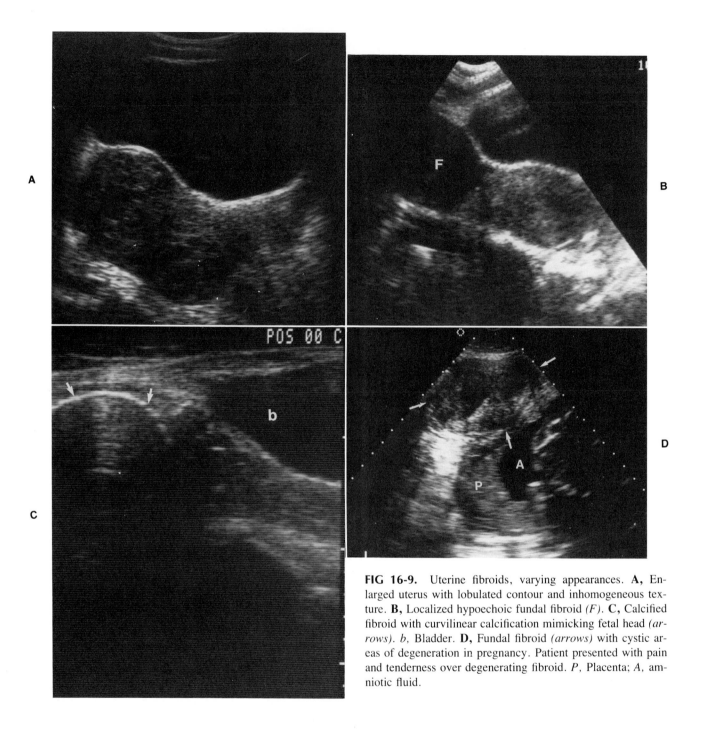

FIG 16-9. Uterine fibroids, varying appearances. **A,** Enlarged uterus with lobulated contour and inhomogeneous texture. **B,** Localized hypoechoic fundal fibroid *(F)*. **C,** Calcified fibroid with curvilinear calcification mimicking fetal head *(arrows)*. *b,* Bladder. **D,** Fundal fibroid *(arrows)* with cystic areas of degeneration in pregnancy. Patient presented with pain and tenderness over degenerating fibroid. *P,* Placenta; *A,* amniotic fluid.

- Intramural: confined to the myometrium
- Submucosal: projecting into the uterine cavity, displacing or distorting the endometrium
- Subserosal: projecting from the peritoneal surface of the uterus

Intramural fibroids are the most common. Submucosal fibroids, although less common, produce symptoms most frequently. Subserosal fibroids may project between the leaves of the broad ligament and are referred to as intraligamentous. Cervical fibroids are uncommon, accounting for less than 3% of fibroids.

Fibroids are estrogen dependent and may increase in size during anovulatory cycles as a result of unopposed estrogen stimulation[27] and during pregnancy, although about half of all fibroids show little significant change during pregnancy.[28] Large fibroids do not interfere with pregnancy and normal vaginal delivery, except when they are located in the lower uterine segment or cervix.

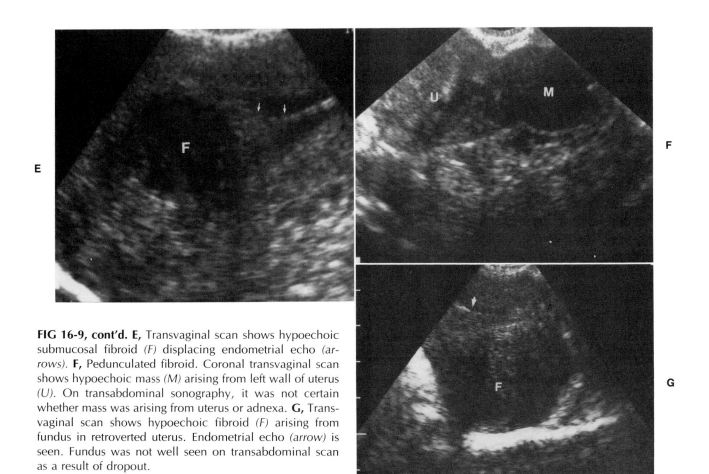

FIG 16-9, cont'd. E, Transvaginal scan shows hypoechoic submucosal fibroid *(F)* displacing endometrial echo *(arrows)*. **F,** Pedunculated fibroid. Coronal transvaginal scan shows hypoechoic mass *(M)* arising from left wall of uterus *(U)*. On transabdominal sonography, it was not certain whether mass was arising from uterus or adnexa. **G,** Transvaginal scan shows hypoechoic fibroid *(F)* arising from fundus in retroverted uterus. Endometrial echo *(arrow)* is seen. Fundus was not well seen on transabdominal scan as a result of dropout.

They rarely develop in postmenopausal women and most stabilize or decrease in size following menopause. Although rare, postmenopausal increase in size should raise the possibility of sarcomatous change.[2]

Sonographically, fibroids have a variable appearance. The uterus may be enlarged with an irregular external contour and inhomogeneous texture. Localized leiomyomata are typically hypoechoic with attenuation of sound caused by the homogeneous composition of fibrous and smooth muscle cells within the tumor. They frequently distort the external contour of the uterus. Minimal contour irregularity at the interface between the uterus and bladder may be a subtle diagnostic sign.[29] **Calcification** may occur in older females, frequently appearing as focal areas of increased echogenicity with shadowing or as a curvilinear echogenic rim, which may simulate the outline of a fetal head.[30] **Degeneration** and **necrosis** produce areas of decreased echogenicity or cystic spaces within the fibroid. This tends to occur more commonly during pregnancy, affecting approximately 7% to 8% of pregnant patients with fibroids, who may present with pain over this area.[28] Submucosal fibroids

may impinge on the endometrium, distorting the lumen. Pedunculated subserosal fibroids may simulate adnexal masses. Transvaginal sonography may be diagnostic by showing the uterine origin of the mass. This technique is also excellent for demonstrating fibroids in the fundus of a retroverted uterus.

Lipomatous Uterine Tumors (Lipoleiomyoma). Lipomatous uterine tumors are uncommon, benign neoplasms consisting of variable portions of mature lipocytes, smooth muscle, or fibrous tissue. Sonographically, the finding of a highly echogenic, attenuating mass within the myometrium is virtually diagnostic of this condition (Fig. 16-10).[31] It is important to identify the lesion within the uterus so as not to confuse it with the more common fat-containing ovarian dermoid. Because lipomatous uterine tumors are usually asymptomatic, they do not require surgery.

Leiomyosarcoma. Leiomyosarcoma is rare, accounting for 1.3% of uterine malignancies, and may arise from a preexisting uterine leiomyoma.[26] Frequently, patients are asymptomatic, although uterine bleeding may occur. This condition is rarely preoperatively diag-

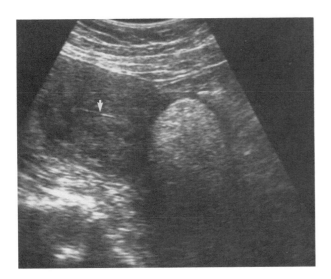

FIG 16-10. Lipoleiomyoma. Sagittal scan shows highly echogenic mass with marked posterior attenuation within myometrium. *Arrow*, Endometrium.

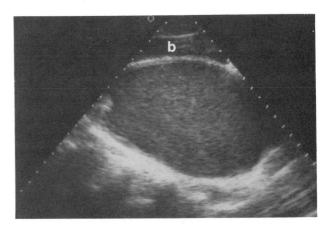

FIG 16-11. Hematocolpos in young patient with imperforate hymen. Sagittal scan shows distended vagina filled with echogenic material compressing bladder *(b)* anteriorly.

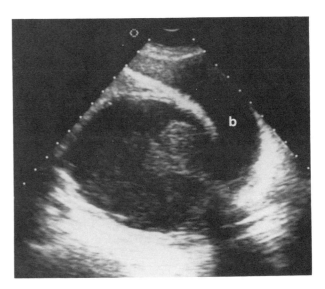

FIG 16-12. Hematometra in patient with cervical stenosis secondary to irradiation. Uterus is distended and filled with echoes of varying intensity as result of blood. *b*, Bladder.

nosed. Sonographically, their appearance is similar to that of a rapidly growing or degenerating fibroid, except when there is evidence of local invasion or distant metastases.

Adenomyosis. Adenomyosis is a form of endometriosis characterized pathologically by the presence of endometrial tissue within the myometrium and uterine enlargement. Adenomyosis is usually most extensive in the posterior wall, leading to thickening of this area. Sonographically, the diagnosis is difficult. It may be suggested if there is diffuse uterine enlargement with a normal contour, normal endometrial, and normal myometrial texture.[32] Thickening of the posterior myometrium, with the involved area being slightly more anechoic than normal myometrium, has also been described.[33] Occasionally, adenomyosis is focal and in these cases is indistinguishable from a leiomyoma. These two conditions frequently occur together.

Abnormalities of the Endometrium

Knowledge of the normal sonographic appearance of the endometrium allows for earlier recognition of endometrial pathologic conditions manifested by endometrial thickening and irregularity or fluid within the endometrial canal. Because of its improved resolution, transvaginal sonography is able to depict subtle abnormalities within the endometrium and clearly define the endometrial-myometrial border.[34]

Hydrometrocolpos and Hematometrocolpos. Obstruction of the genital tract results in the accumulation of secretions, blood, or both within the uterus, vagina, or both—with the location depending on the level of obstruction. Before menstruation, the accumulation of secretions in the vagina and uterus is referred to as **hydrometrocolpos**. Following menstruation, **hematometrocolpos** results from the presence of retained menstrual blood (Fig. 16-11). The obstruction may be congenital and is most commonly due to an imperforate hymen. Other congenital causes include a vaginal septum, vaginal atresia, or rudimentary uterine horn.[35] **Hydrometra** and **hematometra** may also be acquired as a result of cervical stenosis from endometrial or cervical tumors or from postirradiation fibrosis (Fig. 16-12).[36,37]

Sonographically, if the obstruction is at the vaginal level, there is marked distention of the vagina and endometrial cavity with fluid. If seen before puberty, the

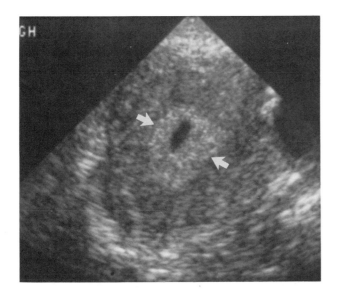

FIG 16-13. Endometrial hyperplasia. Transvaginal scan in postmenopausal patient shows thickened endometrium *(arrows)* with small central fluid collection.

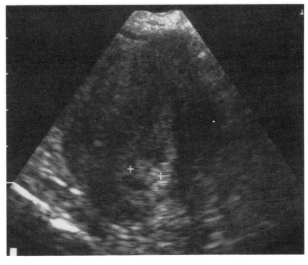

FIG 16-14. Endometrial polyp. Transvaginal scan shows round echogenic polyp (between *cursors*) in endometrial canal.

accumulation of secretions is anechoic. Following menstruation, the presence of old blood results in echogenic material within the fluid. There may also be layering of the echogenic material, resulting in a fluid-fluid level.

Acquired hydrometra usually shows a distended fluid-filled endometrial cavity. Superimposed infection (pyometra) is difficult to distinguish from hydrometra on sonography, and this diagnosis is usually made clinically in the presence of hydrometra.[37]

Endometrial Hyperplasia and Polyps. Hyperplasia of the endometrium is caused by unopposed estrogen stimulation and is the most common cause of uterine bleeding (Fig. 16-13). Endometrial polyps may also cause uterine bleeding in perimenopausal or postmenopausal women, although most are asymptomatic. Malignant degeneration is uncommon. Occasionally, a polyp will have a long stalk, allowing it to protrude into the cervix or even the vagina. Sonographically, these conditions are usually indistinguishable, both showing a thickened endometrium.[38] Occasionally, a polyp may be seen as a discrete mass within the endometrial cavity (Fig. 16-14). Submucosal fibroids may also simulate a polyp, although the use of transvaginal sonography has been helpful in distinguishing these conditions.

Endometritis. Endometritis may occur postpartum or in association with pelvic inflammatory disease (Fig. 16-15). Sonographically, the endometrium may appear prominent, irregular, or both—with or without endometrial fluid.[39] Gas bubbles within the endometrium are diagnostic.

Endometrial Carcinoma. Endometrial carcinoma most commonly occurs in perimenopausal and post-

menopausal women presenting clinically with uterine bleeding. Although the etiologic factors are uncertain, there is a strong association with replacement estrogen therapy.[26] The main sonographic finding is a prominent, thickened endometrium (Fig. 16-16), which usually cannot be differentiated sonographically from endometrial hyperplasia or polyps.[38] Blood within the endometrial cavity, retained products of conception, or an incomplete abortion may produce a similar appearance.[40] Myometrial invasion may be demonstrated with carcinoma.[41,42] Sonography is helpful in staging endometrial carcinoma and distinguishing between tumors limited to the uterus (stage 1 and 2) and those with extrauterine extension (stage 3 and 4).[42,43] Endometrial carcinoma may also obstruct the endometrial canal, resulting in hydrometra or hematometra. In the postmenopausal patient, an endometrium measuring greater than 5 mm should be considered abnormal and warrants further investigation, such as dilatation and curettage.

Intrauterine Contraceptive Devices. Intrauterine contraceptive devices (IUDs) are readily demonstrated on sonography. They appear as a highly echogenic linear structure within the endometrial cavity in the body of the uterus (Fig. 16-17). Several types of IUDs demonstrate a characteristic appearance on sonography, reflecting their gross appearance. One must be able to distinguish the IUD from the normal high-amplitude central endometrial cavity echo. Acoustic shadowing from the IUD is usually demonstrated, and two parallel echoes (entrance-exit reflections), representing the anterior and posterior surfaces of the IUD, may also be observed.[44] Eccentric position of the IUD suggests myo-

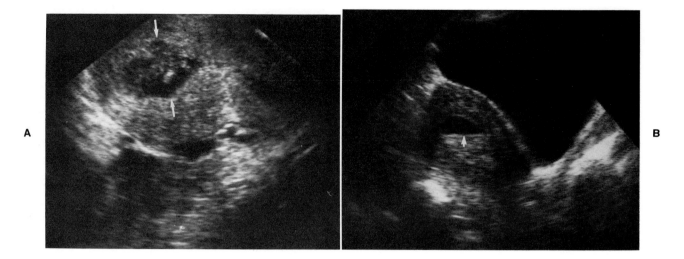

FIG 16-15. Endometritis, varying appearances. A, Transvaginal scan in postpartum patient shows echogenic and anechoic areas within endometrial canal *(arrows)*. B, Sagittal scan in patient with pelvic inflammatory disease shows fluid-fluid level *(arrow)* within endometrial canal. This resolved following antibiotic therapy.

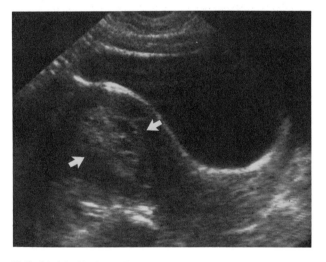

FIG 16-16. Endometrial carcinoma. Sagittal scan in postmenopausal patient with uterine bleeding shows thickened irregular endometrium *(arrows)*.

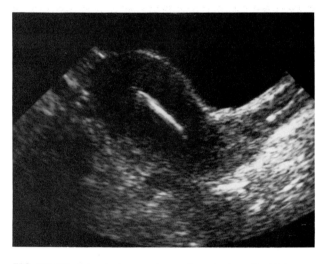

FIG 16-17. Intrauterine contraceptive device. Sagittal scan shows highly echogenic linear structure within endometrial cavity in body of uterus.

metrial penetration. If the IUD is not seen on sonography, a radiograph should be taken to assess whether the IUD is lying free in the peritoneal cavity or is not present, having been previously expelled. The IUD may be hidden by coexisting intrauterine abnormalities such as blood clots or incomplete abortion. When an IUD is present in the uterus in association with an intrauterine pregnancy, the IUD can reliably be seen early in the first trimester, but it is rarely identified thereafter.

Abnormalities of the Cervix

Cervical abnormalities are usually diagnosed clinically. **Retention (nabothian) cysts** of the cervix are commonly seen during routine sonography (Fig. 16-18). They may vary in size from a few millimeters to 4 cm. They may be single or multiple and are usually diagnosed incidentally, but they may be associated with healing chronic cervicitis. Multiple cysts may be a cause of benign enlargement of the cervix.[45]

Cervical carcinoma is usually diagnosed clinically,

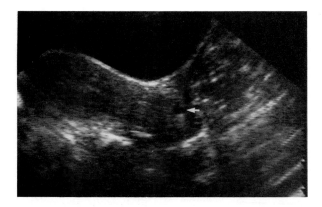

FIG 16-18. Nabothian cyst. Sagittal scan shows small cyst *(arrow)* in cervix.

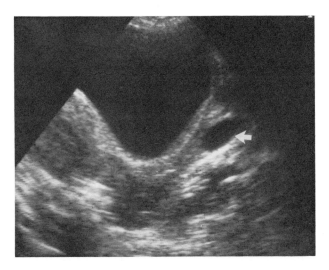

FIG 16-19. Gartner's duct cyst. Sagittal scan shows cystic mass *(arrow)* in vaginal wall.

and patients are rarely referred for sonographic evaluation. Sonography may demonstrate a solid retrovesical mass, which may be indistinguishable from a cervical fibroid. Hydrometra or hematometra caused by obstruction from cervical carcinoma may be seen. Sonography may be used for staging, but computed tomography (CT) and magnetic resonance imaging (MRI) are preferable.

VAGINA

The vagina runs anteriorly and caudally from the cervix between the bladder and rectum. It is best seen sonographically on midline sagittal sections with slight caudal angulation of the transducer. It appears as a collapsed tubular structure with a central high-amplitude linear echo representing the apposed surfaces of the vaginal mucosa (Fig. 16-2). Occasionally, sonography is used to characterize a vaginal mass. **Gartner's duct cysts** are mesonephric duct remnants that form single or multiple cysts along the lateral or anterolateral wall of the vagina (Fig. 16-19). These are the most common cystic lesions of the vagina and are usually found incidentally during sonographic examination. The most common congenital abnormality of the female genital tract is an imperforate hymen, resulting in hematocolpos. **Solid masses** of the vagina are rare (Fig. 16-20). Two cases of neurofibroma of the vagina that appear as solid masses have been described.[46] As in carcinoma of the cervix, sonography is not used for diagnosis of carcinoma of the vagina, but it may play a role in staging.

RECTOUTERINE RECESS (POSTERIOR CUL-DE-SAC)

The **posterior cul-de-sac** is the most posterior and inferior reflection of the peritoneal cavity located between the rectum and vagina and is also known as the *pouch of Douglas*. This is a potential space, and because of its location, it is frequently the initial site for

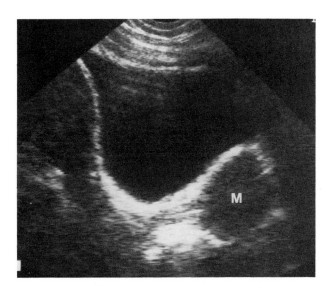

FIG 16-20. Solid mass *(M)* in vagina seen on sagittal scan. At surgery, this was located along anterior wall of vagina and, pathologically, was uterine fibroid.

intraperitoneal fluid collection. As little as 5 cc of fluid has been detected by transvaginal sonography.[47]

Fluid in the cul-de-sac is a normal finding in asymptomatic women and can be seen during all phases of the menstrual cycle. Possible sources have been postulated, including blood or fluid caused by follicular rupture, blood caused by retrograde menstruation, and increased capillary permeability of the ovarian surface caused by the influence of estrogen.[48]

Pathologic fluid collections in the pouch of Douglas may be seen in association with generalized ascites, blood resulting from a ruptured ectopic pregnancy or

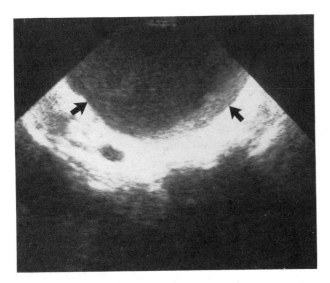

FIG 16-21. Echogenic ascites in cul-de-sac. Transvaginal sonogram in patient with mucinous cystadenocarcinoma of ovary shows fluid with echoes *(arrows)*, which represent mucin.

hemorrhagic cyst, or pus resulting from infection. Sonography may aid in differentiating the type of fluid because blood, pus, and mucin contain echoes within the fluid, whereas serous fluid (either physiologic or pathologic) is usually anechoic. Clotted blood may be very echogenic.[49] Transvaginal sonography can demonstrate echoes within the fluid more frequently because of its improved resolution (Fig. 16-21).

Pelvic abscesses and hematomas can occur in the cul-de-sac, and the sonographic appearance is similar to these conditions elsewhere in the body.

OVARY
Normal Sonographic Anatomy

Uterine location influences the position of the ovaries. The normal ovaries are usually identified laterally or posterolaterally to the anteflexed midline uterus. When the uterus lies to one side of the midline, the ipsilateral ovary often lies superior to the uterine fundus. In a retroverted uterus, the ovaries tend to be located laterally and superiorly, near the uterine fundus. Because of the laxity of the ligamentous attachments, the ovary can be quite variable in position and may be located high in the pelvis or in the cul-de-sac. The ovaries are ellipsoid in shape, with their craniocaudad axes paralleling the internal iliac vessels, which lie posteriorly and serve as a helpful reference (Fig. 16-22). In patients with uterine leiomyomas, the ovaries have been more frequently visualized by transvaginal sonography than by the transabdominal method.[3,8]

The normal ovary has a relatively homogeneous echo texture with a central, more echogenic medulla.

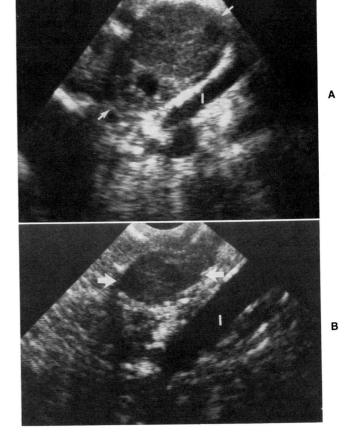

FIG 16-22. Normal ovaries, varying appearance. **A,** Transvaginal scan in menstruating female shows ovary *(arrows)* with single dominant follicle. Internal iliac vein *(I)* is seen posterior to ovary. **B,** Transvaginal scan shows normal postmenopausal ovary *(arrows)*. Note small size and lack of follicles. This ovary measured 1.9 × 1.4 × 1.3 cm, giving volume of 1.8 cc.

Well-defined small anechoic or cystic follicles may be seen peripherally in the cortex. The appearance of the ovary changes with age and phase of the menstrual cycle. During the early proliferative phase, many follicles that are stimulated by both follicle-stimulating hormone (FSH) and luteinizing hormone (LH) develop and increase in size until about day 8 or 9 of the menstrual cycle. At that time one follicle becomes dominant, destined for ovulation, and increases in size, reaching up to 2 to 2.5 cm at the time of ovulation. The other follicles become atretic. A **follicular cyst** develops if the fluid in one of these nondominant follicles is not resorbed. Following ovulation, the corpus luteum develops and may be identified sonographically as a small cystic structure peripherally. The corpus luteum involutes before menstruation.

Because of the variability in shape, ovarian volume has been considered the best method for determining ovarian size. The volume measurement is based on the formula for a prolate ellipse ($0.523 \times$ length $\times$ width $\times$ height). Ovarian volume is less than 1 cc in children under 5 years of age and gradually increases in size until menarche, when the mean volume is 4.2 ± 2.3 cc.[10] In the adult menstruating female, an ovarian volume of 6 cc has been accepted as the upper limit of normal until recently. It has now been shown that the normal ovary may be much larger with a mean volume of 10.0 ± 3.9 cc.[50] A recent study of 866 normal ovaries in this age group reported a mean ovarian volume of 9.8 ± 5.8 cc.[51] Thus a normal ovary may have a volume as large as 15 cc.

Following menopause, the ovary atrophies, with the disappearance of follicles over the next few years, and may be difficult to visualize sonographically. In the postmenopausal patient, the upper limit of ovarian volume has been stated to be 2.5 cc,[52] although a recent study in 220 patients using transvaginal sonography has reported a mean ovarian volume of 2.9 ± 2.2 cc.[53]

Nonneoplastic Lesions

Polycystic Ovarian Disease. Polycystic ovarian disease (PCOD) is a complex endocrinologic disorder resulting in chronic anovulation. An imbalance of LH and FSH results in abnormal estrogen and androgen production.[54] Pathologically, the ovaries contain an increased number of follicles in various stages of maturation and atresia, and there is an increased local concentration of androgens, producing stromal abnormality. The classic Stein-Leventhal syndrome (oligomenorrhea, hirsutism, obesity) is only one form in the spectrum of clinical manifestations of polycystic ovarian disease.

The classic sonographic findings are those of bilaterally enlarged ovaries containing multiple small follicles (Fig. 16-23). The follicles measure from 0.5 to 0.8 cm in size with more than five in each ovary.[55] However, these typical findings are seen in less than half the patients with this condition. Ovarian volume is normal in approximately 30%.[55,56] In one of these studies, discrete follicles could not be seen in slightly less than half of the remaining patients with enlarged ovaries. This was postulated to be due to the tiny size of the follicles, which were beyond the limit of resolution by transabdominal scanning.[56] Because of its superior resolution, transvaginal sonography may, indeed, demonstrate these follicles in a higher percentage of patients. Because ovulation does not occur, the follicles will persist on serial studies. Long-term follow-up is recommended in these patients because the unopposed high estrogen levels appear to be associated with an increased risk of endometrial and breast carcinoma.[54]

Functional Cysts. Functional cysts of the ovary in-

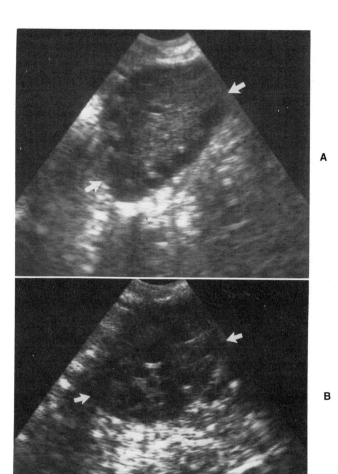

FIG 16-23. Polycystic ovarian disease, varying appearances. **A,** Transvaginal sonography shows enlarged ovary *(arrows)* with multiple peripheral cysts: "string of pearls" sign. **B,** Enlarged ovary *(arrows)* with multiple cysts throughout the ovary.

clude follicular, corpus luteum, and theca-lutein cysts. A **follicular cyst** occurs when a mature follicle fails to ovulate or to involute. Follicular cysts range from 1 to 20 cm in size. However, because normal follicles can vary from a few millimeters to 2 cm and reach up to 2.5 cm at maturity, a follicular cyst cannot be diagnosed with certainty until it is greater than 2.5 cm.[54] They are usually unilateral, asymptomatic, and frequently detected incidentally on sonographic examination. Follicular cysts usually regress spontaneously.

The **corpus luteal cyst** results from the failure of absorption or excess bleeding into the corpus luteum. They are less common than follicular cysts but tend to be larger and more symptomatic. Pain is the major symptom. These cysts are usually unilateral and more prone to hemorrhage and rupture. If the ovum is fertilized, the corpus luteum continues as the corpus luteum of pregnancy, which may become enlarged and cystic. Maximum size is reached at about 8 to 10 weeks and by 16 weeks the cyst has usually resolved.

Sonographically these functional cysts are typically unilocular, anechoic structures with well-defined thin walls and posterior acoustic enhancement. Internal hemorrhage may occur in both types, although it is much more frequently seen in corpus luteum cysts. Hemorrhagic cysts may show a spectrum of findings as a result of the variable sonographic appearance of blood.[57] There may be septations and internal echoes of varying echogenicity (Fig. 16-24). Rupture of a hemorrhagic cyst may mimic a ruptured ectopic pregnancy, both clinically and sonographically.

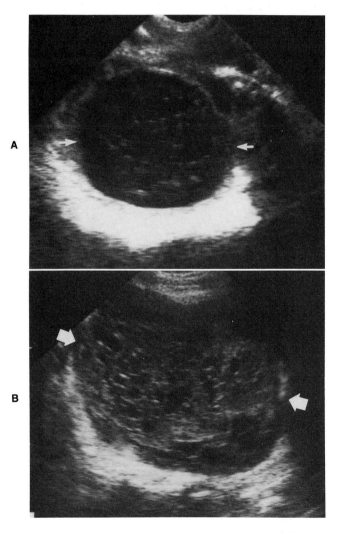

FIG 16-24. Hemorrhagic cysts. **A,** Transvaginal scan shows well-defined adnexal mass *(arrows)* containing low-level internal echoes. There is posterior acoustic enhancement indicating cystic nature of mass. **B,** Transabdominal scan shows large 10-cm echogenic adnexal mass *(arrows)* containing multiple internal echoes interspersed with small cystic spaces. Pathologically, this was large hemorrhagic ovarian cyst.

Functional cysts are the most common cause of ovarian enlargement in young women.[54] Because most functional cysts regress within a short time period the patient should be reexamined at different times of the menstrual cycle or during a subsequent cycle to show a changing appearance or resolution.

Theca-luteal cysts are the largest of the functional cysts and are associated with high levels of human chorionic gonadotropin (HCG). These cysts typically occur in patients with gestational trophoblastic disease but can also be seen in the ovarian hyperstimulation syndrome as a complication of drug therapy for infertility. Sonographically theca-luteal cysts are usually bilateral, multilocular, and very large. They may undergo hemorrhage, rupture, and torsion.

Ovarian Remnant Syndrome. Infrequently, a cystic mass may be encountered in a patient who has undergone bilateral oophorectomy in which a small amount of residual ovarian tissue has been left behind. The surgery has usually been technically difficult because of adhesions from endometriosis, pelvic inflammatory disease, or tumor. The residual ovarian tissue is hormonally stimulated and results in a functional hemorrhagic cyst.[58]

Parovarian Cysts. Parovarian cysts, which account for about 10% of all adnexal masses, are found in the broad ligament and are usually of mesothelial or paramesonephric origin.[59] They vary in size and sonographically have the typical appearance of a cyst. Some cysts may contain internal echoes as a result of hemorrhage.[60] They may undergo torsion and rupture similar to other cystic masses. Parovarian cysts show no cyclic changes. A specific diagnosis is not possible unless a normal ovary is seen separate from the cyst.

Postmenopausal Adnexal Cysts. An adnexal cyst in a postmenopausal woman cannot represent a physiologic cyst because there is no longer sufficient estrogen activity (Fig. 16-25). For many years, their presence had been considered an indication for surgery because a malignant lesion could not be excluded. However, recent studies have shown a low incidence of malignancy in unilocular postmenopausal cysts that measure less than 5 cm in diameter and are without septations or solid components.[61,62] It is now recommended that affected patients be followed by serial sonographic examination without surgical intervention unless there is a change in the size or character of the lesion.[62]

Endometriosis. Endometriosis is defined as the presence of functioning endometrial tissue outside the uterus. Endometriosis most commonly affects the ovary, fallopian tube, broad ligament, and posterior cul-de-sac, but it can occur almost anywhere in the body, including the bladder and bowel. Two forms have been described: diffuse and localized (endometrioma). The diffuse form, which is more common, con-

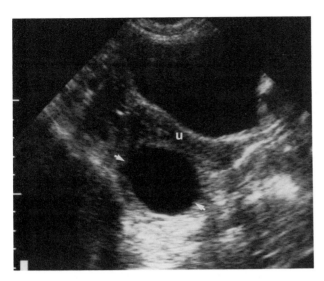

FIG 16-25. Postmenopausal ovarian cyst. Sagittal scan in 75-year-old woman shows 4-cm ovarian cyst *(arrows)* posterior to uterus *(u)*. Cyst contains no internal echoes or septations and had not changed in size over 2 years.

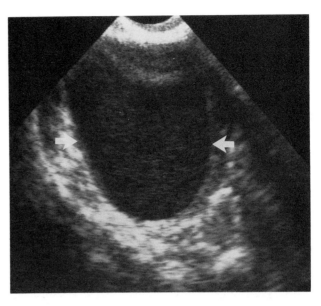

FIG 16-26. Endometrioma. Transvaginal scan shows cystic adnexal mass *(arrows)* filled with low-level internal echoes.

sists of minute endometrial implants involving the pelvic viscera and their ligamentous attachments. The ectopic endometrium is hormonally responsive and undergoes bleeding during the menses, resulting in a local inflammatory reaction with adhesions.[63] This diffuse form is rarely diagnosed by sonography because the implants are too small to be imaged.[64] Clinical symptoms include dysmenorrhea, dyspareunia, and infertility.

The localized form consists of a discrete mass referred to as an **endometrioma,** or chocolate cyst (Fig. 16-26). Endometriomas are usually asymptomatic and may be multiple. The sonographic findings are those of a well-defined predominantly cystic mass, which may contain diffuse low-level internal echoes, frequently located in the dependent portion. Occasionally, a fluid-debris level can be seen. The appearance is similar to a hemorrhagic ovarian cyst because both are cystic masses that contain blood of variable age.[65] Endometriomas showing less typical features may be confused with an ovarian cystadenoma or tuboovarian abscess.

Torsion of the Ovary. Torsion of the ovary is an acute abdominal condition, requiring prompt surgical intervention. It is caused by partial or complete rotation of the ovarian pedicle on its axis. This results in compromise of the arterial supply and venous drainage, causing massive congestion of the ovarian parenchyma and eventual hemorrhagic infarction.[66] Torsion usually occurs in childhood and adolescence and may occur in normal ovaries but is more common in association with ovarian cysts or tumors. Clinically, there is severe pelvic pain, nausea, and vomiting. A palpable mass may be present. Sonographically, the finding of a unilater-

ally enlarged ovary with multiple cortical follicles is considered a specific sign (Fig. 16-27).[66] The multifollicular enlargement is the result of transudation of fluid into the follicles from the circulatory impairment. Duplex Doppler examination may confirm the diagnosis by demonstrating absent blood flow within the ovary.

Massive Edema of the Ovary. This is a rare condition resulting from incomplete torsion of the ovary, causing partial venous and lymphatic obstruction but not arterial occlusion. The few sonographic descriptions show an enlarged hypoechoic ovary secondary to edema.[67]

Neoplasms

Ovarian cancer represents 25% of all gynecologic malignancies, with its peak incidence occurring in the sixth decade of life. It is the third most common gynecologic malignancy, but it has the highest mortality rate as a result of late diagnosis. Because there are few clinical symptoms, approximately 60% to 70% of patients have distant metastases at the time of diagnosis. The overall 5-year-survival rate is 20% to 30%, but with early detection in stage 1, this rises to 80%. Therefore efforts have been directed at developing methods of early diagnosis of this condition. These have focused on transabdominal ultrasound alone[68] and in combination with biologic tumor markers, especially serum CA 125.[69,70] These latter studies have shown that, in a postmenopausal patient, an elevated CA 125 level associated with an ovarian mass is highly specific for malignancy. More recently, transvaginal sonography has been used as a screening method.[53] However, not all

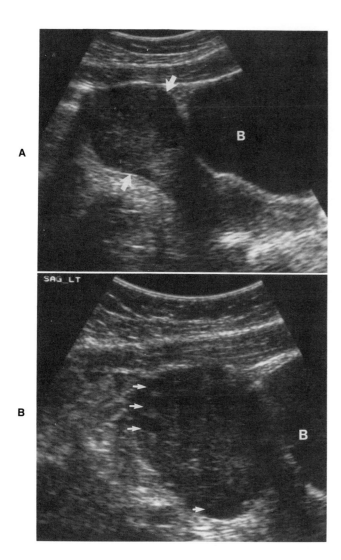

FIG 16-27. Ovarian torsion in 16-year-old girl presenting with acute left-sided lower abdominal pain. **A,** Sagittal scan shows large left-sided adnexal mass *(arrows)*. **B,** Magnified view shows the mass containing multiple peripheral anechoic follicles *(arrows)*. *B,* Bladder.

■ **TABLE 16-1**
Histologic Outline of Ovarian Neoplasms

Type	Incidence (%)	Example
I Epithelial tumors	65-75	Serous cystadenoma (carcinoma)
		Mucinous cystadenoma (carcinoma)
		Endometrioid carcinoma
		Clear cell carcinoma
		Brenner tumor
II Germ cell tumors	15	Teratoma
		Dermoid
		Immature
		Dysgerminoma
		Endodermal sinus tumor
III Sex cord-stromal tumors	5-10	Granulosa cell tumor
		Sertoli-Leydig cell tumor
		Thecoma and fibroma
IV Metastatic tumors	10	Genital primary
		Uterus
		Extragenital primary
		Stomach
		Colon
		Breast
		Lymphoma

postmenopausal ovaries are seen by this method. In a recent study of 67 postmenopausal ovaries, 22% were not visualized by transvaginal sonography.[71]

Histologically, epithelial neoplasms comprise 65% to 75% of ovarian tumors and 90% of ovarian malignancies.[26] The remaining neoplasms consist of germ cell tumors (15%), sex cord-stromal tumors (5% to 10%) and metastatic tumors (10%) (Table 16-1). Sonography reflects the gross morphologic condition of the tumor but not the histology. Therefore it has been difficult to distinguish benign from malignant ovarian tumors by sonography. Well-defined anechoic lesions are more likely to be benign, whereas lesions with less distinct margins, increased echogenicity, and inhomo-geneity favor malignancy. The exception to this is the very echogenic benign teratoma.[72] It has recently been suggested that transvaginal color flow Doppler imaging may be of value in distinguishing malignant from benign lesions, based on neovascularity and a low-pulsatility index.[73]

If a pelvic mass is suspected of being malignant, the abdomen should also be evaluated for evidence of ascites and peritoneal implants, obstructive uropathy, lymphadenopathy, and hepatic and splenic metastases. Hepatic and splenic metastases are uncommon with ovarian carcinoma, but when they occur, they are usually peripheral on the surface of the liver or spleen as a result of peritoneal implants. Hematogenous metastases within the liver or splenic parenchyma may occur late in the course of the disease.

Epithelial Tumors. Epithelial tumors are generally considered to arise from the surface epithelium that covers the ovary and the underlying ovarian stroma. The spread is primarily intraperitoneal, although direct extension to contiguous structures and lymphatic spread are not uncommon. Lymphatic spread is predominantly to the paraortic nodes. Hematogenous spread usually occurs late in the course of the disease.

Serous Cystadenoma and Cystadenocarcinoma. Serous tumors are the most common, comprising 30% of all

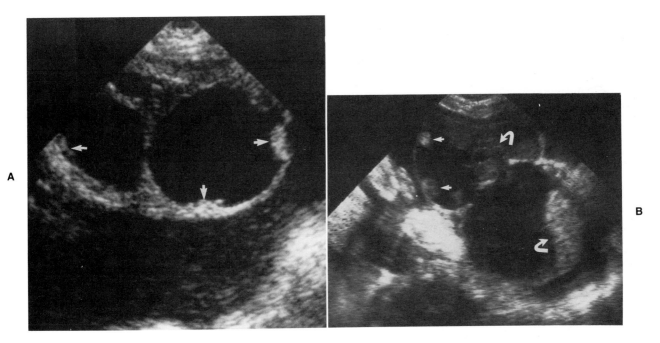

FIG 16-28. Serous cystadenocarcinoma, typical appearances. **A,** Transvaginal scan shows septated cystic mass in right ovary containing multiple small mural nodules *(arrows).* Transabdominal scan showed only septated cystic mass without evidence of nodules. **B,** Transabdominal scan shows large septated ovarian mass containing echogenic mural nodules *(arrows)* and solid areas *(curved arrows).*

ovarian neoplasms. Serous cystadenomas account for 20% of all benign ovarian neoplasms, and serous cystadenocarcinomas account for 40% of all malignant ovarian neoplasms.[26] Approximately 20% of cystadenomas and 50% of cystadenocarcinomas are bilateral. Their size varies greatly, but in general, they are smaller than mucinous tumors.

Sonographically, serous cystadenomas are usually large, thin-walled, unilocular cystic masses, that may contain thin septations. Papillary projections are occasionally seen. Serous cystadenocarcinomas may be quite large and usually present as multilocular cystic masses containing multiple papillary projections, arising from the cyst walls, and septae (Fig. 16-28). The septae and walls may be thick. Echogenic solid material may be seen within the loculations. Papillary projections may form on the surface of the cyst and surrounding organs, resulting in fixation of the mass. Ascites is frequently seen.

Mucinous Cystadenoma and Cystadenocarcinoma. Mucinous tumors are the second most common ovarian epithelial tumor, accounting for 20% of ovarian neoplasms. Mucinous cystadenomas constitute 20% of all benign ovarian neoplasms, and mucinous cystadenocarcinomas make up 6% to 10% of all primary malignant ovarian neoplasms.[26] They are less frequently bilateral than their serous counterparts, with only 5% of the benign and 25% of the malignant lesions occurring on both sides. The benign tumor is approximately seven times as common as the malignant form.

On sonographic examination, mucinous cystadenomas can be huge, measuring up to 15 to 30 cm and filling the entire pelvis and abdomen (Fig. 16-29). Multiple septae are present and low-level echoes caused by mucin may be seen in the dependent portions of the mass. Papillary projections are less frequently seen than in the serous counterpart. Mucinous cystadenocarcinomas are usually large multiloculated cystic masses containing papillary projections and echogenic material and generally have a similar sonographic appearance to serous cystadenocarcinomas (Fig. 16-30).

Penetration of the tumor capsule or rupture may lead to intraperitoneal spread of mucin-secreting cells, which fill the peritoneal cavity with a gelatinous material. This condition, known as **pseudomyxoma peritonei,** is similar sonographically to ascites, although septations and low-level echogenic material may be seen within the fluid (Fig. 16-31). This occurs in 2% to 5% of mucinous cystadenomas, but it can also be seen in cystadenocarcinomas.[74]

Endometrioid Tumor. Endometrioid tumors are nearly all malignant. They are the second most common epithelial malignancy, comprising approximately 20% of ovarian malignancies.[26] Approximately 30% to 50% are

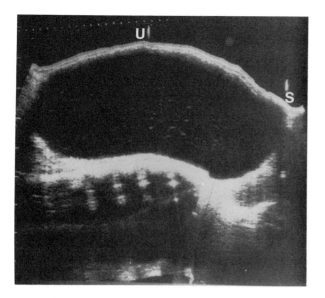

FIG 16-29. Mucinous cystadenoma. Sagittal scan shows huge cystic mass filling pelvis and abdomen. There are multiple low-level echoes seen within dependent portion of mass caused by mucin. *S*, symphysis pubis; *U*, umbilicus.

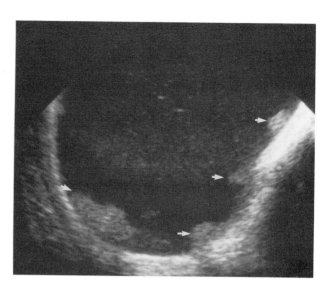

FIG 16-30. Mucinous cystadenocarcinoma. Large adnexal mass containing multiple low-level echoes and solid mural nodules *(arrows)* is seen on transvaginal scan.

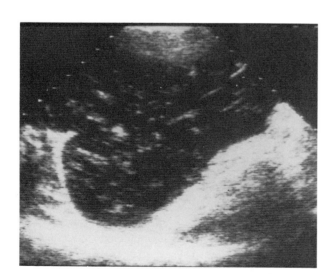

FIG 16-31. Pseudomyxoma peritonei. Transabdominal scan of lower abdomen shows ascites with multiple septations and echoes within ascitic fluid.

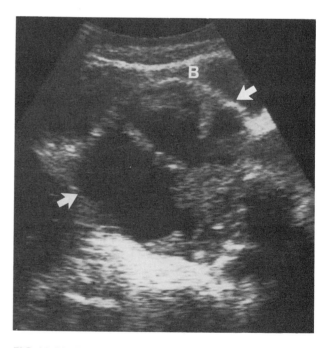

FIG 16-32. Endometrioid carcinoma. Transverse scan shows large complex predominantly cystic mass *(arrows)* compressing bladder *(B)*. Mass contains thick septations and solid echogenic areas.

bilateral. Their histologic characteristics are identical to endometrial adenocarcinoma, and 30% of patients with this condition have associated endometrial adenocarcinoma, which is thought to represent an independent primary tumor. Endometrioid tumors have a better prognosis than other epithelial neoplasms, which is probably related to diagnosis at an earlier stage. Sonographically, they usually present as a cystic mass containing papillary projections (Fig. 16-32), although in some cases a predominantly solid mass is seen, except for areas of hemorrhage or necrosis.[74]

Clear Cell Carcinoma. This tumor is considered to be of müllerian duct origin and a variant of endometrioid carcinoma. It constitutes 5% to 10% of primary ovarian carcinomas and is bilateral in about 40% of patients. Sonographically, it presents as a nonspecific complex mass that can be either cystic or solid.[74]

Brenner Tumor. Brenner tumors are rarely malignant and are uncommon, accounting for 1% to 2% of all ovarian neoplasms. Approximately 6.5% are bilateral. Most patients are asymptomatic, and the tumor is discovered incidently on sonographic examination or at surgery. Thirty percent are associated with cystic neoplasms, usually serous or mucinous cystadenomas or cystic teratomas, frequently in the ipsilateral ovary.[75] Sonographically, Brenner tumors are hypoechoic solid masses (Fig. 16-33) that may contain calcification. Cystic areas may occasionally be seen. Pathologically, they are solid tumors composed of dense fibrous stroma. They appear similar to ovarian fibromas and thecomas or uterine leiomyomas, both sonographically and pathologically.

Germ Cell Tumors

Teratoma. Cystic teratomas make up approximately 10% to 15% of ovarian neoplasms, and 10% to 15% are bilateral. Because ectodermal elements generally predominate, they are virtually always benign and are also called **dermoid cysts.** In contrast to epithelial tumors, they are more commonly seen in the active reproductive

years, but they can occur at any age. They have an extremely variable sonographic appearance (Fig. 16-34). A predominantly cystic mass with an echogenic mural nodule, the "dermoid plug," is considered specific.[76] The dermoid plug usually contains hair, teeth, or fat and frequently casts an acoustic shadow. Correlation with CT images has shown that in many cases the cystic component represents pure sebum, which is liquid at body temperature, rather than fluid.[77] A mixture of matted hair and sebum is highly echogenic because of multiple tissue interfaces and produces ill-defined acoustic shadowing obscuring the posterior wall of the lesion. This has been termed the "tip of the iceberg" sign.[78] A fat-fluid or hair-fluid level may be seen and is also considered specific. An echogenic dermoid may appear similar to bowel gas and may be overlooked. If a definite pelvic mass is clinically palpable and the sonogram appears normal, the patient should be reexamined, looking carefully for a dermoid.

Struma ovarii is a teratoma in which thyroid tissue predominates. Although associated hormonal effects are rare, sonography may be valuable in identifying a pelvic lesion in a hyperthyroid patient when there is no evidence of a thyroid lesion in the neck.[79]

Immature teratomas represent less than 1% of all teratomas and contain immature tissue from all three germ cell layers. They are rapidly growing malignant tumors that most commonly occur in the first two decades of life.

Dysgerminoma. Dysgerminomas are malignant germ cell tumors, constituting approximately 1% to 2% of primary ovarian neoplasms and 3% to 5% of ovarian malignancies.[26] They are composed of undifferentiated germ cells and are morphologically identical to the male testicular seminoma. They are highly radiosensitive with a 5-year-survival rate of 75% to 90%. This tumor occurs predominantly in young women of less than 30 years of age and is bilateral in approximately 15% of cases. The dysgerminoma and the serous cystadenoma are the two most common ovarian neoplasms seen in pregnancy.[74] Sonographically, they are solid masses that are predominantly echogenic but may contain small anechoic areas caused by hemorrhage or necrosis (Fig. 16-35).

Endodermal Sinus (Yolk Sac) Tumor. This rare, rapidly growing tumor with a poor prognosis usually occurs in young females of less than 20 years of age. Increased levels of serum α-fetoprotein (AFP) may be seen in association with this tumor. The sonographic appearance is similar to that of the dysgerminoma.[74]

Sex Cord-Stromal Tumors

Granulosa Cell Tumor. These tumors comprise approximately 2% of ovarian neoplasms and have a low malignancy potential. The majority occur in postmenopausal women, and 95% are unilateral. They are the most

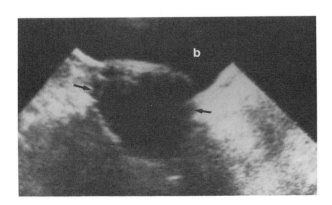

FIG 16-33. Brenner tumor. Sagittal scan shows solid anechoic mass *(arrows)* with posterior attenuation. *b,* Bladder.

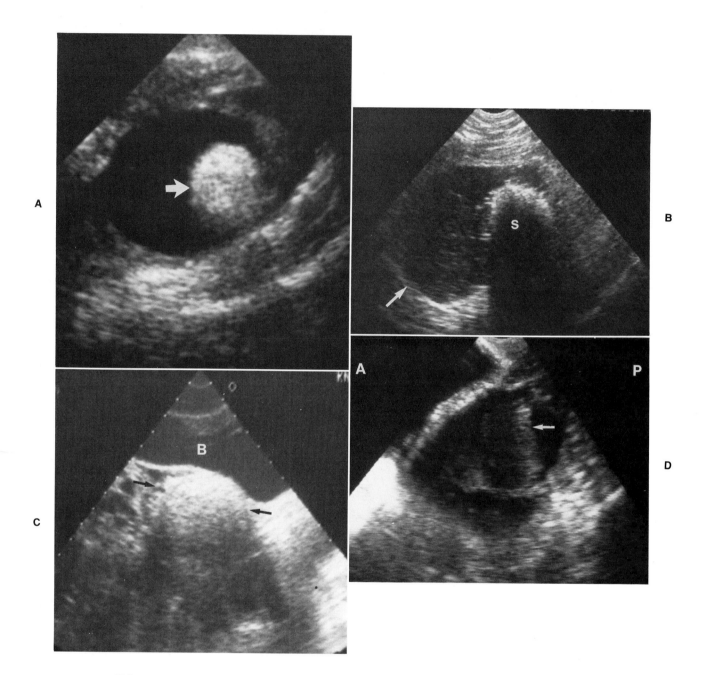

FIG 16-34. Cystic teratomas (dermoid cysts). **A,** Cystic mass with solid echogenic mural nodule *(arrow)*; dermoid plug is seen on transvaginal scan. **B,** Transabdominal scan shows echogenic ovarian mass *(arrow)* containing area of high-amplitude echogenicity with posterior acoustic shadowing *(S)*. **C,** Transabdominal sagittal scan shows highly echogenic mass *(arrows)* with ill-defined posterior shadowing: "tip of the iceberg" sign. Mass shows slight indentation on posterior aspect of bladder *(B)*. This mass could easily be missed and mistaken for bowel gas. **D,** Transvaginal sagittal scan shows mass with hair-fluid level *(arrow)*. Hair-fluid level lies in vertical direction on transvaginal scanning. *A,* Anterior; *P,* posterior.

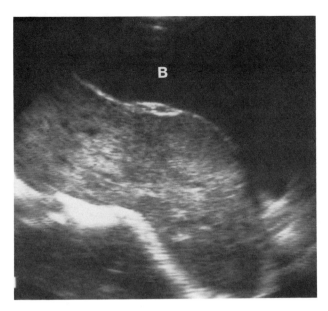

FIG 16-35. Dysgerminoma. Sagittal scan in 16-year-old girl shows large echogenic solid pelvic mass posterior to bladder *(B)*.

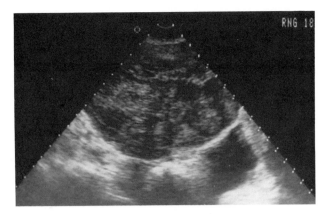

FIG 16-36. Sertoli-Leydig cell tumor. Transabdominal scan shows large inhomogeneous echogenic adnexal mass.

common estrogenically active ovarian tumor.[26] Clinical signs of estrogen production can occur and approximately 10% to 15% of patients with this tumor eventually develop endometrial carcinoma. Sonographically, these tumors vary from small to very large masses. The small masses are predominantly solid, having a similar echogenicity to uterine fibroids. The larger masses are multiloculated and cystic, having a similar appearance to cystadenomas.[74]

Sertoli-Leydig Cell Tumor (Androblastoma). These are rare tumors, constituting less than 0.5% of ovarian neoplasms. They generally occur in women under 30 years of age, and almost all are unilateral. Malignancy occurs in 10% to 20% of these tumors. Clinically, signs and symptoms of masculinization occur in many patients, although others have no endocrine effect or effects may be associated with estrogen production. Sonographically, they have a similar appearance to granulosa cell tumors (Fig. 16-36).

Thecomas and Fibromas. Both these tumors arise from the ovarian stroma and pathologically may be difficult to distinguish from each other. Tumors with an abundance of thecal cells are classified as thecomas, whereas those with fewer thecal cells and abundant fibrous tissue are classified as thecofibromas and fibromas. Thecomas comprise approximately 1% of all ovarian neoplasms and 70% occur in postmenopausal females. They are unilateral, almost always benign, and frequently show clinical signs of estrogen production. Fibromas comprise approximately 4% of ovarian neoplasms, are benign, usually unilateral, and occur most commonly in

menopausal and postmenopausal women. Unlike thecomas, they are rarely associated with estrogen production and therefore are frequently asymptomatic, despite reaching a large size. Ascites has been reported in half the patients with fibromas larger than 5 cm in diameter.[80] **Meigs' syndrome** (associated ascites and pleural effusion) occurs in 1% to 3% of patients with ovarian fibromas but is not specific, having been reported in association with other ovarian neoplasms. Sonographically, these tumors have a characteristic appearance (Fig. 16-37). A hypoechoic mass with marked posterior attenuation of the sound beam is seen as a result of the homogeneous fibrous tissue in these tumors.[80] The main differential diagnosis is that of a Brenner tumor or pedunculated uterine fibroid. Not all fibromas and thecomas show this characteristic appearance, and a variety of sonographic appearances have been noted, probably as a result of the tendency for edema and cystic degeneration to occur within these tumors.[81]

Metastatic Tumors. The most common **origin** of ovarian metastases are tumors of the breast and gastrointestinal tract. The term *Krukenberg tumor* should be reserved for only those tumors containing the typical mucin-secreting "signet ring" cells, usually of gastric or colonic origin. Endometrial carcinoma frequently metastasizes to the ovary, but these may be difficult to distinguish from primary endometrioid carcinoma, as discussed earlier. Sonographically, ovarian metastases are usually bilateral solid masses (Fig. 16-38) but may have a complex appearance and simulate cystadenocarcinoma.[82] Lymphoma may involve the ovary, usually in a diffuse disseminated form, and is frequently bilateral. The sonographic appearance is that of a solid hypoechoic mass similar to lymphoma elsewhere in the body.

FALLOPIAN TUBE

The normal fallopian tube usually cannot be identified by transabdominal or transvaginal sonography, un-

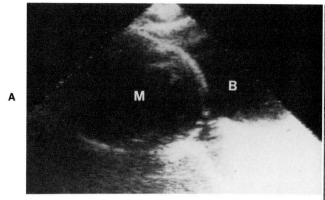

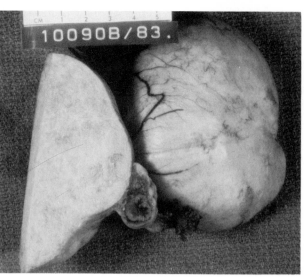

FIG 16-37. Ovarian fibroma. **A,** Sagittal scan shows anechoic solid mass *(M)* with posterior attenuation. Compare attenuation posterior to mass with marked acoustic enhancement posterior to bladder *(B)*. **B,** Pathologic specimen shows the homogeneous solid nature of fibroma.

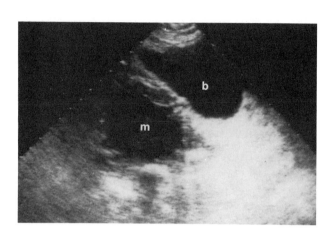

FIG 16-38. Ovarian metastasis from primary breast carcinoma. Sagittal scan shows solid hypoechoic mass *(m)* posterior to bladder *(b)*.

FIG 16-39. Normal fallopian tube. **A,** Transvaginal scan shows echogenic tube *(T)* outlined by ascites *(A)*. There is also complex ovarian mass *(arrows)*, which is ovarian serous cystadenocarcinoma. **B,** Normal fimbrial end of fallopian tube *(T)* outlined by ascites in the same patient. *U,* Uterus.

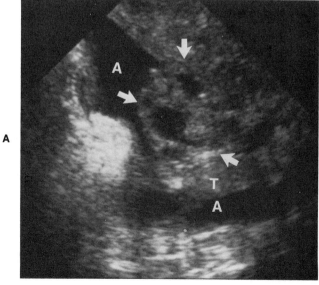

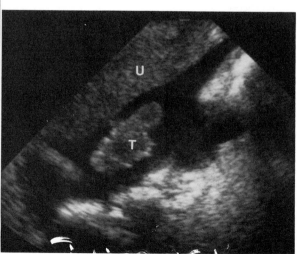

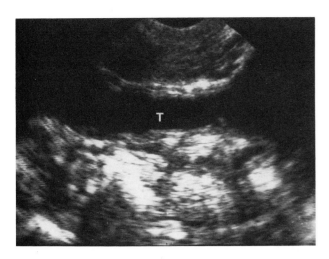

FIG 16-40. Hydrosalpinx. Transvaginal scan in patient with pelvic inflammatory disease shows dilated fluid-filled fallopian tube *(T)*.

less it is surrounded by fluid. The normal fallopian tube is an undulating echogenic structure of approximately 8 to 10 mm in width, running posterolaterally from the uterus to lie within the cul-de-sac near the ovary (Fig. 16-39). The lumen is not seen unless it is fluid filled (Fig. 16-40).[83] Developmental abnormalities of the tube are rare. Abnormalities of the tube include pregnancy (see Chapter 33), infection, and neoplasm.

Pelvic Inflammatory Disease

Pelvic inflammatory disease (PID) is a common condition that is increasing in frequency. It is usually bilat-

eral and caused by sexually transmitted diseases (STDs), most commonly associated with gonorrhea (Fig. 16-41). Other less common causes include appendiceal, diverticular, or postsurgical abscesses that have ruptured into the pelvis and puerperal and post abortion complications. The presence of intrauterine contraceptive devices also increases the risk of PID. These nonvenereal causes are usually unilateral.

Sexually transmitted PID spreads along the mucosa of the pelvic organs, initially infecting the cervix and uterine endometrium (endometritis), the fallopian tubes (acute salpingitis), and finally the region of both ovaries and the peritoneum. A pyosalpinx develops as a result of occlusion of the tube. The diagnosis is usually made clinically, with the patient presenting with pain, fever, and vaginal discharge. A pelvic mass may be palpated.

Sonographically, there are a spectrum of findings.[39] Endometrial thickening or fluid may indicate endometritis. Pus may be demonstrated in the cul-de-sac and contains echogenic material, distinguishing it from serous fluid in this region. On transabdominal sonography, dilated tubes appear as complex predominantly cystic masses that are often indistinguishable from other adnexal masses. However, transvaginal sonography recognizes the fluid-filled tube by its tubular shape with a somewhat folded configuration and well-defined echogenic walls.[84] Low-level echoes may be seen within the fluid as a result of pus. As the infection worsens, tuboovarian abscesses develop, which appear as multiloculated complex masses. Because the ovaries are relatively resistant to infection, areas of recognizable ovarian tissue may be seen within the inflammatory

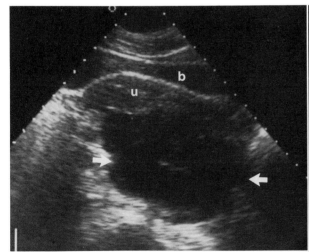

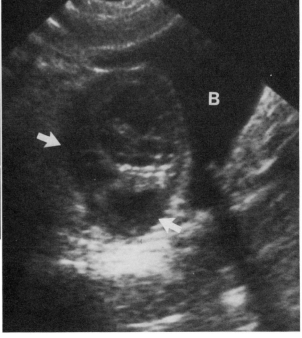

FIG 16-41. Pelvic inflammatory disease, typical appearances. **A,** Sagittal scan shows large predominantly hypoechoic mass with irregular margins *(arrows)* compressing uterus *(u)* and bladder *(b)* anteriorly. **B,** Sagittal scan shows large complex mass *(arrows)*, a tuboovarian abscess. *B,* Bladder.

mass by transvaginal sonography.[47] Sonography is useful in following the response to antibiotic therapy. In chronic PID, extensive fibrosis and adhesions may obscure the margins of the pelvic organs, which blend into a large ill-defined mass. A chronic hydrosalpinx may develop as a result of tubal adhesions and may undergo torsion, with the patient presenting with the abrupt onset of severe pelvic pain. Hydrosalpinx and tubal torsion have also been reported as a late complication in patients undergoing tubal ligation.[85]

Carcinoma

Carcinoma of the fallopian tube is the least common (less than 1%) of all gynecologic malignancies, with adenocarcinoma being the most common histologic type. It occurs most frequently in postmenopausal women in their sixth decade who present clinically with pain, vaginal bleeding, and a pelvic mass. It usually involves the distal end, but it may involve the entire length of the tube. Sonographically, carcinoma of the fallopian tube has been described as a sausage-shaped, discrete, primarily solid adnexal mass that may contain cystic areas caused by necrosis.[86] Transvaginal sonography may show a discrete mass within the tube in this condition.

NONGYNECOLOGIC PELVIC MASSES

Pelvic masses and pseudomasses may be of nongynecologic origin. To make this diagnosis, it is important to visualize the uterus and ovaries separate from the mass (Fig. 16-42). This is frequently not possible because of displacement of the normal pelvic structures by

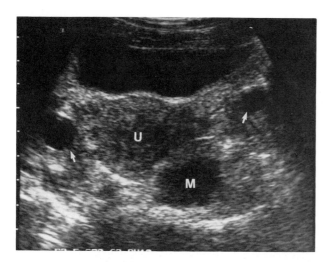

FIG 16-42. Extramedullary hematopoiesis. Transverse scan in 44-year-old asymptomatic woman with thalassemia shows anechoic mass *(M)* to left and separate from uterus *(U)* and both ovaries, which contain cysts *(arrows)*. Diagnosis made by percutaneous biopsy under computed tomography guidance.

the mass. Nongynecologic pelvic masses most commonly originate from the gastrointestinal or urinary tract or may develop after surgery.

Postoperative Pelvic Masses

Postoperative masses may be abscesses, hematomas, lymphoceles, urinomas, or seromas. Sonographically, **abscesses** are ovoid-shaped, anechoic masses with thick irregular walls and posterior acoustic enhancement. Variable internal echogenicity may be seen and high-intensity echoes with shadowing caused by gas may be demonstrated. **Hematomas** show a spectrum of sonographic findings, varying with time.[87] During the initial acute phase, hematomas are anechoic. Following organization and clot formation, they become highly echogenic. With lysis of the clot, hematomas become more complex, until finally, with complete lysis, they are again anechoic. It is frequently not possible to distinguish an abscess from a hematoma sonographically, and clinical correlation is usually necessary.

Pelvic lymphoceles occur following surgical disruption of lymphatic channels, usually after pelvic lymph node dissection or renal transplantation. Sonographically, lymphoceles are cystic, having a similar appearance to **urinomas,** which are localized collections of urine, or **seromas,** which are collections of serum. Sonography-guided aspiration may be necessary to differentiate these conditions.

Gastrointestinal Tract Masses

The most frequent pelvic **pseudomasses** are fecal material in the rectum simulating a complex mass in the cul-de-sac and a fluid-filled rectosigmoid colon presenting as a cystic adnexal mass. A repeat examination with a water enema usually distinguishes the pseudomass from a true mass.[88] **Bowel neoplasms,** especially those involving the rectosigmoid, cecum, and ileum may simulate an adnexal mass. These tumors frequently show the characteristic target sign of a gastrointestinal mass, consisting of a central echogenic focus caused by mucus or gas within the lumen, surrounded by a thickened hypoechoic wall.[89] **Abscesses** related to inflammatory disease of the gastrointestinal tract may also present as an adnexal mass. On the right side, this is most frequently caused by appendicitis or Crohn's disease, whereas abscesses on the left side are usually caused by diverticular disease and are seen in an older age group. Sonographically, they are similar in appearance to postoperative abscesses.

Urinary Tract Masses

A **pelvic kidney** may present as a clinically palpable mass. This is readily recognized sonographically by the typical reniform appearance and the absence of a kidney in the normal location. Occasionally, a marked distended bladder may be mistaken for an ovarian cyst. When a cystic pelvic mass is identified, it is imperative that the bladder be seen separate from the mass. Bladder diverticula may also simulate a cystic adnexal mass. The diagnosis can be confirmed by demonstrating communication with the bladder and a changing appearance after voiding. Dilated distal ureters may simulate adnexal cysts on transverse scans; however, sagittal scans show their tubular appearance and continuity with the bladder.

POSTPARTUM PELVIC PATHOLOGIC CONDITIONS

Pathologic states in the postpartum period are usually the result of infection and hemorrhage. Specific pathologic conditions occurring in the postpartum period include endometritis, retained products of conception, and ovarian vein thrombophlebitis. **Endometritis** is more frequent following cesarean section than vaginal delivery. The most common source of organisms is the normal vaginal flora. The sonographic findings were previously described (see the section on uterus).

Retained Products of Conception

Retained placental tissue following delivery may cause secondary postpartum hemorrhage or may serve as a nidus for infection. Sonographically, the endometrium is thickened and echogenic with some areas of high-intensity echoes (Fig. 16-43, *A*).[90] Large blood clots may show a similar appearance. Occasionally, definitive placental tissue may be identified (Fig. 16-43, *B* and *C*).

Ovarian Vein Thrombophlebitis

Puerperal ovarian vein thrombosis or thrombophlebitis is an uncommon but potentially life-threatening condition (Fig. 16-44). Patients present with fever, lower abdominal pain, and a palpable mass, usually 48 to 96 hours postpartum. The underlying cause is venous stasis and spread of bacterial infection from endometritis. The right ovarian vein is involved in 90% of cases. Retrograde venous flow occurs in the left ovarian vein during the puerperium, which protects this side from bacterial spread from the uterus.[26] This condition may be diagnosed by sonography, CT, or MRI.[91,92] Sonography

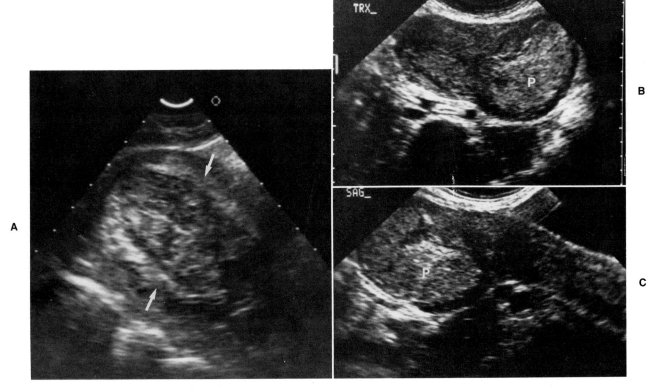

FIG 16-43. Retained products of conception, varying appearances. **A,** Sagittal scan in patient 3 days after therapeutic abortion shows thickened endometrial cavity *(arrows)* filled with echoes of varying intensity. **B,** Transverse scan in patient with persistent bleeding 2 weeks postpartum shows retained placental tissue *(P)*. **C,** Sagittal scan of same patient.
(**B** and **C** courtesy of SR Wilson, M.D., Toronto General Hospital.)

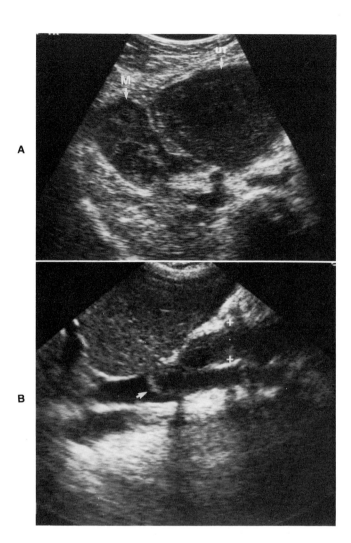

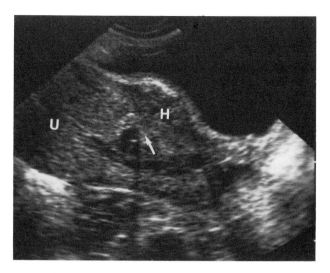

FIG 16-45. Bladder-flap hematoma. Sagittal scan in patient with fever and lower abdominal pain 8 days following cesarean section shows hematoma *(H)* between bladder and cesarean section scar *(arrow)*. *U,* Uterus.
(Courtesy of SR Wilson, M.D., Toronto General Hospital.)

FIG 16-44. Ovarian vein thrombophlebitis. **A,** Transverse scan in patient with fever and right lower abdominal pain 4 days following cesarean section shows mass *(M)* to right of postpartum uterus *(UT)*. **B,** Sagittal scan of abdomen shows echogenic thrombus in distended right ovarian vein (between *cursors*). Thrombus is seen extending into inferior vena cava *(arrow)*.

may demonstrate an inflammatory mass lateral to the uterus and anterior to the psoas muscle. The ovarian vein may be demonstrated as a tubular anechoic structure containing echogenic thrombus. Thrombus in the inferior vena cava may also be seen. Duplex Doppler imaging may demonstrate absence of flow in these veins.[93] Most patients respond to anticoagulant and antibiotic therapy, and follow-up sonography may show resolution of the thrombus and normal flow on duplex Doppler imaging.

Cesarean Section Complications

A lower uterine transverse incision site is commonly used for cesarean section. On sonographic examination, the incision site can be identified as an oval, symmetric region of hypoechogenicity relative to the myometrium, located between the posterior wall of the bladder and the lower uterine segment.[94] Sutures within the incision site may occasionally be recognized as small punctate high-amplitude echoes.

Hematomas may develop from hemorrhage at the incision site **(bladder flap hematomas)** or within the prevesical space **(subfascial hematomas)**. **Bladder flap hematomas** can be diagnosed sonographically when a complex or anechoic mass greater than 2 cm in diameter is located adjacent to the scar between the lower uterine segment and posterior bladder wall (Fig. 16-45). The echogenicity varies depending on the amount of organization within the hematoma.[87] The presence of air within the mass is highly suggestive of an infected hematoma.[95] **Subfascial hematomas** are extraperitoneal in location, contained within the prevesical space, and caused by disruption of the inferior epigastric vessels or their branches during cesarean section. Sonographically, a complex or cystic mass is seen anterior to the bladder. High-frequency, short-focus transducers are frequently necessary to recognize the superficial mass. It is important to identify the rectus muscle to distinguish the **superficial wound hematoma,** which is located anterior to the rectus muscle from the **subfascial hematoma** located posterior to it.[96] Bladder flap and subfascial hematomas may be seen together in the same patient; however, they have different sources of bleeding and should be treated as separate conditions.

REFERENCES
Normal Pelvic Anatomy

1. Williams PL, Warwick R: *Gray's Anatomy*. 37th ed. Edinburgh: Churchill Livingstone; 1989.
2. Jones HW III, Wentz AC, Burnett LS: *Novak's Textbook of Gynecology*. 11th ed. Baltimore: Williams & Wilkins; 1987.

Technique

3. Tessler FN, Schiller VL, Perrella RR, et al: Transabdominal versus endovaginal pelvic sonography: prospective study. *Radiology* 1989; 170:553-556.
4. Mendelson EB, Bohm-Velez M, Joseph N, et al: Gynecologic imaging: comparison of transabdominal and transvaginal sonography. *Radiology* 1988;166:321-324.
5. Lande IM, Hill MC, Cosco FE, et al: Adnexal and cul-de-sac abnormalities: transvaginal sonography. *Radiology* 1988;166:325-332.
6. Leibman AJ, Kruse B, McSweeney MB: Transvaginal sonography: comparison with transabdominal sonography in the diagnosis of pelvic masses. *AJR* 1988;151:89-92.
7. Andolf E, Jörgensen C: A prospective comparison of transabdominal and transvaginal ultrasound with surgical findings in gynecologic disease. *J Ultrasound Med* 1990;9:71-75.

Uterus

8. Coleman BG, Arger PH, Grumbach K, et al: Transvaginal and transabdominal sonography: prospective comparison. *Radiology* 1988;168:639-643.
9. Sample WF, Lippe BM, Gyepes MT: Gray-scale ultrasonography of the normal female pelvis. *Radiology* 1977;125:477-483.
10. Orsini LF, Salardi S, Pilu G, et al: Pelvic organs in premenarcheal girls: real-time ultrasonography. *Radiology* 1984;153:113-116.
11. Nussbaum AR, Sanders RC, Jones MD: Neonatal uterine morphology as seen on real-time US. *Radiology* 1986; 160:641-643.
12. Platt JF, Bree RL, Davidson D: Ultrasound of the normal nongravid uterus: correlation with gross and histopathology. *J Clin Ultrasound* 1990;18:15-19.
13. Miller EI, Thomas RH, Lines P: The atrophic postmenopausal uterus. *J Clin Ultrasound* 1977;5:261-263.
14. Frede TE: Ultrasonic visualization of varicosities in the female genital tract. *J Ultrasound Med* 1984;3:365-369.
15. DuBose TJ, Hill LW, Hennigan HW Jr, et al: Sonography of arcuate uterine blood vessels. *J Ultrasound Med* 1985;4:229-233.
16. Callen PW, DeMartini WJ, Filly RA: The central uterine cavity echo: a useful anatomic sign in the ultrasonographic evaluation of the female pelvis. *Radiology* 1979;131:187-190.
17. Fleischer AC, Kalemeris GC, Entman SS: Sonographic depiction of the endometrium during normal cycles. *Ultrasound Med Biol* 1986;12:271-277.
18. Forrest TS, Elyaderani MK, Muilenburg MI, et al: Cyclic endometrial changes: US assessment with histologic correlation. *Radiology* 1988;167:233-237.
19. Fleischer AC, Kalemeris GC, Machin JE, et al: Sonographic depiction of normal and abnormal endometrium with histopathologic correlation. *J Ultrasound Med* 1986;5:445-452.
20. Farrer-Brown G, Beilby JOW, Tarbit MH: The blood supply of the uterus, II: venous pattern. *Br J Obstet Gynecol Comm* 1970;77:682-689.
21. Pennes DR, Bowerman RA, Silver TM: Congenital uterine anomalies and associated pregnancies: findings and pitfalls of sonographic diagnosis. *J Ultrasound Med* 1985;4:531-538.
22. Fried AM, Oliff M, Wilson EA, et al: Uterine anomalies associated with renal agenesis: role of gray scale ultrasonography. *AJR* 1978;131:973-975.

23. Wiersma AF, Peterson LF, Justema EJ: Uterine anomalies associated with unilateral renal agenesis. *Obstet Gynecol* 1976; 47:654-657.
24. Nicolini U, Bellotti M, Bonazzi B, et al: Can ultrasound be used to screen uterine malformations? *Fertil Steril* 1987; 47:89-93.
25. Reuter KL, Daly DC, Cohen SM: Septate versus bicornuate uteri: errors in imaging diagnosis. *Radiology* 1989; 172:749-752.
26. Kurman RJ: *Blaustein's Pathology of the Female Genital Tract*. 3rd ed. New York: Springer-Verlag; 1987.
27. Smith JP, Weiser EB, Karnei RF Jr, et al: Ultrasonography of rapidly growing uterine leiomyomata associated with anovulatory cycles. *Radiology* 1980;134:713-716.
28. Lev-Toaff AS, Coleman BG, Arger PH, et al: Leiomyomas in pregnancy: sonographic study. *Radiology* 1987; 164:375-380.
29. Gross BH, Silver TM, Jaffe MH: Sonographic features of uterine leiomyomas: analysis of 41 proven cases. *J Ultrasound Med* 1983;2:401-406.
30. Baltarowich OH, Kurtz AB, Pennell RG, et al: Pitfalls in the sonographic diagnosis of uterine fibroids. *AJR* 1988; 151:725-728.
31. Dodd GD III, Budzik RF Jr: Lipomatous uterine tumors: diagnosis by ultrasound, CT and MR. *J Comput Assist Tomogr* 1990;14:629-632.
32. Siedler D, Laing FC, Jeffrey RB Jr, et al: Uterine adenomyosis: a difficult sonographic diagnosis. *J Ultrasound Med* 1987;6:345-349.
33. Bohlman ME, Ensor RE, Sanders RC: Sonographic findings in adenomyosis of the uterus. *AJR* 1987;148:765-766.
34. Mendelson EB, Bohm-Velez M, Joseph N, et al: Endometrial abnormalities: evaluation with transvaginal sonography. *AJR* 1988;150:139-142.
35. Wilson DA, Stacy TM, Smith EI: Ultrasound diagnosis of hydrocolpos and hydrometrocolpos. *Radiology* 1978; 128:451-454.
36. Breckenridge JW, Kurtz AB, Ritchie WGM, et al: Postmenopausal uterine fluid collection: indicator of carcinoma. *AJR* 1982;139:529-534.
37. Scott WW Jr, Rosenshein NB, Siegelman SS, et al: The obstructed uterus. *Radiology* 1981;141:767-770.
38. Johnson MA, Graham MF, Cooperberg PL: Abnormal endometrial echoes: sonographic spectrum of endometrial pathology. *J Ultrasound Med* 1982;1:161-166.
39. Swayne LC, Love MB, Karasick SR: Pelvic inflammatory disease: sonographic-pathologic correlation. *Radiology* 1984; 151:751-755.
40. Rubin D, Graham MF, Cronhelm C, et al: Echogenic hematometra mimicking endometrial carcinoma. *J Ultrasound Med* 1985; 4:47-48.
41. Fleischer AC, Dudley BS, Entman SS, et al: Myometrial invasion by endometrial carcinoma: sonographic assessment. *Radiology* 1987;162:307-310.
42. Cacciatore B, Lehtovirta P, Wahlström T, et al: Preoperative sonographic evaluation of endometrial cancer. *Am J Obstet Gynecol* 1989;160:133-137.
43. Requard CK, Wicks JD, Mettler FA Jr: Ultrasonography in the staging of endometrial adenocarcinoma. *Radiology* 1981;140:781-785.
44. Callen PW, Filly RA, Munyer TP: Intrauterine contraceptive devices: evaluation by sonography. *AJR* 1980;135:797-800.
45. Fogel SR, Slasky BS: Sonography of nabothian cysts. *AJR* 1982;138:927-930.
46. McCarthy S, Taylor KJW: Sonography of vaginal masses. *AJR* 1983;140:1005-1008.

Rectouterine recess (posterior cul-de-sac)

47. Mendelson EB, Bohm-Velez M, Neiman HL, et al: Transvaginal sonography in gynecologic imaging. *Semin Ultrasound CT MR* 1988;9:102-121.

48. Davis JA, Gosink BB: Fluid in the female pelvis: cyclic patterns. *J Ultrasound Med* 1986;5:75-79.

49. Jeffrey RB, Laing FC: Echogenic clot: a useful sign of pelvic hemoperitoneum. *Radiology* 1982;145:139-141.

Ovary

50. Nicolini U, Ferrazzi E, Bellotti M, et al: The contribution of sonographic evaluation of ovarian size in patients with polycystic ovarian disease. *J Ultrasound Med* 1985; 4:347-351.

51. Cohen HL, Tice HM, Mandel FS: Ovarian volumes measured by US: bigger than we think. *Radiology* 1990; 177:189-192.

52. Hall DA, McCarthy KA, Kopans DB: Sonographic visualization of the normal postmenopausal ovary. *J Ultrasound Med* 1986; 5:9-11.

53. Higgins RV, van Nagell JR Jr, Donaldson ES, et al: Transvaginal sonography as a screening method for ovarian cancer. *Gynecol Oncol* 1989;34:402-406.

54. Hall DA: Sonographic appearance of the normal ovary, of polycystic ovary disease, and of functional ovarian cysts. *Semin Ultrasound* 1983;4:149-165.

55. Yeh HC, Futterweit W, Thornton JC: Polycystic ovarian disease: US features in 104 patients. *Radiology* 1987; 163:111-116.

56. Hann LE, Hall DA, McArdle CR, et al: Polycystic ovarian disease: sonographic spectrum. *Radiology* 1984;150:531-534.

57. Baltarowich OH, Kurtz AB, Pasto ME, et al: The spectrum of sonographic findings in hemorrhagic ovarian cysts. *AJR* 1987;148:901-905.

58. Phillips HE, McGahan JP: Ovarian remnant syndrome. *Radiology* 1982;142:487-488.

59. Athey PA, Cooper NB: Sonographic features of parovarian cysts. *AJR* 1985;144:83-86.

60. Alpern MB, Sandler MA, Madrazo BL: Sonographic features of parovarian cysts and their complications. *AJR* 1984; 143:157-160.

61. Hall DA, McCarthy KA: The significance of the postmenopausal simple adnexal cyst. *J Ultrasound Med* 1986;5:503-505.

62. Goldstein SR, Subramanyam B, Snyder JR, et al: The postmenopausal cystic adnexal mass: the potential role of ultrasound in conservative management. *Obstet Gynecol* 1989;73:8-10.

63. Birnholz JC: Endometriosis and inflammatory disease. *Semin Ultrasound* 1983;4:184-192.

64. Friedman H, Vogelzang RL, Mendelson EB, et al: Endometriosis detection by US with laparoscopic correlation. *Radiology* 1985;157:217-220.

65. Athey PA, Diment DD: The spectrum of sonographic findings in endometriomas. *J Ultrasound Med* 1989;8:487-491.

66. Graif M, Itzchak Y: Sonographic evaluation of ovarian torsion in childhood and adolescence. *AJR* 1988;150:647-649.

67. Kapadia R, Sternhill V, Schwartz E: Massive edema of the ovary. *J Clin Ultrasound* 1982;10:469-471.

68. Campbell S, Bhan V, Royston P, et al: Transabdominal ultrasound screening for early ovarian cancer. *Br Med J* 1989; 299:1363-1367.

69. Jacobs I, Stabile I, Bridges J, et al: Multimodal approach to screening for ovarian cancer. *Lancet* 1988;1:268-271.

70. Finkler NJ, Benacerraf B, Lavin PT, et al: Comparison of serum CA 125, clinical impression and ultrasound in the preoperative evaluation of ovarian masses. *Obstet Gynecol* 1988; 72:659-664.

71. Fleischer AC, McKee MS, Gordon AN, et al: Transvaginal sonography of postmenopausal ovaries with pathologic correlation. *J Ultrasound Med* 1990;9:637-644.

72. Moyle JW, Rochester D, Sider L, et al: Sonography of ovarian tumors: predictability of tumor type. *AJR* 1983; 141:985-991.

73. Bourne T, Campbell S, Steer C, et al: Transvaginal colour flow imaging: a possible new screening technique for ovarian cancer. *Br Med J* 1989; 299:1367-1370.

74. Williams AG, Mettler FA, Wicks JD: Cystic and solid ovarian neoplasms. *Semin Ultrasound* 1983;4:166-183.

75. Athey PA, Siegel MF: Sonographic features of Brenner tumor of the ovary. *J Ultrasound Med* 1987;6:367-372.

76. Quinn SF, Erickson S, Black WC: Cystic ovarian teratomas: the sonographic appearance of the dermoid plug. *Radiology* 1985;155:477-478.

77. Sheth S, Fishman EK, Buck JL, et al: The variable sonographic appearances of ovarian teratomas: correlation with CT. *AJR* 1988;151:331-334.

78. Guttman PH Jr: In search of the elusive benign cystic ovarian teratoma: application of the ultrasound "tip of the iceberg" sign. *J Clin Ultrasound* 1977;5:403-406.

79. O'Malley BP, Richmond H: Struma ovarii. *J Ultrasound Med* 1982;1:177-178.

80. Stephenson WM, Laing FC: Sonography of ovarian fibromas. *AJR* 1985;144:1239-1240.

81. Athey PA, Malone RS: Sonography of ovarian fibromas/thecomas. *J Ultrasound Med* 1987;6:431-436.

82. Athey PA, Butters HE: Sonographic and CT appearance of Krukenberg tumors. *J Clin Ultrasound* 1984;12:205-210.

Fallopian tube

83. Timor-Tritsch IE, Rottem S: Transvaginal ultrasonographic study of the fallopian tube. *Obstet Gynecol* 1987;70:424-428.

84. Tessler FN, Perrella RR, Fleischer AC, et al: Endovaginal sonographic diagnosis of dilated fallopian tubes. *AJR* 1989;153:523-525.

85. Russin LD: Hydrosalpinx and tubal torsion: a late complication of tubal ligation. *Radiology* 1986;159:115-116.

86. Subramanyam BR, Raghavendra BN, Whalen CA, et al: Ultrasonic features of fallopian tube carcinoma. *J Ultrasound Med* 1984;3:391-393.

Nongynecologic pelvic masses

87. Wicks JD, Silver TM, Bree RL: Gray scale features of hematomas: an ultrasonic spectrum. *AJR* 1978;131:977-980.

88. Kurtz AB, Rubin CS, Kramer FL, et al: Ultrasound evaluation of the posterior pelvic compartment. *Radiology* 1979; 132:677-682.

89. Salem S, O'Malley BP, Hiltz CW: Ultrasonographic appearance of gastrointestinal masses. *J Can Assoc Radiol* 1980; 31:163-167.

Postpartum pelvic pathology

90. Lee CY, Madrazo B, Drukker BH: Ultrasonic evaluation of the postpartum uterus in the management of postpartum bleeding. *Obstet Gynecol* 1981;58:227-232.

91. Wilson PC, Lerner RM: Diagnosis of ovarian vein thrombophlebitis by ultrasonography. *J Ultrasound Med* 1983;2:187-190.

92. Savader SJ, Otero RR, Savader BL: Puerperal ovarian vein thrombosis: evaluation with CT, US, and MR imaging. *Radiology* 1988;167:637-639.

93. Baran GW, Frisch KM: Duplex Doppler evaluation of puerperal ovarian vein thrombosis. *AJR* 1987;149:321-322.

94. Baker ME, Kay H, Mahony BS, et al: Sonography of the low transverse incision, cesarean section: a prospective study. *J Ultrasound Med* 1988;7:389-393.

95. Baker ME, Bowie JD, Killam AP: Sonography of post-cesarean-section bladder-flap hematoma. *AJR* 1985;144:757-759.

96. Wiener MD, Bowie JD, Baker ME, et al: Sonography of subfascial hematoma after cesarean delivery. *AJR* 1987;148:907-910.

ACKNOWLEDGEMENT

I wish to thank John Lai, RDMS, for his valuable assistance and his contribution to the section on technique.

CHAPTER 17

The Thorax

- William E. Brant, M.D.

Ultrasound is a reliable, efficient, and revealing imaging method to evaluate a wide range of perplexing clinical problems in the chest.[1,2] It can effectively be used to guide a variety of interventional procedures in the thorax. Although the ribs, spine, and air-filled lung may act as barriers to ultrasound visualization of some intrathoracic diseases, the presence of fluid in the pleural space, or tumor, consolidation, or atelectasis in the lung provides ample sonographic windows for evaluation. When film radiography is unable to clarify a chest abnormality, ultrasonography may further characterize the abnormality and limit the differential diagnosis. Sonography can be used to differentiate pleural from parenchymal lesions, to visualize diseased parenchyma hidden by pleural effusion, and to detect pleural septations and other pleural abnormalities not even suspected by other imaging modalities. Ultrasound clearly demonstrates the diaphragm and differentiates subpulmonic effusion from subphrenic abscess.[3] Because ultrasound is portable, it can be readily used at the bedside of critically ill patients, providing safe and accurate guidance for interventional procedures.[4,5] The patient can be examined in any position, minimizing the need for moving patients on life support devices. Cooperative patients can be maneuvered into a variety of positions to optimize sonographic visualization of the mediastinum and deep thoracic structures. Most needle placements can be performed under direct and constant visualization by ultrasound, maximizing safety and accuracy.

PLEURAL SPACE

The pleural space is superficial and readily examined by ultrasound using either a direct or an abdominal approach. A high frequency (5 MHz) linear transducer applied directly to the chest (direct approach) provides a broad near field-of-view that allows excellent visualization of the pleural space (Fig. 17-1, *A*). The lower reaches of the pleural space may be effectively examined by use of a lower frequency (3.5 MHz) sector transducer directed superiorly from the abdomen (abdominal approach). The liver and spleen provide sonographic windows to the thorax. Fluid in the pleural space may allow for examination deep into the thorax. Sector transducers are frequently unsatisfactory for examination of the pleural space when applied directly to the chest (Fig. 17-1, *B*). The sector scanner has a narrow view in the near field and the pleural space is frequently obscured by near field artifact.

Sonographic Appearance

Direct Approach. The normal pleural space is readily recognized when the ribs are used as sonographic landmarks (Fig. 17-2). With the transducer oriented perpendicular to the intercostal spaces, the ribs are displayed as rounded echogenic interfaces with prominent acoustic shadowing. The location and depth of the ribs are noted, and the thickness of the subcutaneous tissues and the overlying muscle are determined. The parietal pleura is located approximately 1 cm deep to the rib interface. The **parietal pleura** lining the bony thorax and the **visceral pleura** covering the lung are seen as thin bright echogenic lines separated by a thin

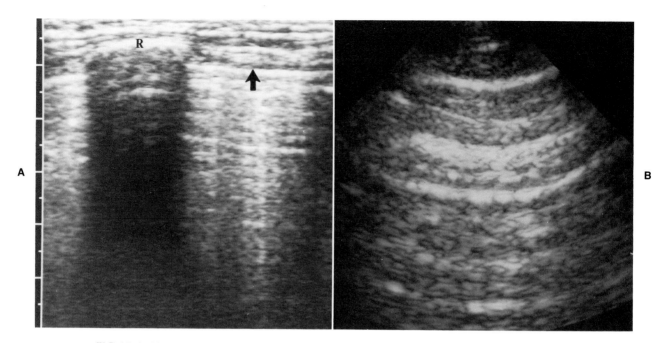

FIG 17-1. Linear array versus sector transducer. **A,** A 5-MHz linear-array transducer applied directly to the chest produces an image of a rib *(R)* and normal visceral pleural-pulmonary interface *(arrow).* The normal pleural space is the hypoechoic line just superficial to the interface. **B,** A 3.5-MHz sector transducer applied directly to the chest produces a confusing image of reverberation artifacts. No anatomic landmarks can be recognized. The normal pleural space is obscured by artifacts in the narrow field close to the transducer surface.

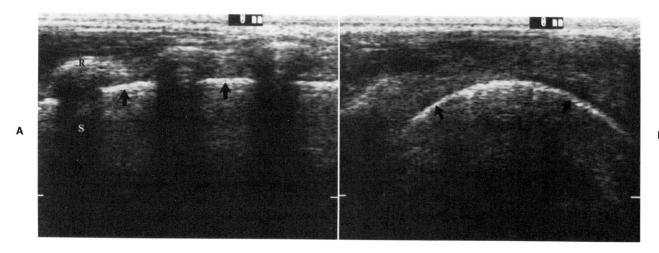

FIG 17-2. Normal pleural space (direct approach). **A,** Longitudinal image from a linear-array transducer applied directly to the chest demonstrates three ribs and the normal pleural space. The ribs produce a bright surface reflection *(R)* and a dense acoustic shadow *(S).* The normal visceral pleural-pulmonary interface *(arrow)* is localized within 1 cm deep to the rib surface. The pleural space is the thin hypoechoic line just superficial to the interface. **B,** A transverse image obtained in an intercostal space with a linear-array transducer demonstrates the curving normal visceral pleural-pulmonary interface *(arrows).* The location of the visceral pleura is confirmed by observing the motion of the lung interface with respiration.

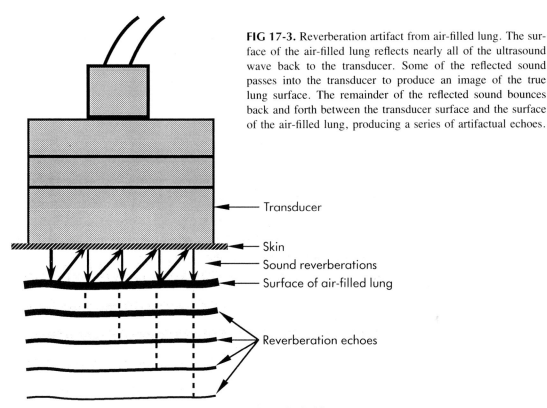

FIG 17-3. Reverberation artifact from air-filled lung. The surface of the air-filled lung reflects nearly all of the ultrasound wave back to the transducer. Some of the reflected sound passes into the transducer to produce an image of the true lung surface. The remainder of the reflected sound bounces back and forth between the transducer surface and the surface of the air-filled lung, producing a series of artifactual echoes.

— Transducer

— Skin

— Sound reverberations

— Surface of air-filled lung

— Reverberation echoes

dark line of normal pleural fluid. Aligning the transducer parallel to and within the intercostal space allows clear demonstration of the pleural surfaces.

Air-filled lung causes a highly reflective interface that blocks transmission of the sound beam into the chest. However, the ultrasound image displays a pattern of bright echoes caused by acoustic reverberation artifact.[6] These echoes are usually bright but formless and diminish in intensity with distance from the transducer (Fig. 17-2). On occasion the echogenic surface of the air-filled lung will be repeatedly duplicated on the image at fixed intervals (Figs. 17-1 and 17-3). The strength of these duplication artifacts also diminishes with increasing distance from the transducer. Although these artifacts may be prominent and confusing on the ultrasound image, they are to be expected and should be recognized as indicators of air-filled lung.

Abdominal Approach. When imaged from the abdomen, the inferior surface of the diaphragm appears as a bright curving interface. On occasion the muscle of the diaphragm may be demonstrated as a thin dark line just above the much brighter echo of the surface. When the lung above the diaphragm is air-filled, the curved surface of the diaphragm-lung interface acts as a **specular** (mirror-like) reflector (Fig. 17-4).[6,7] An artifactual mirror-image reflection of the liver or spleen is displayed above the diaphragm (Fig. 17-5). The presence of this mirror image, although easily recognized as an artifact, should also be viewed as definitive evidence of the absence of pleural fluid.[8,9]

Pleural Fluid

Before embarking upon a search for pleural fluid by ultrasound, the patient's chest radiograph should be reviewed. The location of pleural lesions should be noted for correlation with the ultrasound examination. Areas of suspected loculated pleural fluid or pleural thickening can then be carefully examined.

Direct Approach. Even minute amounts of pleural fluid can be detected by using a high-resolution linear-array transducer applied directly to the chest. Most pleural fluid is relatively anechoic and is easily recognized as an area of echolucency separating the parietal and visceral pleura (Fig. 17-6). The parietal pleura is identified by its position approximately 1 cm deep to the ribs. The visceral pleura is identified by observing motion of the lung as the patient breathes.

Abdominal Approach. Pleural effusions are commonly detected during routine ultrasonographic examinations of the abdomen. The signs of pleural effusion using an abdominal approach include:

- Hypoechoic fluid above the diaphragm
- Visualization of the inside of the thorax through the fluid collection
- Absence of the mirror image reflection of the liver or spleen above the diaphragm (Figs. 17-7 and 17-8).
- Large effusions possibly inverting the diaphragm

Because the air-filled lung will block transmission of sound, the ribs and inside of the bony thorax are not normally visualized above the diaphragm when scan-

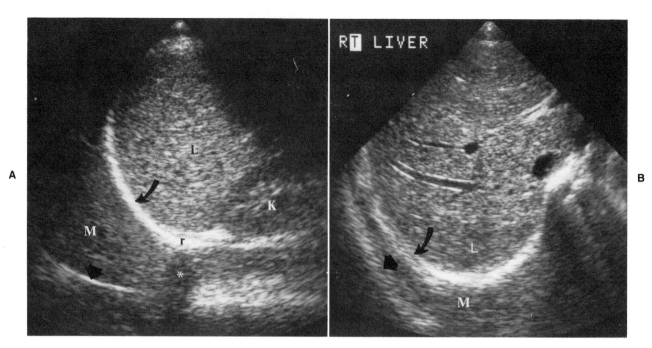

FIG 17-4. Normal pleural space (abdominal approach). **A,** Longitudinal image obtained through the liver *(L)* and kidney *(K)* with a 3.5-MHz sector transducer directed at the diaphragm. The diaphragm-lung surface complex produces a bright curving linear echo *(curved arrow)*. Mirror-image reflections of the liver *(M)* and the diaphragm *(arrowhead)* are displayed above the diaphragm. The limits of the patient's chest are marked by a rib *(r)* identified by its accompanying shadow (*). The image beyond the level of the rib is entirely artifactual. **B,** Transverse image directed through the liver *(L)* shows mirror-image reflections of the liver *(M)* and diaphragm *(arrowhead)*. The curved arrow shows the true diaphragm. The presence of a mirror-image reflection of the liver above the diaphragm is evidence of the absence of pleural effusion.

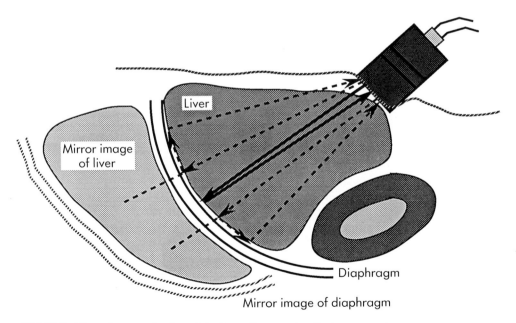

FIG 17-5. Mirror-image reflection of the liver. Because the diaphragm air-filled lung complex is a strong and curving reflector, portions of the ultrasound beam are scattered before being redirected back to the transducer for detection. The time of flight of the echoes is prolonged, causing them to be displayed farther from the transducer. These redirected echoes produce artifactual images of the liver and diaphragm above the level of the true diaphragm.

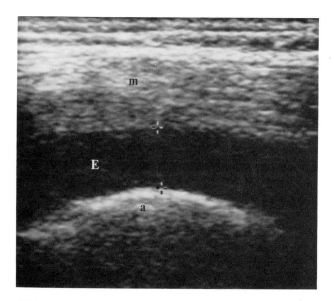

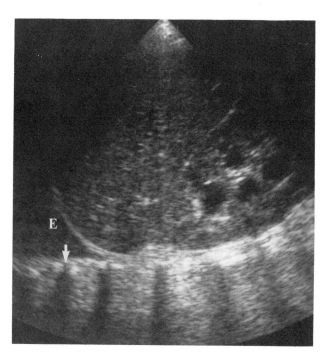

FIG 17-6. Pleural effusion (direct approach). Image obtained in an intercostal space using a linear-array transducer demonstrates a small pleural effusion *(E)* as a band of echolucency separating the parietal and visceral pleura (marked by +). *m,* Intercostal muscle; *a,* Air-filled lung.

FIG 17-7. Pleural effusion (abdominal approach). A longitudinal sector scan through the liver shows a pleural effusion (E) in the costophrenic angle. The patient's chest wall is marked by the ribs (arrow) casting acoustic shadows. The chest wall is visualized above the level of the diaphragm because the pleural effusion allows the transmission of ultrasound waves through it. Compare the appearance of the straight true chest wall seen through the effusion on this image with the curving artifactual duplication of the diaphragm seen in a patient without an effusion in Fig. 17-4, *A.*

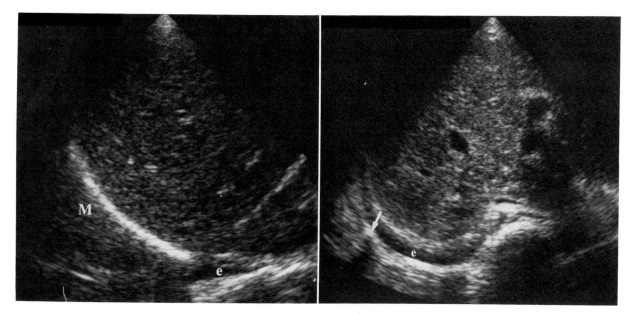

A

B

FIG 17-8. Pleural effusion (abdominal approach). **A,** Longitudinal scan. A small pleural effusion *(e)* is demonstrated in the extreme costophrenic angle. Air-filled lung above the pleural effusion produces the expected mirror-image reflection *(M)* of the liver. **B,** Transverse image through the liver in the same patient again shows the small pleural effusion *(e)*. A rib with its accompanying shadow *(arrow)* marks the limits of the patient's chest wall. Compare to the mirror-image artifacts in Figure 17-4, *B,* which lack the landmarks of the rib and shadow.

ning from the abdomen. The presence of pleural fluid allows transmission of sound and visualization of these structures. Artifactual duplication of the diaphragm must not be mistaken for visualization of the inside of the bony thorax. The inside of the bony thorax forms a straight line, while the artifactual reflection of the diaphragm is curved.

Complex pleural fluid may be difficult to differentiate from solid tissue in the pleural space when it is echogenic. Alternatively, pleural thickening or pleural masses may be hypoechoic and difficult to distinguish from pleural fluid.[10] Some effusions may have floating particulate matter consisting of cells and cellular debris. Other effusions may be gelatinous and move minimally with respiration. Empyemas may be anechoic or echogenic. Prominent septations spanning the pleural space may be demonstrated by ultrasound when their presence is not even suspected by chest radiograph or computed tomography (Fig. 17-9).[11,12] Approximately three quarters of these complex septated effusions are exudative, while the remainder are transudates.[13] Anechoic effusions represent transudative and exudative processes with almost equal frequency.[13] The nature of pleural effusions cannot be accurately determined by their ultrasound appearance alone. Diagnostic thoracentesis is required to determine the composition of pleural fluid. Sonographic features that indicate that a pleural lesion is fluid that can be aspirated include:

- A pleural lesion that changes shape with respiration
- Presence of septations within the pleural lesion that move with respiration
- Echodensities that float and move with respiration within the pleural lesion[14,15]

Pleural Thickening and Pleural Masses

Ultrasound may be used effectively to evaluate pleural abnormalities seen on chest x-rays. Focal pleural lesions may be loculated pleural effusions, thickened fibrous pleural peel, or solid pleural tumors.[10,16] Pleural masses are usually well-circumscribed and hypoechoic or of mixed echogenicity (Fig. 17-10). The presence of internal echoes that do not move with respiration strongly suggests that the pleural lesion is solid. Linear plaque-like calcifications may be seen on the surface of both thickened parietal and visceral pleura. This calcific fibrothorax may result from tuberculous pleurisy, empyema, hemothorax caused by trauma, or asbestosis.[17] Ultrasound may reveal unsuspected chronic effusion in patients with calcific fibrothorax, which indicates a high risk for fistula formation or pulmonic infection and septicemia.[17] Punctate internal calcifications suggest the lesion is solid and likely to be a tumor.[1] Ultrasound can be used to identify areas of solid tumor within pleural effusions and to guide percutaneous needle biopsy of these lesions.[18] Focal areas of pleural thickening can also be localized for pleural biopsy.

Pneumothorax

Pneumothorax is a diagnosis not readily made by ultrasound. Because all air–soft tissue interfaces are nearly completely reflective, the separation of visceral pleura from parietal pleura by air within the pleural space cannot usually be appreciated. However, when

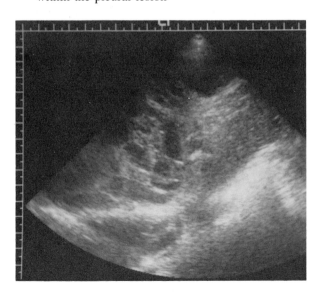

FIG 17-9. Pleural space septations. Complex septations are demonstrated in the pleural space in a patient with malignant pleural effusion.

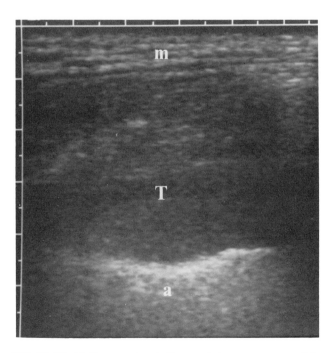

FIG 17-10. Malignant mesothelioma. A heterogeneous solid mass (*T*) occupies the pleural space displacing air-filled lung (*a*) and invading intercostal muscle (*m*).

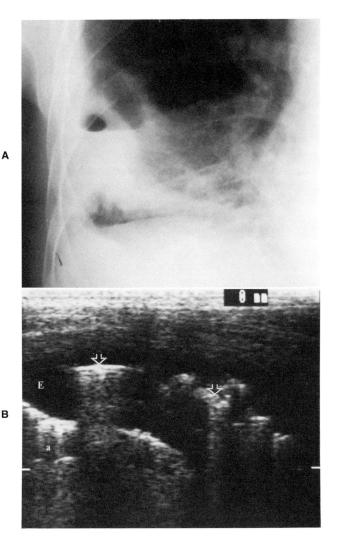

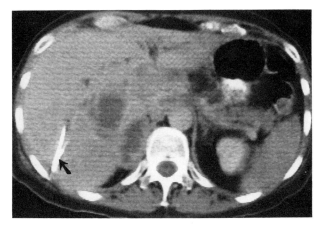

FIG 17-12. Misplaced thoracentesis catheter. A thoracentesis attempted using clinical landmarks alone resulted in the thoracentesis catheter (*arrow*) being sheared off in the liver. Successful thoracentesis was subsequently performed without complication using ultrasound guidance. This patient has metastatic liver disease.

FIG 17-11. Loculated hydropneumothorax. **A,** A loculated hydropneumothorax containing an air-fluid level is seen in the right lower thorax on this PA chest radiograph. **B,** A corresponding sonogram obtained in the intercostal space shows the effusion (*E*) containing loculations of air (*arrows*), which produce bright interfaces with prominent reverberation echoes. The displaced air-filled lung (*a*) has a similar appearance.

both fluid and air are present in the pleural space, pneumothorax can be recognized. Air in any location causes a characteristic bright echo with prominent reverberation artifact caused by nearly complete reflection of the ultrasound beam at the interface between air and tissue (Fig. 17-11).

Invasive Procedures in the Pleural Space

Diagnostic Thoracentesis. Ultrasonographic guidance of diagnostic thoracentesis should be done whenever clinically guided thoracentesis is unsuccessful or is judged to be difficult.[19] Ultrasound guidance adds accuracy and safety to the procedure (Fig. 17-12). It is particularly useful when interpretation of the chest radiograph is difficult, when there is a question of whether the fluid is subpulmonic or subphrenic, and when it is difficult to move the patient into the upright position. After examination of the chest x-ray, the patient is examined sonographically to identify the largest and most accessible pocket of pleural fluid. The location and depth of the fluid and its relationship to the lung are accurately determined. Vital structures such as the heart and aorta are identified and avoided. A safe site for thoracentesis is chosen, based upon careful diagnostic ultrasound examination that uses the direct approach. Actual puncture of the pleural space can then be performed blindly as long as the patient does not change position. Puncture of the pleural space under continuous ultrasound observation is often not possible because the pleural space is so close to the transducer and the needle is difficult to track from the skin surface. The optimal position for diagnostic thoracentesis is the erect sitting position with the patient's arms resting comfortably on a bedside table. However, if the patient is unable to sit, the procedure may be performed with the patient in the lateral decubitus or supine position.

The puncture site is chosen in the intercostal space so that the needle crosses the top of the rib and avoids the neurovascular bundle coursing along the undersurface of the rib. Puncture of the pleural space should be with the needle perpendicular to the chest wall. The puncture site and surrounding area are cleansed with povidone-iodine solution. A local anesthetic, 1% lidocaine solution, is infiltrated subcutaneously at the puncture site. We use a 22-gauge needle attached to a

12-ml syringe for most diagnostic aspirations. Larger syringes are used to obtain 100-ml volumes of fluid or more if cytologic examination is planned. Mild suction is applied while the needle is advanced into the fluid. A characteristic "pop" can usually be felt as the needle punctures the parietal pleura. Care is taken to keep the depth of the needle tip well short of the lung surface. The pleural fluid is inspected for color, clarity, and smell, and is sent to the laboratory for Gram stain, bacterial culture, cell count, cytology, chemistries, and any special studies warranted by the patient's clinical condition.

Occasionally the pleural fluid may be too viscous to aspirate through a 22-gauge needle. When the ultrasonographic diagnosis of pleural effusion is secure but fluid cannot be aspirated, the clinician must first re-examine the patient to determine the accurate location of the fluid, then try larger needles (20- or 18-gauge).

Thoracentesis is an essential part of the evaluation to determine the cause of pleural effusion. **Transudative** pleural effusions are essentially ultrafiltrates of plasma and are caused by an imbalance in the homeostatic forces that control the movement of fluid across pleural membranes. Pleural membranes are usually normal. Common causes of transudative pleural effusions are listed in Table 17-1. **Exudative** effusions are rich in protein and other constituents of whole blood, implying abnormality of the pleural membranes and disruption of the integrity of the pleural blood vessels. The common causes of exudative pleural effusions are listed in Table 17-2.

Numerous laboratory tests may be helpful in determining the cause of pleural effusion.[20] However, the only results that are diagnostic are:

- Presence of malignant cells
- Bacteria on stain or culture
- Presence of lupus erythematosus cells

Exudates generally have a protein content greater than 3 g/dl and a specific gravity equal to or greater than 1.016. Transudates are generally straw-colored and odorless with a white blood cell count less than 1000 per cubic millimeter,[21] but 15% of transudates may be blood tinged. To control costs and maximize diagnostic accuracy, the tests obtained on the pleural fluid must be closely coordinated with the clinical situation and the patient's physician.

Therapeutic Drainage of Symptomatic Effusions.
Large pleural effusions may cause chest pain, dyspnea, or hypoxemia caused by impaired gas exchange. These symptoms can be relieved by drainage of most or all of the pleural fluid. Ultrasound can be used to optimize positioning of the drainage catheter and to measure the completeness of fluid removal. To minimize patient discomfort and risk of infecting the pleural space, complete drainage accomplished as one procedure is preferred to leaving an indwelling catheter. When large pleural effusions are present, the volume of fluid removed at any one setting should not exceed 1 liter. Removal of larger amounts may result in complications of acute mediastinal shift, including acute pulmonary edema, shock, and vasovagal syncope. Therapeutic drainage is accomplished as an extension of diagnostic thoracentesis with placement of a flexible catheter into the pleural space to minimize the possibility of trauma to the lung. Catheter drainage systems are available with flexible catheters that slide over* or through† the

---

*Cook, Bloomington, IN.
†American Pharmaseal, Valencia, CA.

■ **TABLE 17-2**
Common Causes of Exudative Pleural Effusion

Cause	Disorder
Infections	Pneumonia
	Empyema
Neoplasms	Metatatic carcinoma
	Bronchogenic carcinoma
	Lymphoma, leukemia
	Mesothelioma
	Chest wall tumor
Collagen vascular diseases	Rheumatoid arthritis
	Systemic lupus erythematosis
Intra-abdominal diseases	Abdominal surgery
	Pancreatitis
	Subphrenic abscess
Miscellaneous	Pulmonary infarction
	Drug-induced pleural effusion

(Adapted from Jay SJ. Diagnostic procedures for pleural disease. *Clin Chest Med* 1985;6:33-48 and vanSonnenberg E, Nakamoto SK, Mueller PR, et al. Computed tomography and ultrasound-guided catheter drainage of empyemas after chest-tube failure. *Radiology* 1984;151;349-353.)

■ **TABLE 17-1**
Common Causes of Transudative Pleural Effusion

Mechanism	Cause
Increased hydrostatic pressure	Congestive heart failure
	Superior vena cava obstruction
Decreased oncotic pressure	Cirrhosis with ascites
	Peritoneal dialysis
	Acute glomerulonephritis
	Nephrotic syndrome
	Hypoalbuminemia
Miscellaneous	Misplaced venous cathether

(Adapted from Jay SJ. Diagnostic procedures for pleural disease. *Clin Chest Med* 1985;6:33-48 and Chetty KG. Transudative pleural effusions. *Clin Chest Med* 1985;6:49-54.)

needle used to puncture the pleura. The catheter is advanced into the pleural space and the needle is withdrawn. The catheter is connected to a three-way stopcock to which is connected a syringe for aspiration and a bag for fluid collection. This arrangement provides a closed system for repeated aspiration that limits the possibility of contamination of the pleural space. Ultrasonography is used to assess the amount and location of remaining fluid. Then the patient's position can be altered to access remaining fluid. Large loculations of fluid can be removed by separate puncture. When drainage is complete, the needle and catheter assembly are removed. Immediate and 4-hour follow-up chest radiographs should be obtained after all thoracentesis procedures.

Catheter Drainage of Empyema. Numerous studies have documented the advantages of image-directed catheter placement over surgically placed catheters for drainage of empyema.[22-26] Catheter placement with ultrasound guidance is easier, causes fewer complications and less patient discomfort, and has high success rates. Image-guided percutaneous catheter placement is successful in treating empyema in 72% to 92% of cases,[2,22-26] whereas success rates reported with surgically placed chest tubes are 35% to 80%.[26-28]

Empyema is, by definition, the presence of bacteria in the pleural space.[29] The diagnosis is confirmed by the aspiration of gross pus, or the demonstration of bacteria on smear or culture. Most empyemas occur by extension of infection from pneumonia. Trauma, surgery, thoracentesis, esophageal rupture, and subdiaphragmatic abscesses are other causes.

Parapneumonic effusions are exudative pleural effusions; they accompany 40% of cases of bacterial pneumonia.[29,30] They are far more common than empyema, but differentiation is difficult by clinical means other than thoracentesis. Parapneumonic effusions are initially exudative with high protein and white blood cell counts but no bacteria in the pleural fluid. They progress to a fibropurulent stage characterized by fibrin deposition on the pleura with loculation of fluid and formation of limiting membranes. These fibrin membranes are easily demonstrated by ultrasound. The final organization stage produces an inelastic membrane around the lung called a pleural peel.[30] If untreated, pleurocutaneous or bronchopleural fistulas may further complicate the process. Many of these complicated parapneumonic effusions require catheter drainage for resolution even though bacteria do not actually contaminate the pleural space.

Ultrasound is used to identify the largest fluid pocket for catheter placement. Direct puncture of the pleural cavity using the **trocar method** is quicker and easier than using guidewires and catheter exchange techniques. A relatively stiff catheter is needed for the pleu-

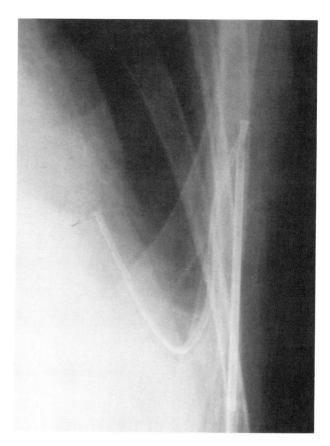

FIG 17-13. Buckled drainage catheter. Placing a flexible catheter in the pleural space for long-term drainage will result in buckling of the catheter because of respiratory motion. This kinked catheter was ineffective and was replaced with a stiff drainage catheter.

ral space because the continued motion of respiration will place traction on the catheter, resulting in buckling and ineffective drainage (Fig. 17-13). Two useful catheters for continuous pleural drainage are the Sacks catheter* available in 5.5, 7.0, 8.2, and 9.4 Fr. sizes, and the Mueller empyema drainage catheter† in 10 and 12 Fr. sizes. Both catheter systems have an inner cannula used to straighten the catheter for insertion and a trocar-pointed stylet that provides a 3- to 4-mm point for puncture.

To introduce the catheter, the puncture site is infiltrated with local anesthetic and a nick is made in the skin with a No. 11 blade. The catheter-cannula-trocar assembly is advanced directly into the pleural space. The trocar is removed and fluid aspiration is attempted. If no fluid is aspirated, the catheter position is adjusted with ultrasound guidance until fluid is easily aspirated. The cannula is directed downward and held firmly in

---

*Electro-Catheter Company, Rahway, NJ.
†Cook, Inc, Bloomington, IN.

place while the catheter is advanced into the most dependent portion of the pleural space. The cannula is removed and the catheter is attached to a three-way stopcock and drainage bag. Aspiration is performed until ultrasound examination confirms that all fluid has been removed. The pleural cavity is then irrigated several times with sterile saline solution to remove particulate matter. The catheter is sutured to the skin and connected to a standard underwater seal pleural drainage system.* The catheter is placed to continuous negative suction (−20 cm water pressure) while the volume of fluid drainage is monitored. When less than 10 ml of fluid drains from the pleural space in 24 hours, the catheter can be removed.

Loculations in the pleural space may prevent complete catheter drainage of pleural fluid. Transcatheter instillation of urokinase or streptokinase has been reported to be useful in lysing fibrin membranes to facilitate drainage.[30,31] Bronchopleural fistula should be suspected in cases that show the presence of both air and fluid in the pleural space, or are slow to resolve after catheter placement. Propyliodone oil suspension† can be injected into the pleural space to perform contrast sinography and detect this complication.[26]

Sclerosis of the Pleural Space. Malignancy is the cause of 40% to 45% of pleural effusions in adults.[32] In 50% to 60% of these patients the effusion is the presenting manifestation causing progressive dyspnea, cough, and chest pain. Treatment is aimed at relieving symptoms. Simple thoracentesis and chest tube drainage may provide temporary relief, but nearly all malignant effusions recur within one month. Chemical pleurodesis is used to induce adhesions of the visceral and parietal pleural surfaces to prevent accumulation of fluid in the pleural space. A wide variety of chemicals have been used; their success rates vary from 25% to 100%, with most being in the range of 60% to 70%.[32-34] Tetracycline is the most common agent used in the United States.

Ultrasound guidance is used to ensure accurate catheter placement for thoracentesis and instillation of the chemical agents, to assess adequacy of drainage and reaccumulation of fluid, and to identify loculated fluid collections. Therapeutic thoracentesis with a small catheter is performed to remove all pleural fluid. Tetracycline, at a dose of 15 to 20 mg/kg body weight, is added to 50 ml of 5% normal saline and injected into the pleural space. The chest catheter is clamped for 24 hours. The patient is instructed to change body position every few minutes to spread the chemical over all pleural surfaces. Ultrasound is used to check for reaccumulation of fluid at 24 hours. If no fluid is present, the

catheter is removed. If fluid has reaccumulated, pleurodesis may be repeated.

Pleural Biopsy. Pleural masses and focal areas of pleural thickening are frequently hidden from fluoroscopic view by accompanying pleural fluid. Ultrasound is effective in demonstrating these lesions and guiding needle placement for biopsy. Pleural masses and thickened pleural areas or those that look abnormal can frequently be biopsied using standard biopsy needles for histologic or cytologic examination. Normal-thickness pleura in areas of loculated pleural effusion can be biopsied using the Cope reverse bevel pleural biopsy needle.* Mueller et al[35] provide an excellent description of the technique of pleural biopsy using the Cope needle.

Complications of Pleural Invasive Procedures. Complications of invasive procedures in the pleural space include pneumothorax, hemothorax from laceration of an intercostal artery, vasovagal reaction, infection of the pleural space, and improper placement of needle or catheter into lung, liver, spleen, or kidney.[20] Removal of large amounts of fluid (more than 1 liter) may cause re-expansion pulmonary edema.

Pneumothorax is the most frequent complication associated with invasive procedures of the thorax. Pneumothorax rates approach 9% for invasive procedures in the pleural space. Most pneumothoraces are small, self-limiting, and produce minimal symptoms. Some pneumothoraces result in progressive loss of lung volume, causing respiratory distress or respiratory failure in patients with underlying lung disease. The physician performing invasive procedures in the thorax must be familiar with the treatment of pneumothorax.

Treatment of Pneumothorax. Tube thoracostomy has been the standard treatment for symptomatic patients with pneumothorax. These tubes are large in size (20 to 40 Fr.) and require surgical placement. Small-caliber catheters, percutaneously placed using fluoroscopic direction, have been shown to be equally effective in treatment of pneumothorax.[36] The smaller catheters, used with a one-way flutter valve, cause less patient discomfort, allow patients to be ambulatory, and are associated with a lower rate of major complications.

A pneumothorax treatment set is available† that includes a 9-Fr. catheter with cannula and trocar, a one-way flutter valve,‡ and a connecting tube with stopcock. The stylet and cannula enter the catheter through a side hole, not through the end of the catheter. The catheter is inserted using the one-step trocar technique. The stopcock is attached to the catheter before puncture to prevent the lung from re-expanding too rapidly. A puncture is made in the second or third anterior inter-

*Pleurevac Company, Queensville, NY.
†Dionosil, Glaxo, Greenford, England.

*Randall, Fachney, Avon, MA.
†Cook, Inc., Bloomington, IN.
‡Heimlich valve, Bard-Parker, Rutherford, NJ.

costal space in the midclavicular line. When the parietal pleura is punctured, the trocar is withdrawn into the cannula. The catheter-cannula assembly is advanced into an anterior and apical position. The cannula and stylet are removed and the flutter valve is attached. The flutter valve allows air and fluid to escape from the pleural space but prevents air and fluid from passing back into the thorax. Opening the stopcock allows slow egress of air and reduction of the pneumothorax. The valve can be connected to a vented drainage bag or underwater seal pleural drainage system.* The average duration for catheter drainage of pneumothorax is 3 to 4 days.[36]

LUNG PARENCHYMA

Air in the periphery of the lung prohibits ultrasound evaluation of parenchymal disease. However, when the peripheral air spaces of the lung are collapsed or filled with fluid, ultrasound examination is possible and can help to determine the nature of the lesion.

---

*Pleurevac Company, Queensville, NY.

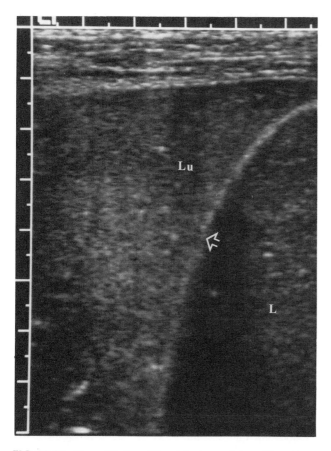

FIG 17-14. Consolidation. The right lower lobe of lung (*Lu*) is densely consolidated, assuming a level of echogenicity greater than that of the liver (*L*). The arrow marks the diaphragm.

Sonographic Appearance

Consolidation and Atelectasis. With consolidation the air spaces of the lung are filled with fluid and inflammatory cells. The highly reflective aerated lung is converted into a firm dense mass with good sound transmission (Fig. 17-14). With atelectasis the alveoli collapse and the lung, or a portion of the lung, becomes airless and capable of good sound transmission.

Consolidated lung is hypoechoic as compared with highly reflective aerated lung and is usually hypoechoic as compared with the liver and spleen because of its high fluid content. The consolidated lung is generally poorly defined and somewhat wedge shaped.[37,38] Air within bronchi surrounded by consolidated lung produced highly reflective linear branching echoes that can be recognized as sonographic air bronchograms.[39] Aerated alveoli surrounded by consolidated lung produce highly reflective globular echoes that can be recognized as sonographic air alveolograms (Fig. 17-15). The high-amplitude echoes produced by trapped air may cause acoustic shadows and reverberation artifacts. Fluid-filled bronchi produce multiple branching anechoic tubular structures within the consolidated lung.[40] Pulmonary vessels can also be recognized as branching tubular structures. Vessels can be differentiated from bronchi by observing their pulsativity, by tracing their origin to the pulmonary artery, or by the use of Doppler.[40] Identification of sonographic air bronchograms, air al-

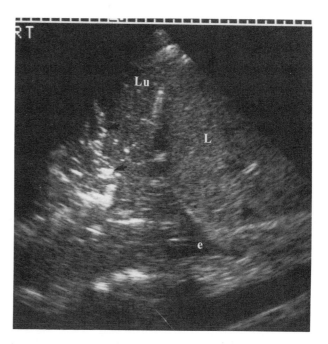

FIG 17-15. Sonographic air alveolograms. The base of the lung (*Lu*) is densely consolidated but the more proximal lung has pockets of aerated alveoli (*arrows*), which produce bright reflections and reverberations. A small pleural effusion (*e*) is also present. *L*, Liver.

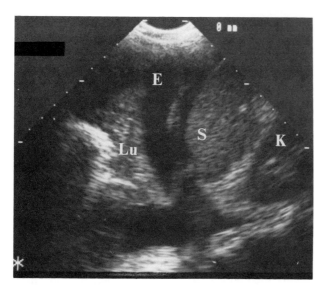

FIG 17-16. Compressive atelectasis. Compressed and collapsed lung (*Lu*) is suspended in pleural effusion (*E*) in this longitudinal sector image obtained in an intercostal space. The lung was observed to move in response to the patient's respiratory efforts. *S*, Spleen; *K*, Left kidney.

veolograms, fluid bronchograms, and pulmonary vasculature helps to differentiate consolidated lung from parenchymal masses and pleural lesions. Ultrasound also is useful to differentiate pneumonia alone from pneumonia with pleural effusion or empyema.

Atelectasis frequently accompanies pleural effusion. The pressure of the pleural fluid produces collapse of the lung. Atelectatic lung appears as a wedge-shaped density moving through the pleural fluid in time with the patient's respirations (Fig. 17-16). Crowding of fluid-filled or air-filled bronchi may be seen within the collapsed portion of the lung.[39]

Lung Tumors. Lung tumors that abut the pleural surface appear as masses partially surrounded by highly reflective aerated lung.[37,38,41,42] The margins of the tumor are often well defined. The tumor stands out in strong relief compared to the surrounding air-filled lung. Echo enhancement is often present deep to the lesion because the tumor is a better sound transmitter than is aerated lung.[38,41] Lesions smaller than 5 cm are usually hypoechoic compared to aerated lung, while lesions larger than 5 cm may be isoechoic compared to aerated lung. The increased echogenicity of larger lesions may be caused by internal hemorrhage or necrosis. Cavitary lesions have hyperechoic walls with central echolucent areas. Foci of calcification within lung masses are easily demonstrated by ultrasonography.[1] Ultrasound may help define tumor extension to pleura and adjacent structures by observing obliteration of the pleural surface echo and lack of gliding movement of the tumor with respiration.[42]

Centrally located lung tumors near the pulmonary hilum may be visualized by ultrasonography when they are associated with lung consolidation.[37] When the lung tumor causes obstruction to the airways, the tumor is visualized as a hypoechoic nodule at the tip of the resulting triangular area of consolidation. Tumors surrounded by consolidated lung appear as hyperechoic masses within hypoechoic fluid-filled lung.

Lung Abscess. A lung abscess is a localized suppurative process characterized by necrosis of lung tissue. Primary lung abscesses are caused by aspiration, necrotizing pneumonia, septic emboli, or a complication of chronic lung disease. These abscesses are amenable to cure by percutaneously placed drainage catheters.[19,43-45] Secondary lung abscesses caused by lung carcinoma, pulmonary sequestration, lung cyst, or bronchoesophageal fistula generally require surgical intervention.

Lung abscesses have thick irregular walls with echogenic debris and air within the internal fluid. Differentiating lung abscess from empyema is frequently a radiographic challenge.[46] Empyemas are confined within the pleural space and tend to have smooth walls of uniform thickness. Lung parenchyma is compressed and displaced. Lung abscesses destroy lung parenchyma, are associated with surrounding areas of lung consolidation, and have irregular walls of varying thickness. With real-time sonography, a lung abscess will demonstrate expansion of its entire circumference with inspiration.[8] In empyema, only the internal wall, the visceral pleura, will show motion with inspiration.

Invasive Procedures in Lung Parenchyma

Lung Biopsy. Percutaneous transthoracic aspiration biopsy using fluoroscopic guidance is a standard method of obtaining tissue diagnosis of pulmonary parenchymal masses.[47] However, fluoroscopic visualization of lung nodules may be difficult when the nodules are pleural based, at the lung apex, in the axilla, or near the diaphragm or mediastinum.[47,48] In comparison, ultrasonographic visualization of lung masses for guidance of biopsy is best in the very areas most difficult to biopsy with fluoroscopic guidance.[38,41,42,49-51] Ultrasound-guided biopsy is quick, convenient, and safe. Because ultrasonography can visualize aerated lung adjacent to pleural-based nodules better than fluoroscopy, the aerated lung can be avoided more easily.[50] The incidence of pneumothorax for biopsy of pleural-based nodules is 2% with ultrasound guidance, as compared to 11% with fluoroscopic guidance.[48,50,52] Both ultrasound and fluoroscopic guidance have a reported 90% to 95% sensitivity for the diagnosis of lung cancer. Ultrasonography is particularly useful in guiding biopsy of peripheral lung tumors obscured by pleural effusion.

Preliminary inspection of the chest x-ray is essential

in planning the approach to ultrasound-guided biopsy. Most lung lesions may be visualized and biopsied through the intercostal space. Lesions at the lung apex may be approached from either above or below the clavicle.[42] Lesions on the diaphragm may be visualized and biopsied using an upward angle through the liver.[48] Once the lesion is visualized, a safe course for the needle is determined. The needle pass into the lesion may be performed either freehand or by use of a needle guide attached to the transducer. The patient is asked to suspend respiration while the needle is being advanced into the lesion. The patient may then resume shallow respiration while the needle is allowed to swing freely. The patient is again asked to stop breathing while the biopsy is taken. Specimens are given to a cytopathologist for immediate examination for adequacy. Biopsies are repeated until diagnostic tissue is obtained. The presence of a cytopathologist in the biopsy suite is essential to maximize diagnostic yield while minimizing the number of needle passes.[47]

Catheter Drainage of Lung Abscess. Most lung abscesses are successfully treated with antibiotics and bronchoscopic internal drainage.[19] Treatment failures are considered candidates for lobectomy. External drainage by catheter was successfully used prior to availability of antibiotics, and has recently been reaffirmed as a successful treatment method with a low complication rate.[43-45] Ultrasound guidance may be used to accurately direct placement of a large-bore surgical tube, or to place a smaller radiologic catheter. The technique for catheter placement is similar to that used for empyema drainage.

Complications of Invasive Procedures in the Lung Parenchyma. Pneumothorax and minor bleeding are the most frequent complications of lung biopsy.[47] The significance of pneumothorax is greatest in patients with severely compromised pulmonary function. The risk of bleeding is increased in patients with coagulopathy. Rare complications include major bleeding, air embolism, and neoplastic seeding of the needle tract.

MEDIASTINUM

Because the mediastinum is surrounded by shadowing bone and reflective lung, it offers a challenge to sonographic evaluation. However, with careful attention to technique and patient positioning, most areas of the mediastinum can be effectively examined.[1,53-56] When abnormalities are detected, ultrasonographic guidance can be used for biopsy.[57] The ability to visualize the needle continually as it courses to the lesion is a significant advantage because this area is so rich with major vascular structures. Detailed knowledge of the three-dimensional anatomy of the mediastinum is critical because the planes of sonographic examination are usually oblique and not readily related to the standard orthogonal planes of **computed tomography (CT)** and **magnetic resonance imaging (MRI).**

Sonographic Appearance

The upper mediastinum is accessible to sonographic investigation by use of a **suprasternal approach.**[53] Patients are examined in a supine position with a pillow placed beneath the shoulders and the neck extended. The transducer is placed at the base of the neck and angled caudally behind the manubrium. Oblique sagittal and coronal plane images can be obtained. The innominate veins, common carotid, brachiocephalic, and subclavian arteries can be examined (Fig. 17-17) and each can be identified by its location and Doppler characteristics. Tortuous vessels causing abnormal widening of the mediastinum, seen on chest x-rays, are easily recognized. Mediastinal masses can be precisely localized and characterized as solid, cystic, vascular, or calcified. The relationship of the mass to cardiac and vascular structures can be defined accurately.

Parasternal scanning of the mediastinum is aided by placing the patient in the appropriate lateral decubitus position.[54] Gravity enlarges the sonographic window by swinging the mediastinum downward. The as-

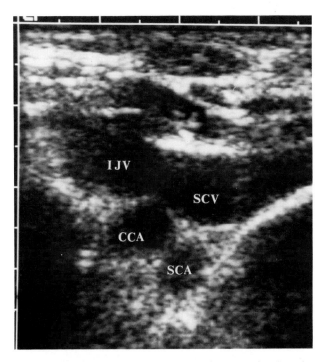

FIG 17-17. Mediastinum—suprasternal approach. An oblique transverse view into the upper mediastinum is obtained by placing a 5-MHz linear-array transducer at the base of the neck and angling downward behind the manubrium. The junction of the left subclavian vein (*SCV*) with the left internal jugular vein (*IJV*) is demonstrated. The left common carotid artery (*CCA*) and left subclavian artery (*SCA*) are also seen. Vessel identification is confirmed by use of Doppler.

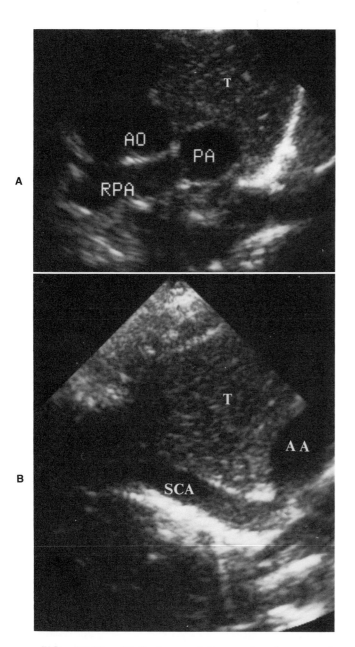

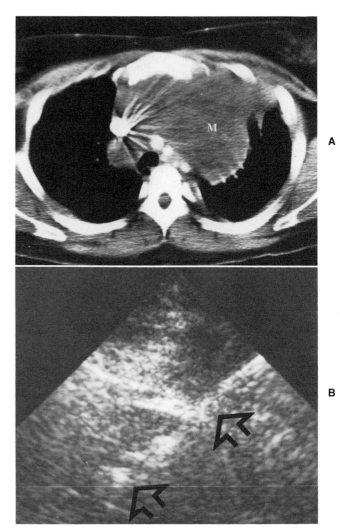

FIG 17-18. Mediastinum—left parasternal approach. **A,** Transverse sector scan obtained in an intercostal space from a left parasternal approach demonstrates a prominent thymus (*T*) in a 2-year-old patient. Also clearly seen are the ascending aorta (*AO*), main pulmonary artery (*PA*) at its bifurcation, and the right pulmonary artery (*RPA*). **B,** Sagittal sector scan obtained in the same left parasternal intercostal space as in **A** demonstrates the aortic arch (*AA*) and origin of the left subclavian artery (*SCA*). T, Thymus.

FIG 17-19. Biopsy of mediastinal lymphoma. **A,** A computed tomography image of the chest 2 cm above the aortic arch demonstrates a large mass (*M*) in the anterior mediastinum displacing the great vessels posteriorly. **B,** Because the patient was pregnant, acutely ill, and required monitoring in the intensive care unit, biopsy was performed using portable ultrasound guidance at the patient's bedside. Tissue samples for histologic diagnosis of non-Hodgkin lymphoma were obtained using a 16-gauge Trucut needle (*arrows*). Constant observation of needle position by ultrasound safely prevented injury of vascular structures by this large needle.
(Courtesy of John P. McGahan, M.D., University of California, Davis Medical Center.)

cending aorta, anterior mediastinum, and subcarinal region are best imaged from a right parasternal approach with the patient lying with the right side down. The pulmonary trunk and left side of the anterior mediastinum are best imaged with a left parasternal approach with the patient in a left lateral decubitus position (Fig. 17-18).

Posterior masses may be imaged from a **posterior paravertebral approach.** Lesions near the diaphragm can be approached from the abdomen *through the liver.* Large masses displace lung and may be imaged *directly* through the intercostal spaces.[1,55]

Invasive Procedures in the Mediastinum

Percutaneous needle biopsy of mediastinal lesions using fluoroscopy or computed tomography for guidance is an accepted and useful diagnostic procedure,[58-63] but the reported experience of using ultrasound guidance for mediastinal biopsy is limited.[47-49,57] However, the simplicity, accuracy, and safety of sonographic guidance are significant advantages for accessible lesions. Lesions in the anterior mediastinum and large lesions that abut the chest wall are most amenable to ultrasound-directed biopsy (Fig. 17-19).

The patient is positioned to optimize ultrasonographic visualization of the lesion. It is preferable to achieve continuous visualization of the needle path with needle direction provided by needle guidance systems that are attached to the transducer. Pneumothorax, hemoptysis, and hemorrhage are the most common complications reported with mediastinal biopsy procedures.

REFERENCES

1. Rosenberg HK. The complementary roles of ultrasound and plain film radiography in differentiating pediatric chest abnormalities. *Radiographics* 1986;6:427-445.
2. O'Moore PV, Mueller PR, Simeone JF, et al. Sonographic guidance in the diagnostic and therapeutic interventions in the pleural space. *AJR* 1987;149:1-5.
3. Landay M, Harless W. Ultrasonic differentiation of right pleural effusion from subphrenic fluid on longitudinal scans of the right upper quadrant: importance of recognizing the diaphragm. *Radiology* 1977;123:155-158.
4. McGahan JP. Aspiration and drainage procedures in the intensive care unit: percutaneous sonographic guidance. *Radiology* 1985;154:531-532.
5. McGahan JP, Anderson MW, Walter JP. Portable real-time sonographic and needle guidance systems for aspiration and drainage. *AJR* 1986;147:1241-1246.

Pleural space

6. Kremkau FW, Taylor KJW. Artifacts in ultrasound imaging. *J Ultrasound Med* 1986;5:227-237.
7. Gardner FJ, Clark RN, Kozlowski R. A model of a hepatic mirror-image artifact. *Med Ultrasound* 1980;4:19-21.
8. Simeone JF, Mueller PR, vanSonnenberg E. The uses of diagnostic ultrasound in the thorax. *Clin Chest Med* 1984;5:281-290.
9. Lewandowski BJ, Winsberg F. Echographic appearance of the right hemidiaphragm. *J Ultrasound Med* 1983;2:243-249.
10. Rosenberg ER. Ultrasound in the assessment of pleural densities. *Chest* 1983;84:283-285.
11. Hirsch JH, Rogers JV, Mack LA. Real-time sonography of pleural opacities. *AJR* 1981;136:297-301.
12. Martinez OC, Serrano BV, Romero RR. Real-time ultrasound evaluation of tuberculous pleural effusions. *J Clin Ultrasound* 1989;17:407-410.
13. Hirsch JH, Carter SJ, Chikos PM, et al. Ultrasonic evaluation of radiographic opacities of the chest. *AJR* 1978;130:1153-1156.
14. Marks WM, Filly RA, Callen PW. Real-time evaluation of pleural lesions: new observations regarding the probability of obtaining free fluid. *Radiology* 1982;142:163-164.
15. Laing FC, Filly RA. Problems in the application of ultrasonography for the evaluation of pleural opacities. *Radiology* 1978;126:211-214.
16. Dershaw DD. Actinomycosis of the chest wall: ultrasound findings in empyema necessitans. *Chest* 1984;86:779-780.
17. Schmitt WGH, Hubener KH, Rucker HC. Pleural calcification with persistent effusion. *Radiology* 1983;149:633-638.
18. Pugatch RD, Spirn PW. Radiology of the pleura. *Clin Chest Med* 1985;6:17-32.
19. Illescas FF. Interventional radiology of the pleural space and lung: small diameter catheters. *Radiology Report* 1989;1:20-31.
20. Jay SJ. Diagnostic procedures for pleural disease. *Clin Chest Med* 1985;6:33-48.
21. Chetty KG. Transudative pleural effusions. *Clin Chest Med* 1985;6:49-54.
22. vanSonnenberg E, Nakamoto SK, Mueller PR, et al. Computed tomography and ultrasound-guided catheter drainage of empyemas after chest-tube failure. *Radiology* 1984;151:349-353.
23. Westcott JL. Percutaneous catheter drainage of pleural effusion and empyema. *AJR* 1985;144:1189-1193.
24. Silverman SG, Mueller PR, Saini S, et al. Thoracic empyema: management with image-guided catheter drainage. *Radiology* 1988;169:5-9.
25. Reinhold C, Illescas FF, Atri M, Bret PM. Treatment of pleural effusions and pneumothorax with catheters placed percutaneously under imaging guidance. *AJR* 1989;152:1189-1191.
26. Merriam MA, Cronan JJ, Dorfman GS, et al. Radiographically guided percutaneous catheter drainage of pleural fluid collections. *AJR* 1988;151:1113-1116.
27. Lemmer JH, Botham MJ, Orringer MB. Modern management of adult thoracic empyema. *J Thorac Cardiovasc Surg* 1985;90:849-855.
28. Grant DR, Finley RJ. Empyema: analysis of treatment techniques. *Can J Surg* 1985;28:449-451.
29. Varkey B. Pleural effusions caused by infection. *Postgrad Med* 1986;80:213-223.
30. Light RW. Parapneumonic effusions and empyema. *Clin Chest Med* 1985;6:55-62.
31. Moulton JS, Moore PT, Mencini RA. Treatment of loculated pleural effusions with transcatheter intracavitary urokinase. *AJR* 1989;153:941-945.
32. Prakash UBS. Malignant pleural effusions. *Postgrad Med* 1986;80:201-209.
33. Zaloznik AJ, Oswald SG, Langin M. Intrapleural tetracycline in malignant pleural effusions: a randomized study. *Cancer* 1983;51:752-755.
34. Ostrowski MJ, Halsall GM. Intracavitary bleomycin in the management of malignant pleural effusions: a multicenter study. *Cancer Treat Rep* 1982;66:1903-1907.
35. Mueller PR, Saini S, Simeone JF, et al. Image-guided pleural biopsies: indications, technique, and results in 23 patients. *Radiology* 1988;169:1-4.
36. Conces DJ Jr, Tarver RD, Gray WC, et al. Treatment of pneumothoraces utilizing small caliber chest tubes. *Chest* 1988;94:55-57.

37. Yang P-C, Luh K-T, Wu H-D, et al. Lung tumors associated with obstructive pneumonitis: ultrasound studies. *Radiology* 1990;174:717-720.

38. Yang P-C, Luh K-T, Sheu J-C, et al. Peripheral pulmonary lesions: ultrasonography and ultrasonically guided aspiration biopsy. *Radiology* 1985;155:451-456.

39. Weinberg B, Diakoumakis EE, Kass EG, et al. The air bronchogram: sonographic demonstration. *AJR* 1986;147:593-595.

40. Dorne HL. Differentiation of pulmonary parenchymal consolidation from pleural disease using the sonographic fluid bronchogram. *Radiology* 1986;158:41-42.

41. Izumi S, Tamki S, Natori H, et al. Ultrasonically guided aspiration needle biopsy in disease of the chest. *Am Rev Respir Dis* 1982;125:460-464.

42. Yang P-C, Lee L-N, Luh K-T, et al. Ultrasonography of Pancoast tumor. *Chest* 1988;94:124-128.

43. Yellin A, Yellin EO, Lieberman Y. Percutaneous tube drainage: the treatment of choice for refractory lung abscess. *Ann Thor Surg* 1985;39:266-270.

44. Weissberg D. Percutaneous drainage of lung abscess. *J Thorac Cardiovasc Surg* 1984;87:308-312.

45. Mengoli L. Giant lung abscess treated by tube thoracostomy. *J Thorac Cardiovasc Surg* 1985;90:186-194.

46. Stark DD, Federle MP, Goodman PC. Differentiating lung abscess and empyema: radiography and computed tomography. *AJR* 1983;141:163-167.

Lung parenchyma

47. Westcott JL. Percutaneous transthoracic needle biopsy. *Radiology* 1988;169:593-601.

48. Pedersen OM, Aasen TB, Gulsvik A. Fine-needle aspiration biopsy of mediastinal and peripheral pulmonary masses guided by real-time sonography. *Chest* 1986;89:504-508.

49. Ikezoe J, Shusuke S, Higashihara T, et al. Sonographically guided needle biopsy for diagnosis of thoracic lesions. *AJR* 1984;143:229-234.

50. Cinti D, Hawkins HB. Aspiration biopsy of peripheral pulmonary masses using real-time sonographic guidance. *AJR* 1984;142:1115-1116.

51. Afschrift M, Nachtegaele P, Voet D, et al. Puncture of thoracic lesions under sonographic guidance. *Thorax* 1982;37:503-506.

52. Berquist TH, Bailey PB, Cortese DA, et al. Transthoracic needle biopsy accuracy and complications in relation to location and type of lesion. *Mayo Clin Proc* 1980;55:475-481.

Mediastinum

53. Wernecke K, Peters PE, Galanski M. Mediastinal tumors: evaluation with suprasternal sonography. *Radiology* 1986;159:405-409.

54. Wernecke K, Potter R, Peters PE, et al: Parasternal mediastinal sonography: sensitivity in the detection of anterior mediastinal and subcarinal tumors. *AJR* 1988;150:1021-1026.

55. Ikezoe J, Morimoto S, Arisawa J, et al. Ultrasonography of mediastinal teratoma. *J Clin Ultrasound* 1986;14:513-520.

56. O'Laughlin MP, Huhta JC, Murphy DJ. Ultrasound examination of extracardiac chest masses in children: Doppler diagnosis of a vascular etiology. *J Ultrasound Med* 1987;6:151-157.

57. Wernecke K, Vassallo P, Peters PE, et al. Mediastinal tumors: biopsy under ultrasound guidance. *Radiology* 1989;172:473-476.

58. Kuhlman JE, Fishman EK, Wang KP, et al. Mediastinal cysts: diagnosis by CT and needle aspiration. *AJR* 1988;150:75-78.

59. Weisbrod GL, Lyons DJ, Tao LC, et al. Percutaneous fine-needle aspiration biopsy of mediastinal lesions. *AJR* 1984;143:525.

60. Linder J, Olsen GA, Johnston WW. Fine-needle aspiration biopsy of the mediastinum. *Am J Med* 1986;81:1005-1008.

61. Moinuddin SM, Lee LH, Montgomery JH. Mediastinal needle biopsy. *AJR* 1984;143:531-532.

62. Gobien RP, Skucas J, Paris BS. Computed tomography-assisted fluoroscopically guided aspiration biopsy of central hilar and mediastinal masses. *Radiology* 1981;141:443-447.

63. Adler OB, Rosenberger A, Peleg H. Fine-needle aspiration biopsy of mediastinal masses: evaluation of 136 experiences. *AJR* 1983;140:893-896.

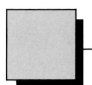

CHAPTER 18

Ultrasound-Guided Biopsy of the Abdomen and Pelvis

- Carl C. Reading, M.D.
- J. William Charboneau, M.D.

Sonographically guided needle biopsy is a rapidly expanding and important aspect of many imaging practices. It has become an accurate, safe, and widely accepted technique for confirmation of suspected malignant masses and characterization of many benign lesions in various intraabdominal locations.[1-6] It also decreases patient costs by obviating operation, decreasing the duration of hospital stay, and decreasing the number of examinations necessary during diagnostic evaluation.[7,8]

Traditionally, sonographically guided needle biopsy has been used for the biopsy of large, superficial, and cystic masses. Currently, however, because of improvements in instrumentation and biopsy techniques, small, deeply located, and solid masses can also be biopsied accurately.

INDICATIONS AND CONTRAINDICATIONS

Most needle biopsies are performed to confirm suspected malignancy before nonsurgical treatment, such as chemotherapy or radiation therapy, is begun. For example, a liver biopsy could be performed to confirm hepatic metastasis in a patient with a known primary malignancy. Less often, needle biopsy is performed to determine the nature of an indeterminate lesion, such as a solitary indeterminate solid hepatic mass in a patient with no history of malignancy. Occasionally, needle biopsy is performed on a mass suspected to be benign. For example, in a patient with recurrent hyperparathyroidism a suspected parathyroid adenoma could be biopsied to confirm the nature of the benign mass before reexploration.

There are three relative contraindications to needle biopsy:

- Lack of a safe biopsy path to the mass without traversing a large vascular structure (such as the inferior vena cava or abdominal aorta)
- An uncooperative patient in whom uncontrolled motion that may lead to difficulty in directing the needle to the mass, causing inadvertent laceration of vessels or vascular organs
- Presence of an uncorrectable coagulopathy

To assess for coagulopathy, the primary information comes from the patient's medical history.[9] If the bleeding history is unremarkable, then most biopsies can be performed without additional laboratory testing. However, if the history suggests a bleeding disorder, a bleeding time or other tests, such as prothrombin time, partial thromboplastin time, and platelet count, should be performed.[10] Mild coagulopathies may occur secondary to the use of aspirin or other drugs, such as carbenicillin, ticarcillin, or beta-lactam antibiotics. If the bleeding time is prolonged, the procedure may be delayed and the drug discontinued until the test becomes normal.[11] Severe coagulopathies are not an absolute contraindication to biopsy. Some coagulopathies can be corrected with vitamin K, fresh-frozen plasma, platelets, or clotting factors. Each patient should be considered individually in regard to whether biopsy is indicated if a coagulopathy exists.

Sonographic guidance can be used for the biopsy of many organs and regions of the body. The technique is optimal for lesions located superficially or at moderate depth in a thin to average-size person. Deep masses or masses in obese patients can be hard to biopsy under sonographic guidance because of the difficulty in lesion visualization resulting from sound attenuation in the soft tissues. Similarly, lesions located within or behind bone or an air-filled lung cannot be visualized for biopsy because of the nearly complete reflection of sound from the bone or air interface. Overlying loops of bowel are usually not a contraindication to needle biopsy if small-caliber needles are used unless sonographic visualization is totally obscured by overlying gas. Theoretically, any mass that is visible sonographically is amenable to needle biopsy.

TECHNIQUE
Guidance Methods

Most sonographically guided biopsies are performed under continuous real-time visualization in a manner analogous to biopsy under fluoroscopic control. Several guidance systems that are designed to facilitate real-time sonographic visualization of the biopsy needle are available. These include dedicated ultrasound biopsy transducers with built-in needle channels or slots within the central or side portions of the transducer that direct the needle in a predetermined angle within the plane of view of the transducer.[12] Some of these systems project computer-generated grids onto the viewing monitor to show the approach and distance to the target. Alternatively, commercially available guides can be fitted to the side of existing transducers. These guides direct the needle to various specific depths from the transducer surface, depending on the preselected angle of the guide relative to the transducer.[13,14] These guides are usually of greater benefit to physicians who do not commonly perform sonographically guided biopsies than to those who have had experience using sonographic guidance.

Many experienced radiologists prefer a "freehand" approach in which the needle is inserted through the skin directly into the plane of view of the transducer, which is used without a guide.[4,6] This approach provides great flexibility to the radiologist by allowing subtle freehand adjustments to be made during the course of the biopsy, thereby compensating for improper trajectory and patient movement. Also, masses that are large and located superficially may not require continuous real-time sonographic needle guidance. In these cases, the location and depth of the mass are determined before the biopsy, and the needle is inserted blindly in that direction to that depth. This technique is similar to that used to perform a biopsy guided by computed tomography.

For sterility, the transducer can be covered with a sterile plastic sheath, but this may degrade image quality and make the transducer more difficult to handle. We prefer to cleanse the transducer with isopropyl alcohol and place it directly on the skin.[6] Sterile gel is used as an acoustic coupling agent. After the biopsy procedure, the transducer is soaked for 10 minutes in a bacteriocidal dialdehyde solution. No complications from infection have been observed or reported from the use of this technique.

Biopsy Needles

A wide variety of needles with a spectrum of calibers, lengths, and tip designs[15-21] are commercially available for use in percutaneous biopsy. Conceptually, needles can be grouped into "skinny" or thin-caliber (20 to 25 gauge) and large-caliber (14 to 19 gauge). Thin-caliber needles are used primarily to obtain specimens for cytologic analysis. However, small pieces of tissue can be obtained for histologic examination. With these needles, masses behind loops of bowel can be punctured with minimal likelihood of infection. Thin-caliber needles are often used to confirm tumor recurrence or metastasis in a patient known to have a previous primary malignancy. Even if the sample is small, the pathologist usually is able to make an accurate diagnosis by comparing the biopsy specimen with the previously obtained tissue.

Large-caliber needles can be used to obtain greater amounts of material for histologic as well as cytologic analysis.[17,20] Their use may be necessary to obtain an adequate histologic specimen to diagnose confidently some types of malignancy (such as lymphoma), many benign lesions, and most chronic diffuse parenchymal disease processes (such as hepatic cirrhosis, renal glomerulonephritis, or renal allograft rejection).[22,23]

Needles may also be categorized according to the configuration of the needle tip. Most needles have either a noncutting, beveled tip (as on conventional injection and spinal needles), or a tissue-cutting tip (as on Menghini needles).[17] Noncutting, beveled tip needles easily penetrate tough soft tissue planes. They are usually used to aspirate fluid and to obtain cytologic specimens. These sharply beveled needles are useful in the biopsy of small masses, such as superficial lymph nodes in the groin or neck, without displacing or deflecting these mobile structures. Needles with a cutting tip are used to obtain a core of tissue when histologic analysis is needed. A variation of the end-cutting needle is the side-cutting (TruCut) needle. This type of needle can be used in conjunction with an automated spring-loaded biopsy gun.[24,25] The automated gun offers several advantages over conventional biopsy needles and techniques:

- A larger core of tissue is obtained consistently.
- A single pass rather than multiple passes is all that is required in most patients. This often decreases discomfort and theoretically makes the procedure safer.
- This biopsy device is easy to learn to operate and can be fired with one hand, allowing the other hand to be used for scanning.

There have been no reports to date of any increased

risk of complications from the use of the automated biopsy gun compared with conventional biopsy techniques.[26-29]

The preference and level of expertise of the pathologist involved in the interpretation of biopsy specimens are a consideration in the selection of needle size and type. Cytopathologists are trained to interpret pathology on the basis of only a few cells and deal well with small specimens. However, many institutions do not have capable cytopathology interpretation. Histopathologists, in contrast, often prefer the largest biopsy specimen possible for interpretation. For example, a large biopsy specimen from a metastatic lesion often allows a more reliable diagnosis of the likely primary site of the malignancy than does either a tiny sample or a cytologic aspiration. Determination of the probable site of primary malignancy is important in that it allows the oncologist to tailor subsequent treatment optimally.

Syringes are attached to the biopsy needles to provide the suction necessary for removing the specimen. Maintaining 10 milliliters of continuous suction throughout the biopsy procedure and during needle withdrawal provides an optimal tissue sample with both large- and thin-caliber needles.[30] Syringes with self-locking plungers are useful because they allow the plunger to be locked in a retracted position to maintain continuous negative pressure within the needle without use of a second hand. This one-hand method frees the other hand to hold the transducer and continuously monitor needle position during the biopsy. We prefer to use needles that also have a central stylet attached to the plunger to prevent the tissue sample from being aspirated into the barrel of the syringe.[6]

Biopsy Procedure

Biopsies are frequently performed on an outpatient basis. Discomfort from the procedure is rarely severe and usually controlled by local anesthesia (1% lidocaine) at the biopsy site after the skin is cleansed and draped. Premedication is usually not necessary. Sedatives and analgesics such as diazepam (Valium), midazolam hydrochloride (Versed), or fentanyl (Sublimaze) can be administered parenterally during the procedure if necessary.[31,32] The psychologic needs of the patient are important and should be addressed. These patients are invariably anxious about the procedure, and the radiologist should be sensitive to their concerns. An explanation of the procedure before and during the biopsy is reassuring and helps to decrease patient anxiety.

Most biopsies are performed by making one or more passes into a mass with a single needle. Occasionally, two needles are used in a coaxial manner whereby a large needle is placed into the mass to be biopsied, the stylet removed, and a longer, thinner-caliber needle is placed through the lumen of the first needle, which serves as a guide. Multiple samples can then be obtained with the smaller needle without the need to reposition the larger needle. The final biopsy specimen is obtained with the large needle before it is removed from the mass. This technique allows a large amount of tissue to be obtained with only one puncture of the capsule of an organ, which may decrease the risk of hemorrhage. In addition, precise needle placement is only performed once, which saves time in the biopsy of lesions in deep or difficult locations.

The aspirate can be stained and processed within 10 minutes after the biopsy specimen is obtained.[33] If the results are inconclusive, a repeat biopsy can be taken until an adequate specimen is obtained. In many laboratories, immediate interpretation of the cytologic specimen is not available. Therefore several samples are often taken to increase the likelihood of a positive result. The specimens are sent to the cytopathology laboratory for interpretation at a later time. After the biopsy the patient is observed for 30 minutes to 2 hours to evaluate for complications, such as hemorrhage.

Needle Visualization

Precise visualization of the biopsy needle by sonography can be a frustrating aspect of biopsy procedures. Several techniques can be used to improve needle visualization. The use of a "bobbing" or in-and-out jiggling movement of the biopsy needle during insertion causes deflection of the soft tissues adjacent to the needle and makes the trajectory of the needle much more discernible within the otherwise stationary field. In addition, the needle must be precisely aligned within the central plane or field of view of the transducer for visualization. When a mechanical guide is used, the needle is usually maintained within the central plane. If the freehand method of guidance is used, the radiologist must frequently check the alignment of the needle with the transducer. When the needle is not visualized it is usually because the needle is misaligned (either initially aligned off-center relative to the central beam of the transducer or angled away from the central beam of the transducer) (Fig. 18-1).

Needle visualization can be improved by increasing the reflectivity of the biopsy needle itself. Large-caliber needles are more readily visualized than thin-caliber needles. Various modifications in needle design that involve roughening or scoring of a portion of the needle to increase sound reflection have been used to increase needle visibility.[34,35] Scoring and Teflon coating of the needle surface slightly improve the reflectivity of the needle in a solid organ. Roughening of the inner stylet seems to be as effective as roughening of the outer needle surface. The use of a screw-type stylet markedly increases reflectivity because the auger-like surface creates many highly reflective acoustic interfaces. This

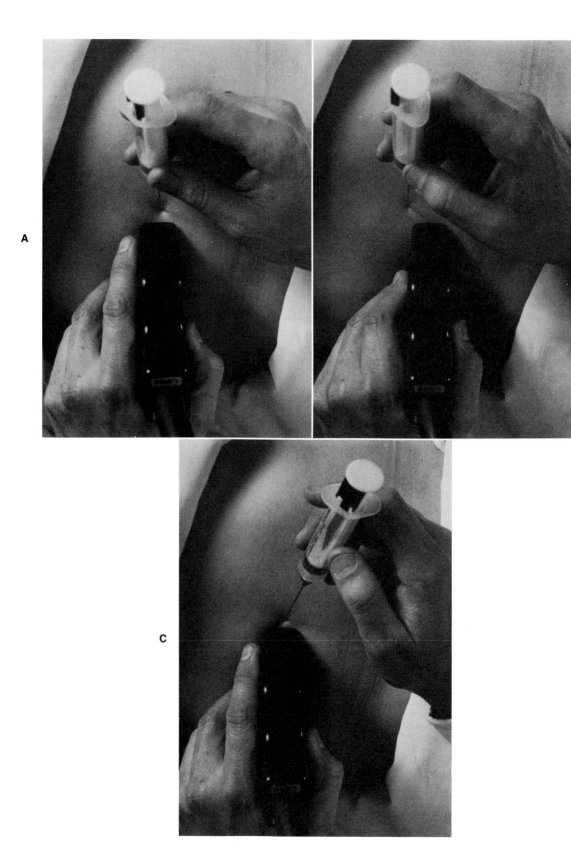

FIG 18-1. Freehand alignment of biopsy needle with the ultrasound transducer. **A,** Correct alignment. Sonographic visualization is optimal. Biopsy needle is aligned precisely within the central plane of the transducer. **B,** Incorrect alignment. Sonographic visualization is poor. Biopsy needle is aligned off-center relative to the transducer. **C,** Incorrect alignment. Sonographic visualization is poor. Biopsy needle is aligned correctly with the center of the transducer but is angled away from the central plane.

stylet was originally designed to increase the amount of cytologic material obtained during fluoroscopically guided biopsy of lung nodules but can be adapted for use in conjunction with sonographically guided biopsies.[36]

The echogenicity of the parenchyma of the organ to be biopsied also affects the visibility of the biopsy needle. If the parenchyma is relatively hypoechoic, such as liver, kidney, or spleen, an echogenic needle can usually be identified. Conversely, if the organ is relatively hyperechoic, it is usually difficult to visualize the echogenic needle tip in this background. This factor is responsible for poor needle visualization in biopsies of retroperitoneal structures or in obese patients.

Linear electronically focused phased-array transducers seem to provide a better image of the biopsy needle than that provided by mechanical-sector transducers.[5,6] The linear transducers also display the subcutaneous tissue in the near field of view to best advantage to allow optimal needle visualization during the beginning of the biopsy so that early adjustments in needle trajectory can be made. Although the linear transducer head is somewhat more awkward to position than a smaller sector transducer, it can generally be manipulated in such a way that both the mass and the biopsy needle can be visualized, even between the ribs during hepatic biopsies. Use of a noncovered but thoroughly cleansed transducer, in direct contact with the skin, also allows better needle visualization than is possible with a plastic-sheathed transducer.

Clear visualization of the biopsy needle is an important element in the success of sonographically guided needle biopsies. The various techniques that have been described can be used to enhance needle visualization. However, considerable real-time scanning experience remains the key factor in the successful performance of biopsies.

REGIONAL BIOPSY TECHNIQUES
Liver

The liver is the most frequently biopsied abdominal organ.[33,34] Hepatic biopsies are usually performed on focal solid masses to confirm metastatic disease in patients with a known primary malignancy. Large masses are more readily accessible than small masses; however, with experience, lesions as small as 0.5 cm can be biopsied (Fig. 18-2).[5,37,38] The location of the mass within the liver does not generally affect the success of a biopsy, although deeply situated lesions, such as those adjacent to the porta hepatis or within the caudate

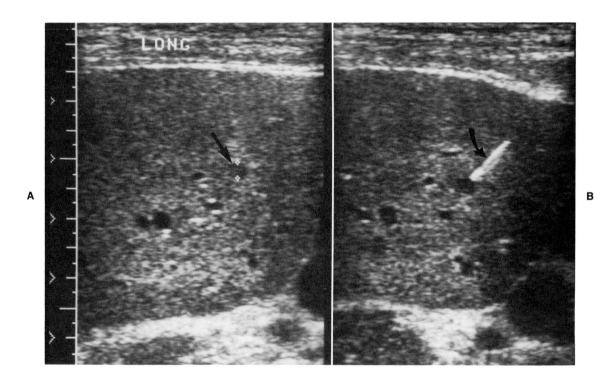

FIG 18-2. Sonographically guided biopsy of a small metastatic lesion in the liver from transitional cell carcinoma of bladder. **A,** Longitudinal sonogram of right lobe of liver shows 0.5 cm mass in midportion *(arrow).* **B,** Coaxial biopsy with an 18-gauge biopsy needle and screw-type stylet *(curved arrow).*

(From Charboneau et al. with permission).

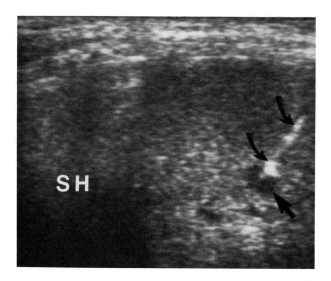

FIG 18-3. Avoidance of lung. Oblique longitudinal sonogram of right lobe of liver showing biopsy needle *(curved arrows)* with 1 cm metastatic lesion *(straight arrow)*. The lung causes posterior acoustic shadowing *(SH)*.

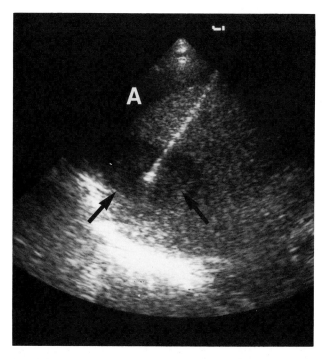

FIG 18-4. Sonographically guided biopsy in the presence of ascites of metastatic lesion from a primary breast carcinoma. Oblique longitudinal sonogram through an intercostal space shows biopsy needle with 3 cm mass *(straight arrows)* in dome of right lobe of liver. *A,* Ascites.

lobe, can be technically more challenging. Masses in the left lobe are usually readily accessible with the transducer on the relatively flat, unobstructed sonographic window of the epigastrium. Lesions in the right lobe of the liver are biopsied from a subcostal approach if they lie in the caudal portion of the liver or from an intercostal approach if they lie in the middle or upper portion of the liver. Although the intercostal approach may transgress the pleural space, the aerated lung is rarely violated because it is well visualized sonographically and can be avoided (Fig. 18-3). Hepatic biopsies have been performed safely under sonographic guidance in the presence of ascites (Fig. 18-4).[39]

Generally, it is not necessary to determine if a hepatic mass is vascular before needle biopsy. Hemorrhagic complications are uncommon even if an 18-gauge needle is used to biopsy a highly vascular mass, such as metastatic carcinoid or islet cell carcinoma.[40] It is probably more important to choose a biopsy route that interposes normal liver between the mass and the liver capsule, if possible, to provide a potential tamponade capability if hemorrhage were to occur.

Benign hepatic lesions, such as atypical cavernous hemangiomas, focal fatty infiltration, and focal areas of normal liver within a fatty-infiltrated liver, can occasionally mimic the appearance of malignancy on prebiopsy imaging studies. These processes can be biopsied under sonographic guidance to exclude malignancy and to confirm their benign nature (Fig. 18-5).[41] A single death has been reported from hemorrhage after the percutaneous biopsy of a large subcapsular hepatic hemangioma with a 21-gauge needle. In this case, it was dif-

ficult to interpose normal liver in the biopsy route.[42] However, in four separate series of 33, 20, 15, and 10 patients who underwent fine-needle biopsy of cavernous hemangiomas, there were no significant complications.[43-46] In addition, my colleagues and I have biopsied more than thirty of these lesions safely.

Pancreas

Solid pancreatic masses that are thought to be unresectable because of metastases or tumor encasement of the mesenteric vessels can be biopsied percutaneously to confirm malignancy and obviate laparotomy (Fig. 18-6). Masses within the body or anterior aspect of the head of the pancreas in a slender to normal-sized person are more accessible to sonographically guided biopsy than are masses in the tail or uncinate process, particularly in obese or large persons. The biopsy success rate is lower in the diagnosis of pancreatic carcinoma than in the diagnosis of malignant lesions in other organs in the abdomen.[1,47,48] Because portions of a visualized pancreatic mass may represent desmoplastic inflammatory change associated with the tumor rather than the tumor itself, the biopsy sample may not demonstrate tumor cells. An increased success rate with sonographic guidance can be expected if the needle is placed into the

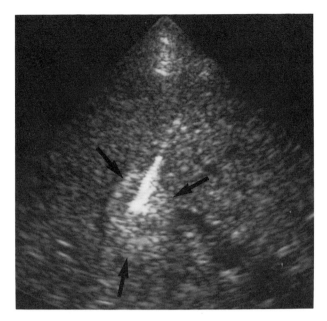

FIG 18-5. Biopsy of 2 cm cavernous hemangioma. Longitudinal sonogram of right lobe of liver showing mass *(straight arrows)* with 21-gauge needle.

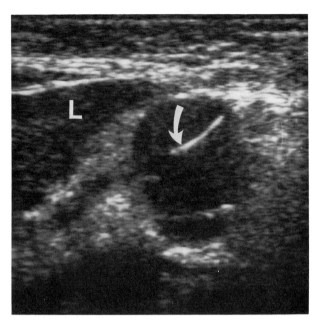

FIG 18-6. Pancreatic biopsy—primary adenocarcinoma. longitudinal sonogram of body of pancreas, showing 18-gauge biopsy needle *(curved arrow)* in 3 cm hypoechoic mass in pancreas. *L,* Left lobe of liver.

hypoechoic central portion of the pancreatic mass, which should represent tumor, rather than into the adjacent echogenic region, which is more likely to be non-malignant pancreatic parenchyma. As carcinoma of the pancreas is often well-differentiated adenocarcinoma, it may be difficult to diagnose from cytologic samples alone,[24,49] because tumors may resemble normal glandular cells. Therefore histologic specimens obtained with cutting needles can be helpful. Cystic pancreatic malignancies are difficult to diagnose accurately by percutaneous biopsy; thus surgical exploration rather than biopsy is recommended for these masses.[3]

Pancreatitis has been reported to be a complication of needle biopsy, as the result of multiple fine-needle passes directed at small pancreatic lesions.[50] One death has been reported from necrotizing pancreatitis after biopsy of a suspected pancreatic mass with a 22-gauge needle; the pancreas was free of tumor at autopsy.[51] In these studies,the authors speculate that it may be more hazardous to biopsy normal pancreas, which has the potential to leak enzymes, than to biopsy a pancreatic adenocarcinoma, which does not form enzymes. Therefore, clear delineation of a hypoechoic pancreatic mass before attempted biopsy may decrease the potential complications as well as improve the biopsy accuracy.

Kidney

Renal masses can be biopsied accurately and safely by using sonographic guidance.[52] The vast majority of solitary solid renal masses represent renal cell carci-

noma. Therefore when a solitary mass is discovered, it is usually removed without prior biopsy. However, if the patient is not a surgical candidate, the mass can be biopsied to obtain tissue confirmation of the presumed malignancy. The rare patient with multiple solid renal masses often undergoes biopsy to differentiate the potential causes of multiple masses, which can be metastases, lymphoma, or multiple renal cell carcinomas (Fig. 18-7). Although these entities can be similar in appearance, their treatments differ widely. Thus accurate diagnosis is necessary.

An atypical cystic renal mass that has internal debris, solid components, or a thick irregular wall can be aspirated and the solid elements biopsied under sonographic guidance in an attempt to differentiate a complicated benign cyst from cystic renal cell carcinoma. The aspiration of grossly bloody fluid raises the suspicion of malignancy, and the recovery of malignant cells is confirmatory. Alternatively, the aspiration of clear, straw-colored fluid and the recovery of benign solid tissue from the wall of the mass supports the diagnosis of a benign atypical cyst.

Sonographic guidance also can be used in the biopsy of kidneys with diffuse parenchymal disease. Insertion of the needle into the lower pole renal parenchyma under continuous real-time guidance, with avoidance of the renal pelvis and major vasculature, has been shown to result in very few complications and produces a tis-

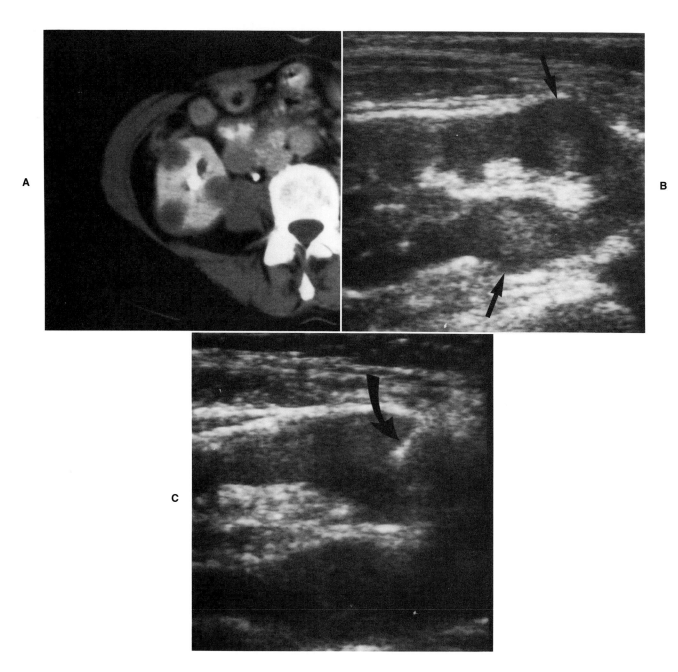

FIG 18-7. Sonographically guided biopsy of kidney containing multiple solid masses—metastasis from lung carcinoma. **A,** Computed tomogram with contrast material shows three small, indeterminate, solid renal masses. **B,** Longitudinal sonogram of right kidney demonstrates two round hypoechoic masses *(arrows)* in the lower pole of the kidney. **C,** Longitudinal sonogram of right kidney shows 18-gauge biopsy needle *(curved arrow)* within anterior mass.

sue sample of excellent quality for microscopic analysis.[53-55] Biopsy of renal transplants with an 18-gauge cutting needle, a spring-loaded biopsy gun, and continuous real-time sonographic guidance has been reported to provide a biopsy specimen that is equivalent in diagnostic quality to the biopsy specimen obtained by the traditional method of blind insertion of a hand-held 14-gauge cutting needle after sonographic localization of the kidney.[56] There were substantially fewer complications with the 18-gauge needle and biopsy gun than with the 14-gauge needle in this series.

Adrenal Gland

The most common indication for adrenal biopsy is to confirm metastatic disease in a patient with an adrenal mass and a known primary malignancy elsewhere. The

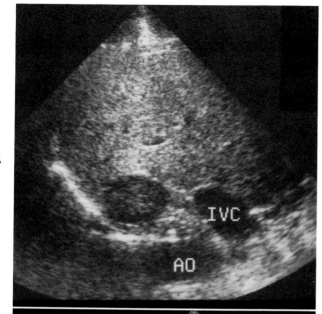

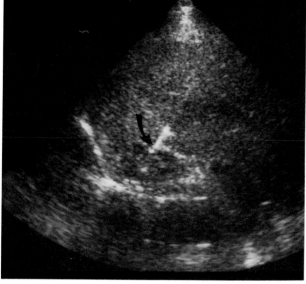

FIG 18-8. Sonographically guided biopsy of right adrenal mass—metastasis from lung carcinoma. **A,** Transverse sonogram through intercostal space and right lobe of liver with patient in the left lateral decubitus position shows a 3 cm solid right adrenal mass. *IVC,* Inferior vena cavas; *AO,* aorta. **B,** Biopsy with 18-gauge needle *(curved arrow).*

right adrenal gland is more accessible to sonographically guided biopsy than the left adrenal gland because of the sonographic window of the right lobe of the liver (Fig. 18-8). For practical purposes, most right adrenal masses need to be at least 2 to 3 cm in diameter to allow adequate visualization and biopsy; most left adrenal masses need to be several centimeters larger. Guidance by computed tomography is often preferable for the biopsy of small adrenal masses.

Brightly echogenic fat-containing adrenal masses and homogeneous, thin-walled, fluid-filled adrenal masses are not biopsied because these should represent benign adrenal myelolipomas and cysts, respectively. The small (<3 cm), homogeneous, smoothly marginated, solid adrenal mass that is discovered incidentally in a patient with no primary malignancy or endocrine abnormality is likely a benign, nonfunctioning, adrenal adenoma and is not biopsied.[57] Follow-up examination in 6 months to 2 years can be performed to confirm lack of change in the size or appearance of the mass. Although benign adenomas can be larger than 3 cm, the likelihood of silent adrenal carcinoma increases significantly if an incidentally discovered mass is larger than 5 cm.[58] However, needle biopsy may not be accurate in these patients because the histologic diagnosis of carcinoma requires the demonstration of adrenal capsular breakthrough or invasion of vascular structures by tumor. Therefore, surgical exploration rather than biopsy is often warranted for asymptomatic adrenal masses larger than 5 cm.[59]

Spleen

The spleen is the abdominal organ least commonly biopsied. Percutaneous splenic biopsy usually is not performed for two reasons. First, it is rare for the spleen to be the only organ in the abdomen involved with a pathologic process such as metastases. In most cases, when a splenic lesion is visualized, there is also concomitant disease in other abdominal organs, such as the liver or lymph nodes, which can be biopsied. Second, the spleen is a highly vascular organ and the risk of hemorrhage from needle biopsy would seem to be high. However, the reported rate of hemorrhage from spleen biopsy is very low.[60-62] In one of these series, there were no significant complications in more than 1000 splenic biopsies.[60]

Further evidence that needle puncture of the spleen is relatively safe comes from past experience with splenoportography. This procedure was performed to opacify the splenic and portal veins before portal or splenic vein surgery. An 18-gauge needle was inserted, often multiple times, into the parenchyma of the spleen, and contrast material was injected. In spite of the fact that these patients were at high risk for hemorrhage from liver disease and associated portal hypertension, the rate of clinically significant hemorrhage was only 2%.

The main clinical reason for performing percutaneous biopsy of the spleen at present is to differentiate a metastasis from recurrent lymphoma in a patient who has a new splenic mass but no disease elsewhere in the abdomen (Fig. 18-9). Recurrent lymphoma can often be diagnosed by comparison of the percutaneous biopsy specimen with tissue previously obtained from the patient. In contrast, needle biopsy of the spleen usually is

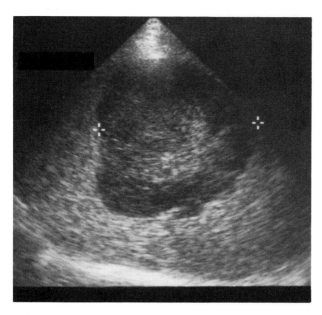

FIG 18-9. Solid, hypoechoic splenic mass on longitudinal sonogram. Recurrent nonHodgkin's lymphoma by needle biopsy.

not performed for the initial, nonoperative diagnosis of lymphoma because of the great difficulty in obtaining an adequate amount of tissue for the complete histopathologic subclassification of lymphoma that is necessary before treatment is begun.

ACCURACY

The accuracy of sonographically guided biopsy has been reported as 66% to 97%, depending on the location, size, and histologic type of the lesions biopsied.* Differences in patient population, technique, and numbers of patients make comparisons of these studies difficult. In our recent series of sonographically guided biopsies of 126 consecutive small (≤3 cm) solid masses in various anatomic locations and of various histologic types, the accuracy of biopsy was 91%.[6] Biopsy results improved with increasing size of the mass in this group of small lesions: Accuracy ranged from 79% in masses of 1 cm or less in diameter to 98% in masses 2 to 3 cm. The accuracy in the liver, where most biopsies were performed, was 96%. On the basis of these results, sonography can be an effective method to guide the biopsy of very small, solid, mobile masses, which can be difficult to sample by biopsy with computed tomographic guidance.

Negative biopsy results are uncommon, but they pose a problem in clinical interpretation. Results that are "negative for malignancy" may be truly negative because of the recovery of normal or benign tissue or may

be falsely negative because of a sampling error, inadequate size of the specimen, or sonographic or pathologic misinterpretation of the images or biopsy specimen. If a false-negative result is suspected, then repeat biopsies, follow-up imaging studies, or surgical exploration may be performed, depending on the level of clinical concern.

COMPLICATIONS

Needle biopsy is associated with rare and usually minor complications. In a review of more than 11,000 needle biopsies with thin-caliber needles, Livraghi et al.[64] found a mortality rate of 0.008%, a major complication rate of 0.05%, and an overall major and minor complication rate of 0.55%. A second review, by Fornari et al.[65] of approximately 11,000 thin-caliber needle biopsies, found a mortality of 0.018% and a major complication rate of 0.18%. A third review of 8000 sonographically guided needle punctures at a single institution, by Nolsoe et al.[66], which included the use of both large-caliber and thin-caliber needles, found a slightly higher mortality, 0.038%, and a major complication rate of 0.187%.

The deaths in these studies were usually secondary to hemorrhage. Two deaths were the result of hemorrhage after biopsies of hepatocellular carcinomas in patients with cirrhotic livers, and one occurred after biopsy of a liver diffusely enlarged with metastatic lesions. Another death was secondary to hemorrhage after biopsy of a hepatic artery aneurysm mistaken for a pancreatic cyst. Doppler evaluation before biopsy would help to exclude aneurysm in a case such as this.[67] If hemorrhage is suspected immediately after biopsy and the patient is hemodynamically stable, the patient should be scanned to evaluate for this complication. Computed tomography, if available, is more accurate than sonography for evaluating for acute hemorrhage. On sonographic examination fresh blood has an echogenicity that is similar to that of surrounding parenchymal organs and tissues and can be overlooked (Fig. 18-10).

Major complications (excluding mortality) in these review series were defined as conditions after biopsy that required medical treatment or surgical intervention. The most common were hemorrhage, bile leakage, pneumothorax, peritonitis, pancreatitis, and needle-tract seeding. Needle-tract seeding is a rare complication, but it often receives a large amount of attention from referring physicians and patients. It has an estimated clinical occurrence rate of approximately 1 in 20,000 biopsies,[68,69] although there have been several reports of needle-tract seeding from biopsy of carcinoma of the pancreas and carcinoma of the prostate.[65,70-73] Single cases of needle-tract seeding have been reported from biopsies of the liver, kidney, pleura, breast, eye, and retroperitoneum.[74-79] Because seeding is such a rare

*References 2, 5, 6, 12, 24, 37, 41, 48, 63.

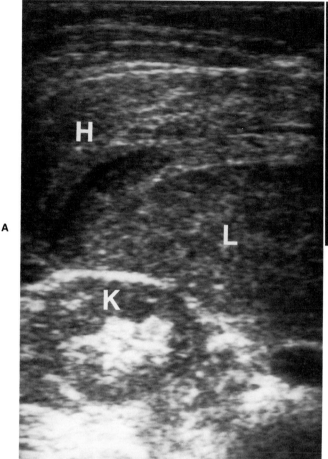

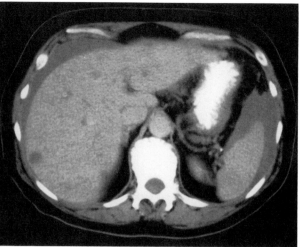

FIG 18-10. Hemorrhage as a complication of liver biopsy. **A,** Transverse sonogram shows echogenic material *(H)* surrounding right lobe of liver *(L).* This echogenic material represents fresh hemorrhage and is difficult to distinguish from the adjacent liver because of similarity in echogenicities of hemorrhage and liver. *K,* Kidney. **B,** Computed tomography with intravenous injection of contrast material clearly shows the fresh intraperitoneal hemorrhage as a crescent of fluid of decreased attenuation that is different from the attenuation of the adjacent spleen and liver, which contains metastasis.

complication, it should not affect the indications for percutaneous biopsy. Fever, transient hematuria, and moderate hemorrhage or pain that did not require treatment except analgesics and observation were considered to be minor complications in these review series.

The differences in the complication rates associated with the use of large-caliber cutting needles and thin-caliber needles may be overstated. One comparative study found complication rates of 0.8% with thin-caliber needles (22 gauge) and 1.4% with large-caliber cutting needles (18 and 19 gauge); this difference was not statistically significant.[80] In a study from our institution, the rate of complications from the use of 18-gauge biopsy needles was 0.3%, which was the same as the rate of complications from the use of 21-gauge needles.[21] This low rate of complications and the recovery of large amounts of histologic and cytologic material with the larger 18-gauge needles have made them the most commonly used biopsy needles in our practice.

Much of the concern regarding larger needles may have arisen initially because of early studies on the use of 14-gauge needles, inserted in a blind manner, for renal and hepatic parenchymal biopsies. The mortality in those series was reported to be as high as 0.1% to 0.17%.[81-85] Under the controlled conditions of continuous real-time sonographic guidance, the risk of using large-caliber needles in biopsy probably is substantially less and lies much closer to the results with thin-caliber needles.

PERCUTANEOUS TUMOR ABLATION WITH ETHANOL

Sonographically guided percutaneous injection of ethanol into hepatic neoplasms was first described as a treatment for small hepatocellular carcinomas in 1983.[86] Since that time other studies have confirmed the safety and value of this procedure in the treatment of both primary and metastatic hepatic lesions.[87-94] Ethanol destroys tissue by cellular dehydration, which produces necrosis and fibrosis, and by vascular thrombosis and occlusion.[95-97] In the treatment of hepatic tumors, percutaneous ethanol injection is usually reserved for patients who are not candidates for other surgical or medical therapy. Currently, the procedure is usually performed on solitary masses that are less than 5 cm in diameter. Rarely, multiple (usually up to three) or large (>5 cm) masses are treated. In most cases, 2 to 8 ml of ethanol is injected into various regions of the mass. The procedure is performed

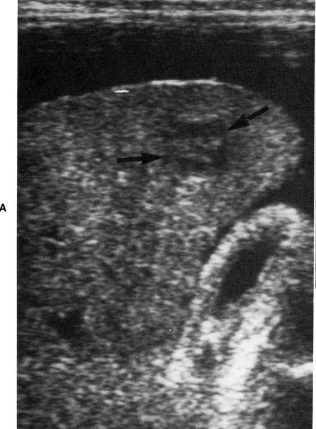

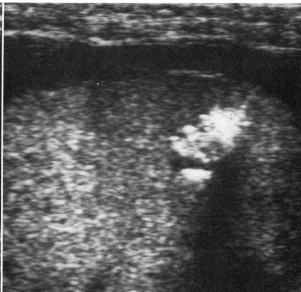

FIG 18-11. Percutaneous ethanol ablation of a hepatoma. **A,** Longitudinal sonogram of right lobe of liver shows ascites with a 1.5 cm hypoechoic solid mass *(arrows),* which proved to be a hepatoma on subsequent needle biopsy. **B,** Ethanol injection through a 21-gauge needle caused the mass to become hyperechoic because of microbubbles of injected fluid.

in the outpatient setting with local anesthesia and is repeated two or three times per week over a period of 1 to 2 weeks.[98] On sonography the region of alcohol injection becomes hyperechoic at the moment of injection. This appearance is probably due to microbubbles in the liquid and often disappears within the first 30 seconds after injection (Fig. 18-11). Complications from the procedure are rare and include transient pain, fever, and alcohol intoxication.[92]

Histopathologic examination of tumors that have been excised after alcohol ablation have shown at least partial necrosis in all masses and total necrosis in most masses.[88-92,94] To date, the longest reported follow-up of patients who have undergone this procedure is 4 years in a series of 59 patients with hepatocellular carcinoma.[93] The survival rate of 79% at 4 years is superior to survival results after hepatectomy in patients with masses of similar size.

REFERENCES

1. Bernardino ME: Percutaneous biopsy. *AJR* 1984; 142:41-45.
2. Grant EG, Richardson JD, Smirniotopoulos JG, et al: Fine-needle biopsy directed real-time sonography: technique and accuracy. *AJR* 1983; 141:29-32.
3. Gazelle GS, Haaga JR: Guided percutaneous biopsy of intraabdominal lesions. *AJR* 1989; 153:929-935.
4. Matalon TA, Silver B: Ultrasound guidance of interventional procedures. *Radiology* 1990; 174:43-47.
5. Charboneau JW, Reading CC, Welch TJ: Computed tomography and sonographically guided needle biopsy: current techniques and new innovations. *AJR* 1990; 154:1-10.
6. Reading CC et al: Sonographically guided percutaneous biopsy of small (3 cm or less) masses. *AJR* 1988; 151:189-192.
7. Mitty HA, Efremidis SC, Yeh HC: Impact of fine-needle biopsy on management of patients with carcinoma of the pancreas. *AJR* 1981; 137:1119-1121.
8. Bret PM, Fond A, Casola G, et al: Abdominal lesions: a prospective study of clinical efficacy of percutaneous fine-needle biopsy. *Radiology* 1986; 159:345-346.

Indications and contraindications

9. Rapaport SI: Preoperative hemostatic evaluation: which tests, if any? *Blood* 1983; 61:229-231.
10. Silverman SG, Mueller PR, Pfister RC: Hemostatic evaluation before abdominal interventions: an overview and proposal. *AJR* 1990; 154:233-238.
11. Rapaport SI: Assessing hemostatic function before abdominal interventions. *AJR* 1990; 154:239-240.

Technique

12. Rizzatto G, Solbiati L, Croce F, et al: Aspiration biopsy of superficial lesions: ultrasonic guidance with a linear-array probe. *AJR* 1987; 148:623-625.
13. Buonocore E, Skipper GJ: Steerable real-time sonographically guided needle biopsy. *AJR* 1981; 136:387-392.

14. Reid MH: Real-time sonographic needle biopsy guide. *AJR* 1983; 140:162-163.

15. Isler RJ, Ferrucci JT Jr, Wittenberg J, et al: Tissue core biopsy of abdominal tumors with a 22 gauge cutting needle. *AJR* 1981; 136:725-728.

16. Wittenberg J, Mueller PR, Ferrucci JT Jr, et al: Percutaneous core biopsy of abdominal tumors using 22 gauge needles: further observations. *AJR* 1982; 139:75-80.

17. Andriole JG, Haaga JR, Adams RB, et al: Biopsy needle characteristics assessed in the laboratory. *Radiology* 1983; 148:659-662.

18. Lieberman RP, Hafez GR, Crummy AB: Histology from aspiration biopsy: Turner needle experience. *AJR* 1982; 138:561-564.

19. Pagani JJ: Biopsy of focal hepatic lesions: comparison of 18 and 22 gauge needles. *Radiology* 1983; 147:673-675.

20. Haaga JR, LiPuma JP, Bryan PJ, et al: Clinical comparison of small- and large-caliber cutting needles for biopsy. *Radiology* 1983; 146:665-667.

21. Welch TJ, Sheedy PF II, Johnson CD, et al: Computed tomography-guided biopsy: prospective analysis of 1,000 procedures. *Radiology* 1989; 171:493-496.

22. Ubhi CS, Irving HC, Guillou PJ, et al: A new technique for renal allograft biopsy. *Br J Radiol* 1987; 60:599-600.

23. Erwin BC, Brynes RK, Chan WC, et al: Percutaneous needle biopsy in the diagnosis and classification of lymphoma. *Cancer* 1986; 57:1074-1078.

24. Jennings PE, Donald JJ, Coral A, et al: Ultrasound-guided core biopsy. *Lancet* 1989; 1:1369-1371.

25. Parker SH, Hopper KD, Yakes WF, et al: Image-directed percutaneous biopsies with a biopsy gun. *Radiology* 1989; 171:663-669.

26. Hopper KD, Baird DE, Reddy VV, et al: Efficacy of automated biopsy guns versus conventional biopsy needles in the pygmy pig. *Radiology* 1990; 176:671-676.

27. Poster RB, Jones DB, Spirt BA: Percutaneous pediatric renal biopsy: use of the biopsy gun. *Radiology* 1990; 176:725-727.

28. Elvin A, Anderson T, Scheibenpflug L, et al: Biopsy of the pancreas with a biopsy gun. *Radiology* 1990; 176:677-679.

29. Parker SH, Lovin JD, Jobe WE, et al: Stereotactic breast biopsy with a biopsy gun. *Radiology* 1990; 176:741-747.

30. Hueftle MG, Haaga JR: obe ect of suction on biopsy sample size. *AJR* 1986; 147:1014-1016,

31. Miller DL, Wall RT: Fentanyl and diazepam for analgesia and sedation during radiologic special procedures. *Radiology* 1987; 162:195-198.

32. Hurlbert BJ, Landers DF: Sedation and analgesia for interventional radiologic procedures in adults. *Semin Interven Radiol* 1987; 4(3):151-160.

33. Miller DA, Carrasco CH, Katz RL, et al: Fine needle aspiration biopsy: the role of immediate cytologic assessment. *AJR* 1986; 147:155-158,

34. Heckemann R, Seidel KJ: The sonographic appearance and contrast enhancement of puncture needles. *J Clin Ultrasound* 1983; 11:265-268.

35. McGahan JP: Laboratory assessment of ultrasonic needle and catheter visualization. *J Ultrasound Med* 1986; 5:373-377.

36. Reading CC, Charboneau JW, Felmlee JP, et al: Ultrasound-guided percutaneous biopsy: use of a screw biopsy stylet to aid needle detection. *Radiology* 1987; 163:280-281.

Regional biopsy techniques

37. Bret PM, Sente JM, Bretagnolle M, et al: Ultrasonically guided fine-needle biopsy in focal intrahepatic lesions: six years' experience. *Can Assoc Radiol J* 1986; 37:5-8.

38. Welch TJ, Reading CC: Imaging-guided biopsy. *Mayo Clin Proc* 1989; 64:1295-1301.

39. Murphy FB, Barefield KP, Steinberg HV, et al: Computed tomography- or sonography-guided biopsy of the liver in the presence of ascites: frequency of complications. *AJR* 1988; 151:485-486.

40. Reubi JC, Kvols LK, Waser B, et al: Detection of somatostatin receptors in surgical and percutaneous needle biopsy of carcinoid and islet cell carcinomas. *Cancer Res* (in press).

41. Spamer C, Brambs H-J, Koch HK, et al: Benign circumscribed lesions of the liver diagnosed by ultrasonically guided fine-needle biopsy. *J Clin Ultrasound* 1986; 14:83-88.

42. Terriff BA, Gibney RG, Scudamore CH: Fatality from fine-needle aspiration biopsy of a hepatic hemangioma, *AJR* 1990; 154:203-204 (letter to editor).

43. Solbiati L, Livraghi T, De Pra L, et al: Fine-needle biopsy of hepatic hemangioma with sonographic guidance. *AJR* 1985; 144:471-474.

44. Nakaizumi A, Iishi H, Yamamoto R, et al: Diagnosis of hepatic cavernous hemangioma by fine needle biopsy under ultrasonic guidance. *Gastrointest Radiol* 1990; 15:39-42.

45. Cronan JJ, Esparza AR, Dorfman GS, et al: Cavernous hemangioma of the liver: role of percutaneous biopsy. *Radiology* 1988; 166:135-138.

46. Caturelli E, Rapaccini GL, Sabelli C, et al: Ultrasound-guided fine-needle aspiration biopsy in the diagnosis of hepatic hemangioma. *Liver* 1986; 6:326-330.

47. Lees WR, Hall-Craggs MA, Manhire A: Five years' experience of fine-needle aspiration biopsy: 454 consecutive cases. *Clin Radiol* 1985; 36:517-520.

48. Hall-Craggs MA, Lees WR: Fine-needle aspiration biopsy: Pancreatic and biliary tumors. *AJR* 1986; 147:399-403.

49. Mitchell ML, Carney CN: Cytologic criteria for the diagnosis of pancreatic carcinoma. *Am J Clin Pathol* 1985; 83:171-176.

50. Mueller PR, Miketic LM, Simeone JF, et al: Severe acute pancreatitis after percutaneous biopsy of the pancreas. *AJR* 1988; 151:493-494.

51. Evans WK, Ho CS, McLoughlin MJ, et al: Fatal necrotizing pancreatitis following fine-needle aspiration biopsy of the pancreas. *Radiology* 1981; 141:61-62.

52. Nadel L, Baumgartner BR, Bernardino ME: Percutaneous renal biopsies: Accuracy, safety and indications. *Urol Radiol* 1986; 8:67-71.

53. Branger B, Oules R, Balducchi JP, et al: Ultrasonically continuously guided renal biopsy. *Uremia Invest* 1985-1986; 9:297-303.

54. Yoshimoto M, Fujisawa S, Sudo M: Percutaneous renal biopsy well-visualized by orthogonal ultrasound applications using linear scanning. *Clin Nephrol* 1988; 30:106-110.

55. Rapaccini GL, Pompili M, Caturelli E, et al: Real-time ultrasound guided renal biopsy in diffuse renal disease: 114 consecutive cases. *Surg Endosc* 1989; 3:42-45.

56. Bogan ML, Kopecky KK, Kraft JL, et al: Needle biopsy of renal allografts: Comparison of two techniques. *Radiology* 1990; 174:273-275.

57. Dunnick NR: Adrenal imaging: Current status. *AJR* 1990; 154:927-936.

58. Dunnick NR, Heaston D, Halvorsen R, et al: Computed tomography appearance of adrenal cortical carcinoma. *J Comput Assist Tomogr* 1982; 6:978-982.

59. Bernardino ME: management of the asymptomatic patient with a unilateral adrenal mass. *Radiology* 1988; 166:121-123.

60. Söderström N: How to use cytodiagnostic spleen puncture. *Acta Med Scand* 1976; 199:1-5.

61. Jansson SE, Bondestam S, Heinonen E, et al: Value of liver and spleen aspiration biopsy in malignant diseases when these organs show no signs of involvement in sonography. *Acta Med Scand* 1983; 213:279-281.

62. Solbiati L, Bossi MC, Bellotti E, et al: Focal lesions in the

spleen: Sonographic patterns and guided biopsy. *AJR* 1983; 140:59-65.

Accuracy*

63. Otto RC: Results of 1000 fine needle punctures guided under real-time sonographic control. *J Belge Radiol* 1982; 65:193-199.

Complications

64. Livraghi T, Damascelli B, Lombardi C, et al: Risk in fine-needle abdominal biopsy. *J Clin Ultrasound* 1983; 11:77-81.
65. Fornari F, Civardi G, Cavanna L, et al: Complications of ultrasonically guided fine-needle abdominal biopsy: Results of a multicenter Italian study and review of the literature. *Scand J Gastroenterol* 1989; 24:949-955.
66. Nolsoe C, Nielsen L, Torp-Pedersen S, et al: Major complications and deaths due to interventional ultrasonography: A review of 8000 cases. *J Clin Ultrasound* 1990; 18:179-184.
67. McGahan JP, Anderson MW: Pulsed doppler sonography as an aid in ultrasound-guided aspiration biopsy. *Gastrointest Radiol* 1987; 12:279-284.
68. Smith EH: The hazards of fine-needle aspiration biopsy. *Ultrasound Med Biol* 1984; 10:629-634.
69. Ryd W, Hagmar B, Eriksson O: Local tumor cell seeding by fine-needle aspiration biopsy. *Acta Pathol Microbiol Immunol Scand* (A) 1983; 91:17-21.
70. Bergenfeldt M, Genell S, Lindholm K, et al: Needle-tract seeding after percutaneous fine-needle biopsy of pancreatic carcinoma. Case report. *Acta Chir Scand* 1988; 154:77-79.
71. Caturelli E, Rapaccini GL, Anti M, et al: Malignant seeding after fine-needle aspiration biopsy of the pancreas. *Diagn Imag Clin Med* 1985; 54:88-91.
72. Haddad FS, Somsin AA: Seeding and perineal implantation of prostatic cancer in the track of the biopsy needle: Three case reports and a review of the literature. *J Surg Oncol* 1987; 35:184-191.
73. Greenstein A, Merimsky E, Baratz M, et al: Late appearance of perineal implantation of prostatic carcinoma after perineal needle biopsy. *Urology* 1989; 33:59-60.
74. Onodera H, Oikawa M, Abe M: Cutaneous seeding of hepatocellular carcinoma after fine-needle aspiration biopsy. *J Ultrasound Med* 1987; 6:273-275.
75. Kiser GC, Totonchy M, Barry JM: Needle tract seeding after percutaneous renal adenocarcinoma aspiration. *J Urology* 1986; 136:1292-1293.
76. Müller NL, Bergin CJ, Miller RR, et al: Seeding of malignant cells into the needle track after lung and pleural biopsy. *Can Assoc Radiol J* 1986; 37:192-194.
77. Fajardo LL: Breast tumor seeding along localization guide wire tracks (letter to editor). *Radiology* 1988; 169:580-581.
78. Glasgow BJ, Brown HH, Zargoza AM, et al: Quantitation of tumor seeding from fine needle aspiration of ocular melanomas. *Am J Ophthalmol* 1988; 105:538-546.
79. Hidai H, Sakuramoto T, Miura T, et al: Needle tract seeding following puncture of retroperitoneal liposarcoma. *Eur Urol* 1983; 9:368-369.

*See also references 2,5,6,12,24,37,41,48.

80. Martino CR, Haaga JR, Bryan PJ, et al: Computed tomography-guided liver biopsies: Eight years' experience. *Radiology* 1984; 152:755-757.
81. Slotkin EA, Madsen PO: Complications of renal biopsy: Incidence in 5000 reported cases. *J Urol* 1962; 87:13-15.
82. Diaz-Buxo JA, Donadio JV Jr: Complications of percutaneous renal biopsy: An analysis of 1,000 consecutive biopsies. *Clin Nephrol* 1975; 4:223-227.
83. Perrault P, McGill DB, Ott BJ, et al: Liver biopsy: Complications in 1000 inpatients and outpatients. *Gastroenterology* 1978; 74:103-106.
84. Terry R: Risks of needle biopsy of the liver. *Br Med J* 1952; 1:1102-1105.
85. Stauffer MH: Needle biopsy of the liver. *Surg Clin North Am* 1967; 47(4):851-860.

Percutaneous tumor ablation with ethanol

86. Sugiura N, Takara K, Ohto M, et al: Percutaneous intratumoral injection of ethanol under ultrasound imaging for treatment of small hepatocellular carcinoma. *Acta Heptol Jpn* 1983; 24:920.
87. Livraghi T, Festi D, Monti F, et al: Ultrasound-guided percutaneous alcohol injection of small hepatic and abdominal tumors. *Radiology* 1986; 161:309-312.
88. Tagawa K, Muto H, Yasuda H, et al: Therapeutic effects of ultrasonically guided ethanol injection for treatment of hepatocellular carcinoma. *Jpn J Med Ultrasonics* 1987; 14:743-744.
89. Shiina S, Yasuda H, Muto H, et al: Percutaneous ethanol injection in the treatment of liver neoplasms. *AJR* 1987; 149:949-952.
90. Sheu J-C, Sung J-L, Huang G-T, et al: Intratumor injection of absolute ethanol under ultrasound guidance for the treatment of small hepatocellular carcinoma. *Hepatogastroenterology* 1987; 34:255-261.
91. Suyama Y, Horishi M, Ebisui S, et al: Ultrasound-guided intratumoral ethanol injection therapy in small liver cancer—clinical evaluation of 20 cases. *Nippon Gan Chiryo Gakkai Shi* 1987; 22:818-826.
92. Fujimoto T: The experimental and clinical studies of percutaneous ethanol injection therapy (PEIT) under ultrasonography for small hepatocellular carcinoma. *Acta Hepatol Jpn* 1988; 29:52-59.
93. Ebara M, Nihei T, Ohto M: Intratumoral injection of absolute ethanol for treatment of small hepatocellular carcinoma. *Naika* 1988; 61:665-669.
94. Livraghi T, Salmi A, Bolondi L, et al: Small hepatocellular carcinoma: Percutaneous alcohol injection—results in 23 patients. *Radiology* 1988; 168:313-317.
95. Yune HY, Klatte EC, Richmond VD, et al: Absolute ethanol in thrombo therapy of bleeding esophageal varices. *AJR* 1982; 138:1137-1141.
96. Ellman BA, Parkhill BJ, Curry TS III, et al: Ablation of renal tumors with absolute ethanol: A new technique. *Radiology* 1981; 141:619-626.
97. Solbiati L, Giangrande A, De Pra L, et al: Percutaneous ethanol injection of parathyroid tumors under ultrasound guidance: Treatment for secondary hyperparathyroidism. *Radiology* 1985; 155:607-610.
98. Shiina S, Tagawa K, Unuma T, et al: Percutaneous ethanol injection therapy for the treatment of hepatocellular carcinoma. *AJR* 1990; 154:947-951.

CHAPTER 19

Ultrasound-Guided Aspiration and Drainage

- John P. McGahan, M.D.

Percutaneous aspiration and drainage procedures have gained wide acceptance in clinical practice because of their safety, simplicity, and effectiveness. While needle puncture and aspiration were first described in 1930,[1] only more recently have percutaneous abdominal aspiration and drainage become popular techniques. The development of newer guidance methods and refinement of catheters have been responsible for this increase.[2,3] Modalities such as sonography and computed tomography (CT) allow for precise needle placement for superficial or deep abdominal fluid or abscess collections.[4]

SELECTION OF GUIDANCE SYSTEMS

Selection of an imaging modality, whether CT, sonography, or fluoroscopy, for aspiration and drainage is influenced by several factors. Considerations include:

- Whether adjacent structures are adequately visualized to plan a safe access route
- Whether the patient can be transported
- The availability of the equipment
- The anatomical area to be aspirated or drained
- Other factors, such as radiation concerns, time requirements, and total cost of the procedure

Two of the most important considerations are the accuracy and safety provided by the guidance system. These outweigh most other considerations, such as expediency or cost of the imaging technology.

Sonographic Guidance Techniques

Sonographic aspiration was initially described using a static scanner with a central hole in the transducer for needle placement.[5,6] Later, ultrasound aspiration techniques most commonly used **indirect ultrasound guidance** for aspiration drainage of abdominal fluid collections (Fig. 19-1).[7] Using this technique, the ultrasound probe is used to select the site of the patient's skin for puncture. The ultrasound probe is removed and the site is marked with pressure from the hub of the needle. The angle and the depth of the puncture are preselected from the ultrasound image and the aspiration or drainage procedure then performed.

Currently, initial needle puncture for abdominal aspiration or drainage procedures uses either the **freehand method** or the use of **biopsy-guided attachments** for needle visualization. Using the **freehand method,** scanning is performed to optimize visualization of both the lesion and the needle. The needle may be positioned either adjacent to the transducer and parallel to the scan plane (Fig. 19-2), or remote from the transducer and perpendicular to the scan plane. Numerous needle-guidance systems are currently available, including attachable biopsy guides that are easily fixed to the transducer or dedicated biopsy transducers with holes or grooves built into the transducer. Attachable needle guides are more commonly used than dedicated biopsy transducers. These guidance systems are designed with slots or grooves sized to needles of different sizes (Fig. 19-3). The angle, direction, and depth of the needle can be continually monitored in real time with the needle guidance systems holding the needle firmly along a predetermined course displayed as a calibrated line on the video monitor of the ultrasound machine. Both of the above methods allow for real-time control of needle puncture in performance of aspiration or drainage procedures.

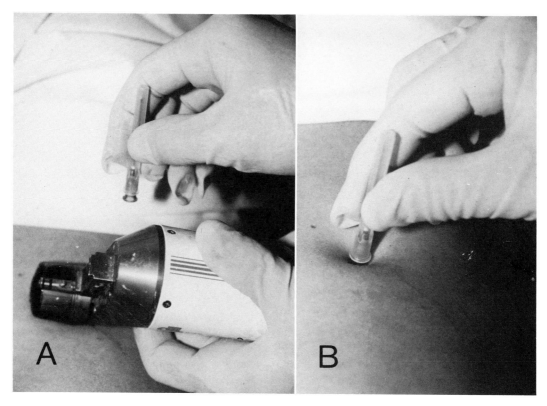

FIG 19-1. Indirect ultrasound guidance. **A,** The skin puncture site, the needle direction, and the depth of puncture are selected by real-time sonography. **B,** The ultrasound probe is removed and the site for puncture is marked by pressure using the needle hub. The site is then prepared and draped for needle insertion.
(From McGahan JP, with permission.)

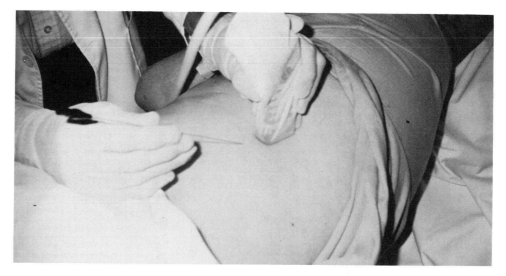

FIG 19-2. Freehand puncture. The needle is inserted to the side of the sterile gloved transducer and advanced under sonographic observation. When the needle can be inserted at a location remote from the transducer, the transducer does not need sterile coverings.
(From McGahan JP, with permission.)

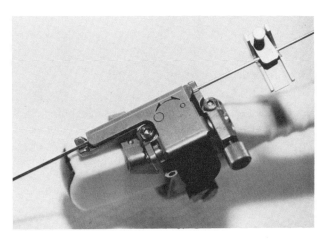

FIG 19-3. Metal biopsy guidance attachments allow for a variety of different needle sizes or catheters to be used for either aspiration/biopsy or drainage procedures. (From McGahan JP, with permission.)

SONOGRAPHIC GUIDANCE OF ABDOMINAL ASPIRATION/DRAINAGE PROCEDURES	
Advantages	Disadvantages
Real-time control	Limitation by air and bowel gas
Needle visualization	Limitation by bone
Precision	Limitation by overlying patient
Expediency	Drains or dressings
Portability	Near-field artifact
Doppler/color flow	
Relatively low cost	
Confirmation of drainage	

Sonographic Advantages and Disadvantages

Sonographic advantages (see box) include real-time visualization of the needle or drainage catheter as it passes into a target area,[8] which allows direct precise needle placement in critical areas with avoidance of intervening structures (Fig. 19-4). Ultrasound-guided aspiration is expedient. The time required for an ultrasound guided paracentesis is not much longer than for routine ultrasound examination. Abdominal drainage procedures often take longer to perform because of the inherent complexity of the procedure, but time requirements are lessened by use of sonographic guidance. Recently, refinements in sonographic instrumentation have allowed ultrasound units to be easily transported to the patient's bedside.[9-11] Thus the critically ill patient need not be moved to the sonographic suite. In review of more than 100 aspiration or drainage procedures performed under ultrasound guidance at our institution, ap-

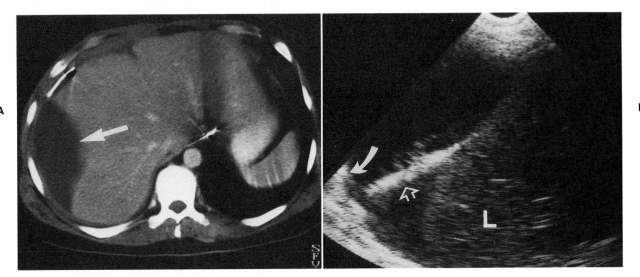

FIG 19-4. Posttraumatic subcapsular hepatic fluid collection—sonographic drainage. **A,** CT shows a subcapsular hepatic fluid collection *(arrow)*. **B,** Using sonographic guidance, a drainage catheter *(open arrow)* was placed within the subcapsular fluid collection using the guidewire exchange technique. *L,* Liver; *curved arrow,* diaphragm.

proximately one third of these procedures were performed portably.[10,11] Although it is inconvenient for the physician and sonographer to leave the ultrasound department, the risk and inconvenience of transporting a critically ill patient must be considered.

Limited reports have demonstrated the utility of pulsed Doppler sonography or color flow imaging as an aid in preventing complications of aspiration or biopsy,[12] by identifying the vascular nature of a mass and in avoiding vascular structures lying within the needle path (Fig. 19-5). Selective use of duplex sonography before abdominal aspiration provides information that should serve to minimize further risk of hemorrhage associated with modern biopsy techniques.

The major disadvantages of sonography, especially in drainage procedures within the abdomen, include poor visualization because of overlying bowel gas, which may obscure the visualization of deeper structures. Near-field artifacts are common with some transducer designs and may prevent visualization of the bowel within the more anterior portion of the abdomen. This bowel could be inadvertently traversed during an aspiration or drainage procedure with catastrophic results.

The advantages and limitations of sonography in performance of aspiration or drainage procedures in specific anatomical areas within the abdomen should be considered for each case. In general, if an abdominal fluid collection or abscess is to be drained with sono-

graphic guidance, it is helpful to have a predrainage CT to evaluate the extent of the abscess and its relation to surrounding anatomical structures.

Sonographic-Fluoroscopic Control

In certain anatomical areas, such as the gallbladder, biliary tract, and liver, combined sonographic-fluoroscopic control for guidance of catheter placement may be preferred. The combined used of sonography for initial needle placement and fluoroscopy for catheter placement, via the guidewire exchange technique, optimizes the advantages of both guidance systems in performance of abdominal drainage procedures. Fluoroscopy may then be used to opacify the area drained and to confirm final catheter placement and the adequacy of drainage.[13] A disadvantage of this combined sonographic-fluoroscopic technique is that the patient must be transported to the radiology department, as the drainage cannot be performed at the patient's bedside.[9,10,13]

Computed Tomography Guidance

One of the inherent advantages of CT scanning is that the entire abdomen is displayed on a cross-sectional image with intravenous and oral contrast defining normal structures from lesions to be biopsied (see box). As such, the area of abnormality can be easily recognized in relation to other intraabdominal structures. Similarly, when performing abdominal aspiration or drainage procedures with CT guidance, the biopsy needle can be

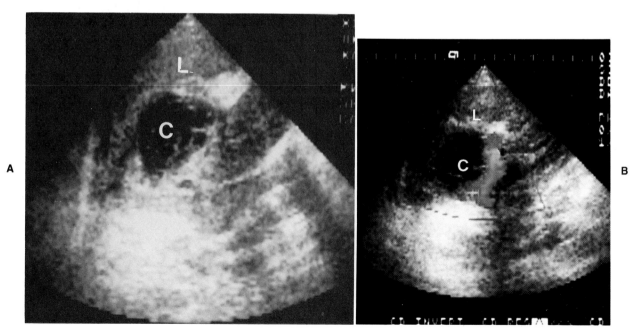

FIG 19-5. Intrahepatic biloma after Kasai procedure for biliary atresia (color flow). **A,** A fluid collection is seen in the liver before aspiration and drainage. **B,** Color flow ultrasound performed before needle puncture demonstrates a large vein along the edge of the cystic collection.

CT GUIDANCE OF ABDOMINAL ASPIRATION/DRAINAGE PROCEDURES

Advantages	Disadvantages
Intravenous contrast	Necessity to transport patient
Visualization of extent of abscess	"Blind" aspiration/drainage
Visualization of bowel, lung, and free air	
Display of entire abdomen	
Visualization through postoperative drains and dressings	
Confirmation of drainage	

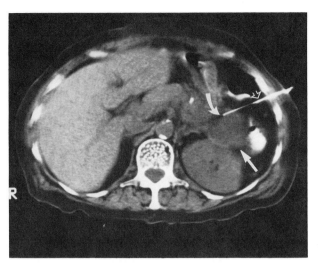

FIG 19-6. Pancreatic pseudocyst—CT drainage. CT scan shows a well-demarcated, cystic area (*straight solid arrow*) in the tail of the pancreas with overlying bowel, which would make sonography-guided drainage difficult. A 22-gauge needle *(curved solid arrow)* followed by an 18-gauge needle *(open arrow)* was passed into the pseudocyst *(straight solid arrow)* under CT guidance avoiding the loop of bowel. A catheter was placed, using the guidewire exchange technique, in the pseudocyst cavity for drainage.

identified, leaving no doubt that the specimen was taken from the correct area.[14]

CT identifies collections of air optimally. These collections may be within an abscess cavity, within overlying bowel, or free in the intraperitoneal space. Identification of air within a fluid collection will help to distinguish this area as an infected abdominal fluid collection or abscess. CT clearly identifies normal overlying bowel. Therefore, when considering percutaneous abscess drainage, especially in the midabdomen, transgression of loops of bowel can be avoided (Fig. 19-6). Avoidance of intervening bowel is necessary not only for abscess drainage but also for aspiration of fluid.[14] Noninfected fluid collections, such as pseudocysts, urinomas, or lymphocysts, may be contaminated by needle passage through overlying loops of large bowel and then into the noninfected fluid collection. Unfortunately, sonography may not always demonstrate a loop of bowel that lies within the needle trajectory.

In the retroperitoneum, CT is clearly superior to sonography in demonstrating abscesses, defining their extent, and showing abnormality of surrounding tissue planes. Involvement of the pancreas, kidney, or psoas areas as well as abscesses secondary to gastrointestinal perforation are best demonstrated with CT. CT provides an anatomical map of the retroperitoneum necessary for planning a safe access route when aspiration or drainage is performed. After the procedure CT may be used to check adequacy of drainage.

Overlying dressings and drains do not interfere with CT visualization as they do with sonographic visualization. Therefore, CT guidance is optimal in postoperative patients.

A major disadvantage of CT guidance is that the patient must be transported to the CT scanner. If the patient is critically ill this is often difficult. A final disadvantage is that after CT localization of an area of fluid collection, the location, angle, and needle trajectory are predetermined, but the needle itself is placed "blindly" without real-time visualization after the patient is removed from the CT gantry. Needle placement must be checked with a repeat scan and possibly changed, thus increasing the time of the procedure. Problems with the drainage procedures, such as guidewire buckling, cannot be evaluated immediately as they can with sonography or fluoroscopy.[14,15]

Selection of CT versus Ultrasound Guidance Methods

The approach to any potentially infected fluid space within the abdomen depends on the anatomical location and the procedure to be performed. For instance, a simple paracentesis is best performed under sonographic guidance. For more complicated drainage procedures in the right upper quadrant, including drainage of the liver, biliary tract, or gallbladder, a combined sonographic-fluoroscopic approach may be preferable (Fig. 19-7). The retroperitoneal areas may be better drained under CT guidance. In some cases, loops of bowel may prevent visualization of intraabdominal abscesses by sonography, making CT the only reliable method of drainage. No single method of guidance or percutaneous drainage is appropriate for all abdominal fluid col-

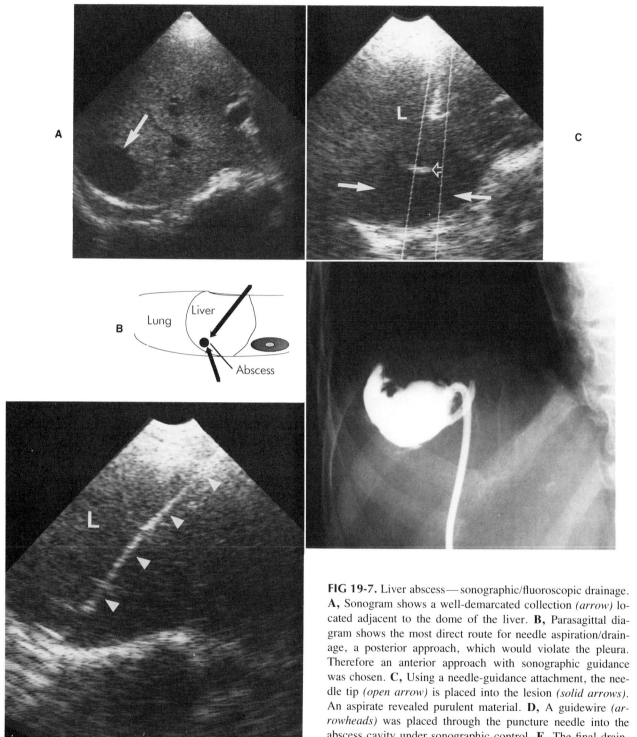

FIG 19-7. Liver abscess—sonographic/fluoroscopic drainage. **A,** Sonogram shows a well-demarcated collection *(arrow)* located adjacent to the dome of the liver. **B,** Parasagittal diagram shows the most direct route for needle aspiration/drainage, a posterior approach, which would violate the pleura. Therefore an anterior approach with sonographic guidance was chosen. **C,** Using a needle-guidance attachment, the needle tip *(open arrow)* is placed into the lesion *(solid arrows)*. An aspirate revealed purulent material. **D,** A guidewire *(arrowheads)* was placed through the puncture needle into the abscess cavity under sonographic control. **E,** The final drainage catheter was placed in the abscess cavity under fluoroscopic control. *L,* Liver.

■ **TABLE 19–1**

Comparison of Guidance Procedure by
Anatomical Region

Anatomical Region	Sonography	Sonography Fluoroscopy	CT
Liver	II	III	III
Biliary tract	I	III	—
Gallbladder	III	III	II
Kidneys (abscess)	I	II	III
Kidney (nephrostomy)	I	III	I
Pancreas	I	II	III
Psoas	I	I	III
Abdominal ascites	III	III	II
Abdominal abscess	I	II	III

I, Least suitable.
II, suitable.
III, Most suitable.

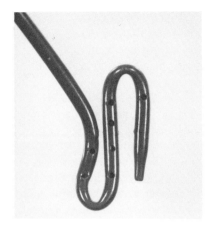

FIG 19-8. Drainage catheter. Hawkins accordion-type catheter for cholecystostomy. Once the catheter is within the gallbladder, the string is pulled to re-form the "accordion," thus preventing catheter dislodgment.
(From McGahan JP, with permission.)

lections or abscesses. Part of the intrigue in implementing abdominal interventional procedures is that each case is different. The approach to any fluid collection or potential abscess must be tailored to the patient, procedure, and specific circumstances (Table 19-1).

SPECIFIC ANATOMICAL AREAS
Gallbladder: Percutaneous Cholecystostomy

Cholecystectomy is the accepted method of treatment of both chronic cholecystitis/cholelithiasis and acute cholecystitis. Although elective cholecystectomy for chronic cholecystitis is associated with a low mortality, there are conflicting reports concerning the management of patients with acute cholecystitis, especially with reference to optimal time for intervention. Some surgeons prefer emergency cholecystectomy, but others advocate delaying cholecystectomy until the patient is less toxic. Emergency cholecystectomy has been shown to have a mortality rate as high as 19%[16] in the elderly. This is most certainly a reflection of not only the cholecystitis but also the poor overall medical condition of these patients. Emergency cholecystostomy has been championed as a life-saving, although temporizing, procedure in the elderly, debilitated, or critically ill patient who presents too great a surgical or anesthetic risk for formal cholecystectomy. Surgical cholecystostomy is a simpler procedure than cholecystectomy, yet it too may be associated with high mortality because of the underlying medical problems in this group of patients.[17] A major advantage of ultrasound-guided cholecystostomy is that the procedure may be performed at the patient's bedside. Thus critically ill patients need not be moved to surgery or the radiology department.

A recent review of 182 percutaneous cholecystostomies indicates the complications are few; there were 1

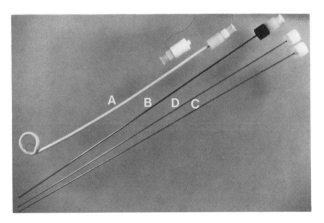

FIG 19-9. McGahan drainage catheter is composed of four components, including a 25-cm long pigtail catheter with *A*, a Cope loop; *B*, a cannula; and *C*, an inner blunted obturator used to straighten the catheter. Once the catheter and cannula are assembled together, the inner blunted obturator is removed and replaced with a sharp inner stylet, *D*, so that the catheter may be inserted via the trocar method.
(From McGahan JP, with permission.)

reported death and 14 technical problems or complications (7%).[11] Many of the technical problems were due to dislodgment of early catheters designed without a securing device.

Newer catheters include some type of securing device. The Hawkins accordion catheter, a self-retaining catheter, may be placed using a coaxial technique after initial puncture with a 22-gauge needle (Fig. 19-8).[18,19] The McGahan drainage catheter set has a distal Cope loop to prevent catheter dislodgment (Fig. 19-9).[19,20]

The catheter is easily placed with ultrasound guidance using a transhepatic route by either the **trocar method** or guidewire exchange technique.

Via the trocar method, a fairly small-diameter catheter, adequate in size to decompress the inflamed gallbladder, fits over a stiffening cannula. A sharp inner stylet is placed within the cannula for insertion. The trocar catheter assembly is advanced transhepatically under sonographic control into the gallbladder. The catheter is pushed from the cannula (Fig. 19-10). The distal loop is re-formed by tightening the attached string to secure the catheter within the gallbladder lumen.

With the **guidewire exchange technique,** the initial puncture needle is placed into the gallbladder. A guidewire is then advanced through the needle and coiled within the gallbladder. The needle is then removed and the guidewire is used as an anchor for passage of a dilator to widen the catheter tract. The catheter-cannula assembly is placed over the guidewire into the gallbladder. Once the catheter is within the gallbladder, the guidewire and the inner cannula are removed while the catheter is simultaneously advanced. The distal Cope loop of the catheter is re-formed to prevent catheter dislodgment (Figs. 19-11 and 19-12).

There are several other applications for percutaneous cholecystostomy, including drainage of the biliary system in patients with failed transhepatic biliary drainage. The cystic duct must be patent to provide a route of drainage for the rest of the biliary system. Furthermore, treatment of cholelithiasis by contact stone dissolution,

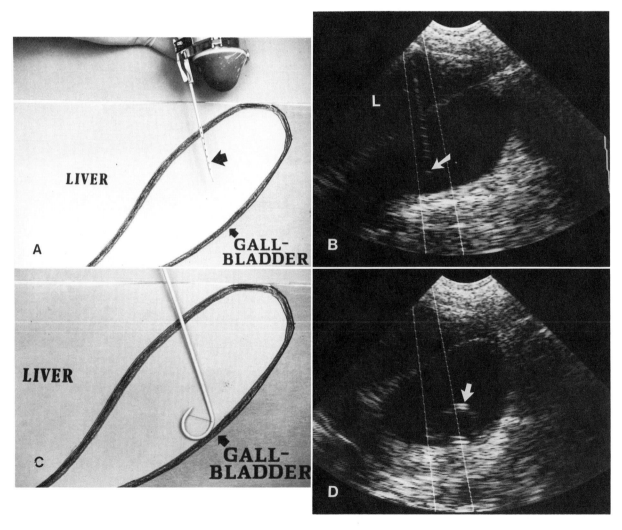

FIG 19-10. Cholecystostomy—trocar method. **A** and **B,** With sonographic guidance, a cholecystostomy catheter *(arrow)* is placed transhepatically via the trocar method into the gallbladder. *L,* Liver. **C** and **D,** Once in the gallbladder, the stylet and the cannula are removed while the catheter is simultaneously advanced into the gallbladder and the distal loop in the catheter *(arrow)* is re-formed.

(From McGahan JP, with permission.)

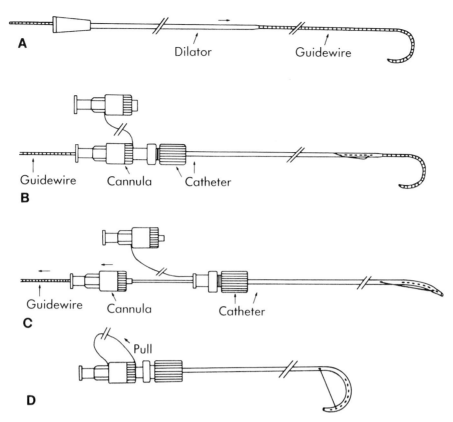

FIG 19-11. Cholecystostomy—guidewire exchange technique. **A,** After needle insertion and placement of a guidewire, a dilator is placed over the guidewire. **B,** The catheter/cannula assembly is then placed over the guidewire into the gallbladder. **C,** Once the catheter is in the gallbladder, the guidewire and inner cannula are removed while the catheter is simultaneously advanced. **D,** The Cope loop of the catheter is re-formed to prevent catheter dislodgment.
(From McGahan JP, with permission.)

basket removal of cholelithiasis, and fragmentation of stones using percutaneously inserted lasers, ultrasound probes, and electrohydraulic or mechanical devices[21-24] may all use percutaneous sonographic guidance to access the gallbladder. Once the stones are removed, the gallbladder potentially could be ablated using a chemical cholecystectomy, by cystic duct occlusion combined with transcatheter sclerosis of the gallbladder.[25] This technique may be used in the future on patients too ill to undergo surgical cholecystectomy.

Biliary Tract: Percutaneous Transhepatic Drainage

Percutaneous transhepatic cholangiography (PTC) and drainage is traditionally performed using "blind" cholangiography with fluoroscopy for initial needle placement. However, the combined use of sonography for the initial needle puncture and fluoroscopy for final catheter placement via the guidewire exchange technique optimizes the advantages of both guidance sys-

tems for performance of PTC, biliary drainage, and other invasive procedures.[13] Selected ducts may be punctured under ultrasound guidance for either PTC or as the site of definitive catheter placement. In patients with segmental biliary obstruction, a "blind" technique allows initial opacification of the biliary system only by chance. However, sonography may allow direct puncture of the appropriate biliary duct. Some authors have advocated the use of ultrasound alone for percutaneous transhepatic biliary drainage.[26]

Liver: Fluid/Abscess Drainage

Hepatic and perihepatic abscesses or fluid collections are usually amenable to percutaneous aspiration and/or drainage. Most commonly, sonography is used for initial needle placement for aspiration of purulent material (see Figs. 19-4 and 19-7) with the catheter placed via the guidewire exchange technique under fluoroscopic control.

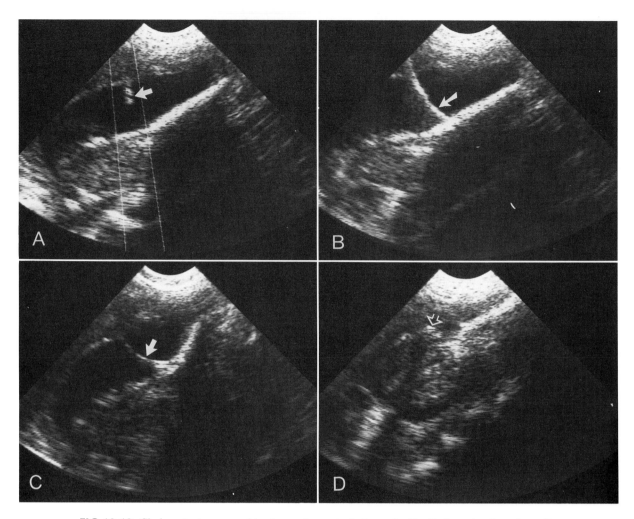

FIG 19-12. Cholecystostomy—guidewire exchange technique. **A,** Needle insertion into the gallbladder *(arrow).* **B,** A guidewire is inserted and the dilator *(arrow)* is placed over the guidewire. **C,** Once the catheter/cannula is within the gallbladder, the guidewire and inner cannula are removed while the catheter is advanced *(arrow).* **D,** After complete aspiration of the gallbladder, only the echogenic catheter is visualized *(open arrow).*
(From McGahan JP, with permission.)

Abdominal Abscesses

Percutaneous catheter drainage of abdominal abscesses has been shown to be a safe and effective alternative to operative drainage, avoiding the morbidity associated with an operation. In many institutions, percutaneous drainage of abscesses is performed before operative therapy is considered.

Patient Selection. There are only a few major contraindications to percutaneous drainage of abdominal abscesses. These include:

- Poorly defined abscesses, such as pancreatic phlegmons, that are not amenable to catheter drainage
- Extensive abdominal abscesses either with multi-

compartment involvement or in multiple locations within the abdomen
- Infected necrotic materials, such as pancreatic necrosis, that would require surgical debridement
- Lack of a safe access route because of overlying bowel or vascular structures
- Major bleeding problems including coagulopathies[27]
- Subdiaphragmatic abscess location preventing catheter placement without transgression of the pleural space

Catheter Drainage. When performing catheter drainage, a safe access route must be determined. The cavity is first aspirated and purulent material obtained.

The catheter is usually inserted via the guidewire exchange technique. Broad-spectrum antibiotics should always be administered before definitive catheter insertion or manipulation of an abscess cavity to minimize bacteremia.

Infected fluid collections may be drained with number 8 to 10 French pigtail-type catheters. More-viscous fluids are best drained with double lumen sump-type catheters. After the procedure, repeat ultrasonography or CT is recommended to check the adequacy of the catheter drainage. The patient is monitored for catheter output, decrease in pain, normalization of temperature, and laboratory parameters. The patient's antibiotics are adjusted according to the results of the culture and sensitivity. To optimize drainage, we usually irrigate the catheter completely after the procedure, although some think that irrigation postdrainage of closed space abscesses causes bacteremia.[27] A follow-up fluoroscopic abscessogram is helpful to identify the size and configuration of the abscess cavity and to note fistulous communications.[28] Most low-output enteric fistulas (less than 50 ml/day) will resolve with a combination of percutaneous drainage and antibiotic therapy alone.[29,30] Those of higher output (over 200 ml/day) may not close with catheter drainage alone. In these cases, hyperalimentation may be useful to decrease enteric secretions and maintain patient nutrition.[27]

Pancreatic Fluid

There are several different terms for pancreatic inflammatory fluid collections or masses.[31] Peripancreatic fluid collections without mature walls may develop during an episode of acute pancreatitis. Many of these disappear spontaneously. Ultrasound needle aspiration may be used to determine if they are infected (Fig. 19-13). After an episode of acute pancreatitis, a mature fibrous wall develops around a fluid collection; this is best termed a **pancreatic pseudocyst**. Needle aspiration may be used to determine if it is sterile or infected.

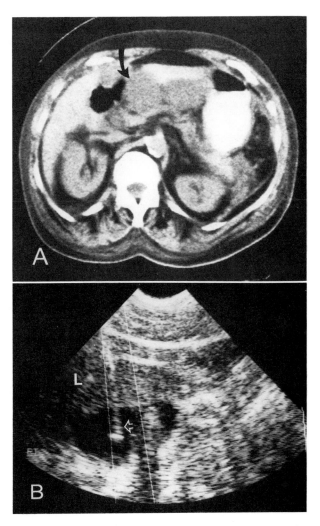

FIG 19-14. Pseudocyst drainage. **A,** CT scan demonstrating bilobed fluid collection *(curved arrow)* anterior to the pancreas and posterior to the fluid-filled stomach. **B,** Under sonographic control using the trocar technique and a transhepatic route, a catheter *(open arrow)* was placed into the pseudocyst, which was successfully drained percutaneously. *L,* liver.
(From Bret PM. In: McGahan JP, editor, with permission.)

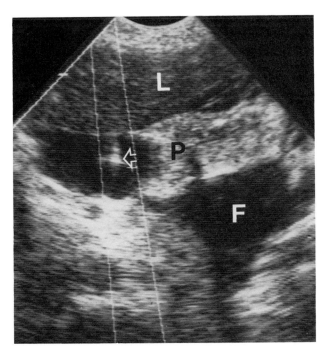

FIG 19-13. Pancreatic aspiration. Transverse scan shows a 22-gauge needle *(arrow)* passed transhepatically into a peripancreatic fluid collection. This and a second fluid collection *(F)* were aspirated with sonographic guidance. *L,* Liver; *P,* pancreas.
(From McGahan JP et al., with permission.)

There is a high reccurrence of pancreatic pseudocysts with simple aspiration. However, vanSonnenberg et al. recently published their experience with percutaneous drainage of pseudocysts with excellent results.[32] The overall cure rate by catheter drainage alone was 90.1%; this includes 48 of 51 infected pseudocysts (94%), and 43 of 50 noninfected pseudocysts (86%). In most of these patients, CT rather than sonography was the primary method of guidance (see Fig. 19-6). Although sonography may be used for guidance of drainage (Fig. 19-14), vanSonnenberg most commonly used the transperitoneal or retroperitoneal route for drainage. Others have advocated use of transgastric drainage of pseudocysts.[31]

Pancreatic necrosis deserves special consideration. Large areas of pancreatic necrosis with surrounding fluid collections require surgical debridement. Percutaneous drainage may be temporizing in drainage of the surrounding fluid collections but are not curative. Pancreatic necrosis phlegmons develop after pancreatic necrosis and inflammation of the pancreatic tissues, and are also not amenable to catheter drainage. Pancreatic abscesses may be treated with percutaneous drainage.[31,32]

Kidney

Renal Cyst. Indications for percutaneous aspiration of a renal cyst include:

- Thick or irregular wall
- Wall calcifications
- Internal echoes or presence of septations
- Presence of a solid mass arising from a wall
- Discrepancy in imaging results as to the cystic or solid nature of a mass.[33]

Ultrasound guided percutaneous fine-needle aspiration of the cyst is simple. Using the aseptic technique, a 22-gauge thin-walled needle may be passed directly into the cyst under ultrasound guidance (Fig. 19-15). Aspirated cyst fluid should be evaluated by culture and sensitivity, lipids (Sudan stain), lactate dehydrogenase (LHD), protein, and glucose. A small amount of protein (less than 2.5 gm/dl) in association with LDH less than 25.5 μ/liter, may be obtained from a simple cyst.[34] Increased LDH is associated with malignancy.[35] Cyto-

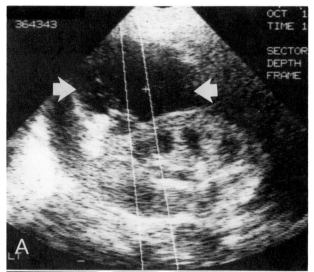

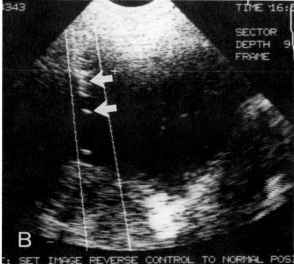

FIG 19-16. Perinephric abscess. **A,** Sonography shows a large perinephric abscess *(arrows)*. **B,** Needle is placed *(arrows)* into the perinephric abscess using an ultrasound biopsy guidance attachment and then exchanged for a drainage catheter.

(From Lindsay DJ et al., with permission.)

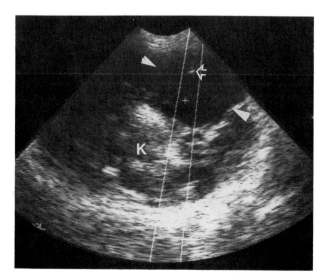

FIG 19-15. Renal cyst aspiration. Renal cyst puncture was performed in this symptomatic patient using a biopsy guidance attachment. The echogenic needle *(arrow)* is noted between the biopsy guidance lines passing into the renal cyst *(arrowheads). K,* Kidney.

(From Lindsay DJ et al., with permission.)

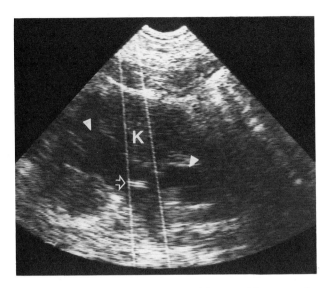

FIG 19-17. Nephrostomy. Using the biopsy guidance attachment, a needle is passed into the hydronephrotic kidney *(K)* with the needle tip *(open arrow)* visualized within the renal collecting structures *(arrowheads)*. Nephrostomy tube was then placed under fluoroscopic control using the guidewire exchange technique.

(From Lindsay DJ et al., with permission.)

logical analysis is important for detection of malignancy.

Perinephric Abscess/Fluid Collections. Fluid collections that occur in the retroperitoneal space include abscesses, urinomas, lymphoceles, and hematomas. CT is usually performed to identify the fluid collection and its extent. Either ultrasonography or CT may be used for aspiration or drainage of these fluid collections. Perinephric fluid aspirations are performed in a fashion similar to renal cyst aspiration. If drainage is needed, the Seldinger technique may be used with sonography for initial needle placement and fluoroscopy for catheter placement (Fig. 19-16). Alternatively, CT may be used to guide fluid or abscess drainage.

Percutaneous Nephrostomy. Recently, sonography has gained wide acceptance as the imaging modality for initial needle placement for percutaneous nephrostomy (Fig. 19-17).[36] After the dilated collecting system is accessed, a catheter is placed via the Seldinger technique using fluoroscopic control.[21]

REFERENCES

1. Blady JV: Aspiration biopsy of tumors in obscure or difficult locations under roentgenoscopic guidance. *AJR* 1939; 42:515-524.
2. Grønvall S, Gammelgaard J, Haubek A, et al: Drainage of abdominal abscesses guided by sonography. *AJR* 1982; 138:527-529.
3. Haaga JR, Alfidi RJ, Havrilla TR, et al: CT detection and aspiration of abdominal abscesses. *AJR* 1977; 128:465-474.
4. McGahan JP, Hanson FW: Ultrasonographic aspiration and biopsy techniques. In: Dublin AB, editor. *Outpatient invasive radiologic procedures: Diagnostic and therapeutic.* Philadelphia: WB Saunders Co; 1989.

Selection of guidance systems

5. Goldberg BB, Pollack HM: Ultrasonic aspiration transducer. *Radiology* 1972; 102:187-189.
6. Holm HH, Als O, Gammelgaard J: Percutaneous aspiration and biopsy procedures under ultrasound visualization. In: Taylor KJW, editor. *Diagnostic ultrasound in gastrointestinal disease.* New York: Churchill Livingstone; 1979.
7. Otto R, Deyhle P: Guided puncture under real-time sonographic control. *Radiology* 1980; 134:784-785.
8. McGahan JP, Brant WE: Principles, instrumentation and guidance systems. In: McGahan JP, editor. *Interventional ultrasound.* Baltimore: Williams & Wilkins; 1990.
9. McGahan JP: Aspiration and drainage procedures in the intensive care unit: percutaneous sonographic guidance. *Radiology* 1985; 154:531-532.
10. McGahan JP, Anderson MW, Walter JP: Portable real-time sonographic and needle guidance systems for aspiration and drainage. *AJR* 1986; 147:1241-1246.
11. McGahan JP, Lindfors KK: Percutaneous cholecystostomy: An alternative to surgical cholecystostomy for acute cholecystitis? *Radiology* 1989; 173:481-485.
12. McGahan JP, Anderson MW: Pulsed Doppler sonography as an aid in ultrasound-guided aspiration biopsy. *Gastrointest Radiol* 1987; 12:279-284.
13. McGahan JP, Raduns K: Biliary drainage using combined ultrasound fluoroscopic guidance. *J Intervent Radiol* 1990; 5(1):33-37.
14. Casola G, vanSonnenberg E: Advantages of computed tomographic guidance, in McGahan JP (ed): *Controversies in ultrasound.* New York, Churchill Livingstone, 1987, pp 225-247.
15. McGahan JP: Advantages of sonographic guidance. In: McGahan JP, editor. *Controversies in ultrasound.* New York: Churchill Livingstone; 1987.

Specific anatomical areas

16. Houghton PW, Jenkinson LR, Donaldson LA: Cholecystectomy in the elderly: A prospective study. *Br J Surg* 1985; 72:220-222.
17. Jurkovich GJ, Dyess DL, Ferrara JJ: Cholecystostomy. Expected outcome in primary and secondary biliary disorders. *Am Surg* 1988; 54:40-44.
18. Hawkins IF Jr: Percutaneous cholecystostomy. *Semin Intervent Radiol* 1985; 2:97-103.
19. McGahan JP: Gallbladder. In: McGahan JP, editor. *Interventional ultrasound.* Baltimore: Williams & Wilkins; 1990.
20. McGahan JP: A new catheter design for percutaneous cholecystostomy. *Radiology* 1988; 166:49-52.
21. Kerlan RK Jr, LaBerge JM, Ring EJ: Percutaneous cholecystolithotomy: Preliminary experience. *Radiology* 1985; 157:653-656.
22. Lux G, Ell C, Hochberger J, et al: The first successful endoscopic retrograde laser lithotripsy of common bile duct stones in man using a pulsed neodymium-Yag laser. *Endoscopy* 1986; 18:144-145.
23. Martin EC, Wolff M, Neff RA, et al: Use of the electrohydraulic lithotriptor in the biliary tree in dogs. *Radiology* 1981; 139:215-217.
24. May GR, Thistle JL: Percutaneous cholecystostomy for gallstone dissolution by methyl tert-butyl ether. *Radiology* 1986; 161(P):90.
25. Becker DC, Quenville NF, Burhenne HJ: Long-term occlusion of the porcine cystic duct by means of endoluminal radio-frequency electrocoagulation. *Radiology* 1988; 167:63-68.
26. Lameris JS, Obertop H, Jeekel J: Biliary drainage by ultrasound-guided puncture of the left hepatic duct. *Clin Radiol* 1985; 36:269-274.
27. Jeffrey RB Jr: Abdominal abscesses: The role of computed to-

mography and sonography. In: McGahan JP, editor. *Interventional ultrasound.* Baltimore: Williams & Wilkins; 1990.

28. Kerlan RV Jr, Pogany AC, Jeffrey RB, et al: Radiologic management of abdominal abscesses. *AJR* 1985; 144:145-149.

29. Kerlan RK Jr, Jeffrey RB Jr, Pogany AC, et al: Abdominal abscess with low output fistula: Successful percutaneous drainage. *Radiology* 1985; 155:73-75.

30. Jeffrey RB Jr, Tolentino CS, Federle MP, et al: Percutaneous drainage of periappendiceal abscesses: Review of 20 patients. *Am J Roentgenol* 1987; 149:59-62.

31. Bret PM: Pancreas. In: McGahan JP, editor. *Interventional ultrasound.* Baltimore: Williams & Wilkins; 1990.

32. vanSonnenberg E, Wittich GR, Casola G, et al: Percutaneous drainage of infected and noninfected pancreatic pseudocysts: experience in 101 cases. *Radiology* 1989; 170:757-761.

33. Lindsay DJ, Lyons EA, Levi CS: Urinary tract. In: McGahan JP, editor. *Interventional ultrasound.* Baltimore: Williams & Wilkins; 1990.

34. Clayman RV, Williams RD, Fraley EE: The pursuit of the renal mass. *N Engl J Med* 1979; 300:72-74.

35. Phillips GN, Kumari-Subaiya S: Renal cyst puncture: LDH as a tumor marker. Presented at the annual meeting of the *Radiology Society of North America,* Chicago, Nov, 1986.

36. Pedersen H, Juul N: Ultrasound-guided percutaneous nephrostomy in the treatment of advanced gynecologic malignancy. *Acta Obstet Gynecol Scan* 1988; 67:199-201.

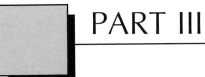

PART III

Intraoperative Sonography

CHAPTER 20

Intraoperative Sonography of the Brain

- Jonathan M. Rubin, M.D., Ph.D.
- William F. Chandler, M.D.

TECHNIQUE
Orientation

The most difficult aspect of intraoperative ultrasound scanning for novices is becoming oriented to the slices that are generated during surgery. Because ultrasound sections are generated at the surgical site, the orientation of the images almost never corresponds to standard anatomic sections. For example, a near-true coronal section of the brain is imaged through the anterior fontanelle of the neonate. From this midline acoustic window, the hemispheres are symmetrically imaged on both sides of the interhemispheric fissure, which is positioned along the central ray of each scanned section. However, neurosurgeons rarely operate directly over the midline because this would necessitate dissecting through the superior sagittal sinus. Instead, they usually try to enter the cranium directly over the area of interest. Images made from such sites produce slices with unusual perspectives (Fig. 20-1). For instance when scanning over the convexities, the falx does not appear

as a line projecting along the midline in coronal sections, but is tipped slightly from the vertical; for parietal craniotomies, this is a slight obliquity, but approaches an angle of 90° from the vertical when scanning on the temporal lobe. Such changes in perspective can be very disorienting for someone with little experience. The inability to recognize the normal anatomy because of these strange perspectives can cause significant consternation and frustration in an environment as tense as an operating room.

To avoid these problems, one should follow a few basic rules. The first is to *begin scanning at a frequency that is low* enough for the sound to traverse the entire brain, generally 3 MHz or less. Although the spatial resolution of scans at these frequencies is not optimal for performing surgical guidance, these images are very useful for orientation. These "whole brain" slices should make it possible to distinguish the anatomy on the abnormal and normal sides of the brain. The choroid plexus, lateral ventricles, falx, and tentorium are very easy to recognize (Fig. 20-1). By identifying these structures, the operator can *produce a slice that corresponds to a standard anatomic section.* This can be done as follows: after placing the transducer in the center of the surgical field, the operator should rotate, *not slide* the scan head until it is possible to see a recognizable relationship between the above structures. There are at least two standard orientations that can be produced from any craniotomy. For example, a sagittal or a coronal slice can be produced from a parietal craniotomy, a transaxial or a coronal slice from a temporal craniotomy, and a transaxial or a sagittal slice from a frontal craniotomy. Once a recognizable section has been produced, the operator should slide the transducer, maintaining the same orientation, from one edge of the craniotomy to the other. By scanning the entire brain in that one orientation, both lateral ventricles, the choroid plexus, the falx, and the tentorium should be visible in standard, well-known relationships. After completing this series of scans, the operator should *rotate the transducer 90° and scan the brain in the orthogonal orienta-*

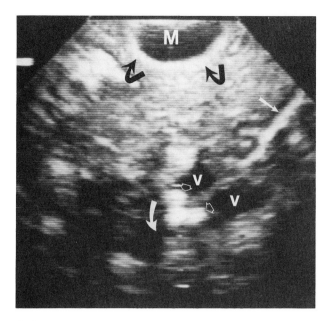

FIG 20-1. Intraoperative sonogram demonstrates tipped field of view. Coronal sonogram on the parietal lobe over a cystic lung carcinoma metastasis *(m)* with echogenic rind of tumor *(curved black arrows)*. Falx *(straight arrow)* projects down in the 2 o'clock position. Lateral ventricles *(v)* with choroid plexus *(open arrows)* are shown entering the third ventricle *(curved white arrow)*. Increased brain echogenicity caused by edema.

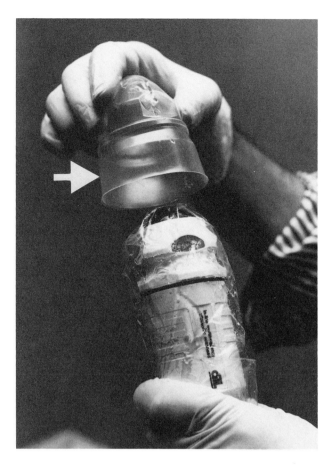

FIG 20-2. Transducer draping procedure. Photograph shows the application of a protective plastic cap *(arrow)* to a draped scan head and cable using a commercially available draping system.
(CIVCO Medical Instruments Company, Kalona, IA 52247.)

tion, again identifying the normal structures. Only after a complete familiarity with the field and its relationship to the craniotomy has been obtained should the search for the lesion begin. The lesion should basically be ignored until all the intracranial relationships relative to the particular craniotomy are understood. *The maxim here is be systematic and avoid random scanning.*

Once the orientation is understood, the transducer should be changed to a *higher frequency, 5 MHz or higher, to interrogate the lesion.* Unless a major error has been made, the lesion of interest will be on the same side of the head as the craniotomy. There is little reason for scanning across the falx once the orientation sequence has been completed. A correctly positioned craniotomy almost always places the area of interest in the near-field of the transducer, usually within 6 cm of the scan head. There is rarely any reason to scan such lesions at frequencies of less than 5 MHz. Therefore the typical case will require a low-frequency transducer (3 MHz or less) for orientation and a higher-frequency transducer (5 MHz or more) for surgical guidance.

Draping the Transducer

Although sterilizable transducers are now available, many scan heads cannot be sterilized and must be

draped for sterility. There are many different draping schemes, and we have covered scan heads with various objects including sterile latex surgical gloves or transparent microscope drapes.[1-4] Each of these works well; the reader could probably devise a draping method that would perform as well. The problem with many of these "home-grown" techniques is that usually they cover the transducer with any thin material that happens to be handy in the operating room at the time. In these cases, the potential for tearing the drape on the rough bony margin of a craniotomy is great. To avoid this hazard, the scan head should ideally be draped with at least two layers of protective material. Alternatively, a commercially marketed draping system can be used (Fig. 20-2). Besides being convenient to use, some commercial draping kits have the additional benefit of a hard, tightly fitting cap that covers both the drape and the scan head. This cap negates the possibility of contamination of the field.

In the operating room, transducer draping requires

two individuals: one who is not scrubbed to manipulate the transducer cord and transducer outside and under the drape, and a second scrubbed individual to control these objects after they are draped. Using a commercial draping system (Fig. 20-2), the transducer and cable are initially covered with a large transparent sterile cover. Having entirely covered the transducer and cord, a plastic cap into which a small amount of sterile contact gel has been added is placed over the draped scan head in a sterile manner. Once draped, the scan head can be touched gently to the dura or directly to the cortex. Experience has shown little difference in image quality whether scanning on the dura mater or the cortex.[4] Saline, dripped onto the surface of the brain, acts as the coupling agent. If necessary, the wound itself can be filled with saline, creating a natural fluid path for scanning.[5]

Time Requirements

One major disadvantage of intraoperative scanning has been the time the radiologist must commit to these procedures. Quencer and Montalvo[6] determined that they spent an average of 52 minutes in the operating room for craniotomies. However, complex cases could last as long as an hour and a half, which is a significant commitment of time. Yet, in our experience, Quencer and Montalvo's numbers are very liberal, and the radiologist's involvement need be nowhere near this great. First, in 18% of their cases, Quencer and Montalvo noted that the radiologist was able to leave the operating room for long periods of time, an average of 48 minutes. Second, we have found that as surgeons become more and more adept at the technique, the radiologist is needed less for the mundane techniques of scanning basics, draping the scan head, and guidance; he or she assumes the role of a consultant. In fact, we have frequently found that it often takes more time to change into operating room attire than it does to monitor a case.

Yet there is often no way that the radiologist can expedite a complex case. A significant time commitment is sometimes necessary for a favorable surgical result.[6] The realization that the radiologist's imaging skills improved the outcome of surgery and the quality of care the patient received is a valuable reward.[7]

TUMORS
High-Grade Gliomas

Tumors in general and high-grade gliomas in particular have very characteristic sonographic appearances. These tumors are almost always more echogenic than the background brain substance (Fig. 20-3).[3,7,8-14] Only

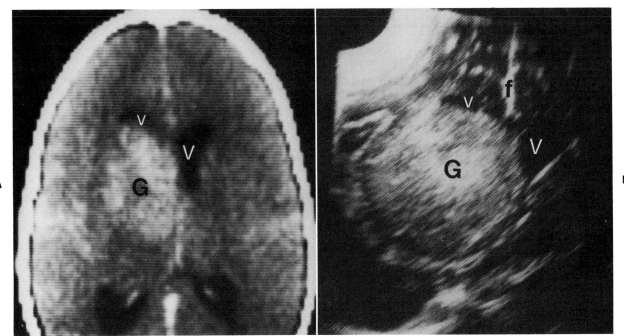

FIG 20-3. Malignant glioma. **A,** CT scan shows a densely enhancing glioma *(G)* that is distorting the lateral ventricles *(V)*. **B,** Coronal sonogram of the highly echogenic glioma *(G)* again shows the compressed ventricles *(V)* and the abutting falx *(f)*.
(From Chandler WF. Use of ultrasound imaging during intracranial operations. In Rubin JM, Chandler WF, eds. *Ultrasound in Neurosurgery*. New York, Raven Press, 1990:67-106.)

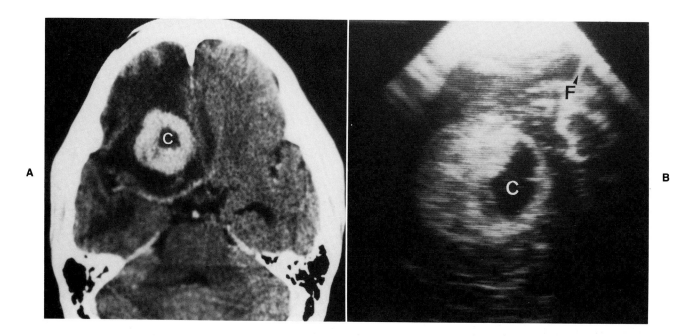

FIG 20-4. High-grade cystic glioma. **A,** CT scan of right frontal enhancing glioma with a cyst *(C)*. **B,** Intraoperative sonogram shows the echogenic ring of tumor around the cyst *(C)*. Falx *(F)*.
(From Chandler WF, Rubin JM. The application of ultrasound during brain surgery. World J Surg. 1987;11:558-569.)

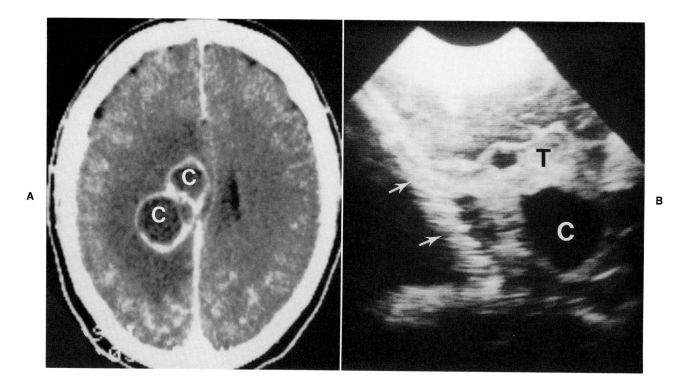

FIG 20-5. Catheter drainage of cystic neoplasm. **A,** CT scan shows a deep tumor with at least two cystic components *(C)*. **B,** Intraoperative sonogram shows a catheter *(arrows)* entering the anterior cyst. Posterior cyst *(C)*. Echogenic tumor *(T)* is lateral to the cysts.

cysts, which frequently arise in these tumors, are hypo-echoic and they have the typical properties of increased through transmission and sharp margins (Fig. 20-4).*At times, it is possible to identify either a tumor nodule within a cyst or a cyst with a hyperechoic ring corresponding to tumor around its edge (Fig. 20-4).

It is clear that ultrasound is the primary imaging modality for cysts.[12,14-16] Both computed tomography (CT) and magnetic resonance imaging (MRI) can have difficulty in distinguishing solid from cystic lesions.[7,12,17-19] Identification of these cysts is crucial because the neurosurgeon may need to drain them in order to decompress the brain before opening the dura mater (Fig. 20-5).[20,21]

Tumor Versus Edema and Necrosis. The distinction between degrees of echogenicity in high-grade gliomas is an interesting one. When performing a biopsy one would like to sample those portions of a lesion containing viable tumor and avoid areas of necrosis or edema. McGahan et al[21] showed that the areas of highest echogenicity in high-grade gliomas usually correspond to areas of necrosis whereas the relatively lower-echogenicity ring immediately around the necrotic area generally represents tumor. Although there is some debate[3,16] and one group[22] has suggested that vasogenic edema is hypoechoic whereas cytotoxic edema is echogenic, edema is now generally thought to be echogenic in the brain and spinal cord (Fig. 20-1).[23,24] This echogenicity is problematic when trying to discriminate tumor margins from edema.[11,22,23] However, edema is more of a problem in identifying and delineating low-grade astrocytomas whose lesions are often more homogeneous than those of high-grade malignancies.[22]

Tumor margins and tumor size on sonography. Although tumor margins are often better seen on ultrasound than CT, comparison of tumor size between modalities seems to vary greatly. Enzmann et al[22] reported that nonenhancing masses on CT scans could appear larger, equal, or smaller on ultrasound. However, lesions enhancing with contrast on CT scans were always less than or equal to the size on the corresponding sonogram. Hypodense or isodense mass margins were seen more clearly on ultrasound than CT; ultrasound more accurately defined tumor extension if there had been no breakdown of the blood-brain barrier.[22] Another group found that CT consistently overestimated tumor size.[16]

An elegant comparative study between ultrasound and CT where CT was the gold standard was performed by LeRoux et al.[25] Twenty-two patients with primary and metastatic brain tumors were evaluated. In patients undergoing surgery for the first time, ultrasound tumor volumes very closely matched CT findings: 101.69% ±

24.7%. However, in patients undergoing subsequent surgeries, ultrasound overestimated the tumor volumes by about 40%. Postoperative gliosis appeared similar to tumor on sonography, thus enlarging the apparent masses. Ultrasound was more likely to improve the delineation of tumor margins relative to CT.

These studies may no longer be relevant now that MRI has become the imaging modality of choice for brain tumors. Lesion size variations and margin definition between ultrasound and MRI are yet to be studied.

In general, high-grade astrocytomas, which generally are large when they are discovered, typically do not present localization problems for neurosurgeons.[15] The value of sonography in these cases lies in *determining the borders of lesions* or in *defining a safe access to a deep tumor*. This localization often can be more accurate and precise than on preoperative imaging examinations such as CT.[22] Sonography can also be useful in *identifying residual tumor* when a total removal has been attempted (Fig. 20-6).[11,12,15] Many of these masses are only biopsied, and although ultrasound certainly can be used to guide biopsies of these lesions, biopsies are now often done under CT guidance.

Pitfalls in Tumor Localization. When scanning across a sulcus, the sulcus can look like a solid mass if the sound beam is parallel to it (Fig. 20-7).[11,26] This fact, which is well-recognized in scans of neonatal heads, can lead to biopsies of normal brain if unrecognized in the operating room. To avoid this pitfall, every suspected mass must be scanned in two orthogonal planes. A mass will look solid in both planes, but a sulcus will look like a line in one of the orientations (Fig. 20-7).

Low-Grade Astrocytomas

Determining the precise location of these slow-growing, infiltrating lesions can be difficult. Even though they may be obvious on CT or MRI, in surgery they may appear very much like normal brain on gross inspection or even on pathologic frozen section.[14,27] Although low-grade astrocytomas may be difficult to visualize sonographically (Fig. 20-8), lesions difficult or impossible to identify on CT scans often are easily seen on ultrasound.[28] Low-grade gliomas are invariably more echogenic than normal brain.[22,28,29] However, the degree of echogenicity in low-grade malignancies is less than for higher-grade malignancies. Tumoral echogenicity can be quite similar to that of edematous brain,[23,29] making the boundary between edema and tumor difficult to identify.

Tumor Versus Edema. A helpful clue for distinguishing tumor from edema is that **tumors invade** whereas edema does not. Therefore tumors usually disrupt or destroy sulcal morphology whereas edema spreads around sulci, sparing them (Fig. 20-9). This

---

*See references 7,8,10,12,14,15.

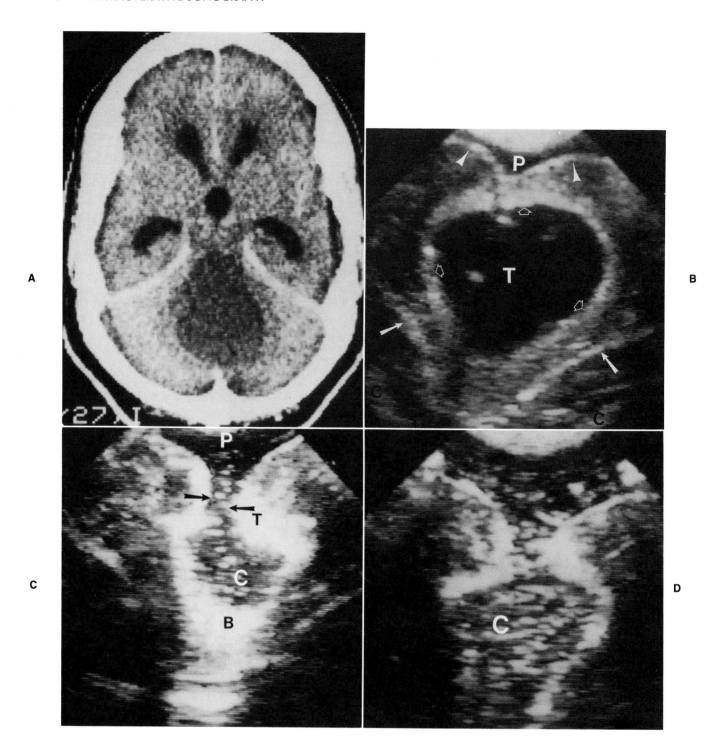

FIG 20-6. Cystic astrocytoma. **A,** CT scan of a hypodense nonenhancing posterior fossa tumor and secondary hydrocephalus. **B,** Transverse scan through saline from the posterior surface of the cerebellum *(arrowheads)*. Large cystic tumor *(T)* is surrounded by an echogenic rind of tumor *(open arrows)*. Tentorium leaves *(arrows)*. Choroid plexus *(C)*. **C,** Transverse scan after "total tumor resection" *(arrows)*. Multiple echoes (air bubbles in the saline) extend from the exterior channel *(arrows)* into the cyst *(C)*. Blood and debris *(B)* are visible. Residual echogenic tumor *(T)* under the overhanging lip of left cerebellar hemisphere. (P-fluid path within the wound). **D,** Final postresection scan shows saline-filled cyst *(C)*. Residual thin echogenic rim of the cavity showed no gross tumor but had rough resected margins.

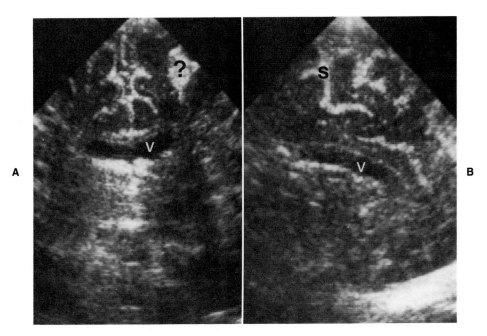

FIG 20-7. Prominent normal sulcus simulating mass. **A,** Coronal neonatal brain ultrasound scan shows an apparent parietal mass. Lateral ventricle *(v).* **B,** 90° rotation of the transducer over the presumed mass produces a line *(S),* proving it is a sulcus. Ventricle *(v).*
(From Bowerman RA. Tangential sulcal echoes. Potential pitfall in the diagnosis of parenchymal lesions on cranial sonography. *J Ultrasound Med.* 1987;6:685-689.)

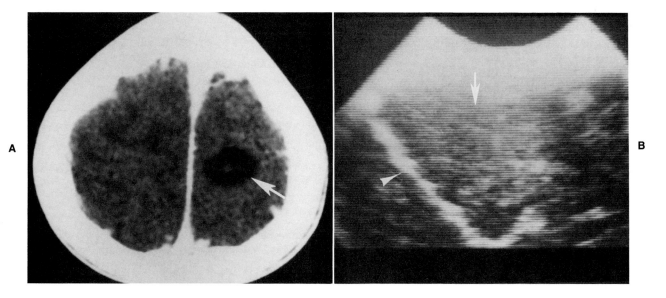

FIG 20-8. Poorly defined low grade astrocytoma. **A,** CT scan shows a well defined, hypodense mass *(arrow)* in the left parietal lobe. **B,** Coronal sonogram shows diffuse, subtle area of increased echogenicity *(arrow)* at the tumor site very similar to edema. Falx *(arrowhead).*
(From Hatfield MK, Rubin JM, Gebarski SS, et al. Intraoperative ultrasound detection of metastatic tumors int the central cortex. *Neurosurgery.* 1982;11:219-222.)

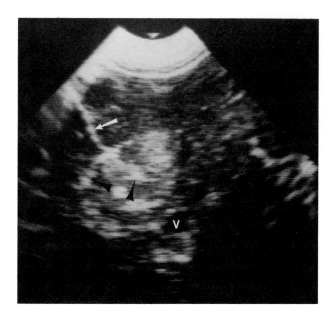

FIG 20-9. Low-grade astrocytoma crossing midline. Coronal scan shows hyperechoic tumor invading the falx *(arrow)* and crossing the midline. Destroyed sulci *(arrowheads)* are within the mass. Lateral ventricle *(v)*.

sign, although generally useful, has been known to fail.[11] In addition, unlike high-grade tumors, *focal areas of increased echogenicity* are more likely to correspond to areas of *viable tumor in low-grade gliomas.*[29] Hence areas of local increased echogenicity can be used to identify viable tumor and often represent prime sites for biopsy.[29]

Unusual Approaches. Before ultrasonography, surgeons had to approach masses from the most direct and often shortest path. If this path transgressed an inviolable portion of the brain such as the motor strip or the primary speech area, an otherwise resectable lesion was considered inoperable. However, using sonography, surgeons can approach lesions from any number of oblique directions. Mapping the motor strip or speech area can be done before a resection while the patient is awake; a surgical path can be designed through a silent area to avoid these essential areas and still intersect the lesion, making an otherwise nonresectable lesion resectable (Fig. 20-10). By avoiding these areas, patients should not have deficits after such operations.

Other Tumors

The entire gamut of brain tumors has been imaged by ultrasound. These lesions have been uniformly more echogenic than the surrounding brain. **Meningiomas** can be detected deep on the falx, at the base of the skull, within the ventricular system, or simply on the convexity.[2] A particularly interesting application is in the evaluation of superior sagittal sinus invasion by a

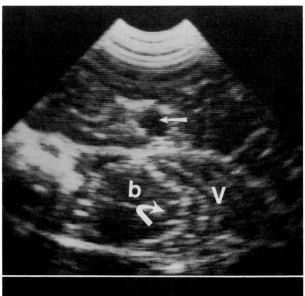

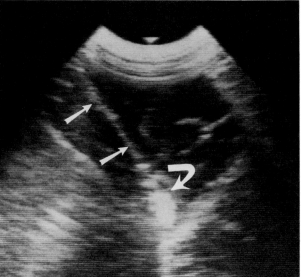

FIG 20-10. Cystic ganglioglioma removed with ultrasound guidance. **A,** Transaxial sonogram shows the cystic mass *(arrow)* lying underneath the primary speech center against the midbrain *(b)* and cerebellar vermis *(V)* (multiple curved folia). Aqueduct of Sylvius *(curved arrow).* **B,** Needle *(straight arrows)* passing through a silent area into the lesion *(curved arrow).* The needle tip has concentric rings etched into it, making it extremely echogenic.

meningioma. Because of the potential for venous infarction, only thrombosed portions of the sinus can be resected. Although color-flow Doppler would be very useful in these circumstances, even with gray-scale scanning alone, blood flow can be seen in the sinus, and the patent portions of the sinus identified. It is then possible for the surgeon to identify and resect only those portions of the sinus that are totally occluded (Figs. 20-11 and 20-12).[2,7]

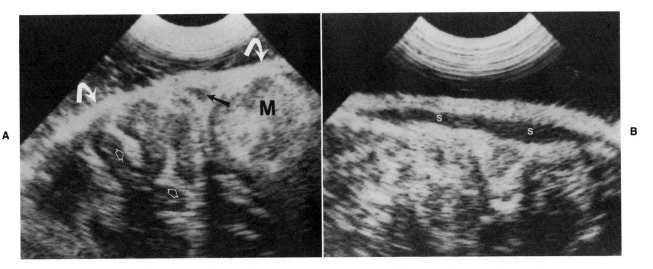

FIG 20-11. Meningioma with patent superior sagittal sinus. **A,** Coronal scan through saline shows triangular superior sagittal sinus *(straight arrow)*. Left parasagittal meningioma *(M)* abuts but does not obstruct the sinus. Dural surface *(curved arrows)*. Multiple sulci *(open arrows)*. **B,** Sagittal scan shows the patent sinus *(s)* with multiple low-level echoes from flowing blood.

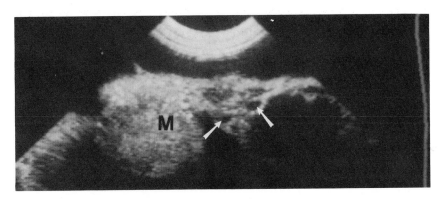

FIG 20-12. Meningioma with superior sagittal sinus invasion. Coronal scan through saline shows a large right parasagittal echogenic mass *(M)* invading the superior sagittal sinus. Two small patent areas of the sinus *(arrows)* show flow, making this area unresectable.
(From Rubin JM, Dohrmann GJ. Intraoperative neurosurgical ultrasound in the localization and characterization of intracranial masses. *Radiology.* 1983;148; 519-524.)

Metastases to the brain can easily be identified.[7,10-14,22,30] Solitary metastases are often resected; typically, they have well-defined margins with surrounding edema. Superficial metastases present few problems, but deep lesions can be very difficult to locate. Sonography can also be valuable for certain superficial metastases by making resection possible. With a lesion near the motor strip, the surgeon can locate a silent area for an approach. With sonographic guidance though the silent area, the lesion becomes resectable (Fig. 20-13).

Small posterior fossa tumors such as **hemangioblastomas, dermoids, epidermoids, ependymomas,** and **medulloblastomas** can easily be seen with sonography, and the solid or cystic nature of a lesion may be accurately determined where CT is not reliable (Fig. 20-14).[27] Multiple closely spaced folia make the cerebellum quite echogenic. The important relationship of a mass to the fourth ventricle can also be made with sonography.

Biopsy

Most ultrasound-guided, intraoperative biopsies are performed using a needle-guidance device attached to the scan head.[31,32] Special biopsy attachments and probes for burr-hole scanning have been designed.[32-35] Two general classes of guides are used. The more com-

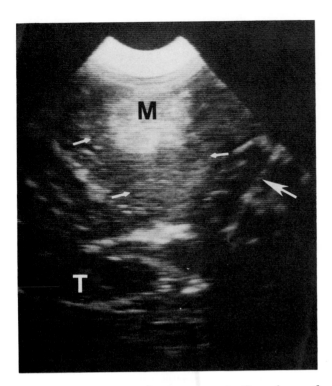

FIG 20-13. Malignant melanoma metastasis. Coronal scan of an echogenic mass *(M)* deep to the right motor strip. Echogenic brain edema surrounds the lesion *(small arrows).* Temporal lobe *(T).* Falx *(large arrow).*

monly used one has a *fixed angle relative to the scan head* with the direction of entry of a needle being altered by rotating the scan head.[31,32] Because of this fixed angle, it is possible to project the needle path on the scanner's video display. The operator need only align the pre-plotted path with the target lesion and pass the needle through the guide into the mass. Besides automated designation of the needle path, the simplicity of such devices is attractive. A limitation is the relatively large contact surface required for scanning, often larger than the usual size of the craniotomy site. This is further complicated by the fact that the transducer must be rotated to such extreme angles in order to biopsy very superficial or very deep lesions that part of the scan has to be sacrificed for the resulting scan to demonstrate the lesion. Such severe transducer angulation removes large portions of the transducer surface from the surface of the brain or dura, diminishing the field of view of the sector image.

The second alternative is to use a *guide with a variable angle to the scan head* in which the depth can be changed. By varying the angle, the point along the central beam of the sector image and hence the depth into the tissue through which the needle passes can be controlled. The distance from the cortex to the mass is de-

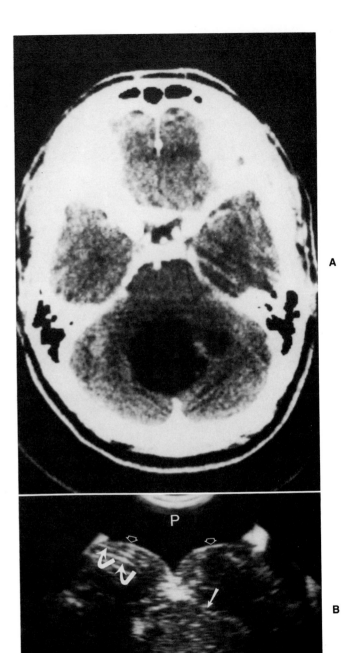

FIG 20-14. Cerebellar epidermoid appears cystic on CT and solid by sonography. **A,** CT scan shows "cystic mass" in the cerebellum. **B,** Transverse intraoperative sonogram: posterior *(P)* through saline shows a large solid, midline cerebellar mass *(straight arrows).* Cerebellar hemispheres *(open arrows).* Folia *(curved arrows).*

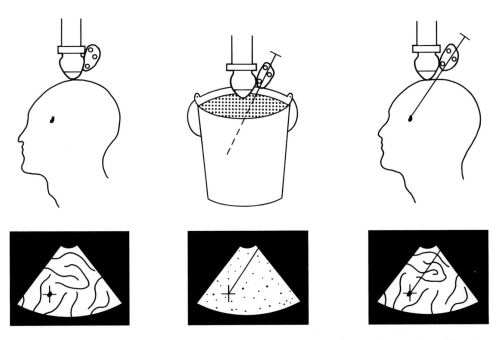

FIG 20-15. Pseudobiopsy. Top line is scanning sequence; bottom line is video monitor. First, the lesion is localized and marked (+). Second, the catheter in the guide is positioned in a fluid bath to pass through the (+) on the screen. The guide is locked in position. Far right, the scanhead is repositioned on the brain or dural surface so that the marked (+) is placed over the target, and the needle is passed.
(From Rubin JM, Carson PL. Physics and techniques. In Rubin JM, Chandler WF, eds. *Ultrasound in Neurosurgery.* New York, Raven Press, 1990:1-67.)

termined ultrasonically by an electronic cursor, the angle of the guide is adjusted to that depth based on preset graduations located on the guide, and a needle is passed. In general, these guides require less contact surface for needle passage than the fixed-angle devices, and the greater flexibility is helpful. However, the prospective needle path cannot be displayed on the video monitor, and the depth settings are only correct if a lesion lies along the central beam of the sector image. If for some reason a lesion cannot be centered in the image, the depth calculations are meaningless.

To avoid this problem, there is a technique called **pseudobiopsy** that one can use (Fig. 20-15).[36] Because lesions are always imaged relative to the scan head, hitting a target on the screen in one field is equivalent to hitting the same target in another field if the speeds of sound in the two fields are the same. Therefore it is possible to pass a biopsy needle or catheter to a preselected target in a saline or water bath, and then pass the probe under ultrasound guidance through the brain intersecting the corresponding intracerebral point. It can be done as follows:

- Identify the lesion of interest sonographically. By definition, this lesion cannot be positioned in the center of the sector image.
- Mark the position of the lesion on the video screen with an electronic cursor.

- Remove the scan head from the surface of the brain or dura and put the tip of the scan head into a beaker of sterile, lukewarm saline or water. The correct temperatures are crucial because the speed of sound in water or saline must closely approximate 1540 m/sec, which is the speed of sound in brain and soft tissue. The correct temperatures are about 38° C for saline and 50° C for water.[37]
- Adjust the needle in the biopsy guide until it passes through the electronic cursor on the video screen, lock the guide into that position, and remove the needle. The depth at which the calibration is set does not relate to the procedure being performed but only indicates the depth at which the biopsy needle will cross the midline.
- Remove the scanhead tip from the fluid and place it back on the brain or dural surface.
- Move the transducer around until the electronic cursor on the video screen again overlies the area of interest, and insert the needle through the guide. The needle will necessarily hit the target (Fig. 20-16).

Needle Visibility. Because the length of the surface of the needle is much larger than a wavelength, it constitutes a specular reflector. Because of this, the angle of reflection is highly dependent on the angle of inci-

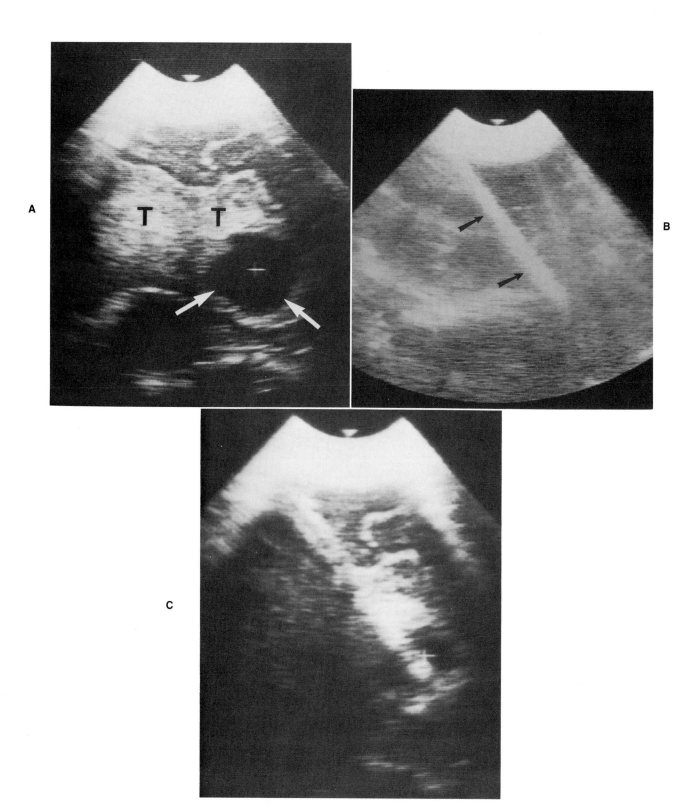

FIG 20-16. Catheter drainage of a cyst using the pseudobiopsy technique. **A,** Transaxial scan shows the cyst marked *(arrows)* that could not be positioned in the center of the sector. Echogenic tumor *(T)*. **B,** Scan of a ventricular catheter *(arrows)* being passed through a saline-filled container. The "+" is obscured by the catheter tip. **C,** Repeat transaxial scan of the brain showing the tip of the catheter intersecting the "+", which has been repositioned over the posterior cyst.

dence. Needle insertion at an oblique angle to the transducer causes most of the sound that strikes the needle to scatter away from the surface of the transducer, decreasing the backscattered energy, which makes the needle and its tip harder to see. One way to prevent this is to roughen or etch the surface of the needle or catheter tip.[38-40] If the roughened surface has irregularities that approximate the size of one wavelength, the backscatter is no longer directionally dependent. Significantly more sound is scattered in the direction of the transducer, which makes it easier to see the needle (Fig. 20-10).

INFECTION

Abscesses of various sizes and in various stages of development can be seen sonographically.[14,15,41] The margins of an abscess are almost always hyperechoic whereas the central echogenicity varies depending on the degree of liquification. The hyperechoic margins in the early stages of an abscess are caused by marked cellular infiltration whereas collagen deposition causes the increased echogenicity later on.[41] Surrounding edema or cerebritis is nearly always echogenic, and distinguishing between the two by ultrasound is difficult if not impossible. Clearly it is possible to aspirate such lesions under ultrasonic guidance.

TRAUMA

Ultrasound has proved to be an extremely useful modality for localizing foreign bodies in the extremities, and it can be very useful in identifying *bone fragments or foreign bodies in the brain* (Fig. 20-17).[42-46] The acoustic impedances of the standard materials that are searched for, such as metal, bone, wood fragments, and glass are different enough from soft tissue to make them readily distinguishable. In general, they all produce bright reflections with or without associated acoustic shadows that help pinpoint their locations. Foreign materials will have backscatter differences: the reflections from wood are less than those from bone or metal.[43] Except for metal, which produces a characteristic "comet-tail" artifact (Fig. 20-18),[43,47,48] the nature of the shadows does not distinguish one material from another. This creates a problem because *one pitfall is air,* which is often present in these wounds along with the foreign bodies. In fact, air can be incorporated directly into wood fragments.[43] Because air also casts shadows, the operator may have difficulty deciding whether a shadow arises from a foreign body or from air in the wound. If the search does not involve finding a large number of fragments, a preoperative CT scan pinpointing the fragment locations can help to limit the search and distinguish air from solid, shadowing materials.

The ultrasound appearance of **intracranial hematomas** is well known from the literature on intraoperative and neonatal neurosonography.[14,15,43,49] Hematomas initially start out as hypoechoic masses during active bleeding, but within a minute after clot formation, the mass becomes quite echogenic with the increased echogenicity caused by red cell aggregation.[50-52] The

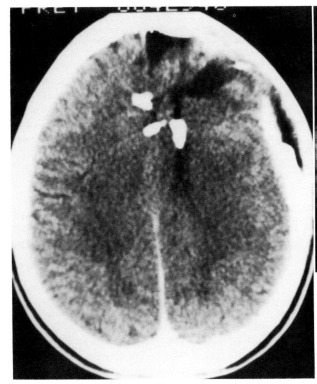

A

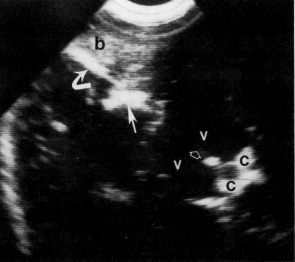

B

FIG 20-17. Foreign body localization. **A,** CT scan showing 3 bone and metal fragments from a gunshot wound to the frontal region. **B,** Coronal sonogram shows a bone fragment *(straight arrow)* that crosses the midline. Falx *(curved arrow).* Lateral ventricles *(v),* septum pellucidum *(open arrow),* and choroid plexus *(c).* Brain *(b)* is highly echogenic consistent with contusion.

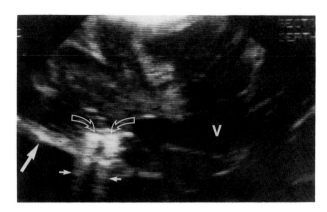

FIG 20-18. Postoperative metallic clips. Transaxial scan shows two highly echogenic clips *(curved arrows)* with comet-tail artifacts behind them *(small arrows)* on feeding vessels of arteriovenous malformation. Falx *(large arrow)*. Ipsilateral lateral ventricle *(V)*.
(From Rubin JM, Carson PL. Physics and techniques. In Rubin JM, Chandler WF, eds. *Ultrasound in Neurosurgery.* New York, Raven Press, 1990:1-67.)

central echogenicity begins to decrease after a period of 3 to 4 days until the hematoma becomes centrally hypoechoic with an echogenic rim. The echogenic rim initially is caused by red cell aggregation, but the rim is eventually collagenized. Histologically, the area of decreased echogenicity corresponds to the breakdown of red blood cells.[53] This decrease in echogenicity continues for about 2 weeks, when the clot starts looking primarily hypoechoic.[53] The upshot of this transition is that hematomas can look different sonographically depending on their time of formation relative to the time of scanning. Thus, it is possible for a hematoma to be isoechoic with the brain, a problem which is more a theoretic than a practical one.

The diagnosis of a hematoma is rarely based on the sonogram alone. A recent history of trauma, a high-density lesion on a CT scan, and a lesion with a high-signal intensity on T1-weighted MRI scans will all help in making the diagnosis. The usefulness of sonography is in localizing the hematoma and monitoring its drainage. These lesions are very easy to locate and, since the diameters of "brain needles" are often on the order of several millimeters, it is usually possible to clearly visualize a needle while decompressing these lesions transdurally (Fig. 20-19). Sonography can also be used for confirming that the hematoma has been totally aspirated without opening the dura.

The development of a hematoma as a surgical complication is a corollary of ultrasound's application in trauma.[8,15,54] Because acute brain swelling during surgery is a potential catastrophe, immediate localization of a developing hematoma is essential. In these circumstances, the surgeon is totally blind without sonography. Ultrasound can immediately locate a developing

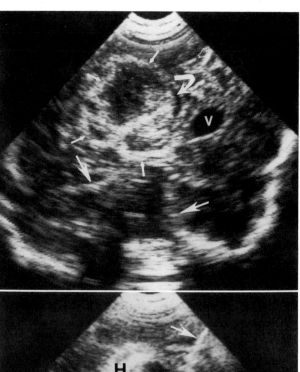

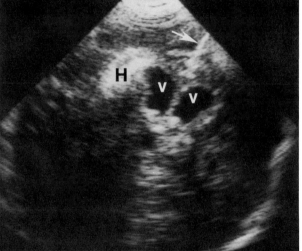

FIG 20-19. Hematoma. **A,** Coronal scan shows a large, complex mass *(small arrows)* in the right cerebral hemisphere that compresses the right lateral ventricle *(curved arrow)*. Left lateral ventricle *(v)*, falx *(open arrow)*, and 2 leaves of the tentorium *(large arrows)*. **B,** Postdrainage coronal scan shows a small residual hematoma *(H)* after drainage. Lateral ventricles *(v)* are both expanded. Falx *(arrow)*.

hematoma, and the lesion can be resected or drained under directed guidance if necessary (Fig. 20-20). If the hemorrhage is entirely intraventricular (Fig. 20-20), only a ventricular catheter is needed for drainage after surgery.

SHUNTS

It has never been much of a feat to introduce catheters into enlarged ventricles; neurosurgeons have been doing so for years. Yet problems can arise even in the most routine cases. For instance, the tip of the catheter

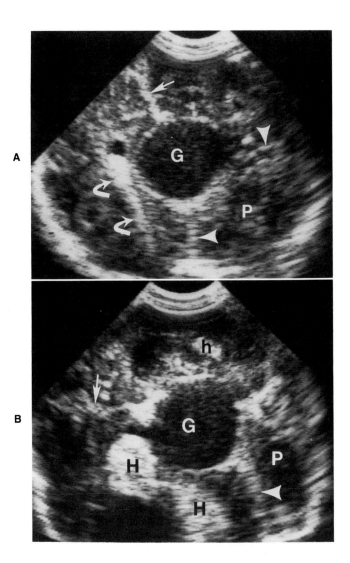

FIG 20-20. Vein of Galen aneurysm. **A,** Coronal sonogram shows a hypoechoic vein of Galen *(G).* **B,** Coronal sonogram more tipped to the right shows two intraventricular hematomas *(H)* and *(h)* that occurred at surgery. Falx *(straight arrow).* Echogenic choroid plexus in the contralateral ventricle *(curved arrows).* Leaves of the tentorium *(arrowheads).* Posterior fossa *(P).*

can pass through the foramen of Monroe and enter the third ventricle (Fig. 20-21). Sometimes the tip can actually become embedded in the thalamus or caudate nucleus, or postshunt bleeding can occur.[54,55] A very common problem is the proximity of the catheter tip to the choroid plexus. It is believed that 80% of proximal shunt obstructions are caused by entanglement of the shunt tip with the choroid plexus.[56] Theoretically, the longevity of shunts would improve if shunt tips could be positioned away from the choroid plexus in the frontal horn of a lateral ventricle.[3,10,20,54,57] Because of the high echogenicity of the choroid plexus on sonog-

raphy, it is easy to place the tips of catheters in portions of the ventricles away from the choroid plexus (Fig. 20-21).[3,10,20,54,57] Furthermore, it is simple to confirm the position of the shunt tip and shunt patency by merely pumping the shunt or injecting small amounts of saline.[3,20,57,58] This maneuver introduces microbubbles that are highly echogenic and easily visible.[58,59] In at least one early series, the longevity of shunts placed under ultrasound guidance was about twice that of non-ultrasound–guided shunts.[54]

Although large ventricles are easy to hit, placing catheters into small ventricles for pressure monitoring or for chemotherapy can be quite difficult.[3,20] In such cases, sonography can be very useful in localizing the ventricle and confirming the position of the catheter.

Two main approaches have been used. In young children with an anterior fontanelle, catheters can be introduced through posterior parietal-occipital trephines or craniectomies while simultaneously monitoring the catheter's progress from the fontanelle.[3,54,57] Because the site of scanning is almost perpendicular to the catheter, the catheter is extremely well seen.

Another approach that has been used in adults is to produce a **keyhole-shaped craniectomy** near the coronal suture.[32] The large portion of the keyhole, generally a small trephine, is for positioning the scan head. A small extension off the trephine is used as a site for introduction of the shunt catheter. The catheter is passed through the smaller hole and monitored under ultrasound guidance. Once the catheter tip has entered the ventricle, the extruding catheter can be attached conveniently to a reservoir positioned over the smaller hole. The reservoir rests on the bone surrounding the smaller hole and stabilizes the position of the catheter.

VASCULAR LESIONS
Arteriovenous Malformation (AVM)

Despite the great success of gray-scale ultrasonography for most neurosurgical applications, its utility for AVMs has been limited, because the gray-scale contrast between large portions of these lesions and the rest of the brain is low.[14,15,54] This is particularly true for the hypoechoic, large, feeding arteries and draining veins, which must be identified for any localizing procedure to have full utility in these instances.[14,15,54]

It is clear that even though portions of AVMs can be imaged in gray-scale,[15,54,60,61] one cannot be certain that the entire lesion with its associated vasculature has been seen.[15,54] In one report, two AVMs were studied; one was seen and the other was termed "subtle", although the associated arteries and veins were seen in both.[54] In another study, a group of 11 AVMs was studied by intraoperative gray-scale alone; only about one half of the lesions could be visualized at all.[15] The identification of draining veins and feeding arteries was

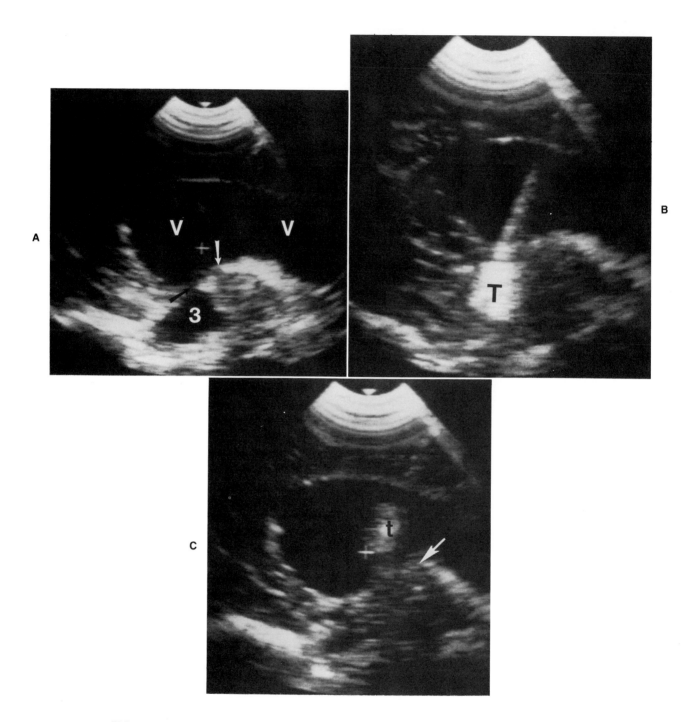

FIG 20-21. Ventricular shunt placement. **A,** Sagittal sonogram shows the anterior margin of the choroid plexus *(white arrow).* **B,** Repeat scan shows the catheter tip *(T)* had migrated through the foramen of Monroe into the third ventricle. **C,** Follow-up scan shows catheter tip *(t)* pulled back into the lateral ventricle. Body of the lateral ventricle *(V).* Foramen of Monroe *(black arrow).* Third ventricle *(3).* The "+" in the lateral ventricle marks the target for the catheter.

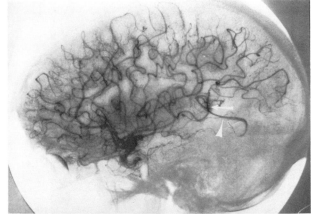

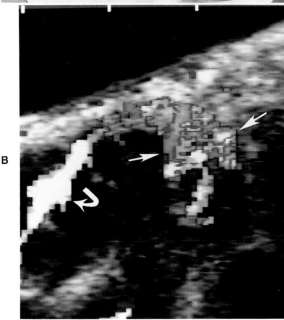

FIG 20-22. Surgically occult AVM. **A,** Preoperative cerebral angiogram with subtraction technique of an AVM *(arrow)* at the posterior aspect of the sylvian fissure that was incompletely resected. Large early draining vein *(arrowhead).* **B,** Color Doppler scan shows small subcortical AVM *(arrows)* with a presumed feeding artery *(curved arrow).*

at best incomplete; however, the ability to distinguish these vessels intraoperatively would be very useful.[60] In particular, the clipping of draining veins too early during surgery can cause a disastrous venous infarction.

Pulsed Doppler seems to have a natural role in these cases.[60,61] It would appear at first glance that the problems of localizing subcortical AVMs and discriminating between feeding arteries and draining veins would be easy by this modality. Yet, considering the complexity of these lesions, the mere mapping of a complex, three-dimensional tangle of vessels with a point sample vol-

ume is daunting if not impossible. Furthermore, the velocity waveforms within these vessels can be very misleading. It is a well-known property of vascular malformations that veins can be "arterialized".[62] Thus, arterial signals can be detected in what are known to be draining veins, although some veins definitely will have venous signals. As a result, the Doppler signals themselves can be misleading, and because these vessels often are barely visible if not invisible on gray scale, the addition of pulsed Doppler offers little to the surgical resection of these lesions.

In contrast, **color flow Doppler** can be an accurate technique to detect and determine the extent of AVMs. The mapping of the lesions themselves is greatly enhanced by the color contrast generated by the high velocity of the blood flowing through them (Figs. 20-22 to 20-24). In particular, high-velocity, multidirectional flows in AVMs are displayed as areas with multiple colors lying side by side in an apparently random fashion. The multiple flow directions and aliasing introduced by the high velocities are responsible for this appearance.

This localized chaotic, turbulent flow is the sine qua non of AVMs; it must be present in order to identify lesions definitively. Vascular lesions can be difficult or impossible to image in cases where there is slow flow, such as venous angiomas, or where there has been an intervention prior to surgery that decreases flow, such as endovascular embolization. Improvements in slow-flow imaging techniques may eventually help in these cases, but any improvement still will require a knowledge of the lesion's approximate position, because any slow-flow technique will produce aliasing and complex signal patterns in neighboring normal vessels, making them look abnormal. These normal vessels could then be mistaken for the lesion itself.

A knowledge of a lesion's approximate position is also necessary when identifying feeding arteries and draining veins. Although in theory one should be able to distinguish arteries from veins by their flow directions relative to the AVM, in practice, because of the complex tangle of vessels, this determination becomes almost impossible to evaluate, even with the use of color. Furthermore, the waveforms themselves can be misleading. However, it should be noted that although an arterial pattern can occur in either arteries or veins, a venous pattern is likely to occur only in veins.

Despite these limitations, color Doppler is still a very useful imaging technique for surgery on AVMs.[63,64] In one report color Doppler was determined to be useful in 8 of 12 intracerebral AVMs.[64] In 3 of the 4 cases in which it was not useful, the cause was either equipment- or procedure-related, and was unrelated to the technique itself. The benefits of the method include:

- Identification of deep or hard to find lesions (Fig. 20-22)

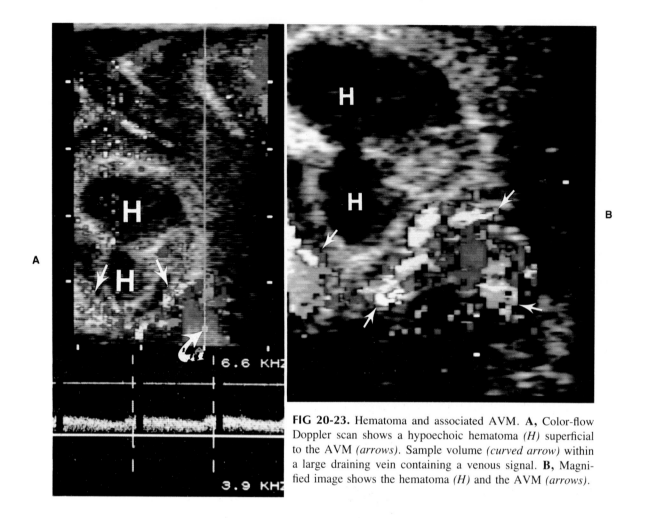

FIG 20-23. Hematoma and associated AVM. **A,** Color-flow Doppler scan shows a hypoechoic hematoma *(H)* superficial to the AVM *(arrows)*. Sample volume *(curved arrow)* within a large draining vein containing a venous signal. **B,** Magnified image shows the hematoma *(H)* and the AVM *(arrows)*.

- Localization of AVMs relative to adjacent hematomas (Fig. 20-23)
- Confirmation of complete resection of lesions that are presumed to have been totally removed (Fig. 20-24).

The latter two advantages are particularly interesting. By removing an AVM-associated hematoma, the surgeon can reduce the intracerebral volume and more easily gain access to the AVM itself. In one case, the intracerebral pressure produced by a hematoma was so high that the AVM only became visible as the hematoma was aspirated.

Color-flow Doppler has proven extremely useful in localizing residual AVMs in certain cases where a total resection had been attempted but not accomplished (Fig. 20-24). A finding of no residual AVM on a postresection scan is conclusive evidence that total removal has been achieved. Without intraoperative confirmation, follow-up surgery may be necessary to remove the portions of an AVM that were missed the first time.[63,64]

Aneurysm

Cerebral aneurysms can also be seen with remarkable clarity using intraoperative ultrasound.[27,65] However, except in certain cases, localization of these lesions is rarely a problem, because aneurysms usually occur at well-defined, easily-localized vascular bifurcations. There are, however, specific examples, such as mycotic aneurysms, where rapid localization of lesions is very difficult without sonography.[14]

In certain circumstances, pulsed Doppler sonography has proved to be useful in aneurysm surgery.[66] In particular, Doppler can be used to evaluate changes in blood flow in the parent artery as the neck of the aneurysm is occluded. A rapidly increasing velocity can herald the onset of spasm in the native vessel. Color-flow Doppler can also be used to evaluate flow in an aneurysm while the neck is being surgically occluded (Fig. 20-25).[63] It can be particularly useful in cases of giant aneurysms where the neck may be wide and difficult to occlude. Although there are only a few such cases, it

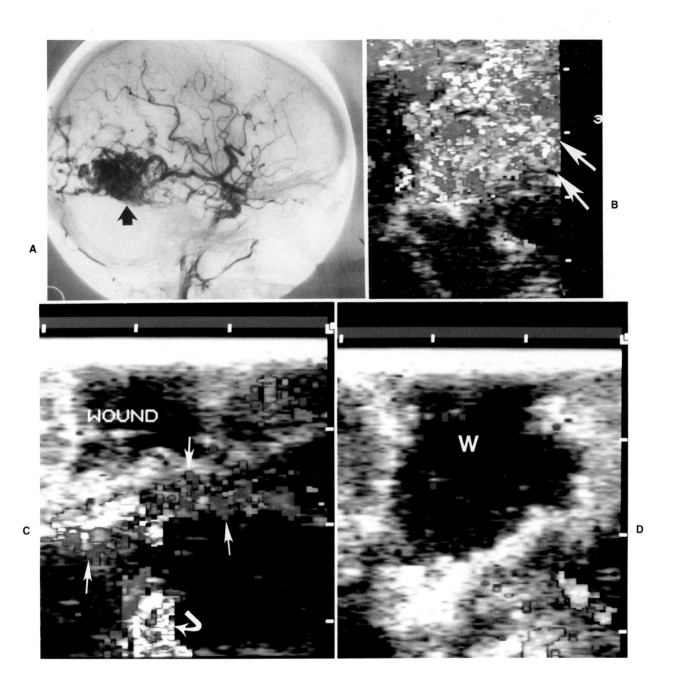

FIG 20-24. Residual AVM. **A,** Cerebral angiogram with subtraction technique shows a large posterior temporal AVM *(arrow)*. **B,** Color Doppler image shows classic turbulent flow of the AVM *(arrows)*. **C,** Initial postresection scan (presumed totally resected) shows at the base of the saline-filled wound, residual AVM with multiple vessels of varied colors *(arrows)* with a high velocity, aliasing vessel *(curved arrow)* deep to the lesion. **D,** Second postresection scan shows no abnormal vessels in the base of the wound *(W)*.

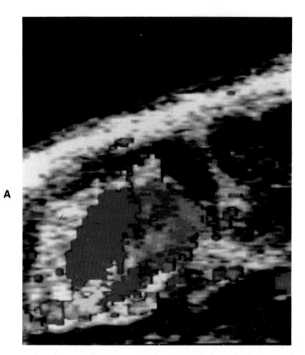
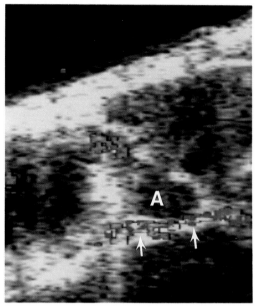

FIG 20-25. Aneurysm of the middle cerebral artery. **A,** Color Doppler image of the giant aneurysm with swirling blood demonstrated by the red-blue color separation. **B,** Post-clipping scan demonstrating no flow in the aneurysm *(A)*. Interestingly, there is probably spasm in the source artery *(arrows)*, which contains multiple and varied colors. These represent either multiple flow speeds or flow directions or both. Such a finding would occur with spasm and/or turbulence.

seems very likely that arterial spasm in the parent vessel could be determined with color Doppler as well.

REFERENCES
Technique

1. Rubin JM, Mirfakhraee M, Duda E, et al. Intraoperative ultrasound examination of the brain. *Radiology* 1980;137:831-832.
2. Rubin JM, Dohrmann GJ, Greenberg M, et al. Intraoperative sonography of meningiomas. *AJNR* 1982;3:305-308.
3. Chandler WF, Knake JE, McGillicuddy JE, et al. Intraoperative use of real-time ultrasonography in neurosurgery. *J Neurosurg* 1982;57:157-163.
4. Gooding GAW, Edwards MSB, Rabkin AE, et al. Intraoperative real-time ultrasound in the localization of intracranial neoplasms. *Radiology* 1983;146:459-462.
5. DiPietro MA, Venes JL. Intraoperative sonography of the Arnold-Chiari malformations. In: Rubin JM, Chandler WF, eds. *Ultrasound in Neurosurgery.* New York, Raven Press, 1990:183-199.
6. Quencer RM, Montalvo BM. Time requirements for intraoperative neurosonography. *AJR* 1986;146:815-818.
7. Rubin JM, Dohrmann GJ. Intraoperative neurosurgical ultrasound in the localization and characterization of intracranial masses. *Radiology* 1983;148:519-524.

Tumors

8. Masuzawa H, Kamitani H, Sato J, et al. Intraoperative application of sector scanning electronic ultrasound in neurosurgery. *Neurol Med-Chir* 1981;21:277-285.

9. Shkolnick A, Tomita T, Raimondi AJ, et al. Work in progress. Intraoperative neurosurgical ultrasound: localization of brain tumors in infants and children. *Radiology* 1983;148:525-527.
10. Knake JE, Chandler WF, McGillicuddy JE, et al. Intraoperative sonography for brain tumor localization and ventricular shunt placement. *AJR* 1982;139:733-738.
11. Pasto ME, Rifkin MD. Intraoperative ultrasound examination of the brain: possible pitfalls in diagnosis and biopsy guidance. *J Ultrasound Med.* 1984;3:245-249.
12. Gooding GAW, Boggan JE, Weinstein PR. Characterization of intracranial neoplasms by computed tomography and intraoperative sonography. *AJNR* 1984;5:517-520.
13. Smith WL, Menezes A, Franken EA. Cranial ultrasound in the diagnosis of malignant brain tumors. *J Clin Ultrasound* 1983;11:97-100.
14. Chandler WF, Rubin JM. The application of ultrasound during brain surgery. *World J Surg* 1987;11:558-569.
15. Rubin JM, Dohrmann GJ. Efficacy of intraoperative ultrasound for evaluating intracranial masses. *Radiology* 1985;157:509-511.
16. Machi J, Sigel B, Jafar JJ, et al. Criteria for using imaging ultrasound during brain and spinal cord surgery. *J Ultrasound Med* 1984;3:155-161.
17. Latchaw RE, Gold LHA, Moore JS Jr, et al. The nonspecificity of absorption coefficients in the differentiation of solid tumors and cystic lesions. *Radiology* 1977;125:141-144.
18. Handa J, Nakano Y, Handa H. Computed tomography in the differential diagnosis of low-density intracranial lesions. *Surg Neurol* 1978;10:179-185.
19. Kjos BO, Brant-Zawadzki M, Kucharczyk W, et al. Cystic intracranial lesions: magnetic resonance imaging. *Radiology* 1985;155:363-369.

20. Rubin JM, Dohrmann GJ. Use of ultrasonically guided probes and catheters in neurosurgery. *Surg Neurol* 1982;18:143-148.
21. McGahan JP, Ellis WG, Budenz RW, et al. Brain gliomas: sonographic characterization. *Radiology* 1986;159:485-492.
22. Enzmann DR, Wheat R, Marshall WH, et al. Tumors of the central nervous system studied by computed tomography and ultrasound. *Radiology* 1985;154:393-399.
23. Smith SJ, Vogelzang RL, Marzano MI, et al. Brain edema: ultrasound examination. *Radiology* 1985;155:379-382.
24. Platt JF, Rubin JM, Chandler WF, et al. Intraoperative spinal sonography in the evaluation of intramedullary tumors. *J Ultrasound Med* 1988;7:317-325.
25. LeRoux PD, Berger MS, Ojemann GA, et al. Correlation of intraoperative ultrasound tumor volumes and margins with preoperative computerized tomography scans: an intraoperative method to enhance tumor resection. *J Neurosurg* 1989;71:691-698.
26. Bowerman RA. Tangential sulcal echoes: potential pitfall in the diagnosis of parenchymal lesions on cranial sonography. *J Ultrasound Med* 1987;6:685-689.
27. Chandler WF. Use of ultrasound imaging during intracranial operations. In Rubin JM, Chandler WF, eds. *Ultrasound in Neurosurgery.* New York, Raven Press, 1990:67-106.
28. Knake JE, Chandler WF, Gabrielsen TO, et al. Intraoperative sonographic delineation of low-grade brain neoplasms defined poorly by computed tomography. *Radiology* 1984;151:735-739.
29. Hatfield MK, Rubin JM, Gebarski SS, et al. Intraoperative sonography in low-grade gliomas. *J Ultrasound Med* 1989;8:131-134.
30. Lange SC, Howe JF, Shuman WP, et al. Intraoperative ultrasound detection of metastatic tumors in the central cortex. *Neurosurgery* 1982;11:219-222.
31. Tsutsumi Y, Andoh Y, Inoue N. Ultrasound-guided biopsy for deep-seated brain tumors. *J Neurosurg* 1982;57:164-167.
32. Tsutsumi Y, Andoh Y, Sakaguchi J. A new ultrasound-guided brain biopsy technique through a burr hole. *Acta Neurochir (Wien)* 1989;96:72-75.
33. Enzmann DR, Irwin KM, Fine IM, et al. Intraoperative and outpatient echoencephalography through a burr hole. *Neuroradiology* 1984;26:57-59.
34. Enzmann DR, Irwin KM, Marshall WH, et al. Intraoperative sonography through a burr hole: guide for brain biopsy. *AJNR* 1984;5:243-246.
35. Berger MS. Ultrasound guided stereotactic biopsy using the Diasonics neuro-biopsy device for deep-seated intracranial lesions. Presented at the Annual Meeting of the American Association of Neurological Surgeons; April 21-15, 1985; Atlanta, GA.
36. Rubin JM, Carson PL. Physics and techniques. In Rubin JM, Chandler WF, eds. *Ultrasound in Neurosurgery.* New York, Raven Press, 1990:1-67.
37. McDicken WW. *Diagnostic Ultrasonics: Principles and Use of Instruments.* New York, John Wiley & Sons, 1976.
38. Rubin JM, Dohrmann GJ. A cannula for use in ultrasonically-guided biopsies of the brain. *J Neurosurg* 1983;59:905-907.
39. Heckermann R, Seidel KJ. The sonographic appearance and contrast of puncture needles. *J Clin Ultrasound* 1983;11:265-268.
40. McGahan JP: Laboratory assessment of ultrasonic needle and catheter visualization. *J Ultrasound Med* 1986;5:373-377.

Infection

41. Enzmann DR, Britt RH, Lyons B, et al. High-resolution ultrasound evaluation of experimental brain abscess evolution: comparison with computed tomography and neuropathology. *Radiology* 1982;142:95-102.
42. Wood JH, Parver M, Doppman JL, et al. Experimental intraoperative localization of retained intracerebral bone fragments using transdural ultrasound. *J Neurosurg* 1977;46:65-71.
43. Enzmann DR, Britt RH, Lyons B, et al. Experimental study of high-resolution ultrasound imaging of hemorrhage, bone fragments, and foreign bodies in head trauma. *J Neurosurg* 1981;54:304-309.
44. Fornage BD, Schernberg FL. Sonographic diagnosis of foreign bodies of the distal extremities. *AJR* 1986;147:567-569.
45. Fornage BD, Schernberg FL. Sonographic pre-operative localization of a foreign body in the hand. *J Ultrasound Med* 1987;6:217-219.
46. Gooding GAW, Gardiman T, Sumers M, et al. Sonography of the hand and foot in foreign body detection. *J Ultrasound Med* 1987;6:441-447.
47. Wendell BA, Athey A. Ultrasonic appearance of metallic foreign bodies in parenchymal organs. *J Clin Ultrasound* 1981;9:133-135.
48. Ziskin MC, Thickman DI, Goldenberg WJ, et al. The comet tail artifact. *J Ultrasound Med* 1982;1:1-7.
49. Grode ML, Komaiko MS. The role of intraoperative ultrasound in neurosurgery. *Neurosurgery* 1983;12:624-628.
50. Lillehei KO, Chandler WF, Knake JF. Real time ultrasound characteristics of the acute intracerebral hemorrhage as studied in the canine model. *Neurosurgery* 1984;14:48-51.
51. Sigel B, Machi J, Beitler JC, et al. Red cell aggregation as a cause of blood-flow echogenicity. *Radiology* 1983;148:799-802.
52. Sigel B, Coelho JC, Spigos DG, et al. Ultrasonography of blood during stasis and coagulation. *Invest Radiol* 1981;16:71-76.
53. Enzmann DR, Britt RH, Lyons BE, et al. Natural history of experimental intracerebral hemorrhage: sonography, computed tomography and neuropathology. *AJNR* 1981;2:517-526.
54. Merritt CRB, Coulon R, Connolly E. Intraoperative neurosurgical ultrasound: transdural and transfontanelle applications. *Radiology* 1983;148:513-517.

Shunts

55. Mahony BS, Gross BH, Callen PW, et al. Intraventricular hemorrhage following ventriculoperitoneal shunt placement: real-time ultrasonographic demonstration. *J Ultrasound Med* 1983;2:143-145.
56. Sekhar LN, Moossy J, Guthkelch AN. Malfunctioning ventriculoperitoneal shunts: clinical and pathological features. *J Neurosurg* 1982;56:411-416.
57. Shkolnik A, McLone DG. Intraoperative real-time ultrasonic guidance of ventricular shunt placement in infants. *Radiology* 1981;141:515-517.
58. Widder DJ, Davis KR, Taveras JM. Assessment of ventricular shunt patency by sonography: a new noninvasive test. *AJR* 1986;147:353-356.
59. Widder DJ, Simeone JF. Microbubbles as a contrast agent for neurosonography and ultrasound-guided catheter manipulation: in vitro studies. *AJR* 1986;147:347-352.

Vascular lesions

60. Nornes H, Grip A, Wikeby P. Intraoperative evaluation of cerebral hemodynamics using directional Doppler technique. Part 1: Arteriovenous malformations. *J Neurosurg* 1979;50:145-151.
61. Fasano VA, Ponzio RM, Liboni W, et al. Preliminary experiences with "real-time" intraoperative ultrasonography associated to the laser and ultrasonic aspirator in neurosurgery. *Surg Neurol* 1983;19:318-323.
62. Helvie MA, Rubin JM. Evaluation of traumatic groin arteriovenous fistulas with duplex Doppler sonography. *J Ultrasound Med* 1989;8: 21-24.
63. Black KL, Rubin JM, Chandler WF, et al. Intraoperative color flow Doppler imaging of AVMs and aneurysms. *J Neurosurg* 1988;68:635-639.

64. Rubin JM, Hatfield MK, Chandler WF, et al. Intracerebral arteriovenous malformations: intraoperative color Doppler flow imaging. *Radiology* 1989;170:219-222.

65. Hyodo A, Mizukami M, Tazawa T, et al. Intraoperative use of real-time ultrasonography applied to aneurysm surgery. *Neurosurgery* 1983;13:642-645.

66. Nornes H, Grip A, Wikeby P. Intraoperative evaluation of cerebral hemodynamics using directional Doppler technique. Part 2. Saccular aneurysms. *J Neurosurg* 1979;50:570-577.

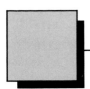

CHAPTER 21

Intraoperative Sonography of the Spine

- Berta Maria Montalvo, M.D.

Clinical outcome of spinal surgery depends not only on accurate preoperative diagnosis, but also on the proper identification and localization of lesions during surgery and their adequate correction. The use of high-resolution sonography in the operating room has provided the spinal surgeon with a new vision. Without sonography, the surgeon had a limited field of view and often had to rely on indirect signs such as transmitted pulsations in order to assess completeness of decompression. With sonography, the contents of the thecal sac are precisely depicted, and a view of the ventral canal is obtained without incurring the risk of retracting delicate neural tissues. The dynamic nature of real-time sonography also affords the surgeon the opportunity to continually monitor the progress and adequacy of the surgical process.

INDICATIONS

Since its introduction in 1982,[1] intraoperative spinal sonography has been used for the intraoperative management of lesions that compress or fix neural elements. These include:

- Herniated disks
- Canal stenosis
- Spine fractures
- Tumors and cysts
- Inflammatory masses
- Congenital anomalies

Sonography has also been used to locate foreign bodies and to guide procedures like biopsies, drainages, and shunt placements. Sonography has significantly improved the effectiveness and precision of each of these applications and its use should be universal.

TECHNIQUE

We use a portable sonographic machine designed for the operating room. It is equipped with preset time-compensation curves, a small 7.5 MHz sector transducer on a long cord, a camera, and a video tape recorder. In the operating room the transducer and cord are draped in a long sterile sheath; sterile gel serves as an acoustic couplet between the transducer and sterile sheath.

The radiologist and the surgeon review the preoperative examinations in order to establish the surgical approach to the case, specifically the level and extent of the surgical exposure. Most patients undergo surgery in the prone position and therefore are examined from a posterior approach. The paraspinal muscles are retracted, the initial laminectomy is performed, and sterile fluid is poured into the wound to serve as an acoustic water path. The tip of the draped transducer is then introduced into the water bath and the surgeon scans the spinal canal and its contents in the transverse and longitudinal planes. Longitudinal scans are oriented so that the cephalad direction will lie to the left of the image; transverse scans are oriented with the left side of the patient on the left, because the patient is prone.

The radiologist and the surgeon review the pertinent findings in the initial scan that may influence the surgical approach. The progress of surgery is monitored with sonography, and the final sonogram documents the results of the surgery.

Limitations

The diagnostic capabilities of intraoperative spinal sonography are limited by the field of view, which is determined by the extent of the laminectomy performed because bone interferes with the transmission of the ultrasound beam. Structures that lie under unresected bone will not be visualized because of acoustic shadowing. A laminectomy that measures at least 1.5 cm by 1 cm is necessary for adequate visualization of the canal and its contents. A laminectomy of this size does not affect spinal stability and in most cases does not require added resection. Sonography cannot be used in microsurgery for disk disease because of the small size of the laminectomy.

Substances other than bone may also interfere with the transmission of sound and will obscure visualization of deeper structures. Specifically, dura mater that is calcified dorsally will interfere with visualization of the thecal sac contents and all other structures that lie ventral to the calcification. Gelfoam, used routinely for hemostasis during surgery, has a characteristic appearance, exhibiting a bright interface and a shadowing artifact of reverberations. In large amounts Gelfoam obscures adjacent structures; in small amounts it may be confused with a pathologic process. Therefore, prior to scanning, it is desirable to remove all Gelfoam from the operative field.

SONOGRAPHIC ANATOMY

The spinal cord and cauda equina are contained within the thecal sac surrounded by anechoic cerebrospinal fluid.[2,3] On transverse views, the cord is oval in shape in the cervical region and round in the thoracic area. The distal cord tapers to the conus medullaris, a characteristic best appreciated on sagittal views. The surface of the cord is brightly reflective, presumably secondary to the pial covering. The parenchyma of the cord is homogeneous and hypoechoic and the gray and white matter are not individually visualized.[2,3] A midline, echogenic structure is seen within the ventral half of the cord. This central echo has a punctate appearance on transverse views and a linear interface on longitudinal sections. The central echo has been shown to represent the central aspect of the anterior median fissure.[4-6] Denticulate ligaments tether the cord laterally and are seen as bright linear interfaces on transverse views. Dorsal arachnoid septations course from the posterior surface of the cord to the dorsal arachnoid and are seen as bright interfaces within the dorsal cerebrospinal fluid (Fig. 21-1).

Dorsal and ventral nerve roots are only rarely seen at the cervical, upper and midthoracic region. They are routinely seen clustering around the conus medullaris as they descend to form the cauda equina. Individual nerve roots typically appear as two parallel bright linear echoes, short on transverse views and long and tubular on longitudinal sections. They are most numerous in the upper lumbar canal where the cauda equina can look like a tangle of spaghetti; at this level it may be difficult to resolve individual nerve roots. The number of spinal

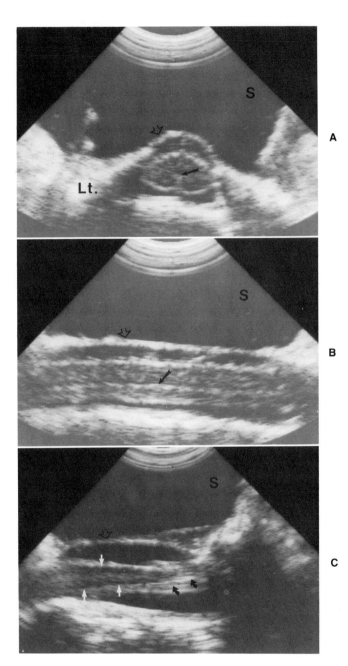

FIG 21-1. Normal spinal cord. Transverse (**A**) and longitudinal (**B**) scans of the cervical cord show an echogenic line *(open arrowhead)* that represents the dorsal dura-arachnoid layer. Spinal fluid surrounds the cord, which is seen as a hypoechoic structure with echogenic boundaries. The central echo of the cord *(straight arrow)* represents the central aspect of the anterior median fissure. (**C**) Longitudinal image of the lower thoracic cord shows the conus medullaris, which is the tapering end of the cord *(white arrows)*. The exiting nerve roots *(black arrows)* are hyperechoic. Saline *(S)*; Left *(Lt)*.
(**A** and **B** from Quencer RM, Montalvo BM. Normal intraoperative spinal sonography. *AJNR*. 1984;5:501-505; 1985;143:1301-1305; **C**, from Montalvo BM and Quencer RM. Intraoperative sonography in spinal surgery: current state of the art. *Neuroradiology*. 1986;28:551-590.)

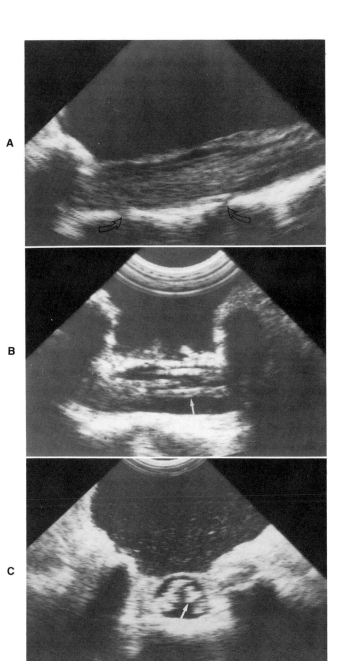

FIG 21-2. Normal cauda equina. **A,** Superior (proximal) cauda equina, longitudinal scan. The nerve roots of the cauda equina are small tubular structures that are difficult to resolve individually in the superior lumbar canal. The dorsal surface of the vertebral bodies is delineated by the highly echogenic lines, which are interrupted by intervertebral disk spaces *(curved arrows).* **B** and **C,** Inferior (distal) cauda equina. Longitudinal *(B)* and transverse *(C)* images at this level show the individual nerve roots *(arrows)* within the subarachnoid space.

nerve roots decreases as the roots exit segmentally, so fewer roots are seen in the distal lumbar region (Fig. 21-2).

The shape of the spinal canal varies at different levels. On transverse images following laminectomy, the canal at the cervical and lumbar regions resembles an open rectangle, while in the thoracic region it approximates the shape of a semicircle. On longitudinal examination, the dorsal aspect of the vertebral body, a characteristically bright interface, is interrupted by the intervertebral space, a structure of medium echogenicity that exhibits acoustic transmission. In the lumbar region, ventral epidural fat is abundant, usually hyperechoic, and symmetrically distributed in the epidural space.

CORD COMPRESSION
Sonographic Criteria for Decompression

Sonography is commonly used to evaluate spinal lesions that compress the spinal cord, thecal sac, or cauda equina. In order to determine the adequacy of surgical decompression, several criteria have been established.[7-9] Lack of displacement of neural elements, is shown by:

- Normal or near normal shape of the spinal cord
- Rounded thecal sac in the lumbar spine
- Normal course of the cauda equina
- Absence of initially identified soft tissue or bony mass
- Normal or near normal shape of the spinal canal
- Open rectangle in the lumbar region
- Space visualized between the thecal sac and the bony canal laterally

Of these, the single most important criterion is the lack of displacement of either the spinal cord or the cauda equina.[7-9]

Herniated Disks

Herniated disks within the spinal canal can be differentiated from surrounding normal and abnormal structures by their typical sonographic appearance. Disks are sharply marginated, exhibit medium echogenicity, can be clearly seen in two views, and are located immediately adjacent to the intervertebral disk space where they compress neural structures (Fig. 21-3). In spondylolisthesis, longitudinal sonograms can establish the presence of a herniated disk when the characteristic soft tissue mass is seen protruding into the canal between the edges of the subluxed vertebrae. Spondylolisthesis without associated disk herniation is seen as a displacement of the normal dorsal vertebral surface (Fig. 21-4). **Ventral epidural fat** should not be confused with a disk as it appears homogeneously hyperechoic, does not displace neural elements, and is symmetrical in distribution. **Scar** on the other hand may be heterogeneous, brightly echogenic and mimic fat, or it

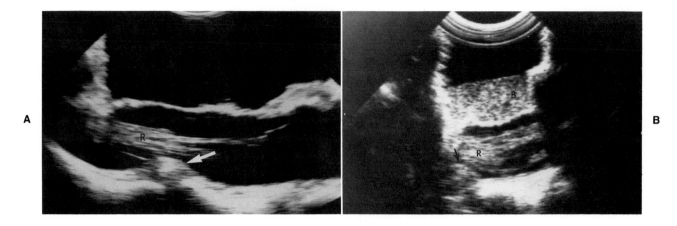

FIG 21-3. Herniated disk, longitudinal scans. **A,** Herniated disk *(white arrow)* is located at the intervertebral interspace. It appears as a sharply marginated soft tissue mass that touches the nerve roots *(R)* in the lumbar region. **B,** When the herniated disk *(black arrow)* is located at the edge of the laminectomy, it may be missed, but compression of the adjacent nerve roots *(R)* helps define the soft-tissue mass. *B,* fresh blood in the saline dorsal to the dura.

may be of medium echogenicity and mimic disk. The identifying characteristic of scar is the absence of a well-defined interface with surrounding tissues (Fig. 21-5). **Swollen roots** are round and well defined on transverse views, but unlike herniated disks, they are poorly defined on longitudinal views.

The ability of sonography to discriminate a disk from other structures has important implications in the surgical management of disk herniation. Because a common cause of failed back surgery is residual disk material,[10] the removal of as much abnormal disk as possible from the spinal canal is a crucial goal of sur-

gery. In our series, 40% of patients examined after routine discectomy were found to have unsuspected residual fragments, which were then removed (Fig. 21-6).[9]

Canal Stenosis

Failure to recognize and adequately treat lateral stenosis is the most common cause of failed back surgery.[10] Sonography provides an immediate evaluation of the effect of bone on adjacent neural tissue during decompression surgery of the lumbar canal for stenosis. Sonography shows when sufficient bone has been removed to result in a decompressed canal. The sac will

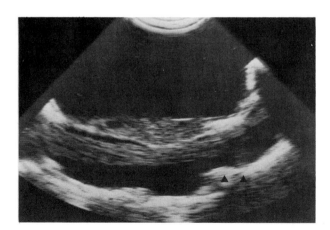

FIG 21-4. Spondylolisthesis. In contrast to a disk, spondylolisthesis is seen as displacement of the normal dorsal surface of the vertebral body *(arrowheads)*, which does not compress neural elements.

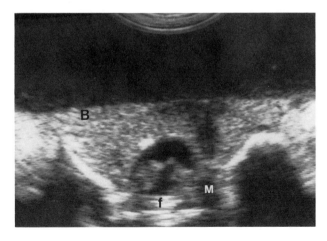

FIG 21-5. Scar. Transverse image shows a poorly marginated mass *(M)* adjacent to the right side of the thecal sac. This poor margination is characteristic of a scar rather than a herniated disk. Note the bright echogenicity of epidural fat *(F)*. *B,* Blood saline layer.

assume a normal rounded configuration and space will be visualized between the sac and the remaining lateral facet. When sonography shows that the thecal sac is encroached laterally by facets at a symptomatic level, the surgeon will extend the facetectomies. (Fig. 21-7). Similarly, if sonography shows that the sac is compressed by a ventral spur, spur resection may be attempted. About 20% of patients examined with sonography after posterolateral decompression for canal stenosis had persistent encroachment of the neural elements by bone and had to undergo further bony removal in order to achieve optimal decompression.[9]

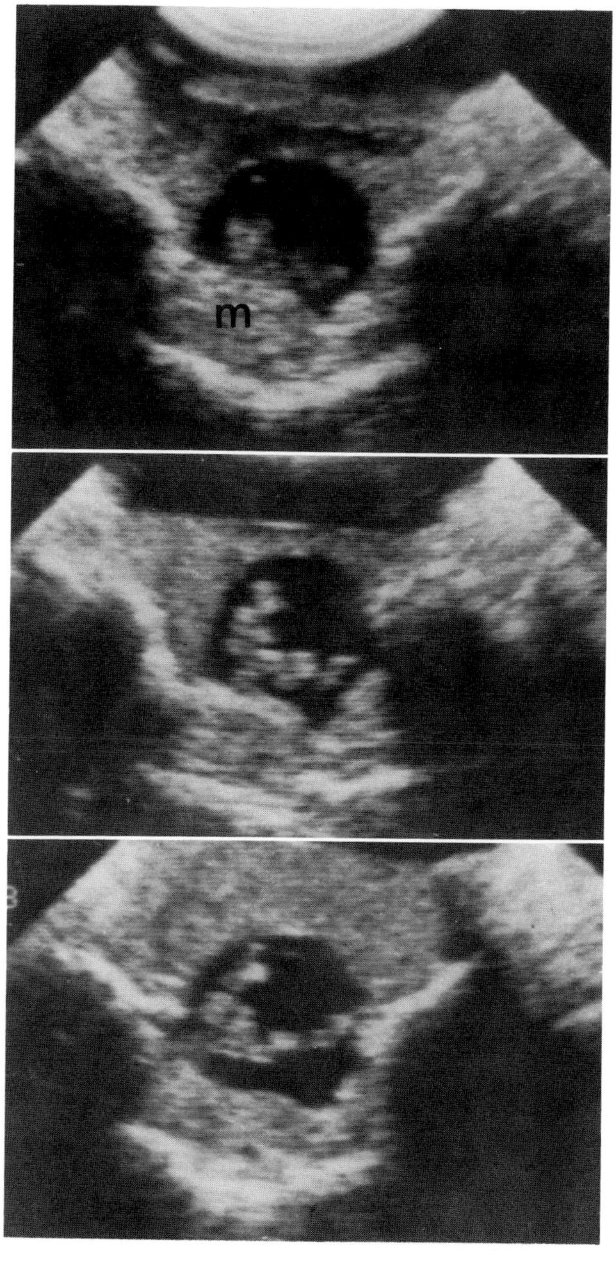

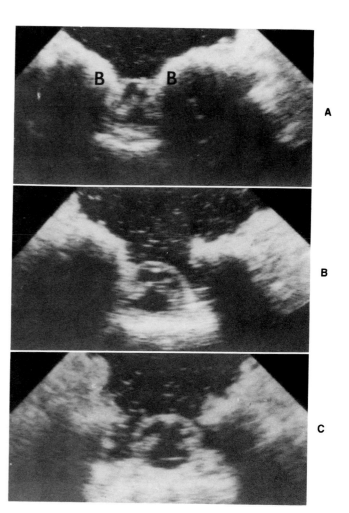

FIG 21-6. Occult residual herniated disk. Transverse images. **A,** After posterior and lateral bone decompression a soft-tissue mass *(M)* with well-defined edges is seen, which deforms the ventrolateral aspect of the thecal sac. This appearance is typical of a disk. **B,** Following diskectomy, residual disk material, which was surgically occult, is visible sonographically, and the thecal sac continues to be deformed. **C,** After the residual occult fragment was removed, no soft-tissue mass remains and the thecal sac is nearly normal in shape. The diskectomy is now judged to be complete.

FIG 21-7. Decompression of spinal canal stenosis. **A,** Transverse image shows inadequate lateral bone decompression following bilateral facetectomies. Residual bony masses *(B)* deform the thecal sac, which is triangular and narrowed. **B,** Extended right facetectomy. The right side of the thecal sac is rounded and there is space between the residual facet and the sac but bony compression persists on the left. **C,** Extended left facetectomy. The left side of the thecal sac is now rounded and there is a wide space between the sac and residual bone.

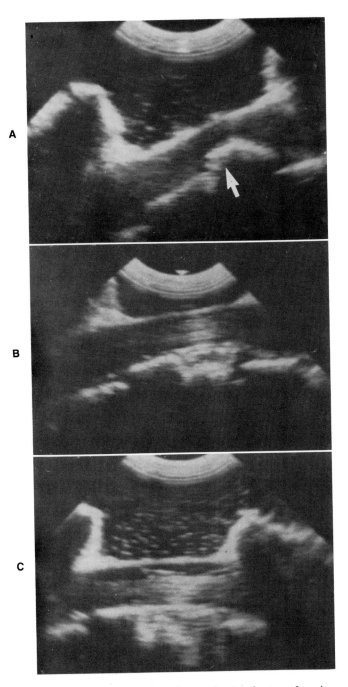

Fractures

Open reduction and stabilization with fusion and metallic rod instruments is the accepted management of patients with unstable thoracic and lumbar fractures because they experience less pain and are mobilized and rehabilitated earlier than when treated with postural reduction alone. The degree of neurologic improvement in patients with incomplete neurologic deficits and bone in the canal may be related to the adequacy of neural element decompression. The bone that compresses the neural elements is usually hidden from view by the spinal cord and thecal sac. "Blind" placement of metallic rods results in inadequate reduction and distraction in a high percentage of cases.[11,12] Mobilizing the spinal cord or thecal sac is risky. Sonography safely provides an accurate view of the ventral canal and evaluates the shape of the spinal canal, the presence of bone in the canal, and the degree of compression of spinal cord or cauda equina (Fig. 21-8). In addition, the extent of intramedullary injuries and the location of the conus medullaris may be assessed.[13-15]

Decompression was inadequate in about half of the 41 patients we studied sonographically who had metallic rod fixation.[15] In this setting, the surgeon may elect to reposition the rods, or to resect or reduce the bone fragment; repeat sonography can document the successful decompression. The use of sonography during metallic rod instrumentation for unstable thoracic and lumbar fractures improves the rate of adequate decompression to about 80%.

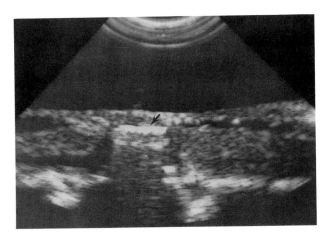

FIG 21-8. Decompression of upper lumbar fracture. Longitudinal images. **A,** Displaced bone fragment *(arrow)* protrudes into the canal, significantly compressing the cauda equina. **B,** Metallic rods were inserted and distracted, and neural compression reduced, but still present. **C,** The bone fragment was removed after posterolateral decompression; vertebral alignment is nearly normal and the cauda equina follows a normal course.

(From Montalvo BM, Quencer RM, Green BA, et al. Intraoperative sonography in spinal trauma. *Radiology.* 1984;153:125-134.)

FIG 21-9. Surgically occult bullet fragment in thoracic cord. Intrathecal bullet fragment *(arrow)* was not palpable because of abundant scar (between cord, bullet, and dura) but was easily identified with sonography by its typical very bright interface with reverberative shadowing. The spinal cord has lost its normal architecture and is uniformly hyperechoic with loss of the normal central echo. These findings are typical of myelomalacia.

(From Montalvo BM, Quencer RM, Green BA, et al. Intraoperative sonography in spinal trauma. *Radiology.* 1984;153:125-134.)

Fragments

Patients who have intracanalicular metallic or bony fragments as a result of recent gunshot wounds undergo surgery to remove these fragments to relieve pain or prevent its development and with the goal of partially reversing any incomplete neurologic deficit that may exist. Sonography has proved to be an effective and fast-localizing tool in these cases and is useful in the evaluation and management of associated lesions, such as intramedullary or subarachnoid cysts (Fig. 21-9).[16]

CYSTIC MYELOPATHY AND SUBARACHNOID CYSTS

Posttraumatic cystic myelopathy is a frequent complication of spinal trauma and it is currently best diagnosed with magnetic resonance imaging. The syndrome presents with pain, spasticity, hyperhidrosis, and ascending motor and sensory loss. The cord lesion is a round or oval cyst that may be lobulated and contain fibroglial scars. It is often associated with myelomalacia of the adjacent cord, cord compression by bone, adhesions that tether the cord, and subarachnoid cysts.[17,18]

Magnetic resonance imaging reliably diagnoses posttraumatic cysts, but sonography is superior to delayed computed tomography myelography in distinguishing intramedullary from subarachnoid cysts and from surrounding myelomalacia. Posttraumatic intramedullary cysts have the typical anechoic appearance of cysts on sonography, occur as small, normal-sized, or enlarged cords, and may be septated (Fig. 21-9). Subarachnoid cysts are seen as anechoic extramedullary collections that displace the cord and may have fibrous septations. Myelomalacia (injured cord) appears as an area of increased echogenicity of the cord that effaces the central echo of the cord (Fig. 21-9).

Surgical management of intramedullary cysts consists of shunting the cyst into the subarachnoid space and lysing the associated adhesions that tether the cord as well as removing other causes of extrinsic cord compression. Surgery prevents further cyst enlargement and frequently reverses recently developed symptoms. Sonography locates the cyst prior to the opening up of the dura; it helps the surgeon to choose the optimal place to enter the cyst with least damage to the intact spinal cord. Intracystic fibroglial scars that may compartmentalize the cyst into separate lobules are identified as thin septa and lysed by the surgeon (Fig. 21-10). Sonography is used after shunting to evaluate adequacy of cyst decompression. If collapse of the cyst is incomplete, the catheter may be repositioned, intracystic scars may be lysed, or a second catheter may be inserted, depending on the cause for the lack of decompression. Persistent cord tethering caused by ventral adhesions can also be seen and the adhesions lysed. Subarachnoid cysts can also be diagnosed and their shunting monitored with sonography (Fig. 21-11).[14-21]

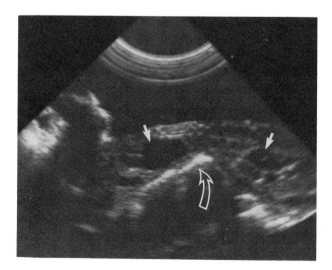

FIG 21-10. Posttraumatic cystic myelopathy. Longitudinal scan shows a large angulated bony fragment *(curved arrow)* that compresses the cord. Multiloculated intramedullary cysts *(arrows)* are observed cranial and caudal to the compression. The compressing bone was removed, and by sonographic guidance, a catheter was inserted to lyse the septations and collapse the cysts.

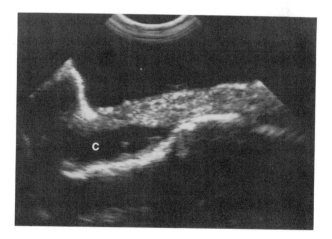

FIG 21-11. Subarachnoid cyst, bone fragment, and myelomalacia. Echogenic, myelomalacic cord is tethered and inseparable from the dorsal dura and is compressed by a posteriorly displaced bone fragment. A large subarachnoid cyst *(C)* displaces the cord cephalad to the site of bone compression. Small intracystic scars are evident as tiny echogenic foci.
(From Quencer RM, Montalvo BM, Green BA, et al. Intraoperative spinal sonography of soft tissue masses of the spinal cord and spinal canal. *AJNR.* 1984;5:507-515;1307-1315.)

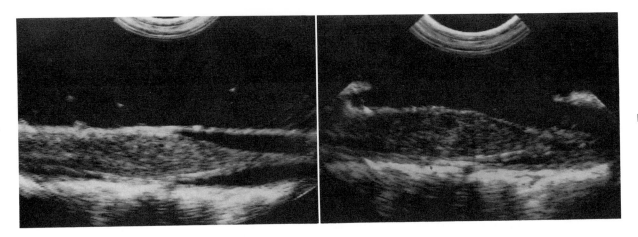

FIG 21-12. Biopsy of intramedullary tumor. Longitudinal scans. **A,** Intramedullary metastatic disease is seen as a slightly hyperechoic area that enlarges the conus medullaris and effaces the central echo. The exact site of the biopsy can be chosen prior to opening the dura. **B,** Following biopsy, a small cystic space confirms that the biopsy was performed in the area of abnormal cord. Notice that the posterior dura is now open.

TUMORS

The sonographic characteristics of intramedullary tumors are nonspecific.[7,22-25] Most tumors enlarge the cord, efface the central echo, and are either isoechoic or hyperechoic compared to normal cord tissue (Fig. 21-12). **Ependymomas, metastases** and **dermoids** are typically well-demarcated hyperechoic lesions. **Astro-**cytomas and ependymomas may also undergo cystic degeneration, which is seen as a cystic region within the tumor. Cord enlargement caused by syringomyelia can be easily differentiated from neoplasm in most cases.[26] Calcification is a nonspecific finding and may be seen with ependymoma, astrocytoma, and dermoid.

For purposes of biopsy, surgeons have traditionally chosen an area of gross cord enlargement; however, the cord may be enlarged secondary to syringohydromyelia, cord edema, or cystic degeneration and biopsies directed at these areas will be nondiagnostic (Fig. 21-13). Sonography determines the optimal site for biopsy by identifying the region of solid cord enlargement where the central echo is absent. Sonography is especially valuable to guide a biopsy of the solid component of a tumor that has associated cystic changes. With the use of sonography, fewer passes are needed for a diagnostic biopsy, unnecessary damage to the cord is avoided, and repeat surgery because of nondiagnostic biopsies is obviated.[23]

Extramedullary masses, such as **metastases, meningiomas, neurinomas, neurofibromas, lipomas,** and **dermoids,** are round or oval in shape, have well demarcated borders, are hyperechoic, and compress the cord or nerve roots in proportion to their size.[7,23] Sonography is valuable in planning surgical resection of these masses. It is used to localize the mass prior to opening the dura, define its craniocaudal and anteroposterior extent, which may not be appreciated visually, and to demonstrate its relationship to normal spinal cord or nerve roots. Sonography can also detect surgically occult residual tumor, which can then be excised, ensuring an optimal result (Fig. 21-14). When tumors are un-

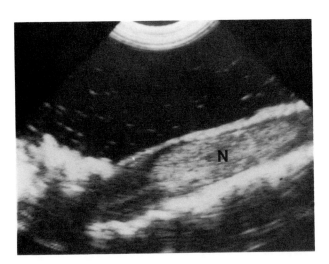

FIG 21-13. Diffuse thoracic cord enlargement with focal astrocytoma. Sonography clearly distinguishes the area of cord enlargement caused by neoplasm (*N,* oval echogenic area) from nonneoplastic enlargement seen superiorly. Note the present of the central echo in the region of the cord free of tumor and the absence of the central echo in the neoplastic region. Areas of cord enlargement do not necessarily represent tumor, as in this case in which a prior nondiagnostic biopsy was performed without the use of sonography.

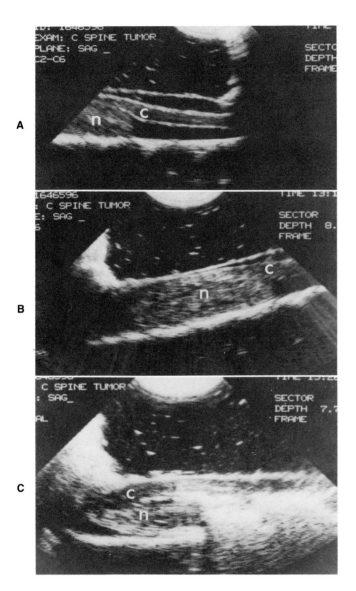

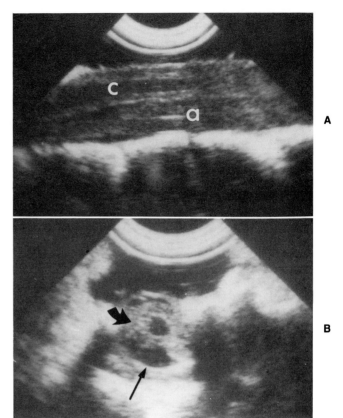

FIG 21-14. Partial resection of neurinoma ventral to cervical cord. Longitudinal scans. **A** and **B,** Prior to resection, sonography defines the ventral location and craniocaudal extent of the neurinoma. **C,** Scan after resection shows residual neurinoma *(N)* in the cranial aspect of the canal. The more caudal region of the canal is partially obscured by acoustic shadow from Gelfoam. Cervical cord *(C).*

(From Quencer RM, Montalvo BM, Naidich TP, et al. Intraoperative sonography in spinal dysraphism and syringohydromyelia. *AJNR.* 1987;8:329-337; 148:1005-1013.)

FIG 21-15. Ventral epidural abscess and meningitis. **A,** Longitudinal view at the level of the conus *(C)* shows an extensive hyperechoic abscess *(A)* elevating the ventral dura and posteriorly displacing the thecal sac, which contains the conus medullaris and cauda equina. **B,** Transverse scan after evacuation. The ventral dura *(straight arrow)* has returned to a normal position confirming adequate drainage. An abundance of diffuse hyperechoic material *(curved arrow)* surrounds the conus and distends the sac. This appearance is typical of meningitis.

resectable, sonography guides the debulking procedures in order to ensure optimal decompression of the spinal cord or cauda equina.

INFECTION

The use of intraoperative sonography is critical in the surgical management of epidural abscesses.[23,27]

Epidural abscesses appear as localized echogenic masses compressing the dural sac. With ultrasound, extradural location, extent in the spinal canal, and their relationship to the spinal cord are clear. Sonography is particularly valuable in the localization of ventral abscesses that are difficult to visualize surgically (Fig. 21-15). Associated meningitis can be distinguished from abscess, and appears as diffuse echogenic material that distends the subarachnoid space and replaces the normal anechoic cerebrospinal fluid (Fig. 21-15). Sonography helps the surgeon to plan the evacuation of epidural abscesses, monitors this process in order to ensure optimal decompression, and prevents unnecessary manipulation of the spinal cord.[27]

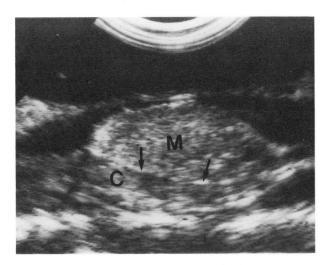

FIG 21-16. Lipoma from conus medullaris. Sonogram prior to opening the dura shows a well-defined, oval, hyperechoic mass *(M)* posterior to the conus *(C)* in a subpial location. The preoperative imaging studies suggested that the mass was within the conus rather than adjacent to it. Note the well-defined interface *(arrows)* between the mass and conus medullaris.

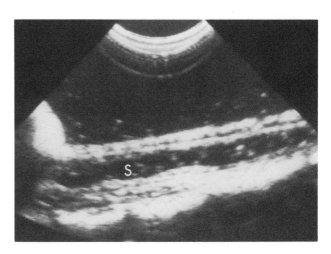

FIG 21-17. Syrinx. Longitudinal image of the cervical cord through an intact dura mater. A long, mostly anechoic cystic space *(s)* is seen within the cord. Note the small echogenic foci, which are most likely scar and are commonly seen in these congenital lesions.

CONGENITAL LESIONS

Spinal dysraphism represents a failure of normal midline fusion and may be associated with multiple lesions, including **congenital tumors, diastematomyelia, syringohydromyelia, meningocele, myelomeningocele,** and **tethered cord.** Each of these anomalies may occur in isolation or in combination with other dysraphic states. Surgery in these cases is performed primarily to free the spinal cord from tethering and to effectively decompress neural tissue. Sonography has proven to be useful in many of these conditions.

As with acquired spinal masses, sonography of congenital tumors defines their extent and their relationship to normal neural tissue. **Lipomas** appear as highly echogenic masses that may be found in the filum terminale (Fig. 21-16). The location and extent of tumor may alter the surgical approach. If sonography demonstrates that the cord is surrounded by tumor and the patient is neurologically normal, the surgeon may take a less aggressive approach and may not completely resect the tumor, particularly if it would require extensive cord retraction.

In **diastematomyelia** sonography can display the cleft of the cord, the site and length of associated bone spurs or fibrous septa, and the nature of any adhesions present, as well as any associated tumors and/or hydromyelic cavities.

Syringohydromyelic cavities are easily detected sonographically and usually managed by shunting to the subarachnoid space or, if small, by fenestration of the cavity (Fig. 21-17). The distal end of the syrinx cavity is identified so that a shunt can be passed into the cavity through the lowest possible portion of the spinal cord, minimizing the risk of neurologic deficit. Any septa that may compartmentalize the syrinx into separate lobules can also be identified with sonography. Successful decompression of the syrinx by a shunt or fenestration can be documented prior to finalizing surgery.[28]

REFERENCES
Indications

1. Dohrmann GJ, Rubin JM. Intraoperative ultrasound imaging of the spinal cord: syringomyelia, cysts and tumors—a preliminary report. *Surg Neurol* 1982;18(6):395-399.

Sonographic anatomy

2. Quencer RM, Montalvo BM. Normal intraoperative spinal sonography. *AJNR* 1984;5:501-505, *AJR* 1984;143:1301-1305.
3. Montalvo BM, Quencer RM. Intraoperative sonography. In: Schnitzlein HN, Murtagh FR, eds. *Imaging Anatomy of the Head and Spine.* 2nd ed. Baltimore, Urban and Schwarzenberg Inc; 1990:443-451.
4. Skaggs PH, Montalvo BM. Sonographic anatomic correlation in the spine. *Radiology* 1984;153(P):326.
5. Montalvo BM, Skaggs PH. The central canal of the spinal cord: ultrasonic identification. *Radiology* 1985;155:535.
6. Nelson MD Jr, Sedler JA, Gilles FH. Spinal cord central echo complex: histoanatomic correlation. *Radiology* 1989;170:479-481.

Cord compression

7. Montalvo BM, Quencer RM. Intraoperative sonography in spinal surgery: current state of the art. *Neuroradiology* 1986;28:551-590.

8. Montalvo BM. The role of intraoperative ultrasonography in the management of spinal lesions. In: Rifkin MD, ed. *Clinics in Diagnostic Ultrasound 22: Intraoperative and Endoscopic Ultrasonography.* New York, Churchill Livingstone Inc; 1987:33-63.

9. Montalvo BM, Quencer RM, Brown MD, et al. Lumbar disk herniation and canal stenosis: value of intraoperative sonography in diagnosis and surgical management. *AJNR* 1990;11:31-40; *AJR* 1990;154:821-830.

10. Burton CV, Kirkaldy-Willis WH, Yong-Hing K. Causes of failure of surgery on the lumbar spine. *Clin Orthop* 1981;157:191-199.

11. Flesch JR, Leider LL, Erickson DL, et al. Harrington instrumentation and spinal fusion for unstable fractures and fracture/dislocations of the thoracic and lumbar spine. *J Bone Joint Surg* 1977;59:143-153.

12. Yosipovitch Z, Robin GC, Makin M. Open reduction of unstable thoracolumbar spinal injuries and fixation with Harrington rods. *J Bone Joint Surg* 1977;59:1003-1015.

13. Montalvo BM, Quencer RM, Green BA, et al. Intraoperative sonography in spinal trauma. *Radiology* 1984;153:125-134.

14. Eismont FJ, Green BA, Berkowitz BM, et al. The role of intraoperative ultrasonography in the treatment of thoracic and lumbar spine fractures. *Spine* 1984;9(8):782-787.

15. Quencer RM, Montalvo BM, Eismont FJ, et al. Intraoperative spinal sonography in thoracic and lumbar fractures: evaluation of Harrington rod instrumentation. *AJNR* 1985;6:353-359; *AJR* 1985;145:343-349.

16. Montalvo BM, Quencer RM, Green BA, et al. Intraoperative spinal sonography in gunshot wounds to the spine. *Radiology* 1984;153(P):260.

Cystic myelopathy and subarachnoid cysts

17. Osborne DRS, Vavoulis G, Nashold BS, et al. Late sequelae of spinal cord trauma. *J Neurosurg* 1982;57:18-23.

18. Quencer RM, Green Ba, Eismont FJ. Posttraumatic spinal cord cysts: clinical features and characterization with metrizamide computed tomography. *Radiology* 1983;146:415-423.

19. Quencer RM, Morse BMM, Green BA. Intraoperative spinal sonography: adjunct to metrizamide computed tomography in the assessment and surgical decompression of posttraumatic spinal cord cysts. *AJNR* 1984;5:71-79; *AJR* 1984;142:593-601.

20. Sklar E, Quencer RM, Green Ba, et al. Acquired spinal subarachnoid cysts: evaluation with magnetic resonance and computed tomography myelography and intraoperative sonography. *AJNR* 1989;10:1097-1104; 153:1057-1064.

21. Gebarski SS, Maynard FW, Gabrielsen TO, et al. Posttraumatic progressive myelopathy. *Radiology* 1985;157:379-385.

Tumors

22. Knake JE, Chandler WF, McGillicuddy JE, et al. Intraoperative spinal sonography of intraspinal tumors: initial experience. *AJNR* 1983;4:1199-1201.

23. Quencer RM, Montalvo BM, Green BA, et al. Intraoperative spinal sonography of soft-tissue masses of the spinal cord and spinal canal. *AJNR* 1984;5:507-515; *AJNR* 1984;143:1307-1315.

24. Platt JF, Rubin JM, Chandler WF, et al. Intraoperative spinal sonography in the evaluation of intramedullary tumors. *J Ultrasound Med* 1988;7:317-325.

25. Post MJD, Quencer RM, Green BA, et al. Intramedullary spinal cord metastases, mainly of nonneurogenic origin. *AJNR* 1987;8:339-346; 1987; *AJR* 1987;148:1015-1022.

26. Hutchins WW, Volgelzang RL, Neiman HL, et al. Differentiation of tumor from syringohydromyelia: intraoperative neurosonography of the spinal cord. *Radiology* 1984;151:171-174.

Infection

27. Post MJD, Quencer RM, Montalvo BM, et al. Spinal infection: evaluation with magnetic resonance imaging and intraoperative ultrasound. *Radiology* 1988;169:765-771.

Congenital lesions

28. Quencer RM, Montalvo BM, Naidich TP, et al. Intraoperative sonography in spinal dysraphism and syringohydromyelia. *AJNR* 1987;8:329-337; *AJR* 1987;148:1005-1013.

CHAPTER 22

Intraoperative Sonography of the Abdomen

- Laurence A. Mack, M.D.
- Robert A. Lee, M.D.
- David A. Nyberg, M.D.

Ultrasound was first used in the operating room for the evaluation of the biliary tree. In the 1960s, investigators reported successful localization of biliary calculi using A-mode probes.[1,2] Because of the difficulty in interpreting these images, the technique did not receive wide acceptance. Improvements in real-time equipment were followed by more widespread use of intraoperative ultrasonography.[3-6] More recently, the development of small, high-resolution transducers has resulted in broad application of this technique.[7] Intraoperative scanning of the liver, pancreas, kidneys, and other viscera have been reported.

GENERAL TECHNIQUES

Commercially available sector transducers that are used for general abdominal scanning can also be used for intraoperative imaging. The large far field of view makes it easier to show the relation of an abnormality to adjacent structures. This is a significant advantage, especially for the inexperienced user. However, these transducers are limited in their near field of view and resolution. Because the transducer is placed directly on the organ to be evaluated, these shortcomings are accentuated during intraoperative ultrasonography. In addition, the relatively large size of conventional sector transducers limits access to the recesses of the peritoneal cavity.

Recently, small linear array transducers designed specifically for intraoperative use have become available.[7] These transducers address many of the problems of sector transducers. They are of higher frequency (typically 7 MHz), which improves resolution. They have a wider near field of view and excellent near-field resolution, which is enhanced by electronic focusing. However, the far field of view and penetration is limited, which makes orientation difficult at times. Many of these transducers are quite small, which permits easy placement into the recesses of the peritoneal cavity.

Sterilization of the transducer may be accomplished in several ways. Gas sterilization allows the transducers to be placed directly into the abdomen without a sterile cover.[8,9] Sterilization by this technique requires 12 to 36 hours, which limits the availability of the transducers. In addition, if the transducer is contaminated, the procedure cannot be continued. A better alternative is the covering of the transducer with a sterile plastic or latex sleeve, which allows for multiple transducer uses each day. A number of commercially available covers are available. Dedicated latex covers that fit specific transducers combined with sterile sleeves have proved most convenient in our experience.

Some "tricks" may be helpful in performing the study. As in the routine sonographic examination, the sonologist should approach the patient from the right side facing the patient's head. Attempts to scan from the left side of the patient may lead to confusion as a reuslt of unfamiliar orientation. Liberal use of warmed saline irrigation solution is helpful in maintaining good transducer-tissue contact. Operative ultrasonography should be regarded as a complementary imaging technique, providing continuity between preoperative diagnosis and operative findings. Therefore all preoperative imaging studies should be reviewed before scanning in the operative room. With this information in mind, operative ultrasound is used to further evaluate previously identified abnormalities and to search for occult lesions.

Successful intraoperative ultrasound examinations are best performed by an experienced sonologist to avoid a lengthy procedure and inconsistent results. One of the major limitations of intraoperative ultrasound is the time it takes, keeping the sonologist away from the radiography department. However, because intraoperative ultrasound often adds significant new information, the time invested usually improves patient care.

BILD DUCTS AND GALLBLADDER
Anatomy

The portal vein and its branches serve as constant anatomic landmarks in intraoperative ultrasound evaluation of the hepatobiliary system. It is important to visualize the extrahepatic biliary ducts in both the transverse and longitudinal planes. By using orthogonal planes, the possibility of confusing bowel gas for calculi is minimized.[10] As the common bile duct is scanned caudally, it courses posteriorly in the head of the pancreas and may be visualized either by scanning through the pancreas or through a compressed, airless duodenum.

The gallbladder can easily be evaluated by intraoperative ultrasound. As in the case of transabdominal sonography, strict adherence to criteria for the diagnosis of calculi is important. Therefore it is important to confirm both acoustic shadowing and stone mobility. The latter is achieved by simply moving the gallbladder and watching small calculi move.

Applications

Sigel et al defined four major uses for intraoperative evaluation of the biliary system:[11]

- Identification of the biliary calculi
- Evaluation of biliary neoplasms
- Evaluation of the gallbladder and its contents
- Localization of the common bile duct and definition of its relation to other structures

Intraoperative ultrasound scanning has been useful to identify biliary calculi.[4,6] Sigel and his colleagues have shown it to be a viable alternative to intraoperative cholangiography (Fig. 22-1). As in transabdominal sonography, the criteria for calculi are echogenic foci, which cast an acoustic shadow. In experienced hands, the sensitivity, specificity, and overall accuracy of operative sonography is equal to or exceeds that of intraoperative cholangiography (Table 22-1). Moreover, the positive predictive value of an intraoperative ultrasound examination is greater (91.8% versus 73.2%) than operative cholangiography.

Intraoperative biliary sonography requires less time than operative cholangiography and can often be completed in less than 10 minutes. This decrease in operative time is even more significant if the cholangiogram requires repeating. Gas bubbles, thick bile, and spasm

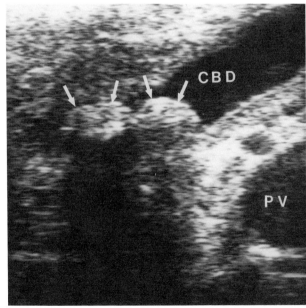

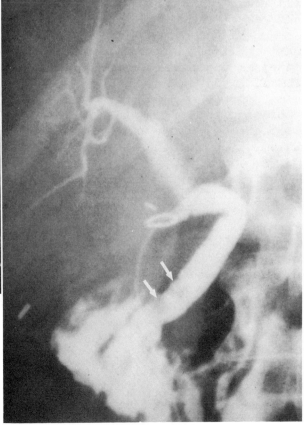

FIG 22-1. Choledocholithiasis. **A,** Intraoperative scan shows mildly dilated common bile duct (CBD). Two calculi *(arrows)* are seen in distal duct. *PV* indicates portal vein. **B,** Operative cholangiogram shows two calculi *(arrows).*
(**A,** From Rifkin MD, Mack LA, Lennard ES et al.: *J Ultrasound* 1986;5:429-433.

■ **TABLE 22-1**

Statistical Comparison of Intraoperative Ultrasonography and Operative Cholangiography to Identify Biliary Tract Calculi

	Intraoperative Ultrasonography	Operative Cholangiography
Sensitivity	93.8	90.0
Specificity	98.6	95.4
Accuracy	98.0	94.8
Positive predictive value	91.8	73.2
Negative predictive value	99.0	98.7

(From Sigel B, Machi J, Beitler JG, et al: *Surgery* 1983;94:715-720.)

of the sphincter of Oddi, all of which can be mistaken for calculi during contrast-enhanced cholangiography, are not a problem during ultrasound imaging. Gas bubbles are not present because the examination is performed before cholecystectomy. Viscous bile does not cast an acoustic shadow and is rarely a diagnostic problem with sonography. The sphincter of Oddi is seen as normal soft tissue around the distal comon bile duct.

Primary tumors of the biliary system may appear as intraluminal papillary-like masses or as a markedly thickened ductal wall. Using intraoperative ultrasound scanning, the level of the neoplasm, its extent, and the location of the normal structures that are to be preserved can be determined. Extension of tumor into adjacent lymph nodes can also be identified.

The gallbladder is usually imaged preoperatively if there is a question of a hepatobiliary pathologic condition. However, for patients undergoing an emergency laparotomy and inpatients in whom a palpable abnormality of the gallbladder is incidentally noted at surgery, intraoperative sonography provides unique diagnostic information (Fig. 22-2).[12] A recent report by Herbst et al suggests that intraoperative sonography also has a role in the evaluation of the gallbladder in patients undergoing bariatric surgery for morbid obesity.[13] In this group of patients, for whom imaging is often poor using the transabdominal route, the authors reported success in intraoperative imaging of the gallbladder in 51 patients with a low false-positive result rate (1.8%) and no false-negative examination findings.

Surgical localization and identification of the common bile duct is rarely a problem.[11] However, the presence of neoplasm or inflammatory changes often makes this task more difficult, and intraoperative sonography may be helpful in identifying the common bile duct and in differentiating it from other structures in the portal region. It can also aid in identifying variations in he-

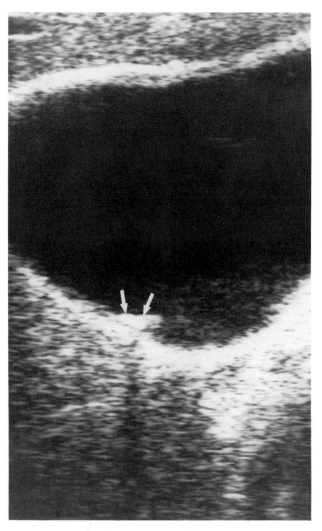

FIG 22-2. Cholelithiasis. Intraoperative scan in patient with palpable abnormality of gallbladder shows small calculus *(arrows)* with distal acoustic shadow. Note small amount of sludge in this fasting patient.
(From Mack LA, Nyberg DA: In: Rifkin MD, ed. *Intraoperative and Endoscopic Ultrasonography*. New York: Churchill Livingstone; 1987.)

patic artery anatomy, which occur in up to 26% of all patients (Fig. 22-3). Intraoperative sonography is helpful in defining these anomalies and thus avoiding damage to the hepatic artery, which may result in hepatic necrosis.

LIVER
Applications

Intraoperative ultrasound of the liver has found its greatest use in patients undergoing surgery for primary or metastatic neoplasms. Three main indications have been identified:

- Intraoperative diagnosis of hepatic masses
- Surgical planning for resection
- Direct subsegmental hepatectomy

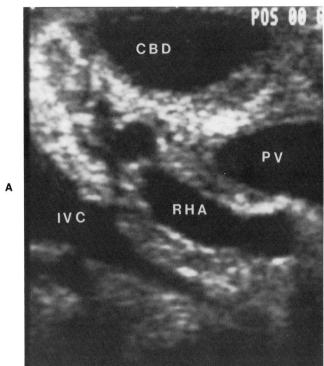

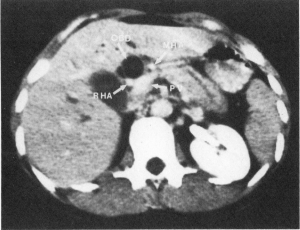

FIG 22-3. Replaced right hepatic artery. **A,** Intraoperative sonogram and, **B,** contrast-enhanced CT through gastrohepatic ligament show replaced right hepatic artery *(RHA)* in characteristic position to right of portal vein *(PV)* and just posterior to dilated common bile duct *(CBD)*. *IVC* indicates inferior vena cava; *MHA,* main hepatic artery.

Preoperative computed tomography (CT) is the technique most widely used to determine the extent of involvement by primary or secondary hepatic tumors. However, several reports have demonstrated that intraoperative sonography is helpful in detecting and diagnosing small lesions that are not visualized by CT. Machi et al found previously unidentified metastases, all of which are nonpalpable, in 12% of patients.[14] Parker et al reported that intraoperative sonography had a far higher sensitivity in detecting malignant hepatic nodules (98%) than did preoperative CT (77%) (Fig. 22-4).[15] Recent advances in CT include injection of contrast directly into the hepatic artery or superior mesenteric artery to provide arterial or portal venous enhancement, respectively. Although these procedures have achieved a high degree of accuracy in identifying focal lesions, false-positive results may result. In our experience, small cysts—many too small to be visualized by transabdominal ultrasound—may cause CT defects indistinguishable from metastases. Intraoperative sonography can readily differentiate small cysts from metastasis (Fig. 22-5).

Even if preoperative studies have confirmed the presence of focal hepatic lesions, the surgeon may not be able to locate the mass. Sheu et al reported that 49% of hepatocellular carcinomas of less than 3 cm in diameter were not palpable or visible.[16] Similar results have been reported by Jin-Chuan et al with 46% of hepatocellular carcinomas not identified by palpation or visual inspec-

tion.[17] In these patients, operative sonography is very important to localize these masses and to plan resection.

Intraoperative ultrasound is also used to influence surgical planning by providing unique information about the relation of known masses to important anatomic structures (Figs. 22-6 and 22-7). Bismuth et al obtained additional information from intraoperative sonography in 33% of patients, which modified the intended procedure in 27%.[18] Information was obtained that demonstrated that the lesion was inoperable in 9%, required a more extensive resection than planned in 3% (Fig. 22-8), and a more abbreviated procedure in 15%. Parker et al found that resection was not possible in 18% of patients based on the findings of intraoperative sonography.[15] Similarly, Rifkin et al reported that, in 19% of patients undergoing hepatic resection, new information that changed the surgical approach was provided by ultrasound.[19] In an additional 14% of cases, new information was provided by ultrasound, but this information did not change the planned operation. Gunven et al reported that, in 31% of patients, intraoperative ultrasound provided unique information which could change the therapeutic approach.[20] Thus intraoperative ultrasound plays an important role in surgical planning.

Ultrasound is also important in directing subsegmental resections of primary hepatocellular carcinoma in patients with compromised liver function.[21,22] In this elegant technique, ultrasound is used to identify portal

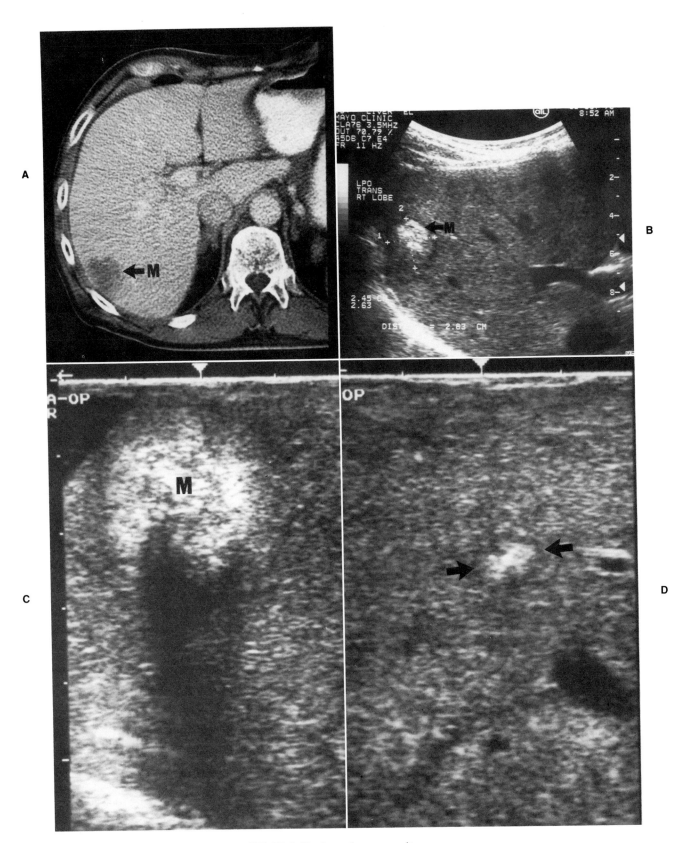

FIG 22-4. For legend see opposite page.

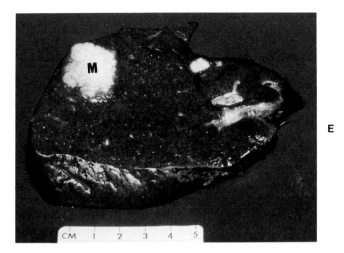

FIG 22-4. Hepatic metastases from adenocarcinoma of colon. **A,** Contrast-enhanced CT scan shows solitary metastasis *(M).* **B,** Transverse preoperative sonogram shows solitary hyperechoic hepatic mass *(M).* **C** and **D,** Intraoperative sonograms show mass previously identified *(M).* Additional small metastasis *(arrows)* was identified. Microcalcification within larger mass is causing acoustic shadowing. **E,** Photograph of gross specimen shows both metastases *(M* and *arrow).*

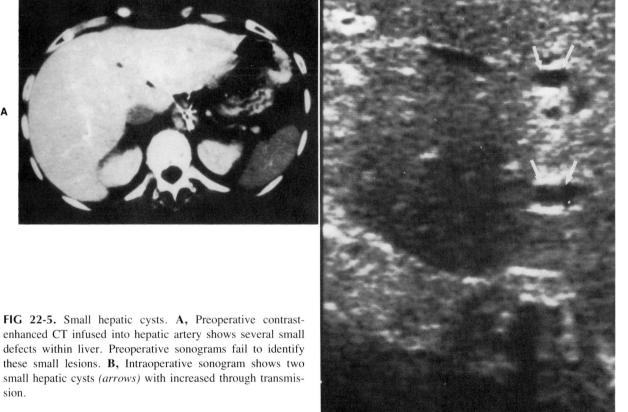

FIG 22-5. Small hepatic cysts. **A,** Preoperative contrast-enhanced CT infused into hepatic artery shows several small defects within liver. Preoperative sonograms fail to identify these small lesions. **B,** Intraoperative sonogram shows two small hepatic cysts *(arrows)* with increased through transmission.

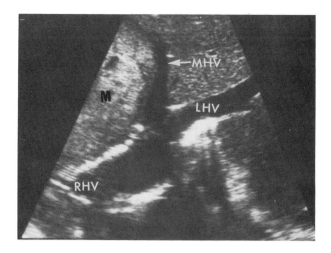

FIG 22-6. Relationship of metastasis to hepatic veins. Transverse intraoperative sonogram in patient with metastases from adenocarcinoma of colon shows relation of hyperechoic metastasis *(M)* to middle hepatic vein *(MHV)*. *LHV* indicates left hepatic vein; *RHV*, origin of right hepatic vein.

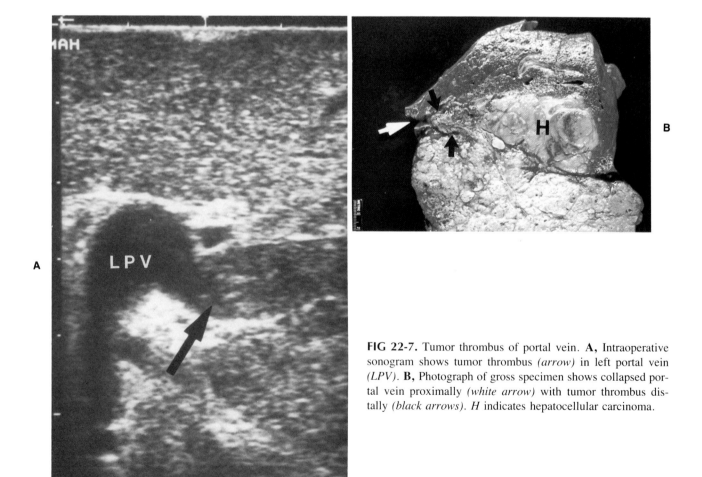

FIG 22-7. Tumor thrombus of portal vein. **A,** Intraoperative sonogram shows tumor thrombus *(arrow)* in left portal vein *(LPV)*. **B,** Photograph of gross specimen shows collapsed portal vein proximally *(white arrow)* with tumor thrombus distally *(black arrows)*. *H* indicates hepatocellular carcinoma.

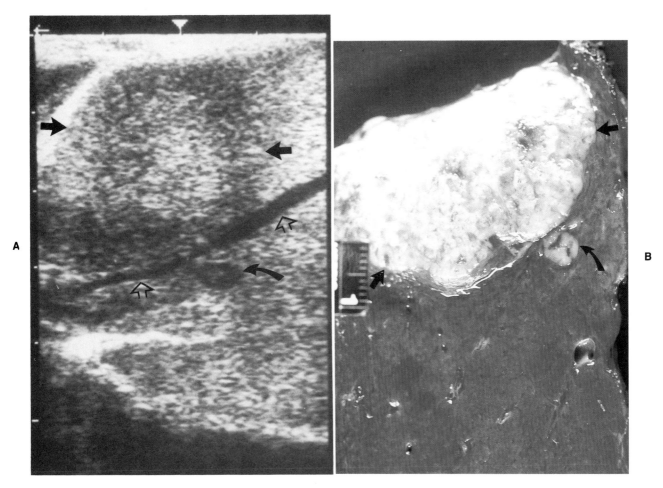

FIG 22-8. Extent of hepatic metastasis provided by operative sonography. **A,** Oblique longitudinal intraoperative scan in patient with metastatic adenocarcinoma of colon shows large metastasis *(black arrows)* adjacent to left hepatic vein *(open arrows).* This mass was identified on preoperative imaging. Second satellite metastasis *(curved arrow)* is identified posterior to hepatic vein. Because of tumor spread beyond left hepatic vein, more extensive hepatic resection was required. **B,** Photograph of gross specimen demonstrating both metastases. *Straight arrow* indicates large metastases; *curved arrow,* satellite metastases.

venous supply to the small areas of the liver containing neoplasm. Colored dye is then injected into the portal branch of the portal vein, identifying ("tattooing") the area to be resected. With this technique, there can be considerable sparing of hepatic parenchyma in patients with already compromised liver function, and the procedure can be accomplished with significantly less blood loss than with conventional resection techniques.

PANCREAS
Carcinoma

Intraoperative sonography is not a replacement of preoperative detection of pancreatic carcinoma. However, in those patients who are thought to have a potentially resectable tumor following preoperative evaluation, intraoperative ultrasonography may be helpful in

three ways:
- Locating a nonpalpable neoplasm
- Staging the neoplasm
- Defining the relation of a mass to adjacent structures

The appearance of a normal pancreatic homogeneous echogenicity can also help to remove suspicion that a carcinoma may be present (Fig. 22-9).[23]

Although most adenocarcinomas are large enough to be easily palpated at the time of surgery, a minority of cases may present at an earlier stage. Ampullary carcinomas may produce biliary obstruction, even when they are small and nonpalpable. In this setting, intraoperative sonography can be helpful in localizing the primary tumor.[24] The echotexture of pancreatic ductal carcinomas is variable when compared with the surrounding

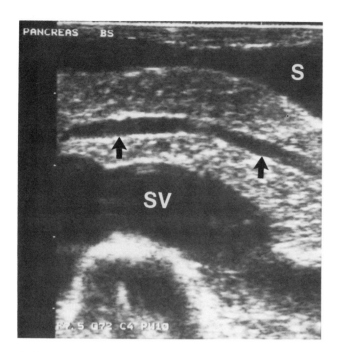

FIG 22-9. Normal pancreatic duct. Transverse intraoperative sonogram of pancreatic body demonstrates pancreatic duct *(black arrows)* and splenic vein *(SV)* with saline *(S)* in peritoneal cavity. Note homogeneous echo architecture of pancreatic body.

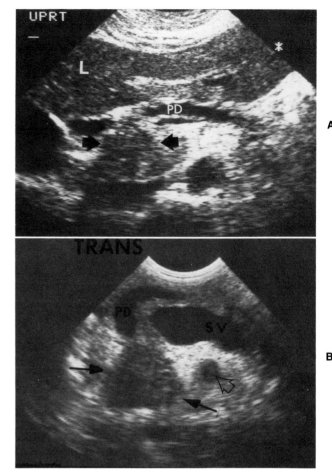

FIG 22-10. Adenocarcinoma of pancreas. **A,** Preoperative transverse sonogram shows hypoechoic mass *(arrows)* in head of pancreas. Pancreatic duct *(PD)* is dilated. *L* indicates left lobe of liver. **B,** Intraoperative sonogram more clearly shows relation of pancreatic mass *(black arrows)* to dilated pancreatic duct *(PD)*. *SV* indicates splenic vein; *open arrow,* superior mesenteric artery.

pancreas. Sigel et al reported that, of 27 adenocarcinomas, only 3 were hypoechoic, whereas 14 were hyperechoic and 10 were nearly isoechoic (Fig. 22-10).[23] If intraoperative needle biopsy is indicated, sonography permits direct guidance of the needle tip into the suspected tumor site, avoiding adjacent vessels and ducts.

In addition to aiding in localizing a pancreatic carcinoma, intraoperative sonography can help define the extent of involvement. Extrapancreatic findings that indicate an advanced and nonresectable tumor may be identified. Venous invasion and liver metastases are important findings that indicate an advance-stage pancreatic carcinoma that precludes surgical resection (Fig. 22-11).[25] Metastases from pancreatic adenocarcinoma are usually hypoechoic.

Pancreatitis

Intraoperative ultrasound scanning of the pancreas is frequently helpful in evaluating complications of pancreatitis. Complications of acute pancreatitis include pseudocysts, abscesses, and vascular thrombosis; complications of recurrent (chronic) pancreatitis may include pancreatic duct dilation, pancreatic insufficiency, and pseudoaneurysms.

Pancreatic and peripancreatic fluid collections may be extremely difficult to localize by direct visualization and palpation during surgery, even when they have been previously delineated by preoperative imaging studies. Surgical evaluation is particularly difficult when the pancreas is inflamed or distorted by pancreatitis. In this situation, intraoperative sonography can rapidly aid in localizing pseudocysts and in ensuring their complete drainage (Fig. 22-12). Multiple pseudocysts can be identified, and small pseudocysts can be distinguished from a dilated pancreatic duct. Intraoperative ultrasound images can demonstrate continuity of pseudocysts with adjacent structures, such as the bowel and stomach, so that determination of the best approach for drainage may be made.

Complications of chronic pancreatitis can be identified on intraoperative ultrasound scans. Typical findings

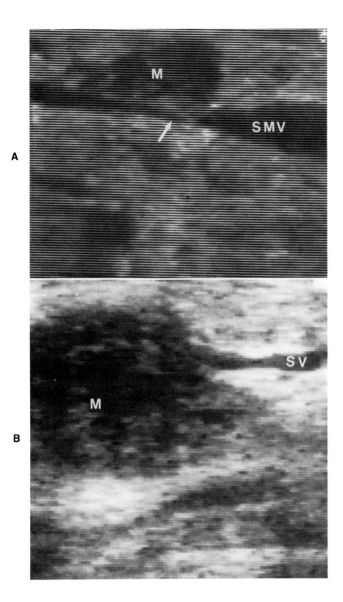

FIG 22-11. Adenocarcinoma of pancreas. **A,** Longitudinal intraoperative scan shows pancreatic mass *(M)* invading *(arrow)* superior mesenteric vein *(SMV)*. **B,** Transverse scan shows tumor mass *(M)* occluding splenic vein *(SV)*.
(From Nyberg DA, Mack LA:In: Rifkin MD, ed. *Intraoperative and Endoscopic Ultrasonography.* New York: Churchill Livingstone; 1987.)

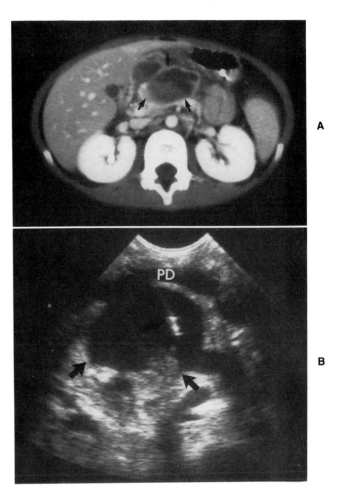

FIG 22-12. Drainage of pseudocyst. **A,** Preoperative contrast-enhanced CT shows pseudocyst *(arrows)* with dependent debris. **B,** Intraoperative sonogram shows pseudocyst *(arrows)* communicating with pancreatic duct *(PD)*. Under ultrasound guidance, needle was placed *(curved arrow)* into pancreatic pseudocyst.

of chronic pancreatitis include a diffusely hyperechoic pancreas, often associated with multiple calculi. The pancreatic duct may be dilated and irregular in contour (Fig. 22-13). Detection of a dilated pancreatic duct is an important finding in patients with chronic pancreatitis who have chronic abdominal pain because a diverting procedure may be performed in these patients. Intraoperative sonography can readily aid in the localization of a dilated pancreatic duct for intraoperative pancreatography and decompression.

Vascular complications of pancreatitis may also be identified on intraoperative ultrasound scans. Splenic or portal venous thrombosis, which may occur in patients with chronic pancreatitis, can be readily detected on these scans. The finding of an intraluminal clot may be indistinguishable from tumor invasion in patients with adenocarcinoma. Occasionally, pseudoaneurysms can also be identified on scans in patients with chronic pancreatitis. This finding is important to recognize, because it is potentially life-threatening.

Islet Cell Neoplasm

Insulinoma. Localization of insulinoma represents a difficult clinical problem. Preoperative imaging for the detection of insulinoma has had limited success. An-

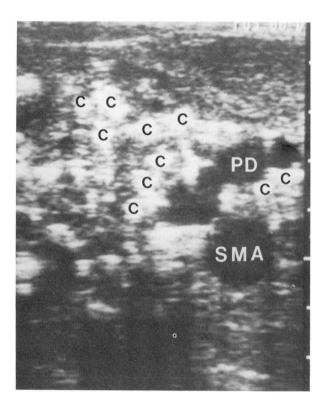

FIG 22-13. Chronic calcific pancreatitis. Transverse intraoperative sonogram shows multiple pancreatic calcifications *(C)*. Pancreatic duct *(PD)* is dilated. *SMA* indicates superior mesenteric artery.

(From Nyberg DA, Mack LA: In: Rifkin MD, ed. *Intraoperative and Endoscopic Ultrasonography*. New York: Churchill Livingstone; 1987.)

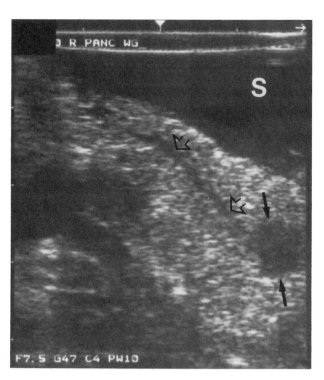

FIG 22-14. Solitary pancreatic insulinoma. Transverse intraoperative sonogram shows 0.8-cm hypoechoic mass *(black arrows)* in pancreatic tail adjacent to pancreatic duct *(open arrows)*. *S* indicates saline.

giography detects these hypervascular lesions with variable success. Sensitivities of 29% to 90% have been reported, with false-positive results noted in up to 57% of cases. Although an experienced surgeon may detect the majority of lesions, 10% to 20% of surgeries are unsuccessful in removing the insulinoma.[26] In one study, CT detected 30% of the insulinomas and preoperative ultrasound identified 61% of the lesions.[27] Therefore intraoperative localization of insulinomas by ultrasound is a crucial step in patient management—the responsibility of which is shared by the radiologist and the surgeon.

Approximately 90% of insulinomas are small, well-defined, round or oval masses that have a fine, hypoechoic echogenicity compared to the normal coarse, hyperechoic echogenicity of normal pancreatic parenchyma (Fig. 22-14). This hypoechoic echotexture is probably due to their homogeneous, smooth internal architecture. Insulinomas as small as 0.3 cm are detectable if they are surrounded by normally echogenic pancreatic parenchyma. Although both benign adenomas and small pancreatic adenocarcinomas may appear hypoechoic, the margins of benign adenomas are well de-

fined because of the presence of a capsule, whereas pancreatic adenocarcinoma has an ill-defined or invisible margin because of infiltration of tissue planes.

Approximately 10% of insulinomas are isoechoic or hyperechoic relative to adjacent pancreatic parenchyma and therefore are poorly visible by ultrasound. This is more common in patients under (approximately) the age of 30 years, possibly because the pancreas is less echogenic in younger patients and the adenomas blend with the normal pancreas. In this setting other findings, including a peripheral halo or a refractive shadow deep to the mass, may be helpful.

Approximately 90% of patients with insulinoma have a solitary adenoma. In a Mayo Clinic review of 22 patients, approximately 85% of solitary insulinomas were visible by using high-frequency intraoperative ultrasonography that was performed by the radiologist without knowledge of the findings by the surgeon (sensitivity 84%).[28] No false-positive results were reported in this series (positive predictive value of 100%). Of the three solitary insulinomas not initially visualized sonographically, two were visible in retrospect after the surgeon identified the location of a palpable abnormality.

Of the 22 solitary insulinomas, 4 (18%) were neither

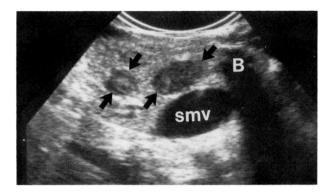

FIG 22-15. Multiple pancreatic insulinomas. Transverse scan in patient with multiple endocrine neoplasia syndrome, type I, shows two hypoechoic insulinomas *(arrows)* within pancreatic head *smv* indicates superior mesenteric vein; *B,* bowel.

palpable nor grossly visible to the surgeon.[28] These tumors were 1.7, 1.5, 1.0, and 0.6 cm in greatest diameter and were located in the head of the pancreas. Two of these patients had persistent hyperinsulinism after failed initial operations. All four of these nonpalpable tumors were visualized ultrasonographically. In addition to detecting occult, nonpalpable insulinomas, intraoperative ultrasound also defines the precise relation of the insulinoma to normal structures that are to be preserved, such as pancreatic ducts, bile ducts, and blood vessels.

Approximately 10% of patients with insulinoma have more than one adenoma, which usually occurs in the multiple endocrine neoplasia (MEN) I syndrome. Patients with this syndrome often have many tiny adenomas that are smaller than 1 cm. In four of these patients with a total of 33 insulinomas, 12 (36%) of these insulinomas were visible sonographically (Fig. 22-15). Five of these twelve masses were nonpalpable. These nonpalpable tumors were 0.3 to 0.7 cm in diameter and were imbedded within the echogenic pancreatic parenchyma. Many small surface masses were missed sonographically, perhaps because they were partially surrounded by the sonolucent fluid path. Fortunately, these surface masses were detectable by palpation or visual inspection.[28]

Gastrinoma

The second most common functioning islet-cell tumor secretes the hormone gastrin, which results in Zollinger-Ellison syndrome. Unlike insulinomas, gastrinomas are likely to be malignant (60% to 90%), are frequently multiple (20% to 40%), and are often located in extrapancreatic tissues, especially the descending duodenum (20% to 40%).[29] Also, unlike patients with insulinoma, many can be safely managed with medical ther-

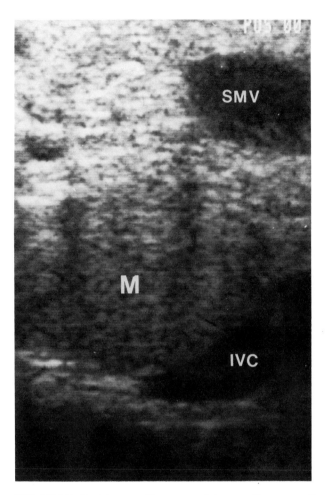

FIG 22-16. Gastrinoma. Transverse intraoperative scan of head of pancreas in patient with Zollinger-Ellison syndrome shows gastrinoma as hypoechoic mass *(M)* in posterior aspect of head of pancreas. *IVC* indicates inferior vena cava; *SMV,* superior mesenteric vein.

apy. Unfortunately, even in the 20% of patients with solitary, nonmetastatic gastrinomas in whom excision could be curative, up to 50% of these tumors are not found at laparotomy.

The sonographic appearance is similar to insulinoma, with the tumors appearing as homogeneous, hypoechoic lesions (Fig. 22-16). Norton et al has suggested that indistinct borders suggest a malignant tumor.[28,30] As with insulinoma, the use of high-frequency intraoperative sonography may aid in localization and may facilitate a curative resection.[31]

REFERENCES

1. Eiseman B, Greenlaw RH, Gallagher JQ: Localization of common duct stones by ultrasound. *Arch Surg* 1965;91:195-199.
2. Knight PR, Newell JA: Operative use of ultrasonics in cholelithiasis. *Lancet* 1963:1023-1025.
3. Lane RJ, Coupland AE: Ultrasonic indications to explore the common bile duct. *Surgery* 1982;91:268-274.

4. Sigel B, Coelho JCU, Nyhus LM, et al: Comparison of cholangiography of ultrasonography in the operative screening of the common bile duct. *World J Surg* 1982;6:440-444.

5. Sigel B, Machi J, Beitler JG, et al: Comparative accuracy of operative ultrasonography of cholangiography in detecting common duct calculi. *Surgery* 1983;94:715-720.

6. Sigel B, Coelho JCU, Machi J, et al: The application of real-time ultrasound imaging during surgical procedures. *Surg Gynecol Obstet* 1983;157:33-337.

7. Rifkin MD, Mack LA, Lennard ES, et al: Intraoperative abdominal ultrasonography: initial experience with a dedicated high-resolution operative transducer. *J Ultrasound Med* 1986;5:429-433.

General technique

8. Gooding GAW: Use of an ultrasound transducer in a sterile field. *Radiology* 1983;147:276.

9. Mittlestaedt Ca, Staab EV, Drobnes WE, et al: The intraoperative uses of real-time ultrasound. *Radiographics* 4:267-282.

Bile ducts and gallbladder

10. Laing FC, Jeffrey RB Jr, Wing VW: Improved visualization of choledocholithiasis by sonography. *AJR* 1984;143:949-952.

11. Sigel B, Machi J, Anderson KW, et al: Operative sonography of the biliary tree and pancreas. *Semin Ultrasound , CT, MRI* 1985;6:2-4.

12. Mack LA, Nyberg DA: Intraoperative ultrasonography of the gallbladder and biliary tract. In: Rifkin MD, ed. *Intraoperative and Endoscopic Ultrasonography*. New York: Churchill Livingstone; 1987:105-120.

13. Herbst CA, Mittlestaedt CA, Staab EV, et al: Intraoperative ultrasonography evaluation of the gallbladder in morbidity obese patients. *Ann Surg* 1984;200:691-692.

Liver

14. Macki J, Isomoto H, Yamashita Y, et al: Intraoperative ultrasonography in screening for liver metastases from colorectal cancer: comparative accuracy with traditional procedures. *Surgery* 1987;101:678-684.

15. Parker Ga, Lawrence WJ, Horsley J III, et al: Intraoperative ultrasound of the liver affects operative decision making. *Ann Surg* 1989;209:569-577.

16. Sheu JC, Lee CS, Sung JL, et al: Intraoperative hepatic ultrasonography: an indispensable procedure in resection of small hepatocellular carcinoma. *Surgery* 1985;97:97-103.

17. Jin-Chuan S, Chue-Shue L, Jeui-Low S, et al: Intraoperative hepatic ultrasonography: an indispensable procedure in resection of small hepatocellular carcinomas. *Surgery* 1987;97-103.

18. Bismuth H, Castaing D, Garden OJ: Use of operative ultrasound in surgery of primary liver tumors. *World J Surg* 1987;11:610-614.

19. Rifkin MD, Rosato FE, Branch HM, et al: Intraoperative ultrasound of the liver: an important adjunctive tool for decision making in the operating room. *Ann Surg* 1987;205:466-472.

20. Gunven P, Makuuchi M, Takayasu K, et al: Preoperative imaging of liver metastases: comparison of angiography, computed tomography scan and ultrasonography. *Ann Surg* 1985; 202:573-579.

21. Makuuchi M, Hasegawa H, Yamazaki S: Ultrasonically guided subsegmentation. *Surg Obstet Gynecol* 1985;161:346-350.

22. Castaing D, Garden JO, Bismuth H: Segmental line resection using ultrasound-guided selective portal venous occlusion. *Ann Surg* 1989;210:20-23.

Pancreas

23. Sigel B, Machi J, Ramos JR, et al: The role of imaging ultrasound during pancreatic surgery. *Ann Surg* 1984;200:486-493.

24. Rifkin MD, Weiss SM: Intraoperative sonographic identification of nonpalpable pancreatic masses. *J Ultrasound Med* 1984;3:409-411.

25. Nyberg DA, Mack LA: Intraoperative ultrasonography of the exocrine pancreas. In: Rifkin MD, ed. *Intraoperative and Endoscopic Ultrasonography*. New York: Churchill Livingstone; 1987:135-150.

26. Galiber AK, Reading CC, Charboneau JW, et al: Localization of pancreatic insulinoma: comparison of pre and intraoperative ultrasound with computed tomography and angiography. *Radiology* 1988;166:405-408.

27. Grant CS, van Heerden J, Charboneau JW, et al: The value of intraoperative ultrasonography. *Arch Surg* 1988;123:843-848.

28. Gorman B, Charboneau JW, James EM, et al: Benign pancreatic insulinoma: preoperative sonographic localization. *AJR* 1986;147:929-934.

29. Charboneau JW, Borman B, Reading CC, et al: Intraoperative ultrasonography of pancreatic endocrine tumors. In: Rifkin MD, ed. *Intraoperative and Endoscopic Ultrasonography*. New York: Churchill Livingstone; 1987:123-134.

30. Norton JA, Cromack DT, Shawker TH, et al: Intraoperative ultrasonographic localization of islet cell tumors. *Ann Surg* 1988;207:160-168.

31. Vinayek R, Frucht H, Chiang H-C, et al: Zollinger-Ellison syndrome: recent advances in the management of the gastrinoma. *Gastroenterol Clin North Am* 1990;19:197-217.

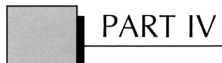

PART IV

Small Parts, Carotid Artery, and Peripheral Vessel Sonography

CHAPTER 23

The Thyroid

- E. Meredith James, M.D.
- J. William Charboneau, M.D.
- Ian D. Hay, M.B., PhD.

Because of the superficial location of the thyroid gland, high-resolution real-time sonography can demonstrate normal thyroid anatomy and pathologic conditions with remarkable clarity. As a result, this technique has come to play an increasingly important role in the diagnostic evaluation of thyroid diseases. Sonography is only one of several diagnostic methods currently available for use in evaluation of the thyroid, so it is important to understand the current capabilities and limitations of this method in order to use it effectively and economically.

INSTRUMENTATION AND TECHNIQUE

Current ultrasound technology provides high-resolution imaging of superficially located structures by using transducers with frequencies between 7.5 and 10 MHz. The theoretic axial resolution of these systems is about 1 mm. No other imaging method can achieve this degree of spatial resolution. Linear-array transducers are preferred to sector transducers because of the wider field of view near the face of the transducer. High-frequency sound waves are attenuated more rapidly in the body tissues, so they cannot be used to image structures that lie deeper than about 5 cm from the skin. Fortunately, in the majority of patients, the thyroid gland is well within this limit and can be imaged completely.

The patient is examined in the supine position with the neck extended. A small pad may be placed under the shoulders to provide better exposure of the neck, particularly in patients with a short, stocky habitus. The examiner usually sits at the head of the table and can steady the transducer by resting an elbow or forearm on the table next to the patient's head. The thyroid gland must be examined thoroughly in transverse and longitudinal planes. Imaging of the lower poles can be enhanced in some patients by asking them to swallow, which momentarily raises the thyroid gland in the neck. Care must be taken to examine the entire gland from upper to lower pole, including the isthmus. The examination should also be extended laterally to include the region of the carotid artery and jugular vein in order to identify enlarged cervical lymph nodes.

In addition to the film images recorded during the examination, we include in the permanent record a diagrammatic representation of the neck showing the location(s) of any abnormal findings (Fig. 23-1). This cervical "map" helps communicate the anatomic relationships of the pathology more clearly to the referring clinician and serves as a useful reference for the radiologist and sonographer on follow-up examinations.

ANATOMY

The right and left lobes of the thyroid gland are situated in the lower part of the neck, along either side of the trachea (Fig. 23-2). They are connected across the midline by the thyroid isthmus, a thin structure draping over the anterior tracheal wall at the level of the junction of the middle and lower thirds of the thyroid gland. The lobes are about equal in size. Normal thyroid parenchyma has a characteristic sonographic appearance of homogeneous medium-to-high level echoes, with little identifiable internal architecture. This uniform background makes detection of focal thyroid lesions relatively easy in most cases.

The strap muscles (sternohyoid and sternothyroid) of the neck are seen as thin sonolucent bands along the anterior surface of the thyroid gland. The larger sternocleidomastoid muscles are located farther anterolaterally. Each thyroid lobe is bounded laterally by the common carotid artery and internal jugular vein, which

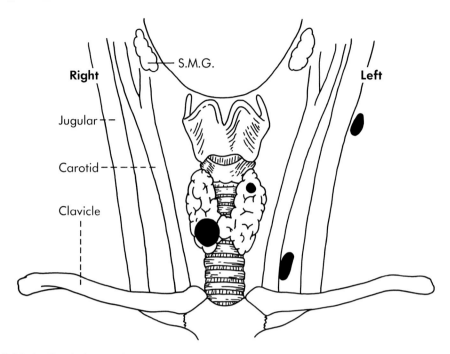

FIG 23-1. Cervical 'map' helps communicate relationships of pathology to clinicians and serves as a reference for follow-up examinations. *SMG,* submandibular gland.

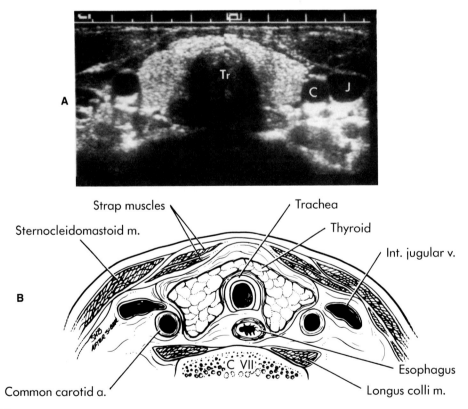

FIG 23-2. Normal thyroid gland. **A,** Transverse sonogram made with 7.5 MHz linear array transducer. **B,** Corresponding anatomic drawing. *Tr,* Tracheal air shadow; *C,* common carotid artery; *J,* jugular vein.

(From James and Charboneau with permission.)

serve as useful anatomic landmarks. The size of the internal jugular vein varies considerably depending on systemic venous pressure and phase of respiration.

Posterior and slightly lateral to each thyroid lobe is the longus colli muscle, which is seen as a wedge-shaped sonolucent structure adjacent to the cervical vertebrae. The minor neurovascular bundle, composed of the recurrent laryngeal nerve and inferior thyroid vessels, lies anatomically between the longus colli muscle and the thyroid gland, but it is rarely identified sonographically as an individual structure. However, small vessels are commonly seen near the surface of the thyroid gland, particularly over the lower pole. Color Doppler imaging demonstrates these surface vessels as well as scattered vessels within the parenchyma. The normal parathyroid glands, which are adjacent to the posterior surface of the thyroid gland, are not usually visible, even with high-resolution ultrasonography.

The air-filled trachea in the midline gives a characteristic curvilinear reflecting surface with associated reverberation artifact. The esophagus, also primarily a midline structure, is hidden from sonographic visualization by the tracheal air shadow. Often, however, a segment of the esophagus may swing laterally, usually toward the left, where it may lie adjacent to the postero-medial surface of the thyroid. The esophagus can be identified by the characteristic sonographic "target" appearance of bowel in the transverse plane. Peristaltic movement also can be visualized within the esophageal lumen when the patient swallows. This laterally located segment of the esophagus should not be mistaken for a thyroid or a parathyroid mass.

NODULAR THYROID DISEASE

Any thyroid disease can manifest itself as one or more nodules. Such nodular thyroid disease remains a common and controversial clinical problem. Epidemiologic studies estimate that between 4% and 7% of the adult population in the United States has palpable thyroid nodules, with women being more frequently affected than men.[1,2] Exposure to ionizing radiation increases the incidence of benign and malignant nodules, with 20% to 30% of a radiation-exposed population having palpable thyroid disease.[3,4]

Although nodular thyroid disease is relatively common, thyroid cancer is rare and accounts for less than 1% of all malignant neoplasms.[5] In fact, the overwhelming majority of thyroid nodules are benign. The clinical challenge is to distinguish the few clinically significant malignant nodules from the many benign ones and, thus, to identify those patients for whom surgical excision is genuinely indicated. This task is complicated by the fact that much of the nodular disease of the thyroid gland is clinically occult (less than 1.5 cm), but it can be readily detected by high-resolution sonogra-

phy. The question of how to manage these small nodules discovered incidentally by sonography is an important one that will be addressed later in this chapter.

Pathologic Features

The most commonly encountered benign thyroid nodules are **colloid** or **adenomatous nodules.** These may not be true neoplasms; they may result instead from cycles of hyperplasia and involution of a thyroid lobule. Hemorrhage or necrosis within these benign nodules is common and results in the most frequently encountered form of the grossly cystic thyroid nodule.

The **benign follicular adenoma** is a true thyroid neoplasm that is characterized by complete fibrous encapsulation. Various subtypes of follicular adenoma include the fetal adenoma, Hürthle cell adenoma, and embryonal adenoma, each distinguished according to the amount and pattern of cellularity.

In most patients with **primary thyroid cancer,** the tumors are of **epithelial origin** and are derived from either the follicular or the parafollicular cells.[5] Malignant thyroid tumors of mesenchymal origin are exceedingly rare, as are metastases to the thyroid. Most thyroid cancers are well-differentiated, and papillary carcinoma (including so-called mixed papillary and follicular carcinoma) now accounts for 75% to 90% of all cases.[5,6] In contrast, medullary, follicular, and anaplastic carcinoma combined represent only 10% to 25% of all thyroid carcinomas currently diagnosed in North America.

Although it can occur in patients of any age, **papillary cancer** is especially prevalent in younger patients.[5] Females are affected more often than males. On microscopic examination, the tumor is multicentric within the thyroid gland in at least 20% of cases.[7] Round laminated calcifications (psammoma bodies) are seen in approximately 25% of cases. The major route of spread of papillary carcinoma is through the lymphatics to nearby cervical lymph nodes. In fact, it is not uncommon for a patient with papillary thyroid cancer to present with enlarged cervical nodes and a palpably normal thyroid gland.[8] Interestingly, the presence of nodal metastasis in the neck does not appear to adversely alter the prognosis for this malignancy. After 20 years, the cumulative mortality from papillary thyroid cancer is only 6%.[8]

Follicular carcinoma is the second subtype of well-differentiated thyroid cancer and accounts for 5% to 15% of all cases of thyroid cancer, affecting females more often than males.[5] Pathologically, follicular cancers are often encapsulated, similar to their benign counterparts, the follicular adenomas. These two tumors may be indistinguishable on gross or microscopic examination. However, the cancers are characterized by microscopic evidence of either capsular or vascular invasion. Follicular cancers tend to spread via the bloodstream rather than via lymphatics, and distant metastasis to lung and bone is more likely than metastasis to cervical lymph nodes. Patients who have follicular carcinoma have a higher cumulative cause-specific mortality than patients with papillary or mixed tumors—approximately 20% to 30% at 20 years.[5,8]

Medullary carcinoma accounts for only about 5% of all malignant thyroid disease. It is derived from the parafollicular or C cells and typically secretes the hormone calcitonin, which can be a useful serum marker. This cancer is frequently familial and is an essential component of the multiple endocrine neoplasia (MEN) type II syndromes. The disease is multicentric or bilateral in about 90% of the familial cases and 20% cases presumed to be sporadic.[5] There is a high incidence of metastatic involvement of lymph nodes, and the prognosis for patients with medullary cancer is considered to be somewhat worse than that for follicular cancer.

Anaplastic thyroid carcinoma is typically a disease of the elderly and represents one of the most lethal human solid tumors. It accounts for less than 5% of all thyroid cancers but carries the worst prognosis, with a 5-year survival rate of only 3.6%.[9] The tumor typically presents as a rapidly enlarging mass extending beyond the gland and invading adjacent structures. It is often inoperable at the time of presentation.

Clinical Workup

Once a thyroid nodule has been detected, the fundamental problem is to determine if it is benign or malignant. Short of surgical excision, several methods for nodule characterization are in common use, including radionuclide imaging, sonography, and fine-needle aspiration (FNA) biopsy. Each of these techniques has advantages and limitations and the one(s) chosen in any specific clinical setting depends to a large extent on available instrumentation and expertise.

It is now generally recognized that FNA is the most effective method for diagnosing malignancy in a thyroid nodule.[10-12] In many clinical practices, FNA under direct palpation is the first diagnostic examination performed on any clinically palpable nodule. Neither isotope nor sonographic imaging is used routinely. Instead, they are reserved for special situations or difficult cases. FNA has had a substantial impact on the management of thyroid nodules because it provides more direct information than any other available diagnostic technique. It is safe, inexpensive, and results in better selection of patients for surgery. The successful use of FNA in clinical practice, however, depends heavily on the presence of an experienced aspirationist and an expert cytopathologist.

Fine-needle thyroid aspirates are classified by the cytopathologist into one of four categories:

- Negative (no malignant cells)
- Positive for malignancy
- Suspicious for malignancy
- Nondiagnostic

If a nodule is classified in either of the first two categories, the results are highly sensitive and specific.[13] The major limitation of the technique is the lack of specificity in the group whose results are "suspicious for malignancy," primarily because of an inability to distinguish follicular or Hürthle cell adenomas from their malignant counterparts. In these cases, surgical excision is required for diagnosis. In addition, up to 20% of aspirates may be nondiagnostic, approximately half of which are so because of cystic lesions from which an adequate cell sample was not obtained. In these cases, repeat FNA under sonographic guidance can be performed with the goal of selectively sampling the solid elements of the mass. Among diagnostic aspirates, the overall accuracy of FNA is about 95%. FNA of the thyroid gland, therefore, is currently the most accurate and cost-effective method for initial evaluation of patients with nodular thyroid disease.

Sonographic Applications

Although FNA has become the primary diagnostic method for evaluating clinically palpable thyroid nodules, high-resolution sonography has three primary clinical applications[14-16]:

- Detection of thyroid and other cervical masses before and after thyroidectomy
- Differentiation of benign from malignant masses on the basis of their sonographic appearance
- FNA guidance

Detection. A basic and practical use of sonography is the establishment of the precise anatomic location of a palpable cervical mass. The determination of whether such a mass is within or adjacent to the thyroid cannot always be made on the basis of the physical examination alone (Fig. 23-3). Sonography can readily differentiate thyroid nodules from other cervical masses such as cystic hygromas, thyroglossal duct cysts, or enlarged lymph nodes. Alternatively, sonography may help confirm the presence of a thyroid nodule when the findings on physical examination are equivocal.

Sonography may be used to detect occult thyroid nodules in patients who have a history of head and neck irradiation during childhood as well as for those with a family history of MEN-II syndrome, because both groups have a known increased risk for development of thyroid malignancy (Fig. 23-4). If a nodule is discovered, a biopsy can be performed under sonographic guidance. It is unknown, however, whether the detection of a thyroid cancer before it becomes clinically palpable will change the ultimate clinical outcome for a given patient.

In the past, when thyroid nodules were evaluated

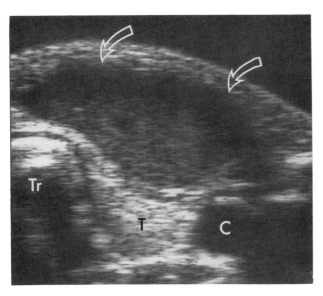

FIG 23-3. Thyroglossal duct cyst. Transverse scan demonstrates a debris-containing cystic mass *(arrows)* anterior to left lobe of thyroid *(T)*. *C,* Left common carotid artery; *Tr,* tracheal air shadow.

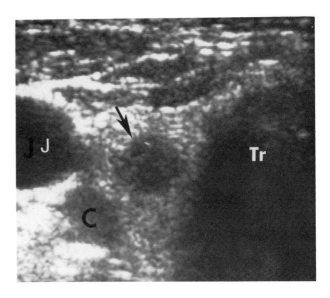

FIG 23-4. Occult papillary carcinoma in patient with previous history of radiation therapy to head and neck. Transverse view of right thyroid lobe demonstrates solid hypoechoic mass *(arrow)* 7 mm in diameter. *C,* Carotid artery; *J,* internal jugular vein; *Tr,* tracheal air shadow.

primarily with isotope scintigraphy, it generally was accepted that a "solitary cold" nodule carried a probability of malignancy of between 15% and 25%, whereas a "cold" nodule in a multinodular gland was malignant in less than 1% of cases.[17] It has been suggested, therefore, that sonography may be used to detect additional occult nodules in patients with a clinically solitary lesion, thereby implying that the dominant palpable mass is benign. Such a conclusion is unwarranted, however, in view of the fact that, pathologically, benign nodules often coexist with malignant nodules. In a recent series of 1500 consecutive patients operated on for papillary carcinoma, 33% had coexistent benign adenomatous nodules or adenomas at the time of surgery.[18] In addition, papillary thyroid cancer is recognized to be multicentric in at least 20% of cases and "occult" (i.e., less than 1.5 cm in diameter) in up to 48% of cases (Fig. 23-5).[7,18] In a recent series, almost two thirds (64%) of patients with thyroid cancer had at least one nodule detected sonographically in addition to the palpable dominant nodule.[19] Pathologically, these extra nodules can be either benign or malignant. Therefore, in patients with a clinically solitary nodule, the sonographic detection of a few additional nodules is not a reliable sign for excluding malignancy.

In patients with known thyroid cancer, sonography can be useful in evaluating the extent of disease, both preoperatively and postoperatively. In most instances a sonographic examination is not performed routinely prior to thyroidectomy, but it can be useful in patients with large cervical masses to evaluate nearby structures such as the carotid artery and internal jugular vein for evidence of direct invasion or encasement by the tumor. Alternatively, in patients who present with cervical lymphadenopathy caused by papillary thyroid cancer but in whom the thyroid gland is palpably normal, sonography may be used preoperatively to detect an occult, nonpalpable primary focus within the gland.

After partial or near-total thyroidectomy for carcinoma, sonography is the preferred method for detecting residual, recurrent, or metastatic disease in the neck.[20] In patients who have had subtotal thyroidectomy, the sonographic appearance of the remaining thyroid tissue may serve as an important factor in deciding whether completion thyroidectomy is recommended. If a mass is identified, its nature can be determined by sonographic-guided FNA. If no masses are seen, the clinician may choose to follow the patient with periodic sonographic studies. For patients who have had total or near-total thyroidectomy, sonography has proved to be more sensitive than physical examination in detecting recurrent disease within the thyroid bed or metastatic disease in cervical lymph nodes (Fig. 23-6).[21] Patients with a history of thyroid cancer often undergo periodic sonographic examinations of the neck to detect nonpalpable recurrent or metastatic disease. When a mass is identified, FNA under sonographic guidance can establish a diagnosis of malignancy and help in surgical planning.

Differentiation. Currently, no single sonographic criterion distinguishes benign thyroid nodules from ma-

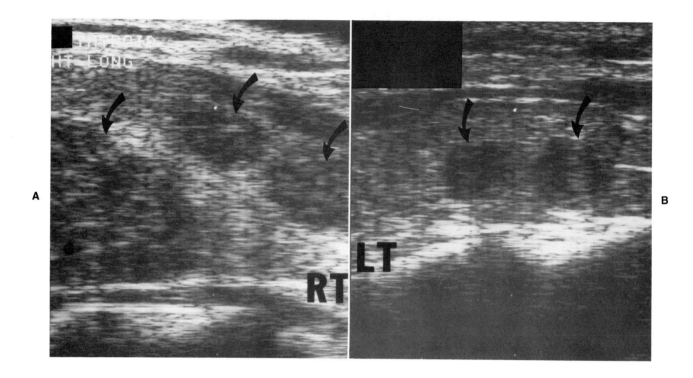

FIG 23-5. Multicentric papillary carcinoma. Longitudinal views of right **(A)** and left **(B)** lobes of thyroid gland show three solid hypoechoic masses in right lobe *(arrows)* and two in the left lobe *(arrows)*.

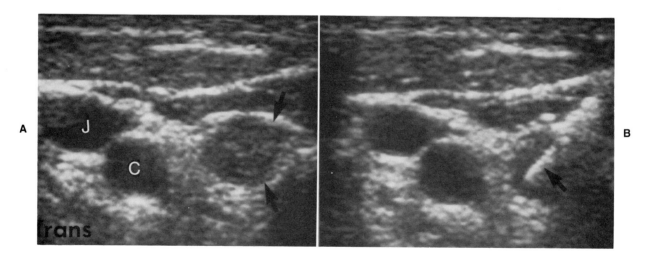

FIG 23-6. Recurrent papillary carcinoma in thyroid bed after previous thyroidectomy for malignant disease. **A,** Transverse view of the right side of the neck shows a 1-cm solid mass *(arrows)* medial to carotid artery *(C)* and jugular vein *(J)*. **B,** Sonographically guided fine-needle aspiration with needle tip within mass *(arrow)*.

■ **TABLE 23-1**
Thyroid Nodules: Sonographic Features versus
Pathologic Diagnosis*

Feature	Pathologic Diagnosis	
	Benign	Malignant
Internal contents		
Solid	I (C)	I (C)
Cystic	P (C)	
Mixed	P (C)	
Echogenicity		
Hypo-	I (C)	I (C)†
Iso-	I (U)	I (U)
Hyper-	P (U)	
Margin		
Well defined	P (C)	
Poorly defined		P (C)
Halo		
Thick/incomplete		P (C)
Thin/complete	P (C)	
Calcification		
Peripheral (eggshell)	P (U)	
Internal		
Coarse	I (U)	I (U)
Fine		P (C)

I, Indeterminate.
P, Probable (>85%).
C, Commonly encountered.
U, Uncommonly encountered.
*Based on Mayo Clinic experience[22] and personal communication from L. Solbiati.
†Although most malignant nodules are hypoechoic, most hypoechoic nodules will be benign because benign nodules are far more common.

lignant nodules with complete reliability.[22,23] Nevertheless, certain sonographic features have been described that are seen more commonly with one type of histology or the other, thus establishing general diagnostic trends (Table 23-1).[23] The fundamental anatomic features of a thyroid nodule on high-resolution sonography are:

- Internal consistency (solid, mixed solid and cystic, or purely cystic)
- Echogenicity relative to the adjacent thyroid parenchyma
- Margination
- Presence and pattern of calcification
- Sonolucent peripheral halo.

Internal Consistency. In our experience, approximately 70% of thyroid nodules are solid, whereas the remaining 30% exhibit various amounts of cystic change. A nodule that has a significant cystic component is usually a benign colloid nodule or an adenomatous nodule that has undergone central degeneration or hemorrhage. When detected by older, lower-resolution

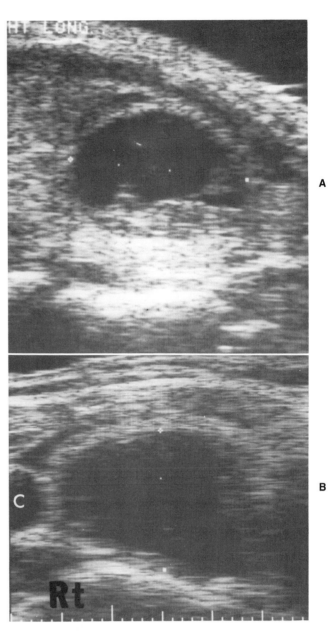

FIG 23-7. Cystic thyroid masses. **A,** Benign, degenerated adenoma. Longitudinal view demonstrates debris-containing cystic mass in right thyroid lobe. **B,** Unusual cystic grade 1 papillary carcinoma. Transverse view of different patient with similarly sized cystic mass in right lobe showing slight wall irregularity. *C,* Carotid artery.

ultrasound machines, these lesions were called "cysts" because the presence of internal debris and a thick wall could not be appreciated. Pathologically, a true epithelium-lined simple thyroid cyst is extremely rare. Virtually all cystic thyroid lesions seen with high-resolution ultrasound equipment demonstrate some wall irregularity and internal solid elements or debris caused by nodule degeneration (Fig. 23-7, *A*).

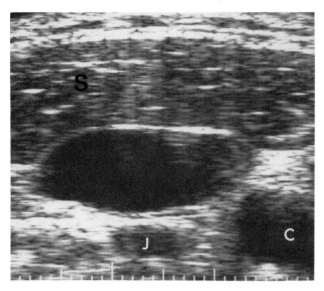

FIG 23-8. Extensive cystic change in an enlarged cervical lymph node containing metastatic papillary carcinoma. Transverse view of right side of neck shows an almost entirely cystic mass located posterior to sternocleidomastoid muscle *(S)* and anterior to the common carotid artery *(C)* and jugular vein *(J)*. The mass contains some solid elements along the medial wall.

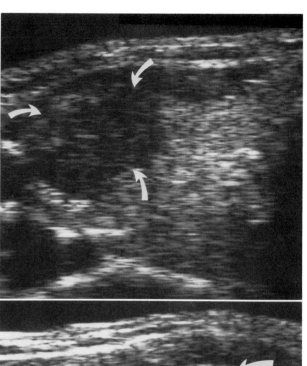

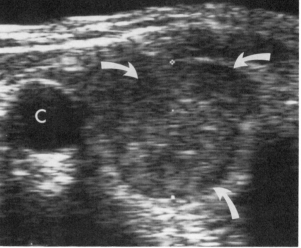

FIG 23-9. Hypoechoic thyroid nodules in two patients. **A,** Papillary thyroid carcinoma. **B,** Adenoma. Transverse view of right thyroid lobe in each case demonstrates a relatively well-circumscribed, uniformly solid hypoechoic mass *(arrows)*. *C,* Carotid artery.

In rare cases, thyroid cancer, particularly the papillary variety, may exhibit varying amounts of cystic change and appear identical to benign degenerated adenomas (Fig. 23-7, *B*).[24] Cervical lymph nodes with metastatic papillary carcinoma may also demonstrate similar cystic morphology although most are solid (Fig. 23-8).

Echogenicity. Thyroid cancers are usually hypoechoic relative to the adjacent normal thyroid parenchyma (Fig. 23-9, *A*). Unfortunately, many benign thyroid nodules are also hypoechoic (Fig. 23-9, *B*). In fact most **hypoechoic nodules** are benign because benign nodules are so much more common than malignant nodules. A predominantly **hyperechoic nodule** is more likely to be benign (Fig. 23-10).[23] The **isoechoic nodule** (visible because of a peripheral sonolucent rim that separates it from the adjacent normal parenchyma) has an intermediate risk of malignancy.

Margination. Benign thyroid nodules tend to have sharp, well-defined margins, whereas malignant lesions tend to have irregular or poorly defined margins. For any given nodule, however, the appearance of the outer margin cannot be relied on to predict the histologic features because many exceptions to these general trends have been identified.

Calcification. Calcification can be detected in 13% of all thyroid nodules but the location and pattern of calci-

fication have more predictive value in distinguishing benign from malignant lesions.[23] Peripheral or eggshell-like calcification is perhaps the most reliable feature of a benign nodule (Fig. 23-11) but occurs in only a small percentage of benign nodules. Scattered echogenic foci of calcification with or without associated acoustic shadows are more common and when these calcifications are large and coarse, the nodule is more likely to be benign. When the calcifications are fine and punctate, however, malignancy is more likely (Fig. 23-12, *A*). Pathologically these fine calcifications may be

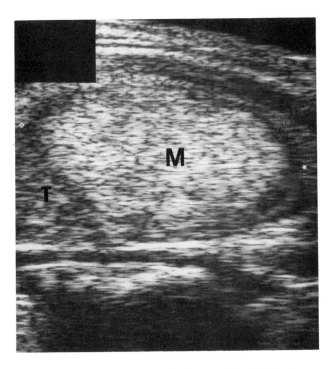

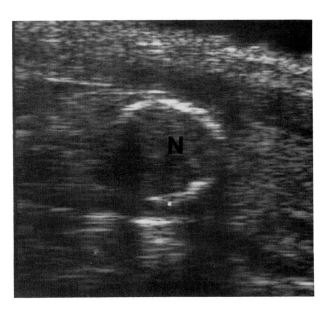

FIG 23-10. Benign Hürthle cell adenoma. Longitudinal scan demonstrates oval-shaped, hyperechoic mass *(M)* involving middle and lower portions of left thyroid lobe *(T)*.
(From James and Charboneau with permission of WB Saunders Co.)

FIG 23-11. Peripheral (eggshell) calcification. Longitudinal image demonstrates 1-cm solid nodule *(N)* with highly echogenic peripheral rim caused by calcification.

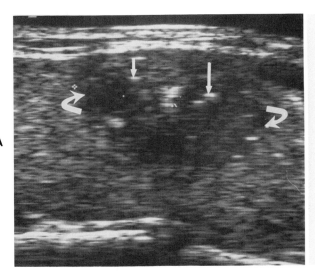

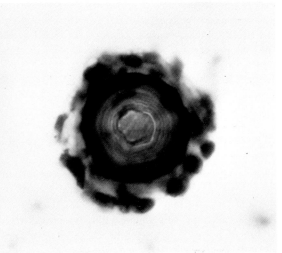

FIG 23-12. Microcalcification in papillary carcinoma. **A,** Longitudinal view of thyroid demonstrates a 1.5-cm oval hypoechoic mass *(curved arrows)* with multiple small punctate echogenic foci *(straight arrows)*. These foci represent psammoma bodies, which are commonly found in papillary carcinoma. **B,** Calcified psammoma body from pathologic specimen.

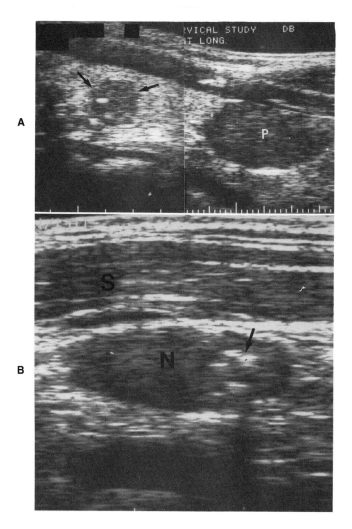

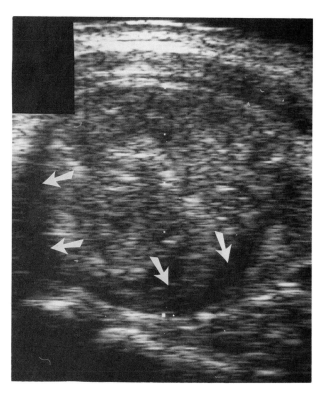

FIG 23-14. Papillary carcinoma with incomplete halo. Longitudinal view demonstrates 2-cm round, heterogeneous, solid mass with an irregular, thick, sonolucent halo *(arrows)* around superior and posterior margins of mass. Fine echogenic foci within mass probably represent psammoma bodies.

FIG 23-13. Medullary thyroid carcinoma and parathyroid adenoma. **A,** Longitudinal view of neck in patient with MEN-II syndrome shows 1-cm hypoechoic solid medullary cancer *(arrows)* containing several small nonshadowing echogenic foci within thyroid gland. Also note large, oval-shaped mass *(P),* which is a parathyroid adenoma inferior to lower pole of thyroid. **B,** Enlarged cervical lymph node *(N)* with calcification due to medullary thyroid carcinoma *(arrow). S,* Sternocleidomastoid muscle.

caused by psammoma bodies (Fig. 23-12, *B*), which are commonly seen in papillary cancers.

Medullary thyroid carcinoma often exhibits bright echogenic foci either within the primary tumor or within metastatically involved cervical lymph nodes.[25] The larger echogenic foci are usually associated with acoustic shadowing. Pathologically, these densities are caused by reactive fibrosis and calcification around amyloid deposits, which are characteristic of medullary carcinoma. In the appropriate clinical setting (e.g., MEN-II syndrome or an increased serum calcitonin level), the finding of echogenic foci within a hypo-

echoic thyroid nodule or a cervical node can be highly suggestive of medullary carcinoma (Fig. 23-13).

Peripheral Sonolucent Halo. A peripheral sonolucent halo that completely or incompletely surrounds a thyroid nodule may be present in 60% to 80% of benign nodules and 15% of thyroid cancers.[15,23,26] Histologically, it is not known what this halo represents; perhaps it represents the capsule of the nodule or compressed thyroid parenchyma. In some cases, color Doppler imaging has shown that the halo is caused by vessels around the periphery of the nodule. More recently, it was suggested that a thin, complete peripheral halo is more likely to be seen with a benign nodule, whereas a thick, incomplete halo is more likely to be indicative of malignancy (Fig. 23-14).[27]

Color Doppler imaging has been reported to show increased vascularity with autonomously functioning thyroid adenomas as well as with thyroid carcinomas (Fig. 23-15).[28,29] Thus, it is not yet possible to define what role, if any, Doppler sonography will have in the evaluation of nodular thyroid disease.

Biopsy Guidance. Sonographically guided percutaneous needle biopsy of cervical masses has become an

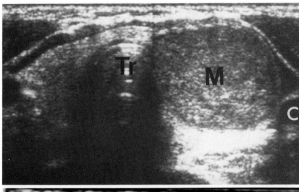

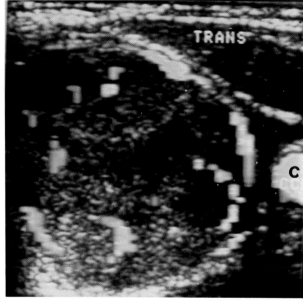

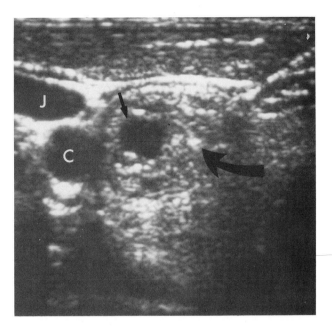

FIG 23-16. Sonographically guided fine-needle aspiration of a benign adenoma. Transverse scan of right thyroid lobe demonstrates needle tip *(curved arrow)* in solid portion of round nodule, avoiding the cystic component *(straight arrow)*. C, Carotid artery; *J,* jugular vein.

FIG 23-15. Large thyroid adenoma with prominent vascularity by color Doppler imaging. **A,** Transverse view of thyroid gland shows large solid mass in left lobe *(M)*. *Tr,* Tracheal air shadow; *C,* carotid artery. **B,** Transverse color Doppler image shows prominent vascularity within the mass.

important technique in many clinical situations. Its main advantage is that it affords continuous real-time visualization of the needle, a crucial requirement for the biopsy of small lesions. The technique of sonographically guided biopsy is described in Chapter 18.

Thyroid nodules that are palpable generally undergo biopsy without imaging guidance. There are three settings, however, in which sonographically guided biopsy of a thyroid nodule is usually indicated. The first is the questionable or inconclusive physical examination when a nodule is suspected but cannot be palpated with certainty. In these patients sonography is used to confirm the presence of a nodule and to provide guidance for accurate biopsy. The second setting is in the patient who is at high risk for developing thyroid cancer and who has a normal gland by physical examination but in whom sonography demonstrates a nodule. Included in this group are patients with a previous history of head and neck irradiation, those who have a positive family history for MEN-II syndrome, and those who have, in the past, undergone subtotal thyroid resection for malignancy. The third group of patients includes those who have had a previous nondiagnostic or inconclusive biopsy performed under direct palpation. Usually about 20% of specimens obtained by palpation guidance are cytologically inconclusive, most often because of the aspiration of nondiagnostic fluid from cystic lesions. Sonography may be used in these cases to selectively guide the needle into a solid portion of the mass (Fig. 23-16).

In patients who have undergone a previous thyroid resection for carcinoma, sonographically guided FNA has become an important method in the early diagnosis of recurrent or metastatic disease in the neck (Fig. 23-17). In our experience with 54 consecutive biopsies of cervical masses, the accuracy of sonographically guided FNA was 94%. Of these 54 sonographically visible masses, 44 were not palpable by clinical examination.[21]

Cervical lymph nodes, both normal and abnormal, can be readily visualized by high-resolution sonography and tend to lie along the internal jugular chain, extending from the level of the clavicles to the angle of the mandible, or in the region of the thyroid bed. Benign cervical nodes usually have a slender, oval shape and

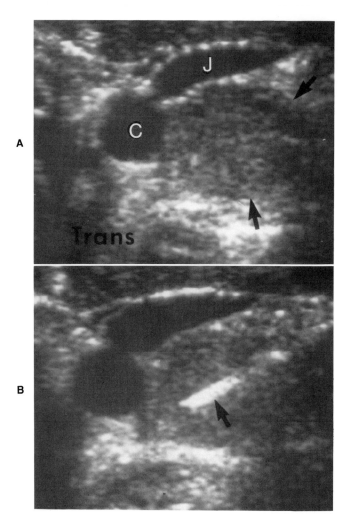

FIG 23-17. Cervical adenopathy caused by metastatic papillary carcinoma. **A,** Transverse view of left side of neck shows 1.5-cm nonpalpable lymph node *(arrows)* adjacent to common carotid artery *(C)* and jugular vein *(J)*. **B,** Sonographically guided fine-needle aspiration with needle tip *(arrow)* within lymph node.

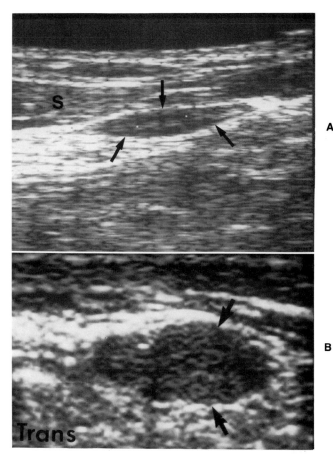

FIG 23-18. Cervical lymph nodes. **A,** Longitudinal view shows typical benign cervical lymph node *(arrows)* with an elongated, slender configuration. Linear echogenic band centrally represents the fatty hilum of the node. *S,* Sternocleidomastoid muscle. **B,** Medullary carcinoma in an enlarged lymph node *(arrows)* with rounder configuration and no central echogenic band.

often exhibit a central echogenic band that represents the fatty hilum (Fig. 23-18, *A*).[30] Malignant nodes, on the other hand, are usually rounder and have no echogenic hilum, presumably because of obliteration by tumor infiltration (Fig. 23-18, *B*). Because these distinctions are not always clear, FNA under sonographic guidance is often used to confirm malignancy. In our experience, biopsy can be done with a high degree of accuracy in cervical nodes that are as small as 0.5 cm.

The Incidentally Detected Nodule

Although using high-resolution sonography to detect small, nonpalpable thyroid nodules may be beneficial in some clinical settings, it may actually introduce problems in other settings. What should one do with the many thyroid nodules detected incidentally during the course of carotid, parathyroid, or other sonographic examinations of the neck (Fig. 23-19)? The goal should be to avoid extensive and costly evaluations in the majority of patients with benign disease, without missing the minority of patients who have clinically significant thyroid cancer. By clinical palpation, the prevalence of thyroid nodules in the United States is 4% to 7% of the general population, but high-resolution sonography has detected thyroid nodules in approximately 41% of a hypercalcemic population.[1,31] Previous studies had shown that patients with hyperparathyroidism have statistically no more nodular thyroid disease than age-matched and sex-matched autopsy controls.[32] Of 1000 consecutive hypercalcemic patients, 410 (41%) had sonographically visible nodules, of which 80 (8%) were clinically palpable. A similarly high prevalence of sonographically de-

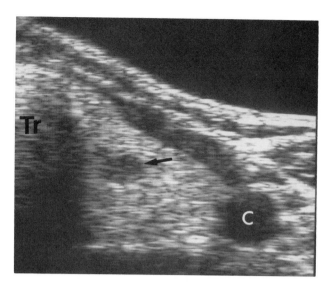

FIG 23-19. Incidentally discovered thyroid nodule. Transverse view of left lobe of thyroid gland, obtained during parathyroid sonographic examination demonstrates 3-mm hypoechoic nodule *(arrow)*. *Tr,* Tracheal air shadow; *C,* carotid artery.

tected thyroid abnormalities was recently reported in Finland.[33] In this study of 101 women with no previous thyroid or parathyroid disease, 35.6% had one or more sonographically visible nodules.

A somewhat higher prevalence of thyroid nodules has been detected at autopsy on patients who had clinically normal thyroid glands (49.5% had one or more grossly visible nodules).[34] Thus, high-resolution sonog-

raphy can detect almost as many nodules as are demonstrated by careful pathologic examination, and both studies showed a direct relationship between the prevalence of thyroid nodules and patient age (Fig. 23-20).

Although these studies have shown a high prevalence of thyroid nodules detected by autopsy and sonography, the prevalence of thyroid malignancy reported in them was only 2% and 4%, respectively, with most (90%) being occult (<1.5 cm) papillary cancers.[31,34] The papillary type of thyroid cancer represents approximately 90% of all thyroid cancers diagnosed in the midwestern United States since 1970.[5,6] The vast majority of patients with occult papillary thyroid cancer have an excellent prognosis, with essentially no reduction in life expectancy and no morbidity from appropriate surgical therapy. Further evidence that most subclinical thyroid cancers have a benign natural history is the fact that the annual incidence of clinically detected thyroid cancer is only 0.005% (5 per 100,000 persons).[5,6]

If nearly 50% of the United States population has subtle evidence of nodular thyroid disease that can be revealed by sonography, yet the annual incidence rate of clinically apparent thyroid carcinoma is only 0.005%, it is clear that only a small minority of patients with thyroid nodules have a risk of harboring clinically significant thyroid cancer (Table 23-2). Furthermore, if 90% of those cancers are papillary and therefore eminently curable after they become clinically apparent, it seems both impractical and imprudent to pursue all of the small nodules detected incidentally by high-resolution sonography for diagnosis. Accordingly, for nonpalpable nodules that are incidentally detected by sonogra-

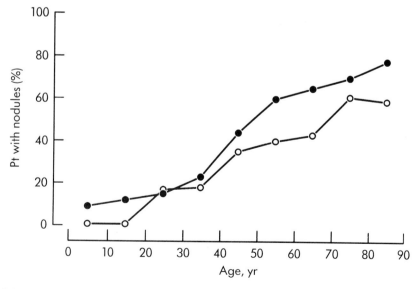

FIG 23-20. Comparison of prevalence of thyroid nodules detected by autopsy *(solid circles;* average 49%, 1955) and sonography *(open circles;* average 41%, 1985), as a function of patient age.
(Modified from Horlocker et al.)

■ **TABLE 23-2**
Prevalence of Thyroid Nodules

Method of Detection	Patients (%)
Autopsy	49
Sonography	41
Palpation	7
Occult cancer (autopsy)	2
Cancer incidence (annual)	0.005

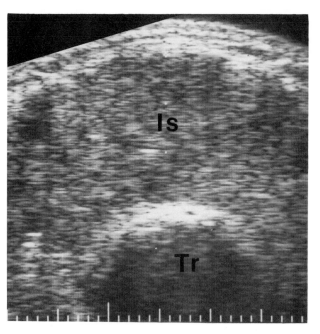

FIG 23-21. Transverse view shows markedly thickened thyroid isthmus *(Is)* in patient with Graves' disease. *Tr,* Tracheal air shadow. The normal isthmus is thin (see Fig. 23-2).

phy and that do not have malignant sonographic features (thick, irregular halo or microcalcification), we simply recommend follow-up by neck palpation at the time of the patient's next routine physical examination. Follow-up sonographic examination, radionuclide imaging, FNA, or surgical excision of such incidental nodules is rarely necessary in our practice.

DIFFUSE THYROID DISEASE

Several thyroid diseases are characterized by diffuse rather than focal involvement. That usually results in generalized enlargement of the gland (goiter), without palpable nodules. Specific conditions that commonly produce such diffuse enlargement include **chronic autoimmune (Hashimoto's) thyroiditis, colloid** or **adenomatous goiter,** and **Graves' disease**—the commonest cause worldwide of thyrotoxicosis (hyperthyroidism). Diagnosis of these conditions is usually made on the basis of clinical and laboratory findings and, on occasion, by FNA. Sonography is seldom indicated. One clinical setting in which high-resolution sonography can be helpful is when the underlying diffuse disease causes asymmetric thyroid enlargement, which raises the possibility of there being a mass in the larger lobe. The sonographic finding of generalized parenchymal abnormality may alert the clinician to consider diffuse thyroid disease as the underlying cause. FNA, with sonographic guidance if necessary, can be performed if a nodule is detected.

Recognition of diffuse thyroid enlargement on sonography can often be facilitated by noting the thickness of the isthmus. Normally, this is a thin bridge of tissue measuring only a few millimeters in anteroposterior dimension. With diffuse thyroid enlargement, the isthmus may be up to 1 cm or more in thickness (Fig. 23-21).

There are several different types of thyroiditis, including acute suppurative thyroiditis, subacute granulomatous thyroiditis (also called de Quervain's disease), and chronic lymphocytic thyroiditis (also called Hashimoto's disease).[35] Each disease has distinctive clinical and laboratory features, whereas sonographic findings are relatively nonspecific. **Acute suppurative thyroiditis** is a rare inflammatory disease that is usually caused by bacterial infection. Sonography can be useful in selected cases to detect the development of a frank thyroid abscess. **Subacute granulomatous thyroiditis** is a spontaneously remitting inflammatory disease that is probably caused by viral infection. No distinctive sonographic findings have been reported in this rare condition.

The most common type of thyroiditis is **chronic lymphocytic (Hashimoto's) thyroiditis.** It typically occurs as a painless, diffuse enlargement of the thyroid gland in a young or middle-aged woman, often associated with hypothyroidism. The typical sonographic appearance of Hashimoto's thyroiditis is diffuse glandular enlargement with a homogeneous but coarsened parenchymal echo texture, generally more hypoechoic than a normal thyroid (Fig. 23-22).[16] No normal parenchyma can be identified. Occasionally, discrete nodules may be seen in a gland affected by Hashimoto's thyroiditis, but the remaining parenchyma will have a diffusely abnormal sonographic appearance. Not infrequently, cervical lymphadenopathy is present, especially the Delphian node above the thyroid isthmus.

Although the appearance of diffuse parenchymal inhomogeneity is quite typical of Hashimoto's thyroiditis, it is not specific. Any of the other diffuse thyroid diseases, most commonly **adenomatous goiter,** may have

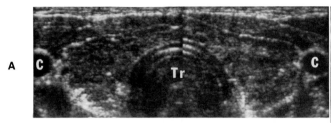

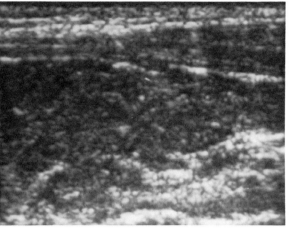

FIG 23-22. Hashimoto's thyroiditis. **A,** Transverse and **B,** longitudinal views of thyroid gland show mild diffuse enlargement with nonhomogeneous, coarsened parenchymal echo-texture. No discrete nodules are discernible. *Tr,* Tracheal air shadow; *C,* carotid artery.

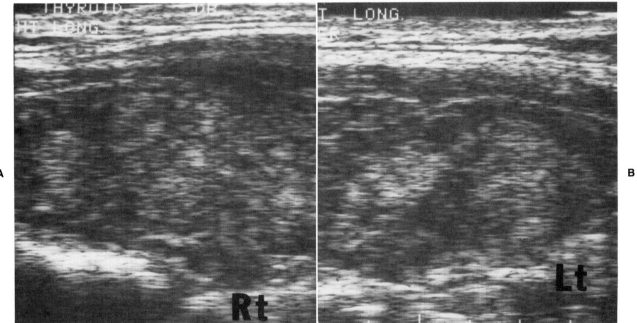

FIG 23-23. Adenomatous goiter. Longitudinal views of right, **A,** and left, **B,** lobes of thyroid show diffuse parenchymal nonhomogeneity without discretely identifiable masses, which is presumably caused by diffuse involvement with small confluent nodules.

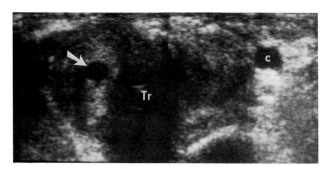

FIG 23-24. Invasive fibrous thyroiditis (Riedel's struma). Transverse view shows diffuse thyroid enlargement, greater on right. Right common carotid artery *(arrow)* is surrounded by this process but left carotid artery *(C)* remains free. *Tr,* Tracheal air shadow.

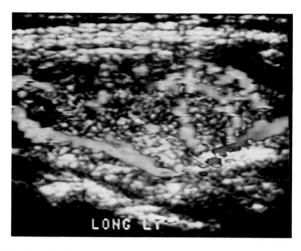

FIG 23-25. Graves' disease. Longitudinal color Doppler image of left thyroid lobe in patient with hyperthyroidism secondary to Graves' disease. Extensive vascularity is seen throughout gland, an appearance that has been called "thyroid inferno."

an identical sonographic appearance. Some patients with adenomatous goiter have multiple discrete nodules separated by otherwise normal-appearing thyroid parenchyma; others have diffuse parenchymal inhomogeneity and mixed echogenicity, with no recognizable normal tissue (Fig. 23-23).

The rarest type of inflammatory thyroid disease is **invasive fibrous thyroiditis,** also called **Riedel's struma.**[35] This disease primarily affects women and tends to progress inexorably to complete destruction of the gland. Some cases may be associated with mediastinal or retroperitoneal fibrosis or sclerosing cholangitis. In the few cases of invasive fibrous thyroiditis examined sonographically, the gland was diffusely enlarged and had an inhomogeneous parenchymal echo texture.[35] The primary reason for sonography was to check for extrathyroid extension of the inflammatory process with encasement of the adjacent vessels (Fig. 23-24). Such information can be particularly useful in surgical planning. Open biopsy is generally required to distinguish this condition from anaplastic thyroid carcinoma. The sonographic findings of these two diseases may be identical.

Graves' disease is a common diffuse abnormality of the thyroid gland and is usually characterized by thyrotoxicosis. As with the other diseases described above, it does not have a distinctive sonographic appearance. Recently, however, Ralls et al described markedly increased vascularity in the thyroid glands of patients with Graves' disease by using color Doppler imaging.[36] This has been called the "thyroid inferno," characterized by multiple tiny areas of flow throughout the entire gland in both systole and diastole (Fig. 23-25). This pattern did not occur in normal subjects or in patients with other thyroid diseases. High-resolution gray scale images did not demonstrate the small vessels within the gland from which the flow signals originated. Several

of the patients in this series also showed a decrease in thyroid vascularity when rescanned after therapy, suggesting that color Doppler imaging could be used to monitor therapeutic response in patients with Graves' disease.

In summary, sonography tends to play a minor role in the diagnosis and management of diffuse thyroid disease. It may be useful in selected patients to determine if asymmetric enlargement is caused by a discrete nodule, to detect abscess formation in rare cases of acute suppurative thyroiditis, and to monitor extraglandular extension of the inflammatory process in Riedel's struma.

REFERENCES
Nodular thyroid disease

1. Rojeski MT, Gharib H: Nodular thyroid disease: evaluation and management. *N Engl J Med* 1985;313:428-436.
2. Van Herle AJ, Rich P, Ljung B-ME, et al: The thyroid nodule. *Ann Intern Med* 1982;96:221-232.
3. Favus MJ, Schneider AB, Stachura ME, et al: Thyroid cancer occurring as a late consequence of head-and-neck irradiation: evaluation of 1056 patients. *N Engl J Med* 1976;294:1019-1025.
4. DeGroot LJ, Reilly M, Pinnameneni K, et al: Retrospective and prospective study of radiation-induced thyroid disease. *Am J Med* 1983;74:852-862.
5. Hay ID: Thyroid cancer. *Curr Ther Hematol Oncol* 1988;3:339-342.
6. Hay ID: Thyroid nodules and thyroid cancer. *Med Int* 1989;63:2601-2604.
7. Black BM, Kirk TA Jr, Woolner LB: Multicentricity of papillary adenocarcinoma of the thyroid: influence on treatment. *J Clin Endocrinol Metab* 1960;20:130-135.
8. McConahey WM, Hay ID, Woolner LB, et al: Papillary thyroid cancer treated at the Mayo Clinic, 1946 through 1970: initial manifestations, pathologic findings, therapy, and outcome. *Mayo Clin Proc* 1986;61:978-996.

9. Nel CJC, van Heerden JA, Goellner JR, et al: Anaplastic carcinoma of the thyroid: a clinicopathologic study of 82 cases. *Mayo Clin Proc* 1985;60:51-58.
10. Gobien RP: Aspiration biopsy of the solitary thyroid nodule. *Radiol Clin North Am* 1979 (12);17:543-554.
11. Miller JM: Evaluation of thyroid nodules: accent on needle biopsy. *Med Clin North Am* 1985 (9);69:1063-1077.
12. Hamberger B, Gharib H, Melton LJ III, et al: Fine-needle aspiration biopsy of thyroid nodules: impact on thyroid practice and cost of care. *Am J Med* 1982;73:381-384.
13. Goellner JR, Gharib H, Grant CS, et al: Fine-needle aspiration cytology of the thyroid, 1980 to 1986. *Acta Cytol* 1987;31:587-590.
14. James EM, Charboneau JW: High-frequency (10 MHz) thyroid ultrasonography. *Semin Ultrasound, CT, MR* 1985;6:294-309.
15. Scheible W, Leopold GR, Woo VL, et al: High-resolution real-time ultrasonography of thyroid nodules. *Radiology* 1979;133:413-417.
16. Simeone JF, Daniels GH, Mueller PR, et al: High-resolution real-time sonography of the thyroid. *Radiology* 1982;145:431-435.
17. Brown CL: Pathology of the cold nodule. *Clin Endocrinol Metab* 1981 (7);10:235-245.
18. Hay ID: Papillary thyroid carcinoma. *Endocrinol Metab Clin North Am* 1990 (9);19:545-576.
19. Hay ID, Reading CC, Weiland LH, et al: Clinicopathologic and high-resolution ultrasonographic evaluation of clinically suspicious or malignant thyroid disease. In: Medeiros-Neto G, Gaitan E, editors. *Frontiers in Thyroidology, vol 2*. New York: Plenum Medical Book Co; 1986.
20. Simeone JF, Daniels GH, Hall DA, et al: Sonography in the follow-up of 100 patients with thyroid carcinoma. *AJR* 1987;148:45-49.
21. Sutton RT, Reading CC, Charboneau JW, et al: Ultrasound-guided biopsy of neck masses in postoperative management of patients with thyroid cancer. *Radiology* 1988;168:769-772.
22. Katz JF, Kane RA, Reyes J, et al: Thyroid nodules: sonographic-pathologic correlation. *Radiology* 1984;151:741-745.
23. Solbiati L, Volterrani L, Rizzatto G, et al: The thyroid gland with low uptake lesions: evaluation by ultrasound. *Radiology* 1985;155:187-191.
24. Hammer M, Wortsman J, Folse R: Cancer in cystic lesions of the thyroid. *Arch Surg* 1982;117:1020-1023.
25. Gorman B, Charboneau JW, James EM, et al: Medullary thyroid carcinoma: role of high-resolution ultrasound. *Radiology* 1987;162:147-150.
26. Propper RA, Skolnick ML, Weinstein BJ, et al: The nonspecificity of the thyroid halo sign. *J Clin Ultrasound* 1980;8:129-132.
27. Solbiati L: Personal communication, 1990.
28. Fobbe F, Finke R, Reichenstein E, et al: Appearance of thyroid diseases using colour-coded duplex sonography. *Eur J Radiol* 1989;9:29-31.
29. Hodgson KJ, Lazarus JH, Wheeler MH, et al: Duplex scan-derived thyroid blood flow in euthyroid and hyperthyroid patients. *World J Surg* 1988;12:470-475.
30. Marchal G, Oyen R, Verschakelen J, et al: Sonographic appearance of normal lymph nodes. *J Ultrasound Med* 1985;4:417-419.
31. Horlocker TT, Hay JE, James EM, et al: Prevalence of incidental nodular thyroid disease detected during high-resolution parathyroid ultrasonography. In: Medeiros-Neto G, Gaitan E, editors. *Frontiers in Thyroidology, vol. 2*. New York: Plenum Medical Book Co; 1986.
32. Lever EG, Refetoff S, Straus FH II, et al: Coexisting thyroid and parathyroid disease - are they related? *Surgery* 1983;94:893-900.
33. Brander A, Viikinkoski P, Nickels J, et al: Thyroid gland: ultrasound screening in middle-aged women with no previous thyroid disease. *Radiology* 1989;173:507-510.
34. Mortensen JD, Woolner LB, Bennett WA: Gross and microscopic findings in clinically normal thyroid glands. *J Clin Endocrinol Metab* 1955;15:1270-1280.

Diffuse thyroid disease*

35. Hay ID: Thyroiditis: a clinical update. *Mayo Clin Proc* 1985;60:836-843.
36. Ralls PW, Mayekawa DS, Lee KP, et al: Color-flow Doppler sonography in Graves disease: "thyroid inferno." *AJR* 1988;150:781-784.

---

*See also references 14,16.

CHAPTER 24

The Parathyroid

- Carl C. Reading, M.D.

High-frequency sonography is a well-established, noninvasive imaging method that is used in the evaluation and treatment of patients with hyperparathyroidism. This technique most commonly is used for the accurate preoperative localization of enlarged parathyroid glands. It also has been used to guide the percutaneous biopsy of suspected parathyroid adenomas, particularly in the setting of persistent or recurrent hyperparathyroidism and for intraoperative localization of abnormal parathyroid glands. Most recently, sonography has been used to guide the percutaneous ethanol ablation of parathyroid adenomas as an alternative to surgical treatment.

EMBRYOLOGY AND ANATOMY

The paired superior and inferior parathyroid glands have different embryologic origins, which aids in un-

derstanding their ultimate anatomic locations.[1] The superior parathyroid glands arise from the fourth branchial cleft pouch, along with the thyroid gland. Minimal migration occurs during fetal development, and the paired superior parathyroids stay close to the posterior aspect of the middle to upper portion of the thyroid. The inferior parathyroid glands arise from the third branchial cleft pouch, along with the thymus.[2] During fetal development these "parathymus glands" migrate caudally along with the thymus, bypassing the superior glands to become the inferior parathyroid glands. These glands are more variable in location than the superior glands. They usually come to rest at the posterior aspect of the lower pole of the thyroid but may fail to dissociate from the thymus and frequently continue to migrate low into the neck tissues with the thymus, caudal to the thyroid (Fig 24-1).

From 1% to 3% of parathyroid glands lie in relatively or frankly ectopic locations in the neck or mediastinum. When located ectopically, the inferior parathyroid gland often has continued to migrate in an anterocaudal direction and usually is in the neck or anterosuperior mediastinum, associated with the thymus.[3] When the superior parathyroid gland is ectopic, it usually either lies far posteriorly in the tracheoesophageal groove or has enlarged and has continued its posterior descent into the posterosuperior mediastinum (Fig. 24-2).[4,5] Less common ectopic positions of the parathyroid glands include intrathyroid and an undescended position high in the neck with a remnant of thymus near the carotid bifurcation, or lower in the neck along the carotid sheath.[6] In rare cases, ectopic glands have been reported low in the mediastinum in the aortopulmonic window, posterior to the carina, posterior to the esophagus, and within the pericardium, or far laterally in the neck within the posterior triangle of the neck.

Most people have four parathyroid glands (two superior and two inferior) each of which measures about 5 × 3 × 1 mm and weighs on average 35 to 40 mg (range 10 to 78 mg).[7] Supernumerary "fifth" glands may result from the separation of parathyroid remnants when the parathyroid glands pull away from the pouch structures during the embryologic branchial complex phase.[8,9] If present, these supernumerary glands are of-

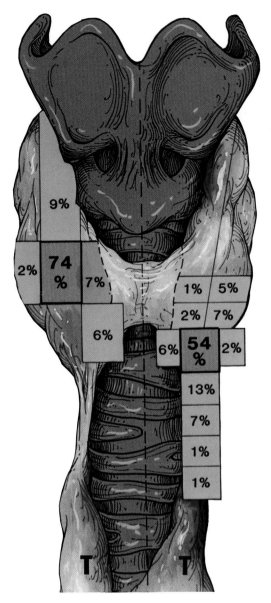

FIG 24-1. Anatomic drawing of the frequency of the location of normal superior and inferior parathyroid glands from 527 autopsies. *T,* Thymus.
(Adapted from Gilmour JR: The gross anatomy of the parathyroid glands. *J Pathol* 1938;46:133-148.)

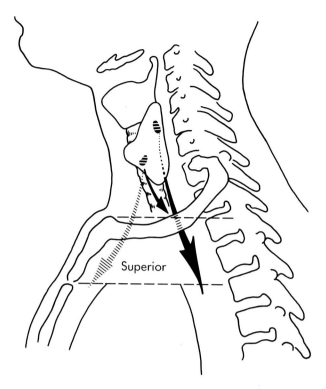

FIG 24-2. Migratory pathways of ectopic parathyroid adenomas. Superior adenomas extend into the posterosuperior mediastinum. Inferior adenomas extend into the anterosuperior mediastinum.

ten associated with the thymus in the anterior mediastinum, suggesting a relationship in their development with the inferior parathyroid glands.[10]

PRIMARY HYPERPARATHYROIDISM
Prevalence

Primary hyperparathyroidism is now recognized as a common disease with a prevalence in the United States of 100 to 200 per 100,000 population.[11] Women have primary hyperparathyroidism two to three times more frequently than men, and it is particularly common after menopause. More than half of the patients with this disease are over 50 years old, and patients rarely are less than 20 years old.

Diagnosis

Hyperparathyroidism is usually suspected because an increased serum calcium level is detected on routine biochemical screening. A serum parathyroid hormone (PTH) level that is "inappropriately increased" for the prevailing serum calcium level confirms the diagnosis. Even when the PTH level is within the upper limits of the "normal range" in a hypercalcemic patient, the diagnosis of primary hyperparathyroidism still should be suspected because hypercalcemia from other causes should suppress parathyroid gland function and decrease the serum PTH level. Most patients are asymptomatic at the time of diagnosis and have no manifestations of hyperparathyroidism, such as nephrolithiasis, osteopenia, subperiosteal resorption, and osteitis fibrosis cystica. However, certain subtle nonspecific symptoms, such as muscle weakness, malaise, constipation, dyspepsia, polydipsia, and polyuria, often are elicited from these otherwise asymptomatic patients by specific questioning.

Pathology

Primary hyperparathyroidism is caused by a single adenoma in 80% to 90% of cases, by multiple gland enlargement in 10% to 20%, and by carcinoma in less than 1%.[12,13] A solitary adenoma may involve any one of the four glands with equal frequency. Multiple gland enlargement can be due to primary parathyroid hyperplasia (most common) or multiple adenomas (less common). Hyperplasia usually involves all four glands asymmetrically whereas multiple adenomas involve two or possibly three glands. Because of this inconsistent pattern of gland involvement and the fact that distinguishing hyperplasia from multiple adenomas can be difficult, histologically these two entities are often considered together as "multiple gland disease."[14]

Multiple parathyroid gland enlargement occurs in more than 90% of patients with multiple endocrine neoplasia, type I (MEN I).[15,16] This condition is an inherited autosomal dominant trait with a high degree of penetrance that causes adenomatous hyperplasia of the parathyroids. Most patients present with hypercalcemia before the third or fourth decade of life. It is likely that all of the parathyroid glands ultimately will be involved in patients with this disease, although not all of the glands may be grossly enlarged at the time of the initial operation.

Carcinoma is a rare cause of primary hyperparathyroidism. The histologic distinction from adenoma is difficult to establish with certainty because both carcinomas and atypical adenomas can exhibit mitotic activity and cellular atypia.[17] The diagnosis usually is made at operation in a patient with a very high calcium level (>14 mg/dl) when the surgeon discovers an enlarged, firm, fibrous gland that is fixed to the surrounding tissues by local invasion.[18-21] Treatment consists of en bloc resection, but in many cases cure may not be possible because of the invasive and metastatic nature of this type of malignancy.

SONOGRAPHIC APPEARANCE
Shape

The most common shape of a parathyroid adenoma is oval (Fig. 24-3). As parathyroid glands enlarge, they dissect between longitudinally oriented tissue planes and acquire a characteristic oblong shape. If this process is exaggerated, they can become more elongated and tubelike. There often is asymmetry in the enlargement, and either the cephalic end or caudal end can be more bulbous, producing a triangular tapering or teardrop shape. Some adenomas have a bilobar shape.[22-24]

Echogenicity

The characteristic hypoechoic echogenicity of parathyroid adenomas is due to the uniform hypercellularity of the gland, which leaves few interfaces for reflecting

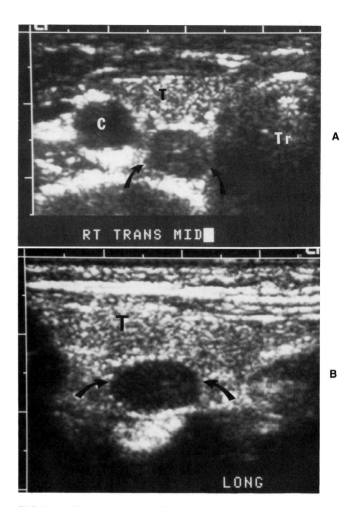

FIG 24-3. Typical parathyroid adenoma. **A,** Transverse, and **B,** longitudinal sonograms of a typical 1 cm oval adenoma *(arrows)* located adjacent to the posterior aspect of the thyroid *(T)*.

sound. The echogenicity of the vast majority of parathyroid adenomas is substantially less than that of thyroid tissue. Four cases of rare functioning parathyroid lipoadenoma have been reported, which are more echogenic than the adjacent thyroid gland because of their high fat content.[25]

Internal Architecture

The vast majority of parathyroid adenomas are homogeneously solid. About 2% have internal cystic components that are due to cystic degeneration (most commonly) or true simple cysts (less commonly (Fig. 24-4).[24,26,27] Rare adenomas may contain focal internal calcification. Color Doppler sonography of an enlarged parathyroid gland may demonstrate a hypervascular pattern with prominent diastolic flow, although further studies will be necessary to verify these findings and to determine if these will be useful in the differentiation of

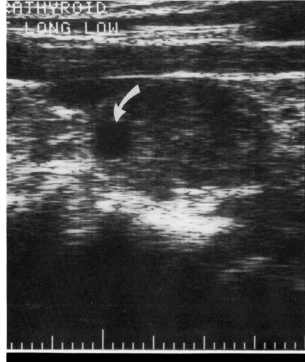

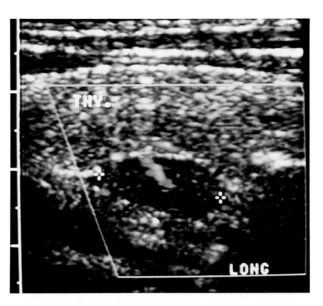

FIG 24-5. Color Doppler image depicting flow in parathyroid adenoma. Longitudinal color Doppler sonogram of a 1 cm parathyroid adenoma that has increased blood flow relative to the normal thyroid. *THY*, Thyroid.

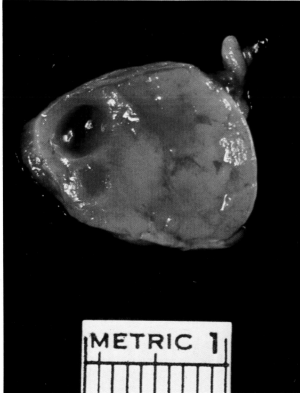

FIG 24-4. Parathyroid adenoma with cystic area. **A,** Longitudinal sonogram showing parathyroid adenoma containing a 3 mm internal cystic component *(arrow)*. **B,** Pathologic specimen.

(From Reading cc, Charboneau JW, James EM, et al: High-resolution parathyroid sonography. AJR 1982;139:539-546.)

parathyroid adenoma from other entities, such as thyroid nodules (Fig. 24-5).[28]

Size

Most parathyroid adenomas are 0.8 to 1.5 cm long and weigh 500 to 1000 mg. The smallest adenomas can be minimally enlarged glands that appear virtually normal at operation but are found to be hypercellular on pathologic examination (Fig. 24-6). The largest adenomas can be 5 cm or more long and weigh more than 10 grams. Preoperative serum calcium levels are usually higher in patients with larger adenomas.[24,29]

Multiple Gland Disease

Multiple gland disease can be due to hyperplasia or to multiple adenomas. Individually, these enlarged glands have the same sonographic appearance as other parathyroid adenomas (Fig. 24-7). However, the glands may be inconsistently and asymmetrically enlarged, and the diagnosis of multiple gland disease often is difficult to make sonographically. The appearance may be misinterpreted as solitary adenomatous disease, or the diagnosis may be missed altogether if the glandular enlargement is minimal.

Carcinoma

Sonographically, carcinomas usually are larger than adenomas. The average carcinoma measures more than 2 cm, in contrast to about 1 cm for adenomas (Fig. 24-8). Carcinomas also frequently have a lobulated contour, heterogeneous internal architecture, and cystic

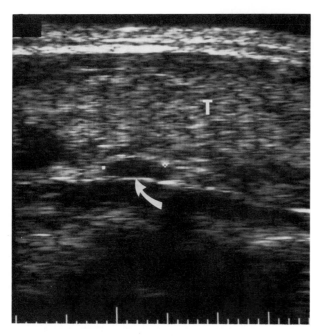

FIG 24-6. Small parathyroid adenoma. Longitudinal sonogram of a minimally enlarged 2 × 6 mm 150 mg superior parathyroid adenoma *(arrow)* adjacent to the posterior aspect of the thyroid. *T,* Thyroid.

components; however, large adenomas also can have these features.[30] In most cases, prospectively carcinomas are indistinguishable sonographically from large benign adenomas.[31] Gross evidence of invasion of adjacent structures, such as vessels or muscles, is the only reliable preoperative sonographic criterion for diagnosis of malignancy, but this is an uncommon finding.

ADENOMA LOCALIZATION

The sonographic examination of the neck for parathyroid adenoma localization is performed with the patient in a supine position. The patient's neck is hyperextended by a pad centered under the scapulae, and the examiner sits at the patient's head. High-frequency (7.5 or 10.0 MHz) real-time transducers are used to provide optimal spatial resolution and visualization in most patients. In obese patients with thick necks or with large multinodular thyroid goiters, use of a 5.0 MHz transducer may be necessary to obtain adequate depth of penetration.

Typical Location

The pattern of the sonographic survey of the neck for adenoma localization can be considered in terms of the

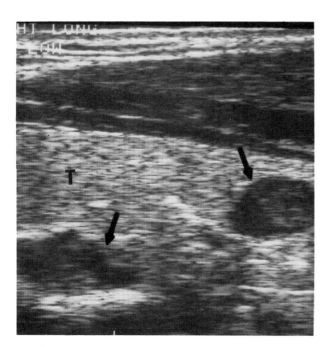

FIG 24-7. Multiple parathyroid gland enlargement. Longitudinal sonogram of the neck, showing superior and inferior parathyroid enlargement *(arrows).* *T,* Thyroid.

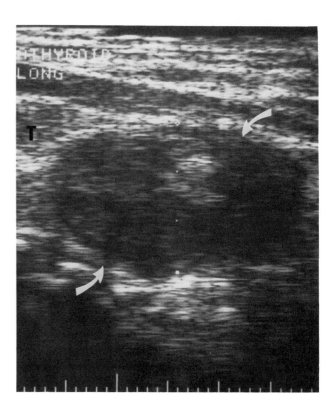

FIG 24-8. Parathyroid carcinoma. Longitudinal sonogram of a 2.5 cm lobulated, parathyroid carcinoma *(arrows)* with a heterogeneous echotexture. *T,* Thyroid.
(From Edmonson GR, Charboneau JW, James EM, et al: Parathyroid carcinoma: high-frequency sonographic features. *Radiology* 1986;161:65-67.)

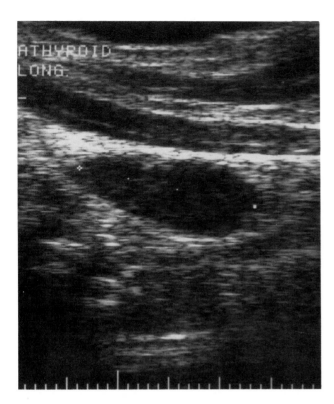

FIG 24-9. Parathyroid adenoma—base of the neck. Longitudinal sonogram, showing a surgically missed 1.5 cm oval parathyroid adenoma in the soft tissues low in the neck just superior to the level of the clavicles.

(From Reading CC, Charboneau JW, James EM, et al: Postoperative parathyroid high-frequency sonography: evaluation of persistent or recurrent hyperparathyroidism. *AJR* 1985;144:399-402.)

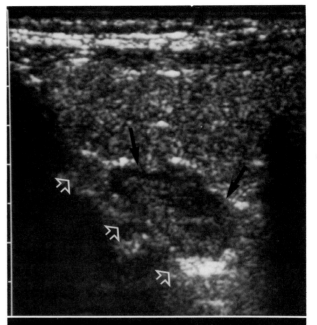

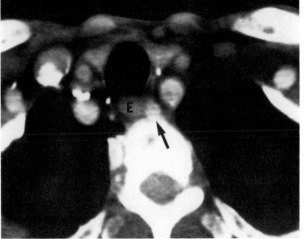

FIG 24-10. Ectopic adenoma—tracheoesophageal groove. **A,** Longitudinal angled parasagittal sonogram, showing a 1.5 cm ectopic superior parathyroid adenoma *(arrows)* deep in the low neck/upper mediastinum adjacent to the cervical spine *(arrowheads)* with posterior acoustic shadowing. **B,** CT scan of the low neck/upper mediastinum, showing the ectopic adenoma *(arrow)* in the left tracheoesophageal groove, adjacent to the esophagus *(E)*.

pattern of dissection and visualization that the surgeon uses in a thorough neck exploration. The examination is initiated on one side of the neck in the region of the thyroid gland. The typical superior parathyroid adenoma usually is adjacent to the posterior aspect of the midportion of the thyroid. The location of the typical inferior adenoma is more variable, but usually it lies close to the caudal tip of the lower pole of the thyroid. Most of these inferior adenomas are adjacent to the posterior aspect, and the rest are in the soft tissues 1 to 2 cm inferior to the thyroid (Fig. 24-9). After one side of the neck has been surveyed, a similar survey is conducted of the opposite side. However, 1% to 3% of parathyroid adenomas are ectopic and will not be found in typical locations adjacent to the thyroid. The four most common ectopic locations will be considered separately.

Retrotracheal Adenoma

The most common location of an ectopic superior adenoma is deep in the neck, posterior or posterolateral to the trachea (Fig. 24-10). Superior adenomas tend to enlarge between posterior tissue planes that extend to-

ward the posterior mediastinum. Acoustic shadowing from air in the trachea can make evaluation of this area difficult. Often, the adenoma protrudes slightly from behind the trachea, and a portion of the mass will be visible. Having the patient turn his or her head to the opposite side will accentuate the protrusion and provide better accessibility to the retrotracheal area. The transducer should be angled medially from the opposite side of the neck to visualize the tissues posterior to the trachea. This process is then repeated from the other side of the neck to visualize the contralateral aspect of the retrotracheal area. This process is analogous to the procedure in which the surgeon runs a fingertip behind the trachea in an attempt to palpate a retrotracheal adenoma.

Maximal turning of the head also often causes the esophagus to move to the opposite side of the trachea as it becomes compressed between the trachea and the cervical spine. If one sees the esophagus move completely to protruding from behind one side of the trachea to

protruding from the opposite side during maximal head turning, it has effectively "swept" the retrotracheal space and would have pushed any parathyroid adenoma in this location out from behind the trachea.

Mediastinal Adenoma

The most common location for ectopic inferior parathyroid adenomas is low within the neck or in the anterosuperior mediastinum (Fig. 24-11).[32] Parathyroid adenomas are sufficiently hypoechoic that they usually can be visualized as discrete structures separate from the thymus and surrounding tissues. To visualize this area optimally, the patient's neck is hyperextended maximally. With this technique and the transducer angled posteriorly and caudal to the clavicular heads, sonographic visualization is often possible inferiorly to the level of the thymus and innominate veins. If the adenoma lies caudal to this level or far anterior, just deep to the sternum, it cannot be visualized sonographically.

When an ectopic superior adenoma lies in the mediastinum, it usually is in the posterosuperior region. These adenomas tend to stay in a more posterior plane than the inferior adenomas and lie quite deep in the low neck or upper mediastinum, requiring use of a 5.0 MHz transducer for maximal penetration. These adenomas may be intimately associated with the posterior aspect of the trachea, and the head-turning maneuver described for retrotracheal adenomas can be applied here as well. With the patient's neck hyperextended and the transducer angled caudally, the posterior mediastinum sometimes can be visualized to the level of the apex of the arch of the aorta. Adenomas caudal to this level cannot be visualized sonographically.

Intrathyroid Adenoma

Intrathyroid adenomas are uncommon and, when present, usually are inferior adenomas.[33-35] Most intrathyroid adenomas are in the posterior half of the middle to lower pole of the thyroid, are completely surrounded by thyroid tissue, and are oriented with their greatest dimension in the cephalad-caudad direction (Fig. 24-12). Intrathyroid adenomas may be overlooked at the time of operation because they are soft and are similar to surrounding thyroid on palpation. A thyroidotomy or subtotal lobectomy may be needed to find an intrathyroid adenoma. Sonographically, however, parathyroid adenomas usually are well visualized because they are hypoechoic, in contrast to the echogenic thyroid parenchyma. The internal architecture and appearance of these adenomas are the same as those of adenomas elsewhere in the neck. Sonographically, intrathyroid parathyroid adenomas can be similar to thyroid nodules in appearance, and percutaneous biopsy often is necessary to distinguish between these entities.

Some superior and inferior adenomas may lie under

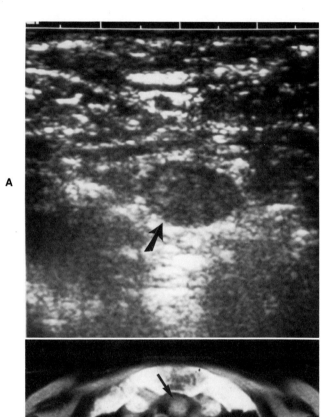

FIG 24-11. Ectopic adenoma—anterosuperior mediastinum. **A,** Transverse sonogram angled caudal to the clavicles showing a 1 cm ectopic inferior oval parathyroid adenoma *(arrow)* in the soft tissues of the anterosuperior mediastinum. **B,** CT scan of the upper mediastinum, showing the ectopic adenoma *(arrow)* in the anterosuperior mediastinum deep to the manubrium, adjacent to the great vessels.

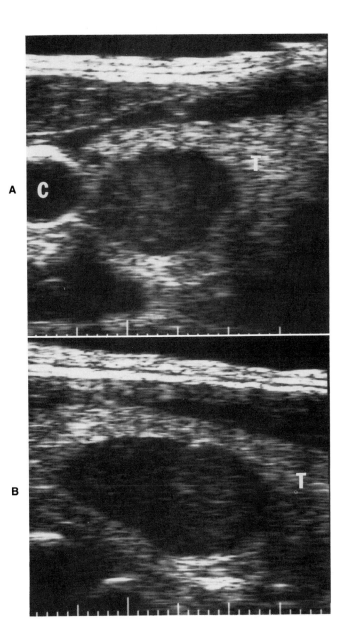

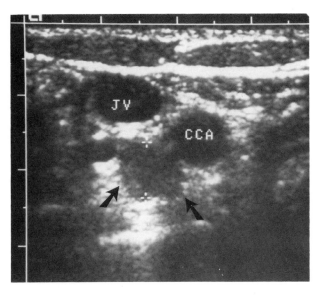

FIG 24-13. Ectopic adenoma—carotid sheath. Transverse sonogram of the right side of the neck, showing an 8 mm ectopic parathyroid adenoma *(arrows)* that was within the carotid sheath at operation, posterior to the internal jugular vein *(JV)* and common carotid artery *(CCA)*.

Carotid Sheath/Undescended Gland

Rare ectopic adenomas can lie in a high position superior and lateral in the neck, near the carotid bifurcation at the level of the hyoid bone or attached to the carotid sheath along the course of the common carotid artery (Fig. 24-13).[36,37] These adenomas probably arise from inferior glands that are embryologically undescended or partially descended and come to reside within or adjacent to the carotid sheath that surrounds the carotid artery, jugular vein, and vagus nerve. These adenomas frequently are overlooked at operation unless the surgeon specifically opens the carotid sheath and dissects within it.[5,6,38] Sonographically, these masses can appear similar to mildly enlarged lymph nodes in the jugular chain, and percutaneous biopsy often is necessary for confirmation.

Treatment

In symptomatic patients with primary hyperparathyroidism the treatment of choice is surgical excision of the involved parathyroid gland or glands. Some controversy exists as to whether asymptomatic patients with minimal hypercalcemia should be treated surgically or followed medically with frequent evaluations of renal function, bone density, and serum calcium level. In one prospective study of 147 asymptomatic patients with a provisional diagnosis of hyperparathyroidism and serum calcium levels less than 11 mg/dl, on clinical follow-up 20% needed operation within 5 years because of progression of their disease.[29,39] Therefore, on the basis of

FIG 24-12. Ectopic adenoma—intrathyroid adenoma. **A,** Transverse and **B,** longitudinal sonograms of the right neck, showing a 2 cm oval intrathyroid parathyroid adenoma completely surrounded by thyroid tissue. This occult adenoma was not palpable at the time of two failed neck operations. *T,* Thyroid; *C,* common carotid artery.

the pseudocapsule or sheath that covers the thyroid gland or within a sulcus of the thyroid, but these are not usually considered to be true intrathyroid adenomas. These adenomas may be difficult for the surgeon to visualize at the time of operation unless this sheath is opened.[7,33] Sonographically, these adenomas appear the same as other parathyroid adenomas that lie immediately adjacent to the thyroid.

this study and others, surgical treatment usually is advised for asymptomatic patients as well as symptomatic patients, as the definitive treatment of hyperparathyroidism.[40,41] The surgical cure rate by an experienced surgeon is greater than 95%, and the morbidity and mortality rates are extremely low.[42]

PERSISTENT OR RECURRENT HYPERPARATHYROIDISM

Persistent hyperparathyroidism is persistence of hypercalcemia after a previous failed parathyroid operation. This is frequently due to an undiscovered ectopic parathyroid adenoma or unrecognized multiple gland enlargement and failure to resect all of the hyperfunctioning tissue at the operation. **Recurrent hyperparathyroidism** is defined as hypercalcemia occurring after a 6-month interval of normocalcemia resulting from the development of a hyperfunctioning parathyroid gland or glands from previously normal glands.[43] It is often seen in patients with unrecognized MEN I. In reoperated patients the surgical cure rate is approximately 10% to 30% lower than initial surgery and, because of scarring and fibrosis from the previous operation, the morbidity of severe postoperative hypocalcemia and recurrent laryngeal nerve damage is up to 20 times higher.[44-49] During the sonographic evaluation of reoperative patients, specific attention is paid to the most likely ectopic parathyroid locations—those associated with a gland that was not discovered at the initial operation.

A small subgroup of patients in whom recurrent hyperparathyroidism develops postoperatively have undergone previous autotransplantation of parathyroid tissue in conjunction with previous total parathyroidectomy.[50-52] In this procedure, a parathyroid gland is sliced into fragments that are inserted into surgically prepared intramuscular pockets in the forearm or sternocleidomastoid muscle. Up to 20% of patients with this type of parathyroid transplantation will develop graft-dependent hypercalcemia.[53] Usually these autotransplanted fragments are too small and too similar in echotexture to the surrounding muscle to be visualized adequately on sonographic examination, but occasionally they can be identified. Regardless of the success of preoperative localization studies, the autotransplanted fragments usually are readily found by the surgeon with the patient under local anesthesia, and a portion of the grafted tissue can be excised to cure the hypercalcemia.

SECONDARY HYPERPARATHYROIDISM

Secondary hyperparathyroidism characteristically is found in patients with chronic renal failure. These patients are unable to synthesize the active form of vitamin D and therefore have chronic hypocalcemia, which results in parathyroid hyperplasia. If untreated, secondary hyperparathyroidism can result in bone demineralization, soft tissue calcification, and acceleration of vascular calcification. Surgical treatment for secondary hyperparathyroidism is uncommon because of the success of dialysis therapy; however, in symptomatic patients who are refractory to dialysis and medical therapy, subtotal parathyroidectomy or total parathyroidectomy with autotransplantation is indicated.[54-57] Sonography is sometimes used in these patients to aid in localization of the enlarged parathyroid glands preoperatively.[58]

ACCURACY

The sensitivity of sonographic parathyroid adenoma localization in primary hyperparathyroidism has been reported to be between 70% and 80%.[24,59-65] Accurate preoperative localization can shorten preoperative evaluation and operative time and thus decrease potential morbidity, particularly in the high-risk patient.[66-69] Parathyroid sonography can be very useful in a patient with severe life-threatening hypercalcemic crisis because prompt visualization of the adenoma can shorten the evaluation necessary before urgent surgery.[69] Finally, when the biochemical diagnosis of hypercalcemia is not clear, the sonographic demonstration of an adenoma helps to confirm the likely diagnosis of hyperparathyroidism.

In persistent or recurrent hyperparathyroidism, the sensitivity of sonography in adenoma localization has been between 36% and 56%.[70-72] Localization studies are clearly indicated because of the lower surgical success rate and the higher morbidity of reoperations. In a recent series[73] of 157 patients who had undergone reexploration for persistent or recurrent hyperparathyroidism, the surgical cure rate was 89%, and it was thought that prospective localization studies contributed to this success. Also, when the adenoma was localized preoperatively, the time of operation was decreased.

Because most persistent and recurrent parathyroid adenomas are accessible in the neck or upper mediastinum via a cervical incision rather than a sternotomy, sonographic examination of the neck is the initial localizing procedure of choice in this setting.[72,74] Other methods that have been used commonly for parathyroid adenoma localization when sonography is negative are CT and thallium 201/technetium-99m subtraction scintigraphy; less commonly used methods are MRI, angiography, and venous sampling.[75-80] In the patient being considered for reoperation, CT and scintigraphy may be useful if sonography is negative, particularly for evaluation of the portion of the mediastinum and retrotracheal areas that are not well seen by sonography. Angiography and venous sampling are more invasive, more expensive, and more technically demanding than CT and scintigraphy and are being used in a decreasing number of centers. These procedures also can be associated with an unacceptably high incidence of complications. MRI is noninvasive but relatively expensive, and it is questionable whether it adds information to what the other localizing methods provide.

PITFALLS IN INTERPRETATION
False-Positive Examination

Normal cervical structures, such as the perithyroid veins, the esophagus, and the longus colli muscles of the neck, can simulate parathyroid adenomas, producing false-positive results during neck sonography.

Perithyroid veins lie immediately adjacent to the posterior and lateral aspects of both lobes of the thyroid and, when one is tortuous or segmentally dilated, it can simulate a small parathyroid adenoma. Scanning maneuvers that help to establish that the structure in question is a vein, not an adenoma, include use of real-time imaging in multiple transverse, longitudinal, and oblique planes to show the tubular nature of the vein, Valsalva's maneuver by the patient, which may cause transient engorgement of the vein, and spectral or color Doppler imaging to show flow within the vein (Fig. 24-14).

The esophagus may partially protrude from behind the posterolateral aspect of the trachea and simulate a large parathyroid adenoma.[81] Turning the patient's head to the opposite side will accentuate the protrusion. Careful inspection of this structure in the transverse plane will show that it has the typical concentric ring appearance of bowel, with a peripheral hypoechoic muscular layer and a central echogenic mucosal/intraluminal contents layer. Using a longitudinal scan plane helps to demonstrate the tubular nature of this structure (Fig. 24-15). Real-time imaging while the patient swallows will cause a stream of brightly echogenic mucus and microbubbles to flow through the lumen, which confirms that the structure is esophagus.

The longus colli muscle lies adjacent to the anterolateral aspect of the cervical spine. If viewed in the transverse plane, it appears as a hypoechoic triangular mass that can simulate a large parathyroid adenoma located posterior to the thyroid gland. However, scanning in the longitudinal plane will show that this structure is long and flat and contains longitudinal echogenic striations that are typical of skeletal muscle (Fig. 24-16). Real-time imaging while the patient swallows can be useful because swallowing will cause movement of the thyroid gland and perithyroid structures, such as a parathyroid adenoma, but the longus colli muscle, which is attached to the spine, will remain stationary. Finally, comparison with the opposite side of the neck will demonstrate similar symmetric findings because the longus colli muscles are paired structures located on both sides of the cervical spine.

Pathologic structures that are potential causes of false-positive results include thyroid nodules and cervical lymph nodes.[24,82] Thyroid nodules can be visualized sonographically in up to 40% of patients undergo-

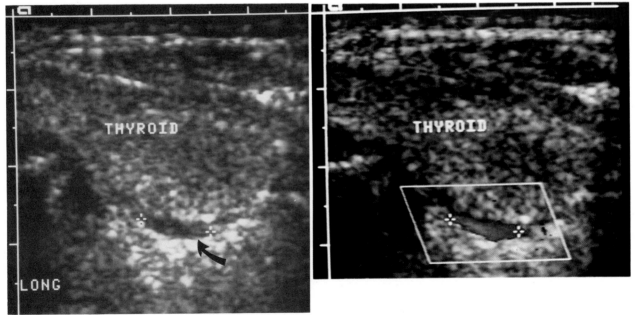

FIG 24-14. Parithyroid vein simulates parathyroid adenoma. **A,** Longitudinal sonogram, showing an 8 mm oval hypoechoic structure *(arrow)* adjacent to the posterior aspect of the thyroid; the structure is suspected to be a parathyroid adenoma. **B,** Color Doppler sonogram, showing flow throughout the lumen of the structure, demonstrating that it is a perithyroid vein.

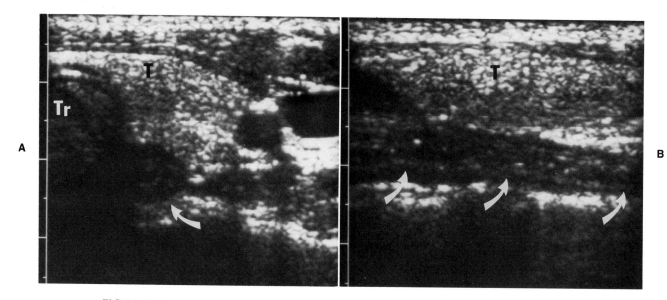

FIG 24-15. Esophagus simulates parathyroid adenoma. **A,** Transverse sonogram of the left neck, showing an 8 mm round hypoechoic structure *(arrow),* located posterior to the thyroid *(T)* and posterolateral to the trachea *(Tr);* the structure is suspected to be a parathyroid adenoma. **B,** Left parasagittal sonogram, showing that the structure is tubular *(arrows)* and contains fluid and echogenic foci in its lumen and therefore is the esophagus. *T,* Thyroid.

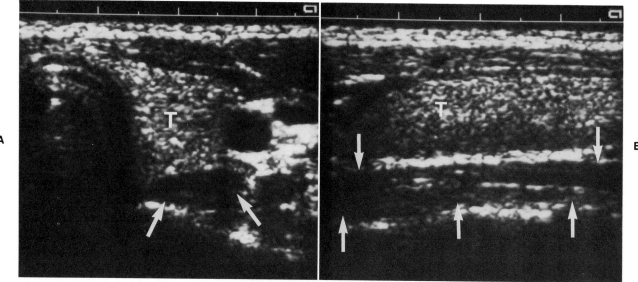

FIG 24-16. Longus colli muscle simulates parathyroid adenoma. **A,** Transverse sonogram of the left neck, showing a 1 cm triangular hypoechoic structure *(arrows)* posterior to the left lobe of the thyroid *(T);* the structure is suspected to be a parathyroid adenoma. **B,** Left parasagittal longitudinal sonogram showing that the structure is elongated and flat with echogenic striations typical of the longus colli muscle *(arrows).*

ing sonographic examinations of the neck for parathyroid disease. If a thyroid nodule protrudes from the posterior aspect of the thyroid, it can simulate a mass in the location of a parathyroid adenoma. One sign that can be useful in this situation is a thin echogenic line that separates the parathyroid adenoma (which arises outside of the thyroid gland) from the thyroid gland itself. Thyroid nodules, which arise from within the thyroid gland, do not show this tissue plane of separation.[59] Morphologically, thyroid nodules unlike parathyroid adenomas are often partially cystic and some are calcified. Also, thyroid nodules often are of a heterogeneous, mixed echogenicity, whereas parathyroid adenomas are of a homogeneous, hypoechoic echogenicity. When a parathyroid adenoma cannot be distinguished from a thyroid nodule by imaging criteria, percutaneous biopsy may be necessary.

Enlarged cervical lymph nodes have an oval, hypoechoic appearance like parathyroid adenomas, but they often also have a central echogenic band or hilum composed of fat, vessels, and fibrous tissue, which is a feature that distinguishes them from parathyroid adenomas.[83] Sonographically visible cervical lymph nodes usually lie laterally in the neck in the internal jugular chain adjacent to the jugular vein away from the thyroid. Occasionally, however, parathyroid adenomas can be found laterally in the neck in the carotid sheath, particularly in the reoperative setting, and percutaneous biopsy may be necessary to distinguish parathyroid adenoma from lymph node.

False-Negative Examination

The three major situations in which examinations give false-negative results are:

- Minimally enlarged adenomas
- Adenomas displaced posteriorly and obscured by a markedly enlarged thyroid goiter
- Ectopic adenomas

Minimally enlarged adenomas are a common cause of error because it can be difficult to distinguish these small masses from thyroid and adjacent soft tissues. Multinodular thyroid goiters interfere with parathyroid adenoma detection in two ways. First, the thyroid gland enlargement displaces structures located adjacent to the thyroid posteriorly, away from the transducer. This can necessitate the use of 5.0 MHz transducers rather than 7.5 MHz transducers to obtain the necessary penetration; this decreases spatial resolution. Second, thyroid goiters have a multinodular contour and irregular echotexture, which hinders the detection of adjacent parathyroid gland enlargement. Some ectopic adenomas, such as retrotracheal adenomas or adenomas located deep in the mediastinum, will be inaccessible and nonvisible because of acoustic shadowing from the overlying air and bone.

INTRAOPERATIVE SONOGRAPHY

Intraoperative sonography occasionally can be a useful adjunct in the surgical detection of parathyroid adenomas, particularly in the reoperative setting.[84,85] Intraoperative scanning can be performed, with a conventional high-frequency (7.5 to 10 MHz) transducer draped with a sterile plastic sheath or with a dedicated sterilized intraoperative transducer. Intraoperative sonography appears to be best suited for the localization of inferior and intrathyroid abnormal parathyroid glands. Superior abnormal glands are more difficult to detect.[85] If intraoperative sonography detects an abnormal parathyroid gland, operative time can be shortened. In most studies, however, intraoperative sonography has not affected the outcome of the operation.

PERCUTANEOUS BIOPSY

Sonographically guided percutaneous biopsy is being used more frequently for preoperative confirmation of suspected abnormal parathyroid glands, particularly in the patient who is a candidate for reoperation.[86-88] This technique has increased the specificity of sonography by permitting the reliable differentiation of parathyroid adenomas from other pathologic structures, such as thyroid nodules and cervical lymph nodes. A positive biopsy reassures the reluctant reoperative patient, in addition to its value to the surgeon.

If the suspected parathyroid adenoma is located in a location remote from the thyroid gland, then the main differential diagnostic consideration is a lymph node. Percutaneous biopsy is performed by using a small caliber, noncutting needle, such as a 25-gauge standard injection needle, to obtain an aspirate that is either parathyroid cells or lymphocytes (Fig. 24-17).[89] If the suspected parathyroid adenoma lies adjacent to the thyroid gland, a larger specimen (histologic specimen rather than cytologic specimen) may be necessary to differentiate parathyroid tissue from thyroid tissue.[90] A histologic specimen can be obtained with a small-caliber (21- to 25-gauge) cutting needle. The smallest caliber cutting needles are sometimes difficult to insert through the tough superficial soft tissue planes of the neck. Such a needle can be readily placed through a larger short noncutting needle inserted as an "introducer" through the superficial tissues. In addition to cytologic and histologic analyses, the aspirated fluid and blood can be diluted with 1 ml of saline and analyzed for PTH by radioimmunoassay.[91] High concentrations of PTH are unequivocal evidence of parathyroid tissue. There have been no reported complications of percutaneous needle biopsy of suspected parathyroid adenomas.

The accuracy of percutaneous biopsy in the differentiation of parathyroid gland from other structures was 87% in one series of 52 cases.[87] Biopsy failures were due to inadequate recovery of tissue.

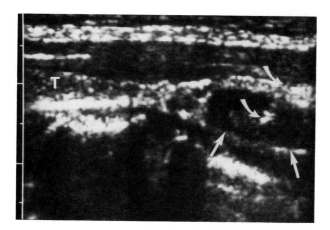

FIG 24-17. Percutaneous needle biopsy of parathyroid adenoma. Longitudinal sonogram, showing a 1.5 cm oval parathyroid adenoma *(straight arrows)* in the soft tissues of the low neck in a patient with recurrent hyperparathyroidism. Needle *(curved arrow)* biopsy obtained parathyroid cells, confirming that this mass was a parathyroid adenoma. *T,* Thyroid.

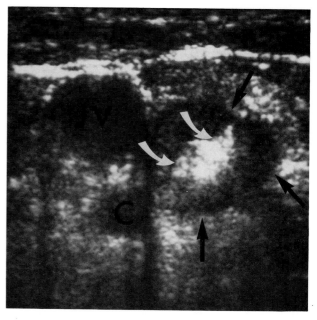

FIG 24-18. Alcohol ablation of parathyroid adenoma. Transverse sonogram, showing a 1.5 cm round parathyroid adenoma *(straight arrows)* low in the right neck in a patient with recurrent hyperparathyroidism who was not a surgical candidate because of poor cardiac function. Under sonographic guidance, ethanol was injected into multiple areas of the adenoma, which caused the tissues adjacent to the needle-tip to become transiently brightly echogenic *(curved arrows). JV,* Jugular vein; *C,* common carotid artery.

ALCOHOL ABLATION

Sonography has been used to guide percutaneous injection of ethanol into abnormally enlarged parathyroid glands for chemical ablation (Fig. 24-18).[92-95] Currently, alcohol ablation is not used routinely in the treatment of patients with primary hyperparathyroidism, but it is reserved as an alternative therapy for patients who are not surgical candidates, who refuse surgery, or who present with life-threatening malignant hypercalcemia in an emergency situation.[96]

Alcohol ablation is performed under local anesthesia after a percutaneous biopsy has confirmed the presence of parathyroid tissue or an increased PTH content in the tissue. A small (22- to 25-gauge) needle is inserted into multiple regions of the mass and 96% ethanol is injected in a volume equal to approximately half the volume of the mass. Under real-time visualization, at the moment of injection the tissue becomes highly echogenic, probably because of microbubbles within the alcohol. This echogenicity slowly disappears over a period of approximately 1 minute. The injections are repeated every other day until the serum calcium level reaches the normal range. In most cases, three to five injections are necessary.

The results of alcohol injection as a treatment for hyperparathyroidism have been promising. In a recent series[94] of 18 patients with primary hyperparathyroidism who underwent percutaneous alcohol ablation, two thirds were cured or showed improvement in their biochemical or clinical status at 6 months or more after the procedure. In one series of 12 patients[95] with secondary hyperparathyroidism, 7 had clinical and biochemical improvement. The adverse effects from ethanol ablation in these two series with a total of 30 patients, were limited to transient vocal cord paralysis in 4 patients and permanent vocal cord paralysis in 1 patient.

REFERENCES
Embryology and anatomy

1. Gilmour JR: The gross anatomy of the parathyroid glands. *J Pathol* 1938;46:133-148.
2. Weller GL Jr: Development of the thyroid, parathyroid and thymus glands in man. *Carnegie Institution of Washington: contributions to embryology,* 1933;24(141):93-139.
3. Akerstrom G, Malmaeus J, Bergstrom R: Surgical anatomy of human parathyroid glands. *Surgery* 1984;95:14-21.
4. Edis AJ: Surgical anatomy and technique of neck exploration for primary hyperparathyroidism. *Surg Clin North Am* 1977;57:495-504.
5. Thompson NW, Eckhauser FE, Harness JK: The anatomy of primary hyperparathyroidism. *Surgery* 1982;92:814-821.
6. Edis AJ, Purnell DC, van Heerden JA: The undescended "parathymus". An occasional cause of failed neck exploration for hyperparathyroidism. *Ann Surg* 1979;190:64-68.
7. Wang C-A: The anatomic basis of parathyroid surgery. *Ann Surg* 1976;183:271-275.
8. Norris EH: The parathyroid glands and the lateral thyroid in man: their morphogenesis, histogenesis, topographic anatomy and prenatal growth. *Carnegie Institution of Washington: Contributions to Embryology* 1937;26(159):247-294.

9. Castleman B, Roth SI: Tumors of the parathyroid glands. In *Atlas of tumor pathology*. Fascicle 14, 2nd series. Washington, DC: *Armed Forces Institute of Pathology;* 1978.

10. Russell CF, Grant CS, van Heerden JA: Hyperfunctioning supernumerary parathyroid glands: an occasional cause of hyperparathyroidism. *Mayo Clin Proc* 1982;57:121-124.

Primary hyperparathyroidism

11. Heath H III, Hodgson SF, Kennedy MA: Primary hyperparathyroidism: incidence, morbidity, and potential economic impact in a community. *N Engl J Med* 1980;302:189-193.

12. Van Heerden JA, Beahrs OH, Woolner LB: The pathology and surgical management of primary hyperparathyroidism. *Surg Clin North Am* 1977;57:557-563.

13. Wang CA: Surgery of the parathyroid glands. *Adv Surg* 1966;5:109-127.

14. Black WC III, Utley JR: The differential diagnosis of parathyroid adenoma and chief cell hyperplasia. *Am J Clin Pathol* 1968;49:761-775.

15. Prinz RA, Gamvros OI, Sellu D, et al: Subtotal parathyroidectomy for primary chief cell hyperplasia of the multiple endocrine neoplasia type I syndrome. *Ann Surg* 1981;193:26-29.

16. Van Heerden JA, Kent RB III, Sizemore GW, et al: Primary hyperparathyroidism in patients with multiple endocrine neoplasia syndromes. *Arch Surg* 1983;118:533-535.

17. Weiland LH: Practical endocrine surgical pathology. In: van Heerden JA, editor. *Common problems in endocrine surgery*. Chicago: Year Book Medical Publishers, Inc; 1989.

18. Schantz A, Castleman B: Parathyroid carcinoma: a study of 70 cases. *Cancer* 1973;31:600-605.

19. Castleman B, Roth SI: Tumors of the parathyroid glands. In *Atlas of Tumor Pathology*. Fascicle 14, 2nd series. Washington DC: Armed Forces Institute of Pathology; 1978.

20. Shane E, Bilezikian JP: Parathyroid carcinoma: a review of 62 patients. *Endocr Rev* 1982;3:218-226.

21. Holmes EC, Morton DL, Ketcham AS: Parathyroid carcinoma: a collective review. *Ann Surg* 1969;169:631-640.

Sonographic appearance

22. Graif M, Itzchak Y, Strauss S, et al: Parathyroid sonography: diagnostic accuracy related to shape, location and texture of the gland. *Br J Radiol* 1987;60:439-443.

23. Randel SB, Gooding GAW, Clark OH, et al: Parathyroid variants: ultrasound evaluation. *Radiology* 1987;165:191-194.

24. Reading CC, Charboneau JW, James EM, et al: High-resolution parathyroid sonography. *AJR* 1982;139:539-546.

25. Obara T, Fujimoto Y, Ito Y, et al: Functioning parathyroid lipoadenoma—report of four cases: clinicopathological and ultrasonographic features. *Endocrinol Jpn* 1989;36:135-145.

26. Lack EF, Clark MA, Buck DR, et al: Cysts of the parathyroid gland: report of two cases and review of the literature. *Am Surg* 1978;44:376-381.

27. Krudy AG, Doppman JL, Shawker TH, et al: Hyperfunctioning cystic parathyroid glands: computed tomography and sonographic findings. *AJR* 1984;142:175-178.

28. Calliada F, Bergonzi M, Passamonti C, et al: Il contributo del color Doppler nello studio ecografico delle ghiandole paratiroidi iperplasiche. *Radiol Med (Torino);* 1989;78(6):607-611.

29. Purnell DC, Smith LH, Scholz DA, et al: Primary hyperparathyroidism: a prospective clinical study. *Am J Med* 1971;50:670-678.

30. Daly BD, Coffey SL, Behan M: Ultrasonographic appearances of parathyroid carcinoma. *Br J Radiol* 1989;62:1017-1019.

31. Edmonson GR, Charboneau JW, James EM, et al: Parathyroid carcinoma: high-frequency sonographic features. *Radiology* 1986;161:65-67.

Adenoma localization

32. Clark OH: Mediastinal parathyroid tumors. *Arch Surg* 1988;123:1096-1099.

33. Thompson NW: The techniques of initial parathyroid exploration and reoperative parathyroidectomy. In: Thompson NW, Vinik AI, editors: *Endocrine Surgery Update*. New York: Grune & Stratton; 1983.

34. Al-Suhaili AR, Lynn J, Lavender JP: Intrathyroidal parathyroid adenoma: preoperative identification and localization by parathyroid imaging. *Clin Nucl Med* 1988;13:512-514.

35. Spiegel AM, Marx SJ, Doppman JL, et al: Intrathyroidal parathyroid adenoma or hyperplasia; an occasionally overlooked cause of surgical failure in primary hyperparathyroidism. *JAMA* 1975;234:1029-1033.

36. Fraker DL, Doppman JL, Shawker TH, et al: Undescended parathyroid adenoma: an important etiology for failed operations for primary hyperparathyroidism. *World J Surg* 1990;14:342-348.

37. Doppman JL, Shawker TH, Krudy AG, et al: Parathymic parathyroid: computed tomography, ultrasound and angiographic findings. *Radiology* 1985;157:419-423.

38. Kurtay M, Crile G Jr: Aberrant parathyroid gland in relationship to the thymus. *Am J Surg.* 1969;117:705.

39. Purnell DC, Scholz DA, Smith LH, et al: Treatment of primary hyperparathyroidism. *Am J Med* 1974;56:800-809.

40. Kaplan RA, Snyder WH, Stewart A, et al: Metabolic effects of parathyroidectomy in asymptomatic primary hyperparathyroidism. *J Clin Endocrinol Metab* 1976;42:415-426.

41. Gaz RD, Wang CA: Management of asymptomatic hyperparathyroidism. *Am J Surg* 1984;147:498-501.

42. Clark OH, Duh QY: Primary hyperparathyroidism: a surgical perspective. *Endocrinol Metab Clin North Am* 1989;18:701-714.

Persistent or recurrent hyperparathyroidism

43. Clark OH, Way LW, Hunt TK: Recurrent hyperparathyroidism. *Ann Surg* 1976;184:391-399.

44. Levin KE, Clark OH: The reasons for failure in parathyroid operations. *Arch Surg* 1989;124:911-914.

45. Cheung PSY, Borgstrom A, Thompson NW: Strategy in reoperative surgery for hyperparathyroidism. *Arch Surg* 1989;124:676-680.

46. Palmer JA, Rosen IB: Reoperative surgery for hyperparathyroidism. *Am J Surg* 1982;144:406-410.

47. Prinz RA, Gamvros OI, Allison DJ, et al: Reoperations for hyperparathyroidism. *Surg Gynecol Obstet* 1981;152:760-764.

48. Grant CS, Charboneau JW, James EM, et al: Reoperative parathyroid surgery. *Wien Klin Wochenschr* 1988;100:360-363.

49. Brennan MF, Marx SJ, Doppman J, et al: Results of reoperation for persistent and recurrent hyperparathyroidism. *Ann Surg* 1981;194:671-676.

50. Wells SA Jr, Ellis GJ, Gunnells JC, et al: Parathyroid autotransplantation in primary parathyroid hyperplasia. *N Engl J Med* 1976;295:57-62.

51. Edis AJ, Linos DA, Kao PC: Parathyroid autotransplantation at the time of reoperation for persistent hyperparathyroidism. *Surgery* 1980;88:588-592.

52. Brunt LM, Sicard GA: Current status of parathyroid autotransplantation. *Semin Surg Oncol* 1990;6:115-121.

53. Brunt LM, Wells SA Jr: Parathyroid transplantation: Indications and results. In: van Herrden JA, editor. *Common Problems in Endocrine Surgery*. Chicago: Year Book Medical Publishers; 1989.

Secondary hyperparathyroidism

54. Wilson RE, Hampers CL, Bernstein DS, et al: Subtotal parathyroidectomy in chronic renal failure: a seven-year experience in a dialysis and transplant program. *Ann Surg* 1971;174:640-652.

55. Diethelm AG, Adams PL, Murad TM, et al: Treatment of secondary hyperparathyroidism in patients with chronic renal failure by total parathyroidectomy and parathyroid autograft. *Ann Surg* 1981;193:777-791.

56. Reid DJ. Surgical treatment of secondary and tertiary hyperparathyroidism. *Br J Clin Pract* 1989;43:68-70.

57. Leapman SB, Filo RS, Thomalla JV, King D: Secondary hyperparathyroidism. The role of surgery. *Am Surg* 1989;55:359-365.

58. Takebayashi S, Matsui K, Onohara Y, et al: Sonography for early diagnosis of enlarged parathyroid glands in patients with secondary hyperparathyroidism. *AJR* 1987;148:911-914.

Accuracy

59. Scheible W, Deutsch AL, Leopold GR: Parathyroid adenoma: accuracy of preoperative localization by high-resolution real-time sonography. *J Clin Ultrasound* 1981;9:325-330.

60. Simeone JF, Mueller PR, Ferrucci JT Jr, et al. High-resolution real-time sonography of the parathyroid. *Radiology* 1981;141:745-751.

61. Kobayashi S, Miyakawa M, Kasuga Y, et al: Parathyroid imaging comparison of 201 TI-99 mTc subtraction scintigraphy, computed tomography, and ultrasonography. *Jpn J Surg* 1987;17:9-13.

62. Buchwach KA, Mangum WB, Hahn FW Jr: Preoperative localization of parathyroid adenomas. *Laryngoscope* 1987;97:13-15.

63. Attie JN, Khan A, Rumancik WM, et al: Preoperative localization of parathyroid adenomas. *Am J Surg* 1988;156:323-326.

64. Erdman WA, Breslau NA, Weinreb JC, et al: Noninvasive localization of parathyroid adenomas: a comparison of x-ray, computed tomography, ultrasound, scintigraphy and magnetic resonance imaging. *Magn Reson Imaging* 1989;7:187-194.

65. Summers GW, Dodge DL, Kammer H: Accuracy and cost-effectiveness of preoperative isotope and ultrasound imaging in primary hyperparathyroidism. *Otolaryngol Head Neck Surg* 1989;100:210-217.

66. Wu DTD, Shaw JHF: The use of pre-operative scan prior to neck exploration for primary hyperparathyroidism. *Aust N Z J Surg* 1988;58:35-38.

67. Brewer WH, Walsh JW, Newsome HH Jr: Impact of sonography on surgery for primary hyperparathyroidism. *Am J Surg* 1983;145:270-272.

68. Russell CFJ, Laird JD, Ferguson WR: Scan-directed unilateral cervical exploration for parathyroid adenoma: a legitimate approach? *World J Surg* 1990;14:406-409.

69. Windeck R, Olbricht TH, Littmann K, et al: Halessonographie in der hypercalamischen Krise. *Dtsch Med Wochenschr* 1985;110:368-370.

70. Levin KE, Gooding GAW, Okerlund M, et al: Localizing studies in patients with persistent or recurrent hyperparathyroidism. *Surgery* 1988;102:917-924.

71. Miller DL, Doppman JL, Shawker TH, et al: Localization of parathyroid adenomas in patients who have undergone surgery. Part I. Noninvasive imaging methods. *Radiology* 1987;162:133-137.

72. Reading CC, Charboneau JW, James EM, et al: Postoperative parathyroid high-frequency sonography: evaluation of persistent or recurrent hyperparathyroidism. *AJR* 1985;144:399-402.

73. Grant CS, van Heerden JA, Charboneau JW, et al: Clinical management of persistent and/or recurrent primary hyperparathyroidism. *World J Surg* 1986;10:555-565.

74. Wang CA: Parathyroid re-exploration: a clinical and pathological study of 112 cases. *Ann Surg* 1977;186:140-145.

75. Sommer B, Welter HF, Spelsberg F, et al: Computed tomography for localizing enlarged parathyroid glands in primary hyperparathyroidism. *J Comput Assist Tomogr* 1982;6:521-526.

76. Stark DD, Gooding GAW, Moss AA, et al: Parathyroid imaging: comparison of high-resolution computed tomography and high-resolution sonography. *AJR* 1983;141:633-638.

77. Okerlund MD, Sheldon K, Corpuz S, et al: A new method with high sensitivity and specificity for localization of abnormal parathyroid glands. *Ann Surg* 1984;200:381-387.

78. Ferlin G, Borsato N, Camerani M, et al: New perspectives in localizing enlarged parathyroids by technetium-thallium subtraction scan. *J Nucl Med* 1983;24:438-441.

79. Krudy AG, Doppman JL, Miller DL, et al: Work in progress: Abnormal parathyroid glands: comparison of nonselective arterial digital arteriography, selective parathyroid angiography, and venous digital arteriography as methods of detection. *Radiology* 1983;148:23-29.

80. Krudy AG, Doppman JL, Miller DL, et al: Detection of mediastinal parathyroid glands by nonselective digital arteriography. *AJR* 1984;142:693-695.

Pitfalls in interpretation

81. Ngo C, Sarti DA. Simulation of the normal esophagus by a parathyroid adenoma. *J Clin Ultrasound* 1987;15:421-424.

82. Karstrup S, Hegedus L: Concomitant thyroid disease in hyperparathyroidism: reasons for unsatisfactory ultrasonographical localization of parathyroid glands. *Eur J Radiol* 1986;6:149-152.

83. Sutton RT, Reading CC, Charboneau JW, et al: US-guided biopsy of neck masses in postoperative management of patients with thyroid cancer. *Radiology* 1988;168:769-772.

Intraoperative sonography

84. Kern KA, Shawker TH, Doppman JL, et al: The use of high-resolution ultrasound to locate parathyroid tumors during reoperations for primary hyperparathyroidism. *World J Surg* 1987;11:579-585.

85. Norton JA, Shawker TH, Jones BL, et al: Intraoperative ultrasound and reoperative parathyroid surgery: an initial evaluation. *World J Surg* 1986;10:631-638.

Percutaneous biopsy

86. Gooding GAW, Clark OH, Stark DD, et al: Parathyroid aspiration biopsy under ultrasound guidance in the postoperative hyperparathyroid patient. *Radiology* 1985;155:193-196.

87. Solbiati L, Montali G, Croce F, et al: Parathyroid tumors detected by fine-needle aspiration biopsy under ultrasonic guidance. *Radiology* 1983;148:793-797.

88. Charboneau JW, Grant CS, James EM, et al: High-resolution ultrasound-guided percutaneous needle biopsy and intraoperative ultrasonography of a cervical parathyroid adenoma in a patient persistent hyperparathyroidism. *Mayo Clin Proc* 1983;58:497-500.

89. Glenthos A, Karstrup S: Parathyroid identification by ultrasonically guided aspiration cytology. Is correct cytological identification possible? *APMIS* 1989;97:497-502.

90. Karstrup S, Glenthoj A, Hainau B, et al: Ultrasound-guided, histological, fine-needle biopsy from suspect parathyroid tumors: success-rate and reliability of histological diagnosis. *Br J Radiol* 1989;62:981-985.

91. Doppman JL, Krudy AG, Marx SJ, et al: Aspiration of enlarged parathyroid glands for parathyroid hormone assay. *Radiology* 1983;148:31-35.

Alcohol ablation

92. Charboneau JW, Hay ID, van Heerden JA: Persistent primary hyperparathyroidism: successful ultrasound-guided percutaneous ethanol ablation of an occult adenoma. *Mayo Clinic Proc* 1988;63:913-917.

93. Karstrup S, Holm HH, Glenthoj A, et al: Nonsurgical treatment of primary hyperparathyroidism with sonographically guided percutaneous injection of ethanol: results in a selected series of patients. *AJR* 1990;154:1087-1090.

94. Karstrup S, Transbol I, Holm HH, et al: Ultrasound-guided chemical parathyroidectomy in patients with primary hyperparathyroidism: A prospective study. *Br J Radiol* 1989;62:1037-1042.

95. Solbiati L, Giangrande A, DePra L, et al: Percutaneous ethanol injection of parathyroid tumors under ultrasound guidance: treatment for secondary hyperparathyroidism. *Radiology* 1985;155:607-610.

96. Karstrup S, Lohela P, Apaja-Sarkkinen M, et al: Non-operative hypercalcemic crisis. *Acta Med Scand* 1988;224:187-188.

CHAPTER 25

Breast Sonography

- Ellen B. Mendelson, M.D.

Mammography is currently the most important breast imaging method. Other diagnostic studies include sonography, spectral and color-flow Doppler imaging, computed tomography (CT), magnetic resonance imaging (MRI), light scanning, and thermography. With the exception of sonography, most of these techniques have limited applications. In the last 10 to 20 years, sonography has secured an important place in the diagnosis and management of breast disease.

There are two different levels of approach to breast evaluation:

- Screening for breast carcinoma
- Diagnosis and management of benign and malignant breast disease

The sole purpose of screening is the identification of breast carcinoma; early detection has resulted in an increased survival rate.[1] The effectiveness of screening programs relies on the sensitivity and accuracy of the examinations, which should be widely available, affordable, and of documented high benefit and low risk.

Breast sonography is unsuited to breast cancer screening, as many studies using both older and state-of-the-art automated and handheld equipment suggest.[2,3] Microcalcifications, an important sign of early breast cancer, are depicted inconsistently, and masses may not be readily differentiated from surrounding isoechoic fat lobules.[4] As a screening examination, breast sonography is also highly operator- and technique-dependent, time consuming, and costly. Most important, sonography is not reliable in detecting occult, nonpalpable breast carcinoma.[3,5]

The breast symptoms of pain and mass are frequently manifestations of normal cyclical changes and benign disease such as cysts, adenosis, and inflammatory processes. These symptoms often are due to physiologic changes and become more worrisome as women enter the age of higher incidence of breast carcinoma. Here, breast sonography makes its greatest contribution in diagnosis and management and is invaluable in identifying lesions and characterizing masses as cystic or solid.

A breast center should have state-of-the-art equipment, and its staff should have the time and ability to integrate the techniques to complete the workup expeditiously. The mammographic studies should be monitored and supplemented with ultrasound and interventional procedures as needed. In deciding to use breast sonography, the radiologist must consider its potential to enhance the mammographic interpretation or alter patient management.[6] Other imaging techniques may also be of value. CT is helpful in demonstrating lesions located far posteriorly and peripherally in the breast and in staging breast cancer by identifying metastatic disease in the thorax and axilla.[7] In the future, MRI may play a role in the evaluation of breast disease.[8,9]

INDICATIONS

The indications for breast sonography are[5,10,11]:

- To characterize mammographic or palpable masses as cystic or solid

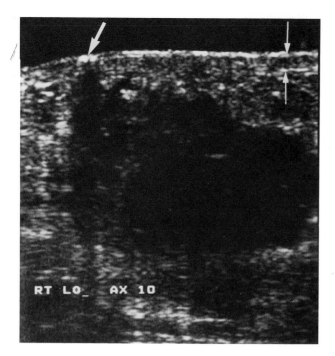

FIG 25-1. Postpartum breast abscess. Hypoechoic, poorly marginated heterogeneous mass within parenchyma of breast. Skin is thickened *(thin arrows)*, and there is small echogenic focus *(arrow)* in subcutaneous tissues consistent with small bubble of gas. Abscess was subsequently drained.

- To evaluate palpable masses in young (under the age of 30 years), pregnant, and lactating patients (Fig. 25-1)
- To evaluate nonpalpable abnormalities for which the mammographic diagnosis is uncertain
- To help exclude a mass in an area of mammographic asymmetric density
- To confirm or better visualize a lesion seen incompletely or on only one mammographic projection (e.g., near the chest wall)
- To guide interventional procedures such as cyst aspiration, fine-needle aspiration biopsy, and presurgical localization

These uses for breast sonography are also applicable to the postsurgical patient and the male breast. Sonography is not used to screen a dense breast in its entirety for a possible mass because of its high-error rate in these patients.[10]

EQUIPMENT

Breast sonography was used as long ago as 1951, when Wild and Reid imaged a 2- to 3-mm tumor with a 15-MHz A-mode transducer.[6] B-mode studies of the breast were subsequently performed with transducers of lower frequency. Currently, there are two types of instruments for breast sonography: automated and hand-

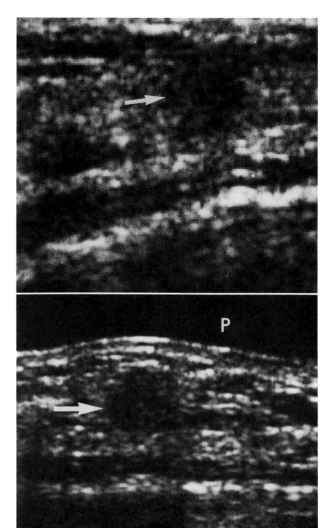

FIG 25-2. Improved near-field imaging with standoff pad. **A,** Without use of standoff pad, there is ill-defined hypoechoic region *(arrow)*, which could be mistaken for artifact. **B,** With 1-cm-thick offset pad *(P)*, mass *(arrow)*, an infiltrating ductal carcinoma, is more clearly visualized because it lies within focal zone of the 7.5-MHz transducer.

held. The advantages of automated breast scanning units include the more reliable display of multiple lesions, which makes comparison with previous examinations easier, and the lower level of operator dependence. Handheld transducers are better suited for the characterization of a known or suspected mass, and the examination is performed more rapidly than with automated units. Guidance of interventional procedures are more easily accomplished with a hand held transducer.

Fear that the ionizing radiation of mammography would induce cancer led to a demand for alternate methods of breast cancer screening, and automated breast ultrasound units were offered in response. The most widely used automated unit currently is a supine scanner that uses a water bag to compress the breast. The bag can be positioned to conform to the breast's curvature. A transducer within the water bag traverses the breast tissue, producing 1- to 2-mm tomographic sections. A modification of this transducer allows for selection from a range of frequencies between 4 and 7.5 MHz. The variable frequency feature can be used to maximize high-resolution imaging of lesions at various locations and depths within the breast.[12]

The use of automated breast ultrasound instruments has decreased, primarily because of the inaccuracy of ultrasound as a screening technique. Bassett reported in 1989 that 53% of 319 radiologists surveyed used breast sonography in their practices. Of this group, 93% used handheld transducers and only 7% used the more costly, cumbersome, and labor-intensive automated scanners.[11]

Handheld ultrasound transducers vary widely in their specifications, design, and quality. Dynamically focused phased array, linear array, and annular array transducers of 7.5 MHz and high resolution 5 MHz are available. Standard-sized transducers and the smaller, intraoperative probes are both appropriate for breast sonography. The focal zones of these high-frequency transducers are 3 cm or less, optimizing the resolution of superficial masses. If the transducer is not focused in the near field, artifactual echoes may occur within cysts. The use of an offset acoustic pad often improves the resolution of near-field lesions (Fig. 25-2).[11] Also suitable for breast ultrasound are high-frequency mechanical sector transducers. Some of these probes have built-in fluid paths, which also help eliminate the artifactual echoes that may appear within cysts. Color-flow and spectral Doppler sonography have recently been used in breast diagnosis, although their value in differentiating benign from malignant solid masses has not been established.[7,13,14]

EXAMINATION TECHNIQUE

The ultrasound study provides an opportunity for physical examination of the breast, and the mammogram should be available for correlation with the sonographic findings. Sonographic evaluation of the breast is most easily performed with the patient in a supine-oblique position. The patient's shoulder and torso of the side to be examined are elevated by a wedge to minimize the thickness of the upper outer quadrant breast tissue. The ipsilateral arm is elevated and flexed at the elbow, with the hand resting comfortably under the neck. The contralateral arm remains at the patient's side. In this supine oblique position, the bulk of breast tissue falls to the contralateral side. Adequate sono-

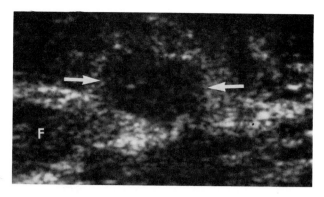

FIG 25-3. Fibroadenoma appearing similar to fat lobule. Oval hypoechoic mass *(arrows)* is small fibroadenoma, which resembles surrounding fat lobules *(F)*.

graphic penetration is assured if the underlying pectoral muscles and ribs are visualized.

Generally, an entire quadrant or area is scanned in sagittal and transverse planes. Suspected abnormalities should be viewed orthogonally so that a pseudomass will be recognized and not misinterpreted as a true lesion. For example, a fat lobule may appear similar to an oval fibroadenoma in one view, (Fig. 25-3). But when the transducer is rotated 90°, the fat lobule often appears elongated rather than rounded.

Imaging the nipple-areolar complex requires special technical maneuvers.[15,16] The nipple creates abrupt changes in surface contour that may result in poor visualization of the deeper tissues. Posterior-acoustic shadowing results from air gaps that form between the irregular skin surface and the transducer surface. Fibrous elements within the nipple may also cause shadowing that obscures the retroareolar region. The tissues beneath the nipple may be imaged by placing the transducer adjacent to the nipple and angling into the retroareolar area (Fig. 25-4). For imaging areas other than the upper outer quadrant, it is preferable to place the patient in the supine position, with her arms at her sides or behind her head.[10] If the purpose of the examination is to evaluate a palpable abnormality and if the lesion is felt only when the patient is seated or standing, the patient should assume that position and locate the site of concern with her fingers. Scanning then should be directed to the region in question.

Sonographic evaluation of multiple lesions may be confusing because a lesion may be counted more than once if viewed from different angles and locations. One approach to counting masses is to try to isolate a lesion manually, pushing it outside of the scanning field. The surrounding parenchyma is then imaged to identify possible additional cysts or solid masses.

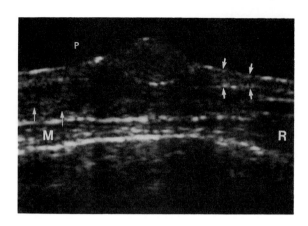

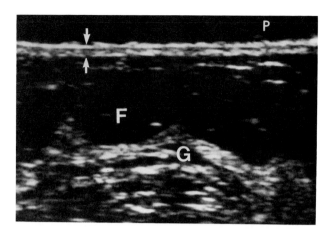

FIG 25-4. Nipple-areolar complex. Using offset pad *(P)* and angling transducer into retroareolar area, tissue beneath nipple can be visualized. Unless probe is angled, its contact with nipple often produces acoustic shadow, obscuring retroareolar area. Periareolar skin is thicker near nipple *(thick arrows)* and thinner near periphery. Small black tubular structures represent mammary ducts *(thin arrows)*. *R* indicates rib; *M,* pectoralis muscle.

FIG 25-5. Normal skin. 7.5-MHz image using standoff pad *(P)* demonstrates two echogenic lines *(arrows)* with thin hypoechoic layer between them. Skin is normally 0.2 cm or less in thickness except in inframammary fold, where it is slightly thicker. Scalloped hypoechoic subcutaneous fat lobules *(F)* are seen. Echogenic layer posterior to fat represents fibroglandular parenchyma *(G)*.

If uncertainty exists in correlating the mammographic or palpable findings with sonographic abnormalities, a small radiopaque marker can be placed on the skin over the lesion as it is evaluated initially. The area is then restudied either by mammography or sonography. Identification of the marker in the expected location will confirm that the identical lesion is being imaged. These maneuvers are unnecessary in most cases, but they can be helpful. If abnormalities are suspected in the skin or superficial subcutaneous tissues, an offset pad or fluid-filled bag can be placed on the skin to improve the resolution of the near-field structures.

SONOGRAPHIC ANATOMY

The anatomic components of the breast and the surrounding structures (skin, ducts, adipose tissue, parenchyma, nipple, blood vessels, retromammary muscles, and ribs) have characteristic sonographic features. The **skin complex** is seen as two thin echogenic lines demarcating a narrow hypoechoic band—the dermis (Fig. 25-5).[17] The normal skin measures up to 0.2 cm in thickness but may be thicker in the lower breast near the inframammary fold.

Fat lobules are oval in one plane of view and elongated in the opposite plane of view. They are hypoechoic relative to the surrounding glandular tissue and may have a central echogenic focus that represents a nidus of connective tissue (Fig. 25-6). Fat lobules located within the breast are usually larger than fat lobules located in the retropectoral area.

The **breast glandular parenchyma** usually appears homogeneously echogenic but may have hypoechoic zones caused by fatty tissue (Fig. 25-7). Not infrequently, the glandular tissue is interlaced with small hypoechoic mammary ducts. The wide range of normal glandular parenchyma seen mammographically can also be appreciated sonographically. Areas of asymmetric density seen by mammography may be due to fibroglandular tissue or a mass. In general, fibroglandular tissue appears echogenic, whereas a mass appears as a hypoechoic or anechoic structure. Found in patients of all ages but a characteristic of the breasts of the very young, extensive homogeneously echogenic tissue often corresponds to mammographically dense breasts, within which radiographic identification of discrete masses may be difficult.

The **mammary ducts,** which are radially arrayed around the nipple, demonstrate progressive luminal enlargement as they converge on the nipple. The ducts are visible as tubular structures that measure 0.1 to 0.8 cm in diameter (Fig 25-8).[11] These ducts become smaller and arborize in the peripheral portions of the breast.

The **nipple** is of medium-level echogenicity and attenuates sound, resulting in a posterior acoustic shadow (Fig. 25-4). The normal nipple may sometimes appear as a well-defined hypoechoic oval structure resembling a superficial adenoma if imaged from an oblique angle.

The mammary tissue is enclosed within a **fascial envelope** composed of a superficial and deep layer.[17] These fascial layers may be seen as a thin line, although they are not usually visible. The superficial layer is

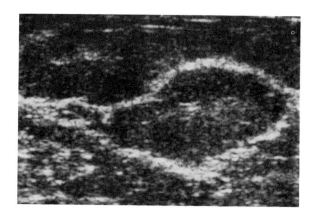

FIG 25-6. Fat lobule. Enlarged view demonstrates oval hypoechoic structure with an echogenic margin of connective tissue. Small echogenic focus in center most likely represents connective tissue. Adipose tissue in breast is typically hypoechoic, unlike echogenic fat in abdominal organs.

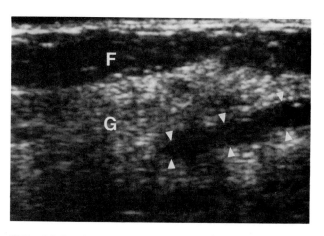

FIG 25-7. Dense fibroglandular parenchyma. Broad echogenic zone of fibroglandular parenchyma *(G)* lies deep to subcutaneous fat layer *(F)*. Linear hypoechoic band *(arrowheads)* represents region of fat within fibroglandular parenchyma.

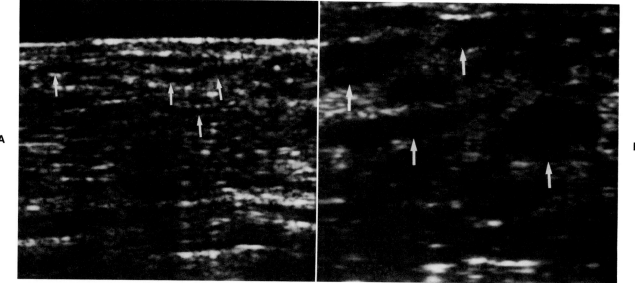

FIG 25-8. Mammary ducts. **A,** Multiple small tubular hypoechoic structures *(arrows)* represent normal mammary ducts in this pregnant patient. Normal ducts measure 0.1 to 0.5 cm in diameter. **B,** Dilated mammary ducts *(arrows)* are seen in patient with duct papillomas.

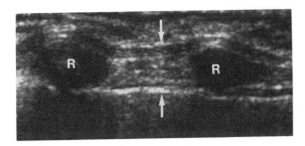

FIG 25-9. Ribs. Longitudinal scan shows oval ribs *(R),* hypoechoic sharply marginated structures that attenuate sound. Intercostal muscles *(arrows)* are identified between ribs.

sometimes seen below the dermis, and the deep layer lies over the retromammary fat and pectoralis muscle. Visualization of the **pectoralis muscle** guarantees that the breast parenchyma has been adequately penetrated at that site. The ribs are oval, hypoechoic, periodic structures behind the pectoralis muscles. They attenuate sound, causing a posterior acoustic shadow (Fig. 25-9).

The **axillary vessels** present as tubular structures, which are often seen pulsating during the real-time examination. Duplex Doppler or color-flow imaging can provide confirmation of their vascular nature. **Lymph nodes** may also be seen in the axilla. Normal lymph

nodes are often elongated and may have an echogenic fatty hilus. Sonographically, small normal lymph nodes may resemble fat lobules or cysts and be indistinguishable from small fibroadenomas.[18] Sonography is not reliable in excluding malignancy within lymph nodes. Normal-sized lymph nodes that are infiltrated with tumor may appear identical to normal nodes. Similarly, enlarged hyperplastic lymph nodes may appear identical to metastatic lymph nodes. Sonography is sometimes useful to confirm a lymph node that may be only partially seen mammographically (Fig. 25-10).

AN APPROACH TO EVALUATING MASSES

Masses detected by mammography that are greater than 1 cm in diameter are commonly visualized sonographically. Cysts of 0.2 to 0.3 cm in diameter can be detected with high-frequency transducers. Solid lesions that measure 0.5 cm in diameter are demonstrable, depending on the frequency of the transducer and its resolution, location of the mass within the breast, and nature of the surrounding parenchyma.[5] Although the sonographic appearances of most solid masses are frequently nonspecific, it is an oversimplification to say that the sole use of breast ultrasound is to differentiate cysts from solid lesions. Sonographic features in conjunction with mammographic appearances and use of more invasive techniques to increase diagnostic speci-

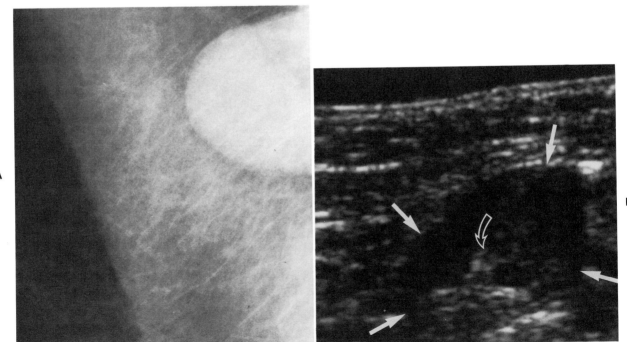

FIG 25-10. Lymph node. **A,** Mammographic view of axilla demonstrates sharply marginated soft tissue density suggestive of enlarged lymph node, which is partially visualized. **B,** Sonogram of this mass depicts the hypoechoic lymph node in its entirety *(straight arrows)* with central echogenic focus caused by fatty hilus *(curved arrow).*

☐ SONOGRAPHIC DESCRIPTION OF BREAST MASSES

Location
Number
Appearance
  Size
  Shape
  Margin
Internal contents
  Solid
  Cystic
  Mixed
Homogeneous or heterogeneous
Parenchymal interface
  Invisible
  Echogenic rim
Posterior sound transmission
  Enhancement
  Shadow
  No change
Skin thickness

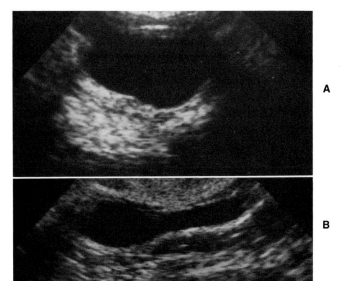

FIG 25-11. Cyst. **A,** Sonogram of the breast demonstrates anechoic mass with well-defined back wall and posterior acoustic enhancement typical of simple cyst. Front wall of cyst is obscured by ring-down artifact and therefore is not sharply defined. **B,** When compression is applied, some simple cysts may change their shapes, becoming elongated. Solid masses do not demonstrate this compressibility.

ficity (e.g., cyst aspiration and fine-needle aspiration biopsy) can provide a reasonable guide to management. Lesion analysis (see the box above) in the context of clinical history, physical findings, patient's age, and risk factors for malignancy can frequently suggest a number of satisfactory conservative approaches.

CYSTS

Breast cysts are common in women in the perimenopausal years of approximately 35 to 50 years of age. Of 593 well-circumscribed mammographic masses over 1 cm evaluated by Moskowitz, 50% were cysts.[4] Following menopause, cysts usually gradually disappear, although they may persist, flourish, or develop in women receiving estrogen or estrogen-progesterone hormonal replacement therapy.[19]

The most important contribution of breast sonography is the confident diagnosis of a simple cyst. No further clinical action is needed when a mass meets the sonographic criteria of a simple cyst unless the patient has pain, the mass interferes with clinical or self examination, or other symptoms are of concern.[16] Consequently, the number of benign breast biopsies has been reduced by 25%.[3,16]

Diagnostic criteria, which should be strictly applied, are the same as those for cysts elsewhere in the body, the lesion should:

- be anechoic
- be round or oval
- be sharply marginated (particularly the posterior walls)
- demonstrate acoustic enhancement posteriorly (Fig. 25-11, A).[10,16]

If a cyst is not under tension, pressure applied to it with the transducer may alter its shape (Fig. 25-11, B). This compressibility is not seen with solid lesions. If there is any doubt, aspiration is indicated.

For dependable diagnosis of cysts, all aspects of sonographic technique require attention.[11] Gain and power settings must be adjusted for each unit and reset for each patient. Focal-zone placement must be appropriate, with an offset pad used for superficial lesions. To demonstrate features of a cyst in lesions deeply seated in the breast or in larger breasts, compression and positional alterations may be necessary. With increased power or time gain compensation (TGC) settings, the anterior portion of a cyst will fill in, but the posterior wall will remain well defined. If all of the criteria are fulfilled, the diagnosis of a cyst can be made with nearly 100% accuracy and only routine follow-up will be necessary.[10,20]

INTERVENTIONAL PROCEDURES
Cyst Aspiration

Any nonpalpable lesion that may represent a cyst but does not fulfill all of the sonographic criteria should be aspirated using sonographic guidance (Fig. 25-12).

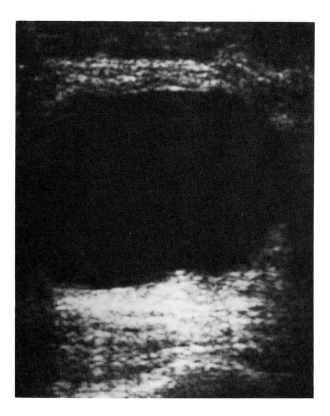

FIG 25-12. Cyst with internal debris. A 3-cm cystic mass with acoustic enhancement posteriorly but poorly defined back wall and fine, low-level, internal echoes. Presence of internal echoes and poorly defined back wall make this lesion indeterminate. Needle aspiration demonstrated thick viscous material was aspirated from benign breast cyst.

Low-level echoes are often present in cysts, and although the lesion will be recognized as a cyst in many instances, aspiration will be required to confirm the diagnosis. Hilton also suggests aspiration of palpable and symptomatic abnormalities.[16]

Once need for the procedure has been established, the efficiency, safety, comfort, and cost of a particular method should be considered. There is no single correct method for performing cyst aspiration, fine-needle aspiration biopsy (FNAB), or presurgical wire localization. Palpable lesions may not require any imaging technique for efficient and economical aspiration or FNAB. Symptomatic nonpalpable cysts should be aspirated using ultrasound guidance. Postaspiration sonography will document complete evacuation or presence of any residual fluid.

Selection of an imaging method to guide the procedure is determined by the location, size, and nature of the lesion. A deeply situated small mass in a large, fatty breast may be aspirated, biopsied, or localized more easily with mammographic fenestrated plate or stereotactic technique than with sonographic guidance. In ad-

dition, masses that are better depicted mammographically than sonographically may be more easily aspirated using mammographic guidance.

Many experienced clinicians suggest that a sterile field is unnecessary.[21] Cleansing of the skin with betadine or alcohol and disinfection of the transducer according to the manufacturer's instructions are adequate preparations. Although all operators wear gloves (predominantly for their own protection), covering the transducer with a sterile sheath is optional.

Several successful techniques have been described for sonographically guided cyst aspirations.[22] The choice of the technique depends on the type of transducer used, the radiologist's experience, and cyst features. With linear transducers, the cyst is imaged at the midposition of the long axis of the transducer face. The needle-tip location can be noted either by jiggling the needle and noting the tissue's movement between the cyst and transducer or by moving the shaft of the needle over the cyst, which continues to be imaged in the midportion of the transducer. The cyst's depth can be measured, and the angle required for the needle's passage into the cyst can be gauged accurately. With experience, the triangulation computation is accomplished without difficulty. Frequently, entry of the echogenic needle tip into the cyst can be visualized, although with this approach, the needle shaft is usually not imaged fully except as a transient tissue derangement (Fig. 25-13). The breast tissue in the area of the cyst should be fixed manually so that the needle penetrates the wall rather than pushes the mobile lesion out of the scan plane. Alternatively, fixation may also be accomplished by firm pressure of the transducer against the breast.

Sonographic visualization of needle passage is possible not only with the freehand method described above but also with transducer-needle guides that clip onto the transducer and hold the needle at a preselected angle appropriate for the depth of the cyst. We do not use needle guides because they are cumbersome and do not ensure visualization of the needle tip.

Another technique for aspiration uses ultrasound to identify a lesion's location by marking the overlying skin. Objects that cause posterior acoustic shadowing, such as a coffee stirrer or needle shaft, are placed between the skin and transducer.[23] When the shadow obscures the cyst deep to it, a marker is placed in that location on the skin and the depth to the mass is measured. The operator fixes the area of the lesion manually and inserts the needle to the predetermined depth. The patient must remain immobile to prevent a shift in the location of the cyst with respect to the skin markers. Small, deeply situated cysts may be difficult to aspirate because even minor movement can alter the alignment of the skin mark and lesion.

A small-caliber (21-gauge) needle may be used ini-

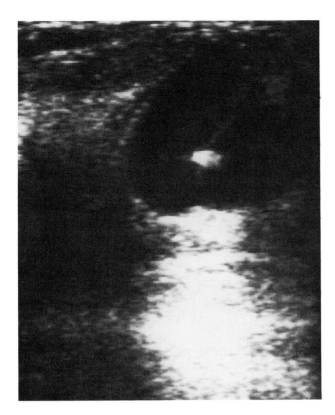

FIG 25-13. Cyst aspiration. A 2-cm cyst with tip of 21-gauge needle visible as echogenic dot within fluid. Only a small portion of the needle shaft can be seen.

tially, and if the cyst contents are of low viscosity, evacuation of the cyst will be rapid and successful. The thin needle may be deflected if a tough, fibrous rind encases the cyst. A stiffer, larger caliber needle will be required to enter thick-walled lesions that resist needle penetration. Larger caliber needles are also required to aspirate cysts that contain viscous fluid. Some authors advocate the use of 18- or 19-gauge needles initially.[17]

Aspiration can be performed using a syringe with or without connecting tubing or by mounting the syringe in an aspirating gun. Suction can be maintained with less exertion if an aspirating gun is used. The transducer is held in one hand and the needle device in the other. If an assistant is available to perform sonography, the radiologist can fix the area of the cyst with one hand and direct the needle into the cyst with the other. During the procedure, manual compression of the cyst increases the completeness of the evacuation. After the procedure, the area of aspiration should be compressed for a short period to help prevent formation of a hematoma, although such collections are rare following cyst aspiration. An ice pack may diminish discomfort. A postaspiration sonogram is obtained to document the reduction or absence of fluid.

There is no consensus regarding what analyses should be performed on the aspirated cyst fluid. For the present, all cyst aspirates from our breast center are submitted for cytologic evaluation, and if the cells are atypical or suggest malignancy, surgical biopsy may be planned. Other radiologists and surgeons discard yellowish serous aspirates and the greenish fluid, which may be associated with fibrocystic changes.[21] Any bloody cyst aspirate or evacuated material of an unusual nature must be analyzed cytologically. If the aspirate is purulent, microbiologic studies (Gram's stain, culture, and sensitivity assays) should be obtained in addition to cytologic studies. If the breast mass is not fluid filled, material from the lesion should be sent for cytologic analysis.

Biopsy

Principles for sonographically guided FNAB are the same as for cyst aspiration. Local anesthetic is not necessary unless multiple passes with a large needle are planned. Needle selections range from a 23-gauge butterfly venipuncture needle to a larger gauge biopsy needle. Needles with etched or coated tips do not significantly improve visualization of the needle within the mass.[22] When the needle tip is visualized within the mass, suction is applied by syringe or aspiration gun, and the needle is moved in and out within the mass. Before needle removal, the suction should be released gently to prevent the aspirate from being sucked into the barrel of the syringe. Two or three entries into different areas of the lesion, including its periphery where viable cells may be present, will be sufficient in most cases. Another sampling method employs a needle unattached to a syringe. Excursion of the needle into the lesion loosens clumps of cells that enter the barrel of the needle.

Injection of a tiny volume of air through the needle into the area of aspiration can mark the site for hardcopy documentation. A bright, linear focus of echoes with posterior acoustic shadowing will denote the site of sampling. The air will also be visible mammographically. If the FNAB is to be followed immediately by surgical biopsy, the air can provide a marker for mammographically or sonographically directed placement of a needle hookwire assembly.

Isolated, small clusters of microcalcifications are occasionally seen with ultrasound. Sonographically guided needle-aspiration biopsy of them probably should not be attempted because of the possibility of obscuring or aspirating an important mammographic marker. In these cases, however, the introduction of a small bolus of air into the tissues with a postprocedural mammogram may provide a landmark for a surgical biopsy should it be required.

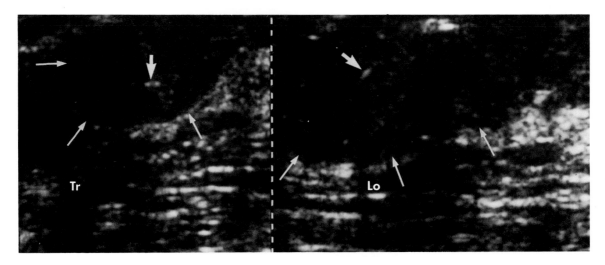

FIG 25-14. Presurgical wire localization of solid mass. Transverse *(Tr)* and longitudinal *(Lo)* images of breast demonstrate short linear echogenic focus *(thick arrows)* representing needle tip near center of hypoechoic mass *(thin arrows)*. Wire is inserted after needle tip has been identified within mass.

Presurgical Needle–Hookwire Localization

Presurgical wire localization is also possible using sonographic guidance, provided the mass is visible.[23,24] One advantage of this technique is that the needle placement occurs with the patient in the same supine position used during the operation. Ultrasound guidance is especially expeditious for lesions located in the far periphery of the breast where mammographic guidance may be difficult.

Any needle-hookwire apparatus, needle alone, or similar device can be adapted to sonographically directed placement. The needle is inserted initially without the hookwire in place (Fig 25-14). If the mass is fluid filled, its contents are aspirated and the evacuation procedure documented. If no fluid is obtained and the needle's location appears certain, the hookwire is inserted and engaged. The needle may be removed at this time or left in place during mammography. Some wires with curved or curled ends cannot be reinserted easily into a needle that has been placed in tissue. Using these devices, sonographically guided presurgical localizations are performed without the initial aspiration attempt. Ninety-degree lateral and craniocaudal views are obtained, confirming accurate placement of the hookwire. Radiographic imaging of the specimen is performed to confirm adequate surgical resection.

Complications

In general, there are few risks from cyst aspiration, FNAB, or presurgical wire localization other than transient minor bleeding into the surrounding tissues. Application of cold packs or an analgesic such as aspirin or acetaminophen relieves discomfort. Rarely, pneumo-thorax may be caused, particularly with lesions located far medially or far laterally, where the distance from skin to pleura may be short and needle entry is perpendicular to the chest wall. A careful determination of needle length, depth of lesion, and distance from skin to chest wall can promote accuracy in aspirating and help prevent inadvertent penetration of the pleura. If the patient complains of sharp pain during respiration, a chest radiograph should be obtained to exclude pneumothorax. Another uncommon risk is local infection.

SOLID AND MIXED MASSES
Nonspecificity of Sonographic Features

Carcinoma of the breast is the leading cause of cancer in women in the United States. The incidence has been increasing, with 175,000 cases anticipated annually.[25] Early detection offers survival benefits.[1] Ideally, breast imaging should be accurate in the diagnosis of carcinoma. Although certain mammographic findings allow specific diagnoses of some malignant and benign abnormalities, there is a wide range of sonographic appearances manifested by neoplastic and nonneoplastic breast lesions.

Ultrasound features of a typical breast carcinoma include:
- Hypoechogenicity
- Irregular borders
- Inhomogeneous echotexture
- Posterior acoustic shadowing
- An echogenic rim of variable thickness that may represent tumor extension or desmoplasia (Fig 25-15)[5]

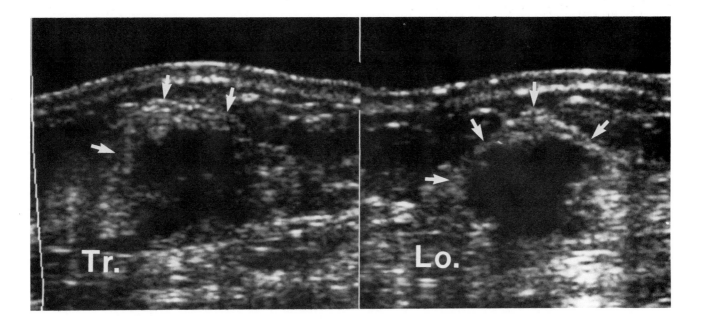

FIG 25-15. Infiltrating ductal carcinoma with echogenic rim. Transverse *(Tr)* and longitudinal *(Lo)* image demonstrates a 2-cm, roughly round, hypoechoic mass with irregular lobulated margins and low-level internal echoes typical of breast carcinoma. Echogenic rim *(arrows)* around mass most likely represents either tumor infiltration or desmoplastic reaction of adjacent tissues.

Although virtually all sonographically visible carcinomas are hypoechoic (relative to adjacent breast parenchyma), many other masses also appear hypoechoic.[5,24]

Posterior acoustic shadowing, which may represent the fibrous response incited by the tumor's presence, is associated with 40% to 60% of carcinomas.[26,27] Benign neoplasms, such as fibroadenomas, may also exhibit posterior acoustic shadowing, and therefore the finding is not specific for malignancy.[5,11] In our experience, posterior acoustic shadows unrelated to calcification occurred in up to 30% of fibroadenomas, particularly with those fibroadenomas that are hyalinized (Fig. 25-16).[28] Posterior acoustic shadows are also seen in association with fat necrosis, postsurgical and traumatic scarring, focal sclerosing adenosis and fibrosis, diabetic fibrosis, and air-containing abscesses (Fig. 25-17).[29,30] Normal tissues may also cause posterior acoustic shadowing as the transducer passes over the curved tissue planes with multiple interfaces of Cooper's ligaments and other connective tissue septa, fat lobules, and breast parenchyma.

The shape of a mass and the appearance of the **borders of the mass** are also unreliable predictors of a benign or malignant nature. Although fibroadenomas are ordinarily oval, carcinomas may be elongated as well as rounded. Benign lesions, such as abscesses, hematomas, and fat necrosis may have jagged margins. Smooth margins, typically seen with fibroadenomas, may also be a sonographic finding in some carcinomas.[31,32]

Skin thickening and edema may signify inflammatory breast cancer but also occur with breast abscess, irradiation therapy, and systemic processes such as congestive heart failure. Although ultrasound does not permit a specific cause to be identified, skin thickening is easy to quantitate with high-resolution sonography (Fig. 25-18). The deeper of the two parallel skin lines usually seen is sometimes interrupted or lost. The thickened dermis—infiltrated, fibrotic, or edematous—often becomes more echogenic compared with the expected hypoechogenicity of this tissue layer (Fig. 25-19). Occasionally, the randomly distributed, engorged lymphatics or interstitial fluid collections can be seen with ultrasound. Subsequent decreasing thickness of the skin can be confirmed sonographically in the patient undergoing radiation therapy whose breast might be difficult to compress fully for mammography. If skin thickening and breast edema are unresolved or cannot otherwise be explained, as in patients with radiation-treated breast carcinoma, breast biopsy with inclusion of dermal lymphatics is indicated to exclude inflammatory carcinoma.[33]

Asymmetric ductal dilation may be an indication of carcinoma or benign lesions such as intraductal papilloma (Fig. 25-20).

Macrocalcifications are well depicted sonographically as echogenic foci, often with posterior acoustic

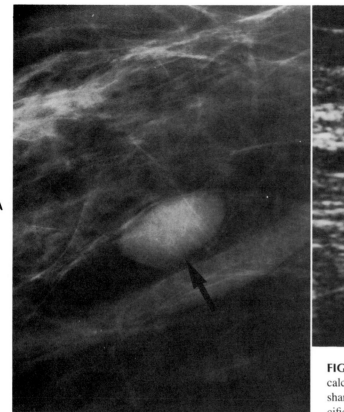

A

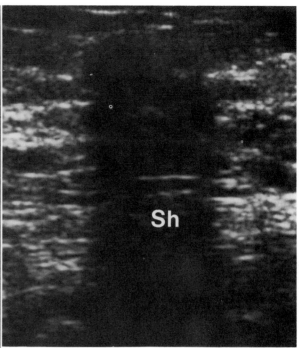

B

FIG 25-16. Posterior acoustic shadowing caused by non-calcified fibroadenoma. **A,** Mammogram demonstrates sharply marginated, oval mass *(arrows),* which is not calcified. **B,** Sonogram of this mass demonstrates marked attenuation of sound, causing posterior acoustic shadow *(Sh).*

FIG 25-17. Calcified cyst causing posterior acoustic shadow. **A,** Magnified mammographic view demonstrates plaque-like, thick calcification of rim of well-defined mass. **B,** Sonogram of this mass demonstrates large acoustic shadow *(Sh)* blocking visualization of internal detail. Portion of calcification is identified as linear echogenic focus anteriorly *(arrow).*

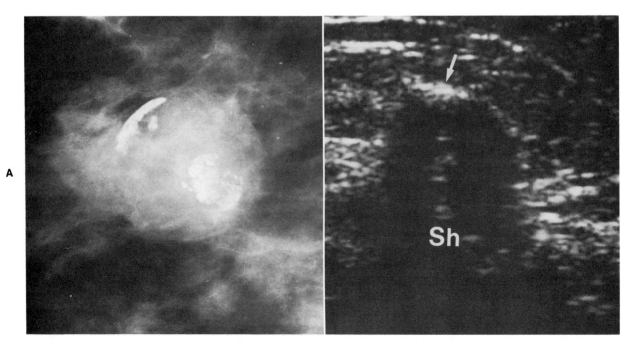

A

B

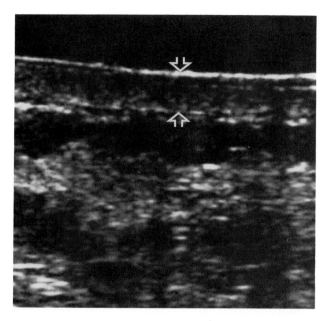

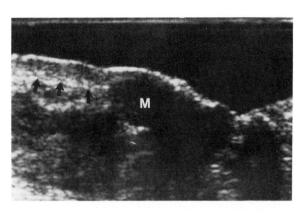

FIG 25-19. Skin thickening caused by inflammatory carcinoma. Sonogram with standoff pad shows deformity of contour of skin caused by underlying, hypoechoic mass *(M)*, which is infiltrative and poorly marginated. Skin superior to mass *(arrows)* is thickened by edema and tumor permeation, measuring approximately 0.7 cm.

FIG 25-18. Skin thickening caused by irradiation. Sonogram with standoff pad demonstrates thickening of dermis to approximately 0.6 cm *(arrows)*. Thickening of the skin complex is a common finding for a year or two after breast conservation therapy (lumpectomy or irradiation).

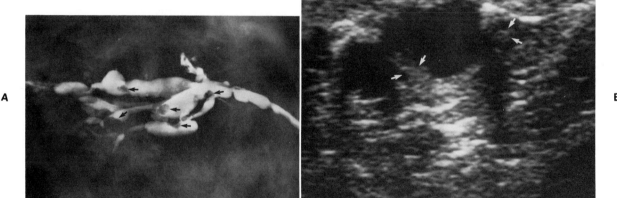

FIG 25-20. Intraductal papillomas with duct dilation. **A,** Galactography shows multiple filling defects *(arrows)* representing papillomas within dilated mammary ducts. **B,** Sonogram of breast shows cystic dilation of mammary ducts, which contain mural echogenic nodules—papillomas *(arrows)*.

shadowing. Popcornlike clumps of calcification are visualized in fibroadenomas. Coarse calcifications are also seen in fat necrosis, areas of scarring, in lymph nodes involved with granulomatous disease, and with other lesions.

Microcalcifications, when clustered, are the most important mammographic marker for nonpalpable cancer, especially intraductal carcinoma.[4] The diameter of

an individual microcalcification measures 0.1 to 0.4 mm. Occasionally, with high-resolution ultrasound equipment, microcalcifications may be seen, especially when they are located within a mass (Fig. 25-21).[5] Microcalcifications, visualized inconsistently, appear as tiny echogenic flecks in the breast parenchyma and are often difficult to distinguish from the many other echogenic surfaces. These microcalcifications usually

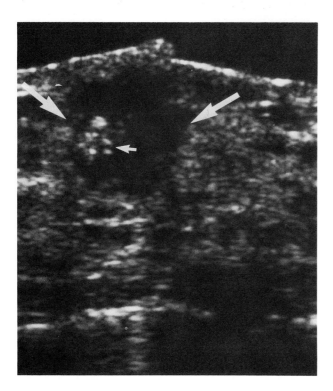

FIG 25-21. Intraductal carcinoma with microcalcification. Sonogram of breast demonstrates hypoechoic mass with lobulated borders *(large arrows)*, containing echogenic foci *(small arrow)* of microcalcification.

do not produce acoustic shadows. Determination of the morphologic features of microcalcifications is beyond the resolution capabilities of current instruments, and estimates of the number and extent of microcalcifications are unreliable.

Malignant Masses

Ductal Carcinoma.   Infiltrating ductal carcinoma accounts for more than 80% of breast cancers.[34] Arising from the ductal epithelium of smaller and medium-sized ductal elements, infiltrating ductal carcinoma may also occur with other histologic types, such as tubular or invasive lobular carcinoma.[35]

On palpation, these masses feel larger than they appear mammographically and sonographically. This well-known clinical phenomenon can be explained by the desmoplastic reaction incited by the tumor. On mammographic examination, these tumors often have irregular and poorly defined margins that reflect the fibrous response and infiltrative behavior of the tumor. Similarly, the majority of infiltrating ductal carcinomas seen sonographically has irregular and ill-defined borders (Fig. 25-22). These tumors are usually heterogeneous, hypoechoic solid masses, which attenuate the acoustic beam. There is, however, a wide range of sonographic appearances of this common type of malig-

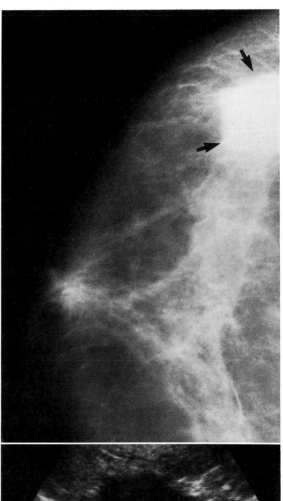

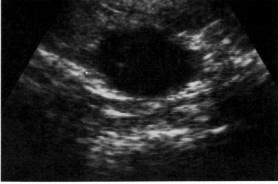

FIG 25-22. Infiltrating ductal carcinoma. **A,** Mammogram demonstrates a dense mass *(arrows)* with spiculation of margin typical of carcinoma. **B,** Sonogram of lesion shows hypoechoic round mass with ill-defined margins, internal echoes, and small amount of posterior acoustic enhancement.

nancy. For example, some infiltrating ductal carcinomas have well-defined margins and do not attenuate sound (Fig. 25-23).

Infiltrating Lobular Carcinoma.   Second in frequency of occurrence but far less common than infiltrating ductal carcinoma is infiltrating lobular carcinoma, contributing 8% to 10% of breast cancers.[36] This tumor's pro-

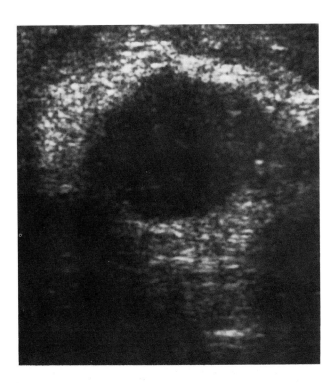

FIG 25-23. Infiltrating ductal carcinoma with posterior acoustic enhancement. Sonogram demonstrates round hypoechoic mass with small amount of posterior acoustic enhancement and thick echogenic rim anteriorly.

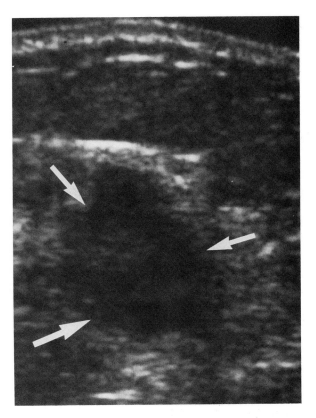

FIG 25-24. Medullary carcinoma. Sonogram depicts lobulated mass *(arrows)* with ill-defined margins, low-level internal echoes, and a small amount of posterior acoustic enhancement.

pensity for bilaterality and multicentricity ranges from 6% to 36%.[37] Although infiltrating lobular carcinoma may be indistinguishable mammographically from the spiculated masses of infiltrating ductal carcinoma, the most common presentation is that of a poorly demarcated, asymmetric, increased density that may be wispy, shaggy, and of low density.[38] The tumor cells travel in a linear pattern through the breast parenchyma without a central tumor nidus. The mammographic appearance reflects these histologic characteristics. Particularly in dense breasts or breasts in which the tumor presents as a subtle area of architectural derangement, ultrasound can be valuable in confirming a mass, sometimes large, that can be hidden but suspected clinically as a vague area of induration. Again, the sonographic appearance is nonspecific— sometimes it is that of the "typical" carcinoma. Occasionally, an extensive, solid, lobulated mass that infiltrates much of the breast is seen.

Medullary Carcinoma. Medullary carcinoma comprises approximately 5% of breast cancers. It occurs with greater frequency in women under the age of 50 years.[39] Mammographically, these tumors, which may be large, are often fairly well circumscribed. The sharp margins and homogeneous internal architecture of medullary carcinoma may result in a sonographic appearance similar to that of a cyst. These tumors may be round, homogeneous, and hypoechoic and may demonstrate posterior acoustic enhancement (Fig. 25-24).[5] Low-level internal echoes of the carcinoma that are most evident at higher gain settings separate these lesions from simple cysts. Some of the margins of the mass may be irregular rather than smooth. These findings may be subtle and aspiration will be necessary to differentiate medullary carcinoma from a cyst or abscess.

Mucinous (Colloid) Carcinoma. Another uncommon form of breast carcinoma, colloid or mucinous, constitutes approximately 1% to 2% of breast cancers. Mucinous carcinoma has a better prognosis than infiltrating ductal carcinoma. This tumor appears similar to medullary carcinoma both sonographically and mammographically, but it usually occurs in older women.[39] The sonographic appearance is of a fairly well-defined hypoechoic mass, with a homogeneous low-level internal echogenicity and a lack of significant posterior acoustic attenuation. These features may reflect the large amount of mucin seen microscopically (Fig. 25-25).

Tubular Carcinoma. Occurring approximately as

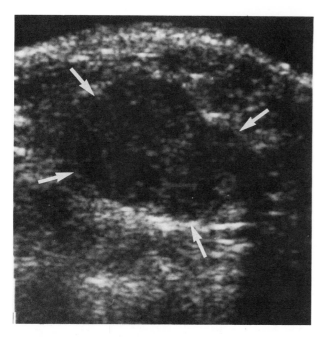

FIG 25-25. Mucinous (colloid) carcinoma. Sonogram shows a 3-cm, hypoechoic, well-marginated, lobulated mass *(arrows)* without a surrounding echogenic rim. Echogenicity is similar to that of adjacent fat lobules with small amount of posterior acoustic enhancement. Appearance of this solid mass might suggest a fibroadenoma, but its large size would prompt surgical or percutaneous biopsy.

frequently as mucinous carcinoma, in pure form these uncommon neoplasms have an excellent prognosis. Mammographically and sonographically, tubular carcinomas may appear as small, well-circumscribed masses. Occasionally on the mammogram, long spicules are seen in association with the small mass (Fig. 25-26), but sonographically, its features are nonspecific.[40] An association between tubular carcinoma and the benign radial scar has been postulated but is not established.[41]

Papillary Carcinoma. Occurring most commonly in postmenopausal women, these rare tumors, which may be well circumscribed mammographically, have a prognosis similar to that of mucinous or tubular carcinomas.[39,42,43] They may be suspected clinically when a bloody nipple discharge is seen, although this sign most often signifies the presence of a benign intraductal papilloma. Sonographically, papillary carcinoma may appear as a cystic mass with solid tissue projecting into the lesion.

Benign Masses

Fibroadenoma. Although they are encountered at all ages, the most common mass in a young woman under 30 to 35 years is a fibroadenoma.[44] Fibroadenomas are multiple in 10% to 20% of cases[45] and bilateral in ap-

proximately 3% or more. Most authors believe that fibroadenomas do not undergo malignant change.

The sonographic features of the fibroadenoma are variable, but in general, fibroadenomas are hypoechoic relative to the fibroglandular parenchyma and isoechoic with fat lobules in the breast (Fig. 25-27).[32] Most of the mass is homogeneous, but homogeneous regions are commonly present. Usually the mass is oval, sharply marginated, and often has a lobulated contour. In the 50 fibroadenomas we reviewed retrospectively, all were oval in at least one projection; no fibroadenoma was round in both projections.[29] The long axis of the fibroadenoma has been noted to lie parallel to the skin surface.[46] The acoustic attenuation pattern is also variable; most fibroadenomas show some posterior acoustic enhancement, but approximately 30% demonstrate posterior acoustic shadowing that is not caused by calcification.[28]

The clinical management of small (< 1.5cm) masses thought to be fibroadenomas depends on the age of the patient and the level of clinical concern.[10,47] In a young patient, observation with follow-up studies in 6 months may be offered as an alternative to excision. Fine-needle aspiration biopsy may add an increased level of confidence if the specimen is interpreted as "consistent with fibroadenoma." A pathologic report of "no malignant cells" may not have the same benign implication because a technical failure, such as missing the mass, can result in the same report.[25,26]

Phyllodes Tumor. A large, well-circumscribed, lobular mass with rapid growth and occurring in a patient over 30 years of age suggests the possibility of phyllodes tumor. Malignant forms, which may metastasize, are identified histologically by mitotic rates exceeding 5 to 10 per high power field.[45] This solid mass has a nonspecific appearance sonographically.

Giant Fibroadenoma. These uncommon neoplasms are also called juvenile fibroadenomas and are characterized by their large size—typically 5 to 10 cm in diameter.[44] These tumors are differentiated from the phyllodes tumor by the younger age range of patients (11 to 20 years of age) and lack of malignant potential, despite their very rapid growth, which may suggest malignancy. Although they may be multiple and bilateral, one tumor is often dominant (Fig. 25-28). The sonographic appearance is similar to that of a large fibroadenoma with low- to medium-internal echogenicity and well-defined margins.

Focal Fibrosis. Focal fibrosis is an uncommon, discrete abnormality that is 10% as common as carcinoma.[21] The cause of focal fibrosis is unknown but may relate to postinflammatory or vascular changes. Mammographically, the lesion is a discoid, well-defined soft tissue density. Often one of its margins is angular, and another seems to merge with the adjacent breast paren-

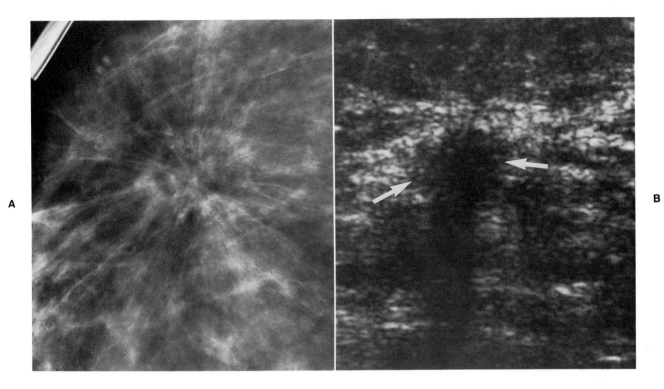

FIG 25-26. Tubular carcinoma. **A,** Magnified mammographic view shows mass with central radiolucent areas and very long radiating spiculations, suggesting radial scar. **B,** Sonogram depicts 0.7-cm, solid, hypoechoic mass with irregular, poorly defined margins *(arrows)* and posterior acoustic attenuation, common features of carcinoma.

chyma.[48] Of the eight cases we reviewed, most appeared sonographically as elliptical, hypoechoic, well-defined lesions with no change in posterior acoustic sound transmission (Fig. 25-29).[48] Another author has reported a case of focal fibrosis that is echogenic with posterior acoustic shadowing.[49]

Fibroadenolipoma. The fibroadenolipoma is a rare

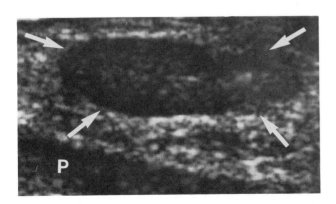

FIG 25-27. Fibroadenoma. This oval, hypoechoic, sharply marginated mass *(arrows)* with low-level internal echoes and slight posterior acoustic enhancement demonstrates typical findings of fibroadenoma. *P* indicates pectoralis muscle.

benign neoplasm composed of fibrous, epithelial, and lipomatous tissues. When large, this lesion may have a lobulated, cauliflower-like appearance. Smaller lesions may be oval, well circumscribed, and contain a foci of fatty tissue. A mammogram that shows an encapsulated and partly or fully radiolucent mass is diagnostic of a fat-containing tumor such as fibroadenolipoma or lipoma. With sonography, fibroadenolipomas are heterogeneous with echogenic components and they may show posterior acoustics attenuation.

Lipoma. Lipomas occur most frequently in older women, and mammographically, they are low-density or radiolucent, thinly encapsulated masses. Unless there is rapid growth, discomfort, or other clinical concern, these benign masses require only routine follow-up. Medium-level, homogeneous echoes characterize these well-defined lesions sonographically (Fig. 25-30), although sonography is not necessary in the diagnostic evaluation of lipoma or other fat-containing masses.

Sebaceous (Inclusion) Cysts. Sebaceous cysts, which are sometimes called inclusion cysts, are usually asymptomatic unless they grow or become infected. They often occur in the intramammary fold, axillary area, or most medial portion of the breasts. On physical

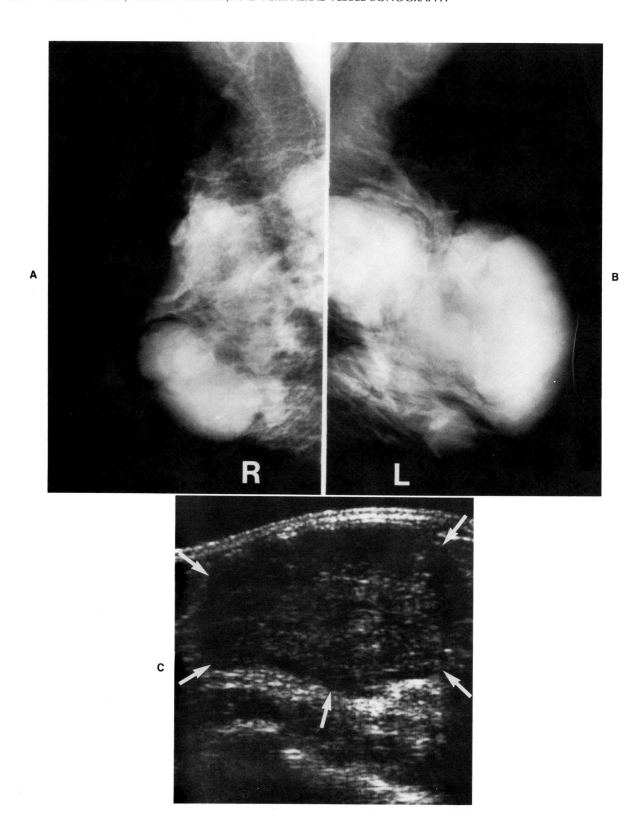

FIG 25-28. Giant (juvenile) fibroadenoma in 15-year-old patient. **A** and **B,** Bilateral mammograms show multiple, large, sharply marginated oval masses and small areas of benign-appearing calcification. **C,** Sonogram of one of the masses demonstrates large, oval, hypoechoic mass *(arrows)* with low-level internal echoes and small amount of posterior acoustic enhancement with normal thickness of the overlying skin.

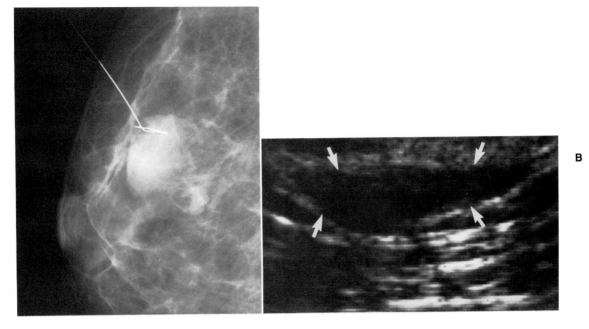

FIG 25-29. Focal fibrosis. **A,** Localization mammogram showing hookwire (*white line* across figure) placed within discoid lesion that has sharp anterior margin and posterior margin that fades into surrounding parenchyma. Perpendicular view may demonstrate flat shape of this lesion. **B,** Sonogram shows well-defined discoid structure *(arrows)* with slight posterior acoustic enhancement.

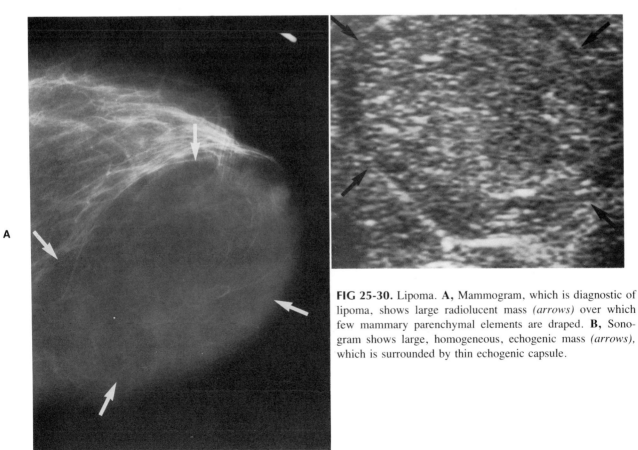

FIG 25-30. Lipoma. **A,** Mammogram, which is diagnostic of lipoma, shows large radiolucent mass *(arrows)* over which few mammary parenchymal elements are draped. **B,** Sonogram shows large, homogeneous, echogenic mass *(arrows),* which is surrounded by thin echogenic capsule.

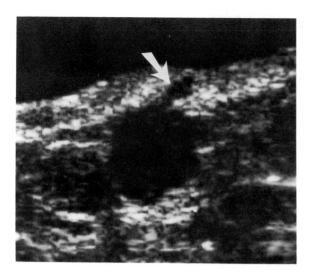

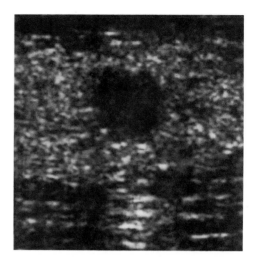

FIG 25-31. Sebaceous (inclusion) cyst. Sonogram demonstrates 1-cm, hypoechoic, lobulated mass with low-level internal echoes and posterior acoustic enhancement. Skin is thickened and small linear sinus tract *(arrow)* extends from mass into skin.

FIG 25-32. Abscess. Round, poorly marginated hypoechoic mass is seen within breast parenchyma with low-level internal echoes and small amount of posterior acoustic enhancement. Percutaneous needle aspiration of this indeterminate mass obtained pus.

examination, an umbilication may be seen in the skin where the tract communicates with the fatty, subcutaneous collection. Mammographically, these lesions are sharply defined and of high-radiographic density. Infected sebaceous cysts may be associated with skin thickening and may resemble superficial carcinomas. Sonographically, these hypoechoic masses are very well defined, and they have scattered low-level internal echoes and posterior acoustic enhancement (Fig. 25-31). In some cases a central echogenic nidus is seen.

Galactocele. Galactoceles are cystic masses that contain milk. They occur during or after lactation. Mammographically, they are well-circumscribed masses of combined soft tissue density and radiolucency that may represent the fatty nature of the milk. A fat-fluid layer may be seen on a mammographic view obtained with a horizontal beam. The sonographic appearance is nonspecific and reports have described galactoceles variably as echogenic lesions and cystic masses with less through transmission than expected for simple cysts.[49,50]

Papilloma. A papilloma is a mass resulting from epithelial proliferation within a lactiferous duct, and papillomas are the most frequent cause of bloody nipple discharge. Mammographically, papillomas may be recognised as beaded soft-tissue densities often associated with dilated ducts in the retroareolar area. Sonographically they may be well-circumscribed solid masses or cystic masses containing solid tissue, similar in appearance to cystic papillary carcinoma (Fig. 25-20).

Abscess. Abscesses most frequently occur in the lactating patient, and *Staphylococcus aureus* is the most common offending organism. Abscesses may be found in older women as a manifestation of periductal mastitis. Abscesses are most commonly located in the retroareolar region, but they may also occur away from the nipple or in women with underlying predisposing abnormalities such as diabetes, corticosteroid administration, and other immunosuppressive conditions. Skin excoriation in severe eczema may provide an entry site for the infectious agent. Sonographic features vary from complex masses with irregular margins to fairly well-circumscribed oval lesions with low-level internal echoes and posterior acoustic enhancement (Fig. 25-32). Needle aspiration can confirm an abscess, and follow-up sonography after treatment should establish resolution. If the lesion has not resolved, biopsy may be indicated to exclude underlying carcinoma.

TRAUMA AND POSTOPERATIVE ALTERATIONS

In breast trauma, for which mammography cannot be performed because of breast contusion and pain, sonography can depict the complex collections of varying echogenicity, depending on the acuteness of injury. If there is need to image the patient, the changes can be tracked sonographically until a mammogram can be performed without severe discomfort. As hematomas resolve, areas of scar and fat necrosis may develop.

Sonography is of particular benefit in the patient who has had surgical augmentation. Mammography may be limited, and ultrasound can be a useful supplement.[51] In addition to parenchymal abnormalities, defects, loc-

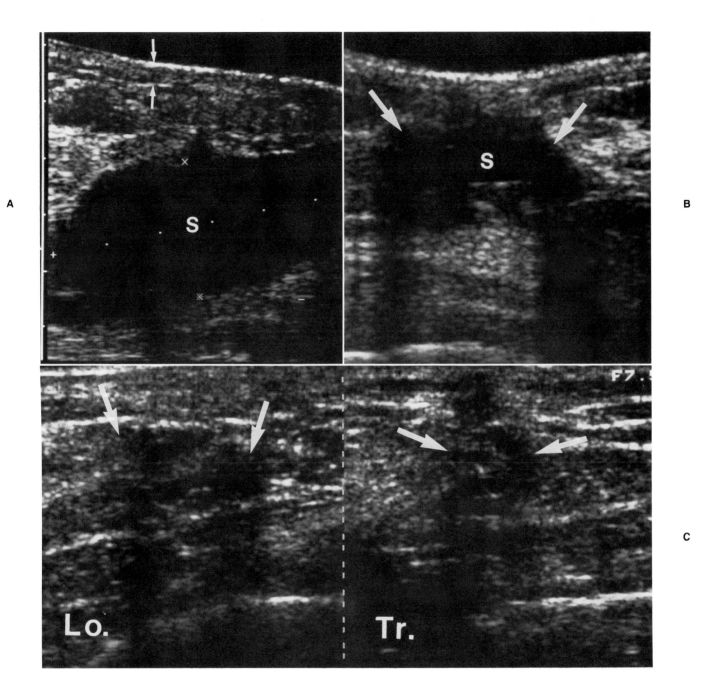

FIG 25-33. Surgically altered breast: resolution of seroma to scar at site of lumpectomy for breast carcinoma. **A,** At 6 months following lumpectomy and radiation therapy, 3-cm anechoic elliptical fluid collection *(S)* seen at lumpectomy site is compatible with seroma. Skin thickening *(arrows)* and increased echogenicity of dermis suggest edema. **B,** At 18 months following lumpectomy and radiation therapy, seroma *(S)* has decreased in size. Margins have become indistinct *(arrows)* and areas of posterior acoustic shadow have appeared, caused by partial scar formation. **C,** At 24 months after lumpectomy and radiation therapy, longitudinal *(Lo)* and transverse *(Tr)* images show that seroma has disappeared, and is replaced by poorly defined, hypoechoic region *(arrows)* with posterior acoustic shadowing. Absence of mass and linear shape on one view and round shape on other view are nonspecific but common sonographic features of scarring. Careful clinical and mammographic correlation is required.

ulations, leakages, and contractures involving the prostheses may be diagnosed with ultrasound.

Along with mammography, sonography is also sometimes used to evaluate the site of a lumpectomy for breast carcinoma. The clinical and mammographic signs of recurrent carcinoma can be similar to postoperative and postirradiation changes, including mass, edema, skin thickening, and calcification.[52] The cavity left by the tumor removal often fills with fluid.[53] These fluid collections resolve over a period of 6 to 18 months, and sonography can be used to confirm that a palpable or mammographic mass is fluid-filled and can document its reduction over time (Fig. 25-33).[54] Later, when scarring occurs, an acoustic shadow will originate from the region. Once the scar has developed, the detection of a new, enlarging, or more nodular mass at that site suggests the possibility of local tumor recurrence.

REFERENCES

1. Tabar L, Fagerberg CJG, Gad A, et al. Reduction in mortality from breast cancer after mass screening with mammography. *Lancet* 1985; 1:829-832.
2. Sickles EA, Filly RA, Callen PW. Breast cancer detection with sonography and mammography: comparison using state-of-the-art equipment. *AJR* 1983; 140:843-845.
3. Bassett LW, Kimme-Smith C, Southland LK, et al. Automated and hand-held breast ultrasound: effect on patient management. *Radiology* 1987; 165:103-108.
4. Moskowitz M. The predictive value of certain mammographic signs in screening for breast cancer. *Cancer* 1983; 51:1007-1011.
5. Jackson VP. Sonography of malignant breast disease. *Semin Ultrasound, CT, MR* 1989; 10:119-131.
6. Dempsey PJ. Breast sonography: historical perspective, clinical applications and image interpretation. *Ultrasound Q* 1988; 6:69-90.
7. Bohm-Velez M, Mendelson EB. Computed tomography, ultrasound and magnetic resonance imaging in evaluating the breast. *Semin Ultrasound, CT, MR* 1989; 10:171-176.
8. Heywang SH, Beck R, Hilbertz T, et al. Magnetic resonance imaging with Gd-DTPA in the breast after limited surgery and radiation therapy. Paper presented at the Radiological Society of North America Annual Meeting, Chicago, IL, Nov, 1989.
9. Schnapf DJ, Dabb R, Wilson D, et al. Magnetic resonance imaging of the reconstructed breast. Paper presented at the Radiological Society of North America Annual Meeting, Chicago, IL, Nov, 1989.

Indications

10. Feig SA. The role of ultrasound in a breast imaging center. *Semin Ultrasound, CT, MR* 1989; 10:90-105.
11. Bassett LW, Kimme-Smith C. Breast sonography: technique, equipment and normal anatomy. *Semin Ultrasound, CT, MR* 1989; 10:82-89.
12. Jackson VP, Kelly-Fry F, Rothschild, et al. Automated breast sonography using a 7.5 MHz PVDF transducer: preliminary clinical evaluation. *Radiology* 1986; 159:679-684.
13. Schoenberger SG, Sutherland CM, Robinson AE: Breast neoplasms: duplex sonographic imaging as an adjunct in diagnosis. *Radiology* 1988; 168:665-668.
14. Jackson VP. Breast neoplasms: duplex sonographic imaging as an adjunct in diagnosis. *Radiology* 1989; 170:578. Letter to the editor.

Examination technique

15. Rubin E, Miller VE, Berland LL, et al. Hand-held real-time breast sonography. *AJR* 1985; 144:623-627.
16. Hilton SVW, Leopold GR, Olson LK, et al. Real-time breast sonography: application in 300 consecutive patients. *AJR* 1986; 147:479-486.

Sonographic anatomy

17. Kopans DB. *Breast Imaging.* Philadelphia: JB Lippincott; 1989:232.
18. Chan TW, Troupin RH, Yeh I-T. Solid axillary masses: attempts at sonographic differentiation of an axillary lymph node from fibroadenoma. *Breast Dis* 1989; 2:187-194.

Cysts

19. Stomper PC, Recht A, Berenberg AL, et al. Mammographic detection of recurrent cancer in the irradiated breast. *AJR* 1987; 148:39-43.
20. Sickles EA, Filly CA, Callen PW. Benign breast lesions: ultrasound detection and diagnosis. *Radiology* 1984; 151:467-470.

Interventional procedures

21. Haagensen CD. *Diseases of the Breast.* 3rd ed. Philadelphia: WB Saunders Co; 1986:267-312.
22. Fornage BD, Sneige N, Faroux MJ, et al. Sonographic appearance and ultrasound-guided fine-needle aspiration biopsy of breast carcinomas smaller than 1 cm³. *J Ultrasound Med* 1990; 9:559.
23. Kopans DB, Meyer JE, Lindors, et al. Breast sonography to guide cyst aspiration and wire localization of occult solid lesions. *AJR* 1984; 143:489-492.
24. D'Orsi CJ, Mendelson EB. Interventional breast ultrasonography. *Semin Ultrasound, CT, MR* 1989; 10:132-138.

Solid and mixed lesions

25. Silverberg E, Boring C, Squires T. Cancer statistics. *CA* 1990; 40:9-26.
26. Cole-Beuglet C, Soriano RZ, Kurtz AB, et al. Ultrasound analysis of 104 primary breast carcinomas classified according to histopathologic type. *Radiology* 1983; 147:191-196.
27. Cole-Beuglet C. Sonographic manifestation of malignant breast disease. *Semin Ultrasound* 1982; 3:51-57.
28. Mendelson EB, Bohm-Velez M, Bhagwanani DG, et al. Sonographic spectrum of fibroadenomas: a guide to clinical management. Paper presented at the Radiological Society of North America Annual Meeting, Chicago, IL, 1988.
29. Harper AP, Kelly-Fry E, Noe JS, et al. Ultrasound in the evaluation of solid breast masses. *Radiology* 1983; 146:731-736.
30. Logan WW, Hoffman HY. Diabetic fibrous disease. *Radiology* 1989; 172:667-670.
31. Cole-Beuglet C, Soriano RZ, Kurtz AB, et al. Sonomammography correlated with pathology in 122 patients. *AJR* 1983; 140:369-375.
32. Jackson VP, Rothschild PA, Kreipke DL, et al. The spectrum of sonographic findings of fibroadenoma of the breast. *Invest Radiol* 1986; 21:31-40.
33. Mendelson EB, Bhagwanani DG, Bohm-Velez M. Imaging the breast treated by segmental mastectomy and irradiation. In: Brunner S, ed. *Recent Results in Cancer Research.* Berlin-Heidelberg: Springer-Verlag; 1990:175-192.
34. Baker RR. Unusual lesions and their management. *Surg Clin North Am* 1990; 70:963-975.
35. Rosen PP. The pathology of breast carcinoma. In: Harris JR, Hellman S, Henderson IC, et al, eds. *Breast Diseases.* Philadelphia: JB Lippincott; 1987:181-185.

36. Howell A, Harris M. Infiltrating lobular carcinoma of the breast. *Br Med J* 1985; 291:1371.

37. Dixon JM, Anderson TJ, Page DL, et al. Infiltrating lobular carcinoma of the breast: incidence and consequence of bilateral disease. *Br J Surg* 1983; 70:513-516.

38. Mendelson EB, Harris KM, Doshi N. Infiltrating lobular carcinoma: mammographic patterns with pathologic correlation. *AJR* 1989; 153:265-271.

39. Baker RR. Unusual lesions and their management. *Surg Clin North Am* 1990; 70:963-975.

40. Feig SA, Shaber GS, Patchefsky, et al. Tubular carcinoma of the breast. *Radiology* 1978; 129:311-314.

41. Fisher ER, Palekar AS, Kotwal N, et al. A non-encapsulating sclerosing lesion of the breast. *Am J Clin Pathol* 1979; 71:239-246.

42. Page DL, Anderson TJ. *Diagnostic histopathology of the Breast*. Edinburgh: Churchill Livingstone; 1987:186-187.

43. Martin JE. *Atlas of Mammography*. Baltimore: Williams & Wilkins; 1982:102-117.

44. Hughes LE, Mansel RE, Webster DJT, et al. *Benign Disorders and Diseases of the Breast*. London: Bailliere Tindall; 1988:59-73.

45. Fechner RE, Mills SE. *Breast Pathology*. Chicago: ASCP Press; 1990:30.

46. Fornage BD, Lorigan JG, Andry E. Fibroadenoma of the breast: sonographic appearance. *Radiology* 1989; 172:671.

47. Brenner RJ, Sickles EA. Acceptability of periodic follow-up as an alternative to biopsy for mammographically-detected lesions interpreted as probably benign. *Radiology* 1989; 171:645-646.

48. Mendelson EB, Bohm-Velez M, Lamas C, et al. Focal breast fibrosis: mimic of breast carcinoma. Paper presented at the American Roentgen Ray Society Annual Meeting, New Orleans, LA, 1989.

49. Adler DD. Ultrasound of benign breast conditions. *Semin Ultrasound, CT, MR* 1989; 10:106-118.

50. Gomez A, Mata JM, Donoso L, et al. Galactocele: three distinctive radiographic appearances. *Radiology* 1986; 158:43-44.

Trauma and postoperative alterations

51. Eklund GW, Busby RC, Miller SH, et al. Improved imaging of the augmented breast. *AJR* 1988; 151:469-473.

52. Paulus DD. Mammography of the treated breast. In: Feig SA, ed. *Breast Imaging: American Roentgen Ray Society Categorical Course Syllabus, 88th Annual Meeting, American Roentgen Ray Society, San Francisco.* 1988:56-57.

53. Fisher B, Bauer M, Margolese R, et al. Five-year results of randomized clinical trial comparing total mastectomy and segmental mastectomy with or without radiation in the treatment of breast cancer. *N Engl J Med* 1985; 312:665-673.

54. Mendelson EB. Imaging of the post-surgical breast. *Semin Ultrasound, CT, MR* 1989; 10:154-170.

CHAPTER 26

The Scrotum

- Rhonda Stewart, M.D.
- Barbara A. Carroll, M.D.

Many imaging modalities have supplemented physical examination in the evaluation of scrotal disease. Since its development in 1974, scrotal ultrasound has proven to be an accurate means of evaluating various scrotal diseases. Technical advancements in high-resolution real-time and color Doppler sonography have led to an increase in the clinical applications of scrotal sonography.

Current uses include:
- Evaluation of the location and characteristics of scrotal masses
- Evaluation of the occult primary tumor in patients with known metastatic disease
- Follow-up of patients with previous testicular neoplasms, leukemia, or lymphoma
- Evaluation of extratesticular pathology
- Evaluation of the acute scrotum
- Evaluation of scrotal trauma

- Localization of the undescended testis
- Detection of varicoceles in infertile men
- Evaluation of testicular ischemia in torsion with color Doppler sonography.[1-7]

IMAGING TECHNIQUE

Thorough palpation of the scrotal contents and history taking should precede the sonographic examination. A direct contact scan is most commonly performed, but a water bath approach may also be employed. Any acoustic coupling gel may be used. The patient is examined in the supine position. The scrotum is elevated with a towel draped over the thighs, and the penis is placed on the patient's abdomen and covered with a towel. Alternatively, the scrotal sac may be supported by the examiner's hand. Patients are asked to localize painful sites and palpable nodules within the scrotum. Palpation of these areas by the sonographer during the examination is often very useful. A 7.5 MHz or 10 MHz transducer is commonly used because it provides increased resolution of the scrotal contents. If greater penetration is needed, a 5 MHz transducer may be used, or with marked scrotal swelling, a 3.5 MHz transducer may be used. Images of both testes are obtained in transverse and sagittal planes. If possible, a transverse scan demonstrating both testes for comparison is obtained. Additional views may also be obtained in the coronal or oblique planes, with the patient upright, or performing the Valsalva maneuver when necessary. Color Doppler examination may also be performed to evaluate testicular blood flow in normal and pathologic states.

ANATOMY

The adult testes are ovoid glands measuring 3 to 5 cm in length, 2 to 4 cm in width, and 3 cm in anteroposterior dimension. Their weight ranges from 12.5 to 19 g. Their size and weight decrease with age.[2,8,9] The testes are surrounded by a dense white fibrous capsule, the tunica albuginea. Multiple thin septations (septula) arise from the innermost aspect of the tunica albuginea and converge posteriorly to form the mediastinum testis (Fig. 26-1). The mediastinum testis forms the support

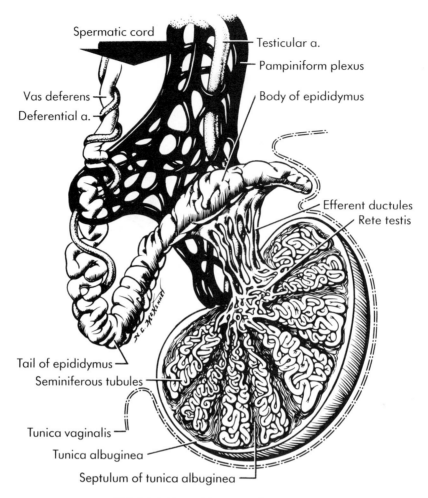

FIG 26-1. Normal intrascrotal anatomy.

for the entering and exiting testicular vessels and ducts. As the septula proceed posteriorly from the tunica albuginea, they form 250 to 400 wedge-shaped lobuli that contain the seminiferous tubules. There are approximately 840 tubules per testis. As the tubules course centrally they join other seminiferous tubules to form 20 to 30 larger ducts, known as the tubuli recti. The tubuli recti enter the mediastinum testis, forming a network of channels within the testicular stroma, called the rete testis. The rete terminate in 10 to 15 efferent ductules at the superior portion of the mediastinum, which carry the seminal fluid from the testis to the epididymis.

Sonographically, the normal testis has a homogeneous granular echo texture composed of uniformly distributed medium-level echoes, similar to that of the thyroid. The mediastinum testis is sometimes seen as a linear echogenic band extending craniocaudally within the testis (Fig. 26-2). Its appearance varies according to the amount of fibrous and fatty tissue present. It is best visualized after age 15 and before age 60.[10] The tunica

albuginea is not normally visualized as a separate structure. The septula testis may be seen as linear echogenic or hypoechoic structures (Fig. 26-3). The rete testis may be visualized as a hypoechoic area adjacent to the head of the epididymis.

The epididymis is a curved structure measuring 6 to 7 cm in length lying posterolateral to the testis. It is composed of a head, a body, and a tail. The head of the epididymis, also known as the globus major, is located adjacent to the superior pole of the testis and is the largest portion of the epididymis. It is formed by 10 to 15 efferent ductules from the rete testis joining together to form a single convoluted duct, the ductus epididymis. This duct forms the body and the majority of the tail of the epididymis. It measures approximately 600 cm in length and follows a very convoluted course from the head to the tail of the epididymis. The body or corpus of the epididymis lies adjacent to the posterolateral margin of the testis. The tail or globus minor is loosely attached to the lower pole of the testis by areolar tissue. The ductus epididymis forms an acute angle at the infe-

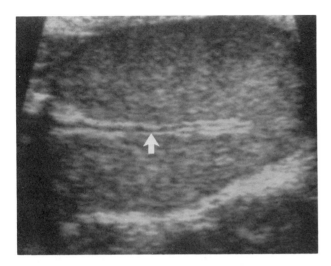

FIG 26-2. Normal mediastinum testis. Longitudinal scan demonstrates the mediastinum testis *(arrow)*, which is seen as an echogenic fibro-fatty tissue surrounding an anechoic vascular structure.

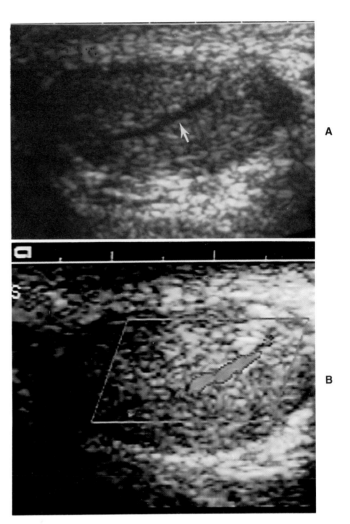

FIG 26-3. Normal testicular band. **A,** Transverse scan of the testis demonstrates a hypoechoic linear intratesticular band. **B,** Color Doppler depicts the vascular nature of this band.

rior aspect of the globus minor and courses cephalad on the medial aspect of the epididymis to the spermatic cord. The appendix testis, a remnant of the Müllerian duct, is a small ovoid structure located beneath the head of the epididymis. The appendix epididymis, representing a detached efferent duct, is a small stalk projecting off the epididymis.

Sonographically, the **epididymis** is normally iso-echoic or slightly more echogenic than the testis, and its echo texture may be coarser. The **globus major** normally measures 10 to 12 mm in diameter and lies lateral to the superior pole of the testis. The **body** tends to be isoechoic or slightly less echogenic than the globus major and testis (Fig. 26-4). The normal body measures less than 4 mm in diameter, averaging 1 to 2 mm. The **tail, appendix epididymis,** and **appendix testis** are not identified routinely as separate structures sonographically unless a small hydrocele is present.

Testicular blood flow is supplied primarily by the **deferential, cremasteric (external spermatic),** and **testicular arteries.** The deferential artery originates from the inferior vesicle artery and courses to the tail of the epididymis, where it divides and forms a capillary network. The cremasteric artery arises from the inferior epigastric artery. It courses with the remainder of the structures of the spermatic cord through the inguinal ring, continuing to the surface of the tunica vaginalis where it anastomoses with capillaries of the testicular and deferential arteries. The testicular arteries arise from the anterior aspect of the aorta just below the origin of the renal arteries. They course through the inguinal canal with the spermatic cord to the posterosuperior aspect of the testis. Upon reaching the testis, the

testicular artery divides into branches, which pierce the tunica albuginea and arborize over the surface of the testis in a layer known as the tunica vasculosa. Centripetal branches arise from these capsular arteries; these branches course along the septula to converge on the mediastinum. From the mediastinum, these branches form recurrent rami that course centrifugally within the testicular parenchyma, where they branch into arterioles and capillaries.[8]

Knowledge of the arterial supply of the testis is important for interpretation of color Doppler sonography of the testis. The color Doppler ultrasound appearance of the normal testis and waveforms of the normal testicular artery have recently been described by Middleton et al.[7] Color Doppler sonography was able to identify accurately the capsular and intratesticular arteries in all cases. The velocity waveforms of the normal capsular

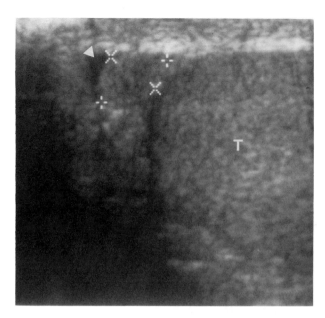

FIG 26-4. Normal head of the epididymitis. Longitudinal scrotal scan demonstrates the head of the epididymitis (xx++) lying superior to the testis *(T)*. A small, normal amount of fluid is seen between the layers of the tunica vaginalis *(arrowhead)*.

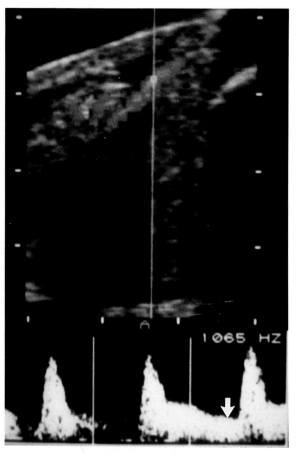

FIG 26-5. Normal color flow and spectral Doppler of the testicular artery. Normal color Doppler scan of the testicular artery demonstrates characteristic low-impedance arterial waveforms with a large amount of end-diastolic flow *(arrow)*.

and intratesticular arteries showed high levels of antegrade diastolic flow throughout the cardiac cycle, reflecting the low vascular resistance of the testis (Fig. 26-5). Supratesticular arteries were also identified in all cases, but their waveforms varied in appearance. Two main types of waveforms were identified: a low-resistance waveform like the capsular and intratesticular arteries, and a high-resistance waveform with sharp, narrow systolic peaks and little or no diastolic flow (Fig. 26-6). This high resistance waveform is believed to reflect the high vascular resistance of the extratesticular tissues. The deferential and cremasteric arteries within the spermatic cord primarily supply the epididymis and extratesticular tissues, but also supply the testis via anastomoses with the testicular artery.

A hypoechoic **intratesticular band** has been described in 10% of normal testes (Fig. 26-3).[11] This well-circumscribed band is most commonly visualized in the middle third of the testicle, nearly perpendicular to the mediastinum on sagittal scans. It measures up to 3 mm in diameter and 3 cm in length. Pulsed Doppler sonography of the band demonstrates a low-resistance waveform characteristic of the normal intratesticular arterial waveform in half the cases. No venous waveforms are obtained, but it is believed that venous flow also contributes to the thickness of the hypoechoic band.

The spermatic cord consists of the vas deferens, the cremasteric, deferential, and testicular arteries; a pampiniform plexus of veins, the lymphatics, and the

nerves of the testis. Sonographically, the normal spermatic cord lies just beneath the skin and is difficult to distinguish from the adjacent soft tissues of the inguinal canal.[12] It may be visualized within the scrotum when a hydrocele is present or with the use of color Doppler sonography (Fig. 26-7).

The layers of the scrotum consist of:

- Skin
- Dartos
- External spermatic fascia
- Cremasteric fascia
- Internal spermatic fascia
- Parietal layer of the tunica vaginalis

The **dartos,** a layer of muscle fibers lying beneath the scrotal skin, is continuous with the scrotal septum, which divides the scrotum into two separate chambers. The walls of the chambers are formed by the fusion of the three fascial layers.

The **tunica vaginalis** is the space between these scrotal fascial layers and the tunica albuginea of the tes-

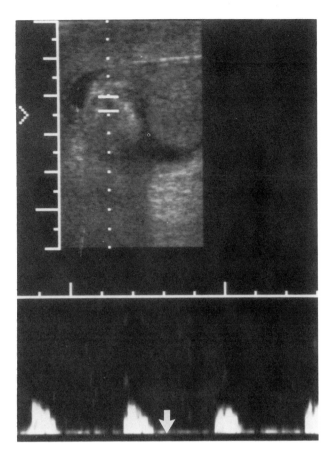

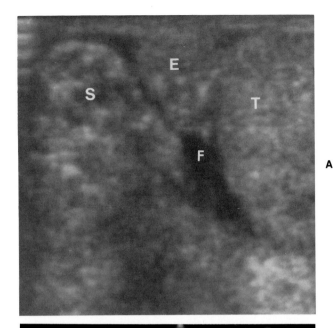

FIG 26-6. Normal extratesticular arterial Doppler tracings. The cremasteric and deferential arteries of the spermatic cord demonstrate a high-resistance waveform without evidence of significant diastolic flow *(arrow).*

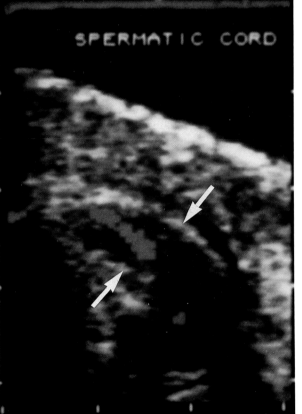

FIG 26-7. Normal spermatic cord. **A,** Longitudinal scan through the scrotum demonstrates the head of the epididymis *(E),* the testis *(T),* a small amount of normal scrotal fluid *(F),* and a prominent spermatic cord *(S).* **B,** Normal color flow within a spermatic cord *(arrows).*

tis. During embryological development, the tunica vaginalis arises from the **processus vaginalis,** an outpouching of fetal peritoneum that accompanies the testis in its descent in the scrotum. The upper portion of the processus vaginalis, extending from the internal inguinal ring to the upper pole of the testis, is normally obliterated. The lower portion, the tunica vaginalis, remains as a closed pouch folded around the testis. Only the posterior aspect of the testis, the site of attachment of the testis and epididymis, is not in continuity with the tunica vaginalis. The inner or visceral layer of the tunica vaginalis covers the testis, epididymis, and lower portion of the spermatic cord. The outer or parietal layer of the tunica vaginalis lines the walls of the scrotal pouch and is attached to the fascial coverings of the testis. A small amount of fluid is normally present between these two layers, especially in the polar regions and between the testicle and epididymis (Fig. 26-7).

The scrotal covering layers are normally inseparable by sonography and are visualized as a single echogenic stripe. If any type of fluid is present in the scrotal wall, the tunica vaginalis may be identified as a separate structure.[2]

SCROTAL MASS

Ultrasound of the scrotum can detect intrascrotal masses with a sensitivity of nearly 100%.[13] It plays a major role in the evaluation of scrotal masses because of its accuracy of 98% to 100% in differentiating intratesticular and extratesticular pathology.[5,14] This distinction is important in patient management because most extratesticular masses are benign, but the majority of intratesticular lesions are malignant.[1,9] All intratesticular masses should be considered potentially malignant until proven otherwise.[2]

Most malignant testicular neoplasms are more hypoechoic than normal testicular parenchyma, however, hemorrhage, necrosis, calcification, or fatty changes can produce areas of increased echogenicity within these tumors. Uniformly echogenic masses are more often benign processes resulting from infectious or vascular abnormalities. Nevertheless, one must still consider even echogenic lesions potentially malignant, as most benign testicular processes, hypoechoic or hyperechoic, are nonspecific in appearance.

Testicular neoplasms account for 1% to 2% of all

■ **TABLE 26-1**
Pathologic Classification of Testicular Tumors

Germ Cell Tumors

Tumors of one histologic type
  Seminoma
    Classical
    Spermatocystic
  Embryonal cell carcinoma
    Adult type
    Infantile type
    Endodermal sinus tumor
  Teratoma
    Mature
    Immature
    With malignant transformation
  Choriocarcinoma
Tumors of more than one histologic type
  Teratoma and embryonal cell carcinoma
  (teratocarcinoma)
  Choriocarcinoma and any other type
  Other combinations

Tumors of gonadal stroma

Leydig cell tumors
Sertoli cell, granulosa cell, theca cell tumors
Tumors of primitive gonadal stroma
Mixtures of the above

Modified from Mostofi FK.

malignant neoplasms in men and are the fifth most frequent cause of death in men aged 15 to 34 years.[15] Approximately 65% to 94% of patients with testicular neoplasms present with painless unilateral testicular masses or diffuse testicular enlargement. From 4% to 14% of patients with testicular neoplasms present with symptoms of metastatic disease,[2,16,17] and 90% to 95% of primary testicular tumors are of germ cell origin and are generally highly malignant.[18] Only 60% of testicular germ cell tumors are of a single histologic type, and the remainder contain two or more histologic types. Gonadal stromal tumors, arising from Sertoli cells or Leydig cells, account for 3% to 6% of testicular masses.[2,9,17] The majority of these mesenchymal neoplasms are benign (Table 26-1).

Malignant Tumors

Germ Cell Tumors. Pure **seminoma** is the most common single-cell-type testicular tumor in adults, accounting for 40% to 50% of all germ cell neoplasms. It is also a common component of mixed germ cell tumors, occurring in 30% of these tumors. Seminomas occur in a slightly older age group when compared with other testicular neoplasms, demonstrating a peak incidence in the fourth and fifth decades.[2,13,19-21] They rarely occur before puberty. They are less aggressive than other testicular tumors and are commonly confined within the tunica albuginea at presentation, although 25% of patients have metastases at diagnosis. As a result of the radiosensitivity and chemosensitivity of the primary tumor and its metastases, seminomas have the most favorable prognosis of the malignant testicular tumors. A second primary synchronous or metachronous germ cell tumor occurs in 1% to 2.5% of patients with seminomas.

Seminoma is the most common tumor type in cryptorchid testes. Between 8% and 30% of patients with seminoma have a history of undescended testes.[17,20,21] The risk of developing a seminoma is substantially increased in an undescended testis, even after orchiopexy. There is also an increased risk for developing malignancy in the contralateral normally located testis, and therefore sonography is sometimes used to screen for an occult tumor in the remaining testis.

Macroscopically, seminoma is a homogeneously solid, firm, round or oval tumor that varies in size from a small nodule in a normal-sized testis to a large mass causing diffuse testicular enlargement.[15] The sonographic features of pure seminoma parallel this homogeneous macroscopic appearance (Fig. 26-8). They are composed predominantly of uniform low-level echoes without calcification or cystic areas.[22] These tumors may be smoothly marginated or ill-defined, but are generally very hypoechoic compared with normally echogenic testicular parenchyma.

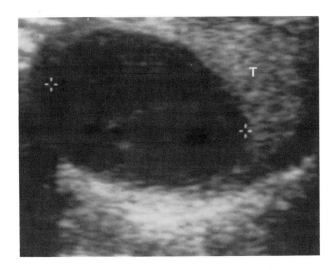

FIG 26-8. Seminoma. A well-circumscribed predominantly hypoechoic intratesticular mass (++) with echogenicity markedly less than that of the normal adjacent testis (T) is characteristic of seminoma.

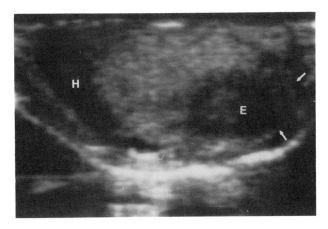

FIG 26-9. Embryonal cell carcinoma. An aggressive poorly marginated embryonal cell carcinoma (E) is seen to invade through the layers of the tunica (arrows). A small hydrocele is also present (H).

Embryonal cell carcinoma is the second most common testicular germ cell neoplasm. It often occurs in combination with other neoplastic germ cell elements, particularly yolk sac tumor and teratoma. It constitutes 20% to 25% of all primary germ cell malignancies. These tumors occur in a younger age group than seminomas, with a peak incidence during the latter part of the second decade and the third decade. It is uncommon before puberty and after the age of 50 years. These malignancies are usually small, replacing part or all of the testis without producing pronounced enlargement. Despite their small size, they tend to be more aggressive than seminomas, frequently invading the tunica albuginea, resulting in distortion of the testicular contour (Fig. 26-9). They frequently cause visceral metastases.[2,21] The infantile form, **endodermal sinus** or **yolk sac tumor,** is the most common germ cell tumor in infants, accounting for 60% of testicular neoplasms in this age group, commonly occurring before the age of 2 years. It is associated with elevated alpha-fetoprotein levels in 95% of infants. Both embryonal cell carcinoma and endodermal sinus tumor are less radiosensitive and chemosensitive than seminomas and have a reported 5-year survival rate of 25% to 35%.[21]

The sonographic features of embryonal cell carcinoma parallel its histology. It is generally more inhomogeneous and poorly marginated than the seminoma. Invasion of the tunica may occur, resulting in distortion of the testicular contour. Cystic areas are present in one third of tumors,[13] and echogenic foci, with or without acoustic shadowing, are not uncommon.

Teratomas constitute approximately 5% to 10% of primary testicular neoplasms.[21] They are defined according to the World Health Organization classification on the basis of the presence of derivatives of the different germinal layers (endoderm, mesoderm, ectoderm). There are three categories of teratomas according to this classification: mature, immature, and teratoma with malignant transformation.[17] One third of teratomas will metastasize, usually via a lymphatic route, within 5 years.[2,21] The reported 5-year survival rate is 70%. The peak age incidence is infancy and early childhood, with another peak in the third decade. Teratomas are the second most common testicular tumor in infants and young children, are most commonly mature and well differentiated, and have a benign course. Occasional cases may contain immature elements, but metastases are rare.[20] Tumors occurring after puberty commonly contain immature and mature elements admixed with other germ cell types. Teratomas in adults are considered malignant.

Sonographically, the teratoma is commonly a well-defined, markedly inhomogeneous mass containing cystic and solid areas of various sizes. Dense echogenic foci causing complete or incomplete acoustic shadowing are common, resulting from focal calcification, cartilage, immature bone, fibrosis, and noncalcific scarring (Fig. 26-10).[22]

Choriocarcinoma is the rarest type of germ cell tumor, constituting only 1% to 3% of malignant primary testicular tumors.[21] It rarely occurs in its pure form; only 18 cases were encountered among more than 6000 testicular tumors registered at the Armed Forces Institute of Pathology.[23] Approximately 23% of mixed germ cell tumors contain a component of choriocarcinoma.[20] The peak incidence is in the second and third decades. These tumors are highly malignant and metastasize early via hematogenous and lymphatic routes. Patients

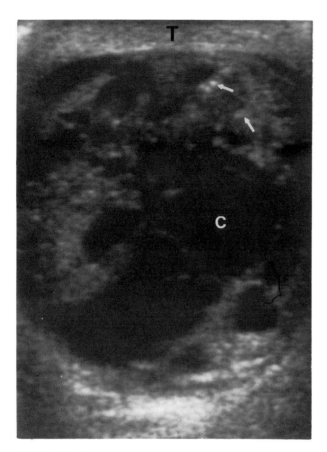

FIG 26-10. Malignant teratoma. A transverse testicular scan demonstrates a large malignant teratoma replacing most of the testis. Cystic *(C)* and solid elements with small echogenic foci *(arrows)* from small calcifications are present. Residual normal testis *(T)*.

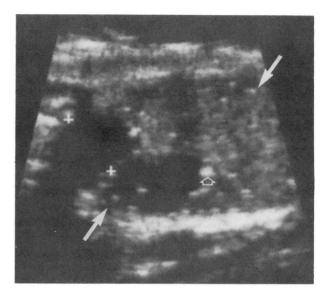

FIG 26-11. Choriocarcinoma. Longitudinal scan demonstrates a testis diffusely involved by choriocarcinoma *(arrows)*. There are large cystic areas of necrosis *(+ +)* and areas of increased echogenicity corresponding to hemorrhage and calcification *(open arrow)*.

often have symptoms resulting from hemorrhagic metastases: hemoptysis, hematemesis, and CNS symptoms. Gynecomastia is common because of the high levels of circulating chorionic gonadotropins.[17] Metastases may be present without any evidence of choriocarcinoma in the testicle. Sonography demonstrates a mass of mixed echogenicity containing areas of hemorrhage, necrosis, and calcification (Fig. 26-11).

Mixed germ cell tumors contain different neoplastic germ cell elements in various combinations. They are the second most common testicular malignancy after seminoma, constituting 40% of all germ cell tumors. They occur in the same age group as nonseminomatous germ cell tumors. The combined teratoma and embryonal cell carcinoma is the most frequent mixed germ cell tumor. It has been called *teratocarcinoma* in the past. It commonly contains both solid and cystic elements, causing its sonographic appearance to be very similar to that of the pure teratoma.

Stromal Tumors. Gonadal stromal tumors account for 3% to 6% of all testicular neoplasms. Approxi-

mately 20% of these tumors occur in children.[15] The term *gonadal stromal tumor* refers to a neoplasm containing Leydig, thecal, granulosa, or lutein cells and fibroblasts in various degrees of differentiation. These tumors may contain single or multiple cell types because of the totipotentiality of the gonadal stroma.[17] Gonadal stromal tumors may also occur in conjunction with germ-cell tumors and may be termed a gonadoblastoma. The majority of gonadoblastomas occur in males with cryptorchidism, hypospadia, and female internal secondary sex organs.[20]

The majority of stromal tumors are Leydig cell tumors. They account for 1% to 3% of all testicular neoplasms and occur predominantly between the ages of 20 and 50 years.[19,20,24] Patients most commonly present with painless testicular enlargement or a palpable mass. Approximately 15% of patients present with gynecomastia resulting from the secretion of androgens, estrogens, or a combination. Impotence, loss of libido, or precocious virilization may also occur in young males. The tumor is bilateral in 3% of cases. From 10% to 15% of tumors demonstrate malignant behavior, invading the tunica at diagnosis. Foci of hemorrhage and necrosis are present in 25% of tumors.[19,24]

These gonadal tumors are usually small, solid, and hypoechoic on ultrasound (Fig. 26-12). Cystic spaces resulting from hemorrhage and necrosis are occasionally seen in larger lesions.[25]

The Occult Primary Tumor. Ultrasound plays an important role in patients with a normal physical examina-

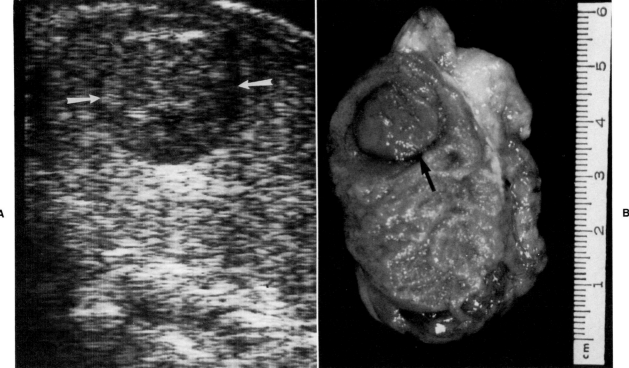

FIG 26-12. Leydig cell tumor. **A,** Longitudinal scan of the superior half of the testis demonstrates a small, solid, homogeneous, and well-circumscribed mass *(arrows).* **B,** Gross pathological specimen confirms the well-circumscribed nature of this Leydig cell tumor *(arrows).*
(Courtesy of J. William Charboneau, M.D., Mayo Clinic, Rochester, Minn.)

tion who present with mediastinal, retroperitoneal, or supraclavicular metastases resulting from metastatic testicular carcinoma.[26-28] The detection of the occult primary tumor is very important in patient management, because if it is not removed, metastases will continue. Ultrasound has been shown to be able to detect impalpable testicular neoplasms. The primary testicular tumor may regress despite widespread advancing metastatic disease resulting in an echogenic fibrous and possibly calcific scar. It has been theorized that this regression is due to the high metabolic rate of the tumor and vascular compromise from the tumor outgrowing its blood supply. Usually no viable tumor cells are identifiable on histologic section in these cases.[15,16] The affected testis is often normal sized or small. The sonographic finding of an echogenic focus with or without posterior acoustic shadowing is not specific for a "burned-out" tumor, but is strongly suggestive of this diagnosis in the context of histologically proven testicular metastases (Fig. 26-13).[29]

Impalpable testicular tumors have also been detected in patients presenting with infertility.[18] In these cases, sonography is also important in surgical localization for intraoperative diagnosis since testicle-sparing resection may be performed if the lesion is benign.

Metastases, Leukemia, and Lymphoma. **Leukemia** and **lymphoma** are the most common metastatic testicular tumors. **Malignant lymphoma** is the most common secondary testicular neoplasm. It accounts for 1% to 8% of all testicular tumors and is the most common testicular tumor in males over 60; still, testicular involvement occurs in only 0.3% of patients with lymphoma.[17,30] The peak age at diagnosis is between 60 and 70 years; 80% of patients are over the age of 50 years at diagnosis. Malignant lymphoma is the most common bilateral testicular tumor, occurring bilaterally either in a synchronous, or more commonly, metachronous manner, in 6% to 38% of cases. One half of bilateral testicular neoplasms are malignant lymphoma.[17,19]

Testicular lymphoma may occur as a site of primary extranodal disease, in association with disseminated disease, or as the initial manifestation of occult nodal

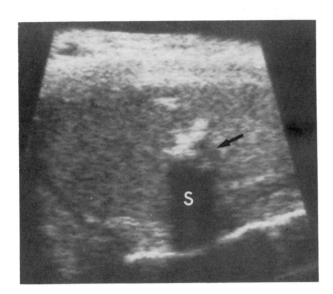

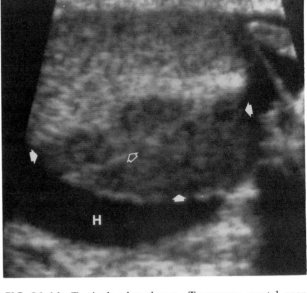

FIG 26-13. Regressed "burned-out" tumor. Longitudinal scrotal scan demonstrates a 0.7 cm, solid, echogenic, calcified mass with acoustic shadowing *(S)* in the midportion of the testis. A small hypoechoic component *(open arrow)* represents either viable residual embryonal cell carcinoma or "burned-out" tumor.

FIG 26-14. Testicular lymphoma. Transverse scrotal scan demonstrates a focal hypoechoic lymphomatous mass *(arrows)* in a patient with diffuse histiocytic lymphoma metastatic to the testis. A small branch of the septula testis is seen *(open arrow)* encased by this lymphomatous mass. *H,* Hydrocele.

disease. Approximately 10% of patients have lymphoma localized to the testis.[17,30] This form of testicular lymphoma has a better prognosis, but systemic lymphoma develops in 25% of patients soon after presentation or after orchiectomy. The remainder of patients with testicular involvement have a uniformly poor prognosis. The 2-year and 5-year survival rates are 4% to 30% and 5% to 20%, respectively. The median survival is 9.5 to 12 months.[31,32]

The clinical presentation of malignant lymphoma is very similar to that of germ cell neoplasms. Most patients present with a painless testicular mass or diffuse testicular enlargement. Approximately 25% of patients have constitutional symptoms of lymphoma, such as fever, weakness, anorexia, or weight loss.[30]

Most malignant lymphomas of the testicle are of the non-Hodgkin's type. Using the Rappaport classification, diffuse histiocytic lymphoma is the most common type of testicular lymphoma, followed by poorly differentiated lymphocytic lymphoma.[17] Hodgkin's lymphoma is extremely rare; only four cases have been reported.[33]

Lymphoma of the testis is often quite large at diagnosis. The tunica vaginalis is usually intact, but extension into the epididymis and spermatic cord is common, occurring in up to 50% of cases.[19] The scrotal skin is rarely involved. Grossly, the tumor is not encapsulated but compresses the parenchyma to the periphery. The

majority of malignant lymphomas are homogeneous and diffusely replace the testis.[17,30] However, focal hypoechoic lesions can occur (Fig. 26-14). Hemorrhage and necrosis are rare.

Leukemia is the second most common metastatic testicular neoplasm. Primary testicular leukemia is very rare, but leukemic infiltration of the testicle during bone marrow remission is common in children.[17,34] It is believed that the testis acts as a sanctuary site for leukemic cells during chemotherapy because of a "blood-gonad barrier" that inhibits concentration of chemotherapeutic agents.[34] The highest frequency of testicular involvement is found in patients with acute leukemia (64%). Approximately 25% of patients with chronic leukemia have testicular involvement.[35] Most cases of testicular involvement occur within 1 year of discontinuation of long-term remission maintenance chemotherapy. The rate of relapse in this setting is nearly 13%.[34]

The sonographic appearance of lymphoma and leukemia is nonspecific. Diffuse infiltration, producing diffusely enlarged, hypoechoic testes, is the most frequent presentation for both processes (Fig. 26-15). Focal, sharply marginated, anechoic masses with through sound transmission and occasional low-level internal echoes have been described in chronic lymphocytic leukemia.[35] Nonlymphomatous metastases to the testes are uncommon, representing only 0.02% to 5% of all testicular neoplasms.[36,37] The most frequent primary

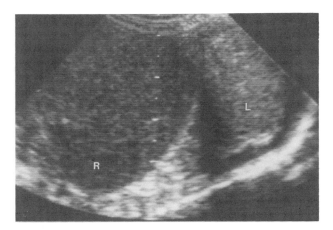

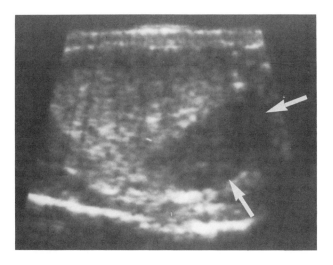

FIG 26-15. Testicular leukemia. Transverse scan showing both the right *(R)* and left *(L)* testes demonstrates diffuse hypoechoic enlargement of the right testis resulting from leukemic infiltrate.

FIG 26-16. Testicular metastasis. Transverse testicular scan demonstrates a hypoechoic lung carcinoma metastasis *(arrows)* to the testis.

sites are the **lung** and **prostate,** accounting for one third and one fifth of testicular metastases, respectively.[19] Other frequent primary sites for metastatic neoplasms include **kidney, stomach, colon, pancreas, and melanoma.**[36,38] Most metastases are clinically silent, being discovered incidentally at autopsy or after orchiectomy for prostatic carcinoma (Fig. 26-16). Testicular metastases are most common during the sixth and seventh decades, and are more frequent than primary germ cell tumors after the age of 50 years.[2,32] They are commonly multiple and are bilateral in 15% of cases.[19] Since primary germ cell tumors may also be multicentric and bilateral, these features are not helpful in distinguishing primary from metastatic testicular neoplasms. Widespread systemic metastases are usually present at diagnosis.[36] Possible routes of metastases to the testis include retrograde venous, hematogenous, retrograde lymphatic, and direct tumor invasion.[30,31] Sites remote from the testis, such as the lung and skin, most likely spread via the hematogenous route. Retrograde venous extension through the spermatic vein has been shown to occur in renal cell carcinoma and may also occur in **bladder** and **prostate** tumors.[39] Neoplasms with metastases to the periaortic lymph nodes may involve the testis through retrograde lymphatic extension. Colorectal carcinoma may also directly invade the testes. Sonographic features of nonlymphomatous testicular metastases vary. They are often hypoechoic, but may be echogenic or complex in appearance.[2]

Benign Intratesticular Lesions

Cysts. Testicular cysts are discovered incidentally on ultrasound in 8% to 10% of the population.[40,41] Cystic testicular lesions are not uniformly benign because testicular tumors may undergo cystic degeneration be-

cause of hemorrhage or necrosis. The differentiation between a benign cyst and a cystic neoplasm is of utmost clinical importance. Benign cysts of the testicle have received much attention in the literature, but cystic neoplasms are not widely reported. Of the 34 cystic testicular masses discovered by ultrasound by Hamm et al.,[40] 16 were neoplastic. Teratomas are the most common tumors to undergo cystic changes; teratomas are usually multiple and vary in size. Solid components are often seen in association with the cystic masses.

There are two types of benign cysts: cysts of the tunica albuginea and intratesticular cysts. **Cysts of the tunica albuginea** are located within the tunica, usually on the anterior and lateral aspects of the testis. They vary in size from 2 to 5 mm and are well defined. They may be solitary or multiple, unilocular or multilocular. They are discovered in patients in their fifth and sixth decades and are commonly asymptomatic. Histologically, they are simple cysts lined with cuboid or low columnar cells and filled with serous fluid. Their etiology is unknown (Fig. 26-17).[42-44] **Intratesticular cysts** are simple cysts filled with clear serous fluid that vary in size between 2 and 18 mm.[45,46] They have sonographic characteristics of benign simple cysts occurring in other organs; they are well-defined, anechoic lesions with thin, smooth walls and posterior acoustic enhancement. Hamm et al.[40] reported that in all 13 of their cases, the cysts were located near the mediastinum testis, supporting the theory that they originate from the rete testis, possibly secondary to posttraumatic or postinflammatory stricture formation (Fig. 26-18).[40,42]

Epidermoid Cysts. The epidermoid cyst is a benign tumor of germ cell origin, representing approximately

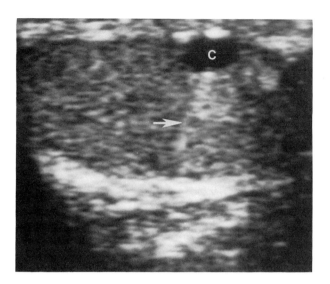

FIG 26-17. Cyst of the tunica albuginea. Longitudinal scrotal scan demonstrates a well-circumscribed peripheral tunica albuginea cyst *(C)* with posterior acoustic enhancement *(arrow)*.

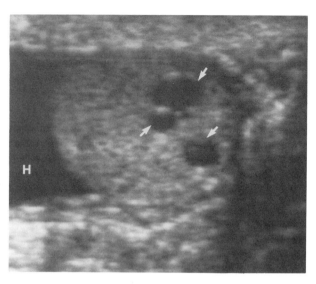

FIG 26-18. Benign intratesticular cysts. Transverse scan demonstrates multiple intratesticular cysts *(arrows)* in the mediastinum testis after multiple episodes of epididymitis. *H,* Reactive hydrocele.

1% of all testicular tumors. These tumors may occur at any age, but are most common during the second to fourth decades.[19,47,48] Patients usually present with a painless testicular nodule, although one third are discovered incidentally on physical examination. Diffuse painless testicular enlargement occurs in 10% of cases.[47,49] These lesions are generally well-circumscribed solid tumors lying beneath the tunica albuginea. Pathologically, the tumor wall is composed of fibrous tissue with an inner lining of squamous epithelium. The cyst is filled with flaky, cheesy-white keratin.

Epidermoid cysts are believed to represent monomorphic or monodermal development of a teratoma along the line of ectodermal cell differentiation.[47,49,50] These benign lesions can only be differentiated from premalignant teratomas through histologic examination. By definition, epidermoid cysts contain no teratomatous elements, and thus have no malignant potential.

Sonographically, epidermoid cysts are generally well-defined, solid, hypoechoic masses, which occasionally are internally hyperechoic. The mass typically has an echogenic capsule (Fig. 26-19).[48,51] Although this appearance is relatively characteristic, malignancy cannot be completely excluded on sonographic findings alone. The proper treatment of these lesions is still debated. A conservative testicle-sparing approach with local excision (enucleation) or simple or radical orchiectomy can be performed. Orchiectomy is usually performed because the diagnosis often cannot be made with 100% certainty clinically, and differentiation from a teratoma can only be made by careful pathologic ex-

amination of the cyst wall and adjacent testis.[47] Orchiectomy results in 100% survival, and no further treatment is necessary.

Cystic Dysplasia. Cystic dysplasia is a rare congenital malformation, usually occurring in infants and young children, although one case has been reported in a 30-year-old man.[52] Only six cases have been described. This lesion is believed to result from an embryologic defect preventing connection of the tubules of the rete testis and the efferent ductules. Pathologically, the lesion consists of multiple, interconnecting cysts of various sizes and shapes, separated by fibrous septae.[17] This lesion originates in the rete testis and extends into the adjacent parenchyma, resulting in pressure atrophy of the adjacent testicular parenchyma. The cysts are lined by a single layer of flat or cuboidal epithelium. Of the reported six patients, two had ipsilateral renal agenesis and one had bilateral renal dysplasia.[53,54] The adult had bilateral renal duplication and obstruction of the upper pole moiety of one kidney.

The sonographic appearance has been reported only once.[52] Examination revealed a large mass containing irregular anechoic spaces varying from 2 to 8 mm. A small amount of normal testicular parenchyma was visualized at the inferior aspect of this mass.

Abscess. Testicular abscesses are usually a complication of epididymo-orchitis; they may also result from missed testicular torsion, gangrenous or infected tumor, or primary pyogenic orchitis. Common infectious causes of abscess formation are **mumps, smallpox, scarlet fever, influenza, typhoid, sinusitis, osteomy-**

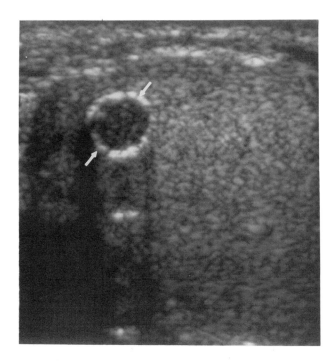

FIG 26-19. Benign epidermoid cyst. Longitudinal testicular scan demonstrates well-circumscribed epidermoid "keratin" cyst with smooth echogenic walls *(arrows)* and echogenic material within it. At surgery a well-encapsulated, benign epidermoid cyst that contained cheesy material was found with calcifications in the capsule. The benign sonographic appearance resulted in testicular sparing.
(Courtesy of Ben Hollenberg, M.D., Presbyterian Hospital, Charlotte, N.C.)

elitis, appendicitis, and many others.[55] The testicular abscess may rupture through the tunica vaginalis, resulting in pyocele formation or fistulous formation to the skin.

Sonography demonstrates, most commonly, an enlarged testicle containing a predominantly fluid-filled mass with hypoechoic or mixed echogenic areas visualized (Fig. 26-20). An atypical appearance has been described in which there was disruption of the testicular architecture with hyperechoic striations separating hypoechoic spaces (Fig. 26-21).[56] The striations were believed to represent fibrous septa that separate the hypoechoic, necrotic testicular parenchyma. There are no diagnostic sonographic features of testicular abscesses, but they can often be differentiated from tumors by clinical symptoms.

Infarction. Testicular infarction may follow torsion, trauma, bacterial endocarditis, polyarteritis nodosa, leukemia, and Henoch-Schönlein purpura.[57,58] The sonographic appearance depends on the age of the infarction. Initially, the infarct is seen either as a focal hypoechoic mass or as a diffusely hypoechoic testicle of normal size. With time, the hypoechoic mass or entire testicle often decreases in size and develops areas of increased echogenicity, representing fibrosis or dystrophic calcification (Fig. 26-22).[9,56,58] The early sonographic appearance may be difficult to differentiate from a testicular neoplasm, but infarcts substantially decrease in size, whereas tumors characteristically enlarge with time.[2]

Sarcoidosis. Sarcoidosis may involve the epididymis, and less commonly, the testis. Genital involvement occurs in less than 1% of patients with systemic sarcoidosis.[2,9] The clinical presentation is one of acute or recurrent epididymitis or painless enlargement of the

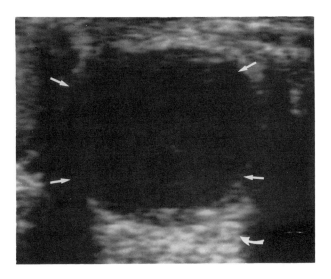

FIG 26-20. Typical testicular abscess. Hypoechoic testicular abscess *(arrows)* is indistinguishable from a tumor. However, enhanced posterior sound transmission *(curved arrow)* suggests that the mass is primarily fluid.

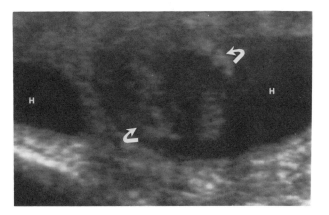

FIG 26-21. Atypical testicular abscess. Atypical appearance of a testicular abscess *(curved arrows)* is noted with echogenic and hypoechoic components. *H,* Bilateral hydroceles.

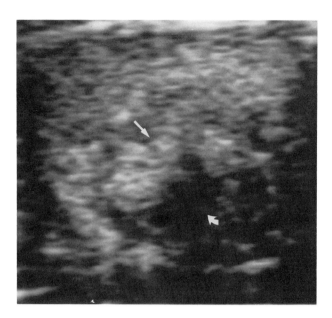

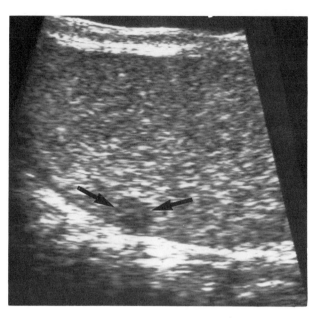

FIG 26-22. Chronic infarction of the testis. Transverse scan through a testis with chronic infarction demonstrates areas of both increased *(arrow)* and decreased *(curved arrow)* echogenicity which is indistinguishable from the appearance of malignancy.

FIG 26-23. Testicular sarcoid. Longitudinal scan of the testis demonstrates a small hypoechoic solid mass *(arrows)* representing sarcoidosis.
(Courtesy of J. William Charboneau, M.D., Mayo Clinic, Rochester, Minn.).

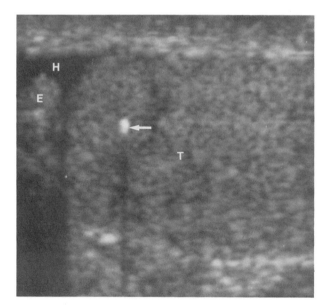

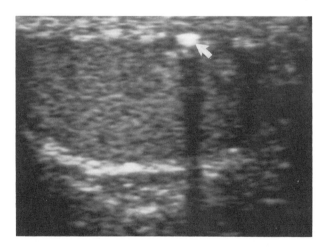

FIG 26-24. Testicular calcification. Longitudinal scrotal scan of an asymptomatic patient reveals a normal-appearing testis *(T)* and epididymis *(E)* as well as a small hydrocele *(H)*. A well-circumscribed focal calcification *(arrow)* was incidentally detected and was probably related to prior inflammatory change or sperm cell granuloma formation because there was no change in 6 months.

FIG 26-25. Calcified plaque from the tunica vaginalis. Longitudinal scan demonstrates calcification of the tunica vaginalis *(arrow)*.

testis or epididymis. Sonographically, sarcoid lesions are irregular, hypoechoic solid masses in the testis or epididymis (Fig. 26-23).[5,59] Occasionally, hyperechoic calcific foci with acoustic shadowing may be seen.[3] Differentiation from an inflammatory process or neoplasm is difficult on sonography, and clinical correlation is necessary. Resection or orchiectomy may be necessary for definitive diagnosis.

Scrotal Calcifications. Scrotal calcifications may be seen within the parenchyma of the testicle, on the surface of the testicle, or freely located in the fluid between the layers of the tunica vaginalis. Testicular microlithiasis is a rare condition in which calcifications are present within the seminiferous tubules.[9,60] Six cases have been reported in the literature. These calcifications occur in normal and cryptorchid testes and have been reported in association with other conditions, including **Klinefelter's syndrome, male pseudohermaphroditism,** and **testicular neoplasms.**[60-62] It is postulated that microlithiasis results from calcification of corpora-amylacea-like bodies that may be found in the seminiferous tubules of both cryptorchid and normally descended testes.[63] Sonography demonstrates innumerable small hyperechoic foci diffusely scattered throughout the testicular parenchyma, causing significant attenuation of the ultrasound beam. Bilateral involvement may occur. No treatment is necessary for testicular microlithiasis. Solitary microlithiasis is a more common, benign condition, possibly related to **inflammatory, granulomatous,** or **vascular calcifications** (Fig. 26-24).

Extratesticular scrotal calculi arise from the surface of the tunica vaginalis and may break loose to migrate about between the two layers of the tunica (Fig. 26-25). They have been called fibrinoid loose bodies or scrotal pearls because of their macroscopic appearance, which is usually round, pearly white, and rubbery. His-

tologically, they consist of fibrinoid material deposited around a central nucleus of hydroxyapatite.[64] They may result from inflammation of the tunica vaginalis or torsion of the appendix testis or epididymis. Secondary hydroceles are common because of inhibition of the normal secretion and absorption by the tunica vaginalis, usually as a result of inflammation. Hydrocele formation facilitates the sonographic diagnosis of scrotal calculi (Fig. 26-26).

Extratesticular Pathology

Hydrocele, Hematocele, and Pyocele. Serous fluid, blood, pus, or urine may accumulate in the space between the parietal and visceral layers of the tunica vaginalis lining the scrotum. The collection is named after the type of fluid that accumulates. These fluid collections are confined to the anterolateral portions of the scrotum because of the attachment of the testis to the epididymis and scrotal wall posteriorly (the bare area) (Fig. 26-27).

The normal scrotum contains a few milliliters of serous fluid between the layers of the tunica vaginalis. Approximately 85% of asymptomatic subjects who underwent scrotal ultrasound had minimal amounts of fluid in one hemiscrotum.[65] A hydrocele represents an abnormal accumulation of serous fluid in this space, and it is the most common cause of painless scrotal swelling.[3]

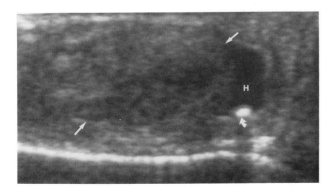

FIG 26-26. Scrotal calculus. Longitudinal scrotal scan demonstrates an inhomogeneous-appearing testis *(arrows)* in a patient with multiple bouts of acute and chronic epididymitis. A small reactive hydrocele *(H)* contains an echogenic free-floating scrotal calculus *(curved arrow)*. This palpable calculus was the reason for the sonogram.

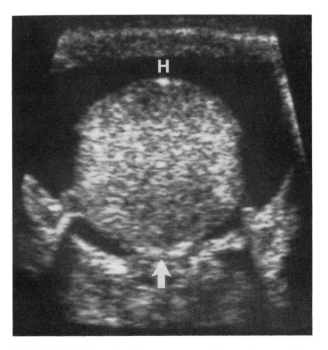

FIG 26-27. Hydrocele. Transverse scrotal scan demonstrates a hydrocele *(H)* surrounding all parts of the testis except the posterior portion *(arrow)* where the testis is attached directly to the scrotal wall.

Hydroceles may be congenital or acquired. The congenital type results from incomplete closure of the processus vaginalis, with persistent open communication between the scrotal sac and the peritoneum. Nearly all congenital hydroceles resolve by 18 months of age.

Acquired hydroceles are often idiopathic. From 25% to 50% of hydroceles are the result of trauma. Large hydroceles are associated with neoplasms in less than 10% of testicular neoplasm cases, whereas small hydroceles occur in 60% of patients with testicular tumors.[2,4,66] Other causes of secondary hydroceles include epididymitis or epididymo-orchitis, torsion, and trauma.[9,21]

Sonography plays an important role in the evaluation of hydroceles. It can detect a potential cause of the hydrocele and permits evaluation of the testicle when a large hydrocele hampers palpation. Hydroceles are characteristically anechoic collections with good sound transmission surrounding the anterolateral aspects of the testis. The fluid provides an excellent acoustic window for imaging the testis. Low-level to medium-level echoes from fibrin bodies or cholesterol crystals may occasionally be visualized moving freely within a hydrocele.[4,13]

Hematoceles and **pyoceles** are much less common than simple hydroceles. Hematoceles result from trauma, surgery, diabetes, neoplasms, torsion, or atherosclerotic disease.[67] Pyoceles result from rupture of an abscess into an existing hydrocele or directly into the space between the layers of the tunica vaginalis. Both hematoceles and pyoceles contain internal septations and loculations (Fig. 26-28). Thickening of the scrotal skin and calcifications may be seen in chronic cases.

Varicocele. A varicocele is a collection of abnormally dilated, tortuous and elongated veins of the pampiniform plexus located posterior to the testis, accompanying the epididymis and vas deferens within the spermatic cord (Fig. 26-29).[3,4,9,68] The veins of the pampiniform plexus normally range from 0.5 to 1.5 mm in diameter, commonly with a main draining vein up to 2 mm in diameter.

There are two types of varicoceles, primary (idiopathic) and secondary. The idiopathic variety is believed to be due to incompetent valves in the internal spermatic vein, which permit retrograde passage of blood through the spermatic cord into the pampiniform plexus. It occurs in 15% to 20% of the general population and is the most common correctable cause of male infertility, occurring in 21% to 39% of men attending infertility clinics.[69-71] Idiopathic varicoceles occur on the left side in 98% of cases and are usually detected in men between 15 and 25 years of age.[9] The left-sided predominance is believed to be due to the fact that the venous drainage on the left side is into the renal vein, as opposed to the right spermatic vein, which drains directly into the vena cava. Idiopathic varices normally distend when the patient is upright or performs a Valsalva maneuver and may decompress when the patient is supine. Primary varicoceles are bilateral in up to 70% of cases.[72] A search for neoplastic obstruction of gonadal venous return must be undertaken in cases of a

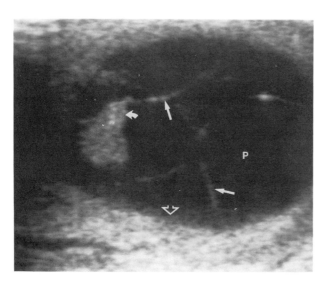

FIG 26-28. Pyocele. Transverse scan through the superior aspect of the right hemiscrotum in a patient with epididymitis and testicular abscess formation demonstrates a pyocele *(P)* with multiple internal septations *(arrow)* and dependent debris *(open arrow).* An enlarged appendix epididymis is also seen *(curved arrow).*

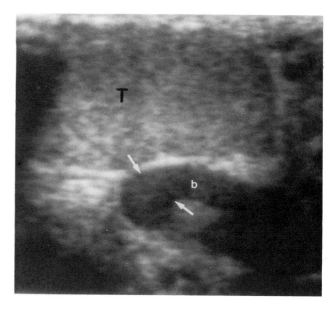

FIG 26-29. Varicocele. Longitudinal scan demonstrates a large serpiginous varix *(arrows)* filled with echogenic material representing slowly flowing venous red blood cells *(b).* T, Testis.

right-sided, nondecompressible or newly discovered varicocele in a patient over the age of 40 years, as these cases are rarely idiopathic.[3] Secondary varicoceles result from increased pressure on the spermatic vein or its tributaries by marked hydronephrosis, an enlarged liver, abdominal neoplasms, or venous compression by a retroperitoneal mass.[4,21] The appearance of secondary varicoceles is not affected by patient position.

Sonography aids in the evaluation of clinically palpable and subclinical varicoceles in infertile men. There is no correlation between the size of the varicocele and the degree of testicular tissue damage leading to infertility. Therefore early detection and treatment of subclinical varicoceles is very important.[71] Sonography also can often elucidate the cause of venous obstruction in secondary varicoceles.

Sonographically, the varicocele appears as multiple serpiginous anechoic structures more than 2 mm in diameter creating a tortuous multicystic collection located adjacent or proximal to the upper pole of the testis and head of the epididymis. Occasionally the varicocele may appear similar to a small septated spermatocele. Differentiation between varicocele and spermatocele may be accomplished using duplex or color Doppler sonography. A high-frequency transducer in conjunction with low-flow Doppler detection settings should be used to optimize slow-flow detection within varices. Slowly moving red blood cells may be visualized with high-frequency transducers, even when flow is too slow to be detected by Doppler. Venous flow can be augmented with the patient in the upright position or during the Valsalva maneuver. In addition, varicoceles, unlike spermatoceles, follow the course of the spermatic cord into the inguinal canal and are easily compressed by the transducer.[2,4,21]

Scrotal Hernia. A scrotal hernia is another common paratesticular mass. Although scrotal hernias are usually diagnosed on the basis of clinical history and physical examination, sonography is useful in the evaluation of atypical cases. The hernia may contain small bowel, colon, and/or omentum.[73] The presence of bowel loops within the hernia may be confirmed by the visualization of valvulae conniventes or haustrations and detection of peristalsis on real-time examination. If these features are absent, differentiation from other extratesticular multicystic masses, such as hematocele and pyocele, may be difficult. The presence of high-amplitude echoes within the scrotum may be due to a hernia-containing omentum or other fatty masses. Sonographic examination of the inguinal canal must also be performed in order to identify the extension of omentum or bowel loops from the inguinal canal into the scrotum.[21,73]

Tumors. Extratesticular neoplasms are rare and usually involve the epididymis. The most common extratesticular neoplasm is the **adenomatoid tumor,** representing 32% of tumors arising in the paratesticular tissues.[16,74] It is most frequently located in the epididymis, especially in the globus minor, but may also arise in the spermatic cord or testicular tunica (Fig. 26-30).[18] This neoplasm may occasionally invade adjacent testicular parenchyma. It may occur at any age, but is most commonly found in patients aged 20 to 50 years.[2,18,75] It is generally unilateral, solitary, well defined, and round or oval shaped, rarely measuring greater than 5 cm in diameter. Occasionally it may appear plaquelike and ill defined. Sonography usually demonstrates a solid, well-circumscribed mass with echogenicity equal to or greater than that of the testis.[2] It may also be hypoechoic.

Other benign extratesticular tumors are very rare, but are more common than benign testicular neoplasms. **Fibromas, hemangiomas, lipomas, leiomyomas, neurofibromas,** and **cholesterol granulomas** have been reported.[18] **Adrenal rests** may also be encountered in the spermatic cord, testis, epididymis, rete testis, and tunica albuginea in approximately 10% of infants.[18] They arise from aberrant adrenal cortical cells that migrate with the gonadal tissues in fetal life. These ectopic adrenocortical cells form small yellow nodules generally less than 1 cm in diameter. Their clinical significance lies in their potential to form tumorlike masses in patients with elevated levels of circulating adrenocorticotropic hormone (ACTH) in cases of **congenital adrenal hyperplasia** and **Cushing's syndrome.** Malignant transformation is rare. These tumors may be hypoechoic and/or hyperechoic with occasional acoustic shadowing (Fig. 26-31).[76]

Papillary cystadenomas of the epididymis may be seen in patients with von Hippel-Lindau disease.[59] Primary epididymal neoplasms include **fibrosarcoma, li-**

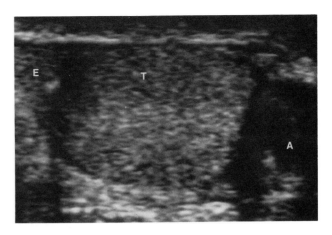

FIG 26-30. Adenomatoid tumor, tail of the epididymis. Longitudinal scrotal scan demonstrates a normal testis *(T)* and head of the epididymis *(E)* with a large well-circumscribed hypoechoic mass *(A)* in the tail of the epididymis.

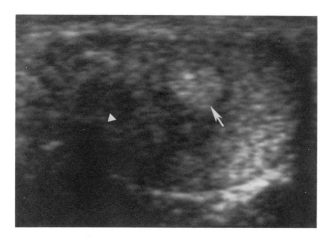

FIG 26-31. Adrenocortical rest cell tumors. Longitudinal scrotal scan demonstrates multiple echogenic *(arrow)* and hypoechoic *(arrowhead)* focal masses in the testis. This appearance is indistinguishable from other malignancies and similar to rest cell tumors in the epididymis or spermatic cord.

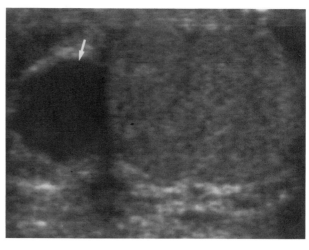

FIG 26-32. Epididymal cyst. Longitudinal scrotal scan demonstrates a large epididymal cyst *(arrow)* involving the head of the epididymis, indistinguishable in appearance from a spermatocele.

posarcoma, and, less commonly, **malignant histiocytoma** and **lymphoma** in adults, and rhabdomyosarcoma in children.

Metastatic tumors to the epididymis are also rare. The most common primary sites include the testicle, stomach, kidney, prostate, colon, and, less commonly, pancreas.[59,74,77,78] Sonography demonstrates focal, echogenic areas of thickening within the epididymis commonly in association with a hydrocele.

Epididymal Lesions

Cystic Lesions. Epididymal cysts and spermatoceles are both cystic masses of the epididymis. Spermatoceles are more common than epididymal cysts. Epididymal cystic structures were seen in 20% to 40% of all asymptomatic patients studied by Leung et al.[65] Approximately 30% of these cysts were multiple. Both epididymal cysts and spermatoceles are believed to result from dilation of the epididymal tubules, but the contents of these masses differ.[3,59] Cysts contain clear serous fluid, whereas spermatoceles are filled with spermatozoa and sediment-containing lymphocytes, fat globules, and cellular debris, giving the fluid a thick, milky appearance.[2,59] Both lesions may result from prior episodes of epididymitis. Spermatoceles have also developed after trauma. Spermatoceles and epididymal cysts appear identical on ultrasound: anechoic, well-circumscribed masses with no or few internal echoes (Fig. 26-32). Loculations and septations are commonly seen (Fig. 26-33). The location of these lesions within the epididymis may suggest their nature, although the differentiation

between spermatocele and epididymal cyst is rarely clinically important. Spermatoceles almost always occur in the head of the epididymis, whereas epididymal cysts arise throughout the length of the epididymis.

Sperm Granuloma. Sperm granulomas are believed to arise from extravasation of spermatozoa into the soft tissues surrounding the epididymis, producing a necrotizing granulomatous response.[2,9,79,80] These lesions are usually asymptomatic, but are frequently associated with prior epididymal infection or trauma. They are most often found in patients after vasectomy. The typical sonographic appearance is that of a solid, hypoechoic mass that is usually located within the epididymis, although they may simulate an intratesticular lesion.[79]

Postvasectomy Changes in the Epididymis. Sonographic changes in the epididymis have been reported in 45% of patients after vasectomy. These findings include epididymal enlargement and inhomogeneity and the development of cysts. It is theorized that vasectomy produces increased pressure in the epididymal tubules, causing tubular rupture with subsequent formation of sperm granulomas. This tubular rupture may protect the testis from the effects of increased back pressure. These sonographic findings are nonspecific and may be seen in patients who have epididymitis. The clinical history and physical examination should differentiate these two entities.[81]

Chronic Epididymitis. Chronic epididymitis may result from incompletely treated acute bacterial epididymitis

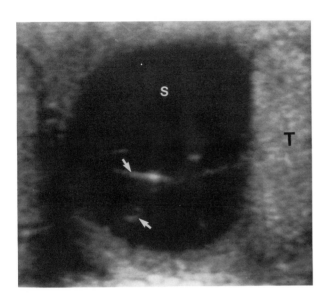

FIG 26-33. Loculated spermatocele. Longitudinal scan of the head of the epididymis demonstrates a loculated spermatocele *(S)* which contains septations *(open arrows). T,* Testicle.

or spread of tuberculosis from the genitourinary tract. Patients with unresolved bacterial epididymitis usually present with a chronically painful scrotal mass, whereas patients with chronic granulomatous epididymitis complain of a hard, nontender scrotal mass.[3] Sonography most commonly demonstrates a thickened tunica albuginea and a thickened, irregular epididymis. Calcification may be identified within the tunica albuginea or epididymis.[2,82] Untreated granulomatous epididymitis may spread to the testes in 60% to 80% of cases.[9] Focal testicular involvement may simulate the appearance of a testicular neoplasm on sonography, whereas diffuse testicular involvement results in an enlarged, irregular testis with diffuse homogeneous hypoechogenicity.

THE ACUTE SCROTUM
Torsion

There is a wide differential diagnosis of an acutely painful and swollen scrotum, including torsion of the spermatic cord and testis, torsion of a testicular appendage, epididymitis and/or orchitis, acute hydrocele, strangulated hernia, idiopathic scrotal edema, Henoch-Schönlein purpura, abscess, traumatic hemorrhage, hemorrhage into a testicular neoplasm, and scrotal fat necrosis.[81] Torsion of the spermatic cord and acute epididymitis or epididymo-orchitis are the most common causes of an acute scrotum. These entities cannot be distinguished by physical examination or laboratory tests in up to 50% of cases.[83] Torsion is more common in children, but represents only 20% of acute scrotal pathology in postpubertal males.[2] Prompt diagnosis is necessary since torsion requires immediate surgery to

preserve the testis. The testicular salvage rate is 80% to 100% if surgery is performed within 5 to 6 hours of the onset of pain, 70% if surgery is performed within 6 to 12 hours, and only 20% if surgery is delayed for more than 12 hours.[84] Immediate surgical exploration has been advised in boys and young men with acute scrotal pain unless a definitive diagnosis of epididymitis/orchitis can be made. This aggressive approach has resulted in an increased testicular salvage rate but also an increase in unnecessary surgical procedures.[85] Radionuclide testicular imaging, real-time sonography, and Doppler sonography have been used to increase the accuracy of differentiation between infection and torsion.

There are two types of testicular torsion, intravaginal and extravaginal. **Intravaginal torsion** is the most common type, occurring most commonly at puberty. It results from anomalous suspension of the testis by a long stalk of spermatic cord, resulting in complete investment of the testis and epididymis by the tunica vaginalis. It has been likened to a "bell and clapper." There is a tenfold greater incidence of torsion in undescended testes after orchiopexy.[86] Anomalous testicular suspension is present in 50% to 80% of contralateral testes.[21]

The **extravaginal** form occurs most commonly in newborns without the "bell and clapper" deformity. It is believed to be due to the motility of the entire vaginalis, resulting in torsion of the testis and its tunica at the level of the external ring. The more compliant veins are obstructed before the arteries in both forms of torsion, resulting in early vascular engorgement and edema of the testicle. A spectrum of gray-scale sonographic changes has been reported within 1 to 6 hours after the onset of testicular torsion.[83,87] The testicle becomes enlarged, inhomogeneous, and hypoechoic compared with the contralateral normal testis (Fig. 26-34). Common extratesticular findings include an enlarged epididymis containing foci of increased and decreased echogenicity, skin thickening, and reactive hydrocele formation. Occasionally, the testicle may appear normal with echogenicity identical to the normal testicle.[88-90] Generalized testicular hyperechogenicity has been reported in two cases of acute torsion in the absence of histologic changes of testicular hemorrhage or infarction.[83,91] During the subacute phase of torsion (1 to 10 days), the degree of testicular hypoechogenicity and enlargement increases within the first 5 days, then diminishes over the next 4 to 5 days. The epididymis remains enlarged but is commonly echogenic. Hydroceles are common in cases of chronic torsion.[87] In a recent report by Vick et al,[91] large echogenic or complex extratesticular masses caused by hemorrhage within the tunica vaginalis, epididymis, or other extratesticular locations were visualized in cases of missed torsion. The gray-scale findings of acute and subacute torsion are not specific and may

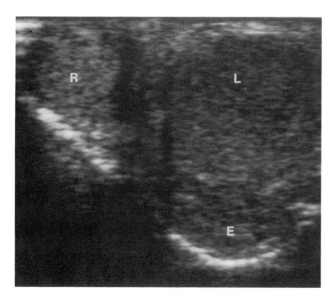

FIG 26-34. Testicular torsion. Transverse scan of the scrotum demonstrates that the left testis *(L)* and epididymis are markedly enlarged and hypoechoic relative to the normal right testis. Similar findings could be seen in a severe case of epididymitis-epididymal-orchitis.

be seen in epididymo-orchitis, testicular infarction secondary to epididymitis, and traumatic testicular rupture or infarction.[92,93]

Pulsed and color Doppler examination of the spermatic cord and testicular vessels in conjunction with gray-scale imaging have been used to help differentiate torsion from epididymo-orchitis.[83,89,94-96] The presence of normal or increased blood flow within the testicle would theoretically exclude the diagnosis of acute torsion. Meticulous scanning of the testicular parenchyma and the use of low-flow detection Doppler techniques is required because testicular vessels are small and have low flow velocities.

The diagnosis of **testicular ischemia** depends on the ability to unequivocally demonstrate the presence of normal blood flow in the normal, contralateral, asymptomatic testicle (Fig. 26-35). Several recent series have reported color Doppler findings in testicular ischemia.[94-96] Using this criterion of presence or absence of intratesticular blood flow on color Doppler, one recent series correctly diagnosed all patients with proven testicular torsion.[96] In addition, torsion of the testicular appendage was correctly diagnosed in five patients so that conservative treatment was undertaken, sparing unnecessary surgery. Another recently published series reported 86% sensitivity, 100% specificity, and 97% accuracy in the diagnosis of testicular torsion using color Doppler sonography.[95] This series reported a single false-negative study with intratesticular blood flow detected in a testis that was subsequently shown at

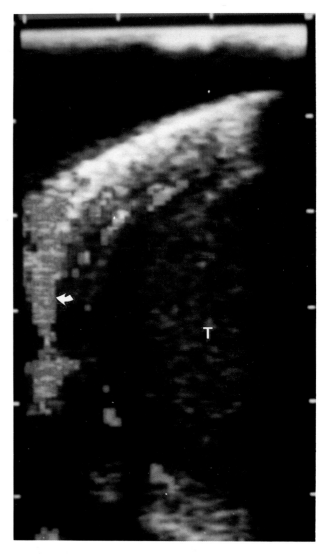

FIG. 26-35. Traumatic avulsion of the testicular artery. Patient with acute swelling and tenderness of the left scrotum, after traumatic avulsion of the testicular pedicle, demonstrates an avascular testis *(T)* on color Doppler examination. Marked hyperemia in the surrounding soft tissues *(curved arrow).*

surgery to be torsed. Interestingly, only a 360-degree torsion of the spermatic cord was present; at least 540 degrees of torsion is considered necessary to completely occlude testicular blood flow. Thus it is possible that with lesser degrees of spermatic cord torsion, minimal residual flow might exist within the testis. Further studies are necessary to determine if changes in the resistivity index might help differentiate such incomplete torsion from normal blood flow. In cases of chronic torsion, color Doppler demonstrates absent intratesticular flow and increased flow in the peritesticular tissues, including the epididymis cord complex and dartos fascia. In cases of detorsion, color Doppler may demonstrate increased testicular and peritesticular flow or normal flow.[94,95] It is important to remember that reactive hyperemia of the testicle, resulting from the resolution of intermittent torsion, may mimic hyperreactive blood flow in epididymo-orchitis on color Doppler sonography. However, clinical findings should help differentiate intermittent torsion and epididymo-orchitis in the acute setting. Torsion of the testicular appendage presents as an avascular hypoechoic mass, adjacent to a normally perfused testis, surrounded by an area of increased color Doppler perfusion.[94] The efficacy of color Doppler sonography in the evaluation of torsion in neonates and children has not yet been assessed in a large series. However, it should be more difficult to detect intratesticular flow in young boys because of the smaller size of both the testes and arteries in children.

Epididymitis and Epididymo-orchitis

Epididymitis is the most common cause of the acute scrotum in postpubertal males, representing 75% of all acute intrascrotal inflammatory processes. It usually results from a lower urinary tract infection and is less commonly hematogenous or traumatic in origin. The common causative organisms are *Escherichia coli*, *Pseudomonas*, and *Aerobacter*.[98] Sexually transmitted organisms causing urethritis, such as *Gonococcus* and *Chlamydia*, are common causes of epididymitis in young men. Less commonly, epididymitis may accompany mumps or syphilitic orchitis. The peak age incidence is between 40 and 50 years. Classically, patients present with the insidious onset of pain, which increases over a period of 1 to 2 days. Fever, dysuria, and urethral discharge may also be present.

Sonography characteristically demonstrates thickening and enlargement of the epididymis, most commonly involving the head.[13] The entire epididymis is involved in 50% of cases. The echogenicity of the epididymis is usually decreased, and its echo texture is often coarse and heterogeneous, probably because of edema and/or hemorrhage (Fig. 26-36). Reactive hydrocele formation is common, and associated skin thickening may be seen.

Color Doppler ultrasound usually demonstrates increased blood flow in the epididymis and/or testis compared with the asymptomatic side. Direct extension of epididymal inflammation to the testicle, called epididymo-orchitis, occurs in up to 20% of patients with acute epididymitis. Isolated orchitis may also occur. In such cases, increased blood flow would be localized to the testis. Testicular involvement may be focal or diffuse. Characteristically, focal orchitis produces a hypoechoic area adjacent to an enlarged portion of the epididymis. If left untreated, the entire testicle may become involved, appearing hypoechoic and enlarged (Fig. 26-37). Testicular involvement may also result from secondary effects of epididymal inflammation. Occasionally, marked edema associated with acute epididymitis may result in occlusion of the testicular blood supply, resulting in ischemia and subsequent infarction. Such changes would be indistinguishable from those associated with testicular infarction secondary to torsion. Resultant ischemia associated with severe epididymitis also predisposes the testicle to infection, which may be

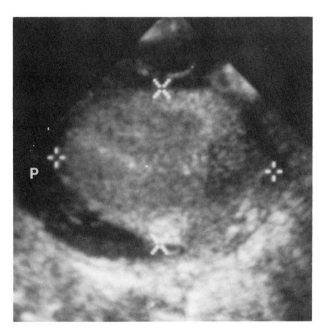

FIG 26-37. Chronic epididymo-orchitis (unresponsive to antibiotic therapy). A diffusely inhomogeneous testis (++) surrounded by a pyocele (P) containing septations and purulent debris. At surgery multiple areas of orchitis and abscess formation were noted within the testis.

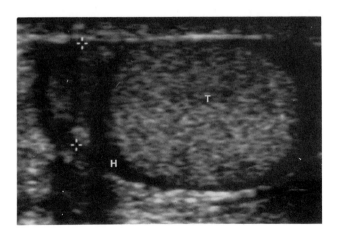

FIG 26-36. Acute epididymitis. Longitudinal scan in a patient with acute epididymitis shows a hypoechoic, enlarged epididymal head (+) and a small reactive hydrocele (H). T, Testis.

in the form of focal orchitis, abscess formation, or diffuse gangrenous epididymo-orchitis.[92] In most cases of epididymo-orchitis, the testicle retains its ovoid and smooth contour.[92,93] Color Doppler sonography may demonstrate focal areas of reactive hyperemia and increased blood flow associated with relatively avascular areas of infarction in both the testis and epididymis in cases of severe epididymo-orchitis. If vascular disruption is extremely severe, resulting in complete testicular infarction, changes would be indistinguishable from those seen in testicular torsion. In such instances, increased blood flow would be seen proximal to the area of vascular disruption because of swelling and edema. The hyperemic blood flow in the dartos and proximal spermatic cord would be in striking contrast to the avascular scrotal contents distal to the point of vascular occlusion.

TRAUMA

Prompt diagnosis of a ruptured testis is of utmost importance because of the direct relationship between early surgical intervention and testicular salvageability. Approximately 90% of testicles can be saved if surgery is performed within the first 72 hours, whereas only 45% may be salvaged after 72 hours.[98,99] Clinical diagnosis is often impossible because of marked scrotal pain and swelling. Jeffrey et al[98] correctly identified 12 out of 12 cases of testicular rupture using sonography. Sonographic features include focal areas of altered testicular echogenicity corresponding to areas of hemorrhage or infarction, and hematocele formation in 33% of patients. A discrete fracture plane was identified in only 17% of cases (Fig. 26-38). The testicular contour is often irregular. Although these features are not specific for a ruptured testicle, they may suggest the diag-

nosis in the appropriate clinical setting, prompting immediate surgical exploration. Vascular disruption may also be demonstrated by color Doppler sonography (Fig. 26-39).

CRYPTORCHIDISM

The testes normally begin their descent through the inguinal canal into the scrotal sac at approximately 36 weeks' gestation. The gubernaculum testis is a fibromuscular structure that extends from the inferior pole of the testis to the scrotum and guides the testis in its descent, which is normally completed at birth.[9] Undescended testis is one of the most common genitourinary anomalies in male infants. At birth, 3.5% of male infants weighing more than 2500 grams have an undescended testis; 10% to 25% of these cases are bilateral. This figure decreases to 0.8% by 1 year since the testes descend spontaneously in most infants. The incidence of undescended testes increases to 30% in premature infants, approaching 100% in neonates who weigh less

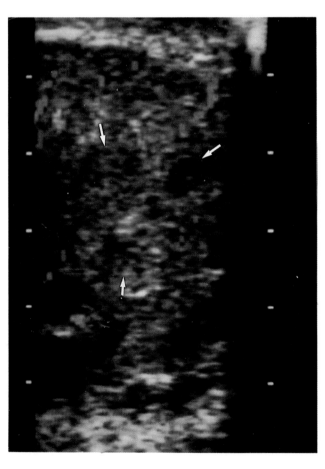

FIG 26-39. Focal posttraumatic testicular edema and hypovascularity. Color Doppler scan through the lower pole of a testis posttrauma demonstrates an area of hypoechogenicity *(arrows)* that is relatively avascular.

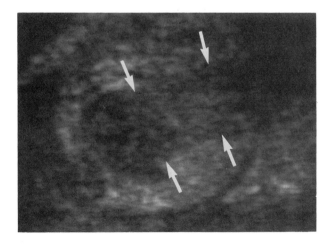

FIG 26-38. Fracture of the testis. Transverse scan through a fractured testis demonstrates a wide hypoechoic linear band *(arrows)* representing the area of testicular fracture.

than 1 kg at birth.[100,101] Complete descent is necessary for full testicular maturation.[100,101]

Malpositioned testes may be located anywhere along the pathway of descent from the retroperitoneum to the scrotum. The majority (80%) of undescended testes are palpable, lying at or below the level of the inguinal canal. Anorchia occurs in 4% of the remaining patients with impalpable testes.[101]

Localization of the undescended testis is important for the prevention of two potential complications of cryptorchidism, infertility and cancer. Infertility results from progressive pathologic changes that develop in both the undescended and contralateral normal testis after the age of 1 year.[101-103] The undescended testis is 48 times more likely to undergo malignant change than the normally descended testis.[2] It is believed that the hormonal deficiency resulting in failure of testicular descent predisposes the patient to malignancy. Approximately 0.04% of patients with an undescended testis will develop carcinoma annually. The lifetime risk of death from a testicular malignancy in men of any age with an undescended testis is approximately 9.7 times the risk in normal men.[102] The most common malignancy is seminoma. The risk of malignancy is increased in both the undescended testis after orchiopexy and the normally descended testis. Therefore, careful serial examinations of both testes are essential.

Because of the superficial location of the inguinal canal in children, sonography of the undescended testis should be performed with a high-frequency transducer and a standoff pad to avoid reverberation artifacts. Sonographically, the undescended testis is often smaller and slightly less echogenic than the contralateral normally descended testis (Fig. 26-40). A specific diagnosis of an undescended testis may be made if the mediastinum testis is identified. A large lymph node or the pars infravaginalis gubernaculi (PIG), which is the dis-

tal bulbous segment of the gubernaculum testis, have been mistaken for the testis, but theoretically, neither of these should contain an internal echogenic band. In reality, visualization of the mediastinum testis in undescended testes is often difficult. In addition, echogenic foci may be visualized within the PIG and lymph nodes, which may lead to a misdiagnosis of undescended testis. After completion of testicular descent, the PIG and gubernaculum normally atrophy. If the testis remains undescended, both structures persist. The PIG is always located distal to the undescended testis, usually in the scrotum, but may be found cranial to the scrotum. Sonographically, the PIG is hypoechoic, a cordlike structure of echogenicity similar to the testis, with the gubernaculum leading to it.[104]

The success of sonography in the localization of undescended testes varies among series. Wolverson et al[105] reported a sensitivity of 88%, specificity of 100%, and accuracy of 91% in the sonographic localization of undescended testes. In a later study, Weiss et al[106] reported a sensitivity of 70% for palpable testes and 13% for nonpalpable testes. Magnetic resonance imaging (MRI) has sensitivity and specificity similar to ultrasound in the evaluation of cryptorchidism.[107,108] MRI shares two main advantages with ultrasound: noninvasiveness and lack of ionizing radiation. An additional advantage of MRI is the ability to obtain multiplanar images of the retroperitoneum and inguinal region. Undescended testes are characteristically hypointense with respect to fat on short TR/TE sequences and hyperintense or isointense with respect to fat on long TR/TE sequences. These signal characteristics of undescended testes are identical to those of scrotal testes. Disadvantages of MRI include cost, long scanning time, frequent need for sedation, and lack of a bowel contrast agent in evaluation of abdominal testes. Because of sonography's lack of ionizing radiation, lower cost, and shorter scanning time, and the fact that it does not require sedation or oral contrast, sonography should be the initial method of evaluation of cryptorchidism. Nonvisualization of an undescended testis on ultrasound or MRI does not exclude its presence, and therefore laparoscopy or surgical exploration should be performed if clinically indicated.

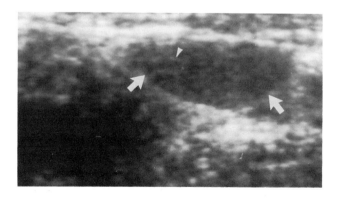

FIG 26-40. Atrophic testis in inguinal canal. Longitudinal scan through the inguinal canal demonstrates an elliptical, small cryptorchid testis *(arrows)* with an echogenic band, representing the mediastinum testis *(arrowhead).*

REFERENCES

1. Carroll BA, Gross DM: High-frequency scrotal sonography. *AJR* 1983;140:511-515.
2. Krone KD, Carroll BA: Scrotal ultrasound. *Radiol Clin North Am* 1985;23:121-139.
3. Vick W, Bird KI, Rosenfield AT, et al: Ultrasound of scrotal contents. *Urol Radiol* 1982;4:147-153.
4. Hricak H, Filly RA: Sonography of the scrotum. *Invest Radiol* 1983;18:112-121.
5. Rifkin MD, Kurtz AB, Pasto ME, et al: The sonographic diagnosis of focal and infiltrating intrascrotal lesions. *Urol Radiol* 1984;6:20-26.

6. Rifkin MD: Scrotal ultrasound. *Urol Radiol* 1987;9:119-126.

7. Middleton WD, Thorne DA, Melson GL: Color Doppler ultrasound of the normal testis. *AJR* 1989;152:293-297.

Anatomy

8. Trainer TD: Histology of the normal testis. *Am J Surg Pathol* 1987;11:797-809.

9. Hill MC, Sanders RC: Sonography of benign disease of the scrotum. In: Sanders RC, Hill MC, editors. *Ultrasound Annual* New York: Raven Press; 1986.

10. Rifkin MD, Foy PM, Goldberg BB: Scrotal ultrasound: acoustic characteristics of the normal testis and epididymis defined with high resolution superficial scanners. *Med Ultrasound* 1984;8:91-97.

11. Fakhry J, Khoury A, Barakat K: The hypoechoic band: a normal finding on testicular sonography. *AJR* 1989;153:321-323.

12. Gooding GAW: Sonography of the spermatic cord. *AJR* 1988;151:721-724.

The scrotal mass

13. Benson CB, Doubilet PM, Richie JP: Sonography of the male genital tract. *AJR* 1989;153:705-713.

14. Rifkin MD, Kurtz AB, Pasto ME, et al: Diagnostic capabilities of high-resolution scrotal ultrasonography: prospective evaluation. *J Ultrasound Med* 1985;4:13-19.

15. Grantham JG, Charboneau JW, James EM, et al: Testicular neoplasms: 29 tumors studied by high-resolution ultrasound. *Radiology* 1985;775-780.

16. Kirschling RJ, Kvols LK, Charboneau JW, et al: High-resolution ultrasonographic and pathologic abnormalities of germ cell tumors in patients with clinically normal testes. *Mayo Clin Proc* 1983;58:648-653.

17. Javadpour N: *Principles and management of testicular cancer.* New York: Thieme Inc; 1986.

18. Goldfinger SS, Rothberg R, Buckspan MB, et al: Incidental detection of impalpable testicular neoplasm by sonography. *AJR* 1986;146:349-350.

19. Talerman A, Roth LM: *Pathology of the testis and its adnexa.* New York: Churchill Livingstone; 1986.

20. Jacobsen GK, Talerman A: *Atlas of germ cell tumors.* Copenhagen: Munksgaard; 1989.

21. Ruzal-Shapiro C, Newhouse JH: Genitourinary ultrasound. In: Taveras JM, Ferrucci JT, editors. *Radiology: diagnosis-imaging intervention.* Philadelphia: JB Lippincott Co; 1986:4.

22. Schwerk WB, Schwerk WNM, Rodeck G: Testicular tumors: prospective analysis of real-time ultrasound patterns and abdominal staging. *Radiology* 1987;164:369-374.

23. Mostofi FK, Price EB Jr: Tumors of the male genital system. In: *Atlas of tumor pathology,* 2nd series, fascicle 8. Washington, D.C.: Armed Forces Institute of Pathology; 1973.

24. Emory TH, Charboneau JW, Randall RV, et al: Occult testicular interstitial-cell tumor in a patient with gynecomastia: ultrasonic detection. *Radiology* 1984;151:474.

25. Cunningham JJ: Echographic findings in sertoli cell tumor of the testis. *J Clin Ultrasound* 1981;9:341-342.

26. Glazer HS, Lee JKT, Melson GL, et al: Sonographic detection of occult testicular neoplasms. *AJR* 1981;138:673-675.

27. Bockrath JJ, Schaeffer AJ, Kies JS, et al: Ultrasound identification of impalpable testicular tumor. *J Urol* 1981;130:355-356.

28. Moudy PC, Makhija JS: Ultrasonic demonstration of a nonpalpable testicular tumor. *J Clin Ultrasound* 1983;11:54-55.

29. Shawker TH, Javadpour N, O'Leary T, et al: Ultrasonographic detection of "burned-out" primary testicular germ cell tumors in clinically normal testes. *J Ultrasound Med* 1983;2:477-479.

30. Doll DC, Weiss RB: Malignant lymphoma of the testis. *Am J Med* 1986;81:515-523.

31. Tepperman BS, Gospodarowicz M, Bush RS, et al: Non-Hodgkin lymphoma of the testis. *Radiology* 1982;142:203-208.

32. Paladugu RP, Bearman RM, Rappaport H: Malignant lymphoma with primary manifestation in the gonad: a clinicopathologic study of 38 patients. *Cancer* 1980;45:561-571.

33. Hamlin JA, Kagan AR, Friedman NB: Lymphomas of the testicle. *Cancer* 1972;29:1532-1536.

34. Rayor RA, Scheible W, Brock WA, et al: High resolution ultrasonography in the diagnosis of testicular relapse in patients with lymphoblastic leukemia. *J Urol* 1982;128:602-603.

35. Phillips G, Kumari-Subaiya S, Sawitsky A: Ultrasonic evaluation of the scrotum in lymphoproliferative disease. *J Ultrasound Med* 1987;6:169-175.

36. Dahnert WF, Rifkin MD, Kurtz AB: Ultrasound case of the day. *Radiographics* 1989;9:554-558.

37. Grignon DJ, Shum DT, Hayman WP: Metastatic tumors of the testes. *Can J Surg* 1986;29:359-361.

38. Werth V, Yu G, Marshall FF: Nonlymphomatous metastatic tumor to the testis. *J Urol* 1981;127:142-144.

39. Hanash KA, Carney JA, Kelalis PP: Metastatic tumors to testicles: routes of metastasis. *J Urol* 1969;102:465-468.

40. Hamm B, Fobbe F, Loy V: Testicular cysts: differentiation with ultrasound and clinical findings. *Radiology* 1988;168:19-23.

41. Gooding GAW, Leonhardt W, Stein R: Testicular cysts: US findings. *Radiology* 1987;163:537-538.

42. Becker J, Arger PH, Wein AJ, Kendall AR: Inclusion cyst of the tunica albuginea: demonstration by ultrasound. *Urol Radiol* 1983;5:127-129.

43. Turner WR, Derrick FC, Sanders P, et al: Benign lesions of the tunica albuginea. *J Urol* 1977;117:602-604.

44. Warner KE, Noyes DT, Ross JS: Cysts of the tunica albuginea testis: a report of 3 cases with a review of the literature. *J Urol* 1984;132:131-132.

45. Takihari H, Valvo JR, Tokuhara M, et al: Intratesticular cysts. *Urology* 1982;20:80-82.

46. Rifkin MD, Jacobs JA: Simple testicular cyst diagnosed preoperatively by ultrasound. *J Urol* 1983;129:982-983.

47. Shah KH, Maxted WC, Dhun B: Epidermoid cysts of the testis: a report of three cases and an analysis of 141 cases from the world literature. *Cancer* 1981;47:577-582.

48. Caravelli JF, Peters BE: Sonography of bilateral testicular epidermoid cysts. *J Ultrasound Med* 1984;3:273-274.

49. Buckspan MB, Skeldon SC, Klotz PG, et al: Epidermoid cysts of the testicle. *J Urol* 1985;134:960-961.

50. Malek RS, Rosen JS, Farrow GM: Epidermoid cyst of the testis: a critical analysis. *Br J Urol* 1986;58:55-59.

51. Cohen EL, Mandel E, Goodman JD, et al: Epidermoid cyst of the testicle: ultrasonographic characteristics. *Urology* 1984;24:79-81.

52. Cho CS, Kosek J: Cystic dysplasia of the testis: sonographic and pathologic findings. *Radiology* 1985;156:777-778.

53. Fisher JE, Jewett TC, Nelson SJ, et al: Ectasia of the rete testis with ipsilateral renal agenesis. *J Urol* 1982;128:1040-1043.

54. Nistal M, Regadera J, Paniagua R: Cystic dysplasia of the testis. *Arch Pathol Lab Med* 1984;104:579-583.

55. Hermansen JC, Dhusid MJ, Sty MR: Bacterial epididymoorchitis in children and adolescents. *Clin Pediatr* 1980;19:812-815.

56. Mevorach RA, Lerner RM, Dvoretsky PM, et al: Testicular abscess: diagnosis by ultrasonography. *J Urol* 1986;136:1213-1216.

57. Vick CW, Bird LI, Rosenfield AT, et al: Scrotal masses with a uniformly hyperechoic pattern. *Radiology* 1983;148:209-211.

58. Blei L, Sihelnik S, Bloom D, et al: Ultrasonographic analysis of chronic intratesticular pathology. *J Ultrasound Med* 1983;2:17-23.

59. Rifkin MD, Kurtz AB, Goldberg BB: Epididymis examined by ultrasound: correlation with pathology. *Radiology* 1984;151:187-190.
60. Doherty FJ, Mullins TL, Sant GR, et al: Testicular microlithiasis: A unique sonographic appearance. *J Ultrasound Med* 1987;6:389-392.
61. Nistal M, Paniagua R, Diez-Pardo JA: Testicular microlithiasis in 2 children with bilateral cryptorchidism. *J Urol* 1979;121:535-537.
62. Vegni-Talluri M, Bigliardi E, Vanni MG, et al: Testicular microliths: their origin and structure. *J Urol* 1980;124:105-107.
63. Breger RC, Passarge E, McAdams AJ: Testicular intratubular bodies. *J Clin Endocrinol Metab* 1965;25:1340-1346.
64. Linkowski GD, Avellone A, Gooding GAW: Scrotal calculi: sonographic detection. *Radiology* 1985;156:484.
65. Leung ML, Gooding GAW, Williams RD: High-resolution sonography of scrotal contents in asymptomatic subjects. *AJR* 1984;143:161-164.
66. Worthy L, Miller EI, Chin DH: Evaluation of extratesticular findings in scrotal neoplasms. *J Ultrasound Med* 1986;5:261-263.
67. Cunningham JJ: Sonographic findings in clinically unsuspected acute and chronic scrotal hematoceles. *AJR* 1983;140:749-752.
68. Wolverson MK, Houttuin E, Heiberg E, et al: High-resolution real-time sonography of scrotal varicocele. *AJR* 1983;141:775-779.
69. Belker AM: The varicocele and male infertility. *Urol Clin North Am* 1981;8:41-44.
70. Gonda RL, Karo JJ, Forte RA, et al: Diagnosis of subclinical varicocele in infertility. *AJR* 1987;148:71-75.
71. Hamm G, Fobbe F, Sorensen R, et al: Varicoceles: combined sonography and thermography in diagnosis and post-therapeutic intervention. *Radiology* 1986;160:419-424.
72. McClure RD, Hricak H: Scrotal ultrasound in the infertile man: detection of subclinical unilateral and bilateral varicoceles. *J Urol* 1986;135:711-714.
73. Subramanyam BR, Balthazar EJ, Raghavendra BN, et al: Sonographic diagnosis of scrotal hernia. *AJR* 1982;139:535-538.
74. Faysal MH, Strefling A, Kosek JC: Epididymal neoplasms: a case report and review. *J Urol* 1983;129:843-844.
75. Pavone-Macaluso M, Smith PH, Bagshaw MA: *Testicular Cancer and Other Tumors of the Genitourinary Tract.* New York: Plenum Press; 1985.
76. Seidenwurm D, Smathers RL, Kan P, et al: Intratesticular adrenal rests diagnosed by ultrasound. *Radiology* 1985;155:479-481.
77. Smallman LA, Odedra JK: Primary carcinoma of sigmoid colon metastasizing to epididymis. *Urology* 1984;23:598-599.
78. Wachtel TL, Mehan DJ: Metastatic tumors of the epididymis. *J Urol* 1970;103:624-626.
79. Dunner PS, Lipsit ER, Nochomovitz LE: Epididymal sperm granuloma simulating a testicular neoplasm. *J Clin Ultrasound* 1982;10:353-355.
80. Ramanathan K, Yaghoobian J, Pinck RL: Sperm granuloma. *J Clin Ultrasound* 1986;14:155-156.
81. Jarvis LJ, Dubbins PA: Changes in the epididymis after vasectomy: sonographic findings. *AJR* 1989;152:531-534.
82. Fowler RC, Chennells PM, Ewing R: Scrotal ultrasonography: a clinical evaluation. *Br J Radiol* 1987;60:649-654.

The acute scrotum

83. Mueller DL, Amundson GM, Rubin SZ, et al: Acute scrotal abnormalities in children: diagnosis by combined sonography and scintigraphy. *AJR* 1988;150:643-646.
84. Hricak H, Lue T, Filly RA, et al: Experimental study of the sonographic diagnosis of testicular torsion. *J Ultrasound Med* 1983;2:349-356.
85. Donahue RE, Cass BP, Veeraraghavan K: Immediate exploration of the unilateral acute scrotum in young male subjects. *J Urol* 1978;124:829-832.
86. Williamson RCN: Torsion of the testis and allied conditions. *Br J Surg* 1976;63:465-476.
87. Finkelstein MS, Rosenberg HK, Snyder HM, et al: Ultrasound evaluation of scrotum in pediatrics. *Urology* 1986;27:1-9.
88. Bird K, Rosenfield AI, Taylor KJW: Ultrasonography in testicular torsion. *Radiology* 1983;147:527-534.
89. Middleton WD, Melson GL: Testicular ischemia: color Doppler sonographic findings in five patients. *AJR* 1989;152:1237-1239.
90. Chinn DH, Miller EI: Generalized testicular hyperechogenicity in acute testicular torsion. *J Ultrasound Med* 1985;4:495-496.
91. Vick CW, Bird K, Rosenfield AT, et al: Extratesticular hemorrhage associated with torsion of the spermatic cord: sonographic demonstration. *Radiology* 1986;158:401-404.
92. Bird K, Rosenfield AT: Testicular infarction secondary to acute inflammatory disease: demonstration by B-scan ultrasound. *Radiology* 1984;152:785-788.
93. Margin B, Conte J: Ultrasonography of the acute scrotum. *J Clin Ultrasound* 1987;15:37-44.
94. Lerner RM, Mevorach RA, Hulbert WC, et al: Color Doppler ultrasound in the evaluation of acute scrotal disease. *Radiology* 1990;176:355-358.
95. Burks DD, Markey BJ, Burkhard TK, et al: Suspected testicular torsion and ischemia: evaluation with color Doppler sonography. *Radiology* 1990;175:815-821.
96. Chen DCP, Holder LE, Kaplan GN: Correlation of radionuclide imaging and diagnostic ultrasound in scrotal diseases. *J Nucl Med* 1986;27:1774-1781.
97. Berger RE, Alexander ER, Harnisch JP, et al: Etiology, manifestations and therapy of acute epididymitis: prospective study of 50 cases. *J Urol* 1979;121:750-754.

Trauma

98. Jeffrey RB, Laing FC, Hricak H, et al: Sonography of testicular trauma. *AJR* 1983;141:993-995.
99. Lupetin AR, King W, Rich PJ, et al: The traumatized scrotum: ultrasound evaluation. *Radiology* 1983;148:203-207.

Cryptorchidism

100. Elder JS: Cryptorchidism: isolated and associated with other genitourinary defects. *Pediatr Clin North Am* 1987;34:1033-1053.
101. Harrison JH, et al: Campbell's Urology. 4th ed. Philadelphia: WB Saunders Co; 1979.
102. Friedland GW, Chang P: The role of imaging in the management of the impalpable undescended testis. *AJR* 1988;151:1107-1111.
103. Kogan SJ: Cryptorchidism and infertility: an overview. *Dialog Pediatr Urol* 1982;4:2-3.
104. Rosenfield AT, Blair DN, McCarthy S, et al: The pars infravaginalis gubernaculi: importance in the identification of the undescended testis. *AJR* 1989;153:775-778.
105. Wolverson MK, Houttuin E, Heiberg E, et al: Comparison of computed tomography with high-resolution real-time ultrasound in the localization of the impalpable undescended testis. *Radiology* 1983;146:133-136.
106. Weiss R, Carter AR, Rosenfield AT: High-resolution real-time ultrasound in the localization of the undescended testis. *J Urol* 1986;135:936-938.
107. Fritzsche PJ, Hricak H, Kogan BA, et al: Undescended testis: value of magnetic resonance imaging. *Radiology* 1987;169:173.
108. Kier R, McCarthy S, Rosenfield AT, et al: Nonpalpable testes in young boys: evaluation with magnetic resonance imaging. *Radiology* 1988;169:429-433.

CHAPTER 27

The Penis

- Bernard F. King, M.D.

The penis is the male genital organ that serves a dual function of erection and as a route of excretion of urine and semen. Imaging of the penis has been limited in the past to plain films, urethrography, and cavernosography. Computed tomography and magnetic resonance imaging have also been advocated as a means of evaluating penile pathology.[1-3] Recently, however, high-resolution ultrasound of the penis with Doppler analysis of the penile blood vessels has offered detailed analysis of the anatomic and vascular structures of the penis. Ready availability and lack of ionizing radiation make ultrasound one of the most promising modalities in evaluating penile pathology.

Sonography can be reliably used for evaluation of penile masses, trauma, and urethral strictures. Peyronie's disease and congenital anomalies of the penis are also adequately evaluated with high-resolution penile sonography.

The most exciting developments in penile sonography have been in the area of impotence. Not only can one obtain gray-scale images of the penis, but, in addition, Doppler analysis of blood flow within the penile arteries can be assessed. This anatomic information and estimation of blood flow within the vessels can aid in the diagnostic evaluation of patients who may have vasculogenic impotence.

ANATOMY

Anatomy of the penis is unique and complex (Fig. 27-1). The penis is composed of three cylindric structures of cavernous tissue. The two **corpora cavernosa** lie in the dorsal two-thirds of the penis and a single **corpus spongiosum** lies in the ventral one-third of the penis. The two corpora cavernosa are the main erectile structures of the penis. Each corpus cavernosum and the corpus spongiosum are enveloped in a thick fascial sheath, the **tunica albuginea.** The urethra travels through the center of the corpus spongiosum. Distally, the penis exhibits a conical extremity, the glans penis. The **glans penis** is formed by an expansion of the corpus spongiosum, which fits over the blunt terminations of the corpora cavernosa. The corpora cavernosa and corpus spongiosum are composed of sinusoidal spaces lined by smooth muscle and endothelium. There is a septum dividing both corpora cavernosa that contains many fenestrations allowing for multiple anastomotic channels that connect the sinusoidal spaces of both corpora cavernosa. These small sinusoidal spaces in the corpora cavernosa distend with blood during an erection. The corpus spongiosum becomes engorged during erection but adds little to the erectile state of the penis.

The blood supply to the penis is primarily via the right and left internal pudendal arteries, which originate from the right and left internal iliac arteries. Each internal pudendal artery gives off a perineal branch, a bulbar branch, and a very small urethral artery before continuing as the artery of the penis. The **right** and **left penile arteries** enter the base of the penis and branch into cavernosal arteries and dorsal arteries. The cavernosal arteries are the primary source of blood flow to the erectile tissue of the penis (Fig. 27-2). Each **cavernosal artery** travels near the center of each corpus cavernosum as it sends small helicine arteries that communicate directly with the sinusoidal spaces, which are not visible sonographically. The paired **dorsal arteries** primarily supply blood to the skin and glans of the penis. However, anastomotic branches occur between the dorsal penile arteries and the deep cavernosal arteries.

Venous drainage of the erectile tissue of the penis primarily occurs via emissary veins, which are not visible sonographically. These emissary veins perforate the thick tunica albuginea and empty into circumflex veins that ultimately travel to the dorsal aspect of the penis and empty into the **deep dorsal penile vein,** which is sonographically visible (Fig. 27-3). The deep dorsal

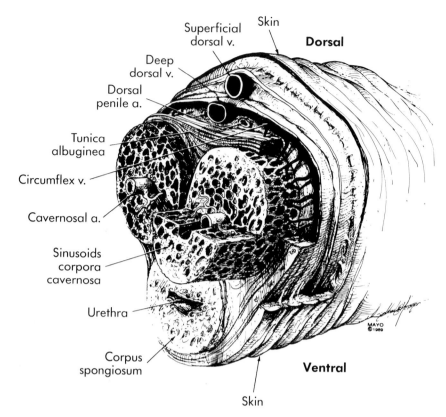

FIG 27-1. Cross-sectional drawing depicting the anatomy of the penis.
(From Quam JP, King BF, James EM et al. Duplex and color Doppler sonographic evaluation of vasculogenic impotence. *AJR* 1989; 153:1141-1147.)

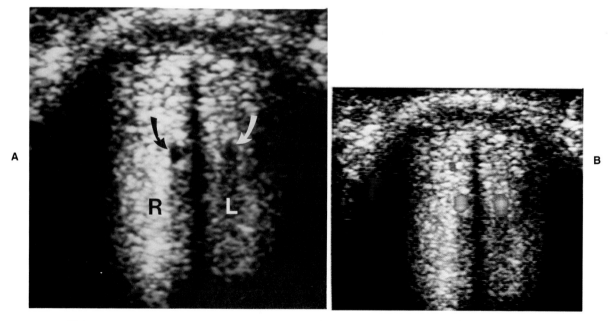

FIG 27-2. Corpora cavernosa. **A,** Transverse sonogram of the penis depicting the right *(R)* and left *(L)* corpora cavernosa. The cavernosal arteries *(arrows)* are seen near the midline of each corpus cavernosum. **B,** Color Doppler sonogram more clearly demonstrates the cavernosal arteries.

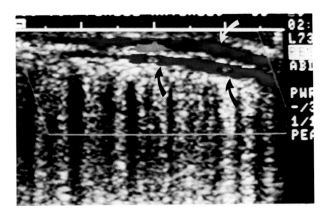

FIG 27-3. Dorsal veins. Longitudinal color Doppler sonogram of the dorsal surface of the penis depicting the deep dorsal penile vein *(black arrows)* that drains the erectile tissue of the penis. Also note the superficial dorsal penile vein *(white arrow)* that drains the skin and glans of the penis.

vein then empties into the retropubic venous plexus. Venous drainage of the corpus cavernosum also occurs through crural veins at the base of the penis. The skin and glans are drained through the superficial dorsal veins.

PHYSIOLOGY

Penile erection results from smooth muscle relaxation in the walls of the sinusoids and the helicine and cavernosal arteries of each corpora cavernosa. As sinusoidal muscle tone diminishes and the sinusoids distend with blood, the small emissary veins become compressed between the peripheral sinusoids and the unyielding peripheral tunica albuginea. This activates a veno-occlusive mechanism that maintains sinusoidal distension and limits venous outflow from the sinusoidal spaces (Fig. 27-4). With continued arterial inflow and limited venous outflow, the sinusoidal spaces distend to such a degree that the cavernosal tissue becomes rigid.[4-15]

The chemical mediators of **sinusoidal relaxation** are poorly understood. Adrenergic mediators appear to inhibit sinusoidal smooth muscle relaxation in the baseline flaccid state. When a psychoerotic stimulus occurs, parasympathetic nerve terminals, mediated by acetylcholine, are stimulated. These cholinergic effects suppress the adrenergic fibers, thus allowing for smooth muscle relaxation. In addition, acetylcholine appears to indirectly stimulate endothelial cells lining the sinusoidal spaces. This cholinergic effect on the endothelial cells is thought to result in the production of **endothelium-derived relaxing factor** (EDRF). This EDRF is believed to directly result in relaxation of the smooth muscle lining the sinusoidal spaces. When the psychoerotic stimulus subsides, the smooth muscle relaxation

and dilatation of the blood vessels supplying the penis diminishes. The sinusoids then shrink, resulting in less compression of the emissary veins and thus allowing venous outflow to again occur unimpeded. The penis then becomes flaccid.[16,17]

EXAMINATION TECHNIQUE

Penile sonographic examination is performed with the patient supine with the penis lying on the anterior abdominal wall (Fig. 27-5). High frequency (7.5 to 10 MHz) linear array ultrasound transducers provide high-resolution images of the penis. The transducer is placed transversely on the ventral surface starting at the level of the glans down to the base of the penis. The two corpora cavernosa are easily identified on transverse images as circular structures adjacent to each other, separated by the septum penis. The cavernosal arteries are visualized near the medial portion of the corpora cavernosa (Fig. 27-2). Rarely one may see collateral vessels either crossing the septum penis from one cavernosal artery to another or from the dorsal penile artery to the cavernosal artery. The two dorsal penile arteries are smaller than the cavernosal arteries and can sometimes be visualized if the dorsal surface of the penis is scanned transversely using color Doppler. The corpus spongiosum is often compressed and difficult to visualize when scanning the ventral aspect of the penis. However, by applying a generous amount of acoustic gel and with gentle compression by the transducer, one can adequately visualize the corpus spongiosum.

The echotexture of the corporal structures should be uniform throughout. The **fascial planes,** including the tunica albuginea, will be seen as a hyperechoic regions surrounding the periphery of the corporal structures. The penis should be scanned to exclude excessive amounts of fibrosis within the corporal bodies and/or in the fascial layers around the corporal bodies. Palpable abnormalities (i.e., Peyronie's plaques) should be scanned to assess the sonographic features of the masses and their exact location with respect to the corporal bodies.

Longitudinal evaluation of each corporal body of the penis should also be obtained from the ventral surface. The cavernosal arteries are seen as small tubular structures with echogenic walls in the center of the corpora cavernosa (Fig. 27-6). Evaluation of the corpus spongiosum and urethra is also performed from the ventral aspect of the penis. Copious amounts of acoustic gel or an acoustic pad on the surface of the penis can be used to optimize visualization and to avoid excessive compression by the transducer. Visualization of the **penile urethra** is optimally performed by distending it. This can be accomplished while the patient is voiding or by injecting the urethra with a viscous lidocaine gel in a retrograde fashion (Fig. 27-7). The latter method is pre-

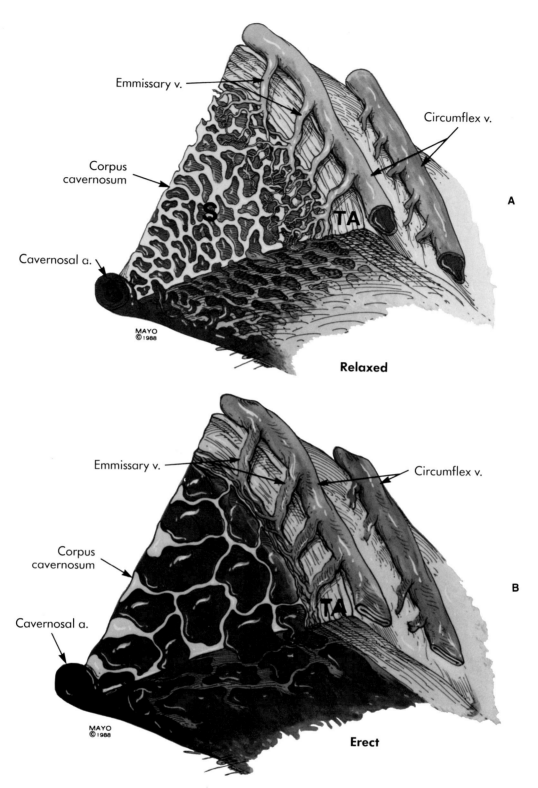

FIG 27-4. Corpus cavernosum in the flaccid and erect state. Cross-sectional wedge drawings of the corpus cavernosum in the flaccid **(A)** and erect **(B)** state. During the erectile process, the cavernosal arteries and sinusoids *(S)* distend with blood and compress the draining venules against the thick and rigid tunica albuginea *(TA)*. The compression and near occlusion of these draining venules prevents venous efflux from the cavernosal tissues and allows for prolonged maximal distension of the cavernosal sinusoids, resulting in an erection.

(From Hattery RR, King BF, Lewis RW, et al. Vasculogenic impotence: duplex and color Doppler. *Radiol Clin North Am* 1991; May.)

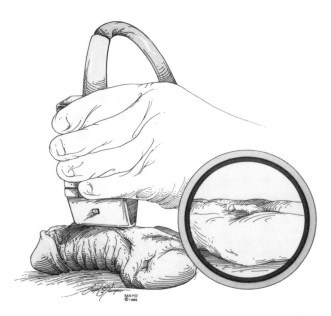

FIG 27-5. Technique of penile sonography. Drawing depicting the technique of penile sonography. The penis is in the anatomic position, lying on the anterior abdominal wall. The transducer is placed on the ventral surface of the penis.
(From Hattery RR, King BF, Lewis RW, et al. Vasculogenic impotence: duplex and color Doppler. *Radiol Clin North Am* 1991; May.)

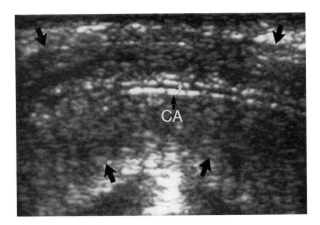

FIG 27-6. Left corpus cavernosum. Longitudinal sonogram of the left corpus cavernosum *(arrows)*. Echogenic walls of the cavernosal artery *(CA)* are seen near the middle of the corpora.

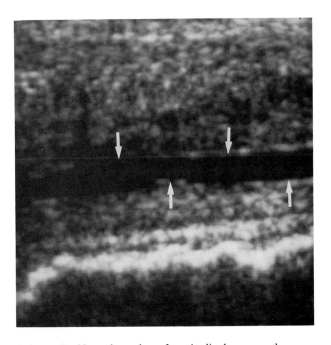

FIG 27-7. Normal urethra. Longitudinal sonourethrogram from the dorsal surface of the penis depicts the normal urethra *(arrows)* distended with lidocaine gel.
(Courtesy of Dr. C.B. Benson, Boston.)

ferred because of optimal distension that can be maintained over a longer period of time. This is accomplished by inserting a tapered tip syringe containing viscous lidocaine jelly into the urethral meatus and then applying a distal penile clamp to maintain distension of the penile urethra.

IMPOTENCE

Until recently it was felt that psychologic factors accounted for most cases or causes of impotence.[18] However, studies using nocturnal penile tumescence have revealed that a majority of cases of impotence have organic causes.[19-23] Subsequent studies have shown that vasculogenic impotence is one of the most frequent causes for erectile failure (Fig. 27-8).[22-26] Vasculogenic impotence may be due to poor arterial inflow into the penis (arteriogenic impotence) or excessive venous leakage of blood from the penis (venogenic impotence), or both.

Noninvasive and Invasive Tests

Many examinations, invasive and noninvasive, have been used to evaluate arterial inflow into the penis and to evaluate for possible excessive venous leakage from erectile tissue.[27-71] Arteriography with selective internal iliac angiography is considered the gold standard in the evaluation of arteriogenic impotence.* However, this technique is invasive and is therefore not suitable as a screening examination. Recently many patients have been screened for vasculogenic impotence by measuring their clinical response to an intracavernosal injection of a vasodilating pharmacologic agent.† Many vasodilat-

*References 27, 29, 30, 38, 43, 44, 50, 54, 63, 66.
†References 5, 20, 31, 32, 55, 56, 72.

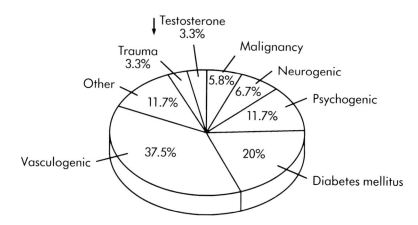

FIG 27-8. Causes of impotence. Pie graph displaying the relative frequencies of the various causes of impotence.
(Modified from Quam JP, King BF, James EM, et al. Duplex and color Doppler ultrasound evaluation of vasculogenic impotence [scientific exhibit]. *Radiol Soc North Am,* Chicago, 1989.)

ing medications have been used, including papaverine, phentolamine, and prostaglandin E-1. By injecting these vasodilators intracavernosally, one can bypass the psychoerotic and neurologic pathways that normally initiate an erection. Most investigators believe that the arterial inflow and veno-occlusive mechanisms are intact if the patient develops an erection after the intracavernosal injection of these vasodilators. Thus a full erection after the intracavernosal injection of a vasodilating agent should indicate an adequate vascular system. Since this method is easy to perform and is reproducible, it offers many advantages as a screening test for vasculogenic impotence. However this technique fails to differentiate arteriogenic from venogenic impotence. This differentiation is important because the treatment for arteriogenic impotence is markedly different from the treatment of venogenic impotence.

The **penile-brachial index** (PBI) was once a very popular screening test for identifying patients who may have arteriogenic impotence.[25,61] The penile-brachial index is calculated by dividing the mean systolic pressure in the penile arteries by the mean systolic brachial artery pressure. In general, a value less than 0.7 suggests arteriogenic impotence. However, studies have shown that there is considerable overlap between normal and abnormal patients using PBI results.

Duplex Doppler Examination

The desire for a more accurate noninvasive test of arterial inflow into the penis led to the development of Doppler pulse wave analysis in patients with possible arteriogenic impotence. With this technique, recording of the **continuous wave Doppler** pattern of the deep cavernosal arteries was used to screen patients for arteriogenic impotence. Early studies with this technique were reportedly more accurate than PBI and

apparently showed good correlation with arteriographic findings. However, later studies with continuous wave Doppler showed inaccuracies because of the inability to differentiate Doppler changes arising in the deep cavernosal artery from changes in the dorsal penile artery.[22,24,28,35,51] In addition, early reports of Doppler analysis were only performed in the flaccid state and therefore functional capability of the penile arteries during erection was difficult to predict. Because of this many have questioned the reproducibility of this method.

Duplex sonography is more accurate than continuous wave sonography because of the ability to visualize the deep cavernosal artery and obtain a reliable pulsed Doppler signal from it. Using real-time gray-scale sonographic visualization, Lue et al showed that precise Doppler sampling and blood velocity measurements of the deep cavernosal arteries could be performed before and after intracavernosal injections of vasodilating agents.[34] In addition changes in diameter of the cavernosal artery could be obtained before and after administration of the vasodilating agent. With knowledge of the blood velocity and change in diameters of the cavernosal arteries after the intracavernosal injection of a vasodilating agent, one can estimate the amount of arterial blood flow available for the corporal erectile tissue of the penis during an artificially induced erection.

The *technique of duplex sonography of the penis* in the evaluation of vasculogenic impotence is still evolving. The examination should take place in a quiet room with minimal distractions and interruptions. Too many external distractions could affect the patient's response to the vasodilating agent and thus alter the velocity parameters. Longitudinal examination of the corpora cavernosa is best accomplished in a parasagittal plane from a ventral approach (Fig. 27-9). In the flaccid state the cavernosal artery can follow a tortuous course and can be

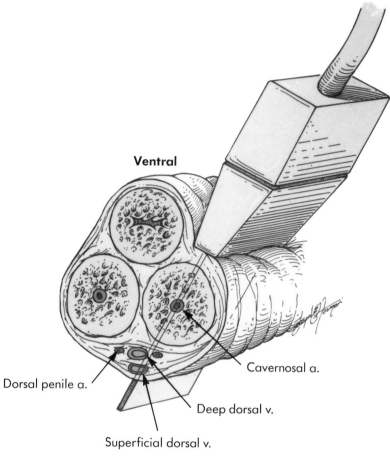

Ventral

Cavernosal a.

Dorsal penile a.

Deep dorsal v.

Superficial dorsal v.

Dorsal

FIG 27-9. Transducer position for Doppler examination of the cavernosal artery. Position on the ventral aspect of the penis. Drawing depicts the medially directed position of the transducer. (From King BF Jr, Hattery RR, James EM, Lewis RW. Duplex sonography in the evaluation of impotence: current techniques. *Semin Intervent Radiol* 1990:7(3-4):215-221.)

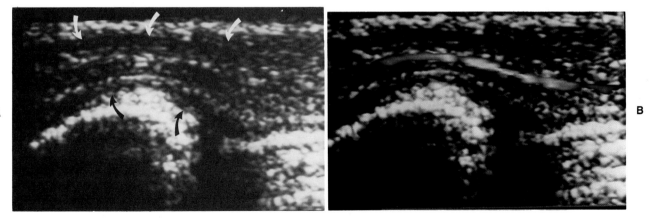

A

B

FIG 27-10. Cavernosal artery. **A,** Longitudinal gray scale sonogram of the corpus cavernosum *(outlined by arrows)*. The cavernosal artery is not identified. **B,** With the addition of color Doppler, the cavernosal artery *(red)* is easily identified.

seen intermittently on longitudinal scans. In the erect state, the cavernosal artery assumes a straighter course. Near the base of the penis the cavernosal artery can be difficult to appreciate on gray-scale imaging. Color Doppler can aid in the identification of the cavernosal artery in this region (Fig. 27-10).

The diameters of the cavernosal arteries can be obtained by measuring the internal lumen (Fig. 27-6). In some patients the cavernosal arteries are too small to accurately measure before the injection of a vasodilating agent. Because of the wide variability, multiple measurements on each side can be obtained and averaged.

Following the measurement of the diameters of the cavernosal arteries, a vasodilating agent is injected. The types and doses of vasodilating agents that are used vary widely. Initially, many investigators use 60 mg of papaverine in 2 ml of solution injected into either the left or right corpus cavernosum.[34] The vasodilating agent easily diffuses from one corpus cavernosum to the other because of the many fenestrations of the septum separating the corpora cavernosa. Other investigators have used a lower dose of papaverine (40 mg) in addition to a second agent such as phentolamine (2.5 mg). Others have used a triple agent consisting of papaverine 4.4 mg, phentolamine 0.15 mg, and prostaglandin E-1 1.5 µg in 0.25 ml to minimize the possibility of priapism, which may occur in 2% to 3% of the patients.[70] It is thought that small doses of these vasodilating agents used together result in an additive effect that al-

lows one to use minimal doses of the vasodilating agent with optimal response and minimal discomfort.

It is important to accurately inject the vasodilating agent into the dorsal two-thirds of the penile shaft so that the agent does not enter into the corpus spongiosum or urethra (Fig. 27-11). Care must also be taken to avoid injecting the vasodilating agent into the subcutaneous tissue, which could result in massive swelling of the skin and possible necrosis. All patients should be informed that if a painful erection occurs or if the erection does not subside after 1 hour, the patient should contact his referring physician or go directly to an emergency room for evaluation and treatment of priapism. Pharmacologic-induced priapism is persistent painful erection of the penis 1 to 3 hours after the intracavernosal injection of a vasodilating agent. Persistent priapism (greater than 1 to 3 hours) could result in ischemic necrosis of cavernosal tissue and resulting fibrosis of this erectile tissue. Patients who are prone to priapism include those who have a history of neurogenic impotence, those with sickle cell disease or trait, and patients on heparin therapy. Small doses or avoidance of vasodilating agents may be warranted in these patients.[55,72-78]

Treatment of priapism usually consists of aspirating approximately 20 ml of blood from a corpus cavernosum. If this fails to relieve the priapism, then 200 µg of phenylephrine HCl (500 µg solution) (Neosynephrine) diluted in 1 ml of normal saline can be injected intracavernosally to facilitate mild vasoconstric-

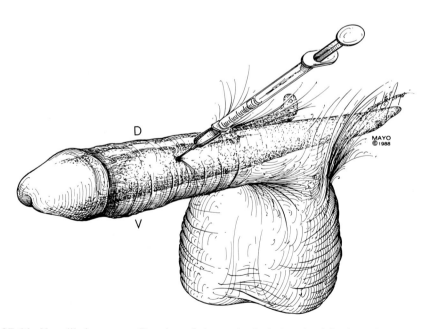

FIG 27-11. Vasodilating agent. Drawing of the penis depicting the injection of a vasodilating agent. Care must be taken to inject the vasodilating agent into the dorsal two-thirds of the shaft of the penis. *D*, Dorsal; *V*, ventral.

tion and cessation of the erection. Treatment of priapism should be carried out by trained and experienced physicians.[70]

Following the intracavernosal injection of a vasodilating agent, the diameters of the cavernosal arteries are again measured and velocity measurements are obtained in these cavernosal arteries. Doppler analysis of blood flow in the cavernosal artery is optimally obtained near the base of the penis where the Doppler angle is the smallest. The smaller the Doppler angle, the more accurate the velocity measurements will be. Spectral Doppler analysis of cavernosal arteries enables one to take **peak systolic** and **end-diastolic velocity** measurements.

Maximal effect of the vasodilating agents is reached about 5 to 20 minutes after the injection in most patients, but the time is highly variable. Therefore most investigators feel that velocity measurements in the cavernosal

arteries should begin approximately 5 minutes after injection. Velocity measurements should then be obtained continuously or at 5-minute intervals for at least 20 to 30 minutes after injection. Peak systolic velocities and end-diastolic velocity measurements should be obtained in both cavernosal arteries at each 5-minute interval. The **post-injection cavernosal artery diameter** measurements should be obtained 5 minutes after injection. The effects of the vasodilating agents may begin to wear off as early as 20 to 30 minutes after the injection.

There appear to be five phases of spectral waveforms in the cavernosal arteries after the intracavernosal injection of vasodilating agents in normal males (Fig. 27-12).[40] These five phases in normal men occur within approximately 5 to 10 minutes after the intracavernosal injection of a vasodilating agent. However, patients with vasculogenic impotence may never complete all

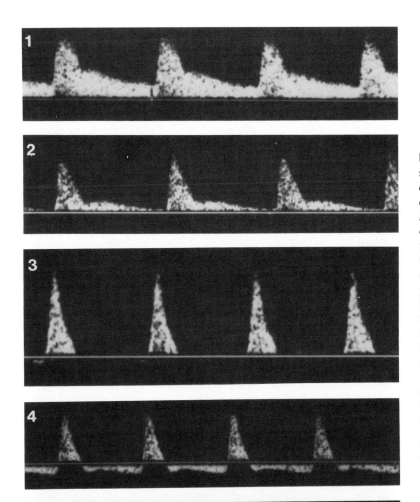

FIG 27-12. Normal spectral waveforms. The spectral waveform in the cavernosal artery undergoes five normal phases following the intracavernosal injection of a vasodilating agent. *Phase 1* occurs during cavernosal and sinusoidal dilatation, resulting in a low-resistance waveform. Forward diastolic velocities are highest in this first phase. *Phase 2* occurs when the sinusoids begin to fill with blood and intrapenile pressure increases. Systolic velocities remain high in this phase, but diastolic velocities begin to approach zero. In *phase 3* full tumescence is reached and intrapenile pressure equals diastolic blood pressure. In *phase 4* full rigidity begins and systolic velocities remain high and intrapenile pressure exceeds diastolic blood pressure and reversal of diastolic flow occurs. In *phase 5* full rigidity occurs and systolic velocities become dampened.
(Modified from Schwartz AN, Wang KY, Mack LA, et al. Evaluation of normal erectile function with color flow Doppler sonography. *AJR* 1989;153:1155-1160.)

normal phases because of abnormal arterial inflow or because of an impaired veno-occlusive mechanism.

Arteriogenic Impotence. Peak systolic velocities following the intracavernosal injection of a vasodilating agent appear to be the most promising parameter when evaluating patients for potential arteriogenic impotence. In a study of normal male volunteers it was found that the **normal average peak systolic velocity** following the intracavernosal injection of a vasodilating agent is approximately 30 to 40 cm/sec.[40] Lue et al found that the majority of patients who have a moderate-to-good response to papaverine clinically have peak systolic velocities of 25 cm/sec or greater.[34] In addition, no patients in their study who had a poor response to papaverine injection had peak systolic velocities of 25 cm/sec or greater. Collins et al also have found that patients who responded sonographically to papaverine had average peak systolic velocities of 26.8 cm/sec.[36] We reported a series of 12 patients with suspected arteriogenic impotence who underwent pelvic arteriography.[38] All five patients with abnormal findings on arteriography also had abnormal peak systolic velocities of less than 25 cm/sec. Six out of seven patients with normal arteriograms had peak systolic velocities in their cavernosal arteries of 25 cm/sec or greater. These studies indicate that when comparing sonographic response of a vasodilating agent to arteriography, a peak systolic velocity of 25 cm/sec or less suggests inadequate arterial inflow to allow for moderate or good erections.

However, Benson et al. have grouped impotent patients into three subgroups based on Doppler ultrasound data.[39] The first subgroup of patients were considered normal and were found to have average peak systolic velocities of 47 cm/sec. The second group of patients, who were felt to have mild-to-moderate arterial insufficiency, had an average peak systolic velocity of 35 cm/sec, and a third group with severe arterial insufficiency were found to have an average peak systolic velocity of 7 cm/sec. The investigators concluded that a cut-off value for normal individuals of 40 cm/sec peak systolic velocity should be used. However, they went on to state that a peak systolic velocity of 30 cm/sec could correctly distinguish all patients with normal cavernosal arteries from those with severe arterial disease.

Arterial blood flow is not only a function of the velocity in a particular vessel but also a function of the cross-sectional area of the lumen of the vessel. Because of this, investigators have advocated measuring the change in diameter of the cavernosal arteries after the injection of a vasodilating agent. These investigators feel that the initial size of the artery is probably not a good indicator of arterial disease and that arterial compliance and ability to dilate are more important.[34] They feel that a 75% increase in vessel diameter is a good indication of normal arterial inflow into the cavernosal artery. However, because of the small size of the cavernosal arteries and the potential error in diameter measurement, one cannot totally rely on diameter changes.

From these data it seems logical to assume that *peak systolic velocities in cavernosal arteries of less than 25 cm/sec after administration of a vasodilating agent should suggest arterial disease* and should lead to a more definite evaluation with selective internal pudendal arteriography if clinically warranted (Fig. 27-13). Values between 25 and 30 cm/sec should be considered borderline. *Peak systolic velocity measurements greater than 30 cm/sec should be considered normal.* However, several exceptions exist. If there is a marked discrepancy between the velocities of the two cavernosal arteries (greater than 10 cm/sec difference), **unilateral arterial disease** of the penis may be present. Adequate blood flow through one cavernosal artery may be all that is needed for adequate erections; however, unilateral arterial disease of the penis may be significant in certain individuals and appropriate arteriography may be need to be pursued. Another exception occurs when the peak systolic velocity is greater than 100 cm/sec. This high velocity has been seen in patients with **diffuse vascular spasm** and/or **small vessel disease.** Such patients demonstrate little or no change in cavernosal arterial diameter measurements before and after the injection of a vasodilating agent. Therefore if extremely high velocities in the cavernosal arteries (greater than 100 cm/sec) are detected, one should closely evaluate the caliber of the cavernosal arteries. If the caliber does not significantly increase following the vasodilating agent, the patient may have diffuse small vessel disease (i.e., diabetes) or diffuse vasospasm (nicotine abuse, medications).

The direction of blood flow in the cavernosal artery may be reversed. It has been shown that reversal of diastolic flow is a normal phenomenon in the latter stages of erection. However, one should *never* encounter reversal of blood flow during systole. Reversal of systolic blood flow is often caused by **proximal penile artery occlusion** with collateral flow in a retrograde fashion into the affected cavernosal artery.[68] Proximal penile artery occlusion can result from trauma, corporal fibrosis, or atherosclerotic vessel disease.

Collateral vessels to the cavernosal artery may be a normal variant. However, collateral vessels from the contralateral cavernosal artery or the dorsal penile artery may also indicate proximal vessel disease in the affected artery. These collateral vessels can often be seen with color Doppler sonography.

Particular attention should be given to the presence of arterial sinusoidal fistulas or arterial venous fistulas within the corporal tissue of the penis in patients who have developed erectile dysfunction following trauma. Color Doppler evaluation can often locate the fistula. Partial priapism is often an accompanying sign in arterial sinusoidal fistulas.

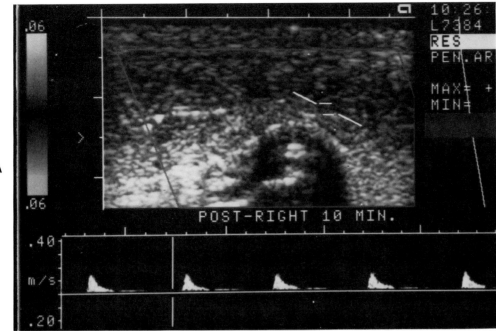

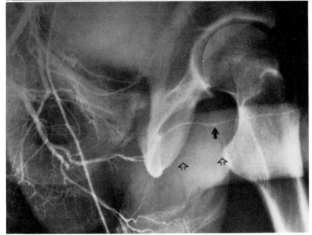

FIG 27-13. Arteriogenic impotence. **A,** Duplex sonogram of the right cavernosal artery following the intracavernosal injection of 60 mg of papaverine revealed a decreased arterial velocity of approximately 15 cm/sec. **B,** Pelvic arteriogram demonstrates no opacification of the cavernosal artery *(open arrows)*. The normal dorsal artery is identified *(black arrow)*.

Venogenic Impotence. Vasculogenic impotence may also be due to excessive venous leakage from the corporal bodies of the penis. Although the exact cause of excessive venous leakage is unknown, it is believed by many investigators to be secondary to stretching of the thick tunica albuginea. This stretching of the tunica albuginea prevents the compression of the emissary veins draining the sinusoids during the erection process. Because of the lack of compression of the emissary veins, venous outflow continues to occur rapidly from the corporal tissues and an erection is never fully obtained.

Traditionally, venogenic impotence has been evaluated with cavernosometry and cavernosography.[4,45-49,53,58] However, these examinations are invasive and are not suitable for screening purposes.

Therefore duplex sonography has been recently used as a screening examination for venogenic impotence.

During the duplex Doppler examination of the cavernosal arteries in the normal patient, there is an increase in diastolic and systolic velocities immediately following the intracavernosal injection of a vasodilating agent. This corresponds to the physiologic dilatation of the cavernosal artery, helicine arteries, and sinusoidal spaces. As the sinusoidal spaces are dilating and filling, resistance in the cavernosal artery is low and forward diastolic flow increases. However, when the veno-occlusive mechanism engages, the sinusoids become maximally distended and intracavernosal pressure increases. At this point, vascular resistance increases and diastolic flow ceases or even reverses. If a patient's veno-occlusive mechanism is not intact, excessive

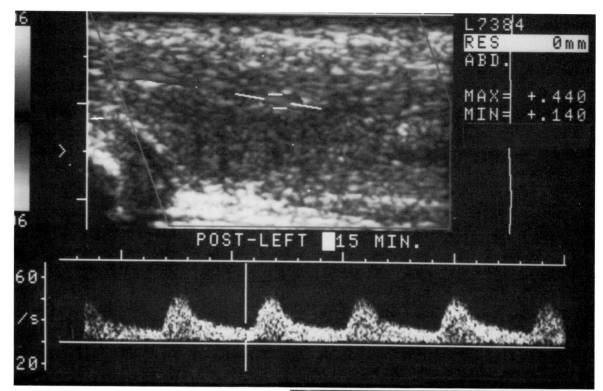

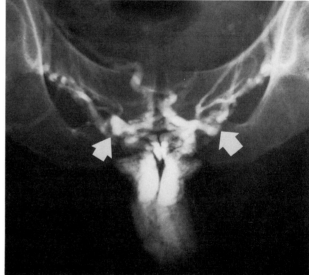

FIG 27-14. Venogenic impotence. **A,** Duplex sonogram of a left cavernosal artery 15 minutes following injection demonstrates a normal peak systolic velocity of 44 cm/sec. However, there is persistent high end-diastolic velocity of 14 cm/sec suggestive of excessive venous leakage. **B,** Cavernosogram reveals massive venous leak into the retropubic venous plexus *(arrows).*

venous leakage will persist and intracavernosal pressures will remain low. The Doppler spectral waveform will continue to exhibit the prominent forward diastolic flow of a low-resistance vascular bed throughout the examination. Therefore patients who continue to have high end-diastolic velocities (over 5 cm/sec) throughout the examination, despite normal arterial inflow (peak systolic velocities 30 cm/sec), may have venogenic impotence[38] (Fig. 27-14). Cavernosometry and cavernosography should be considered in these patients. Patients who demonstrate reversal of diastolic flow in both cav-

ernosal arteries should have an intact venoocclusive mechanism.

The deep dorsal penile vein drains the majority of venous efflux from the corpora cavernosa. Some investigators have recommended velocity measurements in the deep dorsal penile vein as a means of detecting excessive venous leakage. However, early results reveal that normal patients and patients with excessive venous leakage may each have high deep dorsal vein velocities.[71] In addition, it has also been found that some patients who have excessive venous leakage on cavernosometry and cavernosography may leak primarily via the crural veins near the base of the penis and not via the deep dorsal penile vein. Therefore it appears that measuring deep dorsal vein velocities may not be a very helpful parameter for detecting venogenic impotence.

Pitfalls in Duplex Doppler Sonography for Impotence. Although intracavernosal injection of vasodilating agents is supposed to bypass the psychologic stimulus needed for erection, **excessive psychologic overlay** may result in impaired response to these vasodilating agents. Suboptimal peak systolic velocities (<25 cm/sec) can occur in normal patients with excessive anxiety and alpha-adrenergic tone. Occasionally patients become very anxious about an injection into the penis and/or an ultrasound evaluation of the penis. Because of this anxiety, the response to the vasodilating agent may be inhibited. Therefore each patient should be counseled about the safety of the technique, and professional standards should be maintained during the examination. A quiet darkened room may help in allaying fears in certain patients.

Time-Velocity Measurements. Early investigators recommended that velocity measurements should be obtained 5 to 10 minutes after injection. However, recent studies have indicated that the response to the intracavernosal vasodilating agent varies among individuals.[70] Peak systolic velocity in normal males can occur at any time from 5 to 30 minutes after injection. Therefore, in order to detect maximum velocities, the peak systolic velocity measurements should be measured at 5, 10, 15, and 20 minutes after injection.

Because normal individuals will have high end-diastolic velocities early in the examination (5 to 10 minutes after injection), many investigators feel that end-diastolic velocity measurements at the 15-, 20-, and 30-minute time periods should be used in screening patients who may have venogenic impotence. Persistent low-resistance spectral waveforms at these later times (high diastolic velocities greater than 5 cm/sec) indicate persistent and excessive venous leakage as a cause of venogenic impotence.

Proper Injection of Vasodilating Agents. If the vasodilating agent is injected into the corpus spongiosum, the agent will not be available to the sinusoidal tissue in the corpora cavernosa and erection will not occur. In addition, the injection of the vasodilating agent could enter the urethra and be expelled through the urethral meatus.

PEYRONIE'S DISEASE

Peyronie's disease is fibrosis of the fibrous sheaths covering the corpora cavernosa and occurs without known cause, usually in men over 45 years of age. This fibrotic area sometimes does not permit lengthening of the involved surface with erection, so that the erect penis bends toward the involved area. The fibrotic area usually involves the dorsum of the penis but can involve the septum penis and/or lateral aspects of the penis. Because of the fibrotic plaque, the penis bends toward the involved area resulting in a deformity known as a **chordee.** In the early stages of erection it is accompanied by pain and eventually the degree of curvature may preclude coitus. It is believed that the process begins as a vasculitis of the connective tissue beneath the tunica albuginea and then extends to adjacent structures. This leads to fibrosis and at times calcification or even ossification.

Palpation of the shaft reveals a well-demarcated raised plaque of fibrosis that is usually in the midline of the dorsum near the base of the penis, although it may be placed more laterally or distally. Plain film evaluation of the penis may reveal areas of calcification within the indurated area.

Sonographically, the plaques of Peyronie's disease appear as dense hyperechoic areas near the peripheral margin of the corpus cavernosum, usually along the dorsal aspect of the penis.[1,3,51,79-87] In one study, 22% of the plaques identified sonographically were not clinically palpable. In approximately one-third of the patients these plaques will cast an acoustic shadow that is most likely related to the presence of calcification (Fig. 27-15). In rare instances the plaques of Peyronie's disease will be evident as hypoechoic lesions that appear as an enlargement of the pericavernous tissue. This latter presentation is found in the earliest stages of the disease, when fibrosis is scarce and interstitial edema is present. The fibrosis and plaque may extend into the corpus cavernosum and occlude the cavernosal artery. Occlusion of the cavernosal artery may result in arteriogenic impotence.

Sonography can assess the size and location of the plaque for preoperative evaluation. In some individuals sonography may be used to follow patients undergoing medical treatment for evaluation of regression of the plaques.

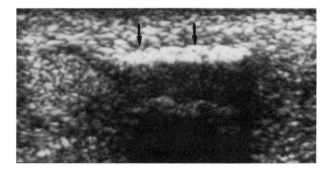

FIG 27-15. Penile plaque. Longitudinal sonogram of the medial aspect of the right corpus cavernosum depicting an echogenic plaque *(arrows)* with posterior acoustic shadow.

PENILE URETHRA

The male urethra consists of the posterior urethra, which includes the prostatic and membranous urethra, and the anterior urethra, which includes the bulbous and penile urethra. The sonographic evaluation of the posterior urethra can be performed using a transrectal ultrasound approach. The anterior urethra can be studied by placing the transducer on the surface of the penis and distending the urethra with fluid or gel.

The indications for sonography of the penile urethra include evaluation of urethral strictures and the detection and localization of foreign bodies or stone material. Sonography has also been used for the evaluation of traumatic urethral disruption and urethral diverticula.[88-92]

Urethral strictures occur most commonly secondary to gonococcal urethritis or trauma. Sonographic evaluation of urethral strictures has several advantages over radiographic studies. Ultrasound does not use ionizing radiation, which is important for younger patients with strictures who may require multiple examinations. During transverse and longitudinal real-time ultrasound the three-dimensional nature of the urethra can be appreciated. The soft tissues surrounding the urethra can also be examined for scarring and other abnormalities. The disadvantage of sonography of the penile urethra is its inability to visualize the posterior prostatic urethra without having to use a transrectal approach. Fortunately, most strictures occur in the anterior urethra.

The normal urethral lumen measures 4 mm or less in diameter and has smooth, thin walls. A stricture of the anterior urethra appears as a segment of narrowed lumen with irregularity and thickening of the urethral wall due to fibrosis and scarring (Fig. 27-16). The length of the stricture can be accurately measured, and dilatation of the urethra proximal to the stricture can also be appreciated. Sonographic guidance of stricture dilatation can be performed when indicated.

Nonradiopaque foreign bodies or **radiopaque stones** may be found in the urethra during ultrasonic evaluation. When looking for a urethral foreign body, the bulbous and penile urethra should be scanned before distension of the urethra to locate the foreign object as it may be dislodged during retrograde filling.

Urethral diverticula in the penile urethra are rare but can occur as a result of previous urethritis. These diverticula appear as fluid-filled outpouchings adjacent to the urethra. Those diverticula that do not fill on retrograde urethrography can be seen sonographically.

PENILE CARCINOMA

Almost all tumors of the penis are of epithelial origin and almost always involve the distal portion of the penis.[85,93,94] The incidence of penile carcinoma is less in those populations where circumcision is common. Stage 1 carcinoma of the penis involves a lesion limited to the glans or foreskin. Stage 2 tumors invade the shaft or corpora cavernosa. Stage 3 tumors are those that invade the shaft and have lymph node involvement. Stage 4 tumors have distant metastases.

Approximately 50% of patients are likely to have metastases in the regional inguinal lymph node chain at

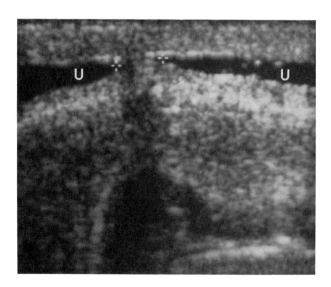

FIG 27-16. Urethral stricture. Longitudinal sonourethrogram depicting a focal urethral stricture *(cursors)*. *U*, Urethra.
(Courtesy of Dr. C.B. Benson, Boston.)

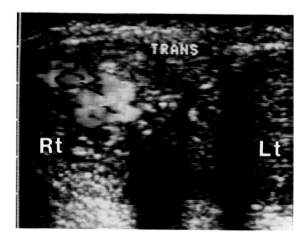

FIG 27-17. Arteriosinusoidal fistula. Transverse color Doppler sonogram shows an area of increased color flow involving a large portion of the right cavernosal tissue consistent with an arteriosinusoidal fistula.
(From Hattery RR, King BF, et al. *Radiol Clin N Am* 1991; 29(3)-629-645.)

the time of recognition because the disease is painless and often hidden within the nonretractable foreskin. Early diagnosis of metastatic nodal involvement remains the best available means for establishing appropriate management and prognosis. Ultrasound-guided fine needle aspiration biopsy of enlarged inguinal lymph nodes can aid in the preoperative assessment in these patients.[94]

High-resolution sonography visualizes the extent of the primary tumor and its involvement in the corporal tissues. Penile cancer can appear hypoechoic or hyperechoic. The margins of the tumor are easily appreciated and the involvement of the corporal tissues can be nicely demonstrated.[85] In penile cancer, a 2-cm margin of tumor-free tissue proximal to the tumor is a prerequisite for penile amputation.

PENILE TRAUMA

Penile trauma can be classified as either penetrating (e.g., knife or bullet) or blunt.[95] Injury to the penis following blunt trauma usually occurs when the penis is erect. Fracture of the penis occurs when there is disruption of the tunica albuginea and corpora cavernosa.[96,97] Penile fractures are often associated with a urethral tear. Although the findings may be clinically obvious, sonography can be helpful for vascular evaluation.[98] In some individuals arterial sinusoidal fistulas occur following straddle injuries. These rare arterial sinusoidal fistulas result in partial tumescence of a portion of the penis.[63,98] Gray-scale sonography of this area may reveal a hypoechoic area due to hematoma in the corpus cavernosum. Color flow Doppler will often more clearly demonstrate an arteriovenous fistula of the cavernosal tissues (Fig. 27-17).

REFERENCES
Anatomy

1. Rollandi GA, Tentarelli T, Vespier M. Computed tomographic findings in Peyronie's disease. *Urol Radiol* 1985;7:153-156.
2. Fisher M, Kricum M. Imaging of the Pelvis. Rockville, MD: Aspen Publishers, Inc; 1989.
3. Hricak H, Marotti M, Gilbert TJ, et al. Normal penile anatomy and abnormal penile conditions: evaluation with MR imaging. *Radiology* 1988;169:683-690.

Physiology

4. Aboseif SR, Lue TF. Hemodynamics of penile erection. *Urol Clin North Am* 1988;15:1-7.
5. Stackl W, Hasun R, Marberger M. Intracavernous injection of prostaglandin E1 in impotent men. *J Urol* 1988;140:66.
6. Fujita T, Shirai M. Mechanism of erection. *J Clin Exp Med* 1989;148:249.
7. Shirai M, Ishii N. Hemodynamics of erection in man. *Arch Androl* 1981;6:27.
8. Tudoriu T, Bourmer H. The hemodynamics of erection at the level of the penis and its local deterioration. *J Urol* 1983;129:741-745.
9. Saenz de Tejada IS, Goldstein I, Krane RJ. Local control of penile erection: nerves, smooth muscle and endothelium. *Urol Clin North Am* 1988;15:9-15.
10. Newman HF, Northup JD, Delvin J. Mechanism of human penile erection. *Invest Urol* 1963;1:350-353.
11. Lue T, Tanagho E. Physiology of erection and pharmacologic management of impotence. *J Urol* 1987;137:829.
12. Saenz de Tejada IS, Goldstein I, Krane RJ. Local control of penile erection: nerve, smooth muscle and endothelium. *Urol Clin North Am* 1988;15:9-15.
13. Shirai M, Ishii N, Mitsukawa S, et al. Hemodynamic mechanism of erection in the human penis. *Arch Androl* 1978;1:345-349.
14. Beutler LE, Gleason DM. Integrating the advances in the diagnosis and treatment of male potency disturbance. *J Urol* 1981;126:338-342.
15. Collins WE, McKendry JBR, Silverman M, et al. Multidisciplinary survey of erectile dysfunction. *Canad Med Assoc J* 1982;128:1393-1399.
16. Lue TF, Tanagho EA. Physiology of erection and pharmacological management of impotence. *J Urol* 1987;137:5:829-836.
17. Lue TF, Zeineh RA, Schmidt RA, et al. Physiology of erection. *World J Urol* 1983;1:194-196.

Impotence

18. Masters WH, Johnson VE. *Human Sexual Inadequacy*. New York: Little, Brown, & Co Inc; 1970.
19. Karacan I, Salis PJ, Williams RL. The role of the sleep laboratory in the diagnosis and treatment of impotence. In: William RL, Karacan I, Frazier SH, eds. *Sleep Disorders: Diagnosis and Treatment*. New York: John Wiley & Sons Inc; 1978.
20. Abber IC, Lue TF, Orvis BR, et al. Diagnostic tests for impotence: a comparison of papaverine injection with the penile-brachial index and nocturnal penile tumescence monitoring. *J Urol* 1986;3-28.
21. Karacan I, Moore CA. Nocturnal penile tumescence: an objective diagnostic aid for erectile dysfunction. In Bennett: AH, ed. *Management of Male Impotence*. Baltimore: Williams & Wilkins; 1982.
22. Krane RJ, Goldstein I, Saenz de Tejada I. Medical progress: impotence. *New Engl J Med* 1989;321:1648-1659.
23. Shabsigh R, Fishman IJ, Scott FB. Evaluation of erectile impotence. *Urology* 1988;32:2:83-90.
24. Mueller SC, Lue TF. Evaluation of vasculogenic impotence. *Urol Clin North Am* 1988;15:65-76.
25. Chiu RC, Lidstone D, Blundell PE. Predictive power of penile/brachial index in diagnosing male sexual impotence. *J Vasc Surg* 1986;4:251-6.
26. Wagner G, Uhrenholdt A. Blood flow by clearance in the human corpus cavernosum in the flaccid and erect states. In: Zorgniotti AW, Rossi G, eds. *Vasculogenic Impotence: Proceedings of the First International Conference on Corpus Cavernosum Revascularization*. Springfield, IL: Charles C Thomas, Publisher; 1980.
27. Forsberg L, Olsson AM, Neglen P. Erectile function before and after aorto-iliac reconstruction: a comparison between measurements of doppler acceleration ratio, blood pressure and angiography. *J Urol* 1982;127:379-82.
28. Velcek D, Sniderman KW, Vaughan ED, et al. Penile flow index utilizing a doppler pulse wave analysis to identify penile vascular insufficiency. *J Urol* 1980;123:669-672.
29. Bookstein JJ. Penile vascular catheterization in the diagnosis and treatment of impotence. *Cardiovasc Intervent Radiol* 1988;11(special issue):183-261.
30. Bookstein JJ, Valji K, Parsons L, Kessler W. Pharmacoarteriography in the evaluation of impotence. *J Urol* 1987;137:333-337.
31. Virag R, Frydman D, Legman M, et al. Intracavernous injection of papaverine as a diagnostic and therapeutic method in erectile failure Angiology. *J Vasc Dis* 1984;35:79-87.

32. Buvat J, Bervat-Hertaut M, Dehaene JL, et al. Is intravenous injection of papaverine a reliable screening test for vasculogenic impotence? *J Urol* 1986;135:476-78.

33. Robinson LQ, Woodcock JP, Stephenson TP. Duplex scanning in suspected vasculogenic impotence: a worthwhile exercise? *Br J Urol* 1989;63:4:432-436.

34. Lue TF, Hricak H, Marich KW, et al. Vasculogenic impotence evaluated by high-resolution ultrasonography and pulsed doppler spectrum analysis. *Radiology* 1985;155:3:777-781.

35. Desai KM, Gingell JC, Skidmore R, et al. Application of Computerized penile arterial waveform analysis in the diagnosis of arteriogenic impotence: an initial study in potent and impotent men. *Br J Urol* 1987;60:5:450-456.

36. Collins JP, Lewandowski BJ. Experience with intracorporeal injection of papaverine and duplex ultrasound scanning for assessment of arteriogenic impotence. *Br J Urol* 1987;59:1:84-88.

37. Krysiewicz S, Mellinger BC. The role of imaging in the diagnostic evaluation of impotence. *AJR* 1989;153:1133-1139.

38. Quam JP, King BF, James EM, et al. Duplex and color Doppler sonographic evaluation of vasculogenic impotence. *AJR* 1989;153:1141-1147.

39. Benson CB, Vickers MA. Sexual impotence caused by vascular disease: diagnosis with duplex sonography. *AJR* 1989;153:1149-1153.

40. Schwartz AN, Wang KY, Mack LA, et al. Evaluation of normal erectile function with color flow Doppler sonography. *AJR* 1989;153:1155-1160.

41. Paushter DM. Role of duplex sonography in the evaluation of sexual impotence. *AJR* 1989;153:1161-1163.

42. Lue TF, Hricak H, Marich KW, et al. Evaluation of arteriogenic impotence with intracorporeal injection of papaverine and the duplex ultrasound scanner. *Semin Urol* 1985;3:1:43-48.

43. Gall H, Barhren W, Scherb W, et al. Diagnostic accuracy of Doppler ultrasound technique of the penile arteries in correlation to selective arteriography. *Cardiovasc Intervent Radiol* 1988;11:4:225-231.

44. Bookstein JJ. Penile angiography: the last angiographic frontier. *AJR* 1988;150:47-54.

45. Lue TF, Hricak H, Schmidt RA, et al. Functional evaluation of penile veins by cavernosography in papaverine induced erection. *J Urol* 1986;135:479-482.

46. Lewis RW. This month in investigative urology: Venous impotence. *J Urol* 1988;140:1560.

47. Bookstein JJ. Cavernosal veno-occlusive insufficiency in male impotence: evaluation of degree and location. *Radiology* 1987;164:175-178.

48. Malhotra CM, Balko A, Wincze JP, et al. Cavernosography in conjunction with artificial erection for evaluation of venous leakage in impotent men. *Radiology* 1986;161:799-802.

49. Lewis RW. Venous surgery for impotence. *Urol Clin North Am* 1988;15:115-121.5

50. Rajfer J, Canan V, Dorey FJ, et al. Correlation between penile angiography and duplex scanning of cavernous arteries in impotent men. *J Urol* 1990;143:1128-1130.

51. Montague D. *Noninvasive Vascular Evaluation in Disorders of Male Sexual Function.* Chicago: Year Book Medical Publishers Inc; 1988.

52. Vickers M, Benson C, Richie J. High-resolution ultrasonography and pulsed wave Doppler for detection of corporovenous incompetence in erectile dysfunction. *J Urol* 1990;143:1125-1127.

53. Datta NS. Corpus cavernosography in conditions other than Peyronie's disease. *J Urol* 1977;118:588-590.

54. Gray R, Keresteci A, St Louis E, et al. Investigation of impotence by internal pudendal angiography: experience with 73 cases. *Radiology* 1982;144:773-780.

55. Lakin M, Montague D, Medendorp S, et al. Intracavernous injection therapy: analysis of results and complications. *J Urol* 1990;143:1138-1141.

56. Virag R, Frydman D, Legman M, et al. Intracavernous injection of papaverine as a diagnostic and therapeutic method in erectile failure. *Angiology* 1984;35:79.

57. Goldstein I, Siroky M, Nath R, et al. Vasculogenic impotence: role of the pelvic steal test. *J Urol* 1982;128:300.

58. Fournier G, Juenemann K, Lue T, et al. Mechanisms of venous occlusion during canine penile erection: an anatomic demonstration. *J Urol* 1987;137:163.

59. Mellinger BC, Vaughan ED Jr, Thompson SL, et al. Correlation between intracavernous papaverine injection and Doppler analysis in impotent men. *Urology* 1987;416-419.

60. Virag R, Bouilly P, Frydman D. Is impotence an arterial disorder? A study of arterial risk factors in 440 impotent men. *Lancet* 1985;1:181-184.

61. Abelson D. Diagnostic value of the penile pulse and blood pressure: a Doppler study of impotence in diabetics. *J Urol* 1975;113:636-639.

62. Nessi R, de Flaviis L, Bellizoni G, et al. Digital angiography of erectile failure. *Br J Urol* 1987;59:584-589.

63. Ginestie JF, Romieu A. *Radiologic exploration of impotence.* Boston: Nijhoff; 1978.

64. Puyau FA, Lewis FW. Corpus cavernosography: pressure, flow and radiography. *Invest Radiol* 1983;18:517-522.

65. Delcour C, Wespes E, Vandenbosch G, et al. Impotence: evaluation with cavernosography. *Radiology* 1986;161:803-806.

66. Maatman TJ, Montague DK, Martin LM. Cost-effective evaluation of impotence. *Urology* 1986;27:132-135.

67. Hattery RR, King BF, Lewis RW, et al. Vasculogenic impotence: duplex and color Doppler. *Radiol Clin North Am* 1991; May.

68. Hattery RR, King BF Jr, James EM, et al. Tenth meeting and postgraduate course of the Society of Uroradiology. Vasculogenic impotence: duplex and color Doppler imaging. *AJR* 1991;156:189-195.

69. Quam JP, King BF, James EM, et al. Duplex and color Doppler ultrasound evaluation of vasculogenic impotence (scientific exhibit). *Radiol Soc North Am,* 1989.

70. King BF Jr, Hattery RR, James EM, Lewis RW. Duplex sonography in the evaluation of impotence: current techniques. *Semin Intervent Radiol* 1990;7(3-4):215-221.

71. King BF Jr. Color Doppler flow imaging evaluation of the deep dorsal penile vein in vascular impotence. *Radiol Soc North Am* 1989: p. 371. Abstract—scientific program.

72. Tanaka T. Papaverine hydrochloride in peripheral blood and the degree of penile erection. *J Urol* 1900;143:1135-1137.

73. Burkhalter J, Morano J. Partial priapism. the role of computed tomography in its diagnosis. *Radiology* 1985;156:159.

74. Abozeid M, Juenemann K, Luo J, et al. Chronic papaverine treatment: the effect of repeated injections on the simian erectile response and penile tissue. *J Urol* 1987;138:1263.

75. Summers J. Pyogenic granuloma: an unusual complication of papaverine injection therapy for impotence. *J Urol* 1990;143:1227-1228.

76. Virag R. About pharmacologically induced prolonged erection. *Lancet* 1985;1:519. Letter to the editor.

77. Hu K, Burks C, Christy W. Fibrosis of the tunica albuginea: complication of long term intracavernous pharmacological self injection. *J Urol* 1987;138:404.

78. Kiely E, Williams G, Goldie L. Assessment of the immediate and long-term effects of pharmacologically induced penile erections in the treatment of psychogenic and organic impotence. *Br J Urol* 1987;59:164.

Peyronie's disease

79. Balconi G, Angeli E, Nessi R, et al. Ultrasonographic evaluation of Peyronie's disease. *Urol Radiol* 1988;10:85-88.
80. Metz P, Ebbehoj J, Uhrenholdt A, et al. Peyronie's disease and erectile failure. *J Urol* 1983;30:1103-1104.
81. Altraffer LF, Jordan JH. Sonographic demonstration of Peyronie's plaques. *Urology* 1981;17:292-295.
82. Fleischer AC, Rhamy RK. Sonographic evaluation of Peyronie's disease. *Urology* 1981;17:290-291.
83. Gelbard M, Sarti D, Kanfman J. Ultrasound imaging of Peyronie's plaques. *J Urol* 1981;125:44-45.
84. Merkle W. Cause of deviation of the erectile penis after urethral manipulations (Kelami syndrome): demonstration of ultrasound findings and case reports. *Urol Int* 1990;45:183-185.
85. Rifkin M. Urethra and penis. In: *Diagnostic Imaging of the Lower Genitourinary Tract*. New York: Raven Press; 1985.
86. Vermooten V. Metaplasia in the penis: the presence of bone, bone marrow and cartilage in the glans. *New Engl J Med* 1933;209:368-369.
87. Frank R, Gerard P, Wise G. Human penile ossification: a case report and review of the literature. *Urol Radiol* 1989;11:179-181.

Penile urethra

88. Benson CB. Sonography of the male urethra. Current status of prostate and lower urinary tract imaging course. AIUM Annual Meeting, March 3-4, 1990, New Orleans.
89. McAninch JW, Laing FC, Jeffrey RB. Sonourethrography in the evaluation of urethral strictures: a preliminary report. *J Urol* 1988;139:294-297.

90. Gluck CD, Bundy AL, Fine C, et al. Sonographic urethrogram: a comparison to roentgenographic techniques in 22 patients. *J Urol* 1988;140:1404-1408.
91. Kauzlaric D, Barmeir E, Peyer P, et al. Sonographic appearances of urethral diverticulum in the male. *J Ultrasound Med* 1988;7:107-109.
92. Merkle W, Wagner W. Sonography of the distal male urethra—a new diagnostic procedure for urethral stricture: results of a retrospective study. *J Urol* 1988;140:1409-1411.

Penile carcinoma

93. Sufrin G, Huben R. Benign and malignant lesions of the penis. In: Gillenwater J, Grayhack J, Howards S, et al, eds. *Adult and Pediatric Urology*. Chicago: Year Book Medical Publishers Inc; 1987.
94. Scappini P, Piscioli F, Pusiol T, Hofstetter A, et al. Penile cancer: aspiration biopsy cytology for staging. *Cancer* 1986;58:1526-1533.

Penile trauma

95. Smith D. *General Urology: Injuries to the Genitourinary Tract*. Los Altos, Calif: Lange Medical Books; 1978:233-252.
96. Grosman H, Gray R, St Louis E, et al. The role of corpus cavernosography in acute "fracture" of the penis. *Radiology* 1982;144:787-788.
97. Ames ES, Newhouse JH, Cronan JJ. Radiology of male periurethral structures. *AJR* 1988;151:321-324.
98. Dierks PR, Hawkins H. Sonography and penile trauma. *J Ultrasound Med* 1983;2:417-419.

CHAPTER 28

The Rotator Cuff

- Laurence A. Mack, M.D.
- Frederick A. Matsen III, M.D.
- Keith Y. Wang, M.D.

Shoulder pain may have a wide variety of etiologies that produce similar symptoms. Tendonitis, cuff strain, and partial-thickness or full-thickness tear may cause pain and weakness on elevation of the arm.[1] Underlying these symptoms in many patients over 40 years of age is rotator cuff fiber failure.[2] Calcific tendinitis, cervical radiculopathy, and acromioclavicular arthritis may also mimic rotator cuff pathology. Contrast arthrography has heretofore been the primary radiologic examination used to distinguish among these various conditions.[3] More recently, high-resolution real-time ultrasound has been shown to be an alternative means of examining the rotator cuff.[4-7]

CLINICAL CONSIDERATIONS

Rotator cuff fiber failure is one of the most common causes of shoulder pain and dysfunction in the patient over 40. Epidemiologic studies by Codman, DePalma, and others have clearly demonstrated that the frequency of rotator cuff fiber failure increases with age.[8-10] Fiber failure demonstrates a sequential progression from partial-thickness tears almost always starting in the supraspinatus, to massive tears involving multiple cuff tendons.

Rotator cuff tearing may occur insidiously and, in fact, unnoticed by the patient, a process termed by some as "creeping tendon ruptures."[11] When a larger group of fibers fails at one time the shoulder demonstrates pain at rest and accentuation of pain on use of the rotator cuff, for example, extension, abduction, or external rotation. When even greater numbers of fibers fail at one time, a process known as "acute extension" of the shoulder may demonstrate sudden onset of substantial weakness in flexion, abduction, and external rotation.

As we age, our rotator cuff becomes increasingly susceptible to tearing with less severe amounts of applied force. Thus, although a major force is required to tear the usual rotator cuff of a 40-year-old, a relatively trivial amount of force may result in tear of the rotator cuff of the average 60-year-old. This is analogous to the predisposition of older patients to femoral neck fractures. Although differences of the acromial shape, abnormalities of the acromial clavicular joint, and other factors may also affect the susceptibility of the rotator cuff to fiber failure, age-related deterioration and loading of the rotator cuff seem to be the dominant factors in determining the failure patterns of the cuff tendons.

Symptoms of rotator cuff fiber failure in the acute phase usually include pain at rest and on motion. Later, subacromial crepitance occurs when the arm is rotated in the partially flexed position, and, finally, arm weakness occurs. When the rotator cuff fails, the humeral head may no longer be stabilized in its normal position with respect to the glenoid. If the humeral head rides superiorly the residual cuff is sandwiched between the head of the humerus and the undersurface of the acromion, giving rise to impingement. As Neer pointed out in 1972 this gives rise to a characteristic traction spur in the coracoacromial ligament and to spurring and sclerosis of the undersurface of the acromion.[12]

TECHNICAL CONSIDERATIONS

Initial reports of rotator cuff sonography employed mechanical sector scanners with frequencies of 5 to 10 MHz. Although these transducers produce high-quality images, their utility is limited by suboptimal superficial resolution secondary to near-field artifact and a narrow superficial image field. In addition, the specular reflection condition can only be met by a small portion of the parallel tendon fibers in the center of the image, which may create an artifactual heterogenous appearance of tendons.

The introduction of high-resolution linear-array transducers has greatly expanded our diagnostic capabilities in the examination of the shoulder as well as other musculoskeletal areas. Clinical experience has demonstrated that 7 MHz transducers are preferable to those of lower frequency. These transducers demonstrate marked improvement in near resolution when compared with other devices. In addition, the broad superficial field of view is helpful in evaluating superficial abnormalities. The specular reflection condition can be met with a greater portion of the parallel tendon fibers. When lower frequency transducers (5 MHz) must be used, an acoustic standoff pad may be helpful to improve the near-field image.

TECHNIQUE

Understanding the complex three-dimensional anatomy of the rotator cuff is crucial to successful rotator cuff sonography. The limits on the acoustic window caused by adjacent bony structures are an additional factor making sonographic evaluation technically difficult (Fig. 28-1). For this reason, comprehensive understanding of normal anatomy gained in the anatomy laboratory or operating room is essential in mastering this technique and accelerating the learning curve.

The patient is scanned while seated on a revolving stool that permits easy positioning during the scanning of both shoulders. The examiner is also seated on a stool, preferably with wheels to enhance mobility. Both shoulders are examined, starting with the less symptomatic side. The following technique for the evaluation of the rotator cuff is used at the University of Washington.[13]

The examination begins with a transverse image of the bicipital groove, which serves as an anatomic landmark to differentiate the subscapularis from the supraspinatus (Fig. 28-2). The groove appears as a concavity in the bright echoes originating from the bony surface of the humerus. The tendon of the long head of the biceps is visualized as a hyperechoic oval structure within the bicipital groove. This view is important in detecting intraarticular fluid, which, even when present in small amounts, may be seen surrounding the biceps tendon (Fig. 28-2).

The transducer is then moved proximally along the

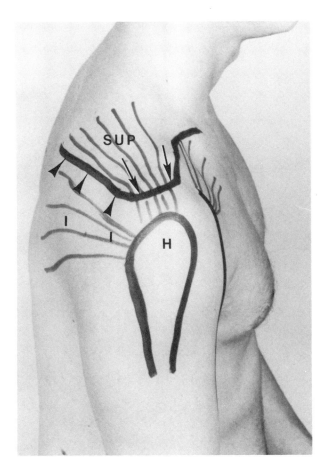

FIG 28-1. General anatomic landmarks. Lateral photograph shows the bony structure, which limits the acoustic window for the examination of the cuff. *Sup,* Supraspinatus muscle and tendon; *I,* infraspinatus muscle and tendon; *arrowheads,* scapular spine; *arrows,* acromion; *H,* humerus.

humerus to visualize the subscapularis tendon, which appears as a band of medium-level echoes deep to the subdeltoid bursa (Fig. 28-3). The subdeltoid bursa is seen as a thin convex echogenic line. When the subscapularis is viewed parallel to its axis, scanning during passive internal and external rotation may be helpful in assessing the integrity of the subscapularis. Turning the transducer 90 degrees will allow scanning perpendicular to the axis of the subscapularis tendon. This view may be helpful in patients with chronic anterior dislocation.

The supraspinatus tendon is scanned perpendicular to its axis (transversely) by moving the transducer laterally and posteriorly. The sonographic window is very narrow, and careful transducer positioning is essential (Fig. 28-4). The supraspinatus tendon is visualized as a band of medium-level echoes deep to the subdeltoid bursa and superficial to the bright echoes originating from the bony surface of the greater tuberosity. It is essential to obtain images that demonstrate the critical

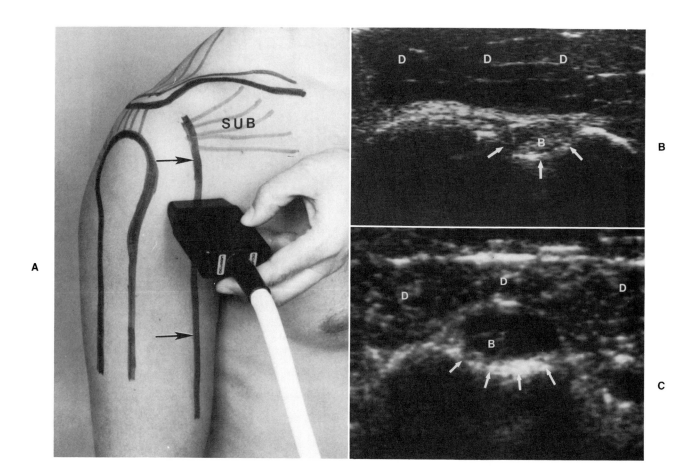

FIG 28-2. Biceps tendon (transverse). **A,** Clinical photograph. **B,** Sonogram shows the biceps tendon *(B)* as a hyperechoic oval structure within the bicipital groove *(arrows)*. **C,** Scan in the same location demonstrates a hypoechoic biceps tendon *(B)* surrounded anteriorly by fluid in a different patient with joint effusion and rotator cuff tear. *D,* Deltoid muscle; *SUB,* subscapularis tendon; *arrows,* bicipital groove.

(From Mack LA et al, with permission.)

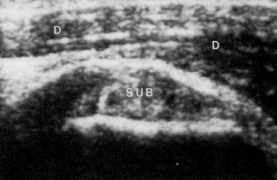

FIG 28-3. Subscapularis tendon. **A,** Clinical photograph and **B,** dual image show the subscapularis tendon *(SUB)* parallel to its axis (longitudinal) in internal and external rotation viewed as a band of medium-level echoes deep to the subdeltoid bursa *(arrowheads). D,* Deltoid muscle; *B,* biceps tendon; *arrows,* humeral surface. **C,** and **D,** Clinical photograph and scan perpendicular to the axis of the subscapularis tendon. *Arrows,* Biceps tendon; *SUB,* subscapularis tendon; *D,* deltoid muscle.

(**A** and **B** from Mack LA et al, with permission.)

zone, which is most susceptible to injury. The critical zone is that portion of the tendon that begins approximately one centimeter posterolateral to the biceps tendon. Failure to adequately visualize this area may cause a false-negative result.

By moving the transducer posteriorly and in the plane parallel to the scapular spine, one may visualize the infraspinatus tendon. It appears as a beak-shaped soft tissue structure as it attaches to the posterior aspect of the greater tuberosity (Fig. 28-5). Passive internal and external rotation may be helpful in examination of the infraspinatus. At this level, a portion of the posterior glenoid labrum is seen as a hyperechoic, triangular structure. The articular cartilage of the humeral head is imaged as a thin, hypoechoic layer superficial to the high-level echoes originating from the bony surface.

By moving the transducer distally on the humerus, the terres minor is visualized as a trapezoidal structure (Fig. 28-6). It is differentiated from the infraspinatus by its oblique internal echoes. Although the terres minor tendon is rarely torn, recent reports have demonstrated that very small intraarticular effusions may be best visualized at this level.[14] Its visualization also ensures that the entire infraspinatus has been scanned.

The transducer is then moved anteriorly and turned 90 degrees so that the biceps tendon is viewed parallel to its axis (Fig. 28-7). Care should be taken to have the transducer parallel to the tendon, or portions of this structure will appear artifactually hypoechoic. Small effusions may be seen as fluid surrounding the hyperechoic biceps tendon, just as they appear on the transverse view.

The transducer is then moved posteriorly so that the supraspinatus tendon is viewed parallel (longitudinal) to its axis (Fig. 28-8, *A* and *B*) The tendon appears as a beak-shaped structure of medium-level echoes extending from under the acromion, which casts an acoustic shadow, to its attachment along the greater tuberosity. The bright linear echoes from the subdeltoid bursa identify the superficial margin of the supraspinatus tendon. Passive abduction-adduction is often very helpful in assessing the integrity of the supraspinatus tendon. Scanning laterally in the same plane may be helpful in visualizing small bursal effusions. As stressed by Crass et al, scanning the supraspinatus tendon with the arm in extension and internal rotation is an important and integral portion of every rotator cuff evaluation (Fig. 28-8, *C* and *D*).[15] This is best achieved by placing the patient's arm behind his back. The supraspinatus may then be scanned perpendicular and parallel to its fibers. In this position, tendons that were obscured by the lat-

Text continued on p. 617.

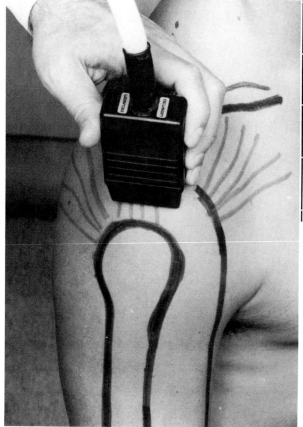

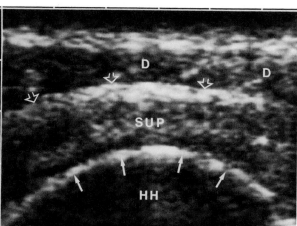

FIG 28-4. Supraspinatus tendon (transverse). **A** and **B,** Clinical photograph and scan show the supraspinatus tendon *(SUP)* as a band of medium-level echoes deep to the subdeltoid bursa *(open arrows). Arrows,* Humeral surface; *D,* deltoid muscle, *HH,* humeral head.
(**B** from Mack LA et al, with permission.)

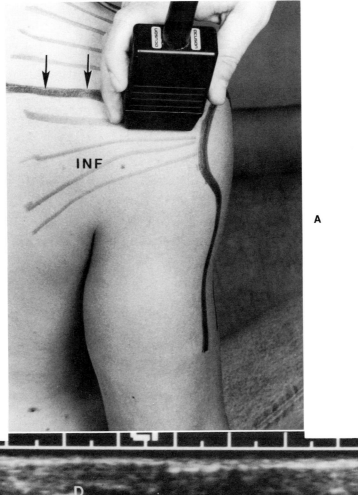

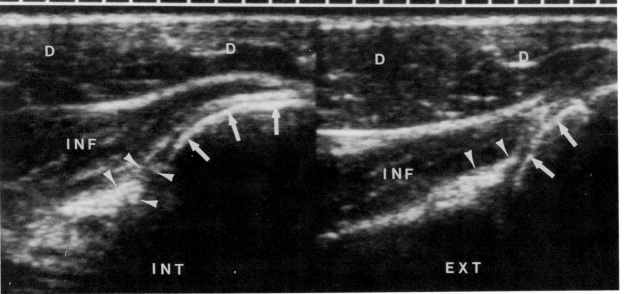

FIG 28-5. Infraspinatus tendon. **A,** Clinical photograph. **B,** Dual image of the infraspinatus tendon *(INF)* in internal *(INT)* and external *(EXT)* rotation. *Black arrows,* Scapular spine; *white arrows,* humeral surface; *D,* deltoid muscle; *arrowheads,* posterior glenoid labrum. (**B** from Mack LA et al, with permission.)

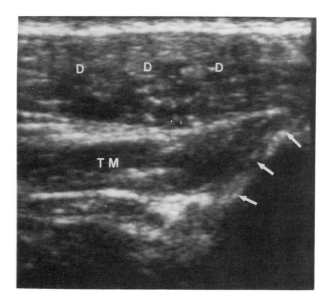

FIG 28-6. Terres minor. The terres minor *(TM)* is visualized as a trapezoidal structure. *Arrows,* Humerus; *D,* deltoid muscle.

(From Mack LA et al, with permission.)

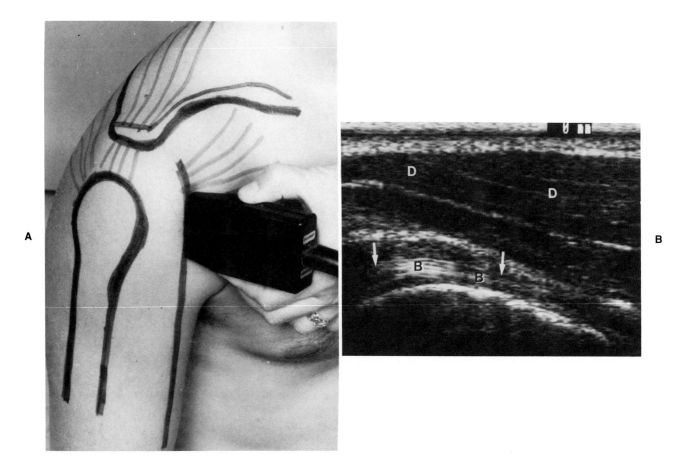

FIG 28-7. Biceps tendon (longitudinal). **A,** Clinical photograph. **B,** Scan shows the biceps tendon *(B)*. Note that the tendon *(arrows)* becomes artifactually hypoechoic as the angle it makes with the transducer diverges from 180 degrees. *D,* Deltoid tendon.

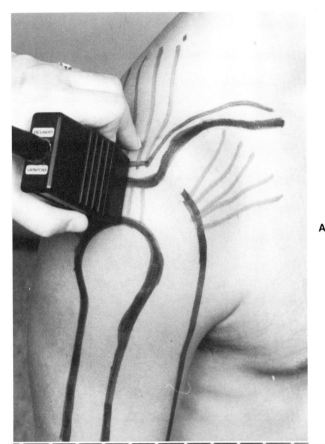

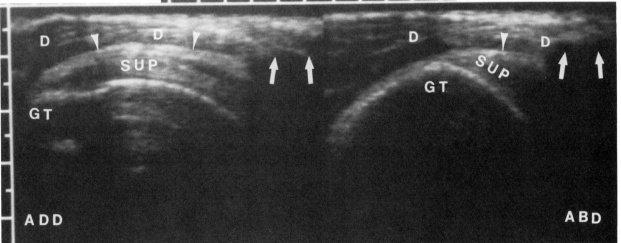

FIG 28-8. Supraspinatus tendon (longitudinal). **A,** Clinical photograph. **B,** Dual image of the supraspinatus tendon *(SUP)* parallel (longitudinal) to its axis in passive abduction *(ABD)* and adduction *(ADD)*. *GT*, Greater tuberosity; *D*, deltoid muscle; *arrowhead*, subdeltoid bursa; *arrows*, acoustic shadow from acromion.
(**B** from Mack LA et al, with permission.)

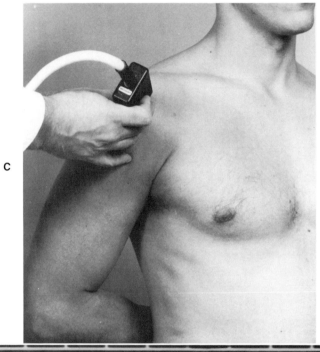

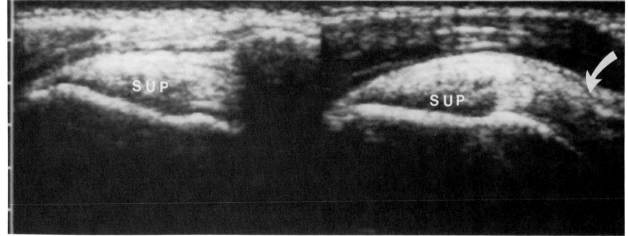

FIG. 28-8, cont'd. C, Transducer position with arm in extension and internal rotation. **D,** Paired longitudinal supraspinatus view in neutral and extension with external rotation demonstrate improved visualization of the supraspinatus tendon *(arrow).*

erally placed acromion may be visualized. Small tears and effusions may also be accentuated with this maneuver.

PREOPERATIVE APPEARANCES
Major Criteria for Tear

Middleton suggested that previously published sonographic criteria for rotator cuff pathology could be categorized into four groups[16]:

- Nonvisualization of the cuff
- Localized absence or focal nonvisualization
- Discontinuity
- Focal abnormal echogenicity.

Nonvisualization of the Cuff. In large rotator cuff tears, no cuff tendon will be visualized and the subdeltoid bursa will directly approximate the surface of the humeral head (Fig. 28-9). In addition, the contour of the bursa will be concave downward rather than convex upward. The bursa may be quite thickened in such patients, often measuring up to 5 millimeters in width. Passive humeral movement is often helpful in such patients to confirm the absence of cuff tendon. Joint and bursal effusion is a common accompaniment to such large tears. The extent of large tears should be reported, as multiple tendons are often involved.

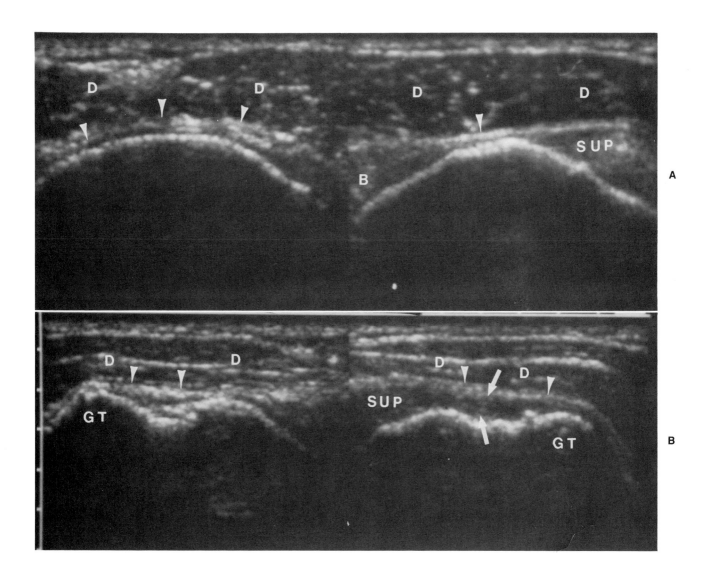

FIG 28-9. Absence of the rotator cuff. **A,** Paired transverse images of the supraspinatus tendon show complete absence of the right supraspinatus and focal absence of the left supraspinatus. Note the apposition of subdeltoid bursa *(arrowheads)* to humeral surface. **B,** Paired longitudinal images of the supraspinatus reveal total absence of the right supraspinatus and partial absence of the left supraspinatus *(arrow)*. *GT,* Greater tuberosity; *D,* deltoid muscle; *Arrowheads,* subdeltoid bursa; *B,* biceps tendon.

Focal Nonvisualization of the Cuff. Smaller tears will appear as localized absence in the cuff. As in very large tears, the subdeltoid bursa will touch the humeral surface (Fig. 28-10). The vast majority of such tears will occur anteriorly in the supraspinatus tendon in the critical zone. Characteristically, a small amount of cuff is preserved surrounding the biceps tendon. Such tears must be confirmed by visualization in two perpendicular scan planes. Tears will be sharply demarcated with abrupt transition from normal to abnormal cuff, in contrast to more diffuse cuff thinning, which is often seen in advanced fiber failure.

Discontinuity. Discontinuity of the cuff is observed sonographically when smaller cuff defects fill with joint fluid or hyperechoic reactive tissue (Fig. 28-11). Such defects may be accentuated by placement of the arm in extension and internal rotation. Often, a small amount of bursal fluid is also present and may be the only sonographic finding with the arm in neutral position.

Abnormal Echogenicity. Cuff echogenicity may be diffusely or focally abnormal. Diffuse abnormalities of cuff echogenicity have proven to be an unreliable sonographic sign for cuff tear (Fig. 28-12). Such findings may be associated with diffuse cuff inflammation or fibrosis, but this finding is only helpful when a clear disparity exists with the contralateral, asymptomatic side.

Focal abnormal echogenicity has been associated with small full-thickness and partial-thickness tears (Fig. 28-13). The area of increased echogenicity is thought to result from granulation tissue, hypertrophied synovium,

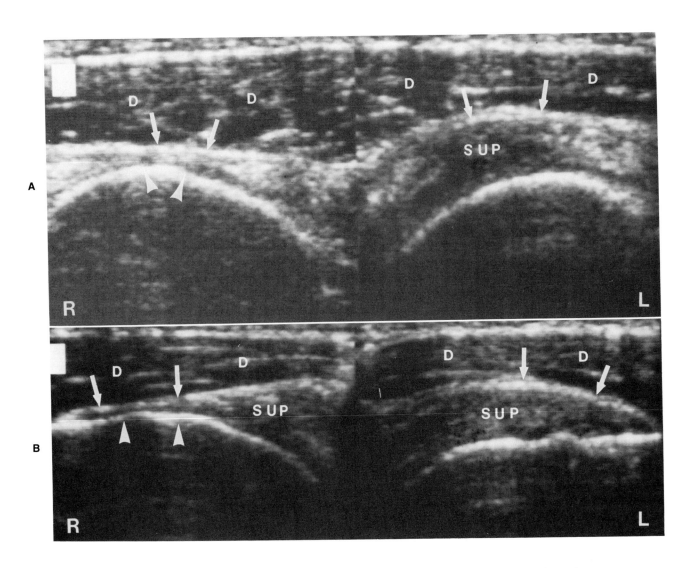

FIG 28-10. Focal nonvisualization of the cuff. **A,** Transverse. **B,** Longitudinal comparison views of the abnormal right and normal left supraspinatus tendons *(SUP)* show focal nonvisualization of the right cuff with approximation of subdeltoid bursa *(arrows)* to the humerus *(arrowheads).* D, Deltoid muscle.

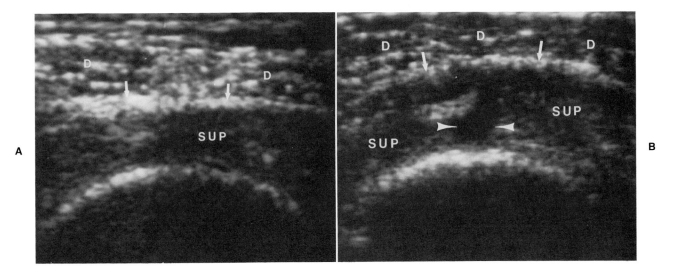

FIG 28-11. Discontinuity of the cuff. Transverse scans of the supraspinatus *(SUP)* in **A,** neutral position and **B,** with the arm in extension and internal rotation show a small tear filled with fluid *(arrowheads)*. Note the tear is only seen with the arm in extension. *D,* Deltoid muscle; *arrows,* subdeltoid bursa.

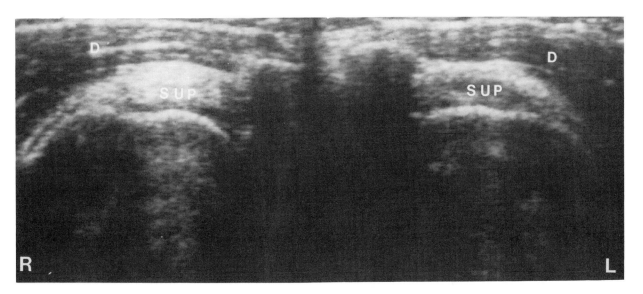

FIG 28-12. Diffusely abnormal echogenicity. Paired longitudinal scans of the supraspinatus *(SUP)* in a patient with acute right-sided tendinitis demonstrate diffusely increased echogenicity. *D,* Deltoid muscle.

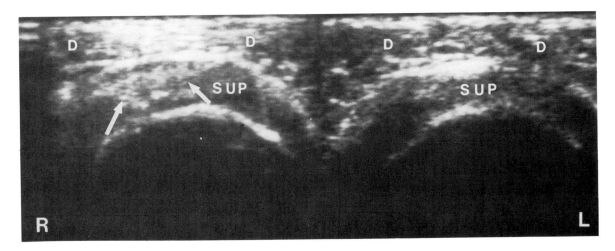

FIG 28-13. Focal increased echogenicity. Paired transverse scans of the supraspinatus tendon *(SUP)* show a focal area of increased echogenicity *(arrows)* on the right side from a partial-thickness tear. *D,* Deltoid muscle.

and hemorrhage. Care must be taken to assure that this finding is real and not secondary to technical artifact.

Minor Criteria for Tear

Subdeltoid Bursal Effusion. Visualization of subdeltoid bursal effusion is the most reliable secondary finding (Fig. 28-14). This may be the only abnormal sonographic finding in patients with small tears. In the presence of an otherwise normal sonogram and appropriate clinical symptoms, visualization of an effusion should

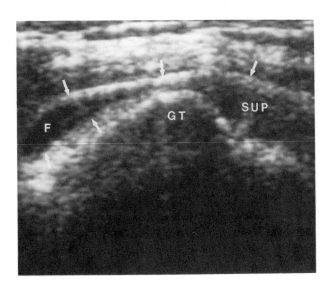

FIG 28-14. Subdeltoid bursal effusion. Longitudinal scan of the supraspinatus *(SUP)* with the transducer placed laterally demonstrates a small subdeltoid bursal effusion *(F)*. *Arrows,* Subdeltoid bursa; *GT,* greater tuberosity.

always be followed by additional evaluation by arthrography or magnetic resonance imaging (MRI).

Concave Subdeltoid Bursal Contour. In the normal patient, the bright linear echoes from the subdeltoid bursa are convex upwards. Concavity of the subdeltoid contour may be noted in medium and large tears, reflecting the absence of cuff tendon.

Humeral Head Elevation. The humeral head may be elevated relative to the acromion when compared with the normal side corresponding to similar plain film findings.

Joint Effusion. Intraarticular effusion has been strongly correlated with cuff pathology.[6] The presence of such fluid should strongly increase the sonographer's suspicion of a full-thickness tear (Fig. 28-2).

POSTOPERATIVE APPEARANCES

Symptomatic patients who are postoperative from acromioplasty or acromioplasty in combination with rotator cuff repair present a difficult diagnostic dilemma. Such symptoms may be caused by tendinitis, impingement, or recurrent rotator cuff tear. Differentiation among these diseases is important in instituting the proper therapy. Arthrography, especially after rotator cuff repair, has been reported to be less reliable than in the preoperative patient, and such studies may be falsely negative or falsely positive.[17] Recent reports in the literature suggest that sonography plays an important role in this group of patients.[18,19] Because surgery may distort sonographic landmarks, sonography in the postoperative patient is rendered more difficult than in the preoperative patient. It is important therefore to understand the surgical procedures used in acromioplasty and cuff repair.

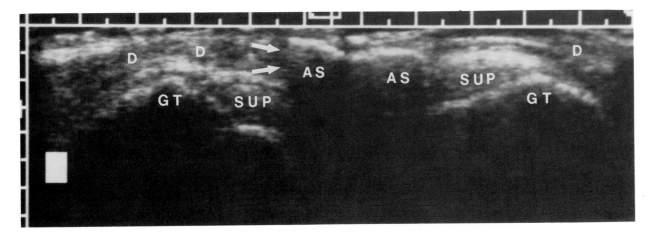

FIG 28-15. Acromioplasty—sonographic appearances. Paired longitudinal supraspinatus *(SUP)* images show the characteristically pointed acromial appearance after acromioplasty *(arrows)*. *D,* Deltoid muscle; *GT,* greater tuberosity; *AS,* acromial shadow.
(From Mack LA et al, with permission.)

In acromioplasty, the anterior, inferior aspect of the acromion is surgically removed. Sonographically, this appears as disruption of the normal, rounded, smooth acromial contour (Fig. 28-15). After surgery, the acromion appears pointed. Because the inferior aspect of the acromion is removed, a greater extent of the supraspinatus may be visualized.

Repair of a cuff tear creates unique sonographic landmarks. The cuff tendons are reimplanted into a trough made perpendicular to the axis of the supraspinatus. The reimplantation trough is placed in the humeral head at a site that provides optimal tendon tension. It therefore may be medial to a variable degree, reflecting the amount of cuff tendon that is preserved. The trough appears sonographically as a rounded defect in the humeral contour best viewed with the transducer longitudinal to the supraspinatus (Fig. 28-16). Suture material may be seen deep in the trough as specular echoes. Scanning the arm in extension and internal rotation may be necessary to visualize this site of tendon reimplantation, especially when it is medially placed (Fig. 28-17). Failure to scan in this position may lead to false-positive diagnosis. Such a maneuver, however, should be used with care, especially in the immediate postoperative period, to avoid reinjury to the friable newly reimplanted tendons.

Sonographic appearances of the cuff tendons never return to normal in the postoperative patient (Fig. 28-18).[18,19] Tendons, especially the supraspinatus, are often echogenic and thinned when compared with the contralateral shoulder. Joint effusions are common and best visualized along the biceps tendon. Because resection of the subdeltoid bursa removes an important landmark, dynamic scanning is especially important in dis-

tinguishing a thin, hyperechoic cuff from adjacent deltoid muscle.

Recurrent Tear

Recurrent cuff tear is common, occurring in up to 40% of patients in whom a small defect was repaired and in 80% of those patients who preoperatively had large tears.[20] Sonographically, recurrent tears most often appear as absence of the cuff. Unless baseline scans are available in the postoperative period, it may be difficult to differentiate small recurrent tears from the appearances created when only a small amount of cuff tendon remains to be reattached. Multiple tendons may be disrupted.

Cuff arthropathy is also commonly seen in this group of patients. Degeneration of humeral cartilage is caused by repetitive, minor trauma and disruption of normal nutrient pathways.[21] Cuff arthropathy appears sonographically as irregularity of the bony surface of the humerus and loss of normal hypoechoic cartilage (Fig. 28-19).

TRAUMA

An emerging application of sonography is the evaluation of subtle greater tuberosity fractures. The clinical examination in acutely injured patients with profound weakness of abduction may be indistinguishable from acute cuff tear. Recent reports suggest that early repair may result in better postoperative results, making this differentiation especially important.[22] For this reason, such patients are often scanned soon after injury.

Greater tuberosity fracture appears as discontinuity in the normally smooth bony surface (Fig. 28-20). Such discontinuities may be subtle and not well visualized on

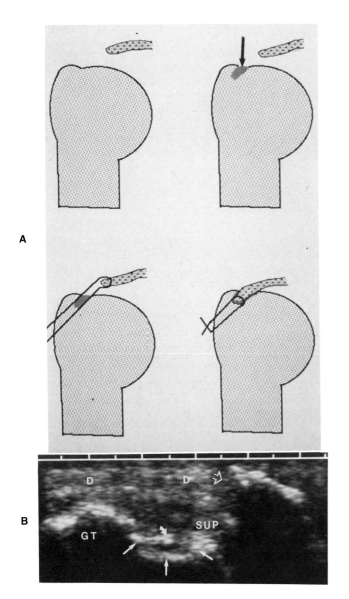

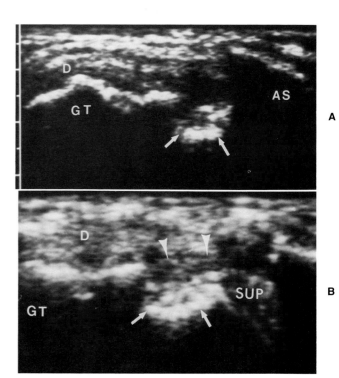

FIG 28-16. Rotator cuff repair—sonographic appearances. **A,** Drawing demonstrating the surgical technique for cuff reimplantation with creation of trough *(arrow)* in the humeral head, reimplantation of the residual tendon within that trough, and characteristic method of suture placement. **B,** Longitudinal supraspinatus *(SUP)* image shows characteristic appearances of reimplantation trough *(arrows)*. Acromioplasty defect *(open arrows)* is also visualized. *GT,* Greater tuberosity; *curved arrow,* reimplantation suture; *D,* deltoid muscle.
(From Mack LA et al, with permission.)

FIG 28-17. Postoperative rotator cuff—importance of examination during extension. **A,** Longitudinal supraspinatus view in standard position of a patient postoperative for repair of full-thickness rotator cuff tear demonstrates the reimplantation trough, but fails to reveal evidence of the supraspinatus tendon, thus suggesting recurrent injury. **B,** Scan with the arm in extension and internal rotation demonstrates that the repair is intact. The residual supraspinatus *(SUP)* is thinned. Note absence of characteristic bright echoes of the subdeltoid bursal *(arrowheads)*. *Arrows,* Reimplantation trough; *GT,* greater tuberosity; *AS,* acromial shadow; *D,* deltoid muscle.
(From Mack LA et al, with permission.)

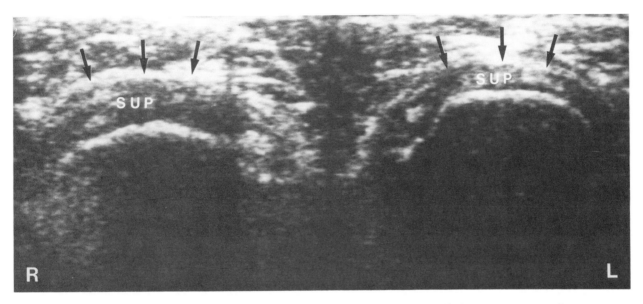

FIG 28-18. Postoperative rotator cuff—abnormal cuff echogenicity. Paired transverse scans of the supraspinatus tendon *(SUP)* after left acromioplasty demonstrate residual thinning and increased echogenicity. *Arrows,* Subdeltoid bursa.
(From Mack LA et al, with permission.)

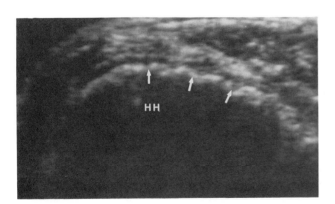

FIG 28-19. Cuff arthropathy. Transverse supraspinatus view in a patient with recurrent cuff tear demonstrates the roughened humeral surface *(arrows)* of cuff arthropathy. *HH,* Humeral head.
(From Mack LA et al, with permission.)

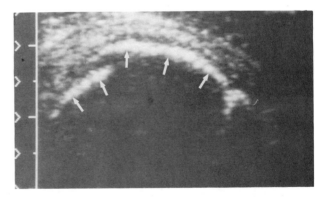

FIG 28-20. Greater tuberosity fracture. Transverse supraspinatus view in patient with a history of trauma and weakness on abduction demonstrates discontinuity of normally smooth humeral surface *(arrows).*

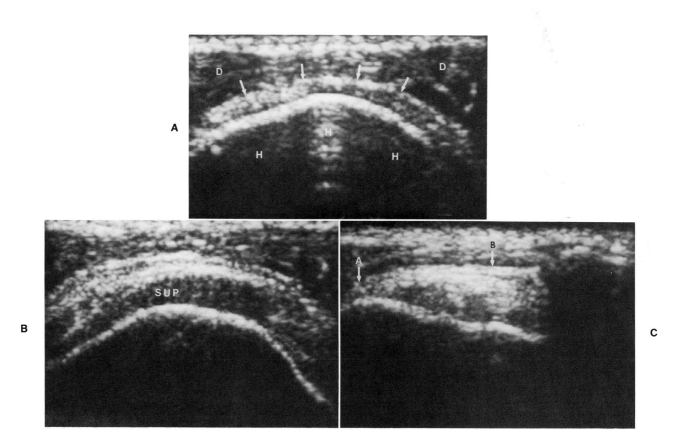

FIG 28-21. False-positive scan—importance of proper transducer position. **A,** Transverse supraspinatus scan suggests rotator cuff tear with apposition of subdeltoid bursa *(arrows)* and humerus *(H)*. **B,** Scan in same patient with transducer placed more medially shows normal supraspinatus *(SUP)* appearances. **C,** Longitudinal scan indicating transducer positions for image **A** and **B.** *D,* Deltoid muscle.

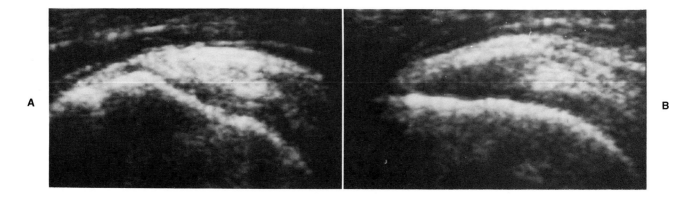

FIG 28-22. Artifactual changes in tendon echogenicity. **A** and **B,** Two views of same supraspinatus tendon demonstrate the considerable changes in echogenicity that may be artifactually created by transducer position and orientation.

initial plain films. Fluoroscopy and computed tomography may be necessary to confirm such lesions. The overlying supraspinatus may be thickened secondary to edema or hemorrhage. Fat may be seen within the joint as a highly echogenic joint effusion that exhibits a characteristic swirling appearance on joint motion. Such findings correspond to a "fat-fluid" level that may be seen on other imaging techniques.

PITFALLS

Inadequate transducer positioning is the most common error in scanning the rotator cuff. False-positive and false-negative results may be produced in this manner. For example, scanning the supraspinatus transversely with the transducer placed laterally may artifactually mimic a rotator cuff tear (Fig. 28-21). More medial placement will demonstrate an intact supraspinatus. For this reason, cuff tears, especially of the supraspinatus, should be viewed in two orthogonal planes whenever possible.

Another cause of error is tendon heterogeneity caused by the geometric relationship of the tendon to the transducer. As demonstrated by Crass et al[23] and Fornage,[24] failure to orient the transducer parallel to the fibers of the tendon may result in artifactual areas of decreased echogenicity (Fig. 28-22). When only a small

area of the tendon is parallel to the transducer, a focal area of increased echogenicity may be produced, mimicking a small partial-thickness or full-thickness tear. This artifact is especially pronounced with sector transducers.

Scans may be limited in obese patients or patients with large subdeltoid bursal effusions. The resulting lateral displacement of the transducer will significantly narrow the sonographic window. Excess soft tissues may also require the use of lower frequency transducers, which will in turn limit the accuracy of the examination.

RESULTS

The published results that have been achieved by rotator cuff sonography vary widely (Table 28-1).[25-29] An analysis of these reports suggests that a number of factors may play an important role in these discrepancies. The sonographic criteria, the patient population, and the desired information are crucial factors.

Reliability of published criteria vary widely. Most authors agree that failure to visualize the cuff has a high predictive value. Focal absence of the cuff is nearly as accurate. Discontinuity is a less accurate finding, with both false-negative and false-positive findings being reported. The least accurate finding is focally increased

■ **TABLE 28-1**
Comparison of Published Results Achieved by Rotator Cuff Sonography

	Mack	Crass	Middleton	Hodler	Brandt Arthrography	Brandt Surgery	Furtschegger Arthrography	Furtschegger Surgery	Miller	Soble Arthrography	Soble Surgery
Sensitivity	91%	93%	93%	100%	75%	71%	91%	91%	58%	92%	93%
Specificity	98%	92%	83%	75%	43%	29%	92%	25%	93%	84%	72%
PPV	98%	84%	78%	90%	55%	56%	94%	95%	88%	75%	78%
NPV	91%	97%	95%	100%	65%	45%	88%	14%	72%	92%	92%
Accuracy	95%	91%	87%	92%	59%	53%	91%	87%	77%	87%	83%
Prevalence	52%	28% (30% of these very small)	60%	27.7%	?	?	58%	94%	48%	43%	50%
Criteria	1,2,3	1,2,3,4a	1,2,3,5	6,1,2,7	1,2,3,4a,5				1,8,9	1,2,4,9	
Gold standard	Surgery	Surgery	Arthro	Surgery	Arthro/Surgery		Arthro/Surgery		Arthro	Arthro	Surgery
Pathology	FT	PT/FT	FT	FT/PT	FT/PT		FT/PT	FT/PT	FT/PT	FT/PT	
Frequency/Equipment	5/7 LA	10 MS	10Ms/75 LA	5/7 LA	7.5 MS 5 LA		5/7 LA		5/7.5 LA	7.5 MS 5.0 LA	

(Data from Mack LA, Gannon MK, Kilcoyne RF, et al: *Clin Orthop* 1988;234:21-27; Middleton WD, Reenus WR, Totty WF, et al: *J Bone Joint Surg* 1986;68:440-450; Crass JR, Craig EV, Feinberg SB. *J Clin Ultrasopund* 1988;16:313-327; Hodler J, Fretz CJ, Terrier F, et al: *Radiology* 1988;169:791-794; Furtschegger A, Resch H: *Europ J Radiol* 1988;8:69-75; Miller CL, Karasick D, Kurtz AB, et al: *Skeletal Radiol* 1989;18:179-183; Soble MG, Kaye AD, Guay RC. *Radiology* 1989;173:319-321; and Brandt TD, Cardone BW, Grant TH, et al: *Radiology* 1989;173:323-327.)
Criteria: *1*, Nonvisualization; *2*, Focal nonvisualization; *3*, Discontinuity; *4*, Abnormal Echogenicity—*a*, Focal; *b*, Diffuse—*5*, Central echogenic band; *6*, Concavity outer border; *7*, Focal flattening RCT; *8*, Marked thinning of RCT; *9*, Distortion of sonographic architecture.
Pathology: *FT*, Full-thickness rotator cuff tear; *PT*, Partial-thickness rotator cuff tear.
Equipment: *LA*, Linear array; *MS*, Mechanical sector.

echogenicity. Middleton recommends its use only when clear asymmetry exists between the shoulders.[16]

The patient population at a given center may also influence results. Patients in a referral center can be expected to have a higher prevalence of pathology and more advanced lesions. Such patient populations, which were the groups studied in the earlier reports, can be expected to have better results than younger patients, who have a higher percentage of small full-thickness tears and partial-thickness tears.

The type of information desired from rotator cuff sonography may vary widely. Clinicians and sonographers must have realistic expectations regarding the utility of this examination. As is the case with MRI and arthrography, sonography cannot realistically be expected to diagnose all lesions of the cuff. In a given patient, it may be necessary to employ a combination of examinations to precisely define the state of the rotator cuff.

In the postoperative patient, reports suggest that sonography is highly reliable. This may reflect the large size of recurrent tears. Mack et al[18] reported sonography was able to confirm all instances of recurrent cuff tear diagnosed at surgery and to confirm 10 of 11 intact tendons. Crass et al[19] reported similar results when sonography was compared with surgical findings.

Rotator cuff sonography thus has the potential to serve as a screening examination for patients with shoulder pain. It will be most useful in patients over 50 years of age who might be expected to have larger lesions. In younger patients with persistent symptoms, negative sonography should be followed by additional examinations. In the postoperative patient, sonography is the best examination in this difficult group of patients.

REFERENCES

1. Matsen FA III, Arntz CT: Subacromial impingement. In Rockwood CA and Matsen FA III, eds: The Shoulder, Vol. II. Philadelphia: W.B. Saunders Company; 1990.
2. Neviaser RJ, Neviaser TJ: Observations on impingement. Clin Orthop 1990;254:60-63.
3. Resnick D: Shoulder arthrography. Radiol Clin North Am 1981;19:243-252.
4. Mack LA, Matsen FA, Kilcoyne JF, et al: Ultrasound evaluation of the rotator cuff. Radiology 1985;157:205-209.
5. Mack LA, Gannon MK, Kilcoyne RF, et al: Sonographic evaluation of the rotator cuff. Accuracy in patients without prior surgery. Clin Orthop 1988;234:21-27.
6. Middleton WD, Reenus WR, Totty WF, et al: Ultrasonographic evaluation of the rotator cuff and biceps tendon. J Bone Joint Surg 1986;68:440-450.
7. Crass JR, Craig EV, Feinberg SB: Ultrasonography of rotator cuff tears: a review of 500 diagnostic studies. J Clin Ultrasound 1988;16:313-327.

Clinical considerations

8. Codman EA: The Shoulder, ed 2. Boston: Thomas Todd; 1934.

9. DePalma AF: Surgery of the Shoulder, ed 2. Philadelphia: Lippincott; 1973.
10. Refior HJ, Kroedel A, Melzer C: Examinations of the pathology of the rotator cuff. Arch Orthop Trauma Surg 1987; 106:301-308.
11. Pettersson G: Rupture of the tendon aponeurosis of the shoulder joint in anterior inferior dislocation. Acta Chir Scand Suppl 1942;77:1-184.
12. Neer CS: Anterior acromioplasty for the chronic impingement syndrome in the shoulder, a preliminary report. J Bone Joint Surg 1972;54A:41-51.

Technique

13. Mack LA, Nyberg DA, Matsen FA III: Sonographic evaluation of the rotator cuff. Radiol Clin North Am 1988;26:161-177.
14. Van Holsbeeck M, Introcaso J, Hoogmartens M: Sonographic detection and evaluation of shoulder joint effusion. Radiology 1990;177(P):214.
15. Crass JR, Craig EV, Feinberg SB: The hyperextended internal rotation view in rotator cuff ultrasound. J Clin Ultrasound 1987;15:416-420.

Preoperative appearances

16. Middleton WD: Status of rotator cuff sonography. Radiology 1989;173:307-309.

Postoperative appearances

17. Calvert PT, Packer WP, Stoker DJ, et al: Arthrography of the shoulder after operative repair at the torn rotator cuff. Br J Bone Joint Surg 1986;68B:147-150.
18. Mack LA, Nyberg DA, Matsen FA III, et al: Sonography of the postoperative shoulder. AJR 1988;150:1089-1093.
19. Crass JR, Craig EV, Feinberg SB: Sonography of the postoperative rotator cuff. AJR 1986;146:561-564.
20. Harryman DDT II, Mack LA, Wang KY, et al: Rotator cuff repair: correlation of functional results with cuff integrity. Accepted for publication in J Bone Joint Surg in press, 1991.
21. Neer CS II, Craig EV, Fukuda H: Cuff tear arthropathy. J Bone Joint Surg 1983;65A:1232-1244.

Trauma

22. Bassett RW, Cofield RH: Acute tears of the rotator cuff: the timing of surgical repair. Clin Ortho 1983;175:18-24.

Pitfalls

23. Crass JB, Van de Vegte GL, Harkavy LA: Tendon echogenicity: ex vivo study. Radiology 1988;167:499-503.
24. Fornage BD: The hypoechoic normal tendon: a pitfall. J Ultrasound Med 1987;6:19-22.

Results

25. Hodler J, Fretz CJ, Terrier F, et al: Rotator cuff tears: correlation of sonographic and surgical findings. Radiology 1988;169:791-794.
26. Brandt TD, Cardone BW, Grant TH, et al: Rotator cuff sonography: a reassessment. Radiology 1989;173:323-327.
27. Furtschegger A, Resch H: Value of ultrasonography in preoperative diagnosis of rotator cuff tears and postoperative follow-up. Europ J Radiol 1988;8:69-75.
28. Miller CL, Karasick D, Kurtz AB, et al: Limited sensitivity of ultrasound for the detection of rotator cuff tear. Skeletal Radiol 1989;18:179-183.
29. Soble MG, Kaye AD, Guay RC: Rotator cuff tear: clinical experience with sonographic detection. Radiology 1989;173:319-321.

CHAPTER 29

The Tendons

- Bruno D. Fornage, M.D.

The tendons of the extremities are particularly well suited for examination by high-frequency (7.5 to 10 MHz) ultrasound transducers because of their superficial location. Disorders of tendons are primarily caused by trauma and inflammation and are usually related to athletic and some occupational activities.

ANATOMY

Tendons are made of dense connective tissue and are extremely resistant to traction forces.[1] The densely packed collagen fibers are separated by a small amount of ground substance with few elongated fibroblasts and are arranged in parallel bundles. The peritenon is a layer of loose connective tissue that wraps around the tendon and sends intratendinous septa between the bundles of collagen fibers.

At the musculotendinous junction, there is an interdigitation between the muscle fibers and the collagen fibrils. The bony insertion of tendons is usually markedly calcified and characterized by the presence of cartilaginous tissue. Tendons have various shapes; they usually attach to tuberosities, spinae, trochanters, processes, or ridges.

Blood supply to tendons is poor, and nutritional ex-

changes occur mostly via the ground substance. With aging, the amount of ground substance and the number of fibroblasts decrease while the number of fibers and fat deposition increase.

In specific areas of mechanical constraint, tendons are associated with additional structures. Fibrous sheaths keep certain tendons close to bony pieces and prevent bowstringing, e.g., the flexor and extensor retinacula at the wrist, the fibrous sheaths of flexor tendons in the fingers, or the peroneal and flexor retinacula at the foot. Sesamoid bones are intended to reinforce a tendon's strength. Synovial sheaths are double-walled tubes with the inner wall in intimate contact with the tendon. The two layers are in continuity with each other at both ends. A minimal amount of synovial fluid allows the smooth gliding of the tendon within its sheath. Synovial bursae are small fluid-filled pouches that are found in particular locations, and act as bolsters to facilitate the play of tendons.

TECHNIQUE OF EXAMINATION

Because of their wider field of view and their better resolution in the near-field, linear-array electronic transducers are best suited for tendon sonography; significant artifacts are generated by mechanical or phased-array sector scanners and convex-array transducers. Images of exquisite resolution are obtained with 7.5 or 10 MHz transducers but the field of view of those probes is usually restricted to a width of 3 to 4 cm. It is recommended that the study of long tendons (e.g., Achilles or patellar tendon) begin with a 5 MHz linear-array transducer, whose 5 to 6 cm wide field of view allows visualization of the whole tendon on a single scan; more detailed images can then be obtained using a higher-frequency probe.

A standoff pad is mandatory to evaluate very superficial tendons (e.g., extensor tendons of the fingers at the dorsum of the hand) or tendons in regions with uneven surfaces.[2] When a standoff material is used, the ultrasound beam should be strictly perpendicular to the region examined in order to avoid artifacts.[3]

The combination of longitudinal and transverse scans provides a three-dimensional approach to the tendon examined. A valuable reference for normal anatomy can be found by scanning the symmetric area in the contralateral extremity or region, although the rare possibility of bilateral tendon injuries should be kept in mind.

Tendons should be examined at rest and during active and passive flexion/extension maneuvers. One advantage of sonography is the ability to perform palpation under real-time monitoring.[3]

NORMAL SONOGRAPHY

All tendons are echogenic and display a typical fibrillar echotexture on longitudinal scans (Fig. 29-1).[3] Although they are easily seen when they are surrounded by hypoechoic muscles, tendons may be less well delineated from adjacent echogenic fat. A key step in the identification of tendons is their mobilization under real-time sonographic monitoring on longitudinal scans. On transverse sections, the reflective bundles of fibers give rise to a finely punctate echogenic pattern (Fig. 29-2). Transverse scans provide the most accurate measurements of tendon thickness.

Sesamoid bones appear as hyperechoic structures that cast an acoustic shadow.[3] When high-frequency transducers are used, synovial sheaths appear as a subtle hypoechoic underlining of the tendon. Large synovial bursae can be seen on sonograms as flattened, fluid-filled structures a few millimeters thick (Fig. 29-3).[4]

The most significant artifact associated with tendon sonography is a false hypoechogenicity resulting from an oblique ultrasound beam. The optimal display of the echogenic fibrillar texture of a tendon requires that the ultrasound beam be strictly perpendicular to the tendon axis. The slightest obliquity causes scattering of the beam, which results in an artifactual hypoechogenicity.[5] Early erroneous descriptions of hypoechoic normal tendons, in particular of the rotator cuff, have probably been caused by this artifact. This artifact constantly affects scans obtained with mechanical, phased-array, and to a lesser extent, curved-array sector scanners, with which only the midline portion of the scan is free of artifacts (Fig. 29-4). When a linear-array transducer is used, the artifact occurs whenever the tendon is not parallel to the surface of the transducer. When the artifact is caused by the tendon's curved course, changing the position of the probe or suppressing the curvature of a tendon through muscle contraction clears the artifact (Fig. 29-5). When a standoff pad is used, it is crucial to verify constantly that the footprint of the transducer is parallel to the tendon's axis. Transverse scans are also affected by false hypoechogenicity artifacts (Fig. 29-6).

Elbow

With the elbow flexed at an angle of 90°, the tendon of the triceps brachii is readily identified on both longi-

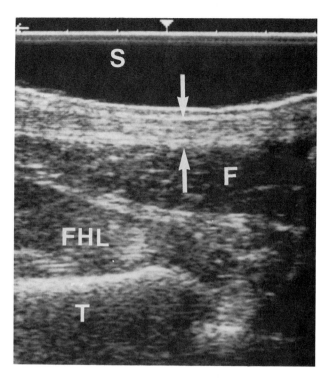

FIG 29-1. Normal Achilles tendon. Longitudinal scan obtained with a 5 MHz transducer shows the echogenic, fibrillar texture of the tendon *(arrows)*. *F*, Kager's fatty triangle; *FHL*, flexor hallucis longus; *S*, standoff pad; *T*, tibia

tudinal and transverse scans. The common tendons of the flexor and extensor muscles of the forearm, arising from the medial and lateral epicondyles, respectively, are also best demonstrated with the elbow flexed at this angle (Fig. 29-7). The tendon of the biceps brachii muscle can also be appreciated at its insertion into the tuberosity of the radius.

Hand and Wrist

In the carpal tunnel, the echogenic flexor tendons of the fingers are surrounded by the hypoechoic ulnar bursa and are best seen when the wrist is moderately flexed (Fig. 29-8).

In the palm, the pairs of superficial and deep flexor tendons are clearly identified. On longitudinal scans, the play of the tendons of a given finger is appreciated in real-time during the flexion/extension of that finger. On transverse scans, the pairs of flexor and superficial tendons appear as echogenic rounded structures, adjacent to the hypoechoic lumbrical muscles (Fig. 29-9).

In the fingers, the flexor tendons follow the concavity of the phalanges and therefore have a hypoechoic artifact along most of their course (Fig. 29-10).[6,7] The examination of the extensor tendons of the fingers requires the use of a standoff pad.

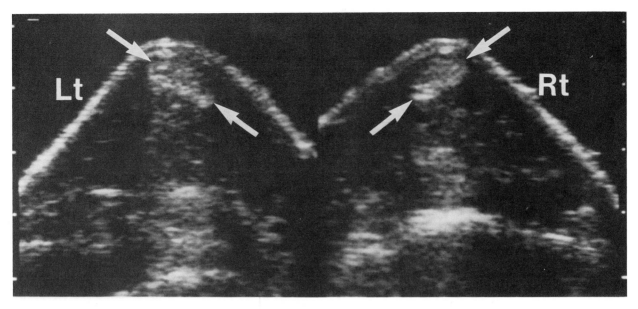

FIG 29-2. Normal Achilles tendons. Transverse scans of the normal echogenic left and right Achilles tendons *(arrows)* demonstrate the oblique orientation of the tendon plane.

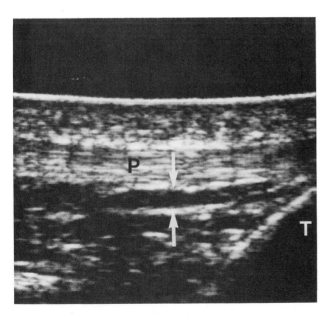

FIG 29-3. Infrapatellar bursa. Longitudinal scan of the knee shows the deep (subtendinous) infrapatellar bursa *(arrows)* posterior to the distal patellar tendon. *T*, Tibia; *P*, patellar tendon.

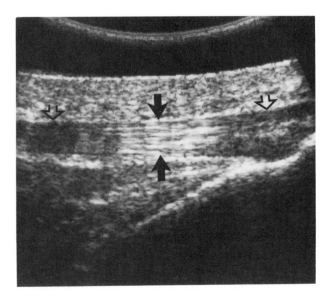

FIG 29-4. False hypoechogenicity of normal tendon caused by curved-array transducer. On this longitudinal scan of the distal patellar tendon obtained with a 10-MHz curved-array sector transducer, the tendon exhibits normal echogenicity *(arrows)* only in the narrow midportion of the scan where the beam is perpendicular to the tendon. On either side, the obliquity of the beam is responsible for the artifactual tendon hypoechogenicity *(open arrows).*

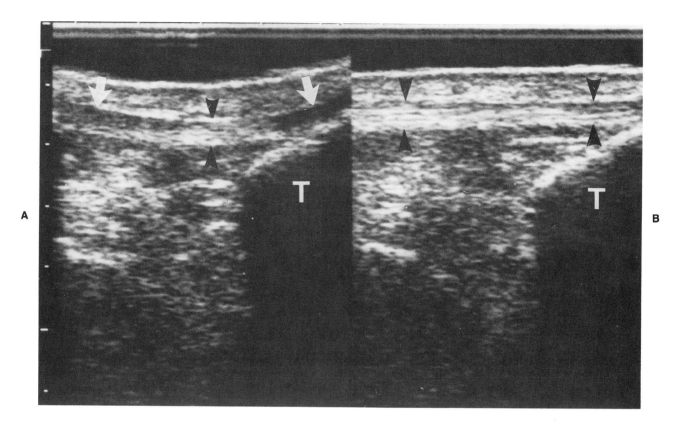

FIG 29-5. False hypoechogenicity of normal patellar tendon caused by the tendon's curved course at rest. **A,** Longitudinal scan at rest shows the curved tendon *(arrowheads)* with the artifact affecting the segments of the tendon that are oblique to the beam *(arrows)*. **B,** Contraction of the quadriceps straightens the tendon *(arrowheads)*, which exhibits normal echogenicity. *T,* Tibia.

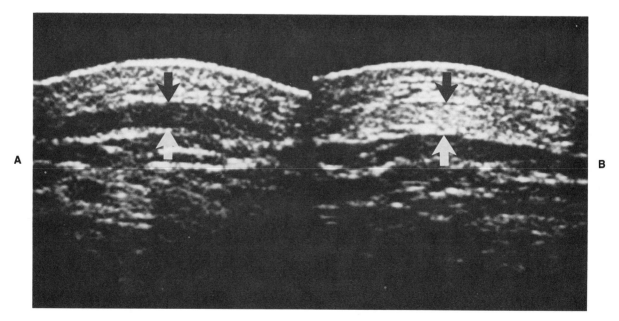

FIG 29-6. False hypoechogenicity of the normal patellar tendon on transverse scans is caused by transducer angulation. **A,** Slightly angled (superiorly or inferiorly) transverse scan shows hypoechoic tendon *(arrows)*. **B,** Transverse scan strictly perpendicular to the tendon axis exhibits normal echogenicity *(arrows)*.

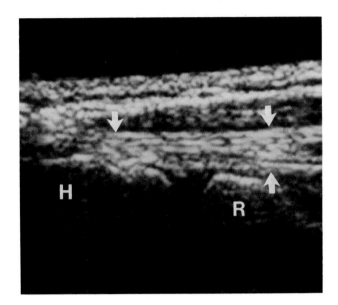

FIG 29-7. Normal elbow. Coronal scan of the lateral aspect of the elbow flexed at an angle of 90° shows the normal echogenic common tendon of the extensor muscles of the forearm *(arrows)* arising from the lateral epicondyle. *H,* Humerus; *R,* radial head.

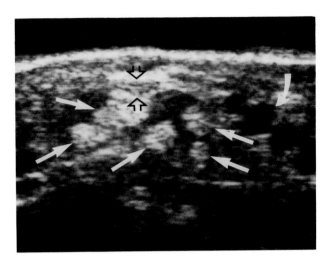

FIG 29-8. Normal wrist. Transverse scan in moderate flexion shows the normal echogenic cross sections of superficial and deep flexor tendons of the fingers *(arrows),* which lie in the hypoechoic ulnar bursa. *Open arrows,* median nerve; *curved arrow,* ulnar artery.

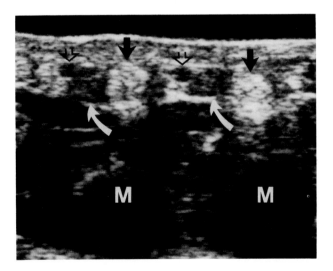

FIG 29-9. Normal palm of hand. Transverse scan shows the normal echogenic, rounded superficial and deep flexor tendons of the third and fourth fingers *(arrows),* adjacent to the hypoechoic lumbrical muscles *(curved arrows). Open arrows,* common palmar digital arteries; *M,* metacarpal bone.

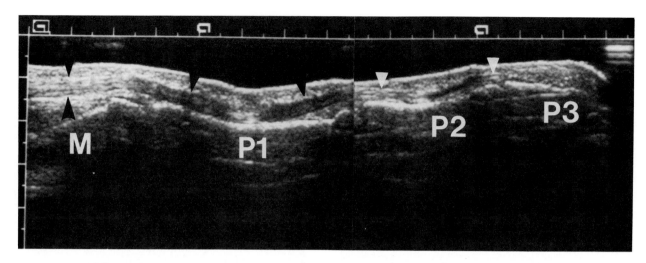

FIG 29-10. Normal finger. Montage of longitudinal scans of the third finger shows the normal superficial and deep flexor tendons *(arrowheads)* coursing along the phalanges. Note that the tendons exhibit normal echogenicity only in the segments in which they are parallel to the linear-array transducer and that they are falsely hypoechoic in the segments in which they lie oblique to the beam. *M*, Metacarpal; *P1*, first phalanx; *P2*, second phalanx; *P3*, third phalanx.

Knee

Sonography is an excellent technique with which to visualize the extensor tendons of the knee.[8-10] Because both the quadriceps and the patellar tendons may be slightly concave anteriorly when the knee is extended and at rest, scans should be obtained during contraction of the quadriceps muscle (or with the knee flexed), which straightens the tendons and eliminates the hypoechoic artifact (see Fig. 29-5).

The quadriceps tendon comprises 4 tendons (the tendon of the rectus femoris superficially, the tendons of the vastus lateralis and vastus medialis muscles, and the tendon of the vastus intermedius), which are not usually distinguished sonographically as separate structures. The tendon lies underneath the subcutaneous fat and anterior to a fat pad and the collapsed suprapatellar bursa (Fig. 29-11). On transverse scans, the tendon is oval.

The patellar tendon extends from the patella to the tibial tuberosity (Fig. 29-12), over a length of 5 to 6 cm. On transverse sections, the patellar tendon is characterized by a convex anterior and flat posterior surface. At its midportion, the tendon is about 4 to 5 mm thick and about 20 to 25 mm wide.[8] The subcutaneous prepatellar and infrapatellar bursae are not visible. The deep (subtendinous) infrapatellar bursa appears as a flattened, anechoic structure, 2 to 3 mm thick (see Fig. 29-3).

Sonography has been used in the evaluation of collateral ligaments, but these ligaments cannot normally be well delineated from the articular capsule and from the surrounding subcutaneous tissues.[11] Despite a few reports claiming its capacity to demonstrate cruciate ligaments, sonography is ineffective for the routine evaluation of these ligaments.[10,12]

Foot and Ankle

The Achilles tendon is formed by the fusion between the aponeuroses of the soleus and gastrocnemius muscles. It inserts into the posterior surface of the calcaneus. In the absence of artifacts, the Achilles tendon is echogenic and exhibits a characteristic fibrillar texture on longitudinal scans (see Fig. 29-1).[13] The termination of the hypoechoic soleus muscle is easily identified anterior to the origin of the tendon. The fatty area known as Kager's triangle that lies anterior to the distal half of the tendon, although most often echogenic, may show some variation in echogenicity. More anteriorly lie the hypoechoic flexor hallucis longus and the echogenic posterior surface of the tibia. The flattened, hypoechoic subtendinous calcaneal bursa is sometimes seen in the angle formed by the tendon and the calcaneus. Occasionally, the tendon fibers at the bony insertion have a short oblique course responsible for an artifactual hypoechogenicity (Fig. 29-13). This pattern should not be misdiagnosed as the subcutaneous calcaneal bursa, which is not normally seen.

On transverse sonograms, the cross-section of the tendon is grossly elliptical and tapers medially. The tendon plane orientation is remarkable in that it is oblique forward and medially (see Fig. 29-2). Because of this configuration, there is a risk of overestimating the thickness of the tendon on strictly sagittal scans of the leg, and measurements should, therefore, be taken from

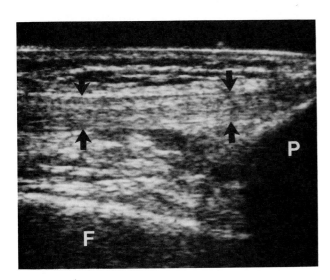

FIG 29-11. Normal quadriceps tendon. Longitudinal scan shows the echogenic tendon *(arrows)* surrounded by fat. *F,* Femur; *P,* patella.

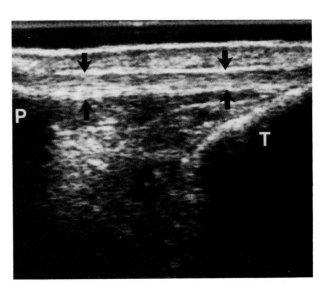

FIG 29-12. Normal patellar tendon. Longitudinal scan shows the echogenic tendon *(arrows)* extending from the patella to the tibial tuberosity. The tendon is about 5 mm thick. *P,* Patella; *T,* tibia.

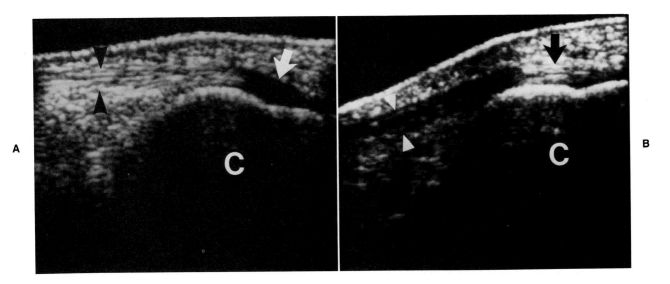

FIG 29-13. False hypoechogenicity of the normal Achilles tendon at its insertion into the calcaneus. **A,** Longitudinal scan with the linear-array transducer parallel to the tendon *(arrowheads)* shows the markedly hypoechoic distal extremity of the tendon *(arrow),* whose course is oblique to the beam. **B,** Placing the transducer parallel to the distal tendon clears the artifact *(arrow),* while the rest of the tendon *(arrowheads)* is now falsely hypoechoic. *C,* Calcaneus.

transverse scans. At 2 to 3 cm above its insertion, the Achilles tendon is 5 to 7 mm thick and 12 to 15 mm wide.[13]

In the ankle, sonography readily demonstrates the tendons of the peroneus longus and brevis laterally and of the tibialis posterior medially. The tendons of the flexor digitorum longus and flexor hallucis longus can also be identified behind the medial malleolus, whereas the tendons of the tibialis anterior, extensor hallucis longus, and extensor digitorum longus are seen at the anterior aspect of the ankle joint. These tendons are enveloped in synovial sheaths. Dynamic examination during specific flexion/extension maneuvers of the ankle and foot is mandatory for definite identification of individual tendons.

In the foot, the examination technique and ultrasound anatomy of the flexor and extensor tendons of the toes do not differ significantly from those of the tendons of the fingers.[7]

PATHOLOGY

Tendon disorders are most often caused either by trauma resulting in tears or by inflammation.

Tears

Tears usually occur on tendons that have been rendered fragile by such factors as aging, presence of calcifications, general or local corticosteroid therapy, and underlying systemic diseases (rheumatoid arthritis, lupus erythematosus, diabetes mellitus, and gout).[14-17] In the absence of those predisposing factors, biopsy specimens taken in the vicinity of the rupture site often demonstrate degenerative changes, sometimes described as "tendinosis."

Complete Tears. Recent complete tendon tears are often correctly diagnosed clinically. However, if delayed, the physical examination may be indeterminate because of inflammatory changes. Sonography can show the full-thickness discontinuity of the tendon. The gap between the torn tendon fragments is filled with hypoechoic hemorrhagic fluid (or clot) or granulomatous tissue, depending on the lesion's age (Fig. 29-14). Also, the gap varies in length, and when the torn fragments are separated by a long distance, the tendon may not be visualized at all. This nonvisualization may occur in complete ruptures of the rotator cuff and of the flexor tendons of the fingers.[18] With the exception of ruptures of the Achilles tendon, in which a hematoma can develop around the whole tendon, ruptures are usually associated with minimal focal hemorrhage. In the case of bone avulsion, the bone fragment appears as a bright echogenic focus with an acoustic shadow (Fig. 29-15).

Incomplete Tears. Incomplete tears are difficult to diagnose clinically and to differentiate from focal tendi-

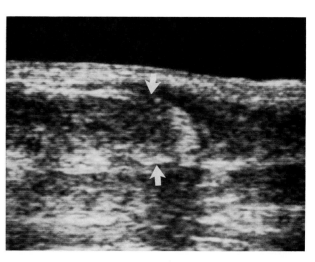

FIG 29-14. Complete tear of the Achilles tendon. Longitudinal scan shows the retracted, swollen, upper fragment *(arrows)*.

nitis. For example, many partial ruptures of the Achilles tendon are diagnosed clinically as nodular tendinitis. Accurate sonographic diagnosis is important because early diagnosis and treatment of a partial tear will prevent a subsequent complete rupture.

Sonographically, recent partial ruptures appear as focal hypoechoic defects in the tendon or at its attachment (Fig. 29-16).[4,19] The three-dimensional evaluation of partial ruptures requires a combination of longitudinal and transverse scans.

A peculiar form of partial rupture of the patellar tendon is the detachment from the patellar apex. Longitudinal scans show the tendon fibers' discontinuity, whereas transverse scans below the patellar apex demonstrate the midline rounded hematoma (Fig. 29-17).

Inflammation

Tendinitis. Tendinitis is mostly associated with athletic or occupational activities. At pathologic examination, there are degenerative changes, often associated with the presence of microcysts. The vascular proliferation and edema are responsible for the increased volume of the tendon. Calcifications are associated with chronic tendinitis. Tendinitis may affect the whole or only part of the tendon. For example, focal tendinitis can be found at either insertion of the patellar tendon.

In acute tendinitis, the tendon is thickened and the margins are ill-defined. There is also a diffuse decrease in echogenicity (Fig. 29-18).[8,13] Because improper scanning technique may result in a falsely hypoechoic tendon, it is crucial to verify that the examination technique is flawless. In addition, comparison with tendons of the unaffected extremity is often valuable.

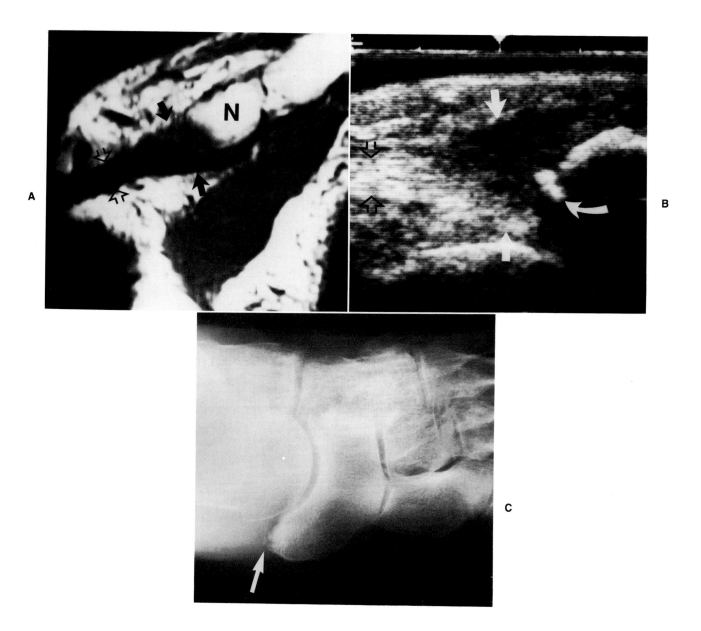

FIG 29-15. Complete tear of the posterior tibial tendon at its insertion into the navicular bone. **A,** Magnetic resonance scan of the foot (oriented to compare with the sonogram) shows the torn ligament *(arrows)*. The open arrows indicate the normal tendon. **B,** Coronal sonogram shows the hypoechoic focal hemorrhage and the tendon discontinuity *(arrows)*. The open arrows indicate the normal tendon. The curved arrow points to the avulsed bone fragment. **C,** Radiograph confirms the bone avulsion at the tendon's insertion into the navicular bone *(arrow)*. *N*, Navicular bone.

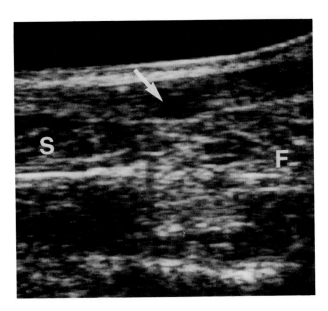

FIG 29-16. Partial rupture of the Achilles tendon. Longitudinal scan of the tendon shows a small focal discontinuity of fibers *(arrow)* at the anterior aspect of the tendon. *F,* Kager's fatty triangle; *S,* soleus.

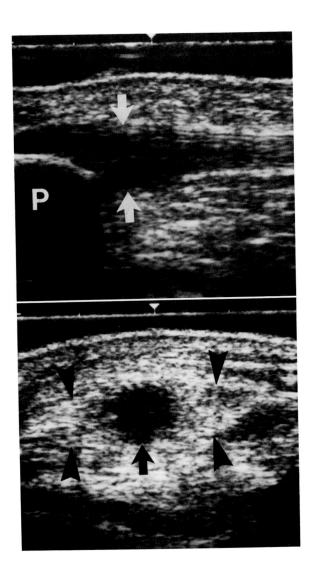

FIG 29-17. Partial detachment of the superior portion of the patellar tendon. **A,** Midsagittal scan shows the hematoma and the tendon discontinuity *(arrows)* at the upper insertion of the tendon. **B,** Transverse scan shows the well-defined, round, hypoechoic midline hematoma *(arrow). Arrowheads,* tendon's margins; *P,* patella.

In chronic tendinitis, the contours of the tendon may be deformed, with a bumpy appearance. High-frequency sonography has proved accurate in the detection of minute intratendinous calcifications, which appear as bright foci with or without acoustic shadowing, occasionally with a comet-tail artifact (Fig. 29-19). However, the size and shape of these calcifications are better appreciated on low-kilovoltage radiographs, preferably obtained with the use of a mammographic unit.[20]

Sonography can also be used to monitor the response to anti-inflammatory therapy. A decrease in size of the tendon and a return to a normal level of echogenicity indicate healing.

Peritendinitis. In peritendinitis, inflammation is limited to the peritenon, the layer of connective tissue that wraps around the tendon. This condition is frequently found in the Achilles tendon. Sonographically, peritendinitis is characterized by a hypoechoic thickening of the peritenon, with the tendon remaining grossly unaffected.

Tenosynovitis. Tenosynovitis is defined as the inflammation of a tendon sheath. Any tendon surrounded by a synovial sheath, especially tendons in the hand, wrist, and ankle, can be affected. Trauma, including repeated microtrauma, and pyogenic infection are mostly responsible for acute tenosynovitis. Sonographically, the diagnosis of acute tenosynovitis is made when fluid in the sheath, even in minimal quantity, is identified (Fig. 29-20).[21,22] Internal echoes representing debris can be seen in suppurative tenosynovitis, a serious condition because of the potential damage to the tendon.[23]

Chronic tenosynovitis is characterized by a hypoechoic thickening of the synovium, most often with little or no fluid. The thickening of the sheath may impair the movement of tendons in narrow passages. In De Quervain's tenosynovitis, the tendons of the abductor pollicis longus and extensor pollicis brevis are constricted by the thickened sheath in the pulley over the radial styloid process. Sonography can demonstrate the hypoechoic thickening of the tendon sheath. Sonogra-

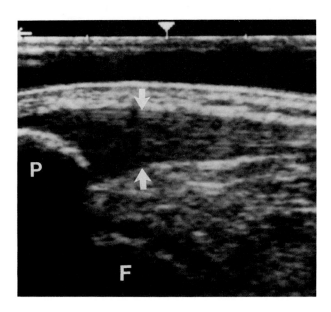

FIG 29-18. Acute patellar tendinitis. Longitudinal scan shows thickening and decreased echogenicity of the superior two thirds of the tendon *(arrows)*. *F*, Femoral condyle; *P*, patella.

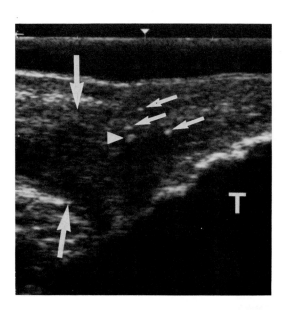

FIG 29-19. Chronic calcified patellar tendinitis. Longitudinal scan of the lower attachment of the tendon shows a markedly thickened, hypoechoic tendon *(long arrows)*, with blurred contours, and tiny hyperechoic calcifications *(short arrows)*, one with a comet tail artifact *(arrowhead)*. *T*, Tibia; *P*, patella.

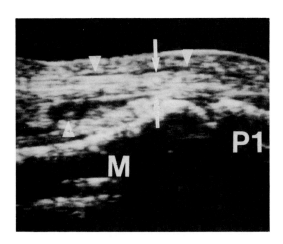

FIG 29-20. Tenosynovitis of the flexor tendons of a finger. Longitudinal scan of the volar aspect of the metacarpophalangeal joint shows the tendon sheath distended by a small amount of fluid *(arrowheads)*. The flexor tendons are normal *(arrows)*. *M*, Metacarpal; *P1*, first phalanx.

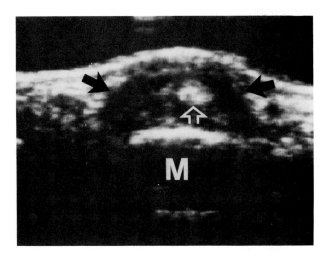

FIG 29-21. Rheumatoid tenosynovitis of the extensor tendon of a finger at the dorsum of the hand. Transverse scan shows the hypoechoic pannus *(arrows)* surrounding the tendon *(open arrow)*. *M*, Metacarpal.

phy can also be used to guide the injection of contrast medium into the sheath for tenography, a study which silhouettes the sheath wall but cannot demonstrate its thickness.

Rheumatoid arthritis has a predilection for synovial tissues, including tendon sheaths in the distal extremities. Sonography has proved effective in the diagnosis of rheumatoid tenosynovitis in the hand.[24] The tendon sheath involved by the pannus is markedly hypoechoic (Fig. 29-21) and, occasionally, fluid is also present in the sheath. Sonographic findings of tendon involvement include thickening and inhomogeneity of the tendon, whose margins are jagged. At a later stage, sonography can demonstrate a partial or complete rupture.

Bursitis. Bursitis occurs most often in the subdeltoid, olecranal, radiohumeral, patellar, and calcaneal bursae. Trauma, and more importantly, repeated microtrauma are thought to play an important role in bursitis, although no initiating factor can be found in many cases. In the early acute stage, when the bursa is filled with fluid, sonograms demonstrate a sonolucent, fluid-filled collection with ill-defined margins. At the chronic stage, a complex sonographic appearance with internal echogenic debris results from the presence of granulomatous tissue, precipitated fibrin, and occasionally, calcification.

Nonarticular Osteochondroses. Osgood-Schlatter and Sinding-Larsen-Johansson diseases are both nonarticular osteochondroses of the knee that occur in ossification centers subjected to traction stress and in which stress to the patellar tendon has been incriminated. Both conditions occur in adolescents, typically in boys practicing athletic activities. Although the diagnosis is strongly suggested by the clinical history, radiographic studies are often performed to confirm the diagnosis. Recently, high-resolution sonography has been used in the evaluation of these two conditions.[25]

Osgood-Schlatter disease is osteochondrosis of the tibial tuberosity. Sonographic findings include swelling of the anechoic cartilage with anterior displacement of subcutaneous tissues; fragmentation of the echogenic ossification center; thickening and decreased echogenicity of the distal patellar tendon; and deep infrapatellar bursitis.

Sinding-Larsen-Johansson disease is osteochondrosis of the accessory ossification center at the lower pole of the patella. In this rare disease, sonography can demonstrate the fragmented, echogenic ossification center and the swollen, hypoechoic cartilage and surrounding soft tissues, including the origin of the patellar tendon.

Postoperative Patterns

After surgery, tendons appear enlarged and heterogeneous with blurred, irregular margins (Fig. 29-22).[4,26]

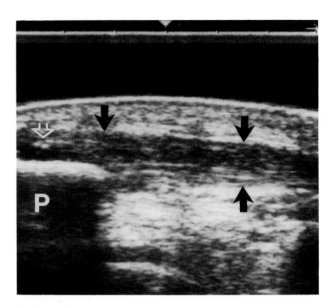

FIG 29-22. Postoperative pattern. Longitudinal scan of the patellar tendon performed 15 months after surgery for tendinitis shows a diffusely thickened, heterogeneous, hypoechoic tendon *(arrows)*, with ill-defined margins, and minute calcifications *(open arrow)*. P, Patella.

This postoperative pattern may last for several months or years and, therefore, sonography cannot reliably differentiate recurrent tears and tendinitis from the postoperative changes. Occasionally, sonography can detect bright echogenic foci caused by residual synthetic suture material or calcification. Doppler studies may demonstrate hypervascularization in tendons postoperatively (Fig. 29-23).

Tumors and Pseudotumors

Benign tumors of tendons or their sheaths include **giant cell tumors** and **osteochondromas.** The giant cell tumor of tendon sheaths is thought to represent a circumscribed form of pigmented villonodular synovitis. It involves preferentially the flexor surface of the fingers and is usually found in young and middle-aged women. Local recurrences may occur after an incomplete excision. Sonographically, these tumors appear as hypoechoic masses, sometimes with lobulated contours.[7] Malignant tumors are rare. **Synovial sarcomas** may arise from a tendon sheath and appear as a hypoechoic mass that may exhibit calcification.

Intratendinous rheumatoid nodules[24] and **xanthomas** in patients with hypercholesterolemia[4] have been reported as hypoechoic masses. Sonography can be used to monitor the effect of therapy on the Achilles tendon's thickness and echotexture in patients who have hypercholesterolemia. Intratendinous tophi appear as highly echogenic foci with acoustic shadowing and,

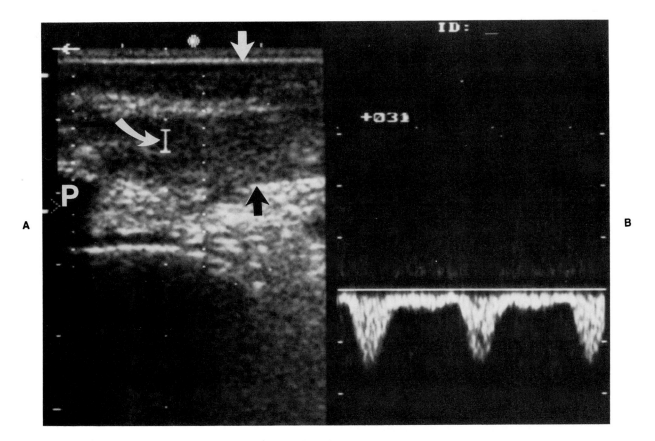

FIG 29-23. Duplex sonography of the patellar tendon 6 months after surgery for acute septic tendinitis. **A,** Longitudinal scan shows markedly hypoechoic, ill-defined tendon *(arrows)*. The curved arrow points to the Doppler gate. **B,** Doppler signal indicates tendon's hypervascularity. *P,* Patella.

therefore, they can be differentiated from intratendinous rheumatoid nodules.[27]

Ganglion cysts most commonly occur in the hand and develop from any joint or tendon sheath. Sonography demonstrates the oval-shaped fluid collection adjacent to the joint space or tendon (Fig. 29-24). Occasionally, chronic cysts or cysts containing a viscous fluid have internal echoes, causing the cyst to appear similar to a hypoechoic solid tumor.

Another cyst that commonly occurs adjacent to a joint is the **popliteal cyst.** These cysts are caused by an abnormal distention of the gastrocnemio-semimembranosus bursa, which frequently communicates with the knee joint through a slit-shaped opening at the postero-medial aspect of the joint capsule. They are frequently found in association with pathologic conditions that cause an increase in the intra-articular pressure through overproduction of synovial fluid, capsular sclerosis, or synovial hypertrophy; among these conditions, rheumatoid arthritis is the most common. Popliteal cysts present clinically as asymptomatic or symptomatic popliteal masses. Large cysts dissecting into the calf or ruptured cysts produce a swollen, painful limb that mimics thrombophlebitis.

A popliteal cyst typically appears as a fluid-filled collection.[28-31] Occasionally, longitudinal scans through the medial gastrocnemius muscle demonstrate a second anechoic area anterior to the muscle (Fig. 29-25) Transverse scans readily confirm that both areas represent sections of the same cyst, which surrounds the muscle. Internal echoes representing fibrinous strands or debris and synovial thickening can be seen in inflamed or infected cysts. In patients with rheumatoid arthritis, the cysts may be completely filled with pannus, thus mimicking solid masses. Osteochondromatosis can also develop in a popliteal cyst, giving rise to hyperechoic loose bodies that cast acoustic shadows when calcified.[32] In a recently ruptured cyst, sonography can demonstrate the leak as a subcutaneous fluid collection extending distally to the lower calf.[29-31] However, when the examination is deferred, sonographic diagnosis may be more problematic because the leaking fluid has resorbed and only an ill-defined hypoechoic residual area remains.[31]

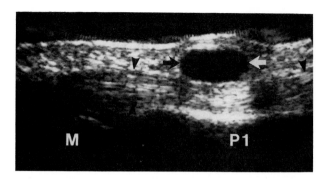

FIG 29-24. Ganglion cyst on the volar aspect of the first phalanx of the second finger. Longitudinal scan shows a well-defined, 0.8 cm cystic structure *(arrows)* anterior to the flexor tendons of the finger *(arrowheads)*. Note the distal acoustic enhancement. *M,* Metacarpal; *P1,* first phalanx.

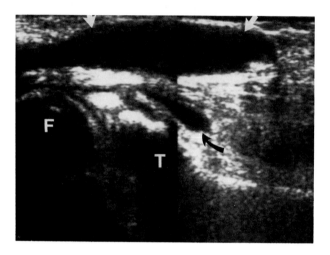

FIG 29-25. Popliteal cyst. Longitudinal scan demonstrates a teardrop-shaped cystic mass *(arrows)* in the soft tissues posterior to the knee joint with a smaller portion *(curved arrow)* anterior to the gastrocnemius medialis muscle. Note the internal echoes due to hypertrophied synovium. *F,* Femoral condyle; *T,* tibia.

SONOGRAPHY VERSUS OTHER IMAGING MODALITIES

For many decades, low-kilovoltage radiography and xero-radiography were the only imaging techniques applicable to tendons. Although they can silhouette tendons, particularly when the tendons are surrounded by fat, these techniques fail to demonstrate the structure of the tendons. However, they are still the best modalities with which to document unequivocally calcifications in tendons or bursae.[20] Tenography is performed by injecting contrast medium into the sheath. This somewhat neglected imaging technique provides detailed, global views of the walls of the sheath but cannot demonstrate the wall per se.[33,34]

Because computed tomography is limited to transverse scans of the extremities in routine practice, it has rarely been used in the evaluation of tendons.[35-37]

Magnetic resonance imaging (MRI) has emerged as an accurate modality for soft-tissue imaging and appears to be a direct competitor of high-frequency sonography in the field of tendon imaging.[38] However, high-frequency sonography is, currently, the only real-time cross-sectional imaging technique, and scans can be quickly obtained along virtually any orientation. High-frequency transducers provide exquisite spatial resolution, and in addition, the cost of the examination is low and equipment is widely available. However, because of the small size of the structures examined and the possibility of technique-related artifacts, tendon sonography, which is operator-dependent, requires considerable experience to obtain accurate results.

REFERENCES
Anatomy

1. McMaster PE: Tendon and muscle ruptures. Clinical and experimental studies on the causes and location of subcutaneous ruptures. *J Bone Joint Surg* 1933;15:705-722.

Technique of examination

2. Fornage BD, Touche DH, Rifkin MD: Small parts real-time sonography: a new "water-path." *J Ultrasound Med* 1984;3:355-357.
3. Fornage BD: *Ultrasonography of Muscles and Tendons.* Examination Technique and Atlas of Normal Anatomy of the Extremities. New York, Springer-Verlag, 1988.

Normal sonography

4. Fornage BD, Rifkin MD: Ultrasound examination of tendons. *Radiol Clin North Am* 1988;26:87-107.
5. Fornage BD: The hypoechoic normal tendon: a pitfall. *J Ultrasound Med* 1987;6:19-22.
6. Fornage BD, Rifkin MD: Ultrasound examination of the hand. *Radiology* 1986;160:853-854.
7. Fornage BD, Rifkin MD: Ultrasonic examination of the hand and foot. *Radiol Clin North Am* 1988;26:109-129.
8. Fornage BD, Rifkin MD, Touche DH, et al: Sonography of the patellar tendon: preliminary observations. *AJR* 1984;143:179-182.
9. Dillehay GL, Deschler T, Rogers, LF, et al: The ultrasonographic characterization of tendons. *Invest Radiol* 1984;19:338-341.
10. Laine HR, Harjula A, Peltokallio P: Ultrasound in the evaluation of the knee and patellar regions. *J Ultrasound Med* 1987;6:33-36.
11. De Flaviis L, Nessi R, Leonardi M, et al: Dynamic ultrasonography of capsulo-ligamentous knee joint traumas. *JCU* 1988;16:487-492.
12. Röhr E: Die sonographische Darstellung des hinteren Kreuzbandes. *Röntgenblätter* 1985;38:377-379.
13. Fornage BD: Achilles tendon: ultrasound examination. *Radiology* 1986;159:759-764.

Pathology

14. Downey DJ, Simkin PA, Mack LA, et al: Tibialis posterior tendon rupture: a cause of rheumatoid flat foot. *Arthritis Rheum* 1988;31:441-446.

15. Ismail AM, Balakrishnan R, Rajakumar MK: Rupture of patellar ligament after steroid infiltration. Report of a case. *J Bone Joint Surg* 1969;51B:503-505.
16. Kricun R, Kricun ME, Arangio GA, et al: Patellar tendon rupture with underlying systemic disease. *AJR* 1980;135:803-807.
17. Morgan J, McCarty DJ: Tendon ruptures in patients with systemic lupus erythematosus treated with corticosteroids. *Arthritis Rheum* 1974;17:1033-1036.
18. Souissi M, Giwerc M, Ebelin M, et al: Exploration échographique des tendons fléchisseurs des doigts de la main. *Presse Med* 1989;18:463-466.
19. Leekam RN, Salsberg BB, Bogoch E, et al: Sonographic diagnosis of partial Achilles tendon rupture and healing. *J Ultrasound Med* 1986;5:115-116.
20. Fornage B, Touche D, Deshayes JL, et al: Diagnostic des calcifications du tendon rotulien. Comparaison échoradiographique. *J Radiol* 1984;65:355-359.
21. Middleton WD, Reinus WR, Totty WG, et al: Ultrasound of the biceps tendon apparatus. *Radiology* 1985;157:211-215.
22. Gooding GAW: Tenosynovitis of the wrist. A sonographic demonstration. *J Ultrasound Med* 1988;7:225-226.
23. Jeffrey RB Jr, Laing FC, Schechter WP, et al: Acute suppurative tenosynovitis of the hand: diagnosis with ultrasound. *Radiology* 1987;162:741-742.
24. Fornage BD: Soft-tissue changes in the hand in rheumatoid arthritis: Evaluation with ultrasound. *Radiology* 1989;173:735-737.
25. De Flaviis L, Nessi R, Scaglione P, et al: Ultrasonic diagnosis of Osgood-Schlatter and Sinding-Larsen-Johansson diseases of the knee. *Skeletal Radiol* 1989;18:193-197.
26. Blei CL, Nirschl RP, Grant EG: Achilles tendon: ultrasonic diagnosis of pathologic conditions. *Radiology* 1986;159:765-767.
27. Tiliakos N, Morales AR, Wilson CH Jr: Use of ultrasound in identifying tophaceous versus rheumatoid nodules (letter). *Arthritis Rheum* 1982;25:478-479.
28. McDonald DG, Leopold GR: Ultrasound B-scanning in the differentiation of Baker's cyst and thrombophlebitis. *Br J Radiol* 1972;45:729-732.
29. Moore CP, Sarti DA, Louie JS: Ultrasonographic demonstration of popliteal cysts in rheumatoid arthritis: A noninvasive technique. *Arthritis Rheum* 1975;18:577-580.
30. Hermann G, Yeh HC, Lehr-Janus C, et al: Diagnosis of popliteal cyst: double-contrast arthrography and sonography. *AJR* 1981;137:369-372.
31. Gompels BM, Darlington LG: Evaluation of popliteal cysts and painful calves with ultrasonography: comparison with arthrography. *Ann Rheum Dis* 1982;41:355-359.
32. Moss GD, Dishuk W: Ultrasound diagnosis of osteochondromatosis of the popliteal fossa. *JCU* 1984;12:232-233.

Sonography versus other imaging modalities

33. Engel J, Luboshitz SW, Israeli A, et al: Tenography in DeQuervain's disease. *Hand* 1981;13:142-146.
34. Gilula LA, Oloff L, Caputi R, et al: Ankle tenography: a key to unexplained symptomatology. Part II: Diagnosis of chronic tendon disabilities. *Radiology* 1984;151:581-587.
35. Reiser M, Rupp N, Lehner K, et al: Die Darstellung des Achillessehne in Computertomogramm. *ROFO* 1985;143:173-177.
36. Mourad K, King J, Guggiana P: Computed tomography and ultrasound imaging of jumper's knee: patellar tendinitis. *Clin Radiol* 1988;39:162-165.
37. Rosenberg ZS, Feldman F, Singson RD, et al: Ankle tendons: evaluation with computed tomography. *Radiology* 1988;166:221-226.
38. Beltran J, Mosure JC: Magnetic resonance imaging of tendons. *CRC Crit Rev Diagn Imaging* 1990;30:111-182.

CHAPTER 30

The Extracranial Cerebral Vessels

- Linda K. Brown, M.D.
- Barbara A. Carroll, M.D.

Stroke secondary to atherosclerotic disease is the third leading cause of death in the United States. From 40% to 50% of these strokes are produced by atherosclerotic disease involving the extracranial carotid arteries, usually within 2 cm of the carotid bifurcation.[1,2] For years, the diagnostic evaluation of the extracranial carotid arterial system consisted of a physical examination and conventional arteriography. More recently intraarterial digital subtraction arteriography (IADSA) has assumed this screening role, but IADSA remains invasive and expensive. Preliminary results suggest that magnetic resonance (MR) angiography can serve as a screening tool for the identification of carotid bifurcation disease,[3] but this modality remains investigational and is not widely available.

Recently, a number of less invasive, less expensive imaging techniques have been developed, which have significantly changed the diagnostic approach to suspected carotid occlusive disease. Indirect noninvasive tests involve evaluation of blood flow in the orbital and ophthalmic vessels as a means of evaluating internal carotid artery occlusive disease. Oculoplethysmography measures arterial systolic pressure in the ophthalmic arteries and analyzes differences in systolic pressures and pulse arrival times. Asymmetry of flow or significant delay in systolic pulse arrival time is indicative of a flow-limiting occlusive lesion. Periorbital bidirectional Doppler uses continuous wave Doppler instrumentation to evaluate flow in the supraorbital and supratrochlear vessels. Evaluation of the direction of flow within these vessels can be useful in defining the presence of severe occlusive disease and collateral flow formation.

Although both of these indirect tests are accurate means of detecting flow-limiting lesions in the internal carotid artery, they cannot localize the site, extent, or number of lesions, detect minimal plaque, or characterize plaque appearance.[2] Transcranial Doppler, using lower frequencies, provides indirect information concerning extracranial carotid occlusive disease and direct evidence for the presence of collateral pathways in the circle of Willis. Other transcranial applications include detection of vasospasm after subarachnoid hemorrhage, assessment of infants undergoing extracorporeal membrane oxygenation or with suspected brain death, and detection of intracranial carotid stenoses.[4-7] These indirect tests lack both the sensitivity and the specificity necessary for a screening test designed to detect a wide spectrum of extracranial carotid arterial plaque disease. Thus such indirect tests are best used in conjunction with direct noninvasive tests when the direct test results are inconclusive or confusing.

Direct noninvasive tests include continuous-wave (CW) and pulsed Doppler imaging techniques, both of which quantify the degree of stenosis present according to the peak frequency shift produced in an area of stenosis. CW Doppler employs two separate transducers, one to send and one to receive the Doppler signal. Because the transmitted Doppler signal is continuous, CW Doppler is not limited by aliasing and thus is particularly useful in detecting a wide range of frequencies. One significant limitation of CW Doppler is a lack of range resolution. If two or more vessels are in the same plane, it is not possible to ascertain with confidence the vessel from which the Doppler signal arises. Pulsed Doppler sonography allows the user to sample discrete locations within the vessel and has improved depth resolution compared with continuous wave Doppler.[2] However, to receive signals from a precise depth, a discrete pulse repetition frequency must be used, limiting the range of detectable frequencies to one half the pulse repetition frequency (PRF). If detected frequencies exceed one half the PRF, aliasing occurs.

"Duplex" ultrasound combines high-resolution real-time gray scale imaging of carotid vessels with physiologic information about blood flow provided by Doppler. There are many possible duplex instrument configurations; however, most currently available systems feature steerable Doppler capabilities and the possibility of "simultaneous" Doppler and imaging examinations. Recently the development of two-dimensional color flow Doppler imaging (CFDI) has generated a great deal of excitement. CFDI provides simultaneous viewing of blood flow and soft tissues over a large anatomic region, with flowing blood acting as a contrast agent to outline vessel flow patterns and pinpoint areas of pathology. In the carotids, as elsewhere, CFDI speeds examination time, enhances confidence of diagnoses, and produces more uniform, reproducible spectral analysis.

Carotid sonography has all the attributes necessary for a valuable screening procedure. It is relatively inexpensive, accurate, and noninvasive. It is readily performed on outpatients, and repeat examinations pose no patient risk. Ultrasound is portable, which allows the study of patients too ill to be transported to the ultrasound suite or those in the operating room. Duplex ultrasound and digital subtraction angiography have been shown to have comparable accuracies in screening for atherosclerotic occlusive disease in patients with hemispheric symptoms. Other carotid ultrasound applications include evaluation of carotid bruits, monitoring progression of known atherosclerotic disease,[8] follow-up during or after endarterectomy,[9] evaluation before major vascular surgery, and evaluation after detection of retinal cholesterol emboli.[10] Nonatherosclerotic carotid diseases can also be evaluated, including carotid dissection,[11-13] fibromuscular dysplasia, malignant carotid artery invasion,[14,15] and carotid body tumors.[16,17]

The most intensively studied application of duplex sonography has been the evaluation of atherosclerotic extracranial carotid disease. The role of vertebral duplex sonography is less well defined and more problematic.

CAROTID ARTERY ANATOMY

The first major branch of the aortic arch is the **innominate** or **brachiocephalic artery,** which divides in-

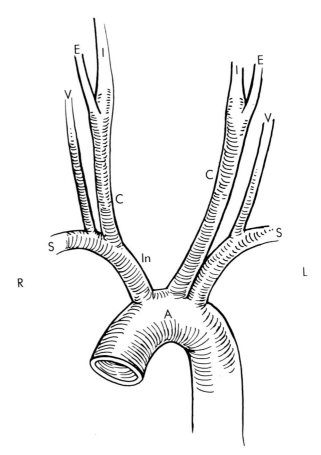

FIG 30-1. Branches of the aortic arch and extracranial cerebral arteries. *A,* Aortic arch. *In,* Innominate artery. *C,* Common carotid artery. *V,* Vertebral artery. *S,* Subclavian artery. *I,* Internal carotid artery. *E,* External carotid artery. *R,* Right side; *L,* left side.

to the **right subclavian** and **right common arteries.** The second major branch is the **left common carotid artery,** which is generally separate from the third major branch, the **left subclavian artery** (Fig. 30-1)

The common carotid arteries (CCA) ascend into the neck posterolateral to the thyroid gland and lie deep to the jugular vein and sternocleidomastoid muscle. At the carotid bifurcation, they divide into the **external carotid artery** (ECA) and the **internal carotid artery** (ICA). The ICA has no branches in the neck. The ECA, which supplies the facial musculature, has multiple branches in the neck.

EXAMINATION TECHNIQUE

Carotid artery examinations are performed with the patient supine, the neck slightly extended, and the head turned away from the side being examined. Some operators prefer to perform the examination at the patient's side, and others prefer to sit at the patient's head. The examination sequence also varies with operator preference. This sequence includes the gray-scale examination, Doppler spectral analysis, and Doppler color flow interrogations. A 5 MHz to 10 MHz transducer is used for imaging, and a 3 MHz to 7.5 MHz for Doppler, the choice depending on the patient's body habitus and technical characteristics of the ultrasound machine.

Gray-scale Examination

Gray-scale examination begins in the transverse projection. Scans are obtained along the entire course of the carotid artery from the supraclavicular notch cephalad to the angle of the mandible (Fig. 30-2, *A* and *B*). Inferior angulation of the transducer in the supraclavicular area images the CCA origin. The left CCA origin is deeper and more difficult to image consistently than the right. The **carotid bulb** is identified as a mild widening of the CCA near the bifurcation. Transverse views of the carotid bifurcation establish the orientation of the external and internal carotid arteries and help define the optimal longitudinal plane in which to perform Doppler spectral analysis. When the transverse ultrasound images demonstrate occlusive atherosclerotic disease, the percentage of diameter stenosis or area stenosis can be calculated directly using electronic calipers and software analytic algorithms available on most duplex instruments.

After transverse imaging, longitudinal scans of the extracranial carotid artery are obtained. The examination plane necessary for optimal longitudinal scans is determined by the course of the vessels demonstrated on the transverse study. In some patients the optimal longitudinal orientation will be nearly coronal, and in others it will be almost sagittal. In the majority of cases, the optimal longitudinal scan plane will be oblique, somewhere between sagittal and coronal. In approximately 60% of patients, both vessels above the carotid bifurcation and the CCA can be imaged in the same plane (Fig. 30-3); in the remainder, only a single vessel will be imaged in the same plane as the CCA. Images are obtained to display the relationship of both branches of the carotid bifurcation to visualized plaque disease, and the cephalocaudal extent of the plaque is measured. Several anatomic features differentiate the ICA from the ECA. In about 95% of patients, the ICA is posterior and lateral to the ECA. This may vary considerably, however.[9] The ICA frequently has an ampullary region of normal mild dilation just beyond its origin and is usually larger than the ECA. One reliable distinguishing feature of the ECA is identification of branching vessels. The superior thyroidal artery is often seen as the first branch of the ECA after the bifurcation. Occasionally an aberrant superior thyroidal artery branch will arise from the distal CCA. The ICA usually has no branches in the neck. In some patients a considerable amount of the ICA will be visible, but in others

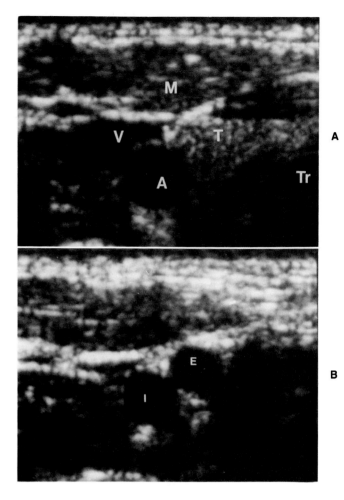

FIG 30-2. Carotid sonographic anatomy. **A,** Right transverse images demonstrate the relationship of the common carotid artery *(A)* to the internal jugular vein *(V)*, thyroid gland *(T)*, and sternocleidomastoid muscle *(M)*. *Tr,* Trachea. **B,** Carotid bifurcation just cephalic to the bulb. External carotid artery *(E)* lies anteromedial to the internal carotid artery *(I)*.

only the immediate origin of the vessel will be accessible. Very rarely, the bifurcation may not be visible at all.[18]

Doppler Spectral and Color Flow Doppler Examination

The extent of the Doppler spectral interrogation required depends on whether color flow Doppler is available. If color flow Doppler imaging (CFDI) is not available, a rapid initial Doppler spectral survey of the entire vessel is made with a wide gate covering the entire width of the vascular lumen. The Doppler gate is then narrowed to a minimum (1.5 cubic mm), and frequency or velocity spectral analysis is performed. Blood flow velocities are obtained and spectral analysis performed

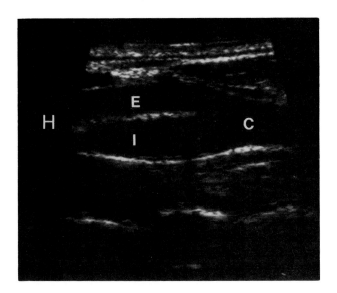

FIG 30-3. Carotid bifurcation. Longitudinal scan through a normal carotid bifurcation demonstrates the common carotid artery *(C)*, internal carotid artery *(I)*, and external carotid artery *(E)*. External carotid artery is the smaller and more anteromedial of the two vessels above the bifurcation in most individuals. *H,* Head of patient.

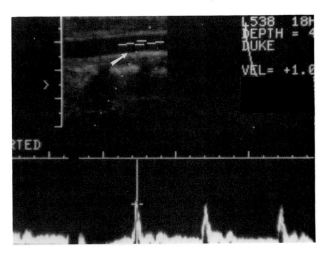

FIG 30-4. Normal Doppler waveform, common carotid artery. Angle theta *(arrow),* between the transducer line of sight *(dotted line)* and the flow vector indicator bar *(aligned parallel to the vascular lumen)* should be between 30° and 60°.

below, at, and just beyond the region of maximum visible stenosis, and at 1 cm intervals distal to the visualized plaque until the vessel becomes intracranial or the signal can no longer be obtained. Positioning the Doppler angle cursor parallel to the vessel walls determines angle theta, which is used to convert frequency information into velocity values (Fig. 30-4). Angle theta is defined as the angle between the Doppler transducer line of sight and the direction of blood flow. The ideal angle theta is 0°, as the cosine of this angle is one, thus resulting in the greatest possible detectable frequency shift. However, this angle is rarely achievable in the clinical setting. Therefore a range of angles from 30° to 60° is considered acceptable for carotid spectral analysis. When angle theta exceeds 60° to 70°, the accuracy of velocity/frequency data declines precipitously to the point where virtually no velocity change is detected at angle theta of 90°. The entire course of the CCA and ICA is interrogated in this manner, with a consistent angle theta maintained throughout the examination when possible. Generally only the origin of the ECA is evaluated, as occlusive plaque here is less common than in the ICA and is rarely clinically significant. A stenosis of the ECA should be noted, however, for it may account for a worrisome cervical bruit when the ICA is normal.[18]

Availability of color flow Doppler imaging (CFDI) technology greatly speeds spectral analysis. CFDI gives real-time flow information over a large cross-sectional area, thus providing a more global overview of areas of flow abnormality. A quick transverse and longitudinal color survey of the extracranial carotid pinpoints areas of high-velocity, disturbed flow, manifested as areas of less saturated, inhomogeneous color. Once areas of abnormal color are identified, one can switch to the duplex mode and place the pulsed Doppler sample volume in an area of color Doppler abnormality. In this fashion, the time-consuming process of pulsed Doppler spectral analysis along the entire course of a vessel can be shortened. In cases where both gray-scale and color Doppler images of an entire carotid artery are normal, only representative spectral traces from the CCA, ICA, and ECA are necessary to complete the examination.

CAROTID ULTRASOUND INTERPRETATION

Each facet of the carotid sonographic examination is valuable in the final determination of the presence and extent of disease. In most instances, the image and Doppler assessments will agree. However, when there are discrepancies between Doppler and image information, every attempt should be made to discover the source of the disagreement. The more closely the image and Doppler findings correlate, the higher the degree of confidence in the diagnosis. Generally speaking, gray-scale images better demonstrate and quantify low-grade stenoses, but high-grade occlusive disease is more accurately defined by Doppler spectral analysis. Color flow Doppler imaging (CFDI) facilitates both imaging and Doppler stenosis determinations and often explains apparent discrepancies between image and spectral Doppler information. If discrepancies cannot be explained, the final analysis should reflect the mismatch between Doppler and image information.

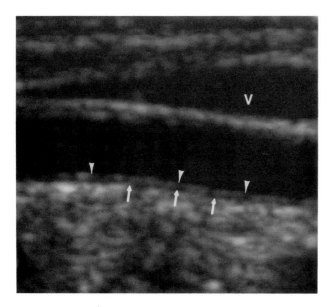

FIG 30-5. Normal common carotid artery wall thickness. Longitudinal scan shows good definition of the far wall layers. The initial bright echo along the far wall *(arrowheads)* defines the lumen-intima interface. The second echogenic line *(arrows)* represents the media-adventitia interface. *V,* Internal jugular vein. A similar set of echoes parallels the near wall.

Visual Inspection of Gray-scale Images

Vessel Wall Thickness. Longitudinal views of the layers of the normal carotid wall demonstrate two nearly parallel echogenic lines, separated by a hypoechoic to anechoic region (Fig. 30-5). The first echo, bordering the vessel lumen, represents the lumen-intima interface; the second echo is caused by the media-adventitia interface. The media is the anechoic/hypoechoic zone between the echogenic lines. The distance between these lines represents the combined thickness of the intima and media. The adventitia appears as an echogenic zone highlighted along its inner margin by the media. Widening of the distance between the lumen-intima interface and the media-adventitia interface above 1.2 mm appears to represent an abnormal finding as does focal plaque, however small, and both correlate with increased risk for subsequent cardiovascular events.[19] Thus either finding should be ranked with, and initiate a search for, other risk factors, such as hypertension, plasma concentrations of high-density lipoproteins, and family history. The clinical utility of the intimal-medial thickness measurement remains investigational, and even the anatomic basis for the double-line pattern is not without controversy; some investigators have raised the concern that this pattern represents an artifact.[19] However, many investigators believe the evaluation of this parameter may become a tool by which progression or regression of early atherosclerosis can be monitored.[20-22]

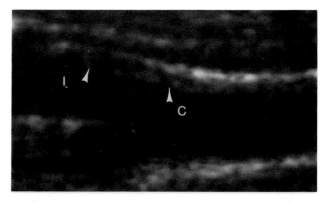

FIG 30-6. Smooth homogeneous plaque. Longitudinal scan at the bifurcation shows wall thickening extending from the common carotid artery *(C)* up into the internal carotid artery *(I) (arrowheads)*. The uniform acoustic texture corresponds pathologically to dense fibrous connective tissue.

Plaque Characterization. Atheromatous carotid plaques should be carefully evaluated to determine plaque extent and location, to assess surface contour and texture, and to measure the diameter and area of stenosis.[23] Several studies have shown that fewer than half of patients with documented transient ischemic attacks (TIAs) have hemodynamically significant carotid stenoses.[24,25] Approximately 50% to 70% of patients may have cerebrovascular symptoms related to ulcerated plaques alone, or in conjunction with hemorrhagic plaque.[26,27] Ulcerated plaques at the carotid bifurcation can be a nidus for emboli that cause both TIAs and stroke.[28,29] Plaque analysis of carotid endarterectomy specimens has implicated intraplaque hemorrhage as an important factor in the development of neurologic symptoms.[20,30-36] However, controversy exists regarding the exact relationship of these changes to symptom onset.[37,38]

Real-time gray-scale imaging is a unique noninvasive method for characterizing atherosclerotic plaque and following changes in plaque morphology.[30,39] An important step in plaque evaluation is classification of plaque texture as homogeneous or heterogeneous.[23,32] **Homogeneous plaques** usually produce a uniform echo pattern and have a smooth surface (Fig. 30-6). The uniform acoustic texture corresponds pathologically to dense fibrous connective tissue. Benign, fibrous plaques are common in asymptomatic older patients. **Calcific plaques** with characteristic acoustic shadowing are also common in the carotid arteries of asymptomatic patients and are generally stable (Fig. 30-7).[18,30] **Heterogeneous plaques,** characteristic of intraplaque hemorrhage, have a complex echo pattern that contains at least one focal sonolucent area (Fig. 30-8). The intimal surface may be smooth or irregular. The complex

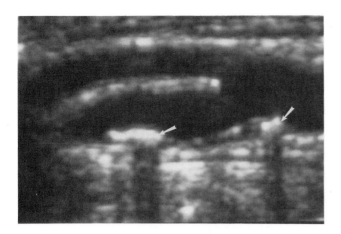

FIG 30-7. Calcific plaques *(arrows)* with acoustic shadowing are common in the carotid arteries of asymptomatic patients and are generally stable.

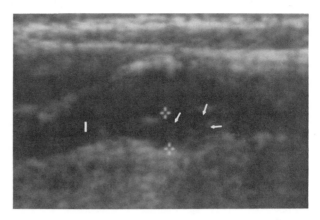

FIG 30-8. Heterogeneous plaque *(between + marks)* near the origin of the internal carotid artery *(I)*. The plaque contains several sonolucent areas *(arrows),* characteristic of intraplaque hemorrhage.

acoustic appearance is associated pathologically with the presence of intraplaque hemorrhage, clot, fibrosis, and irregular calcification. Hemorrhagic plaque is considered unstable and subject to abrupt increase in plaque size after hemorrhage. In addition, virtually all ulcerated plaques are associated with intraplaque hemorrhage. Sonography accurately determines the presence or absence of intraplaque hemorrhage (sensitivity 90% to 94%, specificity 75% to 88%).[30,36,40-42] A false-positive diagnosis of intraplaque hemorrhage may occasionally be made if there are large deposits of lipid within the plaque.[26,32]

The ability of sonography to reliably and reproducibly detect plaque ulceration is controversial.[8,26,43-46] No well-developed universally accepted criteria exist for the sonographic diagnosis of ulceration. Findings that suggest ulceration include:

- A continuous contour showing a focal depression
- A well-defined break in the plaque surface
- An anechoic area within a plaque that extends to the surface (Fig. 30-9)

In general, neither arteriography nor real-time ultrasound is highly accurate in identifying ulcerated plaque.[47,48] It is possible that CFDI may improve sonographic detection of ulceration (Fig. 30-10).[18]

Although the diagnosis of ulceration is controversial, the ability to predict reliably intraplaque hemorrhage with its associated clinical implications underscores the importance of ultrasound plaque characterization. The presence of heterogeneous, irregular plaque should always be noted, as hemorrhagic plaque in a stenosis of less than 50% may be considered a "surgical lesion" in the appropriate clinical setting.

Evaluation of Stenosis. After characterizing plaque texture and surface contour, an attempt should be made

to measure the visible stenosis. Measurements made on longitudinal scans may overestimate the severity of a stenosis by partial voluming through an eccentric plaque. Thus measurements of diameter stenosis and area stenosis should be made in the transverse plane, perpendicular to the long axis of the vessel.[23] Percentage of diameter stenosis and percentage of area stenosis are not always linearly related. Clinical records must state the type of stenosis measured. Asymmetrical stenoses are most appropriately assessed with percentage of area stenosis measurements,[23] although these measurements are

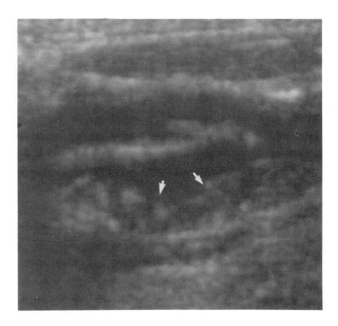

FIG 30-9. Plaque ulceration. Longitudinal view of the internal carotid artery *(I)* shows a focal contour depression *(between white arrows).*

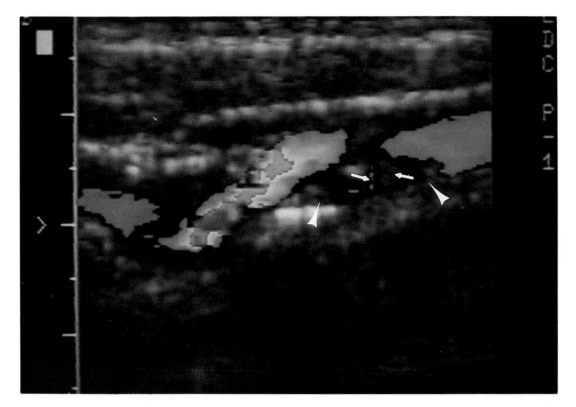

FIG 30-10. Plaque ulceration *(arrowheads)*. Longitudinal color Doppler image near the internal carotid artery *(I)* origin has an irregular contour and contains low-velocity vortices outlined by color *(arrows)* suggesting abnormal flow in ulcerated areas.

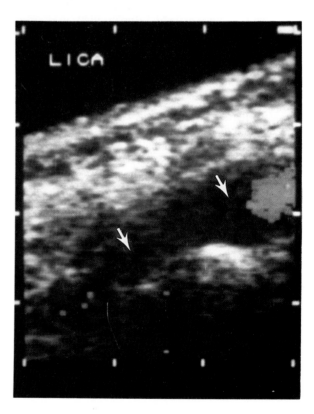

FIG 30-11. Anechoic thrombus. Longitudinal color Doppler image of the internal carotid artery demonstrates proximal flow but no flow distally because of anechoic thrombosis *(arrows)*.

often time consuming and technically difficult. The cephalocaudal extent and length of plaques should be noted as should the presence of tandem plaques.

As the severity of a stenosis increases, the quality of the real-time image deteriorates.[8,49,50] Several factors work against successful image assessment of high-grade stenosis. Plaque calcification and irregularity produce shadowing, which obscures the vessel lumen. "Soft plaque" often has acoustic properties similar to flowing blood, producing anechoic plaques or thrombi that are almost invisible. In the most extreme cases, vessels can show little visible plaque and yet be totally occluded (Fig. 30-11). Color Doppler readily identifies such occlusive phenomena. For these reasons, real-time gray-scale ultrasound is best suited for the evaluation of non–rate-limiting lesions, and not for quantifying high-grade stenoses, which are more accurately determined by spectral and color flow Doppler.[46,51] In fact, sonography is probably the best method for imaging minimal, early atherosclerotic changes, which may go undetected at arteriography.

Spectral Analysis

Normal Doppler Spectrum. The Doppler spectrum is a quantitative graphic display of the velocities and directions of moving red blood cells present in the Doppler sample volume. Although Doppler assessment of carotid occlusive disease can be performed using frequency data, velocity calculations are preferable.[52] Velocity values are potentially more accurate than frequency shift measurements, because angle theta between the transducer line of sight and the blood flow vector (Fig. 30-4) is used to convert a frequency shift to velocity. Frequency shifts vary according to the angle theta and the incident Doppler frequency; velocity measurements take both these factors into account. In addition, velocity values readily translate from transducer to transducer and machine to machine. This allows universal standardization of Doppler spectral analysis.

The Doppler spectral display represents velocities on the *y* axis and time on the *x* axis (Fig. 30-12). By convention, flow toward the transducer is displayed above the zero velocity baseline, and flow away from the transducer is below. For ease of spectral analysis, spec-

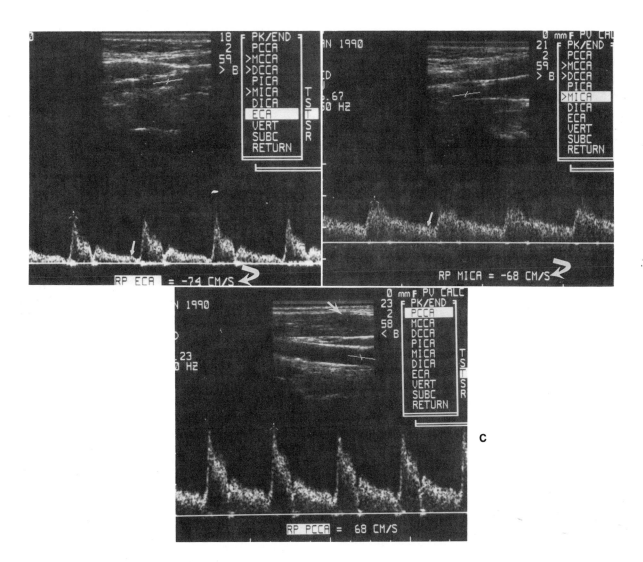

FIG 30-12. Normal Doppler spectral waveforms. **A,** The external carotid artery *(ECA)* shows low-velocity flow in diastole *(arrow),* indicating a high-impedance circulation. **B,** The internal carotid artery *(ICA)* has high diastolic flow *(arrow)* associated with the low impedance of the cerebral vasculature. **C,** Common carotid artery *(CCA)* waveform is a composite of the external and internal carotid arteries. Note that in **C,** flow is toward the transducer *(arrow)* and the Doppler spectrum is plotted above the baseline. In **A** and **B,** flow is directed away from the transducer. Although these spectra have been inverted (placed above the baseline), the negative velocity *(curved arrow)* values remind the operator of the true direction of flow away from the transducer.

tra that project below the baseline are often inverted and placed above the baseline, always keeping in mind the true direction of flow within the vessel. The amplitude of each velocity component [the number of red blood cells (RBCs) with each velocity component] is used to modulate the brightness of the traces. This is also known as a gray-scale velocity plot. In the normal carotid artery, the frequency spectrum is narrow in systole and somewhat wider in early and late diastole. There is usually a black zone between the spectral line and the zero velocity baseline called the "spectral window."[53,54]

The internal carotid (ICA) and external carotid (ECA) branches of the common carotid artery (CCA) have distinctive spectral waveforms. The ECA supplies the high resistance vascular bed of the facial musculature; thus its flow resembles that of other peripheral arterial vessels. Flow velocity rises sharply during systole and falls rapidly in diastole, approaching zero or transiently reversing direction (Fig. 30-12, A). The ICA supplies the low-resistance circulation of the brain and demonstrates flow similar to that in vessels supplying other blood-hungry organs, such as the liver, kidneys, and placenta. The common feature in all low-resistance arterial waveforms is that a large quantity of forward flow continues throughout diastole (Fig. 30-12, B). The CCA waveform is a composite of the internal and external waveforms, but most often the common carotid more closely resembles the internal carotid flow pattern, and diastolic flow is generally above the baseline. Approximately 80% of the blood flowing from the CCA goes through the ICA into the brain, whereas 20% goes through the ECA into the facial musculature. The relative decrease in blood flow through the ECA will cause it to have a generally lower amplitude gray-scale waveform than that found in either the ICA or the CCA.[9]

Spectral Broadening. Atheromatous plaque projecting into the arterial lumen disturbs the normal, smooth laminar flow of erythrocytes. The RBCs move with a wider range of velocities, so the spectral line becomes wider, filling in the normally black spectral window (Figs. 30-13 and 30-14). This phenomenon is termed "spectral broadening." Spectral broadening increases in proportion to the severity of carotid artery stenosis, and a number of schemes have been derived to measure this parameter.[52,55-57] Some duplex machines allow the operator to measure the spectral spread between the maximum and minimum velocities (bandwidth), and thus quantitate spectral broadening. The validity of these measurements remains to be proven, however, and further correlative studies are needed to document the relationship of quantitative spectral broadening parameters to specific degrees of stenosis.[52] Nevertheless, a visible "gestalt" of the amount of spectral window obliteration, as well as color Doppler heterogeneity, provides a useful, if not quantitative, predictor of the severity of flow disturbance.

Pitfalls. "Pseudo-spectral-broadening" can be caused by technical factors, such as too high a **gain setting.** In such instances the background around the spectral

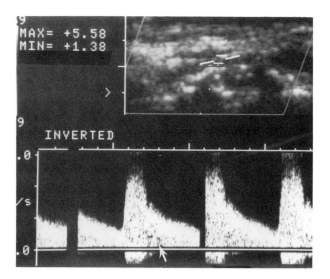

FIG 30-14. Stenosis of 80% to 99% of the internal carotid artery *(ICA)*. Peak systolic velocity is 558 cm/sec. Note obliteration of the spectral window *(arrow)* indicating "turbulence" associated with the more severe stenosis. The diastolic velocity (138 cm/sec) is also abnormally elevated with this severe stenosis. "Inverted" means flow is directed away from the transducer; the spectrum has been inverted and placed above the baseline for ease of spectral analysis.

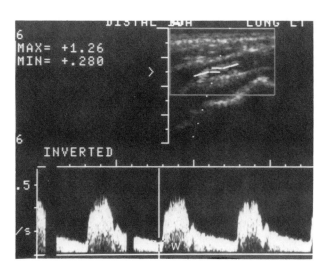

FIG 30-13. Stenosis of 40% to 59% of the internal carotid artery *(ICA)*. High-velocity blood flow patterns in stenotic vessels. High peak systolic velocity (126 cm/sec). Diastolic velocity is normal. *W,* Spectral window.

waveform often contains noise. Whenever spectral broadening is suspected, the gain should be lowered to see if the spectral window clears. Similarly, spectral broadening caused by **vessel wall motion** can occur when the Doppler sample volume is too large or positioned too near the vessel wall. Decreasing the size of the sample volume and placing it midstream should eliminate this potential pitfall.

Altered flow patterns can be found **normally at certain sites** in the carotid system. For instance, it is normal to find flow separation at the site of branching vessels, such as where the CCA branches into the ECA and ICA.[58] Flow disturbances also occur at sites where there is an **abrupt change in the vessel diameter.** For instance, spectral broadening may be encountered in a normal carotid bulb where the CCA terminates in a localized area of dilation as it divides into the ECA and ICA.[9]

The tendency for spectral broadening to occur increases in direct proportion to the velocity of blood flow. For example, it can be observed in normal ECAs, vertebral arteries, and in a CCA that is supplying collateral circulation contralateral to an occluded contralateral ICA. **Increased velocity** may also account for the disturbed flow that is sometimes observed in the normal extracranial carotid arteries of young athletes with normal cardiac outputs or in patients in pathologic high cardiac output states. It is also seen in arteries supplying **arteriovenous fistulas** and **arteriovenous malformations.**[9,59] Postoperative spectral broadening may persist for months **after carotid endarterectomy** in the absence of significant residual or recurrent disease. This may be due to changes in wall compliance.

Tortuous carotid vessels can demonstrate spectral broadening in the absence of plaque disease. Other nonatheromatous causes of disturbed blood flow in the extracranial carotid arteries include **aneurysms, arterial wall dissections,** and **fibromuscular dysplasia.**[9]

Spectral broadening suggests vascular disease; however, correlation with gray-scale and color Doppler images can define the cause of spectral broadening. An awareness of normal flow spectra combined with appropriate Doppler techniques can obviate many potential diagnostic pitfalls.

High-velocity Blood Flow Patterns. Carotid lesions generally begin to reduce blood flow when they decrease vessel diameter by more than 50% (70% cross-sectional area reduction). Flow then decreases gradually until the critical level of 70% diameter reduction (90% area reduction) is reached, beyond which there is a precipitous decrease in flow.[51,60] Clinical investigations suggest that the risk of stroke resulting from compromised blood flow produced by a high-grade stenosis (not embolic stroke) does not increase until stenoses exceed 75% to 80% in diameter. Thus it is important to distinguish these very-high-grade stenoses from other "hemodynamically significant" lesions.[52] It should be noted that the "hemodynamic significance" of a lesion in a supine, resting patient is difficult to ascertain.

In general, flow velocities increase in a stenotic area in proportion to the degree of luminal compromise. These velocity increases are focal and most pronounced in and immediately distal to a stenosis, emphasizing the importance of sampling directly in these regions (Fig. 30-14). As one moves further distal from a stenosis, flow begins to reconstitute and assume a more normal pattern, provided a tandem lesion does not exist distal to the initial site of stenosis. Systolic and diastolic velocity measurements are the foundation for accurate assessment of stenotic lesions by Doppler.[52] **Peak systolic velocity** has proven accurate for quantifying high-grade stenoses.[52,60] The relationship of this parameter to the degree of luminal narrowing is well defined, and it is easily measured and reproducible.[60,61] More recent work suggests that measurements of **peak end diastolic velocity, peak systolic ICA/CCA ratios,** and **peak**

■ **TABLE 30-1**
Doppler Spectrum Analysis

Diameter Stenosis	ICA/CCA Peak Systolic Velocity Ratio	ICA/CCA Peak Diastolic Velocity Ratio	Peak Systolic Velocity	Peak End-Diastolic Velocity
0-40%	<1.5	<2.6	<110 cm/sec > 25 cm/sec	<40 cm/sec
41-59%	<1.8	<2.6	>120 cm/sec	<40 cm/sec
60-79%	>1.8	>2.6	>130 cm/sec	>40 cm/sec
·80-99%	>3.7	>5.5	>250 cm/sec < 25 cm/sec	>80-135 cm/sec
Occlusion			Unilateral damped flow in CCA. No flow or reversed flow proximal to ICA occlusion.	

end diastolic ICA/CCA ratios are also reliable parameters for measurement of hemodynamically significant stenoses.[52,60-62] End-diastolic velocity ratios have proven particularly useful in distinguishing between degrees of high-grade stenosis.[63] Table 30-1 is a composite of numerous published Doppler criteria for determining carotid artery stenoses.[23,57,64-68]

Pitfalls. Although absolute velocity determinations are valuable in assessing the degree of vascular stenosis, there are times when these measurements are less reliable.[52,69] Variations in cardiovascular physiology may affect carotid velocity measurements.[70] For instance, velocities produced by a stenosis in a **hypertensive patient** will be higher than those in a normotensive individual with a comparable narrowing. On the other hand, a **reduction in cardiac output** will diminish both systolic and diastolic velocities. **Cardiac arrhythmias, aortic valvular lesions,** and **severe cardiomyopathies** can cause significant aberrations in the shape of carotid flow waveforms and alter systolic and diastolic velocity readings (Fig. 30-15) These alterations can invalidate the use of standard Doppler parameters to quantify stenoses. **Bradycardia,** for example, produces increased stroke volume, causing systolic velocities to increase, but prolonged diastolic run-off causes spuriously decreased end diastolic values.

Color Doppler can be used to overcome diagnostic dilemmas in these situations, particularly when "cine loop" playback capabilities are present. Cine loop allows the computer to store up to 10 seconds of the previous color flow Doppler recording for playback at the real-time rate or frame-by-frame. This allows one to assess filling of all parts of the vessel lumen. **Obstructive lesions** in one carotid can **affect** velocities in the con-

tralateral vessel. For instance, severe unilateral ICA stenosis or occlusion may cause shunting of increased flow through the contralateral carotid system (Fig. 30-16). This increased flow artificially increases velocity measurements in the contralateral vessel, particularly in areas of stenosis.[71] Conversely, a proximal common carotid or innominate artery stenosis may reduce flow, with consequent reduction of velocity measurements in a stenosis that is distal to the point of obstruction (**tandem lesion**).

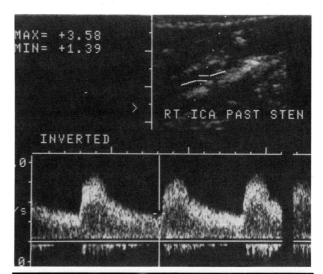

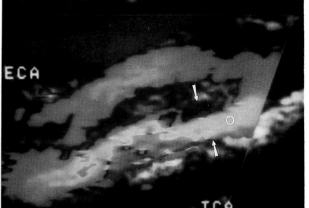

FIG 30-16. High-grade stenosis in left ICA (contralateral) causes spurious velocity elevation in the right ICA. **A,** Markedly elevated peak systolic velocity, just beyond the right internal carotid artery *(ICA)* stenosis (358 cm/sec) corresponds with 80% to 99% stenosis. This velocity value is invalid because the extreme stenosis of the left contralateral ICA increases flow to the right side. **B,** Longitudinal color Doppler image of moderate stenosis of the origin of the right ICA *(O)* demonstrates a moderate atheromatous plaque anteriorly and a residual color-filled lumen *(arrows)*. Color inhomogeneity beyond the stenotic zone shows "turbulence" associated with stenosis and color aliasing because of high velocities. Angiography confirmed right ICA stenosis (40% to 59% range).

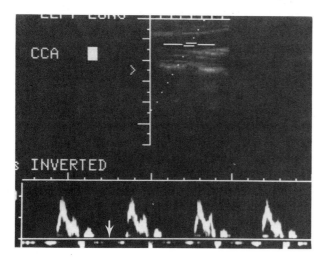

FIG 30-15. Severe aortic insufficiency *(AI)*. Left CCA spectral analysis demonstrates a grossly disturbed pattern with diastolic flow reversal and absent end diastolic flow *(arrow)*.

Velocity ratios that compare velocity values in the ICA to those in the ipsilateral CCA can help avoid some pitfalls.[52] Of particular value are the peak systolic ratio (peak systolic velocity in the ICA stenosis/peak systolic velocity in the common carotid)[57,68] and the end-diastolic ratio (end-diastolic velocity in the ICA stenosis/end-diastolic velocity in the common carotid).[63] Velocity ratios corresponding to specific degrees of vascular stenosis are listed in Table 30-1. Values obtained in the ICA should be obtained at or just distal to the point of maximum visible stenosis and/or at the point of greatest color Doppler spectral abnormality. Values obtained from the CCA should be obtained proximal to the widening in the region of the carotid bulb. Velocity ratios should always be employed when unusually high or low common carotid velociters or significant assemetry of common carotid velocities is detected. As discussed in the previous section on **spectral broadening,** color flow Doppler is invaluable in the avoidance of pitfalls related to spurious Doppler spectral traces.

Although high-grade stenoses usually produce increased velocity in the region of a plaque and distal to it, high-grade intracranial or extracranial occlusive lesions in tandem may reduce anticipated velocity shifts. Vessels should be examined as far cephalad as possible to avoid missing a distal "tandem" lesion. Flow immediately distal to stenosis of over 95% is often damped and decreased in velocity. High-grade vascular narrowings, particularly those of a circumferential nature, that occur over a long segment of a vessel, may also produce damped waveforms without a high-velocity frequency shift (Fig. 30-17). Although no definite velocity elevations are present in such a long circumferential narrowing, spectral broadening and disturbed flow distal to such a narrowing is usually apparent. In addition, the fusiform narrowing is usually detected with the real-time image, particularly if color flow Doppler is employed.

Another source of error in pulsed Doppler ultrasound analysis is **aliasing,** which is caused by the inability to detect the true peak velocity because the Doppler sampling rate (pulse repetition frequency, PRF) is too low. A classic visual example of aliasing can be seen in western films, with the apparent reversal of stage coach wheel spokes when the wagon wheel rotations exceed the film frame rate. The maximum detectable frequency shift can be no greater than half the PRF. With aliasing, the tips of the time velocity spectrum (representing high velocities) are cut off and wrap around to appear below the baseline (Fig. 30-18). If aliasing occurs, **continuous wave probes** used in conjunction with duplex pulsed Doppler can readily demonstrate the true peak velocity shift. Aliasing can also be overcome or decreased by **increasing angle theta** (the angle of Doppler insonation), thereby reducing the detected Doppler shift, or by decreasing the insonating sound beam frequency. **Increasing the PRF** increases the detectable frequency shift, but the PRF increase is limited by the depth of the vessel as well as the center frequency of the transducer.[23,54] One can also **shift the zero baseline** and reassign a larger range of velocities to forward flow to overcome aliasing. It is also valid to **add velocity values above and below the baseline** to obtain an

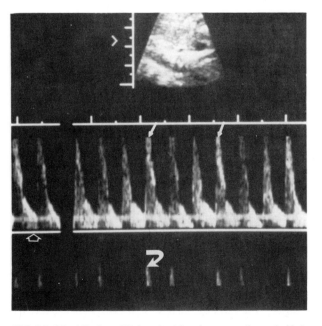

FIG 30-18. Aliasing. High velocities that exceed one half the pulse repetition frequency (PRF) are cut off *(arrows)* and wrapped around *(arrowhead)* to appear below the baseline *(curved arrow)* in reversed direction. The tips of the aliased signals point toward the baseline *(open arrow),* which is the opposite of the waveform for a true flow reversal.

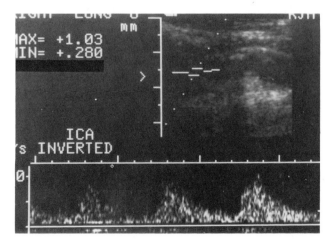

FIG 30-17. Flow distal to a 95% ICA stenosis shows a spectral Doppler trace with an abnormal waveform shapes but no significant velocity elevation.

accurate velocity value, provided multiple wraparounds do not occur, as seen in extremely high velocities. Aliasing may sometimes be useful in color Doppler image interpretation, where color flow Doppler aliasing can accent the severity of flow disturbances as well as define the patent lumen.

Internal Carotid Artery (ICA) Occlusion. Occlusion is diagnosed when no flow is detected in a vessel. A high-grade ICA stenosis or occlusion usually causes an asymmetric, high-impedance signal in the ipsilateral CCA and ICA proximal to the lesion,[72,73] with decreased, absent, or reversed diastolic flow (Fig. 30-19), except when there is ECA collateralization to the intracranial circulation.

Pitfalls. Although accuracy is high for predicting degrees of minimal to severe stenosis, pulsed Doppler and gray-scale sonography are less accurate in differentiating occlusion from severe stenosis.[72,74-76] As a stenosis approaches occlusion, the high-velocity jet is reduced to a mere trickle. Many pulsed Doppler systems are not able to detect this low-amplitude, very slow flow (2 to 4 cm/sec). It may also be very difficult to locate the **small residual lumen,** particularly if the adjacent plaque or thrombus is anechoic, making the residual lumen invisible during real-time examination, or calcified, obscuring visualization. Color flow Doppler systems and use of slower flow rate detection capabilities facilitate more accurate diagnosis of occlusion and allow easier identi-

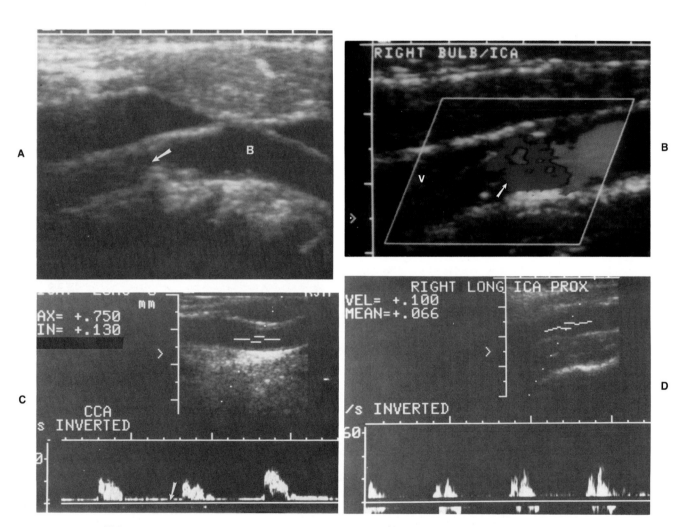

FIG 30-19. Internal carotid artery *(ICA)* occlusion. **A,** Longitudinal gray-scale image of the ICA demonstrates thrombus filling the ICA lumen *(arrow),* suggesting occlusion. *B,* Bulb. **B,** Color Doppler shows flow reversal *(blue)* immediately proximal *(arrow)* to the lesion with no residual channel of flow in the lesion, indicating occlusion. **C,** Damped spectral waveform in the CCA proximal to the occlusion. Note markedly diminished diastolic flow *(arrow),* indicating high resistance. **D,** Damped spectral waveform in ICA proximal to the occlusion, tracing above and below the baseline, indicates bidirectional flow.

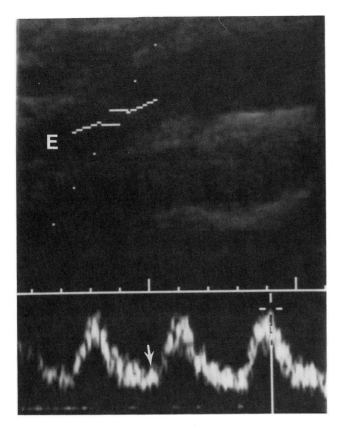

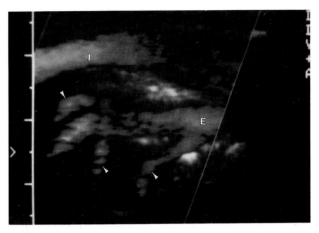

FIG 30-21. The ICA *(I)* and ECA *(E)*, superior to the bifurcation. Longitudinal view color flow Doppler facilitates visualization of ECA branches *(arrowheads)*.

FIG 30-20. Low-resistance flow waveform in an ECA *(E)* that is providing collateral circulation to the brain around an occluded ICA. Note increased end-diastolic flow *(arrow)*.

fication of a residual "string" of flow through a tight stenosis. Still, 100% accuracy is important in this setting as complete ICA occlusion is usually inoperable, but potential for restoration of normal circulation exists if even a small amount of residual flow remains. Thus, angiography is warranted in any person who is an operative candidate who has an apparent ICA occlusion on ultrasound examination.

Another pitfall in the diagnosis of a totally occluded ICA is **mistaking a patent ECA or one of its branches for the ICA.** The situation is especially confusing when ECA/ICA collaterals open in response to longstanding ICA disease and the ECA acquires low-resistance flow characteristics (Fig. 30-20). One technique that can identify the ECA is scanning at the origin of the vessel while simultaneously tapping the temporal artery. This maneuver may alter flow in the ECA, whereas the ICA is unaffected.[49] As discussed previously in this chapter, branching vessels are a unique feature of the ECA that can also assist in its differentiation from the ICA. Color flow Doppler can facilitate the identification of such branching vessels (Fig. 30-21).

Another pitfall in the evaluation of potential ICA occlusion is **transmitted pulsations.** The Doppler cursor must be clearly located in the ICA lumen and pulsatile flow identified. Close attention must be paid to the direction of flow and the nature of pulsations. True center stream sampling should be documented by transverse scanning and the sample volume reduced in size as much as possible. Extraneous pulsations should seldom be transmitted to the center of a thrombus.[49]

Although distal propagation almost invariably occurs with ICA occlusions, CCA occlusions are often localized. Flow may be maintained in the ECA and ICA but must be reversed in one of the two vessels. Most commonly, retrograde flow in the ECA will supply the ICA (Fig. 30-22). Occasionally, the opposite will be encountered.[49,77,78]

Color Flow Doppler Imaging

Normal Color Flow Doppler Examination. Color flow Doppler has been quickly incorporated into routine diagnostic carotid imaging algorithms.[11,79-88] Color flow Doppler imaging displays flow information in real time over the entire image or a selected area. Stationary soft-tissue structures, which lack phase shifts or frequency shifts, are assigned an amplitude value and displayed in a gray-scale format, with flowing blood in vessels superimposed in color.

Color assignment depends on the direction of blood flow relative to the Doppler transducer. Blood flow toward the transducer appears in one color and flow away from the transducer appears in another. Color assignment is arbitrary and is generally set up so that arterial flow is red and venous flow is blue. Color saturation indicates the velocity of blood flow. Deeper shades indicate low velocities. As velocity increases, the shades become lighter. Some systems allow selected frequency

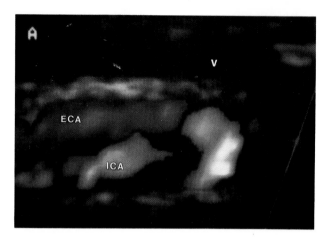

FIG 30-22. Retrograde flow in ECA because of common carotid artery occluded by surgical clamp, used in treating a carotid aneurysm. Longitudinal color Doppler image of the carotid bifurcation demonstrates retrograde flow in the ECA *(blue)* supplying the antegrade ICA *(red)*, flow. *V,* Jugular vein.

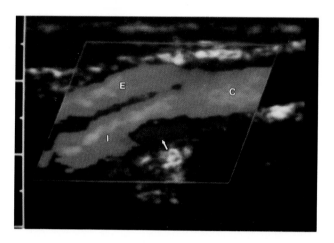

FIG 30-23. Normal longitudinal color Doppler image of the carotid bifurcation. Flow reversal zone blue area *(arrow)* appears at early systole or peak systole and persists variable amounts of time into diastole. *I,* ICA; *C,* CCA; *E,* ECA.

shifts to be featured in a contrasting color, such as green. This "green-tag" feature provides a real-time estimation of the presence of high-velocity flow. Color is a function of the mean frequency shift produced by moving RBCs and angle theta. If a vessel is tortuous or diving, angle theta will change along the course of the vessel, resulting in changing color assignments that are unrelated to a change in RBC velocity. Furthermore, color assignments will reverse in tortuous vessels if their course changes relative to the Doppler transducer, even though the absolute direction of flow is unchanged. If a portion of a vessel parallels the Doppler beam, angle theta is 90°, so little or no frequency shift will be detected and no color will be seen.

Color Doppler studies should be performed with optimal flow sensitivity and gain settings. Color flow should fill the entire vessel lumen but not spill over into adjacent soft tissues. PRF and frame rates should allow visualization of flow phenomena anticipated in a vessel. Frame rates will vary as a function of the width of the area chosen for color Doppler display as well as the depth of the region of interest. The greater the color image area, the slower the frame rate will be. The deeper the posterior boundary of the color image, the slower the PRF. Color Doppler sensitivity should be adjusted to detect anticipated velocities, that is, if slow flow in a preocclusive carotid lesion is sought, low flow settings with decreased sampling rates can be employed. However, the system will then alias at lower velocities because of the decrease in PRF.

With real-time color Doppler imaging, flowing blood becomes in effect its own contrast medium and outlines the patent vessel lumen (Fig. 30-21). This allows deter-

mination of the true course of a vessel with appropriate positioning of angle theta and thus more reliable velocity determinations. Color Doppler allows rapid identification of branches of the external carotid, which facilitates differentiation of the external carotid from the internal carotid, especially if the internal carotid is completely occluded.

As mentioned previously, the laminar flow of blood is disrupted at the carotid bifurcation, and there is normally a transient reversal of flow opposite the origin of the external carotid artery. This normal flow separation is graphically displayed with color Doppler as a blue area located along the outer wall of the bulb, which appears either at early systole or at peak systole and persists for a variable amount of time into the diastolic portion of the cardiac cycle (Fig. 30-23).[87,89] It has been suggested that the absence of this flow reversal is abnormal and may represent one of the earliest changes of atherosclerotic disease. Failure to demonstrate this normal flow reversal should prompt a careful search for subtle plaques at the origin of the internal carotid artery.[87]

Abnormal Color Flow Doppler Examination. Color Doppler delineates the patent vessel lumen. Subtle vessel wall irregularities and hypoechoic plaque are often better visualized with color Doppler than with gray-scale imaging alone (Fig. 30-24). Color Doppler may demonstrate eddying flow in ulcerations within hypoechoic plaques that is not appreciated with conventional gray-scale imaging (Fig. 30-10). Normal flow separation seen in vessel bifurcations, as well as in tortuous vessels, can be readily separated from that associated with plaque disease using color Doppler.

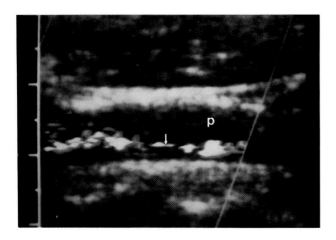

FIG 30-24. High-grade stenosis. Longitudinal color Doppler image of the ICA demonstrates a large amount of plaque *(P)* and a small residual lumen *(arrow)* with white areas indicating high-velocity flow.

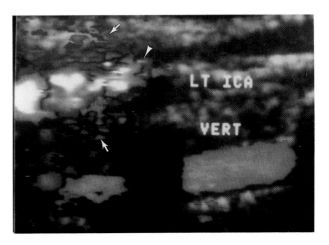

FIG 30-25. Perivascular color artifact distal to ICA stenosis *(arrowhead).* A random localized mixture of red and blue colors in the perivascular soft tissues *(arrows),* resulting from tissue vibration from "turbulent" intravascular blood flow.

Doppler spectral analysis is facilitated by color Doppler because it rapidly identifies flow abnormalities. The highest color shifts can be identified quickly. Then the Doppler gate can be positioned in the region of color abnormality. Color jets define not only the presence of high-velocity flow, but its direction. This facilitates optimal spectral analysis with CFDI-directed angle-theta corrections. The presence of a stenosis can be inferred by color changes in the vessel lumen as well as by visible luminal narrowing. If the stenosis causes a bruit or thrill, the resultant perivascular tissue vibration may actually be visualized with color Doppler as it causes artifactual transient speckles of red and blue color in the tissues adjacent to the stenosis during systole (Fig. 30-25).[79,90] The artifact is most prominent in systole and absent or less prominent in diastole.[90] Preliminary comparisons of color flow Doppler with conventional duplex sampling techniques and angiography show similar accuracy, sensitivity, and specificity.[81-83] However, CFDI improves confidence in diagnosis by clarifying confusing situations, such as those that arise from apparent conflicts between Doppler and gray-scale image information. In addition, use of CFDI to direct Doppler spectral analysis improves the reproducibility of the Doppler examination results.[81]

One must be cautious not to equate color saturation with velocity.[79] The color image is corrected for only one angle regardless of the course of the artery. For instance, white or "green-tagged" flow in a vessel may represent abnormal high-velocity flow or simply may represent a region of flow directed at a more acute angle relative to the transducer. Doppler spectral sampling remains necessary for precise quantification of hemody-namically significant stenoses. Color systems generally compute the mean velocity to produce each color pixel in the image. However, the examiner is usually interested in determining the maximum velocity rather than the mean velocity caused by a stenosis.

Many potential **pitfalls** exist when flow velocity is the primary criterion used in the evaluation for stenoses. Alterations in cardiovascular physiology or obstructive lesions in the ipsilateral or contralateral carotid or vertebral arteries can lead to both overestimates and underestimates of the percentage of stenosis (Fig. 30-16). In such cases, CFDI can provide a direct image of the percentage of stenosis in a fashion analogous to angiography.[84] In fact, since angiography images only the vessel lumen, not the vessel wall, color flow Doppler imaging has the potential to evaluate stenoses even more completely than angiography. Furthermore, since flow patterns are displayed with color Doppler imaging, the local hemodynamic consequences of a lesion can be estimated (Fig. 30-26).[86] Difficulties in determining angle theta in tortuous vessels or vessels that dive deeply can result in inaccurate velocity calculations. Display of the length of the vessel in color allows more accurate selection of the Doppler angle for velocity determinations.

Color Doppler appears to have particular value in detecting small channels of flow in areas of tight carotid stenosis (Fig. 30-27).[81,83,84,86,88] These can be easily missed with duplex scanning if the sample volume is not placed in the precise location of the channel, resulting in the misdiagnosis of complete occlusion when a surgically correctable high-grade stenosis is actually present. In critical high-grade stenosis (90%+), with

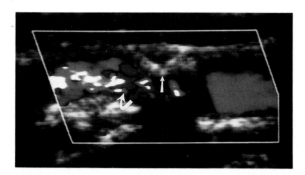

FIG 30-26. Disturbed flow *(curved arrow)* in the ICA distal to a calcified plaque *(straight arrow)* indicates a significant stenosis. Longitudinal color Doppler scan of bifurcation with posterior acoustic shadows, which obscure the vascular lumen at the ICA origin.

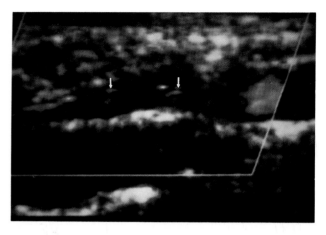

FIG 30-27. Residual "string" of flow *(arrows)* within a long high-grade ICA stenosis. Longitudinal color Doppler scan of the ICA.

markedly damped distal internal carotid artery velocities, standard sensitivity color Doppler settings may fail to demonstrate residual flow. Thus it is always prudent to employ the "slow flow" sensitivity settings to discriminate between critical stenosis and occlusion.[83,84]

Complete occlusion of a vessel is diagnosed when no color flow is identified.[86] Early diastolic flow reversal can be seen at the orifice of an occluded internal carotid artery (Fig. 30-19).[84] The presence of high-grade ICA stenosis or occlusion can often be inferred from inspection of the ipsilateral common carotid artery color Doppler image. This will often show color flow in systole but a conspicuous decrease or absence of color flow in diastole, which is asymmetric compared with the contralateral side.[83,84] The corresponding Doppler waveform shows markedly decreased or completely absent diastolic flow. Experience in the diagnosis of occlusion with color Doppler is limited. Although it promises to facilitate differentiation of high-grade stenosis from occlusion, 100% accuracy has not been documented. Thus, at present, arteriography is still needed to distinguish occlusion from critical stenosis in a patient who is a candidate for operation.

NONATHEROSCLEROTIC CAROTID DISEASE

Nonatherosclerotic carotid disease is far less common than plaque disease. **Fibromuscular dysplasia** (FMD), a noninflammatory process with hypertrophy of muscular and fibrous arterial walls, separated by abnormal zones of fragmentation, involves the internal carotid artery more commonly than other carotid segments. A characteristic "string of beads" appearance has been described on angiography. FMD can be asymptomatic or can result in carotid dissection. In such cases an intimal flap may be seen sonographically. **Arteritis,** resulting from autoimmune processes, such

as Takayasu arteritis or temporal arteritis, or radiation changes can produce diffuse concentric thickening of carotid walls, which most frequently involves the common carotid artery. **Cervical trauma** can produce carotid dissection or aneurysms.

Carotid body tumors, one of several paragangliomas that involve the head and neck, are usually benign, well-encapsulated masses located at the carotid bifurcation. These tumors may be bilateral and are very vascular, often producing a bruit. Some may produce catecholamines, producing sudden changes in blood pressure postoperatively (Fig. 30-28). **Extravascular masses,** such as tumors, hematomas, or abscesses, that compress or displace the carotids can be readily distinguished from primary vascular masses, such as aneurysms.

VERTEBRAL ARTERY

The vertebral arteries supply the majority of the posterior brain circulation. Via the circle of Willis, they also provide collateral circulation to other portions of the brain in cases of carotid occlusive disease. Evaluation of the extracranial vertebral artery seems a natural extension of carotid duplex and color Doppler imaging.[91,92] Historically, however, these arteries have not been studied as intensively as the carotids. The many anatomic variations of normal vertebral arteries, along with the fact that they join to form the basilar artery, make the diagnosis of vertebral disease difficult by any modality. Symptoms of vertebrobasilar insufficiency also tend to be rather vague and poorly defined, compared with symptoms referable to the carotid circulation. It is often difficult to make an association confidently between a lesion and symptoms. Furthermore, there has been relatively limited interest in surgical

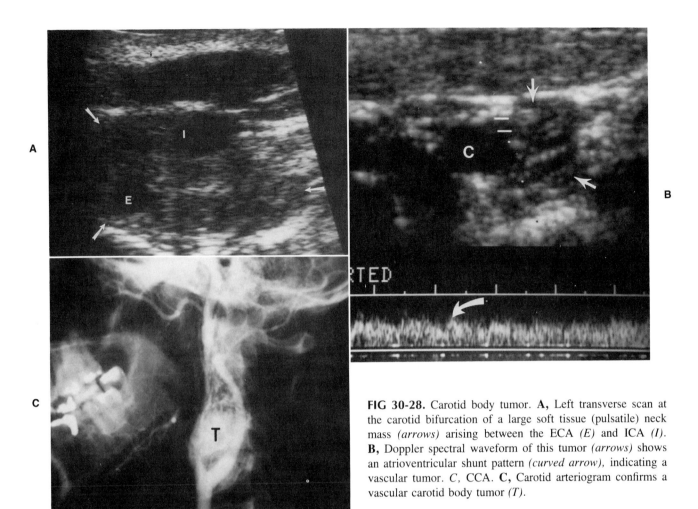

FIG 30-28. Carotid body tumor. **A,** Left transverse scan at the carotid bifurcation of a large soft tissue (pulsatile) neck mass *(arrows)* arising between the ECA *(E)* and ICA *(I)*. **B,** Doppler spectral waveform of this tumor *(arrows)* shows an atrioventricular shunt pattern *(curved arrow)*, indicating a vascular tumor. *C,* CCA. **C,** Carotid arteriogram confirms a vascular carotid body tumor *(T)*.

correction of vertebral lesions.[18] Finally, the small size, deep course, and limited visualization resulting from overlying transverse processes make the vertebral artery more difficult to examine accurately with ultrasound.[92-94] The clinical utility of vertebral duplex scanning remains under investigation. Its role in diagnosing subclavian steal is well established.[18,84,95,96] Less clear cut is the use of vertebral duplex scanning in evaluating vertebral artery stenosis and occlusion.[18,95] Vertebral duplex scanning can also visualize vertebral artery aneurysms and dissections,[97,98] but again, clinical utility has not been established for such applications.

Anatomy

The vertebral artery is usually the first branch off of the subclavian artery (Fig. 30-29). Variation in the origin of the vertebral arteries is common, however. In 6% to 8% of cases, the left vertebral artery arises directly from the aortic arch proximal to the left subclavian artery. In 90% of people, the proximal vertebral artery as-

cends superomedially, passing anterior to the transverse process of C7, and enters the transverse foramen at the C6 level. The remainder of vertebral arteries enter into the transverse foramina at the C5 or C7 level and, rarely, at the C4 level. Size of vertebral arteries is variable, with the left larger than the right in 42% of cases, the two vertebral arteries equal in size in 26% of cases, and the right larger than the left in 32% of cases.[99] One vertebral artery may even be congenitally absent.

Technique and Normal Examination

Vertebral artery visualization with Doppler flow analysis can be obtained in 92% to 98% of vessels.[93,100] Color Doppler facilitates rapid detection of vertebral arteries, but does not significantly improve this detection rate.[101] Vertebral artery duplex examinations are performed by first locating the common carotid in the longitudinal plane. The direction of flow in the common carotid artery and jugular vein is determined. A gradual sweep of the transducer laterally demonstrates the ver-

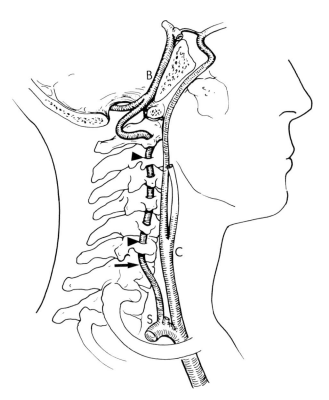

FIG 30-29. Vertebral artery *(arrow)* lateral diagram shows its course through the cervical spine transverse foramina *(arrowheads)* en route to joining the contralateral vertebral artery to form the basilar artery *(B). C,* Carotid artery; *S,* subclavian artery.

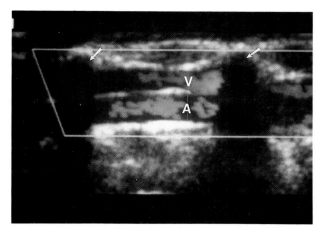

FIG 30-30. Normal vertebral artery *(A)* and vein *(V).* Longitudinal color Doppler shows the vertebral artery and vein running between the transverse processes of C2-C6, which are identified by their periodic acoustical shadowing *(arrows).*

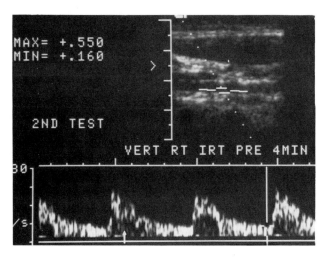

FIG 30-31. Normal vertebral artery Doppler spectral waveform. A low-resistance flow pattern similar to common and internal carotid arteries. Spectral broadening may fill the clear spectral window *(arrow).*

tebral artery and vein running between the transverse processes of C2-C6, which are identified by their periodic acoustical shadowing (Fig. 30-30). Transverse scanning with color Doppler allows the examiner to visualize the carotid artery and jugular vein at the same time and use them as references to determine the direction of flow in the vertebral artery.[95]

Angling the transducer caudad allows visualization of the vertebral artery origin in 60% to 70% of the arteries, 80% on the right side and 50% on the left. This discrepancy may relate to the fact that the left vertebral artery origin is deeper and that it arises directly from the aortic arch 6% to 8% of the time.[93,102]

The presence and direction of flow should be established. Visible plaque disease should be assessed. The vertebral artery supplies blood to the brain and usually has a low-resistance flow pattern similar to that of the common carotid artery, with continuous flow in systole and diastole; however, wide variability in waveform shape has been noted in angiographically normal vessels.[101] Because the vessel is small, flow tends to demonstrate a broader spectrum. The clear spectral window seen in the normal carotid system is usually filled in the vertebrae (Fig. 30-31).[49]

The vertebral vein runs parallel and adjacent to the vertebral artery. Care must be taken not to mistake its flow for that of the adjacent artery, particularly if the venous flow is pulsatile. Comparison with jugular venous flow during respiration should readily distinguish between vertebral artery and vein. At times the ascending cervical branch of the thyrocervical trunk can be mistaken for the vertebral artery. This can be avoided by looking for landmark transverse processes that accompany the vertebral artery and also by paying careful attention to the waveform of the visualized vessel. The ascending cervical branch has a high-impedance waveform pattern similar to that of the external carotid artery.[95]

Subclavian Steal

In the subclavian steal syndrome, the proximal subclavian artery is stenotic or occluded. The ischemic arm "steals" blood from the basilar circulation via retrograde vertebral artery flow during arm exercise, producing symptoms of vertebrobasilar insufficiency (Fig. 30-32). This condition is easily identified by detecting reversed vertebral arterial flow on Doppler spectral tracings and color flow Doppler images (Fig. 30-33). However, some subclavian steals are occult and do not demonstrate reversed flow unless provocative maneuvers are performed. There may be a confusing "partial steal" phenomenon, consisting of retrograde flow in systole and antegrade flow in diastole.[103] These occult steals or partial steals convert to full steals after 5 minutes of ipsilateral arm exercise or after postocclusive hyper-emia[84,103] produced by a 5-minute inflation of a sphygmomanometer to just above systolic pressure. Thus these maneuvers should be a part of the routine evaluation of suspected subclavian steal.

With subclavian steal, color Doppler may show two similarly color-encoded vessels between the transverse processes, representing the vertebral artery and vein.[84] Transverse images of the vertebral artery with color Doppler show reversed flow when compared with the common carotid artery.[92] A Doppler spectral waveform must be produced in all such cases to avoid mistaking flow reversal within an artery for a normal vertebral vein.[84,95] Visualization of only a vertebral vein is very suggestive of vertebral artery occlusion or congenital absence. However, experience with this finding is still preliminary. Demonstration of true flow reversal from any portion of the vertebral artery is sufficient to make the diagnosis. Despite the deep location of the subclavian artery, the corresponding stenosis can occasionally be identified.

Stenosis and Occlusion

Diagnosis of vertebral artery stenosis is more difficult than diagnosis of flow reversal. Most hemodynamically significant stenoses occur at the origin, which is situated deep in the upper thorax and can be seen in only approximately 60% to 70% of patients.[93,100,102] Even if the subclavian-vertebral artery origin is visualized, optimal adjustments of the Doppler angle for accurate velocity measurements may be difficult because of the deep location and vessel tortuosity. No accurate reproducible criteria for evaluating vertebral artery stenosis exist. As flow is normally "turbulent" within the

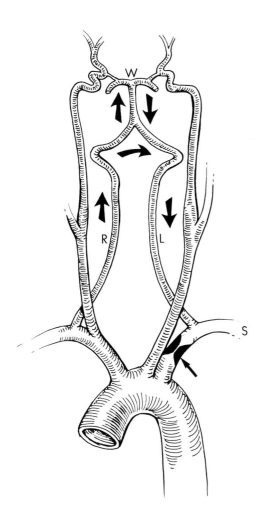

FIG 30-32. Hemodynamic pattern in subclavian steal syndrome diagram. Proximal left subclavian artery occlusive lesion *(small arrow)* decreases flow to the distal subclavian artery *(S)*. This produces retrograde flow *(large arrows)* down the left vertebral artery *(L)* and stealing from the right vertebral artery *(R)* and other intracranial vessels via the circle of Willis *(W)*.

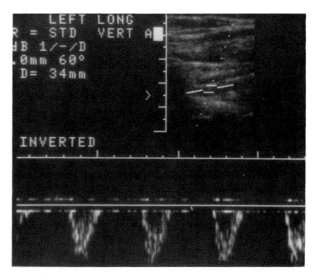

FIG 30-33. Reversed flow in the vertebral artery, diagnostic of subclavian steal. The Doppler spectrum has been inverted, so cephalic flow should project above the baseline.

vertebral artery, spectral broadening cannot be used as an indicator of stenosis. Velocity measurements are not reliable as criteria for stenosis because of the wide normal variation in vertebral artery diameter. Although velocities greater than 100 cm/sec often indicate stenosis, they can occur in angiographically normal vessels. For instance, high flow velocity may be present in a vertebral artery that is serving as a major collateral pathway for cerebral circulation in cases of carotid occlusion.[102] Thus only a focal increase in velocity of at least 50% and/or visible stenosis on gray-scale or color Doppler is likely to indicate significant vertebral stenosis. Variability of resistivity indices (RIs) in normal and abnormal vertebral arteries precludes the use of this parameter as an indicator of vertebral disease.[101]

Diagnosis of vertebral artery occlusion is also difficult. Often, inability to detect arterial flow is due to a small or congenitally absent vertebral artery or a technically difficult examination. Differentiation of severe stenosis from occlusion is difficult for the same reasons. Furthermore, markedly dampened blood flow velocity in high-grade stenoses and a decreased number of red blood cells traversing the area evaluated may result in a Doppler signal with amplitude too low to be detected.[94]

INTERNAL JUGULAR VEIN

The internal jugular veins are the major vessels responsible for return of venous blood from the brain. The most common clinical indication for duplex and color flow sonography of the internal jugular vein is the evaluation of suspected jugular venous thrombosis.[104-111] Other uses include diagnosis of jugular venous ectasia[112-115] and guidance for internal jugular or subclavian vein cannulation,[116-118] particularly in difficult situations where vascular anatomy is distorted.

Technique

The normal internal jugular vein is easily visualized. The vein is scanned with the neck extended and the head turned to the contralateral side. Longitudinal and transverse scans are obtained with light transducer pressure on the neck to avoid collapsing the vein. A coronal view from the supraclavicular fossa is used to image the lower segment of the internal jugular vein and medial segment of the subclavian vein as they join to form the brachiocephalic vein.

The jugular vein lies lateral and anterior to the common carotid artery, lateral to the thyroid gland, and deep to the sternocleidomastoid muscle (Fig. 30-2). The vessel has sharply echogenic walls and a hypoechoic or anechoic lumen. Normally a valve can be visualized in its distal portion.[107,109,119] The right internal jugular vein is usually larger than the left.[114]

Real-time sonography demonstrates venous pulsations related to right heart contractions, as well as

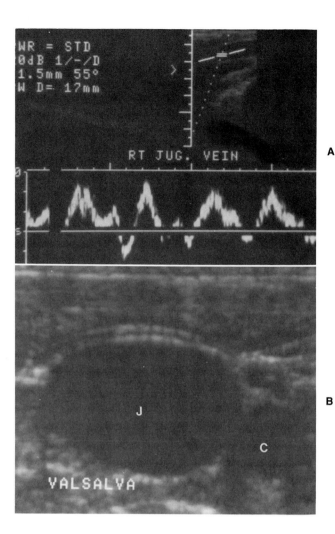

FIG 30-34. Normal jugular vein. **A,** Complex venous pulsations in the jugular vein reflect the cycle of events in the right atrium. **B,** During Valsalva maneuver, increased intrathoracic pressure causes a decrease in the blood return to the heart and the internal jugular vein *(J)* enlarges. *C,* CCA.

changes in venous diameter that vary with changes in intrathoracic pressure. Doppler examination graphically depicts these flow patterns (Fig. 30-34, *A*). On inspiration, negative intrathoracic pressure causes flow toward the heart and the jugular veins decrease in diameter. During expiration and during Valsalva's maneuver, increased intrathoracic pressure causes a decrease in the blood return and the veins enlarge (Fig. 30-34, *B*); little or no flow is noted. Walls of the normal jugular vein coapt completely when moderate transducer pressure is applied. Sudden sniffing reduces intrathoracic pressure, causing momentary collapse of the vein on real-time sonography, accompanied by a brief increase in venous flow toward the heart as shown by Doppler.[106,108-110]

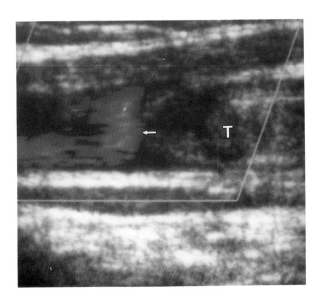

FIG 30-35. Jugular vein thrombosis. Longitudinal color Doppler image demonstrates flow *(arrow)* superior to echogenic thrombus *(T)*.

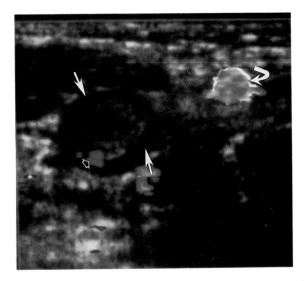

FIG 30-36. Chronic jugular venous thrombosis with increased venous flow in a collateral vein *(curved arrow)*. Transverse color Doppler image. Echogenic thrombus *(arrows)* nearly fills the right jugular lumen. A small recanalized channel shows flow *(open arrow)*.

Thrombosis

Clinical features of jugular venous thrombosis (JVT) include a tender, ill-defined, nonspecific neck mass or swelling. The correct diagnosis may not be immediately obvious.[107] Thrombosis of the internal jugular vein can be completely asymptomatic because of the deep position of the vein and the presence of abundant collateral circulation.[110] This condition was previously diagnosed by venography, an invasive procedure prompted only by a high index of suspicion. With the introduction of noninvasive techniques, such as ultrasound, computed tomography (CT),[120] and magnetic resonance imaging (MRI),[121] JVT is being identified more frequently. Internal jugular thrombosis most commonly results from complications of **central venous catheterization.**[105,109,110] Other causes include **intravenous drug abuse, mediastinal tumor, hypercoagulable states, neck surgery,** and **local inflammation/adenopathy.**[107] Some cases are idiopathic or spontaneous.[108] Possible complications of JVT include suppurative thrombophlebitis, clot propagation, and pulmonary embolism.[107,111]

Real-time examination[104-111] reveals an enlarged noncompressible vein, which may contain visible echogenic intraluminal thrombus. Acute thrombus may be anechoic and indistinguishable from flowing blood; however, characteristic lack of compressibility and absent Doppler or color Doppler flow in the region of a thrombus quickly lead to the correct diagnosis. In addition, there is visible loss of vein response to respiratory maneuvers and venous pulsation. Spectral and color flow Doppler interrogations reveal absent flow (Fig. 30-

35). Collateral veins may be identified, particularly in cases of chronic internal jugular vein thrombosis (Fig. 30-36). Central liquefaction or other heterogeneity of the thrombus also suggests chronicity. Chronic thrombi may be difficult to visualize as they tend to organize and are difficult to separate from echogenic perivascular fatty tissue.[109]

Ultrasound has proved to be a reliable means of diagnosing jugular vein thrombosis and has the advantage over CT and MRI of being inexpensive, portable, and nonionizing, and requiring no intravenous contrast. Ultrasound has limited access and cannot image all portions of the jugular vein, especially those located behind the mandible or below the clavicle. However, knowledge of the full extent of thrombus is not frequently a critical factor in treatment planning.[107,111] Serial sonographic examination to evaluate response to therapy after the initial assessment can be performed safely and inexpensively.

REFERENCES

1. Kricheff II. Arteriosclerotic ischemic cerebrovascular disease. *Radiology* 1987;162:101-109.
2. Carroll BA. "Duplex" Doppler carotid sonography. In: Fleischer AC, James AE, eds. *Diagnostic Sonography: Principles and Clinical Applications.* Philadelphia: W.B. Saunders Company; 1989:762-790.
3. Masaryk TJ, Modic MT, Ruggieri PM, et al. Three-dimensional (volume) gradient-echo imaging of the carotid bifurcation: preliminary clinical experience. *Radiology* 1989; 171:801-806.
4. Glasier CM, Seibert JJ, Chadduck WM, et al. Brain death in infants: evaluation with Doppler ultrasound. *Radiology* 1989;172:377-380.

5. De Bray JM, Joseph PA, Jeanvoine H, et al. Transcranial Doppler evaluation of middle cerebral artery stenosis. *J Ultrasound Med* 1988;7:611-616.

6. Taylor GA, Catena LM, Garin DB, et al. Intracranial flow patterns in infants undergoing extracorporeal membrane oxygenation: preliminary observations with Doppler ultrasound. *Radiology* 1987;165:671-674.

7. Aaslid R, Huber P, Nornes H. Evaluation of cerebrovascular spasm with transcranial Doppler ultrasound. *J Neurosurg* 1984;60:37-41.

8. Ricotta JJ. Plaque characterization by B-mode scan. *Surg Clin North Am* 1990;70(1):191-199.

9. Gerlock AJ, Giyanani VL, Krebs C. *Applications of Noninvasive Vascular Techniques.* Philadelphia: W.B. Saunders Company; 1988:147-159.

10. Taylor KJW: Clinical applications of carotid Doppler ultrasound. In Taylor KJW, Burns PN, Wells PNT, eds. *Clinical Applications of Doppler Ultrasound.* New York: Raven Press; 1988:120-161.

11. Bluth EI, Shyn PB, Sullivan MA, et al. Doppler color flow imaging of carotid artery dissection. *J Ultrasound Med* 1989; 8:149-53.

12. Hennerici M, Steinke W, Rautenberg W. High-resistance Doppler flow pattern in extracranial carotid dissection. *Arch Neurol* 1989;46:670-672.

13. Rothrock JF, Lim V, Press G, et al. Serial magnetic resonance and carotid duplex examinations in the management of carotid dissection. *Neurology* 1989;39:686-692.

14. Gritzmann N, Grasl MCH, Helmer M, et al. Invasion of the carotid artery and jugular vein by lymph node metastases: Detection with sonography. *AJR* 1990;154:411-414

15. Gooding GAW, Langman AW, Dillon WP, et al. Malignant carotid artery invasion: sonographic detection. *Radiology* 1989;171:435-438.

16. Steinke W, Hennerici M, Aulich A. Doppler color flow imaging of carotid body tumors. *Stroke* 1989;20:1574-1577.

17. Tihansky DP, Porter PS. Pulsed Doppler-ultrasonic diagnosis of carotid body tumor. *N Y State J Med* 1989;89:580-582.

Examination Technique

18. Grant EG, Wong W, Tessler F, et al. Cerebrovascular ultrasound imaging. *Radiol Clin North Am* 1988;26:1111-1130.

Carotid Ultrasound Interpretation

19. Nolsoe CP, Engel U, Karstrup S, et al. The aortic wall: an *in vitro* study of the double-line pattern in high-resolution ultrasound. *Radiology* 1990;175:387-390.

20. O'Leary DH, Polak JF. High-resolution carotid sonography: past, present, and future. *AJR* 1989;153:699-704.

21. Poli A, Tremoli E, Colombo A, et al. Ultrasonographic measurement of the common carotid artery wall thickness in hypercholesterolemic patients. A new model for the quantitation and follow-up of preclinical atherosclerosis in living human subjects. *Atherosclerosis* 1988;70:253-61.

22. Pignoli PP, Tremoli ET, Poli A, et al. Intimal plus medial thickness of the arterial wall: a direct measurement with ultrasound imaging. *Circulation* 1986;74:1399-1406.

23. Bluth EI, Stavros AT, Marich KW, et al. Carotid duplex sonography: A multicenter recommendation for standardized imaging and Doppler criteria. *Radiographics* 1988;8:487-506.

24. Carroll BA: Duplex sonography in patients with hemispheric symptoms. *J Ultrasound Med* 1989;8:535-540.

25. Brown PB, Zwiebel WJ, Call GK: Degree of cervical carotid artery stenosis and hemispheric stroke: Duplex ultrasound findings. *Radiology* 1989;170:541-543.

26. O'Donnell TF, Erdoes L, Mackey WC, et al. Correlation of B-mode ultrasound imaging and arteriography with pathologic findings at carotid endarterectomy. *Arch Surg* 1985;120:443-449.

27. Pessin MS, Duncan GW, Mohr JP, et al. Clinical and angiographic features of carotid transient ischemic attacks. *N Engl J Med* 1977;296:358-362.

28. Dixon S, Pais SO, Raviola C, et al. Natural history of nonstenotic, asymptomatic ulcerative lesions of the carotid artery: a further analysis. *Arch Surg* 1982;117:1493-1498.

29. Mohr JP: Asymptomatic carotid artery disease. *Stroke* 1982;13:431-433.

30. Langsfield M, Gray-Weale AC, Lusby RJ. The role of plaque morphology and diameter reduction in the development of new symptoms in asymptomatic carotid arteries. *J Vasc Surg* 1989;9:548-57.

31. Leahy AL, McCollum PT, Feeley TM, et al. Duplex ultrasonography and selection of patients for carotid endarterectomy: Plaque morphology or luminal narrowing? *J Vasc Surg* 1988;8:558-62.

32. Reilly LM, Lusby RJ, Hughes L, et al. Carotid plaque histology using real-time ultrasonography: clinical and therapeutic implications. *Am J Surg* 1983;146:188-193.

33. Persson AV, Robichaux WT, Silverman M. The natural history of carotid plaque development. *Arch Surg* 1983;118:1048-1052.

34. Lusby RJ, Ferrell LD, Ehrenfield WK, et al. Carotid plaque hemorrhage: its role in production of cerebral ischemia. *Arch Surg* 1982;117:1479-1488.

35. Edwards JH, Kricheff II, Gorstein F, et al. Atherosclerotic subintimal hematoma of the carotid artery. *Radiology* 1979; 133:123-129.

36. Imparato AM, Riles TS, Gorstein F. The carotid bifurcation plaque: pathologic findings associated with cerebral ischemia. *Stroke* 1979;10:238-245.

37. Bassiouny HS, Davis H, Massawa N, et al. Critical carotid stenoses: Morphologic and chemical similarity between symptomatic and asymptomatic plaques. *J Vasc Surg* 1989;9:202-12.

38. Lennihan L, Kupsky WJ, Mohr JP, et al. Lack of association between carotid plaque hematoma and ischemic cerebral symptoms. *Stroke* 1987;18:879-881.

39. Rubin JR, Bondi JA, Rhodes RS. Duplex scanning versus conventional arteriography for the evaluation of carotid artery plaque morphology. *Surgery* 1987;102:749-755.

40. Sterpetti AV, Schultz RD, Feldhaus RJ, et al. Ultrasonographic features of carotid plaque and the risk of subsequent neurologic deficits. *Surgery* 1988;104:652-660.

41. Weinberger J, Marks SJ, Gaul JJ, et al. Atherosclerotic plaque at the carotid artery bifurcation: correlation of ultrasonographic imaging with morphology. *J Ultrasound Med* 1987; 6:363-366.

42. Bluth EI, Kay D, Merritt CRB, et al. Sonographic characterization of carotid plaque: detection of hemorrhage. *AJR* 1986; 146:1061-1065.

43. Bluth EI, McVay LV, Merritt CRB, et al. The identification of ulcerative plaque with high resolution duplex carotid scanning. *J Ultrasound Med* 1988;7:73-76.

44. O'Leary DH, Holen J, Ricotta JJ, et al. Carotid bifurcation disease: prediction of ulceration with B-mode ultrasound. *Radiology* 1987;162:523-525.

45. Comerota AJ, Katz ML, White JU, et al. The preoperative diagnosis of the ulcerative carotid atheroma. *J Vasc Surg* 1987;18:1011-1017.

46. Zwiebel WJ, Austin CW, Sackett JF, et al. Correlation of high-resolution, B-mode and continuous-wave Doppler sonography with arteriography in the diagnosis of carotid stenosis. *Radiology* 1983;149:523-532.

47. Eikelboom BC, Riles TR, Mintzer R, et al. Inaccuracy of angiography in the diagnosis of carotid ulceration. *Stroke* 1983;14:882-885.

48. Edwards JH, Kricheff II, Riles T, et al. Angiographically undetected ulceration of the carotid bifurcation as a cause of embolic stroke. *Radiology* 1979;132:369-373.

49. Grant EG: Duplex sonography of the cerebrovascular system. In Grant EG, White EM, eds. *Duplex Sonography.* New York: Springer-Verlag; 1988:7-68.

50. Comerota AJ, Cranley JJ, Cook SE. Real-time B-mode carotid imaging in diagnosis of cerebrovascular disease. *Surgery* 1981;89:718-729.

51. Jacobs NM, Grant EG, Schellinger D, et al. Duplex carotid sonography: criteria for stenosis, accuracy, and pitfalls. *Radiology* 1985;154:385-391.

52. Zwiebel WJ. Spectrum analysis in carotid sonography. *Ultrasound Med Biol* 1987;13:623-636.

53. Taylor KJW, Holland S. Doppler ultrasound: Part I. Basic principles, instrumentation, and pitfalls. *Radiology* 1990;174:297-307.

54. Carroll BA, von Ramm OT. Fundamentals of current Doppler technology. *Ultrasound Quarterly* 1988;6:275-298.

55. Kassam M, Johnston KW, Cobbold RSC. Quantitative estimation of spectral broadening for the diagnosis of carotid arterial disease: method and in vitro results. *Ultrasound Med Biol* 1985;11:425-433.

56. Douville Y, Johnston KW, Kassam M. Determination of the hemodynamic factors which influence the carotid Doppler spectral broadening. *Ultrasound Med Biol* 1985;11:417-423.

57. Garth KE, Carroll BA, Sommer FG, et al. Duplex ultrasound scanning of the carotid arteries with velocity spectrum analysis. *Radiology* 1983;147:823-827.

58. Phillips DJ, Greene FM, Langlois Y, et al. Flow velocity patterns in the carotid bifurcations of young, presumed normal subjects. *Ultrasound Med Biol* 1983;9:39-49.

59. Lichtman JB, Kibble MB. Detection of intracranial arteriovenous malformation by Doppler ultrasound of the extracranial carotid circulation. *J Ultrasound Med* 1987;6:609-612.

60. Robinson ML, Sacks D, Perlmutter GS, et al. Diagnostic criteria for carotid duplex sonography. *AJR* 1988;151:1045-1049.

61. Kohler TR, Langlois Y, Roederer GO, et al. Variability in measurement of specific parameters for carotid duplex examination. *Ultrasound Med Biol* 1987;13:637-642.

62. Moneta GL, Taylor DC, Zierler E, et al. Asymptomatic high-grade internal carotid artery stenosis: is stratification according to risk factors or duplex spectral analysis possible? *J Vasc Surg* 1989;10:475-483.

63. Friedman SG, Hainline B, Feinberg AW, et al. Use of diastolic velocity ratios to predict significant carotid artery stenosis. *Stroke* 1988;19:910-912.

64. Vaisman U, Wojciechowski M. Carotid artery disease: new criteria for evaluation by sonographic duplex scanning. *Radiology* 1986;158:253-255.

65. Jackson VP, Kuehn DS, Bendick PJ, et al. Duplex carotid sonography: correlation with digital subtraction angiography and conventional angiography. *J Ultrasound Med* 1985; 4:239-249.

66. Wetzner SM, Kiser LC, Bezreh JS: Duplex ultrasound imaging: vascular applications. *Radiology* 1984;150:507-514.

67. Dreisbach JN, Seibert CE, Smazal SF, et al. Duplex sonography in the evaluation of carotid artery disease. *Am J Neuroradiol* 1983;4:678-680.

68. Blackshear WM, Phillips DJ, Chikos PM, et al. Carotid artery velocity patterns in normal and stenotic vessels. *Stroke* 1980;11:67-71.

69. Taylor DC, Strandness DE. Carotid artery duplex scanning. *J Clin Ultrasound* 1987;15:635-644.

70. Zbornikova V, Lassvik C. Duplex scanning in presumably normal persons of different ages. *Ultrasound Med Biol* 1986;12:371-378.

71. Hayes AC, Johnston W, Baker WH, et al. The effect of contralateral disease on carotid Doppler frequency. *Surgery* 1988;103:19-23.

72. Bornstein NM, Zlatko GB, Norris JW. The limitations of diagnosis of carotid occlusion by Doppler ultrasound. *Ann Surg* 1988;207:315-317.

73. Bodily KC, Phillips DJ, Thiele BL, et al. Noninvasive detection of internal carotid artery occlusion. *Angiology* 1981;32:517-521.

74. Bridgers SL: Clinical correlates of Doppler/ultrasound errors in the detection of internal carotid artery occlusion. *Stroke* 1989;20:612-615.

75. Fell G, Phillips DJ, Chikos PM, et al. Ultrasonic duplex scanning for disease of the carotid artery. *Circulation* 1981;64:1191-1195.

76. Zwiebel WJ, Crummy AB. Sources of error in Doppler diagnosis of carotid occlusive disease. *AJR* 1981;137:1-12.

77. Bebry AJ, Hines GL. Total occlusion of the common carotid artery with a patent internal carotid artery; report of a case. *J Vasc Surg* 1989;10:469-470.

78. Blackshear WM, Phillips DJ, Bodily KC, et al. Ultrasonic demonstration of external and internal carotid patency with common carotid occlusion: a preliminary report. *Stroke* 1980;11:249-252.

79. Sumner DS. Use of color-flow imaging technique in carotid artery disease. *Surg Clin North Am* 1990;70:201-211.

80. Grant EG, Tessler FN, Perrella RR. Clinical Doppler imaging. *AJR* 1989;152:707-717.

81. Polak JF, Dobkin GR, O'Leary DH, et al. Internal carotid artery stenosis: accuracy and reproducibility of color-Doppler-assisted duplex imaging. *Radiology* 1989;173:793-798.

82. Hallam MJ, Reid JM, Cooperberg PL. Color-flow Doppler and conventional duplex scanning of the carotid bifurcation: prospective, double-blind, correlative study. *AJR* 1989;152:1101-1105.

83. Erickson SJ, Mewissen MW, Foley WD, et al. Stenosis of the internal carotid artery: assessment using color Doppler imaging compared with angiography. *AJR* 1989;152:1299-1305.

84. Erickson SJ, Middleton WD, Mewissen MW, et al. Color Doppler evaluation of arterial stenoses and occlusions involving the neck and thoracic inlet. *Radiographics* 1989;9:389-406.

85. Carroll BA: Carotid sonography: pitfalls and color flow. *Applied Radiology* 1988;October:15-21.

86. Middleton WD, Foley WD, Lawson TL. Color-flow Doppler imaging of carotid artery abnormalities. *AJR* 1988;150:419-425.

87. Middleton WD, Foley WD, Lawson TL. Flow reversal in the normal carotid bifurcation: color Doppler flow imaging analysis. *Radiology* 1988;167:207-210.

88. Merritt CRB: Doppler color flow imaging. *J Clin Ultrasound* 1987;15:591-597.

89. Zierler RE, Phillips DJ, Beach KW, et al. Noninvasive assessment of normal carotid bifurcation hemodynamics with color-flow ultrasound imaging. *Ultrasound Med Biol* 1987;13:471-476.

90. Middleton WD, Erickson S, Melson GL. Perivascular color artifact: pathologic significance and appearance on color Doppler ultrasound images. *Radiology* 1989;171:647-652.

The Vertebral Artery

91. Bendick PJ, Glover JL. Hemodynamic evaluation of vertebral arteries by duplex ultrasound. *Surg Clin North Am* 1990;70:235-244.

92. Lewis BD, James EM, Welch TJ. Current applications of duplex and color Doppler ultrasound imaging: carotid and peripheral vascular system. *Mayo Clin Proc* 1989;64:1147-1157.

93. Visona A, Lusiani L, Castellani V, et al. The echo-Doppler (duplex) system for the detection of vertebral artery occlusive disease: comparison with angiography. *J Ultrasound Med* 1986;5:247-250.

94. Davis PC, Nilsen B, Braun IF, et al. A prospective comparison of duplex sonography vs angiography of the vertebral arteries. *AJNR* 1986;7:1059-1064.

95. Bluth EI, Merritt CRB, Sullivan MA, et al. Usefulness of duplex ultrasound in evaluating vertebral arteries. *J Ultrasound Med* 1989;8:229-235.

96. Walker DW, Acker JD, Cole CA. Subclavian steal syndrome detected with duplex pulsed Doppler sonography. *AJNR* 1982; 3:615-618.

97. Wilkinson DL, Polak JF, Grassi CJ, et al. Pseudoaneurysm of the vertebral artery: appearance on color-flow Doppler sonography. *AJR* 1988;151:1051-1052.

98. Touboul P, Mas J, Bousser M, et al. Duplex scanning in extracranial vertebral artery dissection. *Stroke* 1987;18:116-121.

99. Elias DA, Weinberg PE. Angiography of the posterior fossa. In Taveras JM, Ferrucci JT, eds. *Radiology: Diagnosis-Imaging-Intervention.* Philadelphia: J.B. Lippincott Co.; 1989;3:6-7.

100. Bendick PJ, Jackson VP. Evaluation of the vertebral arteries with duplex sonography. *J Vasc Surg* 1986;3:523-530.

101. Carroll BA, Holder CA. Vertebral artery duplex sonography (abstract). *J Ultrasound Med* 1990;9:S27-28.

102. Ackerstaff RGA, Grosveld WJHM, Eikelboom BC, et al. Ultrasonic duplex scanning of the prevertebral segment of the vertebral artery in patients with cerebral atherosclerosis. *Eur J Vasc Surg* 1988;2:387-393.

103. Kotval PS, Babu SC, Shah PM. Doppler diagnosis of partial vertebral/subclavian steals convertible to full steals with physiologic maneuvers. *J Ultrasound Med* 1990;9:207-213.

The Internal Jugular Vein

104. Williams CE, Lamb GHR, Roberts D, et al. Venous thrombosis in the neck: the role of real time ultrasound. *Eur J Radiol* 1989;9:32-36.

105. Hubsch PJS, Stiglbauer RL, Schwaighofer BWAM, et al. Internal jugular and subclavian vein thrombosis caused by central venous catheters: evaluation using Doppler blood flow imaging. *J Ultrasound Med* 1988;7:629-636.

106. Gaitini D, Kaftori JK, Pery M, et al. High-resolution real-time ultrasonography: diagnosis and follow-up of jugular and subclavian vein thrombosis. *J Ultrasound Med* 1988;7:621-627.

107. Albertyn LE, Alcock MK. Diagnosis of internal jugular vein thrombosis. *Radiology* 1987;162:505-508.

108. Falk RL, Smith DF. Thrombosis of upper extremity thoracic inlet veins: diagnosis with duplex Doppler sonography. *AJR* 1987;149:677-682.

109. Weissleder R, Elizondo G, Stark DD. Sonographic diagnosis of subclavian and internal jugular vein thrombosis. *J Ultrasound Med* 1987;6:577-587

110. De Witte BR, Lameris JS. Real-time ultrasound diagnosis of internal jugular vein thrombosis. *J Clin Ultrasound* 1986;14:712-717.

111. Wing V, Scheible W. Sonography of jugular vein thrombosis. *AJR* 1983;140:333-336.

112. Gribbin C, Raghavendra BN, Ginsburg HB. Ultrasound diagnosis of jugular venous ectasia. *NY State J Med* 1989;9:532-533.

113. Hughes PL, Qureshi SA, Galloway RW. Jugular venous aneurysm in children. *Br J Radiol* 1988;61:1082-1084.

114. Jasinski RW, Rubin JM. Computed tomography and ultrasonographic findings in jugular vein ectasia. *J Ultrasound Med* 1984;3:417-420.

115. Stevens RK, Fried AM, Hood TR. Ultrasonic diagnosis of jugular venous aneurysm. *J Clin Ultrasound* 1982;10:85-87.

116. Lee W, Leduc L, Cotton DB. Ultrasonographic guidance for central venous access during pregnancy. *Am J Obstet Gynecol* 1989;161:1012-1013.

117. Bond DM, Nolan R. Real-time ultrasound imaging aids jugular venipuncture. *Anesth Analg* 1989;68:700-701.

118. Machi J, Takeda J, Kakegawa T. Safe jugular and subclavian venipuncture under ultrasonographic guidance. *Am J Surg* 1987;153:321-323.

119. Dresser LP, McKinney WM. Anatomic and pathophysiologic studies of the human internal jugular valve. *Am J Surg* 1987; 154:220-224.

120. Patel S, Brennan J. Diagnosis of internal jugular vein thrombosis by computed tomography. *J Comput Assist Tomogr* 1981; 5:197-200.

121. Braun IF, Hoffman JC, Malko JA, et al. Jugular venous thrombosis: magnetic resonance imaging. *Radiology* 1985;157:357-360.

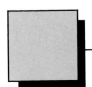

CHAPTER 31

The Peripheral Vessels

▪ Joseph F. Polak, M.D.

As is the case for the extracranial carotid arteries, the vessels of both the upper and lower extremities are easily accessible to sonographic imaging. They are free from the acoustic interference that normally plagues imaging of the abdominal and thoracic vessels and there are enough imaging windows to permit the positioning of the ultrasound transducer directly over the vessel of interest without any loss of signal due to overlying bone. High-resolution ultrasound transducers with frequencies above 5 MHz can be used because the vessels lie close to the skin or can be imaged within depths of less than 6 cm.

Resolution is not the sole factor responsible for the increasing use of sonography for imaging the peripheral vessels. Ultrasound imaging, by itself, is useful for:
- visualizing extravascular masses
- following the development of atherosclerotic deposits
- determining the presence of thrombotic material within veins.

But experience with carotid arteries has shown that it is the addition of Doppler analysis that makes duplex sonography such a powerful diagnostic tool for detecting significant arterial stenoses and assessing perivascular masses. Recently, the dissemination of color Doppler flow imaging has made it possible to directly image blood flow patterns in vivo. When compared to duplex sonography, color flow imaging can survey larger volumes of tissue and longer vascular segments in a shorter period of time. It is, therefore, not surprising that this modality is becoming increasingly popular for imaging the vascular tree.

When compared to venography or angiography, duplex sonography has the advantage of being noninvasive and relatively inexpensive; it is therefore well suited for serial examinations. It has the added advantage of being able to image nonvascular structures in close proximity to the vessels. Computed tomography can also detect structures adjacent to vessels but it is much more expensive, requires contrast material, and, because of poor resolution, cannot be used to detect changes in the lumen of small caliber arteries. Magnetic resonance (MRI) is currently investigational and it offers the promise of imaging not only the extravascular processes, but pathologic changes within the venous and arterial systems as well. Whether MRI proves to be more cost effective than sonography remains to be seen.

INSTRUMENTATION
Gray-scale Imaging

Imaging of the peripheral veins is directed, mainly, to the detection of venous thrombosis or, occasionally, to the preoperative assessment of the saphenous veins before their use as autologous vein grafts. Although transducer imaging frequencies as low as 3.5 MHz can be used to detect thrombi in the femoropopliteal veins, the growing interest in visualization of the calf veins and the accurate determination of vein lumen diameters, favors the use of transducer frequencies of 5-10 MHz. A good compromise is the 5 MHz transducer because it offers overall good resolution while permitting good depth penetration in the thigh. For detailed visualization of smaller diameter veins, a 7 MHz transducer is often substituted. The 10 MHz transducers have been shown to have poor penetration and are rarely used.

The peripheral arteries vary in size from 1 to 6 mm. Accurate visualization of their lumen walls, to determine the presence of atherosclerotic lesions or for the estimation of lumen diameters, requires higher resolution than is possible with 3.5 MHz transducer. As in the venous system, the 5 MHz transducer, with the occasional need for a 7 MHz transducer, is used for the vast majority of the studies.

The linear phased array transducer is ideal for imaging both the veins and arteries of the extremities. The contact surface to the skin is small enough to easily transmit pressure when performing compression ultrasound in the transverse plane. The length of the transducer is sufficient to permit step-by-step longitudinal imaging of a long vascular segment in a minimum of nonoverlapping steps. The absence of any moving parts makes the transducer less apt to malfunction and alleviates the need to continually refill the water path as is the case for mechanically steered transducer scanners.

Doppler Sonography

Mechanical transducers are also ill suited for simultaneous duplex and real-time ultrasound imaging. This might not affect the performance of compression ultrasound since Doppler information is ancillary and is most often used to identify vascular structures.[1] The simultaneous display of Doppler spectral information and gray scale images is, however, a necessity when imaging arteries or arterial bypass grafts. Careful real-time control is often needed to position the Doppler sample gate and to accurately detect sites of maximal blood flow velocity in these small diameter structures. The frequencies used vary between 3 to 5 MHz, tending to be lower than the simultaneous gray-scale image. The pulse repetition rate at these frequencies should rarely cause aliasing of the Doppler spectrum when stenoses are detected.

Color Doppler flow imaging is increasingly used in peripheral vascular sonography. The simultaneous display of moving blood, superimposed on a gray scale image, has made it possible to rapidly survey the flow patterns within the arteries and veins of the extremities.[2] In general, an efficient approach to peripheral vascular sonography relies on color flow Doppler sonography to rapidly identify zones of flow disturbances. Then duplex sonography with Doppler spectral analysis can characterize the type of flow abnormality present. The color Doppler image displays only the mean frequency shift caused by moving structures. Most manufacturers will use lower carrier frequencies for the color flow image than for the gray-scale image. This approach, in part, overcomes the earlier aliasing of the color flow image that occurs at the lower frame rates used for the color display.

The newer curved phased array, or radial array, transducers offer the same advantages as the linear array transducer by combining real-time, gray-scale ultrasound, duplex, and color flow imaging. Their curved geometric design often makes them more difficult to use for imaging the legs and arms although they seem to perform better in visualizing the subclavian vein and artery.

PHYSIOLOGIC MECHANISMS OF DOPPLER FLOW PATTERNS
Normal Arteries

The normal waveform of the arteries at rest is a high resistance pattern reflecting constriction of the small vessels of the muscles distally. This is in sharp contrast to the persistent low resistance profile seen in the internal and common carotid arteries. The typical extremity flow profile shows a triphasic pattern. This consists of a strong forward component of blood flow during systole followed by a short reversal of flow normally corresponding to the dicrotic notch. A return to forward flow of lower amplitude normally follows and lasts for a variable length of diastole. Following exercise, muscular arteries dilate causing a change in the waveform to a monophasic, low-resistance pattern.

Stenotic Arteries

The normal high-resistance pattern disappears when significant arterial disease is present. It is replaced by a low-resistance pattern similar to that of the internal carotid artery. This pattern reflects the opening of collateral vessels and the abolition of the normal arteriolar tone in response to ischemia. It can be seen distal to a significant arterial lesion caused by the loss of normal resting arteriolar tone in response to muscle ischemia. It may also occur proximal to a significant lesion when large collateral vessels have developed.

A localized increase in velocity occurs at the site of a stenosis. This increase is detected as a shift in Doppler frequency proportional to the lumen diameter narrowing across which the blood is flowing.[3-5] This can be shown as an increase in peak systolic velocity on the Doppler spectrum, a decrease in color saturation, or even aliasing on the color map. The motion of blood distal to the stenosis becomes less organized and shows a large variation in both direction and velocity. This zone of turbulence is detected on duplex Doppler sonography as a broadening of the spectral window and as increased variance on color flow imaging.

Normal Veins

The flow pattern in peripheral veins typically shows a constant forward velocity on top of which are superimposed variations caused by respiration. Deep inspiration will normally diminish venous return from the lower extremities because of increased intra-abdominal pressure and cause distension of the vein. In the upper extremity, the negative pressures associated with inspiration will normally increase venous return and cause relative narrowing of the vein diameter. Flow augmentation, caused by squeezing the muscles distal to the vein being imaged, will normally increase venous flow and venous return.

Obstructed Veins

With acute venous obstruction, the normal venous respiratory variations distal and often proximal to the obstruction are lost. Loss of flow augmentation will similarly occur unless a collateral branch has developed or there is partial obstruction. With chronic obstruction, collaterals can develop to the point of reestablishing normal flow patterns distal and proximal to the original lesion.

Venous Incompetence

Venous channels do not, normally, permit retrograde flow. This is because of the protective action of the venous valves, which prevents the transmission of hydrostatic pressures directly into the small veins and capillaries of the feet. This mechanism can be overwhelmed when there has been damage to the valve, either following scarring, or in response to altered flow dynamics. Venous reflux of blood can then be demonstrated during a strong Valsalva maneuver by observing abnormal reversal of venous flow within either or both the superficial and deep veins of the legs.

A recent report has suggested the use of a blood pressure cuff that is inflated proximal to a suspected incompetent vein. Inflation to a standard pressure, with the patient in a semi-upright position, causes reflux of blood whenever a vein is incompetent. Another diagnostic approach is to empty the veins using augmentation of venous return with the subject upright. An abnormal response is return of blood down the incompetent venous channel following the augmentation maneuver.

Arteriovenous Malformations

Arterial venous (A-V) malformations can be classified as **congenital** or **iatrogenic.** Congenital A-V malformations are the abnormal communications between the artery and larger distended venous channels. These are, usually, quite obvious clinically and are located close to the skin surface of the involved extremity. These are normally visualized sonographically as distended venous channels into which feed single or multiple arterial branches. When A-V malformations are small, distended veins may not have had a chance to develop and the abnormality is only seen as an increase in venous blood velocity and turbulence caused by the fistula.

Iatrogenic communications often arise following selective deep arterial or venous catheterization or other penetrating trauma and are not obvious clinically. The actual site of communication can often be visualized by color flow Doppler as a jet of blood, with the draining vein being abnormally distended when compared to the other side. The jet of blood has a high velocity, which can cause vibration of the adjacent soft tissues, resulting in a perivascular Doppler artifact.[6] An important cause of a false positive sonographic diagnosis of A-V fistula is distension of the vein because of a perivascular mass at a more proximal location.

Masses. The differential diagnosis of perivascular masses is dramatically aided by the use of duplex ultrasound. The presence of flow in a mass contiguous to a vessel suggests the diagnosis of pseudoaneurysm. Within the fluid collection is a typical swirling motion or a color yin-yang sign.[7,8] A characteristic to-and-fro Doppler signal occurs at the narrow neck of the pseudoaneurysm. In contrast, a wide neck is more commonly encountered with aneurysms at the anastomosis of synthetic grafts.[9]

Arterial aneurysms are easily recognized by their typical location along the same axis as the artery. Although fusiform aneurysms obey this rule, it may be quite difficult to differentiate a saccular aneurysm from a pseudoaneurysm.[10] An enlarged lymph node is another perivascular mass that can be easily identified by sonography. By color and spectral Doppler sonography, both venous and arterial signals are found radiating from the hilum of the node.

VENOUS THROMBOSIS
Incidence and Clinical Importance

The incidence of venous thrombosis remains an interesting epidemiologic problem. Recent studies suggest that the prevalence of undetected pulmonary emboli in asymptomatic patients dying in the hospital of unrelated causes approaches 30%. There is also data suggesting that the perioperative incidence of venous thrombi, in high-risk populations, can be as high as 30% to 50%.

The incidence of lower-extremity venous thrombosis can be estimated from the annual incidence of fatal pulmonary embolism which, in this country, is close to 50,000 cases. The number of nonfatal symptomatic pulmonary emboli probably reaches up to 600,000 cases a year. Lower-extremity venous thrombosis is thought to occur in up to 95% of such episodes. Asymptomatic occurrences of pulmonary emboli are similarly thought to originate from lower-extremity venous thrombi and are 4 to 5 times more common. A conservative estimate of this problem would, therefore, be close to 2,000,000 cases of venous thrombosis a year.

The source of the vast majority of these emboli is the deep veins of the lower extremities. Data from many clinical studies also suggest that thrombi within the femoropopliteal veins (above the knee), not those limited to the calf veins (below the knee), are more likely to cause pulmonary emboli.[11] This explains why vascular imaging focuses on this portion of the leg. Another factor to consider in patients who have a clinical suspicion of thrombi below the knee is the use of serial ultrasound monitoring at the popliteal vein to document the upward spread of thrombus from below the knee.[12] Many experts believe that it is only when thrombus has spread into the popliteal vein that there is a clinical need to anticoagulate the patient. Proximal spread from thrombi residing in the calf veins is thought to occur in 20% of cases.[13]

At least two patterns of involvement by deep vein thrombosis are thought to occur. The first occurs in patients with symptoms. In these patients, the thrombi are preferentially distributed above the knee and tend to obstruct flow. The second develops in asymptomatic postoperative patients. These patients tend to have nonobstructing thrombi, a much larger proportion of which are located in the deep veins of the calf. These factors come into play when evaluating the diagnostic accuracy of the test.[14]

Lower Extremity

Normal Anatomy. The external iliac vein becomes the common femoral vein at the level of the inguinal ligament. The common femoral vein is medial and slightly deeper than the artery (Fig. 31-1). The first branch of the common femoral vein is the greater saphenous vein, which is a superficially located vein coursing medially towards the foot. The major branching of the common femoral vein into the superficial femoral and deep (profunda) femoral veins occurs just distal to the corresponding branching of the common

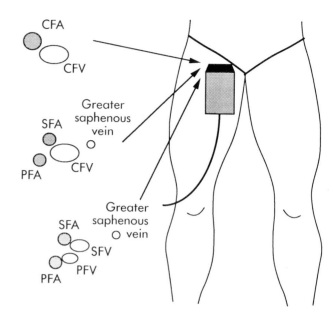

FIG 31-1. Vessel relationships in the groin. Diagram summarizes the relationships between femoral artery and vein in the transverse plane. These bifurcations normally occur within 5 cm of the groin crease. *CFA*, Common femoral artery; *CFV*, common femoral vein; *SFA*, superficial femoral artery; *PFA*, profunda femoral artery.

femoral artery. The deep femoral vein drains the muscles of the thigh while the superficial femoral vein drains the muscles of the lower leg. The superficial femoral vein lies deep or posterior to the superficial femoral artery (Fig. 31-2). Both the artery and vein enter the adductor (popliteal) canal when they cross beneath the adductor fascia in the lower third of the thigh. It may become difficult to compress the superficial femoral vein in the distal thigh as it enters the adductor canal and becomes the popliteal vein. The vein still lies posterior to the corresponding popliteal artery. Because the popliteal vein is normally imaged from the back of the leg rather than from the front, the popliteal vein now lies superficial to the artery. There are two common strategies used to assess vein compressibility. The first is to image from the anterior aspect of the thigh and use a finger placed either beside the transducer or on the posterior thigh at the level of the transducer to transmit pressure. The second is to externally rotate the leg to the frog-leg position and image and compress the posterior thigh.

The lesser saphenous vein originates from the popliteal vein at or slightly above the level of the mid knee and courses posteriorly and then laterally down the leg. The popliteal vein can often be followed to the proximal calf where it separates into the anterior tibial veins and the tibioperoneal trunk. The anterior tibial veins can be followed as they emerge after crossing the

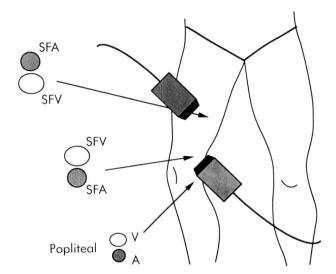

FIG 31-2. Vessel relationships in the mid and distal thigh. In the mid thigh, the superficial femoral artery lies anterior to the vein or veins. (Duplications of the vein occur in up to 20% of patients.) *SFA,* Superficial femoral artery; *SFV,* superficial femoral vein; *V,* vein; *A,* artery.

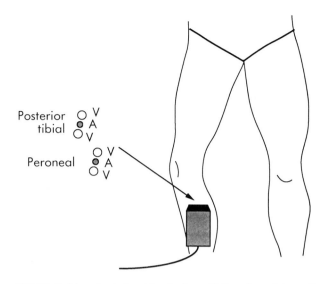

FIG 31-3. Vessel relationships in the calf. Imaging of the calf veins from the medial aspect. The posterior tibial veins and artery lie superficial to the peroneal vessels. Veins are duplicated and visualized to both sides of the arteries.

interosseous membrane and then course as paired veins. The tibioperoneal trunk is difficult to visualize in the upper third of the calf. The posterior tibial paired veins can be imaged as they migrate more superficially at the mid calf and then continue to the back of the medial malleolus (Fig. 31-3). The paired peroneal veins lie deeper and can be difficult to image in the recumbent position. These veins are easier to visualize when the patient is sitting upright with his or her legs in a dependent position. When the transducer is placed over the lateral aspect of the calf, the peroneal veins are identified close to the fibula and can easily be seen from the medial side of the leg. If necessary, the patient can be placed prone and the veins can be scanned from the posterior surface of the leg.

Diagnostic Criteria. Detection of venous thrombi can be made using one or a combination of many different diagnostic criteria. The first and most reliable criterion is the loss of normal vein compressibility.[15-17] This can be determined by holding the transducer in the plane transverse to the artery and vein and gently pushing on the skin until there is apposition of the vein walls. Loss of apposition is normally caused by a venous thrombus. Other possibilities include chronic changes that manifest themselves as wall thickening. Differentiation of the two entities is made by the fact that thrombus tends to be central while wall thickening is clearly seen along the wall, especially on longitudinal imaging (Fig. 31-4). The amount of pressure generated should be less than that necessary to compress the artery.

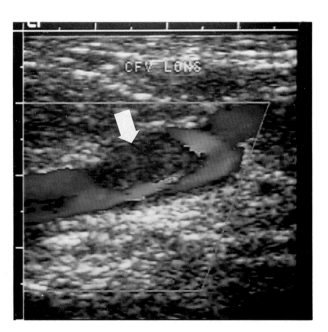

FIG 31-4. Acute common femoral vein thrombosis. Partly obstructive thrombus *(arrow)* involving the femoral vein. Notice that flow is toward the periphery of the vessel. This distinguishes the acute thrombus from chronic deep-vein thrombosis where flow in the vein is more centrally located.

Flow visualization and flow augmentation are used to exclude venous obstruction. Either duplex or color flow sonography can be used to determine whether or not normal respiratory variations are being transmitted.[18] This, in effect, rules out the presence of significant obstruction. The loss of this respiratory phasicity and the loss of increased flow signals, with flow augmentation, are most likely caused by obstructing venous thrombi. An extrinsic obstructing process can cause a similar loss of flow signals. Flow signals in the common femoral vein are routinely used to assess iliac vein patency. Loss of respiratory phasicity or loss of vein distension of the common femoral vein with the Valsalva maneuver are suggestive of iliac vein obstruction.[19,20] The nature of the obstruction cannot be confirmed unless the iliac vein is visualized along its full course.

Echogenic material within the venous lumen is considered to be the most specific of the signs of thrombosis. Various reports have suggested that the clot undergoes serial changes as it ages.[21] Early on, it is sonolucent. Within days, the echogenicity increases. These observations, made mostly in vitro, are not steadfast rules in the patient. There is no accurate way of determining the age of a venous thrombus from the level of its echogenicity. The detection of echogenic material within a vein is only 50% sensitive for the detection of deep vein thrombi because many thrombi are not echogenic.[18]

Venous distension can also be used as evidence of acute venous thrombosis. Over a period of 2 to 6 months after acute thrombosis, the lumen size of the affected vein tends to decrease and may become smaller than the corresponding venous segment in the opposite leg.

The development of collateral veins can be used as evidence of older episodes of thrombosis. One region where collateral veins often develops is in the distal thigh and knee where communicating veins form between the popliteal and profunda femoris veins. Collateral veins may also develop in response to a marked increase of flow in the superficial veins such as the greater saphenous vein.

Diagnostic Accuracy. The diagnostic accuracy of ultrasound is now well accepted. The single criterion of loss of compressibility is 95% sensitive and 98% specific for making the diagnosis of deep vein thrombosis in the popliteal and femoral veins. Changes in the flow dynamics can be viewed as supportive findings, especially for the patient who has symptoms of venous thrombosis.

There are fewer data for the asymptomatic patient who is at high risk for venous thrombosis. Patients who have had neurosurgical or orthopedic procedures have a high incidence of developing venous thrombosis despite remaining asymptomatic. A recent study confirmed the high accuracy of compression ultrasound in such a

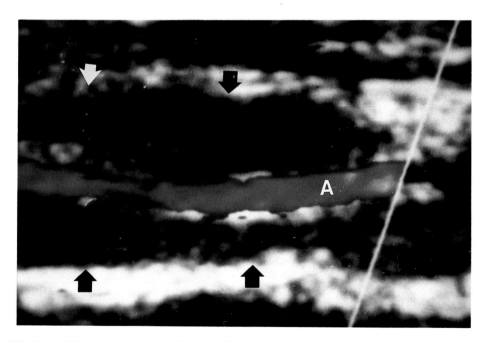

FIG 31-5. Calf vein thrombosis. Thrombus limited to the calf area is shown here as distended paired peroneal veins *(arrows)* without flow signals lying to both sides of the peroneal artery *(A)*.

group despite the nonobstructive nature of the thrombi.[22] Nonobstructive thrombi are less likely to change the Doppler flow pattern in the venous channels proximal or distal to the involved segments.

The increasing use of color flow imaging is unlikely to improve the already impressive accuracy of the examination for determining femoropopliteal vein thrombi.[23] Color flow imaging is likely, however, to improve the imaging of the calf veins (Fig. 31-5). Here, the color flow image can be used as a guide to somewhat confusing anatomy and assist in localizing the paired deep veins.[24] Imaging of the muscular veins can, however, be performed without the aid of color. The current estimate for detecting calf vein thrombosis has increased from earlier estimates of 20% to 30% to as high as 80%. This application is most likely to be used for the gathering of natural history data on the dynamics of venous thrombosis in the calf (Fig. 31-6).

Even if the calf veins are not imaged routinely, it is often worth imaging the site of the calf symptoms because early muscular vein thrombus can frequently be detected.

Serial ultrasound monitoring at the popliteal vein can be used as an alternative to anticoagulation in patients with a high likelihood of calf vein thrombi. The high accuracy of the examination at the popliteal vein makes it very likely that the small subset of patients who show spread can then be detected if they have repeat exams at day 2 and 5 following their first exam.

Venous Insufficiency

Incidence. The incidence of venous insufficiency is difficult to assess but it has been estimated that approximately 6 million people in the United States are af-

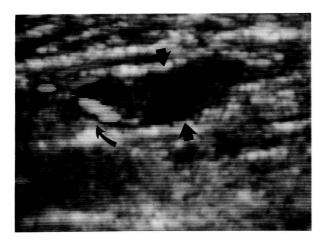

FIG 31-6. Soleal vein thrombus. Longitudinal color Doppler image of the calf area during compression demonstrates that the soleal vein *(arrows)* is distended by sonolucent (fresh) thrombus that is partly obstructive with flow noted at the periphery *(curved arrow)*.

fected. Following acute deep vein thrombosis, venous insufficiency has been shown in at least 60% of the leg veins. This number may actually decrease in the following year to less than 40%. It has also been estimated that up to 60% of patients with obvious clinical venous insufficiency will have a history of deep vein thrombosis.

Patterns and Diagnostic Criteria. In the lower extremity, venous insufficiency is a common sequela of deep venous thrombosis. It may also arise through a combination of pathophysiologic mechanisms which, ultimately, result in the destruction of the venous valves. The final outcome is the loss of the normal protective function of the valves and the direct transmission of elevated hydrostatic pressures into the smaller venules and capillaries of the calf and foot. Often, the patient has chronic skin changes, chronic leg swelling, and stasis ulcers with poor healing. Venous insufficiency in the superficial veins (lesser and greater saphenous) often results in the clinically apparent dilated subcutaneous varicosities.

Changes caused by venous insufficiency of the deep veins can be more indolent and can manifest themselves as chronic swellings of the calf or foot. With time, the perforating veins, which communicate between the deep and superficial veins, frequently become incompetent because of the elevated pressure; the superficial system then becomes involved and subcutaneous varicosities develop.

The diagnosis of venous insufficiency is made by confirming the presence of venous reflux during a set of standard maneuvers. Either duplex sonography or color Doppler imaging can be used. With duplex sonography, reflux in the greater saphenous vein can be shown during the Valsalva maneuver (Fig. 31-7). This same maneuver can be used for the proximal superficial femoral and profunda femoral veins. It is less reliable at the level of the popliteal vein. An alternate approach is compression of the thigh muscles in order to demonstrate reversal of blood flow in the popliteal vein. This technique is referred to as **reverse augmentation.** The popliteal vein valves are the critical sites to assess if vein valve reconstructive surgery is being considered.

Newer methods of quantifying venous reflux with Doppler sonography have recently been proposed. One group has shown that inflation of a compression cuff to a standardized pressure at the thigh can be used to estimate reflux. Another group has proposed the use of distal compression and the appearance of delayed reflux following augmentation. Both approaches are made with the subject upright or semi-upright.[25]

Upper Extremity

Normal Anatomy. Venous imaging of the upper extremity is normally performed from the antecubital

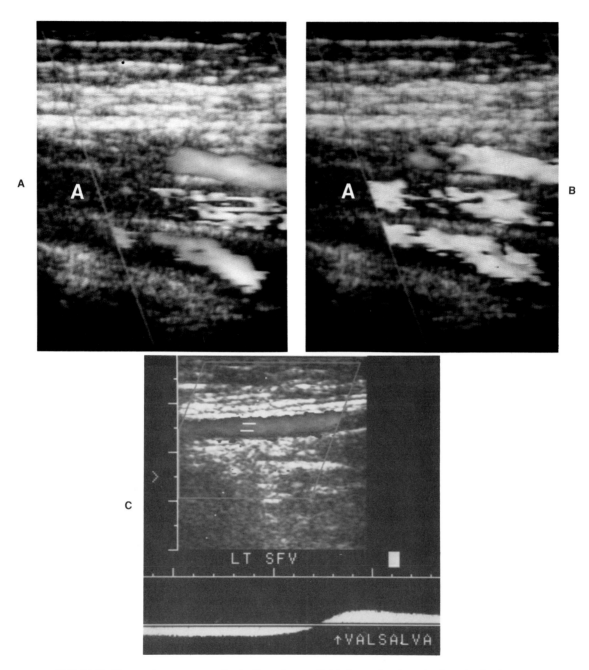

FIG 31-7. Venous incompetence in duplicated superficial femoral veins. **A,** Longitudinal color Doppler image of the duplicated superficial femoral veins *(blue)* near the adductor canal demonstrates that the blood flows in the normal direction, toward the groin, in the resting state. **B,** During Valsalva maneuver there is abnormal reversal of venous blood flow, as demonstrated by the change to red. This reversal is secondary to the development of venous insufficiency following a previous episode of deep-vein thrombosis. **C,** Longitudinal spectral Doppler exam of the SFV of another patient demonstrates reversal of flow during Valsalva maneuver.

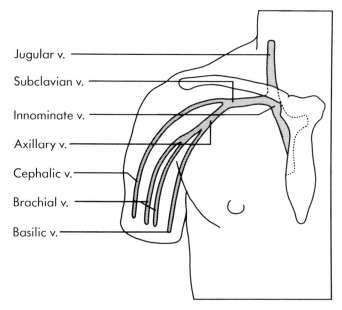

Jugular v.

Subclavian v.

Innominate v.

Axillary v.

Cephalic v.

Brachial v.

Basilic v.

FIG 31-8. Major arm veins. Diagram summarizes the location of the major draining veins of the arm.

fossa to the medial head of the clavicle (Fig. 31-8). The superficially located cephalic and basilic veins are common sites of thrombosis caused by trauma or secondary to intravenous lines. Thrombosis located more centrally is often secondary to effort thrombosis, central catheter placement, or associated with superior vena cava thrombosis.

The basilic vein is a superficial vein identified medially in the superior portion of the arm. This vein, which is often duplicated, joins the more deeply located brachial vein to form the axillary vein. The cephalic vein is a superficial vein found laterally in the arm; it joins the axillary vein as it becomes the subclavian vein. The brachial veins are deeper veins that course parallel to the brachial artery; after it unites with the basilic vein, it continues as the axillary vein superiorly. The subclavian vein can be seen from either above or below the clavicle. When imaged from above, it is seen deeper than the artery while, when imaged from below, it lies superficial to the artery. The subclavian vein joins the internal jugular vein to form the brachiocephalic vein. Imaging is normally possible only to this level with the superior vena cava rarely being imaged.

The internal jugular vein can be followed superiorly from the brachiocephalic vein. It lies lateral and superficial to the common carotid artery and is easily followed to the carotid bifurcation.

Diagnostic Criteria. Exclusion of an obstructing process affecting the more central veins is accomplished by documenting the normal collapse of the subclavian vein with deep, rapid inspiration, or sniffing. As in the

lower extremity, absence or loss of a normal response can be caused by either intrinsic obstruction by thrombus or extrinsic compression of the vein. Loss of compressibility remains the most reliable criterion for the diagnosis of venous thrombosis in the basilic, cephalic, brachial, axillary, and internal jugular veins. A combination of the criteria, discussed above, is used to make the diagnosis of thrombosis within the subclavian vein. For example, the distal third of the vein is accessible to direct visualization and can be compressed. The midportion is often obscured by the clavicle and only total obstruction of the vein can be excluded by confirming normal Doppler flow signals within the distal and proximal thirds of the vein. In the proximal third, the presence of echogenic material and loss of normal Doppler flow signals within the vein can be used as diagnostic criteria.

Diagnostic Accuracy. Despite the difficulties discussed above, the diagnostic accuracy of upper-extremity thrombosis is quite high. Reported series are either too small or did not use a sufficient number of gold-standard examinations (most often venography) to permit an accurate estimate of the sensitivity or specificity of the technique. The accuracy of the technique is quite high in cases of spontaneous effort thrombosis and in instances where indwelling catheters are in place. With concurrent venous obstruction caused by a mediastinal process, the Doppler exam of the proximal portion of the subclavian vein may be less accurate and tends to overestimate the presence and extent of thrombosis.

PERIPHERAL ARTERIAL DISEASE
Incidence and Clinical Importance

Peripheral vascular disease is at least as prevalent as coronary artery disease or cerebrovascular disease. The coexistence of these three processes is also very common. Many patients suffer from peripheral vascular disease for years before seeking medical assistance. This is a reflection of the normal development of collateral channels that often are sufficient to maintain a baseline perfusion to the extremity in the older patient, as long he or she does not exercise or ambulate too vigorously. In general, these patients can go on for years, decreasing their levels of activity as their disease progresses. Disabling claudication is, therefore, more likely to be a presenting symptom in the younger patient.

Other symptoms, which force the patient to seek medical assistance, are the development of chronic changes of arterial insufficiency or poor healing. Additional possibilities include the development of acute embolic events originating from a more proximal arterial lesion, such as ulcerated plaques and thrombosing aneurysms.

The development of arterial bypass surgery has modified the natural history of this disease process. The high patency rates for both arterial bypass surgery and angioplasty have made it possible for patients who would previously have had amputations to keep their extremity until other causes of mortality intercede. Cardiovascular events are likely causes of death in these preselected patients with progressive generalized atherosclerosis.

Duplex sonography is increasingly used to detect evidence of the complications of bypass surgery and to evaluate the success of angioplasty. The use of ultrasound imaging for the preoperative evaluation of saphenous veins to determine their suitability as bypass grafts is also increasing.

Doppler imaging of the leg arteries has become feasible with color Doppler mapping. Although duplex sonography can be used to determine the presence of significant arterial lesions, the task of evaluating the whole leg is labor- and time-intensive. It takes 30 to 60 minutes to map out the arterial tree of each leg using duplex ultrasound. With color Doppler mapping, this task can be accomplished in 15 to 20 minutes.

Lower Extremity

Normal Anatomy and Doppler Flow Patterns. The deep arteries of the leg travel with an accompanying vein (see Figs. 31-1 to 31-3). The common femoral artery starts at the level of the inguinal ligament and continues for 4 to 6 cm until it divides into the superficial and deep (profunda) femoral arteries (Fig. 31-9). The deep femoral artery quickly branches to supply the region of the femoral head and the deep muscles of the thigh. With peripheral arterial disease, collateral pathways often form between this deep femoral artery and the lower portions of the superficial femoral or the popliteal arteries. The superficial femoral artery continues along the medial aspect of the thigh at a depth of 4 to 8 cm until it reaches the adductor canal. It then passes posteriorly in this canal and continues as the popliteal artery. This artery lies posterior to the knee and gives off small geniculate branches that pass around the knee. Finally, the popliteal artery divides into the

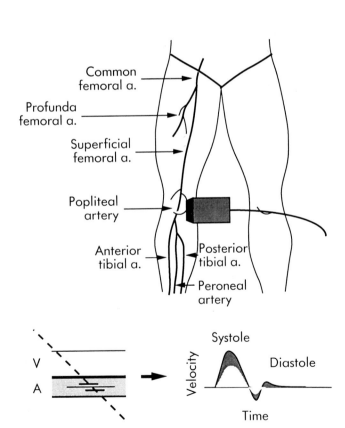

FIG 31-9. Normal leg arterial anatomy and Doppler waveform. The normal Doppler spectrum of flowing blood, in the lower extremity, has a triphasic pattern. There is forward, high-velocity flow in systole, followed by a brief flow reversal in early diastole and, finally, a return to forward, low-velocity flow in mid- and late diastole.

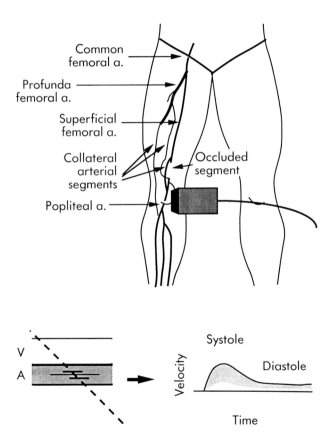

FIG 31-10. Abnormal leg arterial Doppler waveform. With significant arterial disease the Doppler waveform adopts a low resistance pattern normally seen in the internal carotid artery. Flow is in the forward direction during most of diastole. The situation depicted here is that of an occluded segment of the distal superficial femoral artery with collateral vessels supplying the popliteal artery. The Doppler sample is from the popliteal artery distal to the occlusion.

anterior tibial artery and the tibio-peroneal trunk. The anterior tibial artery courses through the interosseous membrane. It finally crosses the ankle joint as the dorsalis pedis artery. The tibio-peroneal trunk gives off the posterior tibial and the peroneal arteries that supply the calf muscles. The posterior tibial artery can be followed down to its typical location behind the medial malleolus.

The normal flow pattern in all of these branches is typically triphasic, which reflects the high resistance of the arteries to muscles (Fig. 31-9). There is an early systolic acceleration in velocity followed by a brief period of low-amplitude flow reversal before returning to antegrade diastolic flow of lower velocity. This pattern is more pulsatile in the deep femoral artery and less pulsatile, with less diastolic flow reversal, in arteries below the knee. The response to exercise (or transient ischemia) is a loss of the normal triphasic pattern and the development of a monophasic pattern with a loss of the period of flow reversal and a higher amplitude of antegrade flow during diastole (Fig. 31-10).

Diagnostic Criteria for Aneurysms. Aneurysms develop as the structural integrity of the arterial wall weakens. Focal enlargement of the artery is more likely to occur at the level of the popliteal or distal superficial femoral artery. They are, often, bilateral and can remain asymptomatic for long periods of time. Ultrasound imaging has become a gold standard in itself for confirming this suspected diagnosis.[26,27] The diagnostic superiority of ultrasound is, in part, because of the progressive thrombosis that fills in the aneurysm frequently makes the lumen appear normal at angiography (Fig. 31-11). Ultrasound can be used to follow these aneurysms, as is done for abdominal aortic aneurysm. There are, unfortunately, no strict size criteria that can be used to determine the patient's suitability for surgery. Current indications for surgery remain the development of symptoms suggestive of distal embolization by an aneurysm of 2 cm or above in diameter.

Doppler techniques are useful in confirming the continued patency of a channel within the thrombosing aneurysm either at presentation or following surgery. A bulge or focal enlargement of 20% of the expected vessel diameter constitutes a simple functional definition of an early aneurysm.

Diagnostic Accuracy with Aneurysms. Direct pathologic verification of ultrasound-diagnosed aneurysms has shown the technique to be quite sensitive, specific, and superior to angiography. The accuracy of Doppler techniques for confirming patency or occlusion has yet to be reported.

Diagnosis Criteria for Stenosis and Occlusion. The diagnosis of peripheral stenosis or occlusion is often made by noting a change in the normal Doppler flow pattern (Fig. 31-12). In cases of less severe arterial stenosis, the period of early diastolic flow reversal decreases and, ultimately, disappears as the lesion becomes more severe. The velocity of the diastolic component also increases with the severity of the lesion (Fig. 31-10). When the lesions are severe, the flow pattern is mainly that of forward flow with the diastolic velocity being quite near that of the peak systolic velocity.

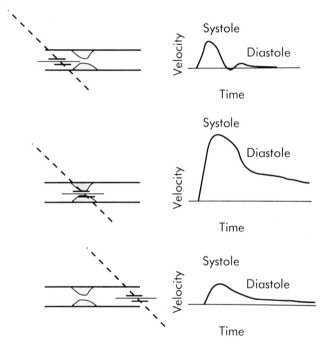

FIG 31-12. Doppler flow patterns relative to location of stenosis. Proximal to the lesion, the flow pattern is normal *(top)*. At the stenosis, the peak systolic velocity increases in proportion to the degree of stenosis *(middle)*. The diastolic portion of the spectrum is affected in different ways dependent on lesion severity and geometry. Distal to the stenosis, the peak systolic velocity has returned to values equal to or lower than those proximal to the stenosis *(bottom)*. If the stenosis is severe, peripheral vasodilation causes an increase in the amount of diastolic flow.

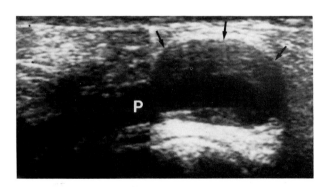

FIG 31-11. Popliteal artery aneurysm. Longitudinal image of the popliteal space demonstrates a 3 × 4 cm aneurysm *(arrows)*, which contains a large amount of thrombus. *P*, Popliteal artery.

One explanation for the development of this pattern is the progressive dilatation of the arterioles within the distant muscle vascular bed, which is caused by the release of metabolites caused by local ischemia. Another is the development of many small collaterals that diminish the effective resistance of the more distally located obstructing lesion. This pattern, although a general finding, may not be seen if the Doppler sample is obtained proximal to high-grade focal lesions (Fig. 31-12). Under such circumstances, the high resistance of the vessel and the absence of collaterals results in forward flow mostly during systole. The peak systolic velocity is, therefore, measured from the Doppler spectrum at the site of a suspected stenosis because it is less likely to vary as a function of peripheral vascular resistance.

A drop in velocity in the femoral artery below 0.9 m/sec normally suggests the presence of a high-grade lesion. Focal areas of doubling of the measured peak systolic velocity have been shown to correspond to lesions of greater than 50% narrowing in the lumen diameter of the artery.[28]

Diagnostic Accuracy with Stenosis and Occlusion. Kohler et al have reported that Doppler sonography has a diagnostic sensitivity of 82% and a specificity of 92% for detecting segmental arterial lesions of the femoropopliteal artery.[29] These authors did, however, remark on the fact that selective sampling had to be performed along the full course of the femoral and popliteal arteries. These segments normally measure 30 to 40 cm so it is not surprising that such a survey takes from 1 to 2 hours to perform.

Color Flow Imaging. For the examination of the carotid arteries, color Doppler sonography has been shown to reduce the examination time by 40% when compared with spectral Doppler alone. A similar effect has been shown when using color flow mapping to detect focal lesions in the femoro-popliteal artery. The diagnostic accuracy of the examination is slightly better than that of noncolor-assisted duplex sonography and the examination time can be reduced to 30 minutes when color Doppler is used.[30]

Upper Extremity

Normal Anatomy and Doppler Flow Patterns. The arterial system of the upper extremity branches that are parallel to the venous system, with the exception that major superficial branches, are absent. The junction of the subclavian artery, with either the innominate or the left brachiocephalic artery, can be identified by using an acoustic window superior to the sternoclavicular joint. The subclavian artery is imaged superficial to the vein when the transducer is placed in the supraclavicular fossa. Near the junction of the mid and proximal third of the clavicle, it is necessary to use an acoustic window with the transducer caudal to the clavicle. From this view, the subclavian artery is seen deep to the subclavian vein. The origin of the axillary artery normally occurs near the junction of the cephalic and the axillary vein. The axillary artery can be traced as it courses medially over the region of the humeral head to become the brachial artery. In most patients, the artery can be followed to the antecubital fossa where it trifurcates into the radial, ulnar, and interosseous branches. The radial and ulnar branches can normally be imaged to the level of the wrist and it is often possible to visualize the smaller digital branches. The normal flow pattern of the large arteries of the arm is similar to the leg arteries with a high-resistance, triphasic appearance.

Pathophysiology. Most clinical interest in the noninvasive evaluation of the upper-extremity arterial branches is directed to the detection of focal stenosis caused by thoracic outlet syndrome, the confirmation of arterial occlusion secondary to emboli or trauma, the evaluation of dialysis shunts, and the detection of complications following coronary arteriography (pseudoaneurysm). There are a few reports in the literature of Doppler evaluation of patients with thoracic outlet syndrome. It is possible to induce stenosis in the subclavian artery by placing the arm in the position that elicits the patient's symptoms. Most patients who have symptoms of thoracic outlet syndrome are symptomatic when their arm is abducted. There is a frequent association between thoracic outlet syndrome and distal arterial embolization. The extent of these acute or chronic occlusions must be mapped out to assess the feasibility of possible bypass surgery before subjecting the patient to angiography. Proximal occlusion of the subclavian artery, sometimes associated with vasculitis, can also be demonstrated.

Complications following arterial puncture for coronary arteriography, such as occlusion, can be rapidly confirmed or excluded. Soft-tissue swelling at the arteriotomy site can be evaluated to differentiate hematoma from pseudoaneurysm. Swirling blood or color flow Doppler is characteristic of pseudoaneurysm, which may arise from the arteriotomy site.

VASCULAR MASSES AND SURGICAL COMPLICATIONS

A major contribution of Doppler sonography to standard gray-scale sonography is its ability to document the presence or absence of blood flow within masses located in close proximity to vessels or vascular prostheses. Although the presence of blood flow within a perivascular mass can be diagnostic of a pseudoaneurysm, the absence of blood flow makes it easier to justify a more conservative approach. In the case of a suspected hematoma, serial follow-up examinations can be used to document resolution of the process. In the instance of a suspected abscess, a needle aspiration can be performed without fear of uncontrolled hemorrhage.

Synthetic Vascular Bypass Grafts

The complications likely to affect the function of synthetic lower-extremity bypass grafts are varied.[31] They depend on the type of bypass graft used and on how much time has elapsed since operative placement. In the first and second years following surgery, graft failure can occur either secondary to technical errors or to the development of fibro-intimal lesions at the anastomoses. Later failures are more likely to be caused by the progression of atherosclerotic lesions in the native vessels proximal and distal to the graft. The late complication of an anastomotic pseudoaneurysm occurs on average 5 to 10 years after graft placement and preferentially affects the femoral anastomosis of aorto-femoral grafts.[32] Infections can develop at any time following graft placement and can be associated with the development of an anastomotic pseudoaneurysm. With time, atherosclerotic changes and fibro-intimal hyperplastic lesions, mixed in with areas of chronic thrombus deposition, can also occur in the synthetic graft conduit.

Masses: Hematoma versus Pseudoaneurysm. Although the accuracy of duplex sonography is more than 95% when making the diagnosis of pseudoaneurysms, no specific waveform patterns have been described when sampling within the pseudoaneurysm.[33,34] The addition of color Doppler imaging can reveal an almost classic appearance of swirling blood in the perivascular mass.[35] However, this sign is not characteristic of only a pseudoaneurysm because saccular aneurysms share similar flow patterns (Figs. 31-13 to 31-16). The diagnosis of pseudoaneurysm is made when careful real-time imaging confirms that the mass is situated beyond the normal lumen of the vessel (Fig. 31-17).

Another sign described on Doppler spectral analysis is the "to-fro" sign detected when sampling the communication between the perivascular collection and the native vessel. The "to-fro" spectral appearance is caused by the blood going into the mass during systole and out of the mass during diastole. Although specific, this jet is often difficult to find and is frequently absent in anastomotic pseudoaneurysms (Figs. 31-17 and 31-18). Color Doppler mapping may be used to help localize this site.

Care must be taken to differentiate perivascular pulsations transmitted within a hematoma from flowing

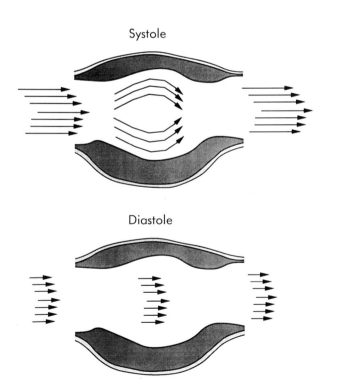

Systole

Diastole

FIG 31-13. Fusiform aneurysm flow pattern. The flow patterns within the lumen of an aneurysm will vary during the different stages of its evolution. Here, with minimal bulging of the wall and a small amount of mural thrombus, flow eddies are established during late systole *(top)*. During diastole, a more normal pattern is reestablished *(bottom)*.

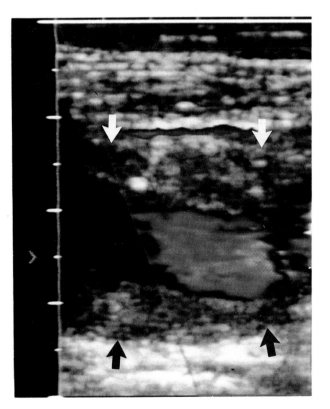

FIG 31-14. Longitudinal color Doppler view of a popliteal aneurysm. Aneurysm with a large amount of thrombus along its wall *(arrows)*. The lumen is straight enough so that there are no significant flow eddies during systole.

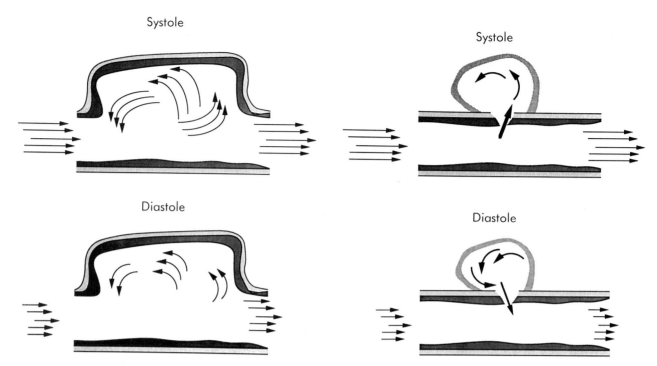

FIG 31-15. Saccular aneurysm flow pattern. A saccular aneurysm has flow eddies during late systole and the major portion of diastole. This corresponds to a "swirling" pattern. Differentiation between a saccular aneurysm and a pseudoaneurysm, arising at the anastomosis of a synthetic graft, can be difficult.

FIG 31-16. Pseudoaneurysm flow pattern. With a pseudoaneurysm, the "swirling" motion of blood is identified, and a small communication between artery and the perivascular collection is visualized, especially when the pseudoaneurysm arises in a native artery. The flow enters the pseudoaneurysm during systole and exits during diastole.

blood. Adjustment of the flow sensitivity of the ultrasound machine can eliminate or minimize this artifact.

Anastomotic Stenosis and Occlusions. The absence of Doppler signals within a graft can be used to diagnose occlusions and to help plan further angiographic access for thrombolysis. The confirmation of an anastomotic stenosis can be made using the flow criteria previously described. There is, however, a normal tendency for turbulent flow to develop at the anastomosis, and increases in velocity because of the geometry of the anastomosis are quite common. Serial monitoring of these sites of disturbed flow may be used with the premise that an increase in velocity, over a few months, is indicative of a developing stenosis.

Autologous Vein Grafts

Two types of venous bypass grafts are currently used for arterial revascularization: the reversed vein and the "in-situ" vein grafts. The reversed vein is a segment of native superficial vein that has been harvested from its normal anatomic location, reversed, and then anastomosed to the native artery segments proximal and distal to the diseased segments. The "in-situ" technique commonly uses the greater saphenous vein, which is left in

its native bed. The valves are lysed and the side branches, which are normally anastomosed to the deep venous system, are ligated. The proximal and distal portions of the vein are mobilized and anastomosed to the selected arterial segments.

Three different failure mechanisms may occur. Early failures are generally ascribed to technical errors and they are likely to result in graft occlusion within the first two months after surgery. These include: poor suture line placement, the opening of unsuspected venous channels in the "in-situ" grafts, poor selection of anastomotic sites, and poorly lysed vein valves. During the first two years after surgery, fibro-intimal or fibrotic lesions can develop, either at the anastomosis or within the graft conduit, most often at the site of a vein valve. Late failures, beyond this two-year period, are thought to be secondary to continued progression of the atherosclerotic process in the native vessels proximal and distal to the anastomoses.

Stenosis. The measurement of graft velocity, either in the early or late postoperative period, can be used to detect grafts with a high likelihood of incipient failure. Bandyk et al have suggested that a peak systolic velocity below 0.4 or 0.45 m/sec can be used to identify

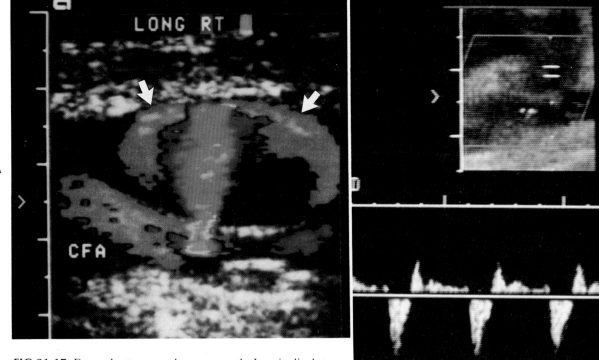

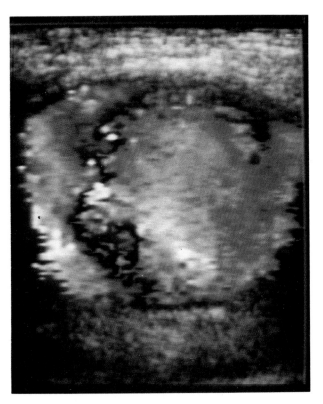

FIG 31-17. Femoral artery pseudoaneurysm. **A,** Longitudinal color Doppler image of the right common femoral artery one day after arteriogram demonstrates an oval mass *(arrows)* anterior to the artery. At real-time, the swirling blood is identified, and the site of leak is seen as a blue jet of color arising from the anterior surface of the artery. **B,** Longitudinal spectral Doppler image with sample gate in the neck of a false aneurysm demonstrates the typical "to and fro" Doppler signal.

grafts that are at risk for failure.[36,37] This criterion can, appropriately, identify the more severely diseased grafts. It does not, however, establish the site of stenoses that are likely to continue to progress until they become flow-restrictive and finally result in graft thrombosis.[38] These lesions are more commonly the outcome of fibro-intimal hyperplasia and their existence and location must be known before they can be monitored for possible progression of severity. Color-assisted Doppler sonography can be used to survey the length of these bypass grafts, which varies from 30 to 75 cm. The site of a suspected stenosis can be quickly identified and Doppler spectral analysis can be used to grade the severity of the stenosis with the use of the peak systolic velocity ratio (Figs. 31-19 and 31-20). This ratio is calculated by dividing the peak systolic velocity measured at the suspected stenosis by that measured in the portion of the graft 2 to 4 cm proximally. A ratio of 2 to 3 is abnormal and corresponds to a 50% to 75% narrowing of the lumen diameter. A ratio above 3 corresponds to a greater than 75% stenosis. Early experience with this

FIG 31-18. Bypass graft aneurysm. Transverse image of a large anastomotic aneurysm at the distal anastomosis of an aortobifemoral bypass graft has within it a typical swirling pattern of blood flow.

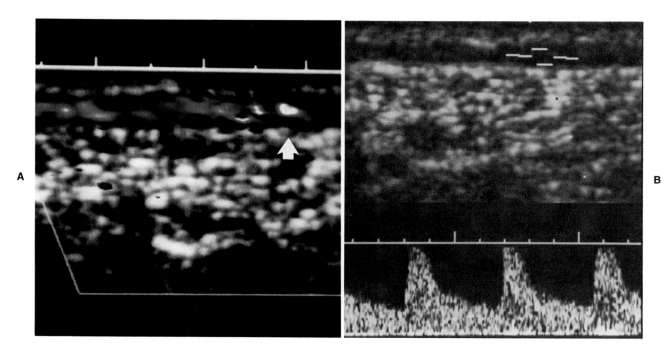

FIG 31-19. Graft stenosis. **A,** This portion of a femoroperoneal "in-situ" bypass graft has a small zone of high-flow velocities indicating stenosis *(arrow)*. **B,** The corresponding Doppler spectrum shows a marked increase in flow velocity at the site of color flow disturbance.

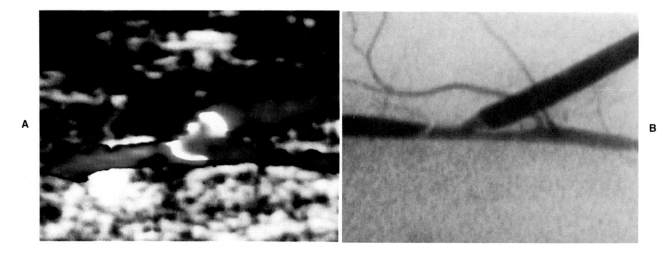

FIG 31-20. Anastomotic stenosis. **A,** This longitudinal image of the anastomosis of a bypass graft to a posterior tibial artery shows a zone of color Doppler aliasing consistent with a significant narrowing. The relatively normal size of the flow lumen is caused by a misregistration of the color signals because of the relative acceleration of the red blood cells. **B,** The corresponding arteriogram confirms the presence of a long stenosis.

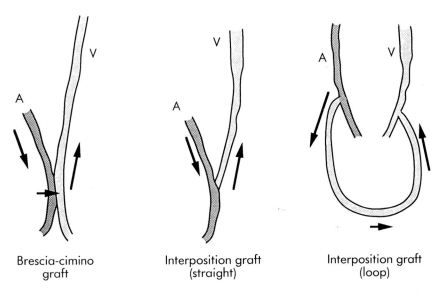

Brescia-cimino graft

Interposition graft (straight)

Interposition graft (loop)

FIG 31-21. Dialysis fistula types. The diagnostic accuracy of (color) duplex imaging is lower for detecting stenoses in the loop type configuration.

method suggest that it is very accurate for the detection and grading of stenoses.[39]

A-V Fistula. This complication is apt to occur with the "in-situ" technique because small A-V fistulas can easily be missed at the time of surgery and may develop immediately after surgery. Color Doppler sonography is a simple and elegant way of documenting their presence. We currently use color Doppler ultrasound preoperatively without angiography to identify sites of A-V communication between the "in-situ" superficial veins and the deeper native veins.

Dialysis Fistula

Ultrasound imaging is also used to evaluate dialysis A-V fistulas.[40,41] These are typically inserted in the forearm and are either synthetic or made of autologous vein (Fig. 31-21). Problems common to dialysis fistula include the development of microaneurysms, larger aneurysms, or stenoses. The accuracy of duplex sonography for stenosis is estimated at 86% with a sensitivity of 92% and a specificity of 84%. False-negative and false-positive results occur because of the turbulent flow patterns set up by the tortuous course these arteriovenous shunts take in the forearm. In the straight segment of the efferent veins, the sensitivity of duplex sonography increases to 95% for a specificity of 97%. The addition of color Doppler does not seem to improve diagnostic accuracy.[42]

Complications of Invasive Procedures

There has been a dramatic expansion in the use of duplex and color Doppler sonography for the evaluation

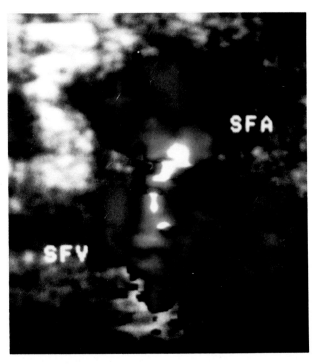

FIG 31-22. A-V fistula. Transverse color flow image of the right leg shows a high velocity jet caused by a fistula between the superficial artery and vein. The patient underwent surgical repair without the need for arteriography because of the clear communication on the color Doppler image.

of patients who have had invasive procedures and in whom the diagnosis of pseudoaneurysm or A-V fistula is suspected. The findings of the sonographic examination are often accepted as conclusive without the need for preoperative angiography.

A-V Fistula. Fistulous communications, following cardiac catheterization or other angiographic procedures, can be quickly detected using color Doppler imaging.[43] In the femoral region, turbulence is seen within either the common femoral or profunda femoral vein with arterialized signals shown on the Doppler waveform. The fistulous communication can often be seen with color Doppler although it may be difficult to localize if duplex sonography is used alone (Fig. 31-22). Another indirect sign of the fistula is dilatation of the vein and poor Valsalva response when compared to the vein in the other extremity.

Pseudoaneurysms. Pseudoaneurysms may develop following trauma or arterial catheterization. Color Doppler will display the typical swirling colors; the likelihood of detecting a direct communication with the vessel is increased if color Doppler imaging is used. The neck of the pseudoaneurysm is frequently small and a spectral tracing from that region will show forward flow in systole and reversed flow in diastole: the "to-fro" sign.

REFERENCES
Instrumentation

1. Barber FE, Baker DW, Nation AW, et al: Ultrasonic duplex echo-Doppler scanner. *IEEE Trans Biomed Eng* 1974;21:109-113.
2. Kasai C, Namekawa K, Koyano A, et al: Real-time two dimensional blood flow imaging using an auto-correlation technique. *Trans Sonics Ultrasound (IEEE)* 1985;SU-32:458-463.

Physiologic mechanisms of Doppler flow patterns

3. Spencer MP, Reid JM: Quantitation of carotid stenosis with continuous wave (C-W) Doppler ultrasound. *Stroke* 1979;10:326-330.
4. Reneman RS, Spencer MP: Local Doppler audio spectra in normal and stenosed carotid arteries in man. *Ultrasound Med Biol* 1979;5:1-11.
5. Ojha M, Johnston KW, Cobbold RS, et al: Potential limitations of center-line pulsed Doppler recordings: an in vitro flow visualization study. *J Vasc Surg* 1989;9:515-520.
6. Middleton WD, Erickson S, Melson GL: Perivascular color artifact: pathologic significance and appearance on color Doppler US images. *Radiology* 1989;171:647-652.
7. Mitchell DG, Needleman L, Bezzi M, et al: Femoral artery pseudoaneurysm: diagnosis with conventional duplex and color Doppler US. *Radiology* 1987;165:687-690.
8. Wilkinson DL, Polak JF, Grassi CJ, et al: Pseudoaneurysm of the vertebral artery: appearance on color flow Doppler sonography. *AJR* 1988;151:1051-1052.
9. Abu-Yousef MM, Wiese JA, Shamma AR: The "to-and-fro" sign: duplex Doppler evidence of femoral artery pseudoaneurysm. *AJR* 1988;150:632-634.
10. Musto R, Roach MR: Flow studies in glass models of aortic aneurysms. *Can J Surg* 1980;23:452-455.

Venous thrombosis

11. Moser KM, LeMoine JR: Is embolic risk conditioned by location of deep venous thrombosis? *Ann Intern Med* 1981;94:439-444.
12. Barnes RW, Nix ML, Barnes CL, et al: Perioperative asymptomatic venous thrombosis: role of duplex scanning versus venography. *J Vasc Surg* 1989;9:251-260.
13. Kakkar VV, Howe CT, Flanc C, et al: Natural history of postoperative deep vein thrombosis. *Lancet* 1969;2:230-233.
14. Lagerstedt CI, Olsson CG, Fagher BD, et al: Need for long-term anticoagulant treatment in symptomatic calf-vein thrombosis. *Lancet* 1985;2:515-518.
15. Cronan JJ, Dorfman GS, Scola FH, et al: Deep venous thrombosis: US assessment using vein compression. *Radiology* 1987;162:191-194.
16. Lensing AW, Prandoni P, Brandjes D, et al: Detection of deep-vein thrombosis by real-time B-mode ultrasonography. *N Engl J Med* 1989;320:342-345.
17. White RH, McGahan JP, Daschbach MM, et al: Diagnosis of deep-vein thrombosis using duplex ultrasound. *Ann Intern Med* 1989;111:297-304.
18. Killewich LA, Bedford GR, Beach KW, et al: Diagnosis of deep venous thrombosis: a prospective study comparing duplex scanning to contrast venography. *Circulation* 1989;79:810-814.
19. Effeney DJ, Friedman MB, Gooding GAW: Iliofemoral venous thrombosis: real-time ultrasound diagnosis, normal criteria, and clinical application. *Radiology* 1984;150:787-792.
20. Polak JF, O'Leary DH: Deep vein thrombosis in pregnancy: noninvasive diagnosis. *Radiology* 1988;166:377-379.
21. Coelho JC, Sigel B, Ryva JC, et al: B-mode sonography of blood clots. *JCU* 1982;10:323-327.
22. Comerota AJ, Katz ML, Greenwald LL, et al: Venous duplex imaging: should it replace hemodynamic tests for deep venous thrombosis? *J Vasc Surg* 1990;11:53-61.
23. Foley WD, Middleton WD, Lawson TL, et al: Color Doppler ultrasound imaging of lower-extremity venous disease. *AJR* 1989;152:371-376.
24. Polak JF, Cutler SS, O'Leary DH: Deep veins of the calf: assessment with color Doppler flow imaging. *Radiology* 1989;171:481-485.
25. Vasdekis SN, Clarke GH, Nicolaides AN: Quantification of venous reflux by means of duplex scanning. *J Vasc Surg* 1989;10:670-677.

Peripheral arterial disease

26. Gooding GAW, Effeney DJ: Ultrasound of femoral artery aneurysms. *AJR* 1980;134:477-480.
27. MacGowan SW, Saif MF, O'Neill G, et al: Ultrasound examination in the diagnosis of popliteal artery aneurysms. *Br J Surg* 1985;72:528-529.
28. Jager KA, Phillips DJ, Martin RL, et al: Noninvasive mapping of lower limb arterial lesions. *Ultrasound Med Biol* 1985;11:515-521.
29. Kohler TR, Nance DR, Cramer MM, et al: Duplex scanning for diagnosis of aortoiliac and femoropopliteal disease: a prospective study. *Circulation* 1987;76:1074-1080.
30. Cossman DV, Ellison JE, Wagner WH, et al: Comparison of contrast arteriography to arterial mapping with color-flow duplex imaging in the lower extremities. *J Vasc Surg* 1989;10:522-529.

Vascular masses and surgical complications

31. Hedgcock MW, Eisenberg RL, Gooding GAW: Complications relating to vascular prosthetic grafts. *J Can Assoc Radiol* 1980;31:137-142.
32. Nichols WK, Stanton M, Silver D, et al: Anastomotic aneurysms following lower-extremity revascularization. *Surgery* 1980;88:366-374.

33. Helvie MA, Rubin JM, Silver TM, et al: The distinction between femoral artery pseudoaneurysms and other causes of groin masses: value of duplex Doppler sonography. *AJR* 1988;150:1177-1180.

34. Coughlin BF, Paushter DM: Peripheral pseudoaneurysms: evaluation with duplex US. *Radiology* 1988;168:339-342.

35. Polak JF, Donaldson MC, Whittemore AD, et al: Pulsatile masses surrounding vascular prostheses: real-time US color flow imaging. *Radiology* 1989;170:363-366.

36. Bandyk DF, Jorgensen RA, Towne JB: Intraoperative assessment of in situ saphenous vein arterial grafts using pulsed Doppler spectral analysis. *Arch Surg* 1986;121:292-299.

37. Bandyk DF, Cato RF, Towne JB: A low flow velocity predicts failure of femoropopliteal and femorotibial bypass grafts. *Surgery* 1985;98:799-807.

38. Grigg MJ, Nicolaides AN, Wolfe JH: Detection and grading of femorodistal vein graft stenoses: duplex velocity measurements compared with angiography. *J Vasc Surg* 1988;8:661-666.

39. Polak JF, Donaldson MC, Dobkin GR, et al: Early detection of saphenous vein arterial bypass graft stenosis by color-assisted duplex sonography: a prospective study. *AJR* 1990;154:857-861.

40. Scheible W, Skram C, Leopold GR: High resolution real-time sonography of hemodialysis vascular access complications. *AJR* 1980;134:1173-1176.

41. Tordoir JH, de Bruin HG, Hoeneveld H, et al: Duplex ultrasound scanning in the assessment of arteriovenous fistulas created for hemodialysis access: comparison with digital subtraction angiography. *J Vasc Surg* 1989;10:122-128.

42. Middleton WD, Picus DD, Marx MV, et al: Color Doppler sonography of hemodialysis vascular access: comparison with angiography. *AJR* 1989;152:633-639.

43. Altin RS, Flicker S, Naidech HJ: Pseudoaneurysm and arteriovenous fistula after femoral artery catheterization: association with low femoral punctures. *AJR* 1989;152:629-631.

Index